Contents

v

The Cervix

To our wives

SECOND EDITION

The Cervix

EDITED BY

Joseph A. Jordan

Birmingham Women's Hospital
Birmingham, UK

Albert Singer

Professor of Gynaecological Research
University of London;
Consultant Gynaecologist
Whittington Hospital
London, UK

ASSOCIATE EDITORS

Howard W. Jones III

Professor of Obstetrics and Gynecology
Director of Gynecological Oncology
Vanderbilt University School of Medicine
Nashville, TN, USA

Mahmood I. Shafi

Consultant Gynaecological Surgeon and Oncologist
Addenbrooke's Hospital
Cambridge, UK

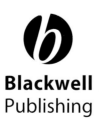

Blackwell
Publishing

© 2006 by Blackwell Publishing Ltd

Blackwell Publishing, Inc., 350 Main Street, Malden, Massachusetts 02148-5020, USA
Blackwell Publishing Ltd, 9600 Garsington Road, Oxford OX4 2DQ, UK
Blackwell Publishing Asia Pty Ltd, 550 Swanston Street, Carlton, Victoria 3053, Australia

First published 1976 by W.B. Saunders Ltd

Library of Congress Cataloging-in-Publication Data

The cervix / edited by Joseph A. Jordan, Albert Singer . . . [et al.]. — 2nd ed.
   p. ; cm.
   Includes bibliographical references.

   ISBN-13: 978-1-4051-3137-7 (alk. paper)
   ISBN-10: 1-4051-3137-3 (alk. paper)

   1. Cervix uteri. 2. Cervix uteri—Diseases.
   [DNLM: 1. Cervix Uteri. 2. Uterine Cervical Neoplasms.
   I. Jordan, Joseph A. II. Singer, Albert.
   WP 470 C419 2006]
   RG310.C45 2006
   618.1′4—dc22

                                2006012844

A catalogue record for this title is available from the British Library

Set in Galliard/Frutiger by Graphicraft Ltd, Hong Kong
Printed and bound in Singapore by COS Printers Pte Ltd

Development Editor: Rebecca Huxley
Commissioning Editor: Stuart Taylor
Production Controller: Kate Charman
Project Editor: Gillian Whytock, Prepress Projects Ltd

For further information on Blackwell Publishing, visit our website:
http://www.blackwellpublishing.com

The publisher's policy is to use permanent paper from mills that operate a sustainable forestry policy, and which has been manufactured from pulp processed using acid-free and elementary chlorine-free practices. Furthermore, the publisher ensures that the text paper and cover board used have met acceptable environmental accreditation standards.

Contributors

Nigel Acheson

MD MRCOG
Consultant Gynaecological Oncologist
Royal Devon and Exeter Hospital
Exeter, UK

Ervin Adam

MD PhD
Professor of Virology and Microbiology
Baylor College of Medicine
Houston, TX, USA

Asif Ahmed

PhD
Professor of Reproductive and Vascular
  Biology
University of Birmingham
Birmingham, UK

Sally Appleton

BSc MB BS
Mater Adult Hospital
Brisbane, Qld, Australia

Katharine Astbury

MB BCh BAO FRCSI MRCOG
Research Fellow in Obstetrics and
  Gynaecology
Coombe Women's Hospital
Dublin, Ireland

Antoni Basta

MD PhD
Professor of Obstetrics and Gynaecology
Head of Department of Gynaecology, Obstetrics
  and Oncology
Jagiellonian University
Krakow, Poland

Peter Blake

MB BS BSc MD FRCR
Consultant Clinical Oncologist
Royal Marsden Hospital
London, UK

Michele Burday

PhD DABMM
Director of Clinical Microbiology
University of Medicine and Dentistry of New
  Jersey
New Jersey Medical School
Newark, NJ, USA

Karen Canfell

BE DPhil
European Scientific Director
Polartechnics Ltd
Sydney, NSW, Australia

Carl Chow

MB BS BSc MRCOG
Consultant Obstetrician and Gynaecologist
Kingston Hospital
Kingston upon Thames, UK

Kasturi Das

MD
Department of Pathology and Laboratory
  Medicine
University of Medicine and Dentistry of New
  Jersey
New Jersey Medical School
Newark, NJ, USA

Alastair R.S. Deery

BSc MB BS FRCPath
Consultant Cellular Pathologist
St George's Hospital
London, UK

Lyndal Edwards

MB BS FRCPA
Staff Specialist, Department of Anatomical
  Pathology
Prince of Wales Hospital
Randwick, NSW, Australia

J. Michael Emens

MD FRCOG
Consultant Gynaecologist
Birmingham Women's Hospital
Birmingham, UK

Sebastian Faro

MD PhD
Clinical Professor
Department of Obstetrics, Gynecology, and
  Reproductive Sciences
University of Texas Houston Health Science Center;
Attending Physician
The Women's Hospital of Texas
Houston, TX, USA

Roy G. Farquharson

MD FRCOG
Clinical Director
Liverpool Women's Hospital
Liverpool, UK

Eduardo L.F. Franco

MPH DrPH
James McGill Professor of Epidemiology and
  Oncology
Director, Division of Cancer Epidemiology
McGill University
Montreal, QB, Canada

Ian H. Frazer

MB ChB MD FAA FTSE FRCP(Ed) FRCPA
Director, Centre for Immunology and Cancer Research
University of Queensland
Woolloongabba, Qld, Australia

Theresa Freeman-Wang

MB ChB MRCOG
Consultant Gynaecologist
Whittington Hospital
London, UK

Raji Ganesan

MB BS MD FRCPath
Consultant Histopathologist
Birmingham Women's Hospital
Birmingham, UK

Harold Gee

MD FRCOG
Consultant Obstetrician
Birmingham Women's Hospital
Birmingham, UK

Cornelius O. Granai
MD
Director, Program in Women's Oncology
Women's and Infants' Hospital;
Associate Professor
Brown University
Providence, RI, USA

Neville F. Hacker
MD FRANZCOG FRCOG FACOG FACS
Professor of Gynaecological Oncology
University of New South Wales;
Director, Gynaecological Cancer Centre
Royal Hospital for Women
Randwick, NSW, Australia

Joseph Hanoch
MD
Department of Gynaecological Oncology
Imperial College Medical School
Hammersmith Hospital
London, UK

Debra S. Heller
MD
Professor of Pathology and Laboratory
    Medicine and of Obstetrics, Gynecology,
    and Women's Health
University of Medicine and Dentistry of New Jersey
New Jersey Medical School
Newark, NJ, USA

Peter W. Hewett
BSc PhD
Lecturer in Reproductive and Vascular Biology
University of Birmingham
Birmingham, UK

Thomas Iftner
PhD
Professor and Head of Section of Experimental
    Virology
University of Tübingen
Tübingen, Germany

Anne M. Jequier
FRCS FRCOG FRANZCOG
Andrologist
Pivet Medical Centre
Leederville, WA, Australia

Howard W. Jones III
MD
Professor of Obstetrics and Gynecology
Director of Gynecological Oncology
Vanderbilt University School of Medicine
Nashville, TN, USA

Joseph A. Jordan
MD FRCOG FRCPI(Hon)
Birmingham Women's Hospital
Birmingham, UK

Raymond H. Kaufman
MD
Professor Emeritus Obstetrics and Gynecology
Baylor College of Medicine
Houston, TX, USA

Henry C. Kitchener
MD FRCS(Glasg) FRCOG
Professor of Gynaecological Oncology
University of Manchester
Manchester, UK

Anita Koushik
PhD
Research Fellow, Department of Nutrition
Harvard School of Public Health
Boston, MA, USA

H. Margot L. Lehman
MB BS FRANZCR GDPH
Staff Specialist, Radiation Oncology
Princess Alexandra Hospital
Brisbane, Qld, Australia

Amali Lokugamage
MB ChB BSc MSc MD MRCOG
Consultant Obstetrician and Gynaecologist
Whittington Hospital
London, UK

David M. Luesley
MA MD FRCOG
Lawson-Tait Professor of Gynaecological
    Oncology
University of Birmingham;
Honorary Consultant Gynaecological
    Oncologist
City Hospital
Birmingham, UK

G. Angus McIndoe
PhD FRCS MRCOG
Consultant Gynaecological Oncologist
Imperial College Medical School
Hammersmith Hospital
London, UK

John M. McLean
BSc MD
Formerly Senior Lecturer in Anatomy and
    Embryology
University of Manchester
Manchester, UK

Donald E. Marsden
BMedSc MB BS FRCOG FRANZCOG CGO
Deputy Director, Gynaecological Cancer Centre
Royal Hospital for Women;
Associate Professor of Obstetrics and Gynaecology
University of New South Wales
Randwick, NSW, Australia

Chris J.L.M. Meijer
MD PhD
Chairman and Director of the Department of
    Pathology
VU University Medical Centre
Amsterdam, The Netherlands

John M. Monaghan
MB ChB FRCOG FRCS(Ed)
Consultant Surgeon
Whitton Grange
Whitton, Morpeth, UK

Anna-Barbara Moscicki
MD
Professor of Pediatrics
University of California San Francisco
San Francisco, CA, USA

Timothy A.J. Mould
MB BS MA DM MRCOG
Consultant Gynaecological Oncologist
University College London Hospital
London, UK

Saloney Nazeer
MD
Consultant Physician and Director of
    Teaching
WHO Collaborating Centre for Research in
    Human Reproduction
Geneva University Hospital
Geneva, Switzerland

Twalib Ngoma
MD
Executive Director
Ocean Road Cancer Institute
Dar es Salaam, Tanzania

Adeola Olaitan
MD FRCOG
Consultant Gynaecological Oncologist
University College London Hospital
London, UK

John J. O'Leary
MD DPhil MSc FRCPath FFPathRCPI
Professor of Pathology
Trinity College Dublin;
Consultant Histopathologist
Coombe Women's Hospital
Dublin, Ireland

Olufemi Olufowobi
MB BS MRCOG
Clinical Research Fellow in Reproductive
    Medicine
Assisted Conception Unit
Birmingham Women's Hospital
Birmingham, UK

The late Andrew G. Östör

MB BS MD FRCPA MIAC
Formerly of the Royal Women's Hospital
Melbourne, Vic, Australia

Julietta Patnick

BA FFPH CBE
Director, NHS Cancer Screening Programmes
Sheffield, UK

Narendra Pisal

MD MRCOG
Consultant Obstetrician and Gynaecologist
Whittington Hospital
London, UK

The late Ellis Pixley

MB BS FAGO FRCOG
Formerly of the King Edward Memorial Hospital
    for Women
Perth, WA, Australia

Walter Prendiville

FRCOG
Associate Professor, Department of Obstetrics and
    Gynaecology
Coombe Women's Hospital;
Chairman, Department of Gynaecology
Tallaght Hospital
Dublin, Ireland

Terence P. Rollason

BSc MB ChB FRCPath
Consultant Histopathologist
Birmingham Women's Hospital
Birmingham, UK

Charles W.E. Redman

MD FRCS(Ed) FRCOG
Consultant Obstetrician and Gynaecologist
University Hospital North Staffordshire
Stoke-on-Trent, UK

Rengaswamy Sankaranarayanan

MD
Head of Screening Group
International Agency for Research on Cancer
Lyon, France

Mahmood I. Shafi

MB BCh MD DA FRCOG
Consultant Gynaecological Surgeon and
    Oncologist
Addenbrooke's Hospital
Cambridge, UK

Khaldoun Sharif

MB BCh MD FRCOG MFFP
Consultant Obstetrician and Gynaecologist
Assisted Conception Unit
Birmingham Women's Hospital
Birmingham, UK

John H. Shepherd

FRCS FRCOG FACOG
Professor of Surgical Gynaecology
St Bartholomew's and the Royal London School of
    Medicine and Dentistry
Queen Mary and Westfield College London
    University;
Consultant Surgeon
Royal Marsden Hospital
London, UK

Michael Sindos

MD
Obstetrician and Gynaecologist
Clinical Research Fellow
Whittington Hospital
London, UK

Albert Singer

PhD DPhil FRCOG
Professor of Gynaecological Research
University of London;
Consultant Gynaecologist
Whittington Hospital
London, UK

Peter J.F. Snijders

PhD
Senior Lecturer and Molecular Biologist
Department of Pathology
VU University Medical Centre
Amsterdam, The Netherlands

Thara Somanathan

MD
Regional Cancer Centre
Medical College Campus
Trivandrum, Kerala State, India

Andrea R. Spence

MSc
Research Associate, Division of Cancer
    Epidemiology
McGill University
Montreal, QB, Canada

Margaret A. Stanley

PhD
Professor of Epithelial Biology
University of Cambridge
Cambridge, UK

Frank Stubenrauch

PhD
Assistant Professor of Experimental Virology
University of Tübingen
Tübingen, Germany

Sun Kuie Tay

MB BS MD FRCOG
Senior Consultant Obstetrician and Gynaecologist
Singapore General Hospital;
Clinical Associate Professor of Medicine
National University of Singapore
Singapore

Gillian M. Thomas

BSc MD FRCPC
Staff Radiation Oncologist
Sunnybrook Regional Cancer Centre;
Professor of Radiation Oncology and Obstetrics and
    Gynaecology
University of Toronto
Toronto, ON, Canada

Richard W. Todd

MD MRCOG
Consultant Gynaecological Oncologist
University Hospital North Staffordshire
Stoke-on-Trent, UK

René H.M.Verheijen

MD PhD
Professor of Gynaelogical Oncology
VU University Medical Centre
Amsterdam, The Netherlands

Patrick G. Walker

MD FRCOG
Consultant Gynaecologist
Royal Free Hospital
London, UK

Thomas C. Wright Jr

MD
Department of Pathology
Columbia University College of Physicians and
    Surgeons
New York, NY, USA

Preface to the first edition

The physiological and pathological conditions affecting the cervix are amongst the most commonly discussed topics in contemporary obstetrics and gynaecology. Problems such as the place of cytological screening programmes in the detection of cervical precancer and the cost-effectiveness of such procedures; the neoplastic potential of the stilboestrol-induced atypical vaginal and cervical epithelium in the adolescent; the increasing clinical use of prostaglandins; the positive or negative aspects of the active management of labour — all of these concern the practising gynaecologist and obstetrician in his everyday work. Again, not only the clinicians, but the physiologist, biochemist, pathologist and epidemiologist are concerned with the various functional parameters of this small and central genital organ.

In the early 1970s, we asked ourselves where, as clinicians, we would look for up-to-date information about the management of problems related to the cervix; as teachers, was there a comprehensive text that we could recommend to our students, both undergraduates and those studying for higher degrees; as research workers, where could we find details of current research work on the cervix? No single text existed which fulfilled these criteria. We made a list of all that we, as clinicians, teachers and research workers, would wish to know about the cervix, and the result was the chapter framework of this book.

We believe that the text discusses in a critical and detailed manner the many controversial topics related to the cervix. Forty-three authors have contributed to this book and so it comes as no surprise to find many of them questioning long-established and accepted dogmas; and in some instances novel and unique ideas have been substituted. Writing in their individual styles, they have not only attempted to stress past and present knowledge but have also considered future trends in their subjects, and many of them have reviewed new, unpublished data.

In a major undertaking of this kind much direct and indirect support demands our grateful acknowledgement. Special thanks must go to Professor Hugh McLaren, who first stimulated the interest of J.A.J. in the cervix and who unselfishly encouraged the development of a colposcopy service in his department and later the research programme using the scanning electron microscope. Over the years, technical assistance in Birmingham has been freely given by Dennis Williams and Miss Josephine Allen and their help has been of particular value in the preparation of this text. The technique of colposcopy was taught to J.A.J. by Per Kolstad in 1967, since which time he has been a constant source of help and encouragement; his assistance and friendship are gratefully acknowledged.

The training and initial interest in the study of the cervix was given to A.S. 12 000 miles away from the accepted centres of cervical study. In Sydney, Australia, Bevan Reid and Malcolm Coppleson nurtured and disciplined the ideas and concepts that are expressed in this text. Their contributions in this field are momentous and both of us feel privileged to have been associated with them. The art of colposcopy was also taught in Sydney to A.S. by Dr Henry Frant whose comprehensive European training so easily blended over the years with that of his new environment. The Cancer Detection Clinic at the King George V Hospital, Sydney, provided perfect surroundings for the detailed and concentrated study of the cervix. To its staff of Mrs Rose Gorski and Betty Taggart and Miss A. Heenan and Miss D. Arnold go special thanks, as also to a fellow clinical colleague, Dr Peter Child, whose critical comments contributed so much to the understanding of the basic changes in the pregnant cervix. A special acknowledgement is due to Mr Robert Markham for his assistance and expert advice in many of the cellular and tissue studies. Dr Ellis Pixley of Perth, Western Australia, allowed A.S. to study and review his unique material relating to the fetal, neonatal and prepubertal cervix. He gave freely of his knowledge on this subject and this greatly assisted A.S. in the formulation of the conclusions which are based on this material and described in Chapter 8.

In Oxford, Professor Sir John Stallworthy extended hospitality to A.S. which enabled a continuation and development of the initial Australian studies relating to the high-risk cervical cancer female. His encouragement and assistance, wisely leavened with critical insight, were always positive, well-meaning and helpful, and always appreciated. In Sheffield, Professor Ian Cooke created the milieu in which the aspirations to produce

The Cervix came to fruition. His unobtrusive encouragement has been a great stimulus to both of us.

A final acknowledgement is due for secretarial assistance: in Sheffield to Mrs Jennifer Haydn-Smith and in Birmingham to Miss Sandra Bullock. The illustrations in some of the text were produced by the Department of Medical Illustrations, Royal Hospital, Sheffield, under the able direction of Mr Alan K. Tunstill; Miss Sue Hunter expertly drew the line figures that appear in Chapters 2, 5, 8, 18 and 25.

Both of us feel that this text could not have been completed so painlessly or so rapidly without the friendly and sincere advice, encouragement and cajoling of Mr David Inglis of W.B. Saunders and his two able and charming subeditors, Mrs Maggie Pettifer and Miss Pat Terry.

Joseph A. Jordan, Birmingham
Albert Singer, Sheffield
June 1976

Preface to the second edition

It was nearly three decades ago that two young research fellows, recently having completed their MD and PhD degrees respectively, asked 43 of their mainly senior colleagues to contribute to an all-encompassing text dealing with the cervix in health and disease. Indeed, they were anxious that a certain amount of youthful temerity would result in their colleagues' refusal to join such an ambitious project, but few declined and so became *The Cervix*, first published in 1976.

Now 30 years later a second edition is, following a 4-year gestation and much anxiety from the current contributors and editors, about to be delivered. Numerous delays have been encountered in its development, mainly as a result of the editors' wish to incorporate the latest information that flows in ever-increasing torrents from meetings, seminars and workshops around the world. The IARC (WHO) meeting in Lyon in 2004, which critically reviewed all aspects of cervical cancer screening, the biennial International HPV meetings and, finally, the triennial EUROGIN conference, held in April 2006, are all covered but their inclusion did inevitably cause delay.

Since the first edition was published much has happened in virtually every aspect of this subject. In many instances, where there was doubt there is now certainty, and where there was certainty there is now doubt. Who would have contemplated human papillomavirus being the cause of lower genital neoplasia and molecular markers challenging the all-powerful and seemingly certain method of screening in the form of exfoliative cytology? One could only have dreamt of these changes in 1976. What has developed, not surprisingly, over those years is a more certain understanding of the fundamental mechanisms of carcinogenesis, and so the editors have recruited experts in these fields to give a comprehensive and up-to-date report on this rapidly evolving and exciting area.

Balancing this new knowledge with clinical practice has been challenging, not only in fields related to oncology but also in those relating to benign diseases and conditions affecting the cervix. The emotional problems of women with malignant and non-malignant disease have also been acknowledged and their important place in clinical practice discussed.

The understanding of the basic structure and function of the cervix has evolved at just as rapid a pace. These new concepts have been described and clarified by the generous contributions of illustrations from some colleagues who are not authors. The editors have therefore been able to produce what they feel will be an authoritative and visually attractive text for the reader. The style of textual presentation has been kept uniform throughout and repetition kept to a minimum by cross-referencing wherever appropriate.

Great professionalism has been shown by the response of many of the contributors whom we asked to update their original contributions at a late stage, in many cases resulting in references as recent as 4–5 months before publication being included in their chapters. We can only admire and thank them most sincerely. Andrew G. Östör was a close friend and internationally recognised pathologist who sadly passed away after he had submitted a draft of his chapter. It has been brought to completion by his colleagues as Chapter 22. Ellis Pixley died some years ago but his chapter is regarded by the editors as a classic and is reproduced in its original form. Both are remembered with fondness and respect.

The production of such a text needs many hands on board. The two original editors invited two colleagues, Howard Jones III of Nashville, TN, USA, and Mahmood Shafi of Cambridge, UK, to assist with its production: we are most grateful to them for their help and support. The huge task of organising and retyping most of the raw material for the book, correction of text and liaison with contributors was undertaken in the first instance by Madeline and Joost Cohen of Textpertise in London, whose contribution was invaluable. The expertise of Rebecca Huxley of Blackwell Publishing in Oxford in coordinating the production meant that the post-submission tasks for the editors were clearly set out and their work thereby immeasurably facilitated. Although she despaired over delays occasioned by our additions to supposedly completed chapters in order to incorporate the newest research, without her ingenuity and forbearance this book would not be the state-of-the-art resource that it has become. The final stages of production were taken in hand by Gillian Whytock and her team at Prepress Projects, who assisted the editors in resolving the remaining issues and produced this beautiful, polished volume. Again, their contribution to the final success of this publication is inestimable.

Our wives and families have had to endure many years of missed events and absent partners and have been, effectively, wedded to this project. We hope that they appreciate that through their support (for the second time in their married lives) they have contributed to a piece of work that will benefit all womankind, who will, it is hoped, benefit from the knowledge and expertise that is incorporated in *The Cervix*.

Joseph A. Jordan, Birmingham
Albert Singer, London
June 2006

PART 1

Basic structure and function of the cervix

CHAPTER 1

Morphogenesis and differentiation of the cervicovaginal epithelium

John M. McLean

INTRODUCTION

Although the study of prenatal life dates back to antiquity, the first attempt to describe human prenatal development, utilising only human material, was the *Manual of Human Embryology* published in two volumes by Kiebel and Mall in 1910 and 1912. The Carnegie collection, established by Mall in 1915 with 813 human embryos, is now, with its several thousand specimens, the most important and most thoroughly studied collection of human embryos in the world.

As neonates of placental mammals must be capable of sustaining extra-uterine life, all essential organs are developed and functional at birth. This prerequisite for survival is achieved during markedly different periods of gestation. An interval of 14–16 days between fertilisation and parturition is sufficient for the hamster, 20–23 days suffice for mice and rats while the comparable period for elephants is 22 months and for humans is approximately 38 weeks. The first 8 weeks of prenatal human life constitute the embryonic phase and the remaining 30 weeks the fetal phase. During embryogenesis, all essential organ systems develop and, with the exception of the lungs, are functional while the recognisable form of the human infant is established. The majority of congenital anomalies arise as a result of defective morphogenesis during the later part of embryogenesis and early part of the fetal period.

Because development is a continuous process, various means have been used to identify and tabulate the progression of events during normal human embryogenesis. The founder of the Carnegie collection, Mall, was the first to introduce staging into human embryology. Mall's observations, together with those of his successor, Streeter, form the basis upon which the first 8 weeks of human development are described in 23 Carnegie stages. Using the Carnegie collection and other human embryos, including some fertilised *in vitro*, O'Rahilly (1973) produced the first comprehensive and authoritative account of the prenatal period from fertilisation to the end of the third week of gestation (Carnegie stages 1–9). In 1987, with Muller as co-author, the 1973 publication was revised and extended to cover the whole of embryogenesis (Carnegie stages 1–23).

Generally, the crown–rump length of larger embryos and all fetuses should be stated in preference to, or at least in addition to, the supposed age (O'Rahilly and Muller, 1987) but, in this account, the reference point will be the postovulatory age, i.e. the length of time since the last ovulation, related, when appropriate, to the Carnegie stage. As ovulation and fertilisation are closely related in time, the postovulatory interval is an adequate measure of embryonic age. Embryonic age, length and stage are all interrelated. Age, however, conveys an immediate meaning as it is a familiar yardstick, but it must be recognised that prenatal ages are only as useful as postnatal ages, because they are reference points for the usual pattern or range of developmental events.

Much of the available information on human embryogenesis is derived from traditional embryological studies. However, with the advent of assisted conception and the establishment of the Human Fertilisation and Embryology Authority, direct observation of the human embryo *in vitro* has provided an additional source of information on the preimplantation phase of human embryogenesis. Furthermore, the use of sophisticated computer technology in association with specifically designed three-dimensional transvaginal probes allows more detailed *in vivo* three-dimensional ultrasound reconstructions of embryos and early fetuses. The results obtained using these techniques correspond well to those obtained from classical human embryology (Blaas *et al.*, 1998).

EARLY EMBRYOGENESIS

The embryo, at fertilisation, initiates, sustains, directs and controls its own development. Embryogenesis begins with fertilisation, Carnegie stage 1, and is followed by a phase of preimplantation development, Carnegie stages 2 and 3. Implantation begins on day 6 and is completed on day 12, Carnegie stages 4 and 5. During these few days, the embryo enters into an intimate vascular relationship with the mother and becomes dependent on her for continued existence. Significant events are also taking place within the embryo during this period: continuous cell division and differentiation; the formation of the blastocyst within which is the embryonic pole; the appearance of the amniotic cavity within the embryonic pole on day 7 and, with it, the formation of two basic cell types, ectoderm and endoderm, establishing the bilaminar embryo; the appearance of the primitive umbilical cord on day 11; and, during Carnegie stage 6, days 13–15, the formation of the primitive streak and the conversion of the embryo into a trilaminar structure of ectoderm, intraembryonic mesoderm and endoderm.

The central nervous system and the skin, together with its appendages, arise from ectoderm; endoderm gives origin to the gastrointestinal tract, the respiratory tract and the urogenital sinus, while the remaining body structures are formed from intraembryonic mesoderm, within which the pericardial, pleural and peritoneal cavities also develop. The flat trilaminar early embryo, however, remains bilaminar at two sites, the buccopharyngeal membrane at the rostral end of the embryo and the cloacal membrane at its caudal end.

FLEXION

The neural tube, derived from ectoderm, is enclosed within the intraembryonic mesoderm during Carnegie stages 9–13, days 19–28. The rapid growth of the neural tube causes the flat trilaminar embryo to fold along its longitudinal and transverse axes, creating a marked dorsal convexity and ventral concavity and forming head, tail and lateral folds (Fig. 1.1a and b).

The endoderm is drawn into the ventral concavity of the embryo and is subdivided into foregut, midgut and hindgut. The hindgut is caudal to the rostral limit of the allantoic diverticulum and also dorsal and rostral to the cloacal membrane (Fig. 1.1a). The intraembryonic mesoderm in the midembryo region (Fig. 1.1b) is subdivided into paraxial mesoderm, lateral mesoderm and intermediate mesoderm. The paraxial mesoderm surrounds the neural tube and is the site of somite formation. The lateral mesoderm, so named because of its location in the flat trilaminar embryo, is carried ventrally by the formation of the lateral folds. The lateral mesoderm accommodates the primitive peritoneal cavity, which divides it into splanchnopleuric mesoderm, associated with endoderm and destined to form the visceral muscle of the gut tube and bladder, and somatopleuric mesoderm, associated with ectoderm and destined to participate in the formation of the body wall.

The intermediate mesoderm extends the length of the body cavity. It is lateral and ventral to the paraxial mesoderm and adjacent to the midline, dorsal mesentery of the gut tube. At the caudal end of the primitive peritoneal cavity, the intermediate mesoderm is in continuity with the mesoderm investing the terminal portion of the hindgut and, ventral to the hindgut, with the urorectal septum (Fig. 1.2). Within the intermediate mesoderm, structures involved in the morphogenesis of the urinary and reproductive systems develop.

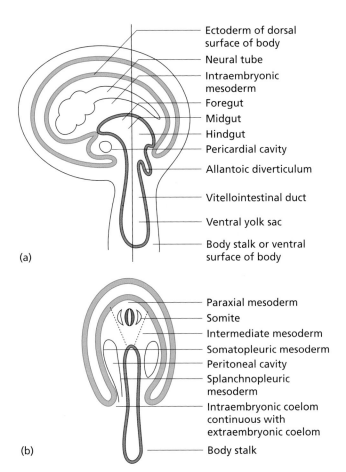

(a)

Labels: Ectoderm of dorsal surface of body; Neural tube; Intraembryonic mesoderm; Foregut; Midgut; Hindgut; Pericardial cavity; Allantoic diverticulum; Vitellointestinal duct; Ventral yolk sac; Body stalk or ventral surface of body

(b)

Labels: Paraxial mesoderm; Somite; Intermediate mesoderm; Somatopleuric mesoderm; Peritoneal cavity; Splanchnopleuric mesoderm; Intraembryonic coelom continuous with extraembryonic coelom; Body stalk

Fig. 1.1 (a) A midline section of the embryo after formation of the head and tail folds. (b) A transverse section of the midembryo region after formation of the lateral folds.

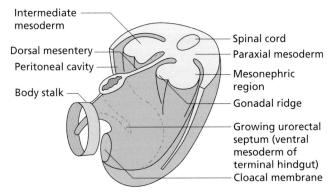

Labels: Intermediate mesoderm; Dorsal mesentery; Peritoneal cavity; Body stalk; Spinal cord; Paraxial mesoderm; Mesonephric region; Gonadal ridge; Growing urorectal septum (ventral mesoderm of terminal hindgut); Cloacal membrane

Fig. 1.2 The caudal half of the embryo showing the gonadal ridge and mesonephric region of the intermediate mesoderm which, at its caudal limit, is continuous with the mesoderm investing the hindgut.

The urorectal septum

The hindgut, established during the process of flexion, is the endoderm enclosed within the tail fold of the embryo. It lies caudal to the rostral limit of the allantoic diverticulum and

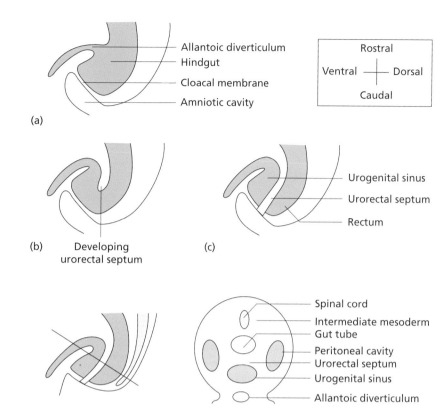

Fig. 1.3 (a) The primitive hindgut is enclosed within the embryonic tail fold. (b) The developing urorectal septum grows dorsally and caudally from the rostral limit of the allantoic diverticulum. (c) The fusion of the urorectal septum with the cloacal membrane divides the hindgut into urogenital sinus and rectum.

Fig. 1.4 A transverse section through the embryonic pelvis demonstrates the continuity of the intermediate mesoderm with the mesoderm of the urorectal septum.

dorsal and rostral to the cloacal membrane (Fig. 1.3a). The mesoderm at the rostral limit of the allantoic diverticulum extends dorsally and caudally in the line of the tail fold curvature, as the urorectal septum, dividing the hindgut into ventral and dorsal parts. As the division proceeds, the two parts of the hindgut remain in continuity with each other caudal to the advancing mesoderm of the urorectal septum (Fig. 1.3b). The mesoderm reaches the cloacal membrane at 30–32 days as the Carnegie stage moves from 13 to 14 (O'Rahilly and Muller, 1987). As the urorectal septum fuses with the cloacal membrane, the embryonic hindgut is completely divided into the ventral urogenital sinus and dorsal rectum (Fig. 1.3c).

The urorectal septum, interposed between the dorsal gut tube and the ventral urogenital sinus, is in direct continuity across the wall of the gut tube with the intermediate mesoderm (Fig. 1.4).

The mesonephric ducts

The first indication of the urinary system in the human embryo appears at 21 days when mesonephric vesicles develop within the intermediate mesoderm (O'Rahilly and Muecke, 1972). These vesicles associate medially with branches of the dorsal aorta and laterally with a solid rod of cells developing within the lateral part of the intermediate mesoderm at 24 days. This solid rod of cells acquires a lumen at 26 days and forms the mesonephric duct. The mesonephric vesicles open into the mesonephric duct as it extends caudally through the intermediate mesoderm. Skirting the gastrointestinal hindgut, the mesonephric duct enters the urorectal septum to reach the posterior (dorsal) surface of the urogenital sinus into which it opens at 28 days during Carnegie stage 13 (O'Rahilly, 1977). At 30–32 days (O'Rahilly and Muller, 1987), the urorectal septum completes the separation of the urogenital sinus from the rectum. The functioning mesonephros produces an increase in pressure in the closed urogenital sinus and ruptures the ventral part of the cloacal membrane, allowing urogenital sinus endoderm to come into apposition with body wall ectoderm and the urogenital sinus to communicate with the amniotic cavity (Ludwig, 1965).

In 1759, Caspar Friedrich Wolff described a symmetrical pair of paravertebral swellings in the chick embryo as the precursors of the kidneys. The adjective Wolffian is therefore often used to describe the duct and vesicles of the mesonephros (Stephens, 1982). The mesonephros has only a transient renal function in the human embryo, but the mesonephric duct is crucial to the subsequent morphogenesis of the kidney and female reproductive tract. As the urorectal septum reaches the cloacal membrane at 30–32 days, the caudal end of each mesonephric duct, having already opened into the urogenital sinus, gives origin to the ureteric bud and begins to be incorporated into the posterior wall of the urogenital sinus (Keith, 1948; Davies, 2001). The portion of the mesonephric duct incorporated into the urogenital sinus subsequently forms the

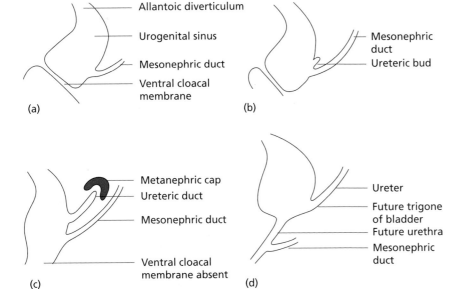

(a)
— Allantoic diverticulum
— Urogenital sinus
— Mesonephric duct
— Ventral cloacal membrane

(b)
— Mesonephric duct
— Ureteric bud

(c)
— Metanephric cap
— Ureteric duct
— Mesonephric duct
— Ventral cloacal membrane absent

(d)
— Ureter
— Future trigone of bladder
— Future urethra
— Mesonephric duct

Fig. 1.5 (a) The mesonephric duct, within the urorectal septum, opens into the urogenital sinus. (b) The caudal limit of the mesonephric duct gives origin to the ureteric bud. (c) The metanephric cap forms at the growing end of the ureteric bud or duct. (d) Tissue of mesonephric origin is incorporated into the posterior aspect of the urogenital sinus between the ureter and the mesonephric duct.

trigone of the bladder and the posterior wall of the urethra (Fig. 1.5). The ureteric bud, arising from the mesonephric duct, ascends the duct's path of descent and, acquiring a lumen, eventually forms the collecting system and ureter of the ipsilateral kidney (Davies, 2001) with the metanephric cap forming renal tissue.

The paramesonephric ducts

Johannes Müller (1830), describing genital development, identified another cord of cells on the outer aspect of the mesonephric or Wolffian cord. He concluded that, although the two cords were either attached or adjacent to each other, they were 'two quite different things'. These Müllerian ducts, now termed paramesonephric ducts, appear in the human embryo between Carnegie stages 16 and 17 at 37–41 days (O'Rahilly and Muller, 1987). Each duct appears as an invagination of the peritoneal epithelium on the lateral aspect of the intermediate mesoderm at the cephalic end of the mesonephros (Felix, 1912; Faulconer, 1951). Initially, each paramesonephric duct extends caudally as a cord of cells in the intermediate mesoderm, in close association with, and initially lateral to, the mesonephric duct (Fig. 1.6). The mesonephric duct has been shown experimentally both to induce the paramesonephric duct (Didier, 1973a,b) and to guide its descent (Gruenwald, 1941); indeed, the growing caudal tip of the paramesonephric duct lies within the basement membrane of the mesonephric duct (Frutiger, 1969). As the paramesonephric cord of cells continues its descent, a lumen appears in its cranial portion and extends caudally behind the growing tip of the paramesonephric cord, converting it into a duct. During descent, the paramesonephric duct passes ventral to the mesonephric duct and completes its journey to

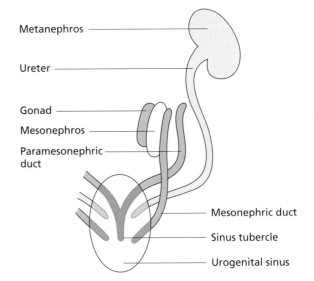

Metanephros —
Ureter —
Gonad —
Mesonephros —
Paramesonephric duct —
— Mesonephric duct
— Sinus tubercle
— Urogenital sinus

Fig. 1.6 The indifferent human embryo possesses mesonephric and paramesonephric ducts. The terminal paramesonephric ducts fuse within the urorectal septum and reach the urogenital sinus at the sinus tubercle situated between the openings of the two mesonephric ducts.

the posterior aspect of the urogenital sinus within the urorectal septum on the medial aspect of the mesonephric duct and in close apposition to the contralateral paramesonephric duct (Fig. 1.6). Indeed, as soon as the paramesonephric ducts come into close contact with each other, they begin to fuse even before their growing ends reach the urogenital sinus (Koff, 1933). The external surfaces of the medial walls, initially in apposition, begin to fuse and eventually the duct lumina are separated only by a median septum (O'Rahilly, 1977).

At 49 days, before the paramesonephric ducts reach the urogenital sinus, a tubercle appears on the internal aspect of its posterior wall, between the openings of the mesonephric ducts. This tubercle is not formed by the paramesonephric ducts but identifies the site at which the common paramesonephric duct fuses with the posterior wall of the urogenital sinus at 56 days (Glenister, 1962; Josso, 1981).

Sexual determination and differentiation

The sex of an individual is determined at fertilisation with sexual dimorphism being brought about by subsequent differentiation. The genetic or chromosomal sex of the zygote determines the gonadal sex of the embryo, which itself regulates the differentiation of the internal and external genital apparatus and hence the sexual phenotype of the individual. At puberty, the development of secondary sexual characteristics reinforces the phenotypic manifestations of sexual dimorphism, which achieves its biological fulfilment in successful procreation.

Both male and female embryos possess the same indifferent gonadal and genital primordia. The indifferent gonad differentiates as a testis under the influence of 'a battery of genes on the Y chromosome . . . and certain genes on other chromosomes' (Mittwoch and Burgess, 1991; Slaney *et al.*, 1998). In placental mammals, sexual dimorphism is mediated by the testis and its secretions and takes place in an environment of high estrogen and progestogen concentrations. However, it has long been recognised that these differentiating processes are regulated by numerous specific genes, located on sex chromosomes and autosomes, that act through a variety of mechanisms, including organising factors, sex steroid and peptide secretions and specific tissue receptors (Grumbach and Conte, 1981). More recently, 79 genes have been identified as being specifically expressed in the developing gonad and sex ducts, and 21 of the gonad-specific genes showed sexual dimorphic expression, suggesting a role in sex determination and/or gonad differentiation (Wertz and Herrmann, 2000).

GENITAL DUCT DIFFERENTIATION

During Carnegie stage 14, at 32 days, the gonadal ridge begins to form on the medial aspect of the mesonephros (O'Rahilly and Muller, 1987). Until approximately 42 days, Carnegie stage 17, this ridge forms the indifferent gonad, and male and female embryos are morphologically indistinguishable (Fig. 1.7). The transformation of the indifferent gonad into an embryonic testis or ovary takes place over the following 14 days, during Carnegie stages 18–23.

At the end of the embryonic period, with the completion of Carnegie stage 23, the fetus has either testes or ovaries, but possesses both mesonephric and paramesonephric duct systems (Fig. 1.7). Subsequent sexual differentiation of these ducts is governed by fetal testicular hormones (Jost, 1947), which cause regression of the paramesonephric ducts and

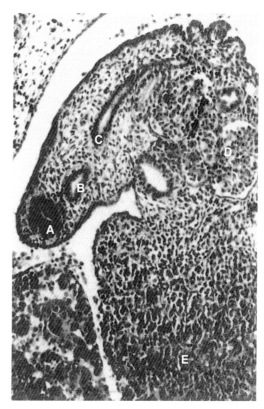

Fig. 1.7 A transverse section of the right side of the upper abdomen of a 42-day embryo showing: A, the paramesonephric duct with a barely discernible lumen; B, the mesonephric duct; C, a mesonephric tubule; D, the mesonephros; E, the gonad. H&E × 325.

stabilisation of the mesonephric ducts. In the female fetus, the absence of testicular hormones allows regression of the mesonephric ducts and stabilisation of the paramesonephric ducts.

Male differentiation

Paramesonephric duct

In the male paramesonephric duct, regression begins at 56–60 days (Jirasek, 1977). Once initiated, regression extends caudally and cranially and is complete at 70 days (Jirasek, 1971). Remnants survive bilaterally: the closed cranial portion is associated with the testis as its appendix (hydatid of Morgagni), and the caudal ends participate in the formation of the prostatic utricle.

Regression of the male paramesonephric ducts is caused by anti-Müllerian hormone (AMH), a glycoprotein produced by Sertoli cells (Blanchard and Josso, 1974; Price, 1979), first identified in the fetal testes at 60 days (Jirasek, 1977). AMH is capable of causing paramesonephric duct regression for a limited time during intrauterine life and, unless its action is initiated early in the fetal period and rapidly completed, the paramesonephric ducts become resistant to its inhibitory effect (Josso *et al.*, 1977). Persistence of paramesonephric ducts has been observed in otherwise normal human males and in some animals (Jost, 1965; Josso, 1979). This abnormality is X-linked (Sloan and Walsh, 1976) and may be due to a defect in AMH production or a block to its action. The gene for human AMH has been localised to the short arm of chromosome 19 (Cohen-Haguenauer *et al.*, 1987).

The morphological evidence of AMH's action on the para-mesonephric ducts indicates dissolution of the basal membrane and mesodermal condensation around the duct (Josso and Picard, 1986). Recent work has confirmed these observations. In transgenic mice of both sexes, overexpression of the human AMH gene is associated with increased apoptosis in the Müllerian epithelium, while in AMH-deficient male mice, there is decreased apoptosis (Allard *et al.*, 2000). Although apoptosis is the decisive event in Müllerian duct regression, the epitheliomesenchymal interaction is required for its completion (Allard *et al.*, 2000). The fetal and post-natal testis continues to produce AMH, and its serum concentration begins to decline only with the onset of puberty (Hudson *et al.*, 1990). Its role during this period is unknown, but it has been suggested that it is involved in the process of testicular descent and the suppression of meiotic maturation of male germ cells (Josso and Picard, 1986). Post-natally, granulosa cells also secrete AMH (Ueno *et al.*, 1989), resulting in serum concentrations in pubertal girls and women that are similar to those in men (Gustafson *et al.*, 1992). These authors observed increased concentrations of AMH in a patient with an ovarian sex cord tumour. A more recent immunohistochemical study of AMH expression in human prenatal and postnatal gonadal tissue confirmed its restriction to Sertoli and granulosa cells and provided evidence of ovarian expression just before birth (Rajpert-DeMetys *et al.*, 1999).

Mesonephric duct

The second aspect of male differentiation is the integration of the mesonephric duct into the genital system when the metanephric kidney begins to function at 50 days (Potter and Osathanondh, 1966). The cranial mesonephric tubules establish continuity with the rete testis to become the vasa efferentia, the mesonephric duct forms the epididymis and vas deferens, while its closed cranial end persists as the appendix of the epididymis.

The persistence of the mesonephric duct and its incorporation into the genital system of the male fetus is testosterone dependent. Testosterone production by Leydig cells of the testis begins at 56 days (Siiteri and Wilson, 1974) under the control of maternal chorionic gonadotrophin (Hudson and Burger, 1979). Stabilisation of the mesonephric ducts occurs between 56 and 70 days in synchrony with the degeneration of the paramesonephric ducts (Price *et al.*, 1975). Mesonephric

ducts in young female embryos can be stabilised by exposure to testosterone before the end of the 'critical period' for sex differentiation. In man, this critical period embraces the end of embryogenesis and the beginning of early fetal life. Thereafter, exposure of the female fetus to testosterone does not prevent the degeneration of the mesonephric ducts (Josso, 1981) but will cause varying degrees of virilisation of the external genitalia (Grumbach and Ducharme, 1960).

Female differentiation

As male differentiation of the paramesonephric and mesonephric ducts occurs in the XY fetus, the comparable structures in the XX fetus are already irreversibly committed to female organogenesis (Josso *et al.*, 1977). Female organogenesis involves regression of the mesonephric ducts and stabilisation of the paramesonephric ducts.

Mesonephric duct

The mesonephric duct has been shown experimentally to induce the paramesonephric duct (Didier, 1973a,b) and to guide its descent (Gruenwald, 1941). The caudal end of each mesonephric duct gives origin to the ureteric bud and is incorporated into the urogenital sinus to form the trigone of the bladder and the posterior wall of the urethra (Fig. 1.5). As the metanephric kidney begins to function at 50 days (Potter and Osathanondh, 1966), the female mesonephric system becomes redundant, although it has been suggested that the mesonephric ducts contribute to the formation of the uterus (Witschi, 1970) and the vagina (Forsberg, 1965).

Towards the end of embryogenesis, the mesonephric vesicles begin to degenerate together with the mesonephric ducts. The lumen of the mesonephric duct is obliterated at 75 days and only remnants persist at 105 days (Josso, 1981). A number of mesonephric derivatives may be located in the adult female. A constant finding is the epoophoron associated with the ovary and derived from the cephalic mesonephric duct and adjacent vesicles (Duthie, 1925). A more caudal portion of the mesonephros may be encountered in the broad ligament as the paroophoron, while remnants of the terminal mesonephric duct may persist lateral to the uterus and vagina or incorporated into the cervix (O'Rahilly, 1977; Buntine, 1979). Adjacent to the lower genital tract, such remnants are referred to as Gartner's ducts.

Paramesonephric duct

Uterine tube

The upper segment of each paramesonephric duct develops fimbriae at its cephalic end and subsequently forms the uterine tube. The transverse lie of the uterine tube is established by the descent of the ipsilateral ovary into the pelvis. The uterotubal junction is demarcated by an abrupt increase in the diameter of the uterine segment.

Uterus

The morphogenesis of the uterus begins as the para-mesonephric ducts come into apposition within the urorectal septum and begin to fuse. At the end of the embryonic period, the caudal segment of the common paramesonephric duct reaches the posterior wall of the urogenital sinus and fuses with the sinus tubercle (Fig. 1.8a), situated between the openings of the two mesonephric ducts (Glenister, 1962; O'Rahilly, 1977; Josso, 1981). At 63 days, the body and the cervix are distinguishable by the presence of a constriction between them (Hunter, 1930). Linear extension of the cavity occurs by further fusion of the paramesonephric ducts rostrally and by their continued growth caudally (O'Rahilly, 1977). This growing caudal end in contact with the posterior wall of the urogenital sinus induces additional cellular proliferation, essential to the development of the vagina.

Sinuvaginal bulb

After the common paramesonephric duct fuses with the sinus tubercle, in the posterior wall of the urogenital sinus, two dorsal projections from the sinus are identified which unite to form the midline sinuvaginal bulb (Fig. 1.8b). As the sinuvaginal bulb arises following the fusion of the common paramesonephric duct with the urogenital sinus, at a site between the openings of the two mesonephric ducts, it has been variously suggested that the vagina, through the contribution made to it by the sinuvaginal bulb, arises from the paramesonephric ducts (Felix, 1912), the mesonephric ducts (Forsberg, 1973), the urogenital sinus (Bulmer, 1957; Fluhmann, 1960) or from a combination of paramesonephric and mesonephric tissue (Witschi, 1970), paramesonephric and mesonephric tissue (Witschi, 1970), paramesonephric and

sinus tissue (Koff, 1933; Agogue, 1965), or mesonephric and sinus tissue (Forsberg 1973), with the relative contributions of each tissue an additional matter for controversy (O'Rahilly, 1977).

Vaginal plate

Subsequent proliferation of the lining epithelium of the sinuvaginal bulb converts it into a midline solid tissue projection, displacing the genital canal, at the caudal limit of the common paramesonephric duct, in a dorsal direction (Fig. 1.8c). The solid sinuvaginal outgrowth and the solid caudal end of the genital canal together form the vaginal plate identified in the fetus at 87 days (Fig. 1.8c). The formation of the vaginal plate is followed immediately by its caudal extension towards the cloacal vestibule. As this caudal extension occurs, desquamation of cells from the vaginal plate establishes the utero-vaginal canal (Fig. 1.8d), opening into the cloacal vestibule at 14 weeks (Terruhn, 1980).

Uterine cervix and vagina

The cervix, which forms the distal two-thirds of the fetal uterus (Pryse-Davies and Dewhurst, 1971), is of paramesonephric origin (Koff, 1933; Forsberg, 1965; Witschi, 1970) with its epithelium probably derived from the urogenital sinus (Fluhmann, 1960). The solid sinovaginal bulb and the caudal portion of the common paramesonephric duct together form the vaginal plate, which establishes the vagina after canalisation.

For many years, the conflicting opinions expressed concerning the morphogenesis and differentiation of the cervicovaginal epithelium were of little more than academic interest.

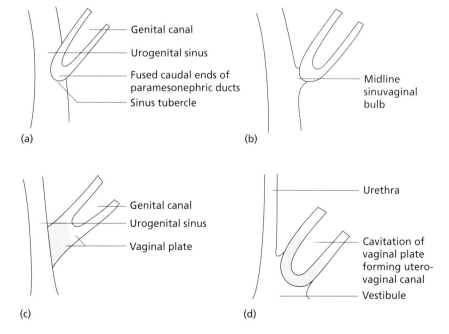

Fig. 1.8 (a) The fused paramesonephric ducts form the genital canal, the solid caudal end of which abuts the posterior wall of the urogenital sinus at the sinus tubercle. (b) Cellular proliferation of the sinus epithelium generates the sinuvaginal bulbs, which fuse and displace the genital canal dorsally. (c) Further cellular proliferation converts the sinuvaginal bulb into a solid tissue projection which participates in the formation of the vaginal plate. (d) Extensive caudal growth of the vaginal plate brings its lower surface into the primitive vestibule.

However, since the early 1970s, many publications have associated the occurrence of cervical and vaginal ridges, vaginal adenosis, ectropion and clear cell carcinoma of the vagina in young adult females with prenatal exposure to diethylstilbestrol (Greenwald *et al.*, 1971; Herbst *et al.*, 1971, 1972, 1974; Fetherston *et al.*, 1972; Hill, 1973; Pomerance, 1973; Barber and Sommers, 1974). The drug was considered to have had a teratogenic effect on the developing lower genital tract. Uterine synechiae and hypoplasia in 60% of exposed females indicate that the teratogen also affects the upper genital tract (Kaufmann *et al.*, 1977). In addition, some 20% of exposed males demonstrate some abnormality of their reproductive tracts such as epididymal cysts, hypoplastic testes, cryptorchidism and spermatozoal deficiencies (Gill *et al.*, 1976).

Differences of opinion concerning the interpretation of the morphological evidence of vaginal development may indicate a variation in the sequence of events involved in its morphogenesis. Nevertheless, it is reasonable to assume that the sinuvaginal bulb, arising from the urogenital sinus (Koff, 1933; Bulmer, 1957), forms the lower part of the vagina. The occurrence of certain congenital anomalies strongly supports this interpretation; otherwise, the presence of a rectovaginal fistula would be difficult to explain, as would the opening of a misplaced ureter into the vagina (Bremer, 1957) and the foreshortening of the vagina in the congenital absence of paramesonephric ducts.

When the vaginal opening reaches the vestibule at 14 weeks (Terruhn, 1980), the sinus and paramesonephric elements both contribute to the vaginal canal, with the sinus portion exhibiting stratified squamous epithelium and the paramesonephric portion pseudostratified columnar epithelium. At this stage, the genital canal has a cervical dilatation which marks the region of the vaginal fornices (Koff, 1933), while at 17 weeks the future os is identified as the site of the squamocolumnar junction (Bulmer, 1957). During this interval, the pseudostratified columnar epithelium of the paramesonephric component of the vagina has been transformed into stratified squamous epithelium (Bulmer, 1957; Davies and Kusama, 1962). It has been variously reported that, at 22 weeks, the cervical canal is lined with stratified squamous epithelium with an entropion present (Eida, 1961), while from 22 weeks to term the squamocolumnar junction is said to be situated some distance external to the os, producing the congenital ectropion (Davies and Kusama, 1962).

A possible interpretation of the evidence is that the cervix and the upper segment of the vagina are initially lined by paramesonephric tissue, which subsequently undergoes apoptosis to be replaced by sinus tissue. In explanation of the teratogenic effect of diethylstilbestrol, it has been suggested that the drug delays or limits this apoptosis and replacement and adversely affects the persisting paramesonephric tissue (Ulfelder and Robboy, 1976). Certainly, the occurrence of upper genital tract abnormalities associated with prenatal exposure to diethylstilbestrol (Kaufmann *et al.*, 1977) supports these suggestions.

In the newborn, the stratified squamous epithelium of the vagina shows evidence of a marked estrogen response. The site of the junction between the cervical and vaginal epithelia is variable and there is a range of normal appearances.

Role of p63

Apoptosis, programmed cell death, is an integral part of all biological systems and occurs in response to cascades of signals that are highly conserved throughout the animal kingdom. The protein p53, first described in 1979, is the gene product of *TP53*, which maps to chromosome 17p12. p53 has several functions in the cell and is often described as 'the guardian of the genome' because of its role in preventing replication of cells with damaged DNA. Loss or mutation of *TP53* is probably the commonest single genetic change in cancer (Strachan and Read, 1999).

p63 is a recently characterised p53 homologue (Reis-Filho and Schmitt, 2002). p63 protein, the gene for which maps to chromosome 3q27, is required for cutaneous development and is expressed in immature squamous epithelium and reserve cells of the cervix (Ince *et al.*, 2002). As humans with p63 mutations exhibit defects in genitourinary development (Ince *et al.*, 2002), its role in female genital tract development has been investigated in mice. In mice, the transformation of vaginal paramesonephric pseudostratified columnar epithelium to stratified squamous epithelium takes place during the first week of neonatal life (Forsberg, 1963).

In the reproductive tract of the adult female mouse, p63 is highly expressed in basal cells of the vaginal and cervical epithelium but not in uterine epithelium (Kurita and Cunha, 2001). These investigators, although unable to detect p63 in embryonic paramesonephric epithelium, demonstrated its expression in the differentiated vaginal epithelium during the first week of postnatal life. They further demonstrated that neonatal exposure to diethylstilbestrol induced irregularities in p63 expression and epithelial differentiation during the first week of postnatal life. They concluded that such exposure disturbs uterine and vaginal epithelial differentiation by perturbing epithelial expression of p63 during development.

REFERENCES

Agogue M (1965) Dualite embryologique du vagin humain et origine histologique de sa muqueuse. *Gynecologie et Obstetrique* 64: 407–414.

Allard S, Adin P, Gouedard L *et al.* (2000) Molecular mechanisms of hormone-mediated Müllerian duct regression: involvement of beta-catenin. *Development* 127: 3349–3360.

Barber HRK, Sommers SC (1974) Vaginal adenosis dysplasia and clear-cell adenocarcinoma after diethylstilbestrol treatment in pregnancy. *Obstetrics and Gynecology* 43: 645–682.

Blaas HG, Eik-Nes SH, Berg S *et al.* (1998) In-vivo three-dimensional ultrasound reconstructions of embryos and early fetuses. *Lancet* 352: 1182–1186.

Blanchard MG, Josso N (1974) Source of the anti Müllerian hormone synthesized by the fetal testes: Müllerian inhibiting activity of fetal bovine Sertoli cells in tissue culture. *Pediatric Research* 8: 968–971.

Bremer JL (1957) *Congenital Anomalies of the Viscera.* Cambridge: Harvard University Press.

Bulmer D (1957) The development of the human vagina. *Journal of Anatomy* 91: 490–509.

Buntine DW (1979) Adenocarcinoma of the uterine cervix of probable Wolffian origin. *Pathology* 11: 713–718.

Cohen-Haguenauer O, Picard JY, Mattei MG *et al.* (1987) Mapping of the gene for anti-Müllerian hormone to the short arm of human chromosome 19. *Cytogenetics and Cellular Genetics* 44: 2–6.

Davies J (2001) Intracellular and extracellular regulation of ureteric bud morphogenesis. *Journal of Anatomy* 198: 257–264.

Davies J, Kusama H (1962) Developmental aspects of the human cervix. *Annals of the New York Academy of Science* 97: 534–550.

Didier E (1973a) Recherches sur la morphogenese du canal de Muller chez les oiseaux. I. Etude descriptive. *Wilhelm Roux Archives* 172: 287–302.

Didier E (1973b) Recherches sur la morphogenese du canal de Muller chez les oiseaux. II. Etude experimentale. *Wilhelm Roux Archives* 172: 287–302.

Duthie GM (1925) An investigation of the occurrence, distribution and histological structure of the embryonic remains in the human broad ligament. *Journal of Anatomy* 59: 410–431.

Eida T (1961) Entwicklungsgeschichtliche Studien über der Verschiebung der Epithelgrenze an der Portio vaginalis cervicis. *Yokohama Medical Bulletin Supplement* 12: 54–63.

Faulconer RJ (1951) Observations on the origin of the Müllerian groove in human embryos. *Contributions to Embryology* 34: 159–164.

Felix W (1912) The development of the urogenital organs. In: Keibel F, Mall FP (eds) *Manual of Human Embryology.* Philadelphia: Lippincott, pp. 752–979.

Fetherston WC, Meyers A, Speckhard ME (1972) Adenocarcinoma of the vagina in young women. *Wisconsin Medical Journal* 71: 87–93.

Fluhmann CF (1960) The developmental anatomy of the cervix uteri. *Obstetrics and Gynecology* 15: 62–69.

Forsberg JG (1963) *Derivation and Differentiation of the Vaginal Epithelium.* Lund: Hakan Ohlssons Boktryckeri.

Forsberg JG (1965) Origin of vaginal epithelium. *Obstetrics and Gynecology* 25: 787–791.

Forsberg JG (1973) Cervicovaginal epithelium: its origin and development. *American Journal of Obstetrics and Gynecology* 115: 1025–1043.

Frutiger P (1969) Zur Fruhentwicklung der Ductus paramesonephrici und des Mullerschen Hugels beim Menschen. *Acta Anatomica* 72: 233–245.

Gill WB, Schumacher GFB, Bibbo M (1976) Structural and functional abnormalities in the sex organs of male offspring of women treated with diethylstilbestrol. *Journal of Reproductive Medicine* 16: 147–152.

Glenister TW (1962) The development of the utricle and of the so called 'middle' or 'median' lobe of the human prostate. *Journal of Anatomy* 96: 443–455.

Greenwald P, Barlow JJ, Nasca PC *et al.* (1971) Vaginal cancer after maternal treatment with synthetic estrogens. *New England Journal of Medicine* 285: 390–392.

Gruenwald P (1941) The relation of the growing Müllerian duct to the Wolffian duct and its importance for the genesis of malformations. *Anatomical Record* 81: 1–19.

Grumbach MM, Conte FA (1981) Disorders of sex differentiation. In: Williams RH (ed.) *Textbook of Endocrinology,* 6th edn. Philadelphia: Saunders, pp. 423–514.

Grumbach MM, Ducharme JR (1960) The effects of androgens on fetal sexual development, androgen-induced female pseudohermaphroditism. *Fertility and Sterility* 11: 157–180.

Gustafson ML, Lee MM, Scully RE *et al.* (1992) Müllerian inhibiting substance as a marker for ovarian sex-cord tumor. *New England Journal of Medicine* 326: 466–471.

Herbst AL, Ulfelder H, Poskanzer DC (1971) Adenocarcinoma of the vagina: association of maternal stilbestrol therapy with tumor appearance in young women. *New England Journal of Medicine* 284: 878–881.

Herbst AL, Kurman RJ, Scully RE (1972) Vaginal and cervical abnormalities after exposure to stilbestrol in utero. *Obstetrics and Gynecology* 40: 287–298.

Herbst AL, Robboy SJ, Scully RE *et al.* (1974) Clear-cell adenocarcinoma of the vagina and cervix in girls: analysis of 170 registry cases. *American Journal of Obstetrics and Gynecology* 119: 713–724.

Hill EC (1973) Clear cell carcinoma of the cervix and vagina in young women: a report of six cases with association of maternal stilbestrol thereby and adenosis of the vagina. *American Journal of Obstetrics and Gynecology* 116: 470–484.

Hudson B, Burger HG (1979) Physiology and function of the tests. In: Shearman RP (ed.) *Human Reproductive Physiology,* 2nd edn. Oxford: Blackwell Scientific Publications.

Hudson PL, Douglas I, Donahoe PK *et al.* (1990) An immunoassay to detect human Müllerian inhibiting substances in males and females during normal development. *Journal of Clinical Endocrinology and Metabolism* 70: 16–22.

Hunter RH (1930) Observations on the development of the human female genital tract. *Contributions to Embryology* 22: 91–108.

Ince TA, Cviko AP, Quade BJ *et al.* (2002) p63 coordinates anogenital modelling and epithelial cell differentiation in the developing female urogenital tract. *American Journal of Pathology* 161: 1111–1117.

Jirasek JE (1977) Morphogenesis of the genital system in the human. In: Blandau RJ, Bergsma D (eds) *Morphogenesis and Malformation of the Genital System.* New York: Liss, pp. 13–39.

Josso N (1979) Development and descent of the fetal testis. In: Bierich JR, Giarola A (eds) *Cryptorchidism.* London: Academic Press, pp. 7–20.

Josso N (1981) Differentiation of the genital tract: stimulators and inhibitors. In: Austin CR, Edwards RG (eds) *Mechanisms of Sex Differentiations in Animals and Man.* London: Academic Press, pp. 165–203.

Josso N, Picard JY (1986) Anti-Müllerian hormone. *Physiological Reviews* 66: 1038–1090.

Josso N, Picard JY, Tran D (1977) The anti-Müllerian hormone. In: Blandau RJ, Bergsma D (eds) *Morphogenesis and Malformation of the Genital System.* New York: Liss, pp. 59–84.

Jost A (1947) Recherches sur la differentiation sexuelle de l'embryon de lapin. *Archives d'Anatomie Microscopic et Morphologie Experimental* 36: 271–315.

Jost A (1965) Gonadal hormones in the sex differentiation of the mammalian fetus. In: de Haan RL, Ursprung H (eds) *Organogenesis*. New York: Holt Reinhart & Winston, pp. 611–628.

Kaufmann RH, Binder GL, Grav PM Jr *et al.* (1977) Upper genital tract changes associated with exposure in utero to diethylstilbestrol. *American Journal of Obstetrics and Gynecology* 128: 51–56.

Keith A (1948) *Human Embryology and Morphology*, 6th edn. London: Arnold.

Keibel F, Mall FP (1910–1912) *Manual of Human Embryology*, 2 vols. Philadelphia: Lippincott.

Koff AK (1933) Development of the vagina in the human fetus. *Contributions to Embryology* 24: 59–90.

Kurita T, Cunha GR (2001) Roles of p63 in differentiation of Müllerian duct epithelial cells. *Annals of the New York Academy of Science* 948: 9–12.

Ludwig E (1965) Uber die Beziehungen der Kloakenmembran zum Septum urorectale beimenschleichen Embryonen von 9 bis 33 mm. *Zeitschrift für Anatomie und Entwicklungsgeschichte* 124: 401–413.

Mittwoch U, Burgess AMC (1991) How do you get sex? *Journal of Endocrinology* 128: 329–331.

Müller J (1830) *Bildungsgeschichte der Genitalien aus anatomischen Untersuchungen an Embryonen des Menschen und der Tiere*. Dusseldorf: Arnz.

O'Rahilly R (1973) *Developmental Stages in Human Embryos* Part A: *Embryos of the First Three Weeks (Stages 1–9)*. Washington, DC: Carnegie Institution of Washington, Publication 631.

O'Rahilly R (1977) The development of the vagina in the human. In: Blandau RJ, Bergsma D (eds) *Morphogenesis and Malformation of the Genital System*. New York: Liss, pp. 123–136.

O'Rahilly R, Muecke EC (1972) The timing and sequence of events in the development of the human urinary system during the embryonic period proper. *Zeitschrift für Anatomie und Entwicklungsgeschichte* 138: 99–109.

O'Rahilly R, Muller F (1987) *Development Stages in Human Embryos*. Washington, DC: Carnegie Institution of Washington.

Pomerance W (1973) Post-stilbestrol secondary syndrome. *Obstetrics and Gynecology* 42: 12–18.

Potter EL, Osathanondh V (1966) Normal and abnormal development of the kidney. In: Mostofi FK, Smith E (eds) *The Kidney*. Baltimore, MD: Williams & Wilkins, pp. 1–16.

Price D, Zaaijer JJP, Ortiz E *et al.* (1975). Current views on embryonic sex differentiation in reptiles, birds and mammals. *American Zoology* 15: 173–195.

Price JM (1979) The secretion of Müllerian inhibiting substance by cultured isolated Sertoli cells of the neonatal calf. *American Journal of Anatomy* 156: 147–158.

Pryse-Davies J, Dewhurst CJ (1971) The development of the ovary and uterus in the foetus, newborn and infant: a morphological and enzyme histochemical study. *Journal of Pathology and Bacteriology* 103: 5–25.

Rajpert-De Meyts E, Jorgensen N, Graem N *et al.* (1999) Expression of anti-Müllerian hormone during normal and pathological gonadal development: association with differentiation of Sertoli and granulose cells. *Journal of Clinical Endocrinology and Metabolism* 84: 3836–3844.

Reis-Filho JS, Schmitt FC (2002) Taking advantage of basic research: p63 is a reliable myoepithelial and stem cell marker. *Advances in Anatomical Pathology* 9: 280–289.

Siiteri PK, Wilson JD (1974) Testosterone formation and metabolism during male sexual differentiation in the human embryo. *Journal of Clinical Endocrinology and Metabolism* 38: 113–125.

Slaney SF, Chalmers IJ, Affara NA *et al.* (1998) An autosomal or X-linked mutation results in true hermaphrodites and 46, XX males in the same family. *Journal of Medical Genetics* 35: 17–22.

Sloan WR, Walsh PC (1976) Familial persistent Müllerian duct syndrome. *Journal of Urology* 115: 459–461.

Stephens TD (1982) The Wolffian ridge: history of a misconception. *ISIS* 73: 254–259.

Strachan T, Read A (1999) *Human Molecular Genetics*, 2nd edn. Oxford: Bios Scientific Publishers.

Terruhn V (1980) A study of impression moulds of the genital tract of female fetuses. *Archives of Gynaecology* 229: 207–217.

Ueno S, Takahashi M, Manganaro TF *et al.* (1989) Cellular localisation of Müllerian inhibiting substance in the developing rat ovary. *Endocrinology* 124: 1000–1006.

Ulfelder H, Robboy SJ (1976) Embryologic development of human vagina. *American Journal of Obstetrics and Gynecology* 126: 769–776.

Wertz K, Herrmann BG (2000) Large-scale screen for genes involved in gonad development. *Mechanisms of Development* 98: 51–70.

Witschi E (1970) Development and differentiation of the uterus. In: Mack HC (ed.) *Prenatal Life*. Detroit, MI: Wayne State University Press, pp. 11–35.

Wolff CF (1759) Theoria generationis. Quoted by Adelman HB (1966) *Marcello Malpighi and the Evolution of Embryology*. New York: Cornell University Press.

CHAPTER 2

The functional anatomy of the cervix, the cervical epithelium and the stroma

Albert Singer and Joseph A. Jordan

This chapter will endeavour to define the anatomy of the cervix and its epithelium under three sections. These are:

1 gross anatomy;
2 subepithelial stroma;
3 dynamic epithelial anatomy.

GROSS ANATOMY

The cervix is the lower part of the uterus and, as such, is divided from the upper part, or corpus, by a fibromuscular junction, the internal os separating this fibrous cervix from the muscular corpus. There is the formation of a sphincter at this junction which may cause weakness in later life, resulting in incompetence and miscarriage during pregnancy. This weakness may be either of a congenital or of a traumatic nature and is discussed in Chapter 15.

The cervix, projecting as it does through the anterior vaginal wall at the vaginal vault, means that there is an upper supravaginal portion and a lower vaginal portion of approximately the same length. The vaginal mucosa is reflected around the front, back and sides of the cervix, thereby forming the vaginal fornices. The cervix is basically cylindrical, although the overall shape is extremely variable and it is such that, in the nullipara, it is cylindrical, being some 3 cm in length and 2 cm in diameter. Changes in the shape and structure of the cervix are due to an increase in its overall size and eversion of the epithelial contents of the lower endocervical canal, and this occurs predominantly in pregnancy (Chapter 7) but also to a lesser extent at puberty (Chapter 6). During delivery and labour, further alterations may occur as a result of injury. This results in the multiparous cervix having a characteristic appearance that is more bulbous, with the cervix itself larger than that found in the nullipara. The external os is horizontal in the former where it is circular in the latter.

The passage between the uterine cavity and the vagina is via the endocervical canal, which is continuous with the endometrial cavity above at the level of the internal os and with the vagina below at the external os. The endocervical canal is fusiform in shape and approximately 3 cm long, and it is flattened from front to back and measures some 7 mm at its widest point. However, it is a dynamic structure with the diameter of the external os being influenced by cyclical changes, with alterations resulting in the dimensions of the canal itself, in tissue vascularity and in the quantity and biophysical characteristics of the mucus secreted from the endocervix (Chapter 11) (Hafez, 1981, 1982). Increases in vascularity, congestion and oedema as well as in the secretions of mucus are predominant during the early (proliferative) phase of the cycle, with these changes reaching a peak at ovulation, providing the ideal circumstances for sperm transport as discussed in Chapter 12.

Anteriorly, the supravaginal portion of the cervix is separated from the bladder by a distinct layer of connective tissue (parametrium), which also extends to the sides of the cervix and laterally between the layers of the broad ligaments. The uterine arteries are contained within this tissue and, on each side of the cervix, the ureter runs downwards and forwards within the parametrium at a distance of about 2 cm from the cervix. During the latter part of its course, the ureter runs downwards towards the bladder between the anterior and posterior layers of the broad ligament in the ureteric tunnel. Posteriorly, the supravaginal cervix is covered with peritoneum that continues down over the posterior vaginal wall to be reflected on to the rectum, so forming the rectouterine pouch or pouch of Douglas.

The cervix is held in position by its ligaments, namely the uterosacral and lateral ligaments (Fig. 2.1a). The uterosacral ligament runs from the supravaginal portion of the cervix and upper third of the vagina in a posterior direction to the second, third and fourth sacral vertebrae. The ligament consists mainly of fibrous tissue and some smooth muscle and also contains within it nerves, blood vessels and lymphatics. It is thought to hold the cervix in its normal position, i.e. back towards the rectum and, in so doing, helps to maintain the uterus in its anteverted position.

The lateral ligaments, which are also known as the transverse cervical ligaments or the cardinal ligaments of Mackendrodt, lie at the base of the broad ligament where there are well-defined fascial ligaments also containing connective tissue and smooth muscle. They form an inverted U-shaped attachment

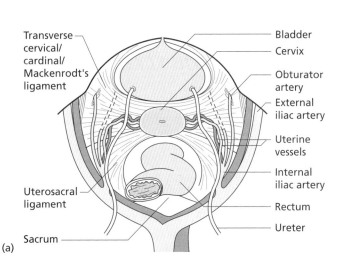

(a)

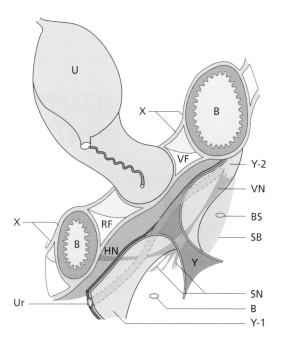

(d)

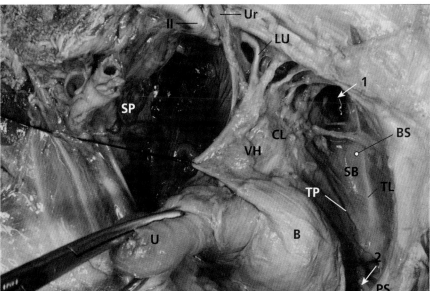

(b)

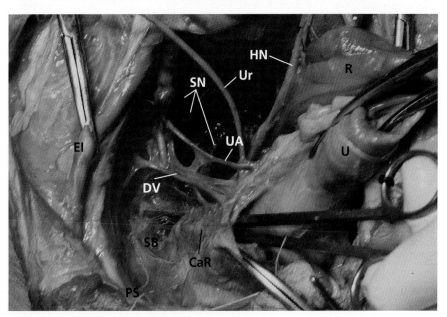

(c)

Fig. 2.1 (a) Diagrammatic representation of a section taken horizontally through the pelvis at the level of the cervical internal os. It shows the arrangement of the principal cervical ligaments, blood vessels and ureter. (b) Photograph of the left paravesical space. There is a hollow (arrowhead 1) between the transverse cervical ligament (CL) and the short fibrous bundle (SB), leading to the caudal chamber of the pararectal space. The area around the genital hiatus (arrowhead 2) is the true pelvic floor. Ur, ureter; U, uterus; B, bladder; SP, sacral promontory; Il, internal iliac artery; VH, vesicohypogastric fascia; LU, lateral umbilical artery/ligament; TP, tendinous arc of pelvic fascia; TL, tendinous arc of levator ani muscle; PS, pelvic symphysis; BS, paravesical space. (c) Paravaginal space and caudal chamber of the pararectal space. U, uterus; B, bladder; Ur, ureter; SB, short fibrous bundle; PS, pubic symphysis; R, rectum; CaR, caudal reflection of lateral ligament of pubis; UA, uterine artery; DV, deep uterine vein; HN, hypogastric nerves; SN, pelvic splanchnic nerves; EI, external iliac artery. (d) Schematic illustration of the pelvic connective tissue. U, Uterus; B, bladder; Ur, ureter; SN, pelvic splanchnic nerve; HN, hypogastric nerve; VN, vesical nerve branch; SB, short fibrous bundle; BS, paravesical space; VF, vesicouterine space; RF, rectouterine space; X, pubovesical ligament, superficial layer of the vesicouterine ligament, rectouterine ligament, and rectococcygeal ligament; Y-1, mesoureter, etc; Y-2, deep layer of the vesicouterine ligament, etc.; X, suspensory system; Y, supporting system; Y-1, cranially reflected bundle; Y-2, caudally reflected bundle. From Yabuki *et al.* (2005), with permission.

medially to the anterior, superior and posterior marginal walls of the supravaginal cervix and laterally and below to the white line and fascia of the levator ani muscle. The lateral ligaments therefore provide the principal means of support to the cervix. In any description of the gross anatomy, the lymphatic drainage, nerve and blood supply should also be discussed. Recently Yabuki *et al.* (2005) presented excellent illustrations of pelvic anatomy that seem to highlight discrepancies arising between classic descriptions of pelvic anatomy and those of pelvic structures derived from clinical observations by gynaecological oncological surgeons. Such an example is seen in Figures 2.1b–d, which show extensive dissections of the pelvis, outlining in particular the development of the vesicohypogastric fascia and Mackenrodt's ligament, as well as a detailed description of the pelvic connective tissue (Fig. 2.1d).

THE SUBEPITHELIAL STROMA

The covering cervical epithelium has an underlying stroma that is composed predominantly of elastic tissue with a small amount of smooth muscle. The elastic tissue is composed of collagen and elastin, and its ultrastructure has only recently (Leppert and Yu, 1991) been defined. Using scanning electron microscopy (SEM), the elastic fibres of both uterine body and cervix have been shown to be composed of two distinct structures, fibrils and thin sheets of elastic membranes. The fibrils are arranged into fishnet-like structures while within the thin elastic membranes there are fenestrations and pits with diameters of some 3–5 μm. In the study by Leppert and Yu (1991), the concentration of the insoluble elastin was found to be approximately 1.4% of the dry, defatted tissues of the cervix, while the total collagen was estimated to be between 64.3% and 72.4%.

Orientation of the elastic fibres within the cervix has been described in detail by Leppert *et al.* (1986), who showed that they are orientated from the external os to the periphery and from there in a band upwards towards the internal os, where they become sparse in that area of the cervix that contains the greatest amount of smooth muscle, just below the internal os.

Rotten *et al.* (1998) assessed the evolution of the elastic fibre network in the cervix during and after pregnancy with biopsies obtained and stained with a polyphenolic compound to elastic fibres exclusively, which enabled an automatic image analysis to be done. This showed that the elastic fibre network was made up in two specific patterns, the first being with fibres running parallel to the basement lamina of the epithelium and the second of thinner, perpendicular fibres. They showed a decline in the cervical elastin content as pregnancy progressed, with a constant decline, dissociation and disorganisation of these fibres becoming more clearly evident as gestation progressed. In the postpartum period (5–7 weeks), the elastic fibre network had become completely restructured, and these findings supported a role for elastin in the process of cervical maturation and reconstruction during pregnancy and after delivery.

Smooth muscle constitutes only 10–15% of cervical tissue, as documented by Danforth (1947). The distribution of the smooth muscle is predominantly in the outer one-third to one-quarter of the cervix with variable amounts of muscle located closer to the endocervical mucosa (Hughesdon, 1952). In one study, Tiltman (1998) has described the presence of a different group of smooth muscle bundles, found within the endocervical submucosa. These fibres are morphologically and immunohistochemically distinct from the inherent muscle deeper in the cervix. They possess more cytoplasm, are arranged in bundles unseparated by collagen and lack estrogen and progesterone receptors. These bundles are found in approximately 25% of uterine cervices, usually residing in the region of the transformation zone. At present, their significance remains a source of speculation.

The tensile strength and firmness of the cervix is derived from the collagen that is the predominant protein of the extracellular matrix of the cervix. Minamoto *et al.* (1987) described four types of collagen within the dense fibrous tissue of the cervix, which are broken down by the enzyme collagenase during labour. It would seem that the cells involved in this degradation during the process of cervical dilatation are not resident fibroblasts, as had previously been assumed, but rather polymorphonuclear leucocytes that migrate from blood vessels within the cervix (Osmers *et al.*, 1992). Not surprisingly, there is an elevation in serum collagenase levels during the ripening process at term and in active labour it increases still further (Granstrom *et al.*, 1992).

It also seems that smooth muscle within the cervix might play a role in ripening of the cervix prior to the onset of labour, as described in Chapter 13. It has been demonstrated that smooth muscle cells undergo a process of apoptosis or programmed cell death during the ripening process. Apoptosis is a genetically timed event, and pharmacological agents aimed at this process could potentially play an important role in the prevention of preterm labour and also in the management of post-term pregnancy.

Assessment of the biochemical and muscular contractile ability of the cervix has shown no significant difference in these physical properties (Petersen *et al.*, 1991) between tissues taken from the distal and proximal parts of the cervix or between the circular and longitudinally arranged elastic tissues. Petersen *et al.* (1991) concluded that the passive mechanical strength of the cervix markedly exceeds its active muscular contractile ability, and this is explained by a high collagen concentration and a low content of smooth muscle within the cervical tissues. This is discussed in more detail in Chapter 13.

DYNAMIC EPITHELIAL ANATOMY

The transformation zone

In late fetal life, the original columnar epithelium of the Müllerian duct covers the uterine cavity and extends

1. Original epithelia

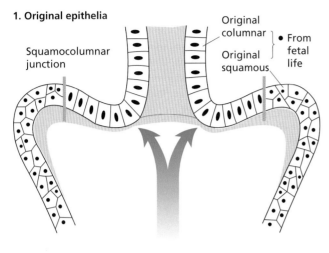

2 **Metaplastic squamous epithelium**
Typical transformation zone

- Late fetal life
- Adolescence
- Pregnancy

3 **Abnormal (atypical) epithelium**
Atypical transformation zone

- Adolescence
- Pregnancy
- ? Other times

Includes (immature metaplastic squamous epithelium)
Cervical intraepithelial neoplasia 1–3, early invasion

Fig. 2.2 Types of cervical epithelium.

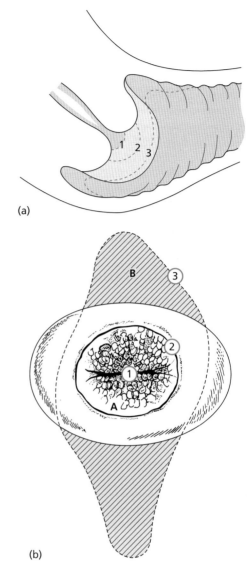

(a)

(b)

Fig. 2.3 (a) The position of the original squamocolumnar junction. (1) shows the junction within the endocervix, (2) shows it at a mid-distance point between the endocervix and vaginal fornix and (3) shows an extensive transformation zone with the squamocolumnar junction extending on to the vaginal fornix. (b) Reprographic representation of the positions of the original squamocolumnar junction as represented in (a).

downwards into the cervical canal, where it comes into contact with the original squamous epithelium from the vagina, the principal contribution of the urogenital sinus (Forsberg, 1976). This process is also discussed in Chapters 1 and 5.

During late fetal life and in adolescence, but mainly in the first pregnancy, the more caudal of the original columnar epithelium is partially or completely replaced with squamous epithelium by the physiological process of squamous metaplasia. This change introduces an element of instability to this junctional interface between the two original epithelial types, and it has been suggested that this process may be concerned with the later development of cervical neoplasia (Reid 1982).

There are therefore present in the adolescent and adult cervix three types of epithelium, each with an easily recognisable and characteristic histological and morphological appearance (Fig. 2.2).

These types are:

1 original (sometimes called native) squamous or columnar epithelium;

2 metaplastic squamous epithelium;

3 atypical epithelium, comprising pathological epithelia grouped together under this title, some of which may have malignant potential.

The original epithelia that are laid down during intrauterine development persist into adult life. The boundary between the original columnar and squamous epithelium, as has been described within the fetal cervix, occurs at an easily recognis-

able point called the original squamocolumnar junction. The position of this permanent junction may be at any point across the ecto- or endocervix, or in the vaginal fornix (Figs 2.3–2.6).

During certain periods of life, alterations occur within the original columnar epithelium which result in the formation by a process of metaplasia of the second type of epithelium, called metaplastic squamous. It is a physiological process occurring over a short period that is measurable in days or weeks. The introduction of the colposcope with its magnified and illuminated vision has enabled the natural history of this process to be

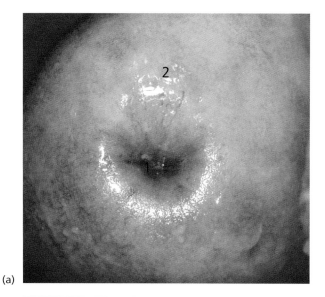

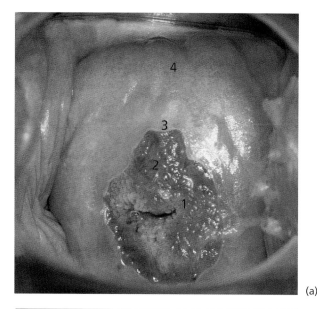

(a)

(a)

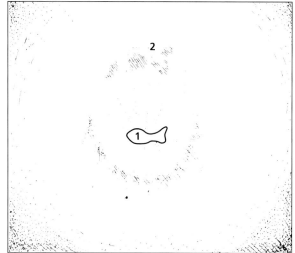

(b)

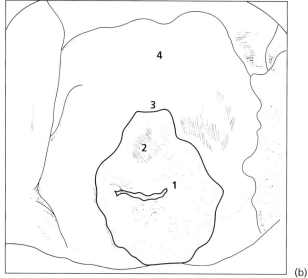

(b)

Fig. 2.4 The cervix showing the squamocolumnar junction (1) in the endocervix, with original squamous epithelium (2) covering the ectocervix.

Fig. 2.5 The original squamocolumnar junction (3) is at the mid-distance point between the endocervix and the vaginal fornix. The original columnar epithelium is at (1), with a small island of metaplastic squamous epithelium at (2). Original squamous epithelium is at (4).

studied. Metaplasia, as it occurs in late fetal life, adolescence and pregnancy, will be discussed below in relation to the appropriate epithelia (see Chapters 6 and 7).

It soon became apparent that, within the area medial to the original squamocolumnar junction, there occurred all the dynamic, physiological and pathological processes that are found in the human cervix. This area has been called the transformation zone by the colposcopist: when normal metaplasia occurs within its boundaries, it is labelled the physiological transformation zone (Fig. 2.7).

It has been suggested (Reid 1992) that, during the early stages of metaplasia, the epithelium is vulnerable to genetic change that may result in the tissue acquiring neoplastic potential. This third type of epithelium has distinctive morphological characteristics and possesses the same topo-

graphical arrangement within the transformation zone as the physiological epithelium (i.e. original and metaplastic) (Fig. 2.7). The transformation zone in this situation is called the atypical transformation zone and within its area will reside the precursors of squamous cervical cancer.

The original squamous epithelium

Histological appearance

This epithelium, of the stratified type similar to that in the vagina, covers the vagina and joins the original columnar

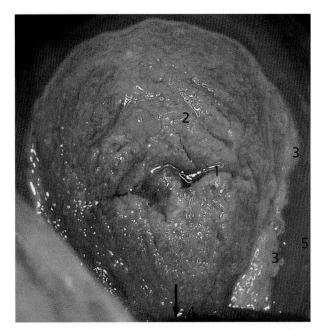

(a)

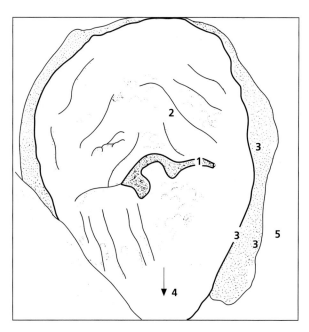

(b)

Fig. 2.6 Colpophotograph showing an extensive transformation zone. The endocervical canal is at (1) with islands of metaplastic epithelium at (2) within areas of original columnar epithelium. The original squamocolumnar junction is at (3) with a small longitudinal strip of immature squamous metaplastic epithelium (stippled) medial to this line, and extends posteriorly in the 6 o'clock position into the posterior vaginal fornix (towards 4). The original squamous epithelium is at (5). This appearance of the transformation zone is also called an ectropion or ectopy.

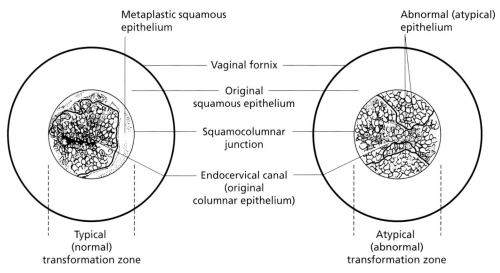

Fig. 2.7 Distribution of epithelium within the cervix.

epithelium at the fixed point of the original squamocolumnar junction. Containing variable amounts of glycogen, it is distinguished microscopically by its five distinct layers or zones (Fig. 2.8). These are:

Zone 1 The lowest layer, consisting of a single row of small cylindrical cells with relatively large nuclei that are sometimes referred to as basal cells or stratum cylindricum (1 in Fig. 2.8).

Zone 2 This consists of several layers of polyhedral cells with fairly large nuclei and distinct intercellular bridges. It is some-

times referred to as the parabasal cell layer, prickle cell layer or stratum spinosum profundum (2 in Fig. 2.8). Mitotic figures are occasionally found in these first two layers.

Zone 3 Cells in this zone begin to flatten and have glycogen-rich cytoplasm with frequent vacuolation. These cells are known as the intermediate, navicular, clear or stratum spinosum superficiae cells (3 in Fig. 2.8).

Zone 4 This layer is of variable thickness and is often not recognisable. Consisting of a number of closely packed

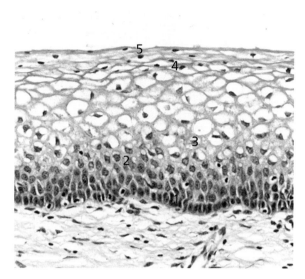

Fig. 2.8 Histological section of original squamous epithelium.

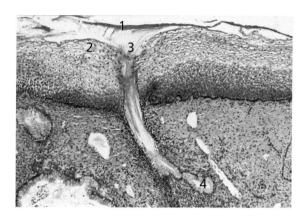

Fig. 2.9 Photomicrograph of mature squamous metaplastic epithelium showing a layer of keratinised cells (1) above the superficial epithelial layer (2). A gland opening is seen as (3), connecting to glands situated in the stroma (4).

polyhedral cells with a keratohyaline granular structure, it is referred to as the intraepithelial zone or the condensation zone (4 in Fig. 2.8).

Zone 5 This zone comprises the superficial layer of cells that are elongated, flattened with small pyknotic nuclei and contain a large amount of cytoplasm. They represent keratinisation and are most plentiful at times of high estrogen levels. This layer is referred to as the stratum corneum (5 in Fig. 2.8).

The squamous epithelium is separated from the fibrous stroma by a basement membrane that can be readily demonstrated by electron microscopy. The thickness of the epithelium depends upon the hormonal status of the subject. In young girls and elderly women, the epithelium is not usually stimulated, is only a few cell layers thick (atrophic epithelium) and is largely undifferentiated with absent glycogen. During the sexually mature period, all layers respond differentially to hormonal stimulation with estrogens, producing proliferation, complete maturation of all the layers of the epithelium and desquamation. In contrast, progesterone acts on the intermediate layer causing thickening, but does not lead to complete maturation. When the ratio of progesterone to estrogen is increased, as occurs during pregnancy and in the second phase (secretory) of the menstrual cycle, then the intermediate cells predominate. When this ratio is reversed, as occurs during the first (proliferative) phase of the menstrual cycle or when exogenous estrogens are given, then there is a predominance of the superficial cell layers (Konishi *et al.*, 1991).

Occasionally, a process of keratinisation (Fig. 2.9) is seen above the superficial cells. This distinct morphological change occurs when cells synthesise large amounts of cytoplasmic keratin while the nucleus of the cell becomes pyknotic, dies and disappears, leaving the anucleate structure of the cell behind

(anucleate squames). Keratin is a chemical substance, a fibrous protein that occurs in epidermal tissues such as hair and nails. It occurs in cells in the form of long bundles of fibres that are related in origin to keratohyaline bodies in the cytoplasm. Synthesis of these fibres begins when cells are still in the basal layers. As epithelial cells differentiate and begin to migrate to the upper layers of an epithelial surface, increasing amounts of keratin may be synthesised. The amount of keratin in a cell may be related to how rapidly the cell differentiates and the type of epithelium in which it occurs (Smedts *et al.*, 1993).

Ultrastructural appearance: as seen with transmission electron microscopy (TEM)

The ultrastructural appearances of the various epithelial types of the cervix are usually determined from study of biopsy material obtained at colposcopy or from hysterectomy specimens. The material is prepared in a standard fashion and the method is described elsewhere (Lawrence and Shingleton, 1980). This epithelium has distinctive ultrastructural appearances.

A transmission electron micrograph of a basal cell of a normal squamous epithelium is seen in Figure 2.10. The nuclei are oval with some indentations of the membrane, with chromatin being condensed along the membrane and coarsely clumped in other areas. The nucleoli in Figure 2.10 are prominent and within the cytoplasm are numerous ribosomes and mitochondria. There are peripheral tonofilaments and numerous desmosomes with interdigitating microvilli. The basement membrane is well defined and many hemidesmosomes are evident.

The basal cells are elongated with their long axes perpendicular to the plane of the epithelial stromal junction. The cells rest on an undulating basement membrane approximately 300 Å in thickness separated from the plasma membrane

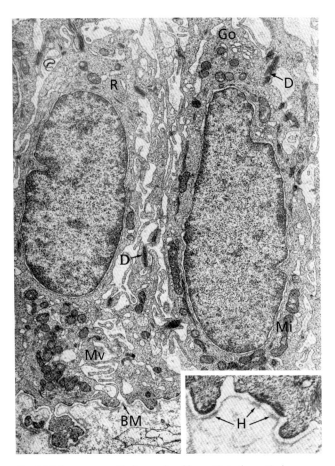

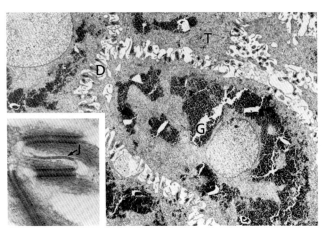

Fig. 2.11 Squamous epithelium — intermediate layer. Note the oval, inactive nuclei, peripheral tonofibrils (T) and glycogen lakes (G). Numerous microvilli and desmosomes (D) are present at cell borders (× 5400). Inset: desmosomes and gap junctions (J) connect adjacent cell processes. Numerous tonofilaments converge on attachment plates (× 56 000).

Fig. 2.10 Squamous epithelium — basal layer. Note the vertical orientation of cells, convoluted basement membrane (BM), interdigitating microvilli (Mv) and desmosomes (D) at surfaces. The cytoplasm contains ribosomes (R), mitochondria (Mi) and Golgi zones (Go). Nuclear heterochromatin is peripherally located (× 15 000). Inset: note hemidesmosomes (H) along the basement membrane (× 50 000).

by an electron-lucent zone approximately 300 Å wide. Hemidesmosomes are spaced at frequent intervals along the convoluted foot processes of the basal epithelial cells; these attachment plates are characterised by focal condensations of the plasma membrane paralleled by a thin electronic-dense line and fine filaments extended to the basement membrane. Microvillous projections of the plasma membrane extend into the intercellular spaces, and adjacent cell membranes are joined at intervals by desmosomes. These structures are composed of matched dense plates of adjacent cell membranes joined by an amorphous substance that is bisected by a slender immediate line. Dense aggregations of tonofilaments in the peripheral cytoplasm converge on the attachment plates of the desmosomes. The cytoplasm is rich in free ribosomes, and occasional profiles of rough-surfaced endoplasmic reticulum are present. Mitochondria are numerous, especially in the

subnuclear areas, and an occasional Golgi complex is seen. The nucleus occupies a large portion of the cell, with the nuclear membrane occasionally being thrown into shallow folds. The nuclear chromatin is coarsely distributed and a single nucleus is present, although double nuclei may occasionally be seen.

The cells from the parabasal layer contain nuclei that are oval with a fine chromatin distribution. The cytoplasm here is more abundant than in the basal cells and contains numerous ribosomes, mitochondria and bundles of tonofilaments. There are numerous desmosomal attachments between the cells.

Cells of the intermediate layer contain nuclei that are more rounded, smaller and inactive with cytoplasmic organelles that are less conspicuous but which contain large glycogen lakes that are visible within the abundant cytoplasm (Fig. 2.11). There are numerous microvilli and desmosomes at the cell borders. The superficial squamous cells (Fig. 2.12) contain nuclei that are pyknotic, with the cell being flattened and the remnants of the glycogen lakes just visible. The cell borders consist of short microvilli and small desmosomes. The cells of the superficial layer (see Fig. 2.15) characteristically present a markedly flattened cytoplasm, the rims of which exhibit tonofilaments and surround glycogen pools. Nuclei which are shrunken and pyknotic are another feature of this layer. Short microvillous projections of cell membranes extend between cells and on the surface of the most superficial cells. The surface ultrastructure when viewed by scanning electron microscopy (SEM) shows quite clearly that the so-called villi are in fact ridges seen in cross-section. The desmosomes appear shortened and less numerous, possibly in preparation for exfoliation.

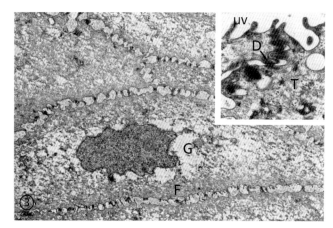

Fig. 2.12 Squamous epithelium — superficial layer. Note the flattened cells, pyknotic nucleus, remnants of glycogen lakes (G) and feltwork of cytoplasmic filaments (F) (×5400). Inset: surface details. Note stubby microvilli (μv), shortened, small desmosomes (D) and tonofilaments (T) (×25 000).

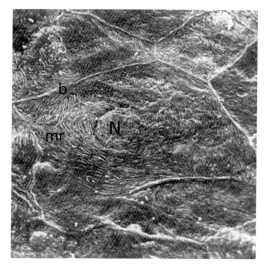

Fig. 2.14 Cell from squamous epithelium showing microridges. mr, microridges; b, cell boundary; N, nucleus (×1260).

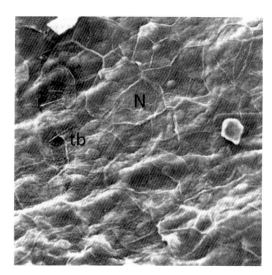

Fig. 2.13 Pavement-like appearance of squamous epithelium. tb, terminal bars; N, nucleus (×412).

Ultrastructural appearance: as seen by scanning electron microscopy

The original squamous epithelium, as seen in SEM, appears smooth with the cells being flattened and polygonal with a central raised nuclear area with raised terminal bars being seen between adjacent cells (tb in Fig. 2.13). At higher magnification, the surfaces of the cells show a typical pattern of microridges (mr in Fig. 2.14) that are approximately 0.15 μm wide with spaces of about 0.25 μm between them. There is variation in the length of these microridges (the longest are up to 40 μm in length) and they show anastomoses. Microridges less than 1 μm long rarely occur on normal squamous cells.

The microridges show no particular orientation towards each other at the centre of the cells but peripherally they are often arranged parallel to the cell boundaries. The prominent terminal bars (about 0.5 μm high) seem to be formed by folding over and interdigitation of the edges of adjacent cells.

The original columnar epithelium

Gross morphological appearance

This epithelium lines the endocervix, and occasionally the ectocervix, with coarse secretory cells that utilise both apocrine and merocrine methods of secretion. When observed colposcopically, the gross appearance of the epithelium is seen to exist in two forms (Figs 2.15–2.17). The first, called rugae, are relatively coarse subdivisions appearing as two or three mounds or cushions on the cervical lips (Z in Fig. 2.16), their longitudinal extensions into the endocervix being referred to as plicae palmatae or arbor vitae (Figs 2.16 and 2.17). The second form (1 in Figs 2.15 and 2.18 (a) and (b) in Fig. 2.27) appears as bunches of small 'grapes' composed of the basic subunit of the epithelium, the villus. This structure is usually ovoid, about 1.5 × 0.15 μm in diameter, and can appear as a flattened mound. Each villus is separated from the others by the intervillous space.

Histological examination suggests that the subepithelial stroma contains glands that connect with the surface. However, Fluhmann (1957, 1961) showed, by constructing a three-dimensional model of this area, that the so-called glands are in reality part of an extensive cleft-like system (Fig. 2.20). They can also be seen in Figures 2.18 and 2.19.

These clefts frequently become occluded by the metaplastic squamous process, with the result that they appear as tunnels

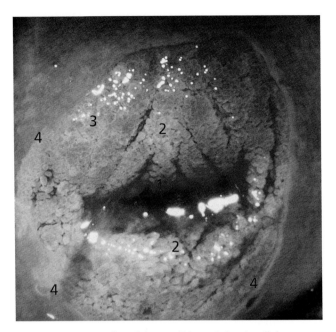

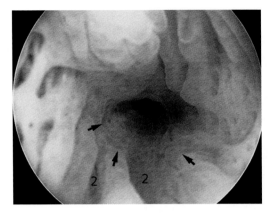

Fig. 2.17 The metaplastic process extending to the region of the internal os (1). Its upper extent is arrowed, with the columnar epithelium appearing at this point and in the intervening so-called crypt spaces (2).

Fig. 2.15 The cervix of an adolescent (16 years) showing all the stages of squamous metaplasia. The endocervix with its original columnar epithelium is at (1). The coarse subdivisions of the epithelium appearing as two or three mounds or cushions around (2) on the anterior (upper) cervical lip are called rugae. Also around position (2) is seen stage 2 of squamous metaplasia development (see below) with fusion of the villi and, at (3), this has extended to fusion of all the villi. Immature squamous epithelium is present, adjacent and medial to the original squamocolumnar junction at (4).

Histological appearance

This epithelium lines the endocervical canal and occasionally extends on to the ectocervix. Histologically, the cells of this epithelium appear tall, slender and elongated and are uniformly arranged in one layer and closely packed in a 'cobble-stone' pattern (Fig. 2.22). The nuclei are round or oval and generally situated in the lower third of the cell: during active secretion, as in pregnancy and at ovulation, they are found in the middle or base of the cells (Fig. 2.22). The bases of the columnar cells are attached to the basement membrane by hemidesmosomes. There are two types: non-ciliated secretory cells and kinociliated cells.

The secretory cells that utilise both apocrine and merocrine methods of secretion have a dome-shaped raised surface covered with many short microvilli measuring 2×0.2 μm wide. Secretory cells stain deeply with periodic acid–Schiff (PAS) during the peak of the biosynthesis stage and become engorged with heterogeneous secretory granules. Fibrillary bodies are frequently noted in the cytoplasm of mucus-secreting endocervical cells and reflect a storage form of glycoprotein (Phillip, 1975). Cyclical changes in the histochemical and ultrastructural characteristics of the secretory granules correspond to changes in estrogen levels (Wolf *et al.*, 1978). It has also been suggested that there are changes within the epithelium during the menstrual cycle. There seems to be an admixture of secretory and ciliated cells within the endocervix, which alters with the phase of the menstrual cycle or as a result of hormonal influences. Occasionally, areas of columnar epithelium do not show the typical microvilli and appear relatively smooth.

The ciliated cells are covered with kinocilia that beat rhythmically towards the cervical canal and vagina. Ciliated cells are more frequent in the endocervical columnar epithelium, and are particularly high in the endocervical canal near the endometrial junction. They are rarely seen on the

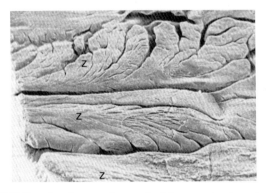

Fig. 2.16 Scanning electron micrograph of the opened endocervical canal demonstrating the 'arbor vitae'.

or blind tubes (Fig. 2.20). When total occlusion of secretions occurs, it results in a localised mucus collection and the development of an epithelial cystic structure that is recognisable clinically as a Nabothian follicle. The exit to the surface from many of these tunnels is easily recognisable colposcopically and is referred to as a gland opening (arrowed structure in Figs 2.18 and 2.21).

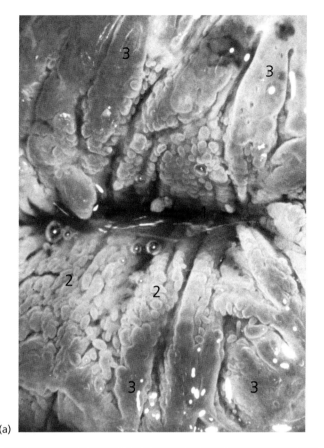

(a)

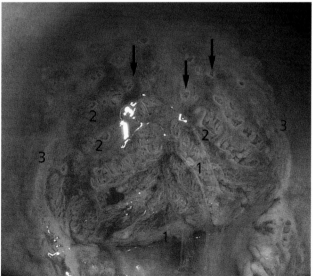

(b)

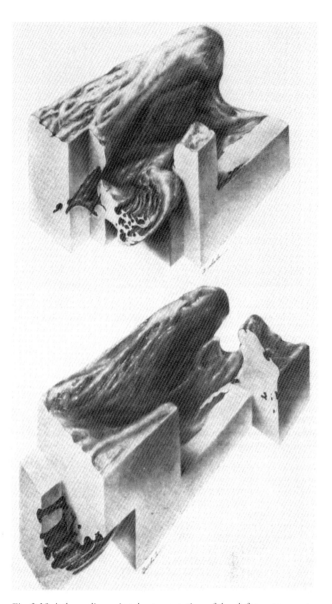

Fig. 2.19 A three-dimensional representation of the cleft arrangement existing within the endocervix. From Fluhmann (1961).

Fig. 2.18 (a) The villi, being the structures of the basic subunit of the original columnar epithelium, are seen at (1) and (2). Immature squamous metaplastic epithelium exists at (3). The longitudinally running folds running towards the internal os are obvious. (b) Colpophotograph (× 15) of the anterior cervical lip showing the rugae arrangement (1) of the columnar epithelium. Individual villi are seen (2), with fusion between some of them already evident at (3), indicating the initiation of metaplastic transformation. Gland openings are seen arrowed.

ectocervix. The ciliated cells have round or oval nuclei with fine chromatin distribution; the cytoplasm is characterised by numerous mitochondria, free ribosomes, occasional lysosomes and profiles of rough and smooth endoplasmic reticulum. Ciliated cells also have surface microvilli interspersed with kinocilia. The function of the ciliated cells is not clear, although it is assumed that they are involved in the clearance of secretory macromolecules from the adjacent secretory cells.

Ultrastructural appearance: as seen with transmission electron microscopy (TEM)

A single layer of tall slender cells rests on a basement membrane more even than that of squamous epithelium but

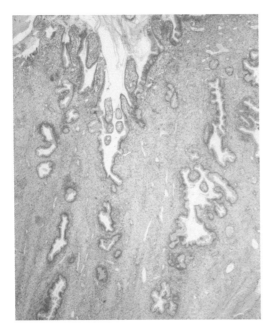

Fig. 2.20 Photomicrograph of endocervical columnar epithelium showing it arranged in what appears to be a typical glandular system. It is, in fact, organised in a cleft-like arrangement, as seen in Figure 2.19.

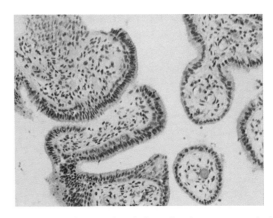

Fig. 2.22 Benign endocervical epithelium showing mucus-producing columnar endocervical epithelium.

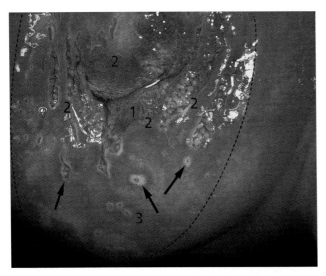

Fig. 2.21 Colpophotograph of a mature transformation zone in a 38-year-old woman. The native columnar epithelium is at (1) within the endocervix, and the new squamocolumnar junction can easily be seen at (2). Mature metaplastic squamous epithelium is present at (3) (see below). Within this area are small gland openings (arrowed). The dotted line marks the original squamocolumnar junction, and the native squamous epithelium is lateral to this line.

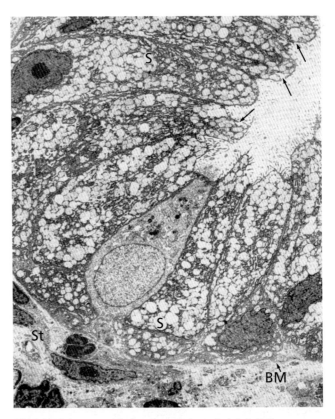

Fig. 2.23 Columnar epithelium in an endocervical cleft. Tall secretory cells have basilar, active nuclei and numerous secretory droplets (S). Merocrine secretion is demonstrated (arrows). A single ciliated non-secretory cell is present. A flattened basement membrane (BM) separates the epithelial cells and adjacent stroma (St) (× 5000).

otherwise with the same substructure (Fig. 2.23). The base of the cells is attached to the base of the membrane by hemidesmosomes and, on the lateral surface, the cells are closely approximated to the plasma membranes, which are often thrown into complex interdigitating folds. Desmosomes connect adjacent cells with close junctions, especially prominent near the luminal surface. The nuclei are quite irregular in outline and exhibit coarsely distributed chromatin and conspicuous nucleoli; in the cytoplasm, the mitochondria are numerous, especially in the subnuclear position.

In Figure 2.23, a typical tall secretory cell within columnar epithelium is seen, containing numerous secretory droplets (S). The nuclei of the cells are small, are located at the base and have a dense chromatin pattern. The basement membrane (arrowed) separates the cells from the stroma. The luminal border of the cells has well-developed microvilli (Mv). Also in Figure 2.23, the single non-secretory cell has cilia at the luminal border, and numerous mitochondria are present in the cytoplasm of this cell, which also has a round nucleus with finely distributed chromatin.

Ultrastructural appearance: as seen with scanning electron microscopy

As described above, the basic unit of the columnar epithelium is the small ovoid villus. Each villus is separated from its neighbour by the intervillous space. Ultrastructurally, each villus is covered by columnar cells, the exposed surface of which is small (about 4 μm in diameter), irregular, polygonal and of uniform size. The villi are closely packed, so that they present a regular cobblestone appearance (Fig. 2.24). The surface of the cells is slightly raised and covered with many short microvilli that are approximately 2 μm long. Occasionally, areas of epithelium do not show the typical villus or clefts and appear relatively smooth. Examination of these areas will show invagination of the epithelium lined with columnar cells. These have been discussed and are seen to be the so-called cervical clefts. The surface representation of the surface aperture of the subepithelial glandular components is sometimes called a gland opening (Figs 2.18 and 2.21). They have a distinctive SEM (Fig. 2.24b) and histological appearance (Fig. 2.24c).

Metaplastic squamous epithelium

The transformation zone, that area in which squamous metaplasia occurs, is obvious in 90% of postmenarchal cervices, being a physiological process occurring in late fetal life, at the menarche and during pregnancy. It transforms columnar to squamous epithelium in a matter of days and weeks. The epithelium, once formed, does not revert to its original glandular state. The mechanisms inducing its development are related essentially to the increasing exposure of the columnar epithelium to the vaginal pH (Chapter 7).

Colposcopic appearance

When the transformation zone is observed by the illuminated and magnified vision allowed by colposcopy during periods of active metaplasia, it can be seen that a stepwise progression of changes develops from the grape-like configuration of the columnar epithelium to the smooth surface of the definitive squamous epithelium (Figs 2.25 and 2.26). The metaplastic transformation process is usually incomplete, such that the resultant epithelia that have been exposed to it have varied morphological appearances. The process, as seen colposcopically, can be divided into five stages. These are displayed diagrammatically in Figure 2.27.

Stage 1 The first recognisable colposcopic manifestation of this change is pallor within the grape-like epithelial villus (2 in Fig. 2.26; (stage 1 in Fig. 2.27). The redness of the stromal capillaries, as observed through the overlying translucent columnar epithelium, is replaced by a glazed appearance which, after a short time that may be measured in weeks or days, gives rise to a pale pink surface. This is coincidental with the

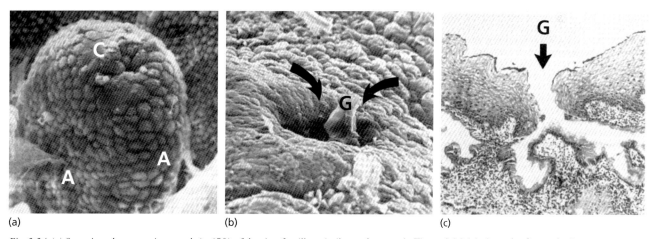

(a) (b) (c)

Fig. 2.24 (a) Scanning electron micrograph (× 650) of the tip of a villus, similar to that seen in Figure 2.10 (a). A patch of metaplastic squamous epithelium (C) has appeared at the most exposed part of this structure, i.e. the apex. Columnar cells (A) occupy the sides and depths of the intervening clefts and intervillous spaces. (b) A scanning electron micrograph showing a gland opening (G) in an area of metaplastic squamous epithelium. (c) A histomicrograph (× 65) of a longitudinal section taken through the centre of the gland opening (G) as seen in Figures 2.18 and 30.2.

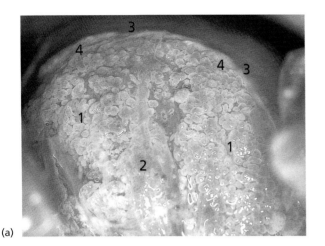

(a)

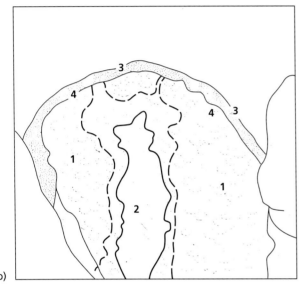

(b)

Fig. 2.25 Colpophotograph showing the stages of a metaplastic transformation process with individual villi with opaque apices indicating stages 1 and 2 present in area (1). In the area marked (2), there are already fused villi with a smooth surface, indicating stages 3 and 4; areas (3) and (4) also indicate stages of maturing metaplastic epithelium.

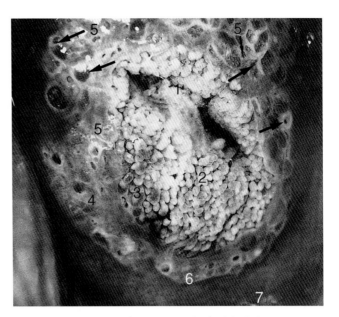

Fig. 2.26 Colpophotographic montage of a physiological transformation zone. The original squamous epithelium (7) and the columnar epithelium (1) are separated by sheets of metaplastic squamous epithelium at various stages of development. Early metaplastic transformation is visible at (1) and (2) while the more advanced stages are present at (3) and (4). In the more mature epithelium in the region of (5), there are many gland openings (arrowed). The squamocolumnar junction is at (6).

Stages 4 and 5 Over time, the epithelium matures and the stromal cores disappear (4 in Fig. 2.26; stages 4 and 5 in Fig. 2.27).

The process can be arrested at any stage so that the resultant appearance of the transformation zone is usually that of metaplastic epithelium in any one of the five stages that have been described. The original columnar epithelium can still occasionally be seen on the ectocervix, where small openings to the surface exist. These are referred to as gland openings (Fig. 2.21, and 5 and arrowed in Fig. 2.26). The original squamocolumnar junction can usually be clearly seen (6 in Fig. 2.26).

The process has a typical topographical distribution within the transformation zone, being confined predominantly to the summits of the rugae (Figs 2.17 and 2.18), the tips of the villi (2 in Fig. 2.26) and the peripheral borders of the transformation zone adjacent to the squamocolumnar junction (6 in Fig. 2.26). As will be discussed below, these are areas that are most exposed to the vaginal environment and, when exposure occurs, predominantly during pregnancy, the process spreads to the spaces in between the rugae and down into and along the sides of the villus. The process is topographically a variable one, with occasional islands of villous tissue existing adjacent to large sheets of smooth metaplastic epithelium (2 in Fig. 2.25 and 5 in Fig. 2.26). The rim of this tissue existing around the margins of the transformation zone has led some

histological appearance of a multilayered undifferentiated sheet of cells towards the top of the villus (stage 2 in Fig. 2.27).

Stage 2 As the process progresses and the new squamous epithelium commences to grow down the side of the villus, so the individual villi become attached; their original form is still discernible (3 in Fig. 2.26, stage 2 in Fig. 2.27, Fig. 2.28).

Stage 3 The fusion of the villi now becomes complete, resulting in the smooth squamous surface (stage 3 in Fig. 2.27). Histologically, this now appears as a multilayered epithelium with the stromal core of vessels indicating the original position of the fused villi.

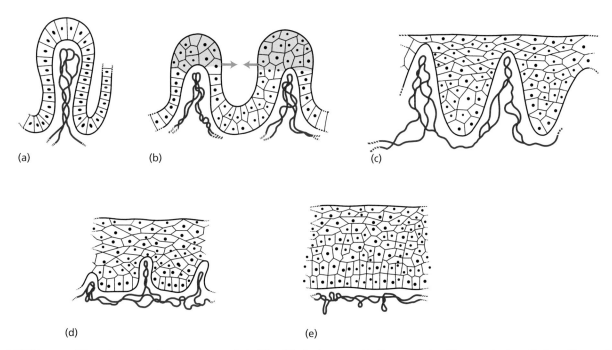

Fig. 2.27 The normal Stage is process of squamous metaplasia. The villi of columnar epithelium are replaced by metaplastic epithelium. The capillary structures of the stroma in the villi are compressed and reduced in height, ultimately forming a network under the epithelium; this is ndistinguishable from the capillary network of normal squamous epithelium (modified from Kolstad and Stafl, 1982).

investigators to propose that ingrowth of squamous epithelium occurs from the margins of the squamocolumnar junction by a process called squamous epithelialisation (Ferenczy and Winkler, 1994). Sequential colposcopic monitoring of the cervix during pregnancy clearly shows that ingrowth is a very uncommon phenomenon (Singer, 1976).

The process is most active during late fetal life (Chapter 6), during adolescence (Jacobson *et al.*, 1999) and in pregnancy (Chapter 7), with the last producing the most dramatic alterations in cervical morphology. All these stages will be discussed in later chapters. This is as a result of the conversion of large areas of original columnar to squamous epithelium by the metaplastic process. Exposure of the former from its endocervical position to the acidic pH of the vagina most probably stimulates this change, the lower pH of the ectocervix most probably destroying the buffering action of the mucus that protects the columnar cells. Exposure is produced by the process of eversion, where the surface epithelium of the endocervix is transported to an ectocervical position (see Fig. 7.1). This process, most active in the primigravida, results from an increase in the size of the cervix, resulting in downward prolapse of the endocervical tissue. In the multigravid cervix, metaplasia also occurs but the mechanism is different, in that there is very little eversion but much opening up or gaping of the lower part of the cervix, facilitating entry of acidic vaginal secretions into the upper reaches of the endocervix (Riedewald *et al.*, 1990; see Fig. 7.1).

Metaplasia also occurs in the pubertal and adolescent cervix in a similar manner to that operating in pregnancy and is most probably caused by exposure of the original columnar epithelium to the vaginal pH. For example, at puberty, a time of increasing and novel hormone secretion, an increase in cervical volume and acidification of the vagina occurs, with resultant eversion of the endocervical columnar epithelium and eventual metaplastic transformation (Singer, 1975). It would seem as though this process is most active when the progesterone/estrogen ratio is high, as during late fetal life and pregnancy and in women using oral contraception (Maqueo *et al.*, 1966).

Histological appearance

Corresponding with the colposcopic appearances are definite histological features that account for the varied histology associated with this process. Like its colposcopic counterpart, the histological changes can essentially be divided into five stages.

Stage 1 In the first phase, which corresponds with the pallor at the tip of the villus, the columnar epithelial cells seem to lose their mucous coat and are reduced in height and increased in width (Figs 2.29 and 2.30). Coppleson and Reid (1967) further describe the enlargement and eventual disruption of the nuclei of these cells, which probably corresponds with the liberation of hydrolytic enzymes, resulting in cell death and the inability of the cells to produce mucin. The subepithelial region (2 in Fig. 2.29, Fig. 2.30), which is composed of stromal cells, is the site of much activity during this stage. It was proposed

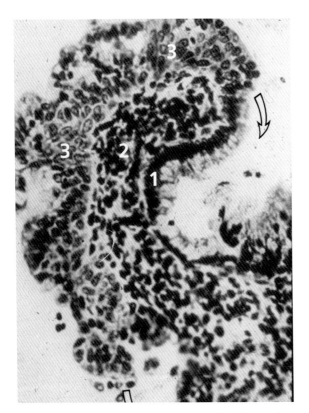

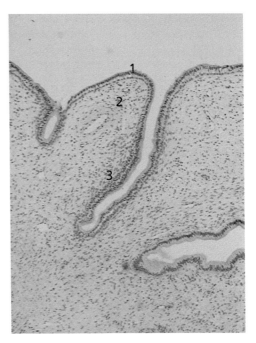

Fig. 2.29 Photomicrograph of punch biopsy from a villous surface projection showing the earliest stage of squamous metaplasia with a single layer of columnar epithelium (1), a cellular stroma (2) and a small area of multilayered undifferentiated squamous cells at (3).

Fig. 2.28 Photomicrograph from a punch biopsy of a villous surface projection showing the earliest stage of metaplasia with a single layer of columnar cells (1) overlying an extremely cellular and active stroma (2). An area with a multilayered undifferentiated sheet of epithelial cells is seen at (3). This process will quickly descend into the clefts between the adjacent villi (arrowed) with fusion of their opposed surfaces following rapidly. When the tip of this villus is fused colposcopically, it will already have lost its typical translucent appearance, as seen at (2) in Figure 2.27 and (2) in Figure 2.26.

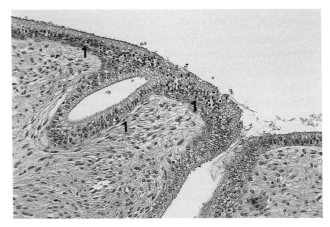

Fig. 2.30 A single layer of 'reserve cells' appearing conspicuously beneath the columnar mucinous endocervical cells (1). The origin of these cells is uncertain but, at this stage, their detailed keratin signature already identifies them as parabasal or suprabasal squamous cells. They are present over the papillary surface and within the endocervical crypts or troughs. Their monotypic single layer occurrence at one moment suggests a threshold crossed or a switch tripped over.

by Coppleson and Reid (1967) and Reid *et al.* (1967) that an activation process is initiated among these cells, which results in their transformation into the progenitor cells of the new squamous epithelium.

Stage 2 In the second phase, it appears that there is active formation of a new basement membrane, which follows the degeneration of the one underlying the columnar epithelium at the outset of the metaplastic transformation. A single layer of 'reserve cells' now appears beneath the columnar epithelial cells (Figs 2.30 and 2.31).

Stage 3 In the third phase of the metaplastic transformation process that is seen colposcopically as the progressive fusion of adjacent villi (Fig. 2.32), the eventual disappearance of the villous structure occurs, except for the retention of variable amounts of columnar epithelium in the depths of crypts and tunnels (Fig. 2.33). In these sites, they appear to be insulated from the vaginal pH, which seems to be the stimulus to metaplasia. The distinctive surface apertures of the subepithelial

glandular components are called gland openings (Figs 2.21 and 2.26). Histologically, this stage presents difficulties for the pathologist because there is a mixture of both columnar and metaplastic elements. This is clearly seen in Figure 2.33, in which the outline of the original villi can be seen. The metaplastic

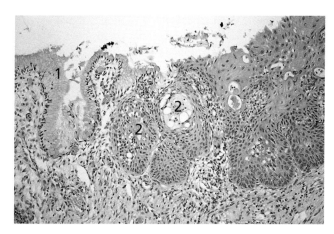

Fig. 2.31 A later stage of still incomplete squamous metaplasia with normal endocervical epithelium on the left at (1). Within the developing squamous epithelium, there are residual columnar-lined surfaces (2) with endocervical cells.

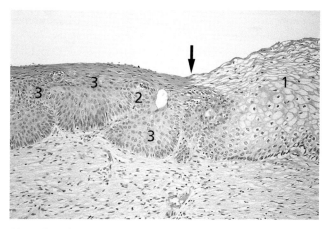

Fig. 2.32 As the metaplastic process continues, the epithelium loses its columnar surface and the mature squamous epithelium appears. Solid arrow separates the original squamocolumnar junction (1) with its usual pale glycogenated squamous layers from the metaplastic endothelium (2). There is striking epithelial scalloping or irregularity of the lower half of the epithelium (3) as a result of the intercalated stromal papillae which were originally sited between the endocervical crypts and still contain capillary vascular channels. The new epithelium is very often darker with reduced glycogen levels and may remain so.

process has extended to the tips of these villi, although there are still remnants of columnar epithelium.

Stage 4 This stage is characterised colposcopically by smooth patches of immature metaplastic epithelium. These appearances correspond histologically to an epithelium that has a predominantly smooth-surfaced appearance, with occasional stromal papillae projecting into it (Fig. 2.32; see also Fig. 2.35). These represent the original stromal cores of the fused villi. In many instances, the original columnar epithelium can be seen underlying the new metaplastic epithelium (Fig. 2.34). It is also common to find metaplastic epithelium within the clefts

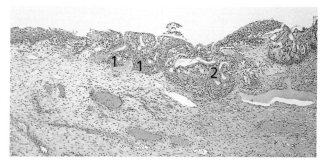

Fig. 2.33 Photomicrograph showing an incomplete metaplastic epithelium at (1) with underlying degenerate columnar endocervical cells at (2). The glandular architecture is still visible in this area.

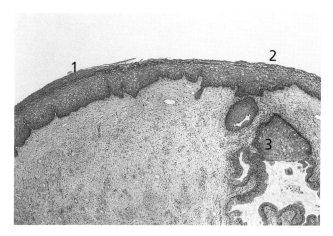

Fig. 2.34 A histological section showing the border between the original squamous epithelium (1) and recently formed squamous metaplasia on the right at (2). The metaplastic epithelium is of a mature type and involves superficial gland crypts with metaplasia (3) occurring within them. These changes are in the area of the original squamocolumnar junction.

and tunnels of the columnar epithelium. It has been postulated that there are three mechanisms by which it is found in this position. First, a direct invasive process into the cleft by the metaplastic epithelium from the surface; this has clearly been shown to occur in the second stage of metaplasia. Second, it has been postulated that metaplasia occurs in the actual depths of the columnar epithelium by less well-differentiated epidermoid-type cells. Third, it has also been suggested that metaplasia arises from proliferation of reserve or indifferent cells that reside beneath the normal columnar cells (Fig. 2.30).

Stage 5 This is represented by mature squamous epithelium with occasional crypt occlusion by underlying immature metaplastic squamous epithelium causing the development of an occlusion cyst full of mucous secretions; this structure is called a Nabothian follicle (Fig. 2.35).

The finding of metaplastic epithelium within the tunnels and clefts gives rise to an appearance called epidermisation. The entire gland lumen may be filled, with occasionally the

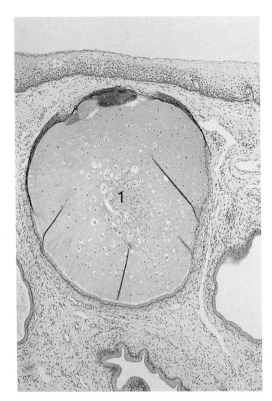

Fig. 2.35 Histological section revealing occasional crypt occlusion by immature metaplastic squamous epithelium with the formation of a Nabothian follicle (cyst) which contains mucus cell secretions (1).

small central gland-like mucin-filled cavity remaining as the residuum of the pre-existing tall columnar epithelium.

This multilayered epithelium seen in stages 3–5 can now reach maturity and, at this stage, it may sometimes be difficult to differentiate histologically from the original squamous epithelium of the ectocervix [Figs 2.21 (colposcopic view) and 2.34]. It is still possible, even with this maturing epithelium, to see evidence of the pre-existing endocervical gland-like arrangements within the basal layer, with its undulating appearance (Fig. 2.32). The residuum of the original mucus-secreting epithelium is usually seen as tiny basophilic-staining central cores.

Between the development of a final mature multilayered epithelium and the earliest origins of the metaplastic process lie a number of histological appearances that are the cause of much confusion among pathologists. It has to be realised that the process can be arrested at any point within or between the three stages described above. It also appears that progression towards a mature squamous epithelium may be resumed at any stage after such an arrest. Reference to Figures 2.31 and 2.33 shows the admixture of the different epithelial stages within the metaplastic transformation zone that exist simultaneously within the same cervix. It is no wonder that pathologists have given at least 50 different terms to the histological representation of these arrested stages (Coppleson *et al.*, 1971).

Of even more importance is the confusion that may develop between the physiological changes described above and those of neoplasia. Superficial evaluation may lead to the erroneous diagnosis of squamous or glandular intraepithelial neoplasia, adenocarcinoma, adenosquamous cancer or the common squamous carcinoma. Conversely, it must be recognised that all these conditions may arise in the cervix and, therefore, the pathologist has to study the individual cells carefully for any signs of neoplastic change. It is suggested that the common squamous carcinomas arise within the areas of metaplastic transformation. It is accepted that both precancerous and cancerous squamous lesions of the cervix arise within the transformation zone and are bounded by the squamocolumnar junction.

Variations of the metaplastic process: the congenital transformation zone

These histological appearances within this multilayered epithelium have sometimes been called the congenital transformation zone (Anderson *et al.*, 1992). Some authors also refer to these changes as the vaginal transformation zone (Coppleson and Reid, 1986). They have a characteristic colposcopic appearance (Figs 2.36–2.39), are considered to be variants of squamous metaplasia and have many histological features in common.

The epithelium in some cases may also be acanthotic, indicating an increase in cells within the prickle or basal layer as identified in Figures 2.40 and 2.41. Maturation within the squamous epithelium may not be fully complete and, sometimes, there may even be other disorders of maturation with an excessive maturation on the surface, as exemplified by keratinisation, while there is delayed and incomplete maturation of the deeper layers. As seen in Figures 2.40 and 2.41, there may be irregularity of the epithelial–stromal junction with apparent incursions of squamous epithelium, so-called stromal papillae, into the stroma. Very often, the tips of these processes appear to be separate from the overlying epithelium, giving the impression of invasive buds (Fig. 2.41). This is a typical finding of the so-called congenital transformation zone.

The epithelium within this zone gives rise to specific colposcopic and histological appearances, the latter of which have been described above. Colposcopically, it can be seen in the cervices of many young women in which there exists epithelium, usually situated on the caudal side of a more recently formed transformation zone, which stains intensely white with acetic acid and has a fine and regular mosaic or punctate appearance (Figs 2.36–2.39). This epithelium is non-glycogenated and seems to represent a form of immature squamous metaplasia. Some authors believe it to represent metaplasia occurring in late fetal life (Linhartova, 1970; Pixley, 1976a; Coppleson and Reid, 1986; Borgno *et al.*, 1988) and have therefore called the area within which this epithelium

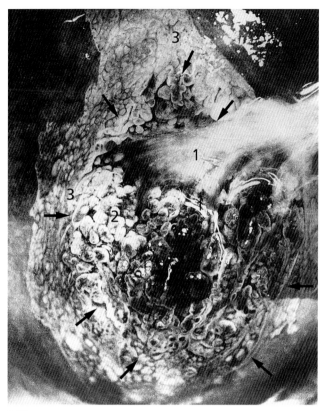

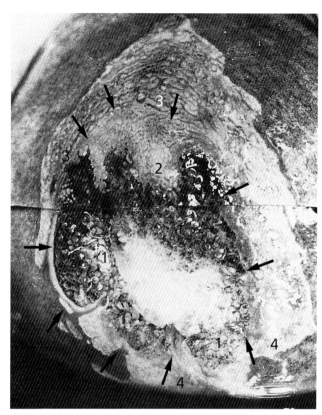

2.36

2.37

Figs 2.36 and 2.37 The first pattern of the congenital transformation zone shows regular fine mosaic epithelium that extends anteriorly and posteriorly on to the vaginal fornices. In Figure 2.36, the endocervical canal is at (1), and early metaplastic epithelium is developing within the original columnar epithelium at (2). The original transformation zone with its concentric boundary, identified as the original squamocolumnar junction, is arrowed. The fine and regular mosaic epithelium of the congenital transformation zone (3) is caudal to this line and extends anteriorly, laterally and posteriorly on to the vaginal fornices. In Figure 2.37, original columnar epithelium exists at (1) and the original squamocolumnar junction, marking the lateral boundaries of the transformation zone, is arrowed. At (2), there is an area of acetowhite smooth epithelium, indicative of immature metaplasia. Caudal to the original squamocolumnar junction are elements of the congenital transformation zone. On the anterior lip at (3), there exists a fine, regular mosaic and punctated area that extends laterally and posteriorly in the form of patchy keratotic tissue. Biopsies from these tissues in areas (3) and (4) show a very acanthotic type of epithelium. This is characterised by markedly elongated stromal papillae with the classic stromal ridges subdividing the surface epithelium into discrete fields, resulting in the mosaic appearance. Keratinisation is seen on the surface, particularly in area (4).

is found the congenital transformation zone (Anderson *et al.*, 1992). It has many similarities to squamous metaplasia later in life, with maturation of the squamous epithelium being incomplete and with disorders of maturation that can occur in the form of excessive surface maturation either with accompanying keratinisation or with delayed and incomplete maturation of the deeper layers.

Most of these lesions are benign, but their very bizarre nature can be disconcerting to the inexperienced colposcopist and pathologist, who may falsely interpret these changes as representing cervical precancer or cancer. Because they may also contain colposcopic features of abnormal or atypical epithelium (i.e. acetowhiteness, punctation and mosaic vascular changes), the transformation zone is designated as atypical. Some examples of the various patterns are shown in Figure 2.38,

in which congenital transformation zones are seen. Sometimes, these changes may also be associated with subclinical human papillomavirus (HPV) infection, and it is not uncommon in young women and adolescents to find the two types of epithelium co-existing.

Origin of the metaplastic cells

For over 60 years, controversy has centred upon the origin of the metaplastic epithelial cell. There are, at present, three major views as to its origin. Two of these insist that the new cells arise from structures present within the epithelium; the third places the origin of the progenitor cell in the subepithelial stroma.

Mayer (1910) and many other pathologists after him (as summarised by Singer 1976) believe that a primitive cell

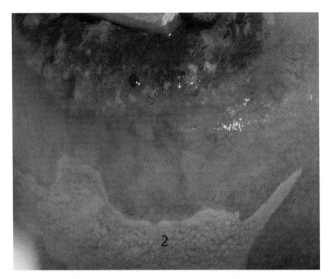

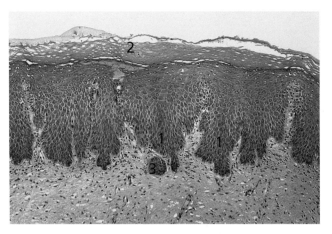

Fig. 2.40 A punch biopsy from an area of mosaic epithelium similar to that seen in Figure 2.36. It shows the typical acanthotic appearance (1) of the congenital transformation zone. The epithelium also shows some mild parakeratosis (2). The stromal papillae are elongated, and vessels extend between them and towards the surface, giving rise to the fine mosaic pattern seen colposcopically. Buds of squamous epithelium are visible at (3).

Fig. 2.38 An area of very fine and irregular epithelium (2) that is most probably related to the transformation zone seen at (1). However, the epithelium at (2) is in an area of original squamous epithelium, and it may be that this is another form of the congenital transformation zone. It would need to be differentiated from vaginal intraepithelial neoplasia (VAIN), and the only method of diagnosis is by punch biopsy and the resultant pathology (see Chapter 41).

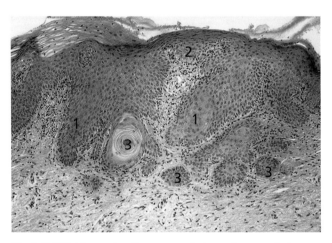

Fig. 2.41 This biopsy taken from an area designated a congenital transformation zone shows acanthotic rete pegs (1) with parakeratosis at (2). The epithelium is completely benign. Epithelial buds with pearl formation are present at (3).

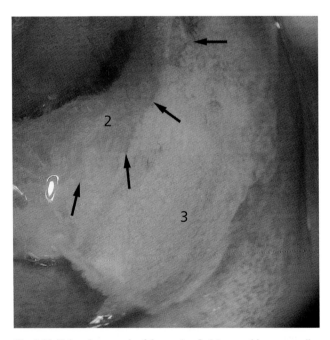

Fig. 2.39 Colpophotograph of the cervix of a 14-year-old non-sexually active female, showing the endocervical original columnar epithelium (1) with some early metaplasia already developing at (2). The lateral boundaries (arrowed) of the transformation zone are in the form of the original squamocolumnar junction; caudal to this, a large patch of fine and regular mosaic epithelium (3) exists. This area represents a form of the congenital transformation zone.

present in relation to the columnar epithelium has the potency to develop squamous elements. This cell, the reserve cell, exists between the columnar cells and the basement membrane and is believed to be a component of most cervices (Fig. 2.30). The second theory, propounded by Fluhmann (1961), insists that subcolumnar basal cells are derived directly from columnar cells and have the potential to develop into columnar or squamous epithelium. However, after destruction of the overlying epithelium by electrodiathermy, it is possible to witness the regeneration of the new metaplastic epithelium from cells beneath the previously present and destroyed epithelium (Singer 1976).

A number of studies have attempted to confirm Fluhmann's hypothesis of the basal cell or the reserve cell origin of the new epithelium. Peters (1986), using histological, immuno-histological and ultrastructural methods, suggested that these cells originated from T lymphocytes, with a predominance of T-cytotoxic and -suppressor cells. A more heterogeneous inflammatory cell population was present in the cervical epithelium, which was believed by Peters (1986) to be quite distinct from the cells commonly referred to as reserve cells (reserve cell hyperplasia) and which have specific epithelial characteristics. The author believed that the reserve cell arose within the epithelium and represented an early sign of squamous metaplasia.

Studies involving the intermediate filament proteins (cytokeratins) have presented evidence that would indicate that the reserve cell is a common progenitor of both immature squamous metaplasia and endocervical columnar cells. Smedts and his group, in a comparison of the keratin expression patterns between reserve cells and endocervical columnar cells (Smedts *et al.*, 1993b), showed that many of the keratins found in reserve cells are also found in columnar cells, albeit to a lesser degree. As endocervical columnar cells are in an end-stage of differentiation and probably display very little metaplastic activity, it would seem that these cells are derived from reserve cells, most of which lose expression of the specific keratins 5, 6, 14 and 15 during differentiation into columnar cells and, for some unexplained reason, initiate the expression of a specific keratin, number 4. It was found that, when reserve cells proliferate and transform into squamous metaplastic epithelium, the keratins found in simple epithelia ceased to be expressed and that the synthesis of keratins that are characteristic of non-keratinising epithelia, such as keratins 4 and 13, is initiated. This gave rise to the premise that both immature squamous metaplasia and endocervical columnar cells were indeed derived from a common progenitor source, i.e. the reserve cell.

Likewise, in their studies of mature squamous metaplastic epithelium, Smedts *et al.* (1993b) found that the keratin expression was identical to that found in ectocervical epithelium with the exception of keratin 17, which is sporadically expressed in the basal cell layers of ectocervical epithelium. Furthermore, keratin expression is not compartmentalised as strictly as in the ectocervical non-cornifying epithelium. This probably means that the mature squamous metaplastic epithelium, even though it seems mature on morphological criteria, is not yet fully mature as judged by its keratin phenotype.

Tsutsumi *et al.* (1993) have provided further evidence that the endocervical epithelia may give rise to squamous metaplasia. They cultured normal human endocervical cells and showed that they formed epithelia that resembled squamous metaplasia *in vivo*. They tested for cytokeratin, mucin expression and morphological features of the endocervical cells in monolayer cultures and in implants beneath the skin of nude mice. Human endocervical cell implants in nude mice morphologically formed epithelia similar to immature squamous metaplasia and showed variable CK18 cytokeratin expression. They also showed homogeneous CK13 expression through all layers and expressed mucin and CK7 in the suprabasal cells. They believed that this evidence supported the likely view that human endocervical cells are bipotential cells and undergo differentiation readily and reversibly to give rise to mucosecretory 'columnar cells' and native reserve cell types 'in culture'.

Zwillenberg (1998) also presented evidence that suggested that the true stem cell (the new squamous epithelium) was not the basal cells but the parabasal cells.

The third hypothesis is that the underlying stroma gives rise to the progenitor cells of the new epithelium. Reid *et al.* (1967) produced tissue destruction to a depth of 5–10 μm in the human cervix and then followed the subsequent regeneration process by tissue biopsy and colposcopy. They suggested that the major source of metaplastic tissue was mononuclear cells that had migrated into the acellular area within 24–48 hours after injury. Very soon after this, these cells formed a new squamous epithelium. Singer *et al.* (1968) further demonstrated that labelled peritoneal monocytes reinjected into the peritoneal cavity of a rat whose uterine lining had been destroyed by cauterisation were capable of migrating into the regenerated squamous-lined lumen. Song (1964) has also postulated that stromal cells give rise to the new epithelium, while Lawrence and Shingleton (1980), although disagreeing with some of the observations of Coppleson and Reid (1967), maintain that 'from a histological viewpoint, the most likely origin for the sub-columnar progenitor cell appears to be the subepithelial stromal cell'. Their observations were based on detailed light and electron microscopic observations.

Smedts *et al.* (1993b) have presented evidence indicating that stromal cells cannot play a part in the formation of the new metaplastic squamous epithelium. Stromal cells were shown to be devoid of keratin, in contrast, to reserve cells, which have a highly sophisticated and complex keratin composition. Vimentin has not been observed in reserve cells, whereas it is a component of stromal cells. It is also well known that transition from one type of epithelium to another, as occurs in squamous metaplasia, is associated with gradual keratin change. It would therefore seem from this evidence that it is highly unlikely that stromal cells, migrating as they do through a basement membrane, would initiate the expression of up to 10 different keratins while they are in a transitional phase within the endocervical stroma, especially as they contain no cytoskeletal proteins of the keratin type.

A process called squamous epithelialisation has been suggested as a possible mechanism for the 'remodelling' of the ectocervix, especially after the removal of the overlying epithelium. Originally suggested by Mayer (1910) and then revised by Ferenczy and Winkler (1994), it suggests that tongues of squamous epithelium from the original native squamous epithelium of the vaginal portion ride beneath the adjacent columnar epithelium which has been sloughed off, for example in the erosive process after delivery (Chapter 7). Ferenczy and Winkler insist that it is a reactive change due to inflammation and regeneration and that the epithelial cells do not originate from the subcolumnar cells as in metaplasia, but would possibly grow in from the original squamous epithelium. Jacobson *et al.* (2000) are unsure as to which process, squamous metaplasia or epithelialisation, independently modifies the area of 'ectopy', and they are again unsure as to which process, an acidic pH change, hormones, trauma, chronic irritation, semen or chronic infection, stimulates each of these processes 'independently'. Chronic infection induced by *Chlamydia trachomatis*, for example, may induce these changes, especially if there is a large area of 'erosion' or 'ectopy' visible on the ectocervix. However, the authors believe that the process of squamous epithelialisation is indeed very rare, but examination of sequential colpophotographs of a pregnancy study, as listed in Chapter 7, may be examples of this process. The area C in Figures 7.6 and 7.7 and area (4) in Figures 7.3 and 7.4 could be examples of this limited ingrowth process.

Functional cells of the epithelium (see also Chapter 4)

The cervical epithelium, exposed as it is to multiple biological, chemical and mechanical insults, has developed an extensive immune surveillance and regulating system. The most important cells in this respect are the antigen-presenting cells, which are concerned with the collection of antigens encountered in the epithelium and the transportation of this antigenic message to the underlying dermis. The cells primarily concerned with this antigen-presenting mechanism are the epithelial Langerhans cells (LC), which are Birbeck granule-containing bone marrow-derived cells and are located mainly in the suprabasal layer of the epidermis. They are a type of immature dendritic cell. Their role has been documented by many groups (Morelli *et al.*, 1992, 1993; Teunissen, 1992; Woodworth and Simpson, 1993; Wira *et al.*, 2000; Giannini *et al.*, 2002). Langerhans cells are readily identified by their strong expression of CD1a and major histocompatibility complex (MHC) class II antigens. They possess the ability to activate T lymphocytes and also have the ability to migrate from the epithelium to the regional lymph nodes. Their numbers can be diminished in a number of situations, especially, for example, when HPV infection is present (Tay *et al.*, 1987; Hussain *et al.*, 1992; Morelli *et al.*, 1993); Barton *et al.* (1988) also showed a dose–response relationship between the number of cigarettes smoked and the diminution of LC counts, identifying the cells by immunocytological staining for S-100 protein and T6 (CD1) antigen.

T lymphocytes are present in the cervix and their immune role has been investigated (Morris *et al.*, 1983; Tay *et al.*, 1987; Morelli *et al.*, 1993). It has been shown, especially by Tay *et al.* (1987) using monoclonal antibodies to pan-T

(CD4) and T8 (CD8) antigen as well as introducing an improved quantitative method for expressing cell counts, that in histologically normal cervices, the T4 (CD4) and T8 (CD8) populations are present in a similar proportion to that found in the peripheral circulation. When HPV and cervical intraepithelial neoplasia exist within the epithelium, however, there is a progressive reduction in the number of T lymphocytes and a reversal of the normal T4 (CD4)/T8 (CD8) ratio. These observations and others (Miller *et al.*, 1992) provide a morphological basis for the existence of a mucosa-associated lymphoid tissue system within the cervical epithelium.

Macrophages are found in most tissues within the body and perform a variety of functions, including non-specific phagocytosis, antigen presentation, direct cytotoxicity to virally infected or tumour cells and the inhibition of lymphocyte proliferation. There are very few published studies of the role of macrophages within the cervix, but Tay *et al.* (1987), using two monoclonal antibodies, E9 and E11, to detect total macrophages and a subpopulation of activated macrophages respectively, have shown that these cells are scarce in the normal cervix with few active cells present. When HPV or cervical intraepithelial neoplastic lesions are present, however, there is a progressive epithelial infiltration of macrophages, particularly activated ones. It would seem that these cells are specifically directed against viral antigens. Much interest has been expressed in the role of these cells in cervicovaginal human immunodeficiency virus (HIV) transmission (Hussain *et al.*, 1992).

Two other types of cells of a functional nature have been found within the epithelium: natural killer cells and B lymphocytes. Their role is essentially that of exerting a cytotoxic effect against virally infected and neoplastic tissue or of facilitating phagocytosis (Parr and Parr 1991). As well as functional cells within the cervical epithelium, there are specific lymphokines that recruit and activate immune cells at the site of infection; these have been reviewed by Woodworth and Simpson (1993).

Effect of sex hormones on the transformation zone

The effect of sex hormones on the transformation zone and the surrounding issues has been extensively studied and summarised recently by Remoue *et al.* (2004). They have shown that the expression of receptors, both estrogenic and progestogenic, is significantly higher in the transformation zone than in the ectocervix, and immunohistochemical studies indicate that hormone receptor-positive cells are mainly observed in the parabasal and intermediate layers in both the transformation zone and the ectocervical epithelium. They also demonstrated that immature squamous metaplastic epithelium showed a significantly higher density of hormone receptor-positive cells than the more mature metaplastic epithelium found within the ectocervical area. They also suggested that this was a reason for the raised risk of neogenesis in the transformation zone as a result of this higher sensitivity to sex hormones.

The squamous epithelium is stimulated by estrogens in respect of its proliferation and maturation. This is in contrast to progesterone, which inhibits maturation. Receptors for estrogens and the estrogen-responsive or estrogen-regulated proteins are found in variable amounts in the basal, parabasal and intermediate cells throughout the cycle and during pregnancy. There also seems to be a small increase in the receptors in the first part of the menstrual cycle (follicular phase) (Ciocca *et al.*, 1956; Dresler *et al.*, 1986; Nonogaki, 1990; Ferenczy and Wright, 1994). Parabasal cells tend to have progesterone receptors, especially during the second phase of the cycle (luteal) and pregnancy.

Induction of metaplasia may well have a hormonal basis. Jacobson *et al.* (2000) believe that the subcolumnar reserve cells and other cells undergoing this process are most likely to be responsive to both estrogen and progestogen, with estrogen receptors and estrogen-responsive proteins being found in the reserve cells and those undergoing metaplasia throughout the menstrual cycle and pregnancy. They suggest that the reason why metaplasia is so pronounced in pregnancy is because of an interaction of both estrogen and progestogen with the estrogen-responsive protein and progesterone receptors, both being pronounced in the tissues during pregnancy.

Progesterone tends to be bound in endocervical columnar cells at high levels during the first part of the menstrual cycle (follicular). Sanborn *et al.* (1976) initially showed that women on high-dose combined oral contraceptive pills had binding of progesterone at levels equal to or above that in the second phase of the menstrual cycle (secretory). These cells also have a high number of estrogen receptors that do not seem to vary during the menstrual cycle, but estrogen-responsive or estrogen-regulated protein is not found in this tissue at all in the menstrual cycle. However, the type of mucus production changes with exposure to estrogens.

The locally immune microenvironment of the cervix would also seem to be exquisitely sensitive to hormonal changes, and Giannini *et al.* (2002) insist that this is as a result of their effect on the keratinocytes and the Langerhans cells mentioned above. Production of cytokines/chemokines is important in maintaining a balanced turnover of LC. This process is most probably influenced by the complex differentiation state of keratinocytes, which would seem to be altered in metaplastic areas of the transformation zone and possibly during the development of cervical neoplasia (Smedts *et al.*, 1992, 1993a; Hubert, 1999).

Both Schurrs and Verheul (1990) and Wira *et al.* (2000) have shown that sex hormones seem to be involved in the regulation and the production of cytokines/chemokines and, therefore, may influence the migration and function of these LC. It would therefore seem possible that these hormones are involved in the neoplastic process by altering the cytokine/chemokine-dependent interaction between keratinocytes and the LC. This in turn could have an influence on the role of HPV in cervical neoplasia development; this effect is particularly evident in the transformation zone because of a high level of sex hormone receptor expression in that area compared with the ectocervix (Remoue *et al.*, 2004).

SUMMARY

The cervical epithelium undergoes dramatic changes in its structure many times during life. These alterations commence as early as fetal life and continue to the menopause; the result is a dynamic epithelium of varied morphology. The essential element of change involves the development of a new squamous epithelium within the columnar epithelium that lines the cervical canal and ectocervix. This process, named metaplasia, is primarily a physiological one; it also seems to be central to the development of epithelial neoplasia in the cervix.

ACKNOWLEDGEMENTS

The authors wish to thank the publishers of the first edition, W.B. Saunders Co., for their kind permission in allowing the reproduction of many of the figures that appeared in the first edition of *The Cervix* (edited by J.A. Jordan and A. Singer, London, 1976).

Professor H. Shingleton and Dr J. Allen of Birmingham, AL, USA, kindly provided the transmission electron micrographs that appear in this chapter. Dr A.R.S. Deery of the Royal Free Hospital, London, has provided many of the colour digital images.

The authors appreciate the generosity of Professor Y. Yabuki for allowing the reproduction of Figures 2.1b,c and d, which originally appeared in the *American Journal of Obstetrics and Gynecology*.

REFERENCES

Anderson MC, Jordan J, Morse A, Sharpe F (1992) Congenital transformation zone. In: Anderson MC *et al.* (eds) *Text and Atlas of Integrated Colposcopy.* London: Chapman & Hall Medical, p. 78.

Barton SE, Maddox PH, Jenkins D *et al.* (1988) Effect of cigarette smoking on cervical epithelial immunity; a mechanism for neoplastic change. *Lancet* 2: 652–654.

Borgno G, Bersani R, Micheletti L *et al.* (1988) Colposcopic findings before sexual activity. *The Cervix and the Lower Female Genital Tract* 2: 69–74.

Ciocca D, Puy L, Lo Castro G. (1956) Localization of an estrogen-responsive protein in the human cervix during the menstrual cycle, pregnancy, and menopause and in abnormal cervical epithelia without atypia. *Obstetrics and Gynecology* 155: 1090–1096.

Coppleson M, Reid B (eds) (1967) *Preclinical Carcinoma of the Cervix Uteri.* Oxford: Pergamon Press.

Coppleson M, Reid B (1986) The vaginal transformation zone. In: Coppleson M, Reid B (eds) *Colposcopy*, 3rd edn. Springfield, IL: Charles C. Thomas, p. 408.

Coppleson M, Pixley E, Reid B (eds) (1971) *Colposcopy: a Scientific Approach to the Cervix in Health and Disease.* Springfield, IL: Charles C. Thomas, p. 121.

Danforth DN (1947) The fibrous nature of the human cervix and its relation to the isthmic segment in gravid and non-gravid uteri. *American Journal of Obstetrics and Gynecology* 53: 541–557.

Dressler L, Ramzy I, Sledge G *et al.* (1986) A new marker of maturation in the cervix: the estrogen-regulated 24K protein. *Obstetrics and Gynecology* 68: 825–831.

Ferenczy A, Winkler B (1994) Benign diseases of the cervix. In: Kurman R (ed.) *Blaustein's Pathology of the Female Genital Tract.* New York: Springer-Verlag, pp. 203–227.

Ferenczy A, Wright TC (1994). Anatomy and histology of the cervix. In: Kurman R (ed.) *Blaustein's Pathology of the Female Genital Tract.* New York: Springer-Verlag, pp. 185–201.

Fluhmann CF (1957) The nature of development of the so-called glands of the cervix. *American Journal of Obstetrics and Gynecology* 74: 753–768.

Fluhmann CF (1961) *The Cervix Uteri and its Diseases.* Philadelphia: Saunders.

Forsberg JG (1976) Morphogenesis and differentiation of the cervicovaginal epithelium. In: Jordan J, Singer A (eds) *The Cervix.* London: Saunders, p. 3.

Giannini SL, Hubert P, Doyen J *et al.* (2002) Influence of mucosal epithelium microenvironment on Langerhans' cells: implications for the development of squamous intraepithelial lesions of the uterine cervix. *International Journal of Cancer* 97: 654–659.

Granstrom LM, Ekman GE, Malmstrom A *et al.* (1992) Serum collagenase levels in relation to the state of the human cervix during pregnancy and labor. *American Journal of Obstetrics and Gynecology* 167: 1284–1288.

Hafez ES (1981) Surface ultrastructure and functional histology of the uterine cervix. *Reproduction* 4: 243–249.

Hafez ES (1982) Structural and ultrastructural parameters of the uterine cervix. *Obstetrical and Gynecological Survey* 37: 507–516.

Hubert P, van de Brule F, Giannini SL *et al.* (1999) Colonization of in vitro formed cervical human papillomavirus-associated (pre)neoplastic lesions with dendritic cells: role of granulocyte/macrophage colony-stimulating factor. *American Journal of Pathology* 154: 775–784.

Hughesdon PE (1952) The fibromuscular structure of the cervix and its changes during pregnancy and labour. *Journal of Obstetrics and Gynaecology of the British Empire* 59: 763–776.

Hussain LA, Kelly CG, Fellowes R *et al.* (1992) Expression and gene transcript of Fc receptors for IgG, HLA class II antigens and Langerhans cells in human cervico-vaginal epithelium. *Clinical and Experimental Immunology* 90: 530–538.

Jacobson DL, Peralta L, Farmer M *et al.* (1999) Cervical ectopy and the transformation zone measured by computerized planimetry in adolescents. *International Journal of Gynaecology and Obstetrics* 66: 7–17.

Jacobson DL, Peralta L, Graham NM *et al.*(2000). Histologic development of cervical ectopy: relationship to reproductive hormones. *Sexually Transmitted Diseases* 27: 252–258.

Kolstad P, Stafl A (1982) *Atlas of Colposcopy,* 3rd edn. Edinburgh: Churchill Livingstone.

Konishi L, Fujii S, Nonogaki H *et al.* (1991) Immunohistochemical analysis of estrogen receptors, progesterone receptors, Ki-67 antigen, and human papillomavirus DNA in normal and neoplastic epithelium of the uterine cervix. *Cancer* 68: 1340–1350.

Lawrence DW, Shingleton HM (1980) Early physiologic squamous metaplasia of the cervix; light and electron microscopic observations. *American Journal of Obstetrics and Gynecology* 137: 661–671.

Leppert PC, Yu SY (1991) Three-dimensional structures of uterine elastic fibers; scanning electron microscopic studies. *Connective Tissue Research* 27: 15–31.

Leppert PC, Cerreta JM, Mandl L (1986) Orientation of elastic fibers in the human cervix. *American Journal of Obstetrics and Gynecology* 155: 219–224.

Linhartova A (1970) Congenital ectopy of the uterine cervix. *International Journal of Obstetrics and Gynaecology* 8: 653–655.

Maqueo M, Azuela I, Calderon J *et al.* (1966) Morphology of the cervix in women treated with synthetic progestins. *American Journal of Obstetrics and Gynecology* 96: 994–998.

Mayer R (1910) Die Epithelentwicklung der Cervix und Portio vaginalis uteri. *Archiv Gynaekologica* 91: 579–586.

Miller CJ, McChesney M, Moore PF (1992) Langerhans cells, macrophages and lymphocyte subsets in the cervix and vagina of rhesus macaques. *Laboratory Investigation* 67: 628–634.

Minamoto T, Arai K, Hirakawa S *et al.* (1987) Immunohistochemical studies on collagen types in the uterine cervix in pregnant and non-pregnant states. *American Journal of Obstetrics and Gynecology* 156: 138–144.

Morelli AE, Di Paola G, Fainboim L (1992) Density and distribution of Langerhans cells in the human uterine cervix. *Archives of Gynecology and Obstetrics* 252: 65–71.

Morelli AE, Sananes C, di Paola G *et al.* (1993) Relationship between types of human papillomavirus and Langerhans cells in cervical condyloma and intraepithelial neoplasia. *American Journal of Clinical Pathology* 99: 200–206.

Morris HHB, Gatter KC, Stein H *et al.* (1983) Langerhans cells in human cervical epithelium; an immunohistological study. *British Journal of Obstetrics and Gynaecology* 90: 400–411.

Nonogaki H, Fujii S, Konishi I *et al.* (1990) Estrogen receptor localization in normal and neoplastic epithelium of the uterine cervix. *Cancer* 66: 2620–2627.

Osmers WD, Raff MW, Alderman-Grill BC (1992) Origin of cervical collagenase during parturition. *American Journal of Obstetrics and Gynecology* 166: 1455–1460.

Parr MB, Parr EL (1991) Langerhans cells and T lymphocyte subsets in the murine vagina and cervix. *Biology and Reproduction* 44: 491–498.

Peters WM (1986) Nature of 'basal' and 'reserve' cells in oviductal and cervical epithelium in man. *Journal of Clinical Pathology* 39: 306–312.

Petersen LK, Oxlund H, Uldbjerg N *et al.* (1991) In vitro analysis of muscular contractile ability and passive biomechanical properties of uterine cervical samples from nonpregnant women. *Obstetrics and Gynecology* 77: 772–776.

Phillip E (1975) Normal cervical epithelium. *Journal of Reproductive Medicine* 14: 188–191.

Pixley E (1976) Morphology in the fetal and prepubertal cervicovaginal epithelium. In: Jordan J, Singer A (eds) *The Cervix.* London: Saunders, p. 75.

Reid B (1982) Carcinogenesis. In: Coppleson M (ed.) *Gynecologic Oncology.* London: Churchill Livingstone, p. 36.

Reid B, Singer A, Coppleson M (1967) The process of cervical regeneration after electrocauterization. *Australian and New Zealand Journal of Obstetrics and Gynaecology* 7: 125–135.

Remoue F, Jacobs N, Miot V *et al.* (2004) High intraepithelial expression of estrogen and progesterone receptors in the transformation zone of the uterine cervix. *American Journal of Obstetrics and Gynecology* 189(6): 1660–1665.

Riedewald S, Kreutzmann IM, Heinze T *et al.* (1990) Vaginal and cervical pH in normal pregnancy and pregnancy complicated by preterm labour. *Journal of Perinatal Medicine* 18: 181–186.

Rotten D, Gavignet C, Colin MC *et al.* (1988) Evolution of the elastic fibre network of the human uterine cervix before, during and after pregnancy. A quantitative evolution by automated image analysis. *Clinics in Physiology and Biochemistry* 6(5): 285–292.

Schurrs AH, Verheul HA (1990) Effects of gender and sex steroids on the immune response. *Journal of Steroid Biochemistry* 35: 157–172.

Sanborn B, Held B, Kuo H. (1976) Hormonal action in human cervix. II. Specific progesterone binding proteins in human cervix. *Journal of Steroid Biochemistry* 7: 665–672.

Singer A (1975) The uterine cervix: from adolescence to the menopause. *British Journal of Obstetrics and Gynaecology* 82: 81–89.

Singer A (1976) The anatomy of the cervix. In: Jordan J, Singer A (eds) *The Cervix*. London: Saunders, p. 13.

Singer A, Reid B, Coppleson M (1968) The role of peritoneal mononuclear cells in the regeneration of the uterine epithelium of the rat. *Australian and New Zealand Journal of Obstetrics and Gynaecology* 8: 163–170.

Smedts F, Ramaekers F, Troyanovsky M *et al.* (1992) Basal-cell keratins in cervical reserve cells and a comparison to their expression in cervical intraepithelial neoplasia. *American Journal of Pathology* 140: 601–613.

Smedts F, Ramaekers FCS, Vooijs PG (1993a) The dynamics of keratin expression in malignant transformation of cervical epithelium; a review. *Obstetrics and Gynecology* 82: 465–474.

Smedts F, Ramaekers F, Leube RE *et al.* (1993b) Expression of keratins 1, 6, 15, 16 and 20 in normal cervical epithelium, squamous metaplasia, cervical intraepithelial neoplasia and cervical carcinoma. *American Journal of Pathology* 142: 403–412.

Song J (1964) *The Human Uterus: Morphogenesis and Embryological Basis for Cancer*. Springfield, IL: Thomas.

Tay K, Jenkins D, Maddox P *et al.* (1987) Subpopulations of Langerhans cells in cervical neoplasia. *British Journal of Obstetrics and Gynaecology* 94: 10–15.

Teunissen MBM (1992) Dynamic nature and function of epidermal Langerhans cells in vivo and in vitro; a review, with emphasis on human Langerhans cells. *Histochemical Journal* 24: 697–716.

Tiltman AJ (1998) The significance of smooth muscle bundles in the endocervical submucosa. *British Journal of Obstetrics and Gynaecology* 105: 113–116.

Tsutsumi K, Sun Q, Yasumoto S *et al.* (1993) In vitro and in vivo analysis of cellular origin of cervical squamous metaplasia. *American Journal of Pathology* 143: 1150–1158.

Wira CR, Rossol RM, Kaushic C (2000) Antigen-presenting cells in the female reproductive tract: influence of estradiol on antigen presentation by vaginal cells. *Endocrinology* 141: 2877–2885.

Wolf DP, Blasco L, Khan MA *et al.* (1978) Human cervical mucus, viscoelasticity and sperm penetrability during the ovulatory menstrual cycle. *Fertility and Sterility* 30: 163–169.

Woodworth CD, Simpson S (1993) Comparative lymphokine secretion by cultured normal human cervical keratinocytes, papillomavirus-immortalized, and carcinoma cell lines. *American Journal of Pathology* 142: 1544–1555.

Yabuki Y, Sasaki H, Hatakeyama N *et al.* (2005) Discrepancies between classic anatomy and modern gynecologic surgery on pelvic connective tissue structure: harmonization of those concepts by collaborative cadaver dissection. *American Journal of Obstetrics and Gynecology* 193: 7–15.

Zwillenberg LO (1998) At 40 years of the 'Golden Chain'. *Gynecological and Obstetric Investigations* 46(4): 247–251.

CHAPTER 3

The vascular, neural and lymphatic anatomy of the cervix

Timothy A.J. Mould and Carl Chow

The cervix is part of the uterus, so it is not surprising that their vascular and nerve supplies are interrelated. However, in terms of lymphatic anatomy, the cervix tends to behave as a separate entity, utilising a system of drainage more or less distinct from that of the rest of the uterus.

This chapter describes the vascular and nerve supply initially, looking particularly at the relation of the innervation and nerve-sparing radical surgery. Following this, the lymphatic anatomy and the anatomical position of the sentinel node are described in detail in relation to their vital importance in the spread of cervical neoplasia.

VASCULAR ANATOMY

The blood supply to the cervix is arranged bilaterally with the arterial supply being directed from three main sources: directly from the uterine artery and its cervicovaginal branch and from the vaginal artery (Fig. 3.1).

The cervicovaginal branch of the uterine artery, the main source, leaves the uterine artery at about the level of the internal os and runs down the lateral margin of the cervix, where it

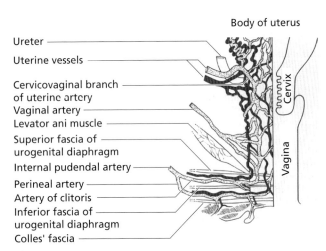

Fig. 3.1 Diagrammatic view of the blood supply of the cervix and vagina.

Body of uterus

Ureter

Uterine vessels

Cervicovaginal branch of uterine artery

Vaginal artery

Levator ani muscle

Superior fascia of urogenital diaphragm

Internal pudendal artery

Perineal artery

Artery of clitoris

Inferior fascia of urogenital diaphragm

Colles' fascia

Cervix

Vagina

gives off branches which pass medially and anastomose with branches of the vaginal artery.

Two important features characterise the anatomical arrangement of this arterial supply. First, the main stream of flow is along the margins of the cervix, allowing considerable haemostasis to be achieved during surgery (e.g. cone biopsy) by the insertion of high laterally placed sutures. Second, there is a profuse anastomotic potential maintaining blood flow with two separate branches of the internal hypogastric artery (i.e. uterine and vaginal) as well as a direct connection between the uterine and ovarian arteries. In addition, there is extensive potential for anastomosis bilaterally.

Zinser and Rosenbauer (1960) studied the details of this arterial arrangement and concluded that the endocervical canal is supplied mainly by branches coming directly from the uterine artery, while the portio vaginalis cervicis is supplied predominantly by its cervico-uterine branch. They also categorised the terminal vessels within the cervix into four zones:

1 The deepest comprises a plexus of freely anastomosing vessels lying in the stroma.

2 Arising from the deepest zone, a zone of palisade-like vessels runs perpendicularly or obliquely towards the epithelial surface.

3 The palisade zone terminates near the epithelium in a basal network parallel to the surface.

4 From the basal plexus, terminal capillaries of the subepithelial tissue arise and form capillary loops just below and indenting the epithelium.

The third and fourth zones are visible colposcopically, and their characteristic arrangement is discussed elsewhere. Examples of the terminal vascular bed are shown in Figures 3.2 and 3.3.

The venous drainage flows laterally into a rich plexus on either side of the cervix, with subsequent drainage by vessels analogous to the arterial supply.

NERVE ANATOMY

Many gaps exist in our current knowledge about the neural connections of the cervix. Although there is a substantial body of information concerning the various pathways of uterine innervation, there is no clear picture as to the role played

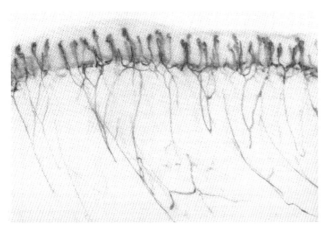

Fig. 3.2 Section of squamous epithelium and stroma stained for alkaline phosphatase to demonstrate the capillary system. The palisade arrangement of stromal capillaries can be seen running perpendicular to the surface and ending in an extensive capillary network just below the squamous epithelium. From the subepithelial network, the capillary loops of dermal papillae protrude upwards into the epithelium (× 75).

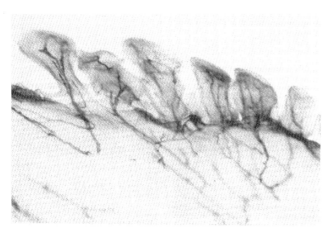

Fig. 3.3 Section of columnar epithelium and stroma stained for alkaline phosphatase, demonstrating capillary loops within endocervical papillae (× 75).

by the nervous system in cervical or uterine function. However, the same autonomic plexuses supply the bladder and rectum, the function of which can be severely affected by the surgical treatment of cervical cancer.

Cervical supply

The cervix is much more richly innervated in the region of the internal than the external os (Krantz, 1959; Coupland, 1962; Krantz and Phillips, 1962; Rodin and Moghissi, 1973). This is not surprising as much of the uterine innervation is directed to the muscle tissue (Bell, 1972) and, within the cervix, the amount of smooth muscle relative to fibrous tissue diminishes sharply from above downwards.

Krantz (1959) described a rich neural plexus surrounding the blood vessels and underlying endocervical clefts. Coupland (1962) observed that nerve fibres positive for cholinesterase-specific staining were most numerous in relation to cervical glands, arterial vessels and strands of smooth muscle. Nakanishi and Wood (1971) found that cholinesterase-positive nerve fibres were abundant in the cervix in contrast to their uncommon presence in the body of the uterus.

Rodin and Moghissi (1973) employed differential staining techniques to distinguish adrenergic (sympathetic) from cholinergic (parasympathetic) fibres. They demonstrated an extensive adrenergic network at the internal os where smooth muscle is abundant and throughout the cervix in relation to blood vessel walls. In their experience, the distribution of cholinergic fibres was much the same, although the cholinergic supply was less profuse. In contrast to previously mentioned studies, they did not find dense plexuses around endocervical clefts. They also made the interesting observation that extensive networks of the nerve fibres were not present in the postmenopausal cervix.

The function of these neural networks is unclear. Considerable work has been done, especially during pregnancy and parturition, on the relationship of the autonomic innervation to myometrial activity. However, assembling the pieces of this puzzle is proving to be a very difficult task. To compound the problem, it must be remembered that the cervix takes an opposite course from the body of the uterus during labour: the cervix thins and stretches whereas the wall of the body of the uterus contracts.

The sensory nerve supply of the cervix is intimately related to its autonomic supply. Although it has been suggested that the sensory outflow travels via the parasympathetic and that from the body of the uterus via the sympathetic (Cleland, 1933), this probably seems to be too rigid a division. Krantz (1973) stated that the sensory nerves were related to both sympathetic and parasympathetic tracts and therefore reached the spinal cord at both the thoracolumbar and the sacral levels. It appears unlikely that there exist many highly specialised sensory nerve endings within the cervix. Krantz (1959) described some lamellar corpuscles in the endocervix and isthmic regions, but Coupland (1962) found no specialised sensory nerve endings in the mucous membrane of the ectocervix.

Simple clinical observation provides some clues to the type of sensory apparatus within the cervix. Stretching of the endocervix, particularly the internal os, is sometimes painful. In contrast, extremes of temperature, either cold (cryocautery) or heat (electrical cautery), do not usually produce more than minor discomfort. Grasping the ectocervix with a tenaculum produces a burning sensation in some women.

These observations suggest that the sensory system of the skin covering the ectocervix is much less sophisticated than that covering other exposed areas of the body.

Uterine supply

The uterus derives its nerve supply via pathways of the autonomic nervous system, with both sympathetic and parasympathetic divisions contributing (Fontaine and Herrmann, 1932; Davis, 1933; Krantz, 1959; Bonica, 1967).

The sympathetic supply originates at the T5 to L2 level, sending out fibres which synapse at one of the many plexuses lying either on the posterior abdominal wall or in the pelvis. Thus, fibres that eventually reach the uterus are predominantly postganglionic. Parasympathetic (splanchnic nerve) fibres originate at the S2 to S4 level, run over piriformis lateral to the rectum and synapse in the same plexuses. Plexuses can be found bilaterally on the lateral pelvic sidewall at the level of the recto-uterine peritoneal reflection. They are seen as a 3-cm flat mesh of nerves at the terminal branches of the internal iliac vessels which stretches from an area anterior and lateral to the rectum, lateral to the cervix and vaginal fornix, to the bottom of the pelvis at the base of the bladder and anorectal junction (Hoffman, 2004) (Fig. 3.4).

The majority of uterine nerves converge peripherally and pass anteriorly away from the posterior abdominopelvic wall in the uterosacral fold of the peritoneum. This anatomical point was emphasised by Doyle (1955), who felt that the uterosacral ligament was the obvious area to interrupt in attempting to treat uterine pain.

Close to the uterine end of the uterosacral folds lie the major pelvic plexuses. These major pelvic plexus are variably referred to as the uterovaginal plexus, cervical ganglion or the ganglion of Frankenhauser. The proximal part of the plexus lies along the lateral aspect of the uterosacral ligaments and supplies branches to the rectum. The middle part of the plexus passes through the caudal posterior–lateral cardinal ligament entering the uterus at about the level of the internal os. The distal portion is found in the paracolpium and lateral aspect of the vesicovaginal ligament and supplies fibres to the bladder.

Nerve-sparing radical hysterectomy

Clearly, the neural supply of the uterus and cervix that is described above will be interrupted at radical hysterectomy. The pelvic autonomic nerve supply to the other pelvic structures such as the bladder (Fig. 3.5a and b) and rectum has also commonly been damaged at radical surgery for the treatment of cervical cancer.

Nerve-sparing surgical techniques have been developed in order to minimise this collateral damage. Identification and careful dissection of the pelvic plexuses described above is the cornerstone of nerve-sparing techniques.

The proximal part of the plexus must be dissected off the lateral part of the uterosacral ligament in order to preserve the fibres to the rectum. This is achieved by careful dissection of the prerectal and pararectal spaces to identify clearly the uterosacral ligaments before dissecting the lateral aspects of the ligament (Sakamoto and Takizawa, 1988).

The distal or lateral part of the plexus supplying the bladder must be preserved to prevent damage to bladder function. In order to do this, the cardinal ligaments are carefully dissected along with the origin and deep path of the uterine vein. The plane between the paracolpium and the pelvic plexus can be identified (Fig. 3.6a and b).

The uterine branches of the pelvic plexus are cut, enabling dissection of the paracolpium without interruption of the distal portion of the plexus that supplies the bladder (Figs 3.7–3.10).

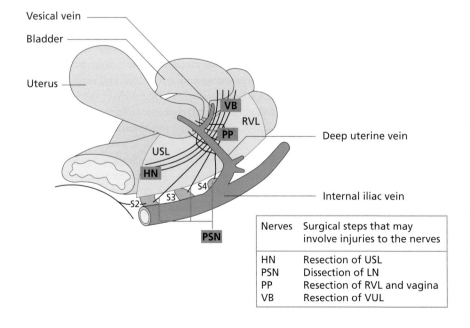

Nerves	Surgical steps that may involve injuries to the nerves
HN	Resection of USL
PSN	Dissection of LN
PP	Resection of RVL and vagina
VB	Resection of VUL

Fig. 3.4 The autonomic nerves innervating the pelvic structures. HN, hypogastric nerves; PSN, pelvic splanchnic nerves; PP, pelvic plexus. This plexus is composed of the fusion of two nerve fibres that intermingle and are derived from the sympathetic nerves —mainly the hypogastric nerves—and the parasympathetic nerves—pelvic splanchnic nerves. The bladder is innervated by these nerve fibres branching from the pelvic plexus. VB, vesical branch of the pelvic plexus; USL, uterosacral ligament; RVL, rectovaginal ligament.

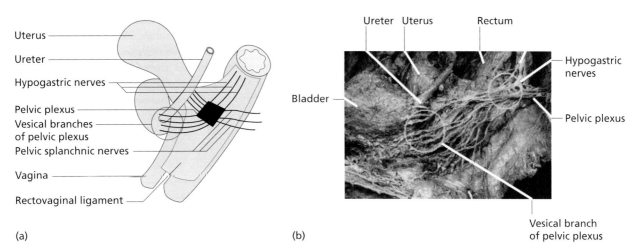

Fig. 3.5 (a) Illustration of autonomic nerves that control bladder function. (b) Anatomical distribution of autonomic nerves in cadavers.

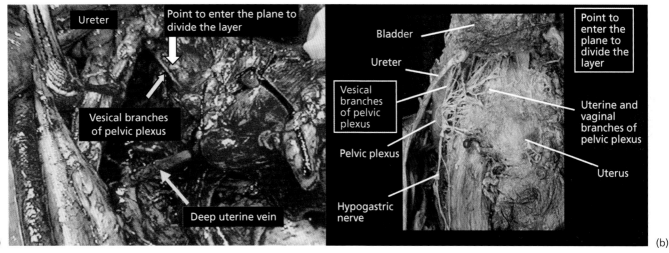

Fig. 3.6 (a) Vesical branches of the pelvic plexus after detection of the vesicouterine ligament and the point at which the plane must be entered to divide the vesical branch of the pelvic plexus and the paracolpium. (b) The same point at which the plane must be entered to divide the layers in the cadaver.

This technique has significant advantages in that the postoperative surgical bladder morbidity usually associated with this technique is dramatically reduced, as described by Sakaragi *et al.* (2005). In their recent publication, there was no difference in survival, blood loss or operation time, with significant advantages, as mentioned above, in the postsurgical bladder mortality rate.

LYMPHATIC SYSTEM ANATOMY

Isolated references to the lymphatic system date back to ancient Greek medicine, with its modern study generally being attributed to Assellius, who, in 1622, described the lacteals in the mesentery of dogs. His discovery attracted the attention of anatomists, who then produced detailed descriptions of the lymphatic drainage in many species, including man. An under-

standing of the function of this system developed less rapidly, but it is clear that, by the early nineteenth century, there was an awareness of the importance of lymph nodes as a site of cancer metastases. This awareness was heightened by Virchow, who, in 1860, set out a theory to explain this relationship of lymphatics and neoplasia. He postulated that cancer spread along lymphatic pathways to the regional lymph nodes, where it became trapped and held in check. The node was seen as a barrier to cancer dissemination, which in time became overwhelmed and a source of further malignant spread.

Virchow's barrier theory of lymph node function became an important part of the rationale underlying the trend towards a more aggressive approach to the treatment of malignant tumours. It was appreciated that treatment of cancer should, where possible, be extended to include not only the primary neoplastic site but also the regional nodes draining this site,

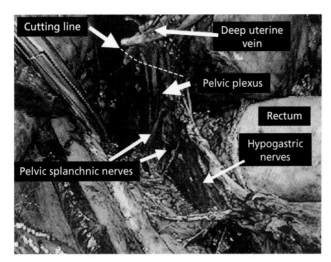

Fig. 3.7 The cutting line between the pelvic plexus and its uterine branch, which is shown after resecting and pulling upward of the deep uterine vein.

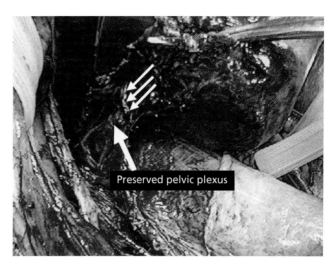

Fig. 3.9 Separated and retracted pelvic plexus after the autonomic nerve preservation procedure.

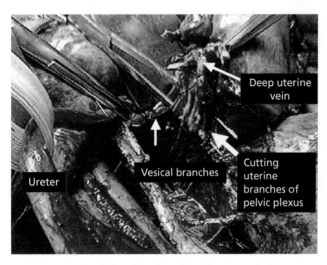

Fig. 3.8 Separation of the pelvic plexus from the rectovaginal ligament.

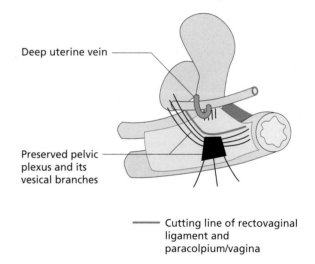

Fig. 3.10 Illustration of systematic autonomic nerve preservation and the cutting line of the rectovaginal ligament, paracolpium and vagina as described by Sakaragi *et al.* (2005).

in the hope that early metastases would be removed with resulting improvement in survival rate This view was put into practice in gynaecology in the late nineteenth century, when pelvic lymphadenectomy was employed as an adjunct to hysterectomy in the treatment of cervical carcinoma. Although radiotherapy has replaced surgery as the treatment of choice in many centres, the principle of extending treatment to include regional lymph nodes has remained in the form of external irradiation to the pelvic sidewalls in cases of cervical malignancy.

The modern management of cervical carcinoma has begun to use the concept of the sentinel lymph node to guide the use of radiotherapy in an attempt to minimise side-effects.

Cervical lymphatics at the capillary level

The cervix has a rich lymphatic supply (Rusznyak *et al.*, 1967; Yoffey and Courtice, 1970), but it is difficult to identify with precision the arrangement of its lymphatic capillary bed. The current view, summarised by Plentl and Freidman (1971), is that there is a three-layer arrangement of beds (Fig. 3.11).

A rather irregularly arranged bed underlies the epithelium of the endocervical clefts and drains into the stroma, whence it continues outwards in a series of perforating lymphatic capillaries which pass to the outer areas of the stroma. These perforating vessels receive drainage from a second capillary bed also located in the stroma. At the periphery of the cervix,

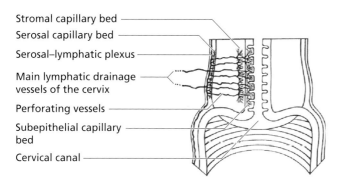

Stromal capillary bed

Serosal capillary bed

Serosal–lymphatic plexus

Main lymphatic drainage vessels of the cervix

Perforating vessels

Subepithelial capillary bed

Cervical canal

Fig. 3.11 Diagrammatic representation of the lymphatic capillary drainage of the cervix.

the lymphatic drainage opens out into a coarse network, the serosal lymphatic plexus, which retains its designation even though the bulk of the organ is not covered by serosa. This plexus receives a third capillary bed that arises on the outer surface of the cervix. The combined drainage system merges into several main vessels which fan out either laterally in the base of the broad ligament or posterolaterally in the uterosacral folds. Lymph flow from the cervix and body of the uterus is arranged horizontally rather than vertically (Rusznyak *et al.*, 1967) so, inevitably, at the junction between these two regions, there is some overlap reflecting the anatomically imprecise distinction between them.

The structure of the lymph capillaries is of particular interest as cancer has a marked affinity for passage along them. It is generally accepted that they begin as closed endothelial tubes that do not open directly into extracellular spaces (Patek, 1939; Casley-Smith and Florey, 1961). However, electron microscopic studies have demonstrated that their walls contain certain structural peculiarities when compared with the capillary wall of the blood vascular system. These differences have been summarised by Pressman *et al.* (1967) and are:

1 Lymphatic capillaries lack the well-developed basement membrane found in blood capillaries.

2 The attachment zones between the endothelial cells of lymphatic capillaries are poorly developed or even absent.

3 Lymphatic capillaries have a wider lumen than blood capillaries.

4 The endothelial cells of the lymphatic capillaries have a much more attenuated cytoplasm than those of blood capillaries.

5 Lymphatic capillaries lack pericytes.

6 The endothelial cell nucleus of the lymphatic capillary extends into the lumen to a greater extent than does the nucleus of an endothelial cell in the blood capillary.

Thus, the lymph capillary appears on electron microscopy to be a very thin-walled structure. Some workers (French *et al.*, 1960; Casley-Smith, 1964; Leak and Burke, 1968), by studying the passage of particles into its lumen, suggest that gaps between endothelial cells exist or may form in response to

certain stimuli, thereby allowing particles up to cellular size to enter the lumen.

It is tempting to speculate that the thin and porous nature of the lymph capillary wall explains the accessibility of the lymphatic system as a pathway for cancer spread. However, more information is needed before a clearer picture of the early steps in this process is available. One of the problems encountered in studying lymphatic capillaries is that the structure of the capillary walls varies from tissue to tissue with little data available at present specifically related to their appearance in the cervix.

Lymph drainage of the cervix

Lymph channels

The lymph flow converges in a radial and lateral direction to leave the cervix via collecting channels. According to Eichner *et al.* (1954), there is some anastomosis across the midline posteriorly, but none anteriorly. Zeit and Wilcoxon (1950) found that India ink, injected into the cervix laterally, drained mainly to unilateral nodes, but noted that some material appeared in contralateral nodes. The various reports on the course of the major lymph vessels draining the cervix via afferent vessels to pelvic nodes (Poirier *et al.*, 1903; Leveuf and Godard, 1923; Rouvière, 1932; Canela, 1934; Nesselrod, 1937; Henriksen, 1949) are contradictory. The consensus is that three main pedicles, each composed of several lymph vessels, emerge from either side of the cervix.

The most anterior runs laterally, at first closely related to the uterine artery, crossing the ureter and then ascending on the pelvic sidewall to reach the external iliac group of nodes. A second pedicle arising at the same level, but slightly posterior to the first, follows the uterine artery back towards its origin to reach the nodes of the internal iliac group. The third pedicle leaves the cervix posterolaterally and progresses in the uterosacral fold, reaching nodes situated over the sacrum. The fact that Eichner *et al.* (1954) emphasised the pedicle leading to the internal iliac nodes while Nesselrod (1937) could not demonstrate it highlights the inherent difficulties in applying neat anatomical divisions to a system as diffuse and variable as the pelvic lymphatics.

Lymph nodes

The pelvic nodes (Fig. 3.12) can be categorised into three broad groupings; one is related to the external iliac vessels and is the continuation of the lymphatics of the lower extremities, while the second group is related to the internal iliac artery and its various branches. The two systems merge at the level of the common iliac arteries, where they drain into a third group, the common iliac nodes (Figs 3.13 and 3.14).

External iliac system

The main lymph flow from the lower extremities becomes

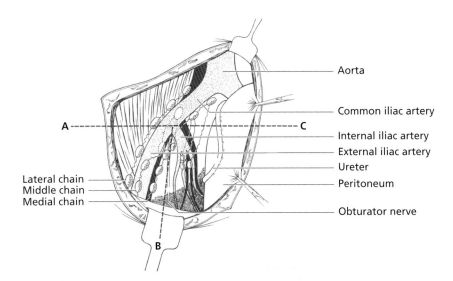

Fig. 3.12 Diagrammatic representation of the lymph nodes of the right half of the pelvis in relation to the main arteries. The broken lines divide the nodes into three main groups; within the area A to B, external iliac lymph nodes; within B to C, internal iliac lymph nodes; above A to C, common iliac nodes.

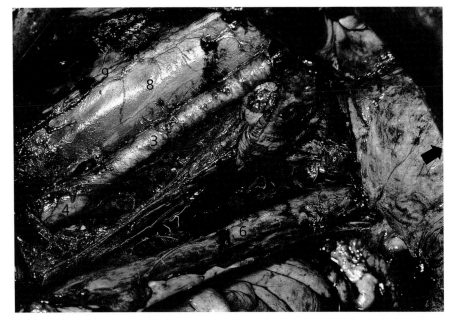

Fig. 3.13 Large vessels in the pelvic sidewall exposed in order to show the situation of draining lymph glands. The lateral and medial chains of the external iliac glands (1) have been displaced medially during the operation with the main mass of fat and glands seen at (2); the common iliac (4), the external iliac (3) and the internal iliac (5) are now displayed. The ureter (6) is well medial near the peritoneal edge at (7). The psoas muscle is at (8) and the genitofemoral nerve at (9).

closely related to the femoral vessels in the upper thigh and passes upward beneath the inguinal ligament to enter the pelvis in close relation to the external iliac artery and vein. The lymph vessels and nodes at this level are arranged in three chains: lateral, middle and medial. The lateral chain, lying on the psoas muscle, runs along the lateral aspect of the external iliac artery. The middle chain, the most superficial, lies on the external iliac vein or is slightly tucked in between the vein and the external iliac artery. The medial chain runs just below and is often partly hidden by the internal iliac vein, where some of the nodes of the chain may come to lie very close to the obturator nerve. Each chain consists of one or more lymph vessels interrupted by a variable number of nodes. Fuchs (1969) described an average of one to four nodes in each of the lateral and middle chains, and slightly more in the medial chain. A prominent node or group of nodes situated midway along the

medial external iliac chain has been referred to in some anatomical descriptions as the obturator node (or nodes). This designation has been justifiably criticised on the grounds that it is confusing to give a separate name to a portion of the chain; this discrepancy in terminology unfortunately still exists in the literature. In this chapter, the term obturator lymph node will be used to refer only to a small node or nodes of the internal iliac system positioned in close relation to the obturator artery.

Internal iliac system

The internal iliac nodes are related to the various branches of the internal iliac artery and tend to be considerably smaller in size. They are therefore less obvious than those of the external iliac system. Nevertheless, they are an important part of the lymphatic drainage of the pelvic organs, and of the musculoskeletal system of the hip region.

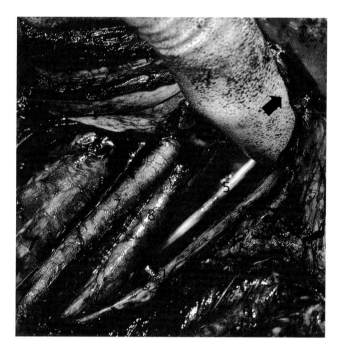

Fig. 3.14 Completion of removal of the pelvic lymph glands shows the arrangement of the vessels that had previously been overlaid and encompassed by the lymph glands and lymphatic drainage systems. The angle between the external iliac vein (1) and the internal iliac artery (2) is held open by the surgeon's forefinger and is seen to be quite clear for the glands and fat. The external iliac artery is at (3) and the ureter is seen at (4). The obturator nerve is at (5).

Poirier *et al.* (1903) described the internal iliac nodes as being close to the origin of the different branches of the internal iliac artery, but Fuchs (1969) pointed out that there were nodes situated more peripherally along the arterial branches supplying the pelvic organs. The various internal iliac lymph nodes are listed below.

Obturator nodes When they occur, true obturator lymph nodes are small and related to peripheral branches of the obturator artery.

Superior gluteal nodes These nodes are inconsistent and, when present, are situated at the origin of the superior gluteal artery.

Inferior gluteal nodes These nodes, like the superior gluteal nodes, are not found regularly. When present, they lie at the origin of the inferior gluteal artery.

Lateral sacral nodes These nodes are situated along the course of the lateral sacral artery and therefore are in close relationship to the lateral margin of the sacrum.

Visceral nodes Visceral nodes have been described in relation to the bladder, rectum and uterus. Of these, a node or group

of nodes may occur just lateral to the cervix, very closely related to the uterine artery as it crosses the ureter; various names, such as parametrial, ureteral and juxtacervical, have been attributed to this node or group of nodes, but the frequency of its occurrence is not clear.

The importance of the parametrial nodes is disputed. A parauterine node at the junction of the uterine artery and the ureter has been described (Plentl and Friedman 1971) and Burghardt and Girardi (1993) described nodes throughout the parametrium. Javert (1954) and Kolbenstvedt (1973) reported that neoplastic involvement of these parametrial nodes almost invariably means widespread metastatic spread to other pelvic nodes. Burghardt and Girardi (1993), however, stated that positive parametrial nodes are found in 23% of patients with stage IIb disease.

Common iliac system Common iliac nodes and vessels are basically a direct continuation of the external iliac system and retain the three-chain arrangement found there. The lateral chain continues in a position lateral to the common iliac artery. The middle chain moves posteriorly to lie behind the artery and veins, while the medial chain lies medial to the artery and vein. As the vessels of opposite sides converge superiorly, lymph nodes of the bilateral medial chains converge to form a small cluster just below the aortic bifurcation. This cluster of medial chain nodes is sometimes referred to as the nodes of the sacral promontory. Those of the common iliac system, in addition to being a continuation of the external iliac system, also receive much of the efferent lymph flow from nodes of the internal iliac group. Thus, the external and internal iliac portions of the pelvic lymphatic system merge, and the combined flow from the common iliac level proceeds towards the thoracic duct via para-aortic channels.

It is important not to adopt an excessively compartmentalised view of pelvic lymphatics. Anastomotic connections are common within the main chains of lymph flow along the external iliac system and between nodes of the internal and external iliac system (Jackson, 1967).

Lymphatic pathways from the cervix to the pelvic lymph nodes

It is now possible to link the lymph drainage of the cervix to the specific groups of pelvic nodes. This flow is via several main collecting vessels which are grouped into three pedicles on each side, with each tending to travel to different lymph node groups. The first pedicle takes a lateral course and then ascends on the pelvic sidewall to enter the external iliac nodes. Of the three chains of the external iliac group, the middle one is the major recipient of flow from the anterior pedicle (Canela, 1934). Any of the three nodal chains may receive a portion of this flow. The second pedicle travels laterally and rather posteriorly from the cervix along the uterine artery to become the afferent vessels to nodes situated at the division of the internal iliac artery. The third pedicle takes a much more posterior course along the uterosacral folds to reach the lateral sacral nodes.

It must be emphasised, however, that there are many exceptions to this general pattern (see 'The concept of the sentinel node' below). Not infrequently, lymph vessels from the cervix pass directly to nodes belonging to the common iliac group. In a minority of women, vessels from the cervix may take an upward course in the broad ligament to join others flowing from the body of the uterus and proceed to nodes at para-aortic level (Poirier *et al.*, 1903). This anatomical fact explains the occasional occurrence of primary para-aortic lymph node metastases from cervical carcinoma (Javert, 1954; Fuchs, 1969).

It is obvious that a wide variety of nodes act as primary sites for cervical lymph drainage. Consequently, potential first node sites of cervical carcinoma spread are widely spaced in the pelvis, with anomalous drainage patterns extending this area even further into the lower abdomen. This fact has a significant bearing on the overall approach to the treatment of cervical cancer.

The concept of the sentinel lymph node (see also Chapter 39)

The sentinel lymph node is defined as the first draining lymph node of an anatomical region and, therefore, the histological examination and disease status of that lymph node would be representative of all the non-sentinel nodes. The status of the sentinel node may be used to guide the surgical treatment of cervical cancer, avoiding radical surgery in those nodal-positive patients who would be better served by the alternative treatment modality of chemoradiation.

The recent evidence for the identification of sentinel nodes in respect of the metastatic spread of cervical cancer comes from the work of a number of authors (Dargent *et al.*, 2000; O'Boyle *et al.*, 2000; Verheijen *et al.*, 2000; Malur *et al.*, 2001) using techniques of preoperative lymphoscintigraphy, an intraoperative gamma probe and a blue dyeing agent. (Fig. 3.15).

These techniques result in the identification of a sentinel node in over 90% of cases. The exact location of the sentinel node varies between patients, and evidence for this can be drawn from one of the largest case series by Levenback *et al.* (2002). This study, which involved 39 patients with stage I–IIA cervical cancer, was able to demonstrate a 100% detection rate of sentinel nodes. The detection methods involved preoperative lymphoscintigraphy using injection of a radio-isotope, technetium-99, into the cervical tumour and intra-operative injection of a vital dye (isosulfan blue) (Fig. 3.15), again intracervically. An intraoperative gamma probe was used to trace the nodal chains under evaluation in a systematic manner. Positive nodes were taken to be those that turned blue with the dyeing agent and nodes that demonstrated a 10-fold increase in the radiation count relative to the background levels.

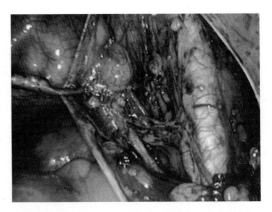

Fig. 3.15 Blue nodes clearly visible in the obturator fossa after injection of peritumoral blue dye. The first draining nodes are thereby identified by this colouring technique. From Buist *et al.* (2003) with permission.

A total of 132 lymph nodes were identified as being sentinel nodes at the time of surgery. Some 80% of these were found at three node sites within the pelvis: obturator, iliac below the bifurcation of the common iliac artery and parametrial. The most common locations for sentinel nodes were the interiliac and obturator basins. Of interest, 12 sentinel nodes (9%) were found in the para-aortic region. This finding introduces a dilemma; is the lymphatic drainage pattern of the cervix always sequential or could there be direct drainage from the cervix to the common iliac or even para-aortic lymph nodes? The available mapping techniques used so far do not allow this question to be answered definitively, but other evidence suggests that the sequential model is the more likely in most patients.

We can also look for evidence of the nature of lymphatic spread of disease by careful examination of surgical specimens. Benedetti-Panici *et al.* (1996) conducted an in-depth study of anatomical and pathological specimens from 225 cases of radical hysterectomies with both systematic and aortic lymphadenectomy in patients with stage IB–IV cervical cancer. They were able to show that lymphatic metastases through paracervical tissues seemed to occur less commonly (29% of cases). In fact, most of their detected cases of positive lymph node involvement occurred in the superficial obturator area (86%). They were able to conclude from their study that parametrial nodes were mainly located in the cardinal and vesico-uterine ligaments and that, in terms of nodes affected by disease, the superficial obturator, external iliac, common iliac, paracaval, intercavoaortic and para-aortic nodes seemed to be the groups most frequently involved.

In another earlier study by Dargent *et al.* (2000), sentinel lymph nodes were identified laparoscopically in patients with early-stage cervical cancer. Thirty-five patients were recruited into their study, and systematic node dissection was performed on 69 pelvic sidewalls.

Among the 63 identified sentinel nodes, 53 were located in contact with the external iliac vein, lateral to the inferior vesical artery and ventral to the origin of the uterine artery, seven were located close to the origin of one of the collaterals of the internal iliac artery, and three were adjacent to the left common iliac vein. The rate of identification failure appeared to be dependent on the quantity of injected blue dye.

Similar work by Malur *et al.* (2001) identified sentinel lymph nodes in 78% of their patients (39/50). They discovered that para-aortic sentinel lymph nodes were more often located in the paracaval region (12 out of 18 lymph nodes, 66%) than in the para-aortic region (6 out of 18, 33%). The pelvic sentinel node (*n* = 39 patients) was located in 26% (27/105 lymph nodes) at the origin of the uterine artery and in 25% (26/105 lymph nodes) at the division of the common iliac artery. In 12% (13/105), the node was present in the parametrium.

It appears from the results obtained in this study and others that the anatomical position of the sentinel node is variable. The optimal success rates in identification of sentinel nodes rely on the use of a combination of markers rather than each being used in isolation.

ACKNOWLEDGEMENTS

A major portion of this chapter has remained unchanged since it appeared in the first edition, in which it was written by Dr R.C. Gustafson, MD, FRCOG, who was then lecturer in the Department of Obstetrics and Gynaecology at the University of Birmingham. Mr T.A.J. Mould and Mr C. Chow have edited the chapter and added the section on the anatomical position of the sentinel lymph nodes.

Figures 3.4–3.10, which appeared originally in the *International Journal of Gynecological Cancer*, have been kindly given to the authors and the editors by Professor N. Sakaragi of the Department of Obstetrics and Gynaecology, Hokkaido University School of Medicine in Sapporo, Japan, and his co-workers, Drs Todo, Kudo and Yamamoto. Professor T. Sato of the Department of Functional Anatomy, Tokyo Medical and Dental University School of Medicine, Tokyo, Japan, kindly gave permission for the photographs of cadaver dissections in Figures 3.5b and 3.6b to be used. Figures 3.13 and 3.14 are from the *Colour Atlas of Gynaecological Surgery*, edited by Mr D. Lees and Professor A. Singer, and published by Mosby Wolfe, London. Figure 3.15 has kindly been provided by Dr Buist.

REFERENCES

Bell C (1972) Autonomic nervous control of reproduction: circulatory and other factors. *Pharmacological Reviews* 24: 677–736.

Benedetti-Panici P, Maneschi F, Scambia G *et al.* (1996). Lymphatic spread of cervical cancer: an anatomical and pathological study based on 225 radical hysterectomies with systematic pelvic and aortic lymphadenectomy. *Gynecological Oncology* 62: 19–24.

Bonica JJ (1967) *Principles and Practice of Obstetric Analgesia and Anaesthesia*, Vol. 1, Ch. 5. Philadelphia: Davis.

Buist MR, Pijpers RJ, van Lingen A *et al.* (2003) Laparoscopic detection of sentinel lymph nodes followed by lymph node dissection in patients with early stage cervical cancer. *Gynecological Oncology* 90: 290–296.

Burghardt E, Girardi F (1993) Local spread of cervical cancer. In: *Surgical Gynecological Oncology*. New York: Thieme, pp. 203–212.

Canela L (1934) Quel est le premier relai ganglionnaire normal du pedicle iliaque externe des collecteurs lymphatiques cervico-uterins. *Annales d'Anatomie Pathologique* 11: 740–741.

Casley-Smith JR (1964) Endothelial permeability. The passage of particles into and out of diaphragmatic lymphatics. *Quarterly Journal of Experimental Physiology* 49: 365–383.

Casley-Smith JR, Florey HW (1961) The structure of normal small lymphatics. *Quarterly Journal of Experimental Physiology*, 46, 101–106.

Cleland JGP (1933) Paravertebral anaesthesia in obstetrics. *Surgery, Gynecology and Obstetrics* 57: 51–62.

Coupland RE (1962) Histochemical observations on the distribution of cholinesterase in the human uterus. *Journal of Obstetrics and Gynaecology of the British Commonwealth* 69: 1041–1043.

Dargent D, Martin X, Mathevet P (2000) Laparoscopic assessment of the sentinel lymph node in early stage cervical cancer. *Gynecologic Oncology* 79: 411–415.

Davis AA (1933) The innervation of the uterus. *Journal of Obstetrics and Gynaecology of the British Empire* 40: 481–497.

Doyle JB (1955) Paracervical uterine denervation by transection of the cervical plexus for the relief of dysmenorrhea. *American Journal of Obstetrics and Gynaecology* 70: 1–16.

Eichner E, Goldberg I, Bove ER (1954) In vivo studies with direct sky blue of the lymphatic drainage of the internal genitals of women. *American Journal of Obstetrics and Gynaecology* 67: 1277–1287.

Fontaine R, Herrmann LG (1932) Clinical and experimental basis for surgery of the pelvic sympathetic nerves in gynecology. *Surgery, Gynecology and Obstetrics* 54: 133–163.

French JE, Florey HW, Morris B (1960) The absorption of particles by the lymphatics of the diaphragm. *Quarterly Journal of Experimental Physiology* 45: 88–103.

Fuchs WA (1969) Normal anatomy. In: Fuchs WA, Davidson JW (eds) *Recent Results in Cancer Research; Lymphography in Cancer*. Berlin: Springer-Verlag, Ch. 5.

Henriksen E (1949) The lymphatic spread of carcinoma of the cervix and of the body of the uterus. *American Journal of Obstetrics and Gynecology* 58: 924–940.

Hoffman MS (2004) Extent of radical hysterectomy: evolving emphasis. *Gynecologic Oncology* 94: 1–9.

Jackson RJA (1967) Lymphographic studies related to the problem of metastatic spread from carcinoma of the female genital tract. *Journal of Obstetrics and Gynaecology of the British Commonwealth* 73: 339.

Javert CT (1954) The lymph nodes and lymph channels of the pelvis. In: Meigs JV (ed.) *Surgical Treatment of Cancer of the Cervix*. New York: Grune and Stratton, Ch. 2.

Kolbenstvedt A (1973) A critical evaluation of foot lymphography in the demonstration of the regional lymph nodes of the uterine cervix. *Gynecologic Oncology* 2: 24–38.

Krantz KE (1959) Innervation of the human uterus. *Annals of the New York Academy of Science* 15: 770–784.

Krantz KE (1973) The anatomy of the human cervix, gross and microscopic. In: Blandau RJ, Moghissi KS (eds) *The Biology of the Cervix*. Chicago: University of Chicago Press, Ch. 4.

Krantz KE, Phillips WP (1962) Anatomy of the human uterine cervix, gross and microscopic. *Annals of the New York Academy of Science* 97: 551–563.

Leak LV, Burke JF (1968) Electron microscopic study of lymphatic capillaries in the removal of connective tissue fluid and particulate substances. *Lymphology* 1: 39–52.

Levenback C, Coleman RL, Burke TW *et al.* (2002) Lymphatic mapping and sentinel node identification in patients with cervix cancer undergoing radical hysterectomy and pelvic lymphadenectomy. *Journal of Clinical Oncology* 20: 688–693.

Leveuf J, Godard H (1923) Les lymphatiques de l'uterus. *Revue de Chirurgie* 61: 219–248.

Malur S, Krause N, Kohler C *et al.* (2001) Sentinel lymph node detection in patients with cervical cancer. *Gynecologic Oncology* 80: 254–257.

Nakanishi H, Wood C (1971) Cholinergic mechanisms in the human uterus. *Journal of Obstetrics and Gynaecology of the British Commonwealth* 78: 716–723.

Nesselrod JP (1937) An anatomic restudy of the pelvic lymphatics. *Annals of Surgery* 104: 905–916.

O'Boyle JD, Coleman RL, Bernstein SG *et al.* (2000) Intraoperative lymphatic mapping in cervix cancer patients undergoing radical hysterectomy: a pilot study. *Gynecologic Oncology* 79: 238–243.

Patek P (1939) The morphology of the lymphatics of the mammalian heart. *American Journal of Anatomy* 64: 203–249.

Plentl AA, Friedman EA (1971) Lymphatic system of the female genitalia. The morphologic basis of oncologic diagnosis and therapy. *Major Problems in Obstetrics and Gynecology* 2: 1–223.

Poirier P, Cuneo B, Delamere G (1903) *The Lymphatics.* London: Archibald Constable.

Pressman JJ, Dunn RF, Burtz M (1967) Lymph node structure related to direct lymphaticovenous communications. *Surgery, Gynecology and Obstetrics* 124: 963–973.

Rodin M, Moghissi KS (1973) Intrinsic innervation of the human cervix: a preliminary study. In: Blondau RJ, Moghissi KS (eds) *The Biology of the Cervix.* Chicago: University of Chicago Press, Ch. 5.

Rouvière H (1938) *Anatomy of the Human Lymphatic System.* Michigan: Edwards Bros.

Rusznyak I, Foldi M, Szabo G (1967) *Lymphatics and Lymph Circulation; Physiology and Pathology.* Oxford: Pergamon Press.

Sakamoto S, Takizawa K (1988) An improved radical hysterectomy with fewer urological complications and with no loss of therapeutic results for invasive cervical cancer. *Ballière's Clinical Obstetrics and Gynecology* 2: 953–962.

Sakaragi K, Todo Y, Kudo M *et al.* (2005) A systematic nerve-sparing radical hysterectomy technique in invasive cervical cancer for preserving post-surgical bladder function. *International Journal of Gynecological Cancer* 15: 389–397.

Verheijen RH, Pijpers R, van Diest PJ *et al.* (2000) Sentinel node detection in cervical cancer. *Obstetrics and Gynecology* 96: 135–138.

Virchow R (1860) *Cellular Pathology.* New York: Robert M. de Wit.

Yoffey JM, Courtice FC (1970) *Lymphatics, Lymph and Lymphomyeloid Complex.* London: Academic Press.

Zeit PR, Wilcoxon G (1950) In vivo coloring of pelvic lymph nodes with India ink. *American Journal of Obstetrics and Gynecology* 59: 1164–1166.

Zinser UK, Rosenbauer KA (1960) Untersuchungen uber die Angioarchitektorik der normalen und pathologisch veranderten Cervix uteri. *Archiv für Gynäkologie* 194: 73–112.

CHAPTER 4

Immunochemistry and immunology of the cervix

Margaret A. Stanley

The cervix uteri is a fascinating organ from the cell biological point of view. The stratified non-keratinising squamous epithelium of the ectocervix meets the mucus-secreting columnar epithelium of the endocervix in the transformation zone at an abrupt point, the squamocolumnar junction. This apparent clash of cellular cultures is made more intriguing by the fact that the progenitor cell of both epithelia is almost certainly the same — the reserve cell. Furthermore, cancerous transformation in the cervix initiated by oncogenic genital human papillomaviruses (HPVs) occurs in that very same transformation zone in and around the squamocolumnar junction. Issues of fundamental importance with generic implications are therefore the regulation of epithelial differentiation and the maintenance of tissue architecture in this organ and the corruption of these processes during carcinogenesis. This chapter addresses some of these issues and describes how immunochemistry, a powerful analytical tool in pathobiology, has contributed to our understanding of the structure, organisation and host defences of the cervical mucosae.

IMMUNOCHEMISTRY

Immunochemistry is the identification of a tissue constituent *in situ* by means of a specific antigen–antibody reaction tagged by a visible label; it is a powerful technology of value in both research and diagnosis. Covalent linking of antibody molecules with other molecules (dyes) was first attempted in the 1930s, and what emerged from these experiments was the observation that such chemical labelling did not disrupt the antigen–antibody interaction. Immunocytochemistry came into its own, however, when A.H. Coons and his colleagues at the Harvard Medical School had the notion of localising substances in tissues by means of specific antibodies labelled with a fluorescent dye, fluorescein isothiocyanate. Immunofluorescence remains a popular and effective technology because of its speed and simplicity, and the use of confocal microscopy has enlarged the applications dramatically. However, there are disadvantages to immunofluorescence; the need for specialised microscopes, a high background and the fact that the preparations are not permanent resulted in a search for different labels, and enzyme labels, particularly peroxidase and alkaline phosphatase, became the workhorse of the immunohistologist. Enzyme labels are developed histochemically at the end of the antigen–antibody reaction and yield intensely coloured end-products that can be viewed in the conventional light microscope. The specificity of the signal depends upon the exquisite specificity of the antigen–antibody interaction, but the sensitivity of the technology has been increased by technical developments that amplify the label signal.

Immunochemistry is widely used and unfortunately often abused because, regrettably, the cardinal rules for the technology, the use of appropriate controls and the authentication of reagents are too often forgotten. The primary antibody should be specific and of high affinity, avidity and titre, and the optimal dilution for the tissues under analysis must be determined by titration for each batch of antibody (even from the best commercial sources). More than one antibody directed against the antigen of interest should be used (particularly important for monoclonal antibodies) as specific epitopes may be masked or lost during tissue preparation. Controls are absolutely critical because cross-reactivity and non-specific staining must be excluded. Each staining batch should include a positive control, a negative control in which the primary antibody is excluded and, if possible, an absorption control in which the primary antibody has been preabsorbed with pure antigen.

CYTOSKELETON AND CELL ADHESION

Keratin expression in cervical epithelia

Keratins are the major structural proteins of epithelia and, together with actin microfilaments and tubulin microtubules, make up the cytoskeleton of the vertebrate epithelial cell. Keratins belong to the superfamily of intermediate filament (IF) proteins forming α-helical coiled-coil dimers that associate laterally and end-to-end to form 10-nm filaments. Human epithelial keratins comprise a large family of IF proteins numbered 1–20 distributed in a tissue-specific and differentiation-related fashion (Moll *et al.*, 1982). They are subdivided into two sequence types, type I (acidic) and type II (basic), and these are typically expressed as specific pairs with complex expression patterns. The expression pattern of these molecules in different epithelia can be defined by immunostaining using polypeptide-specific monoclonal antibodies that recognise only a specific keratin isotype.

In the ectocervix, keratins 5 and 14 decorate all cells of the basal and parabasal layers and occasional cells in the suprabasal layers but are rarely detected in the superficial layers (Moll *et al.*, 1983). This keratin pair is characteristic of the proliferative compartment of stratified squamous epithelium. Keratin 19 stains the basal layer strongly but is detected only sporadically in the parabasal and suprabasal layers (Dixon and Stanley, 1984). K19 is characteristic of 'wet' mucosae and is not detected in epidermis. The differentiation-specific keratins that decorate the suprabasal and superficial cells of the ectocervix are K4, K10 and K13. Overall, ectocervical epithelium expresses type II keratins 4, 5 and 6 and type I keratins 13, 14, 15 and 19 with sporadic expression of keratins 2, 8, 11, 16 and 17 (Smedts *et al.*, 1990).

Endocervical columnar cells contain keratins 7, 8, 16, 18 and 19 with variable expression of 4, 6, 15 and 20. The keratin expression in reserve cells is quite complex (Smedts *et al.*, 1992). Keratins 8, 14, 16, 17, 18 and 19 are present in all reserve cells; 5, 6 and 15 are often but not always detected. Keratin 13 is present in a subpopulation of reserve cells (Levy *et al.*, 1988). Reserve cell keratin expression is informative about the potential differentiation programmes of these cells (Levy *et al.*, 1988). It is clear that most keratins found in reserve cells (with the exception of 4 and 7) are also detected in endocervical columnar cells, but the expression level of most of these keratins is very low. Smedts and colleagues (1992) speculate that, during the differentiation of reserve cells into columnar cells, expression of K4 and K7 is initiated, and expression of keratins 5, 6 14, 15 and 16 is lost but that of K18 increases.

In immature and mature squamous metaplasia, all the reserve cell keratins are expressed (Gigi Leitner *et al.*, 1986). Keratins 8 and 18 are quite strongly expressed in immature squamous metaplasia (Dixon and Stanley, 1984), quite clearly identifying the histogenesis from the reserve cell. However, in mature squamous epithelia, K8 and K18 expression is downregulated, and the pattern of expression closely resembles that of ectocervical epithelium with basal/parabasal expression of keratins 5, 14, 15, 16, 17 and 19 and suprabasal expression of the differentiation-specific keratins 4 and 13 (Smedts *et al.*, 1993). The expression of K15 is of interest as this keratin is a marker of certain squamous epithelial differentiation programmes, e.g. oesophagus. K15 is variably expressed in reserve cells, and Smedts and colleagues speculate that this may reflect differences in the differentiation status of the reserve cells, with those expressing K15 predestined for metaplasia.

Cervical intraepithelial neoplasia grades I and II (CIN1,

CIN2) have a keratin expression pattern essentially similar to that of ectocervical epithelium with the presence of keratins 19, 5, 14, 15, 4, 13, 6 and 16. These lesions can be distinguished from CIN3 because of the expression in CIN3 of the reserve cell keratins 8, 17 and 18, a phenomenon that probably reflects the loss of differentiation that characterises CIN3. Cervical carcinomas have complex and heterogeneous keratin expression patterns (Ivanyi *et al.*, 1990). Keratinising squamous cell carcinomas express keratins 4, 10, 13, 15, 16, 8 and 18 but not K7. Keratin 7 is present in non-keratinising squamous cell carcinomas, but keratins 4, 10, 13, 15 and 16 are absent (Smedts *et al.*, 1993). Adenocarcinomas exhibit a remarkable similarity to the reserve cell keratin phenotype with a consensus keratin expression pattern of keratins 7, 8, 14, 15, 17, 18 and 19 plus sporadic expression of keratins 4, 6 and 5. Overall, the keratin expression pattern in high-grade CIN and carcinomas strongly suggests that the progenitor cell of these lesions is the reserve cell and gives support to the view that most, if not all, high-grade CIN and cervical carcinomas arise at the squamocolumnar junction in a focus of squamous metaplasia.

Cell–cell adhesion molecules

Cell–cell adhesion is a defining feature of epithelia. The major class of cell adhesion molecules (CAMs) is the cadherins, a large gene family that includes among its members the classical cadherins of the adherens junction and the desmosomal cadherins. These molecules support calcium-dependent adhesion that mediates cell–cell recognition events that, together with organisation of the cytoskeleton, bring about the morphological transitions that maintain tissue organisation in the adult organism. The classical cadherins are transmembrane protein homodimers. The ectodomain of the dimer mediates binding, while the cytoplasmic domain associates with β- and α-catenin and, via these molecules, to the actin cytoskeleton. Stable cell adhesion requires the complete cadherin–catenin complex, and loss of or change in the structure of a member of the complex will disrupt adhesion and the signalling events associated with the complex.

In the ectocervix, E cadherin (E cad) is the dominant CAM, located predominantly at the lateral margins of cells in the basal, parabasal and suprabasal layers (Vessey *et al.*, 1995; de Boer *et al.*, 1999). Some cytoplasmic E cad can be detected in para- and suprabasal layers and probably reflects the active recycling of adherens junctions in these layers. P cadherin (P cad) is expressed only in the basal layers of the ectocervix. In the endocervix, E cad decorates the lateral margins of cells with no detectable intracellular staining: P cad is absent from endocervical columnar cells. Interestingly, E cad is absent from the reserve cell and P cad is the dominant reserve cell cadherin. However, actively dividing cells in immature squamous metaplasia are characterised by E cad expression, both at the lateral boundaries of cells and intracellularly. P cad expression is dramatically increased in immature squamous metaplasia. Mature squamous metaplasia is characterised by an E cad expression similar to that of ectocervix. P cad expression in mature squamous metaplasia closely reflects the degree of squamous maturation, eventually being confined to the basal layer.

E cad expression is significantly reduced in CIN3, with almost complete absence in the basal layers, and parallels the expression of the differentiation-associated markers such as involucrin. This may be related to HPV infection as expression of HPV 16 E6 in basal keratinocytes inhibits E cad expression (Matthews *et al.*, 2003). P cad expression, in contrast, increases from the lower to the upper cell layers in CIN3, suggesting that cell–cell adhesion mediated via the adherens junctions is P cad dependent in CIN3. These data support the notion that the cellular phenotype in CIN3 reverts to that of the primitive progenitor cell, the reserve cell.

As effective cell adhesion and signalling are mediated by the complete cadherin–catenin complex, the expression of α- and β-catenins in the CIN spectrum is of interest. Immunocytochemical studies reveal only a slight decrease in β-catenin in CIN3 but a dramatic decrease in α-catenin, although the number of biopsies studied is small (de Boer *et al.*, 1999). The functional consequences for adhesion in CIN3 of the loss of α-catenin are not clear. The normal role of this molecule is to anchor the actin cytoskeleton at the adherens junction. It may be that other molecules can take over this role, but the properties of the junction would be changed. It is important to remember that adhesion is not just sticking plaster between cells, but these junctions are relay stations for signalling, and changes in signalling could have profound implications.

The other strong adhesion complexes of epithelia are the desmosomes, also members of the cadherin superfamily. The desmosomal transmembrane proteins are the desmogleins 1, 2 and 3 and the desmocollins. They link into the cytoplasmic proteins, desmoplakins I and II, plakoglobin (a homologue of β-catenin) and plakophyllin. In normal ectocervical epithelium, pericellular staining for desmocollins 1, 2 and 3 is usually seen throughout the epithelium (de Boer *et al.*, 1999; Alazawi *et al.*, 2003); a similar distribution is seen in CIN1 but a variable distribution in CIN3. Desmogleins 1 and 3 are distributed throughout the epithelium, but there is a significant reduction in desmoglein in CIN3 (Fig. 4.1). Desmoplakin expression is reduced in CIN3 in most cases. Cell adhesion complexes are dramatically reduced in CIN3, and these changes are not simply a reflection of increased proliferation because desmosomal complexes are unaltered in immature squamous metaplasia (de Boer *et al.*, 1999). They are more likely to be a consequence of neoplastic transformation and the genetic instability that characterises CIN3.

Cell–matrix adhesion

Interactions between epithelial cells and their underlying basement membrane and matrix proteins are critical in the maintenance of tissue architecture influencing cell polarity, cell fate and cell determination. The differentiation programme is specified in the basal layer, and key elements in this are the signals from the matrix. The integrins are an important class of molecules that mediate both cell–cell and cell–matrix interactions. They are heterodimers composed of an α- and a β-chain that mediate interactions with the cytoskeleton. Normal cervical squamous epithelium expresses α2β1, α3β1, α6β4 and, occasionally, α6β1 integrins (Hughes *et al.*, 1994). The β1-, β4-, α2-, α3-, α6- and αv-chains are strongly expressed in the basal layer of normal and koilocytic epithelium, but lost in the more superficial layers. Integrin expression is retained in

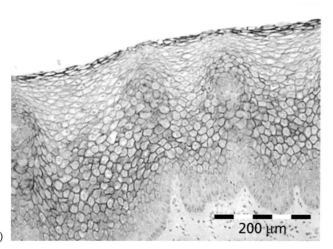
(a)

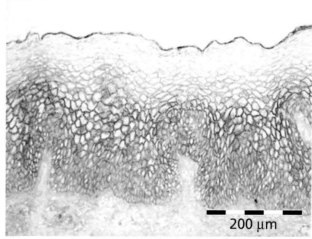
(b)

Fig. 4.1 Desmoglein 1 and 3 expression in normal cervical epithelium (a) and CIN3 (b). Courtesy of Dr Will Alazawi and Dr Nick Coleman.

CIN and invasive carcinoma, but there is heterogeneity of expression, and this is particularly marked for α6β4, with focal loss or overexpression at the tumour–stroma interface in invasive carcinoma. Other matrix molecules and their receptors also show changes during cervical neoplastic progression, with increased expression of laminin chains (Nordstrom *et al.*, 2002) and laminin receptors (al Saleh *et al.*, 1997) associated with invasiveness.

PROLIFERATION

Proliferation markers

The balance of cell proliferation, differentiation and death in tissues is dependent upon the tight control of the cell cycle – a set of stages, defined on the basis of DNA replication, through which the dividing somatic cell proceeds (Fig. 4.2). The replication of chromosomal DNA in the S phase of the cell cycle is an irrevocable step under very tight regulation. Markers of DNA replication that can be used to identify cells in cycle and/or the deregulation of this could therefore be important diagnostic reagents. Two of the most widely used markers have been PCNA (proliferating cell nuclear antigen) and Ki-67. PCNA is a nuclear protein that is an auxiliary protein for DNA polymerase δ, an enzyme involved in both DNA replication and DNA repair. Numerous studies have shown a correlation between Ki-67 expression and the size of the proliferating

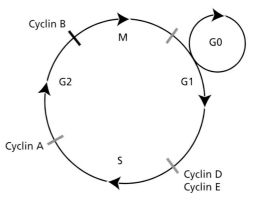

Fig. 4.2 The cell cycle. The cycle is divided into four phases: G1, a period of intense metabolic activity when many cellular components are duplicated – the duration varies in response to external factors such as growth factors and hormones; S, the phase of DNA synthesis; G2, preparing for phase M, chromosome condensation, segregation and the separation of the two daughter cells. The coordination of this progression depends upon the cyclins, so named because their concentrations rise and fall in a regular pattern through the cell cycle.

compartment (Brown and Gatter, 1990). The function of the Ki-67 antigen is not clear, and it is possible that the molecule is not essential for proliferation. However, it is a reliable and robust reagent that gives a good indication of the size of the proliferating compartment and its dysregulation during neoplastic progression (Fig. 4.3).

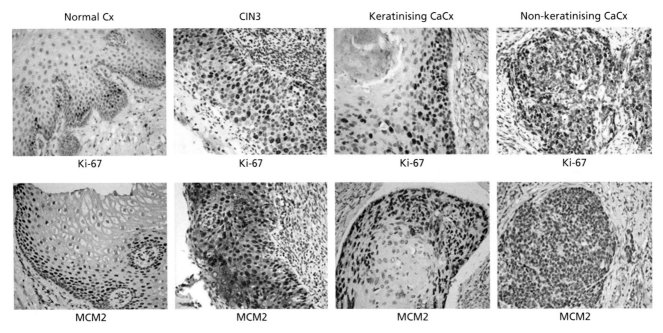

Fig. 4.3 Expression of the proliferation markers Ki-67 and MCM2 in normal and neoplastic cervical epithelium. In normal epithelium, cycling cells are confined to the parabasal layers, and only occasional cells in the basal layer are in cycle. In CIN3, cycling cells occupy the full thickness of the epithelium. In invasive carcinoma, the proportion of cells in cycle reflects the degree of differentiation, but all cells at the tumour edge are in cycle.

One group of proteins that appear to be very accurate biomarkers of proliferation are the minichromosome maintenance proteins (MCMs). This family of proteins form a prereplication complex that binds to the sites on DNA at which replication will be initiated and effectively 'licenses' the cell to replicate DNA. Importantly, these proteins are present only during the cell cycle, being lost during quiescence and differentiation; they can therefore be used as specific markers of proliferation. In normal cervical epithelium, MCM staining is restricted to the nuclei of parabasal cells; basal cells are occasionally positive and superficial cells are completely negative (Fig. 4.3). Interestingly, metaplastic cells have been reported as showing staining only in the basal layer, but in CIN expression correlated well with the degree of dysplasia, with 50% of cells in the superficial layers of CIN1 being positive compared with > 90% in CIN3 and invasive cancer (Freeman *et al.*, 1999). The MCMs have some advantages as biomarkers of proliferation: the antibodies are robust and effective on formalin-fixed tissue, they are specific for cells in cycle and do not detect cells undergoing DNA repair.

Cyclins and cyclin-dependent kinases

The intrinsic regulation of the cell cycle depends upon the interaction of molecules that accelerate progression, the cyclin-dependent kinases (cdks) and their substrates, the cyclins, and those that act as brakes on progress, the cyclin-dependent kinase inhibitors (cdkis). Specific cyclins appear for brief periods at specific periods in the cycle, are phosphorylated by the relevant cdk and then rapidly degraded after completion of the relevant cell cycle stage (Fig. 4.2). The expression of these molecules has been examined in normal and neoplastic cervical epithelium. Cyclins A, B, D, and E can be detected in the basal and parabasal cells of normal epithelium, and this is independent of the menstrual cycle (Kanai *et al.*, 1998). In high-grade CIN, cyclin and cdk expression occurs throughout the full thickness of the epithelium, and overexpression of these molecules occurs in invasive carcinoma (Fig. 4.4).

Cyclin-dependent kinase inhibitors

The cdkis negatively regulate cell cycle progression, and the expression of these regulators in normal and neoplastic epithelium may have diagnostic utility. The inhibitor p16^{INK4a} binds to cdk4 or cdk6 and, in so doing, blocks the phosphorylation of pRb and the entry into S phase. Infection with oncogenic HPVs and deregulation of the HPV E6/E7 oncogenes are inexorably associated with high-grade CIN and carcinoma. In this situation, HPV E7 binds to pRb and overrides the checkpoint controlling entry into S phase. As a consequence, p16^{INK4a} builds up in the cell and is overexpressed (Sano *et al.*, 1998). Using a panel of p16^{INK4a}-specific monoclonal antibodies, Klaes and colleagues (2001) have demonstrated overexpression of p16^{INK4a} specifically in CIN lesions associated with high-risk HPV and in carcinomas, but not in normal cervix or inflammatory lesions. p27 is a negative regulator of the G1 phase of the cell cycle associating with cyclinA/E–cdk2 complexes and blocking the G1–S phase transition. In normal cervical epithelium, p27 is strongly expressed in intermediate and superficial cells, but only weakly expressed in basal and parabasal cells. The subcellular location is predominantly nuclear (Dowen *et al.*, 2003), but cytoplasmic staining has been reported (Shiozawa *et al.*, 2001). In CIN and invasive carcinoma, p27 immunoreactivity is lost or reduced, and loss is associated with poor prognosis in invasive cancer (Huang *et al.*, 2002).

The essential feature of cell cycle regulators is the controlled expression and degradation of the key molecular players. Degradation is usually achieved by ubiquitin-mediated proteolysis, and one important mediator of this is the SCF^{skp2} ubiquitin ligase complex, which promotes proteolysis of the cdkis p21 and p27 as well as cyclins and transcription factors. In normal cervical epithelium, skp2-expressing cells are confined to the basal and parabasal compartment — the inverse of p27 expression. Increased expression is seen in high-grade CIN and, again, an inverse correlation with p27 expression is evident (Fig. 4.5), although the number of cases of CIN in this particular study

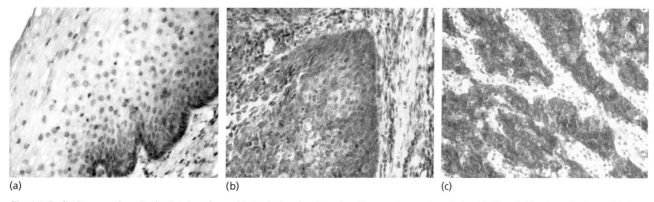

(a) (b) (c)

Fig. 4.4 Cyclin D expression. Cyclin D is just detectable in the basal and parabasal layers of normal cervical epithelium (a) but is easily detectable in CIN3 (b) and highly expressed in invasive cervical carcinoma (c).

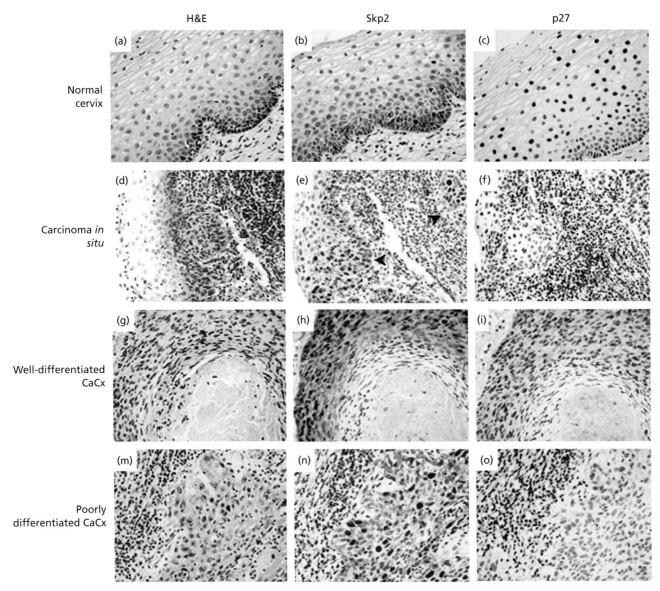

Fig. 4.5 Expression of the cdk inhibitor p27 and the F box protein skp2 in normal cervix (a–c), CIN3 (d–f) and invasive cervical carcinoma (g–i and m–o). The inverse relationship between the expression of p27 and skp2 is lost in invasive carcinomas.

(Dowen *et al.*, 2003) were small. The distribution of skp2 and the correlation with p27 expression vary in invasive cancer. Poorly differentiated and small cell carcinomas of the cervix invariably exhibit high skp2 expression, but well-differentiated keratinising carcinomas have significantly lower levels of expression (Fig. 4.5). In normal epithelium, skp2 expression is nuclear, but in carcinomas both nuclear and cytoplasmic protein can be detected. The topographical separation of p27 and skp2 expression is lost in invasive carcinomas and, in approximately 50% of cases, p27 is expressed, albeit at low level, in the presence of skp2. In other cancers, skp2 overexpression is associated with poor prognosis, but whether a similar association occurs in cervical cancer remains to be shown.

IMMUNOCYTES AND IMMUNE FUNCTION

T-cell subsets

The immune cell that predominates in the normal cervix is the T lymphocyte (McKenzie *et al.*, 1991; Poppe *et al.*, 1998; Stanley, 2001); B cells are rarely detected, although plasma cells identified by the CD38 surface marker are found in the subepithelial stroma (Johansson *et al.*, 1999). T lymphocytes are present in both epithelium and stroma, with most studies showing that CD4+ cells predominate in the stroma and CD8+ cells in the epithelium (Fig. 4.6a and b). The great majority of these lymphocytes express the CD45RO marker (Fig. 4.6f)

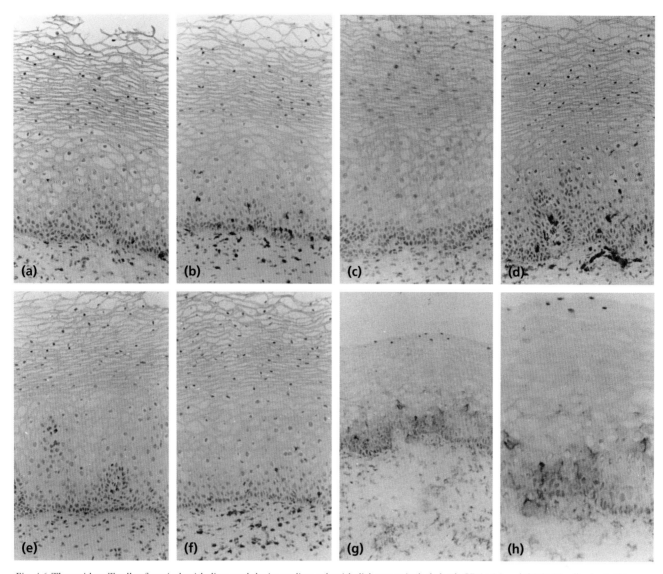

Fig. 4.6 The resident T cells of cervical epithelium and the immediate subepithelial stroma include both CD4+ (a) and CD8+ T-cell subsets (b). These cells are antigen 'experienced', and expression of the CD45RO marker (f) is evident, but expression of CD45RA, a marker of antigen-naive T cells, is not detectable (e). Macrophages identified by the CD14 marker occur in the stroma but are not detectable in the epithelium (c). HLA-DR expression is not seen on keratinocytes but occurs on mononuclear and dendritic cells in both epithelium and stroma (d). CD1a expression, a marker of Langerhans cells, is detectable on cells with a dendritic morphology, with cell bodies located in the parabasal layers (g and h). Magnification (a–g) × 120, (h) × 250 (Coleman, 1993).

and are antigen experienced or memory cells with relatively few naive CD45RA cells being detected (Coleman, 1993). About 10% of the mononuclear cell population of the cervix are macrophages, as determined by the expression of the CD14 receptor. CD14+ cells are almost exclusively confined to the stroma and are rarely detected intraepithelially (Fig. 4.6c).

Several studies have documented T-cell numbers in both low- and high-grade CIN but with differing results. A significant reduction in intraepithelial T-cell numbers, particularly the CD4+ subset, was found in all grades of CIN by Tay and colleagues (1987), but in other studies an increase in

the intraepithelial CD8+ subset was documented with equal numbers of CD4 and CD8 cells in the stroma (Viac *et al.*, 1990). Fluorescence-activated cell sorting (FACS) analysis of lymphocytes isolated from normal and CIN lesions (Bell *et al.*, 1995) revealed a significant depression of CD4+ cells in CIN lesions but an increase in the CD8+ population (Fig. 4.7), a phenomenon also observed by McKenzie and colleagues (1991) in an immunohistochemical analysis.

Paradoxically, more CD8+ cells are recruited into invasive carcinomas than to high-grade CIN (Edwards *et al.*, 1995) and, furthermore, these lymphocytes are activated, expressing

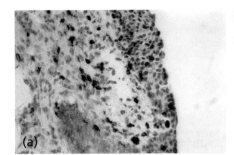
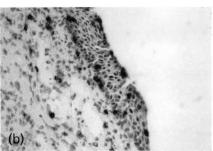

Fig. 4.7 Cells expressing the T-cell marker CD3 dominate the stromal and epithelial compartment in CIN3 (a). The majority of the T cells in these lesions are CD8+ (b). Magnification × 400.

cytotoxic factors such as granzyme B (Bontkes *et al.*, 1997). However, when the cytokine profile of the tumour-infiltrating lymphocytes (TILs) is determined, these cells belong to the T cytotoxic-2 subset and secrete interleukin (IL) 4, IL-5 and IL-10, which generate an immunosuppressive tumour milieu and block the cytotoxic potential of the TILs (Sheu *et al.*, 2001). The role of HPV antigen-specific CD8+ T cell responses has been critically reviewed (Man, 2005).

In a comprehensive analysis of the cervical microenvironment, Kobayashi and colleagues (2004) have shown clearly that strong pro- and anti-inflammatory responses are both present in high-grade squamous intraepithelial lesions (HGSILs). In particular, a robust Th1 response with abundant expression of interferon (IFN) γ by CD4, CD8 and natural killer (NK) cells could be demonstrated but, despite this, HPV-infected HGSIL persists, a phenomenon that may be related to the immunosuppressive environment with the recruitment of regulatory T cells together with the acquisition of resistance to apoptosis induced by cytokines such as type I interferons and tumour necrosis factor (TNF) α.

An important group of cytotoxic effector cells that includes the NK subset have the morphology of large granular lymphocytes (LGLs) and form a minor compartment of normal cervical immunocytes (McKenzie *et al.*, 1991). LGLs with the NK phenotype CD56+, CD16+, CD3–, CD2^{variable}, CD57^{variable} are rarely found within either normal cervical epithelium or CIN but are found in the stroma, particularly in the endocervix. A separate subset of LGLs with the phenotype CD56+, CD16–, CD3+, CD2+ is found within the ectocervical epithelium, and this subset dominates the intraepithelial population in high-grade CIN (McKenzie *et al.*, 1991) (Fig. 4.8).

It has been shown in *in vitro* studies that cells with a phenotype CD8+, CD56+ can be generated after exposure of peripheral blood mononuclear cells (PBMCs) to HPV 16 or 18 E7 pulsed dendritic cells (Santin *et al.*, 2001). These cells have a high cytolytic activity against HPV 16- or 18-containing tumour cells *in vitro*, but whether they are equivalent to the CD56+ LGLs that dominate some CIN3 remains unknown.

In order to recruit immunocytes to tissues, the endothelium of the stromal capillaries must express the appropriate adhesion molecules that act as ligands for the homing receptors on the cells. Intercellular adhesion molecule-1 (ICAM-1) (Coleman and Stanley, 1994a), vascular adhesion protein-1

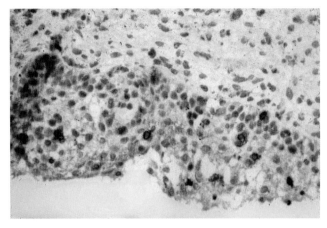

Fig. 4.8 In CIN3, intraepithelial lymphocytes expressing the CD56 marker are frequent and have the morphology of large granular lymphocytes. Magnification × 400 (McKenzie *et al.*, 1991).

(VAP-1) and P selectin (Johansson *et al.*, 1999) are constitutively expressed on the endothelial cells of stromal capillaries in normal cervix. These molecules preferentially mediate the recruitment of Th1 rather than Th2 lymphocytes into tissues, and their expression is consistent with the immunophenotypes that have been described for the T-cell subsets in normal cervical epithelium (al Saleh *et al.*, 1998; de Gruijl *et al.*, 1999).

Antigen-presenting cells

The antigen-presenting cells of the cervix include Langerhans cells (LCs) and stromal dendritic cells. Cells with the morphology and immunophenotype of LCs are found in the epithelium of the ectocervix and in squamous metaplasia, and their frequency has been estimated as between 64 and 343 cells/mm^2 epithelium. The cell bodies of LCs are generally oriented basally within the normal ectocervical epithelium, from where the dendritic processes extend superficially (Fig. 4.6g and h). When antigen-presenting cell numbers are analysed, low-grade cervical lesions (CIN1, LGSILs) are, overall, immunologically quiescent, with decreased numbers of morphologically altered LCs (Hawthorn *et al.*, 1988). It is possible that this decrease simply reflects the normal egress of antigen-carrying LCs from the epidermis to the draining node for antigen presentation. However, virtually all cervical squamous intraepithelial lesions

(SILs) arise in the transformation zone (TZ), often associated with squamous metaplasia, and there is evidence that LC numbers are reduced in squamous metaplasia (Roncalli *et al.*, 1988) and in the TZ, where these LC have an immature phenotype (Giannini *et al.*, 2002). The reduced numbers of LCs in SILs may simply reflect the histogenesis. High-grade cervical lesions (CIN2/3) also exhibit a decrease in LC numbers intraepithelially (Viac *et al.*, 1990), a phenomenon that may be related to neoplasia as there is *in vitro* evidence that immortalised HPV-infected cervical cells inhibit LC recruitment (Hubert *et al.*, 1999). However, expression of HPV 16 E6 in basal keratinocytes inhibits E cadherin expression and, as LC/keratinocyte adhesion is mediated via cadherin–cadherin interactions, this could reduce LC retention in squamous epithelium (Matthews *et al.*, 2003). One factor that does seem to be associated with LC depletion is smoking. Early studies showed a relationship between LC number in cervical epithelium and smoking (Barton *et al.*, 1988), and the results from a recent intervention study (Szarewski *et al.*, 2001) show an association between reduction in cervical LC, CD4 and CD8 subsets and cigarette smoking.

MHC class II expression

MHC class II glycoproteins present antigen to CD4+ T cells: these molecules are constitutively expressed only on profes-

sional antigen-presenting cells such as dendritic cells, B cells and macrophages. The keratinocytes of the squamous epithelium of the genital tract do not express MHC class II antigens under normal conditions, but can be induced to do so by pro-inflammatory cytokines such as IFN-γ and TNF-α (Coleman and Stanley, 1994b). A variable expression of class II antigens is seen in low-grade CIN ranging from no (Warhol and Gee, 1989) to patchy focal expression (Coleman and Stanley, 1994b). Class II expression is seen in high-grade CIN (Fig. 4.9c) and is predominantly in an extensive, diffuse staining pattern (Cromme *et al.*, 1993a; Coleman and Stanley, 1994b).

At least 80% of cervical cancers express class II antigens on the malignant keratinocytes (Cromme *et al.*, 1993a; Glew *et al.*, 1993). It is likely that the expression of class II antigens on neoplastic keratinocytes is induced rather than constitutive. Increased numbers of T cells are observed in the stroma underneath HLA-DR-positive CIN (Coleman and Stanley, 1994b), and there is an increase in tumour-infiltrating lymphocytes in DR-positive regions of carcinomas (Hilders *et al.*, 1994). A significant proportion of CIN3 express ICAM-I as well as HLA-DR, although the expression of these molecules is not coordinated (Stanley *et al.*, 1994). Evidence from *in vitro* studies suggests that expression of ICAM-I in immortal HPV 16-expressing keratinocytes is constitutive rather than induced (Coleman *et al.*, 1993), probably as a consequence of neoplastic transformation.

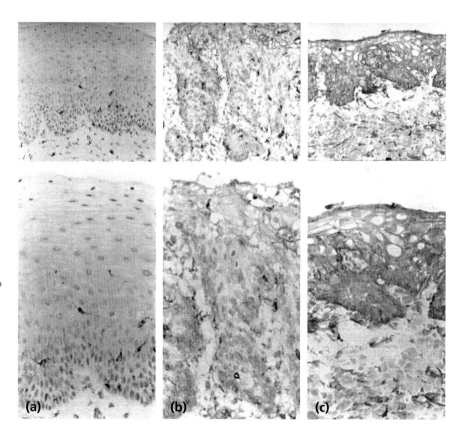

Fig. 4.9 Patterns of expression of HLA-DR in normal and neoplastic cervix. In the normal ectocervix (a), staining is confined to Langerhans cells in the epithelium and mononuclear cells in the stroma; the keratinocytes are negative. In low-grade CIN (b), there is focal, moderately strong, surface staining of basal keratinocytes and koilocytes. Intense cytoplasmic staining of the abnormal epithelium is seen in high-grade CIN (c). Magnification: top, × 100; bottom, × 200.

MHC class I expression

MHC class I glycoproteins present antigen to CD8+ T cells and are constitutively expressed on all normal cells except red blood cells. Normal cervical epithelial cells express class I, but loss of expression of these molecules is a phenomenon associated with malignant progression (Cromme *et al.*, 1993b). Loss of class I expression occurs in CIN and may be associated with clinical progression (Bontkes *et al.*, 1998). There is evidence from *in vitro* studies that HPV 16 E7 gene expression can downregulate class I expression when HPV 16 sequences are integrated into the host genome, but this effect is lost if the virus is present as the episome (Bartholomew *et al.*, 1997). Integration of the HPV genome is frequent in invasive cervical carcinoma, and downregulation of MHC class I expression in cervical squamous cell carcinomas has been well documented (Glew *et al.*, 1993). These changes have been shown in a proportion of tumours to be post-transcriptionally regulated (Cromme *et al.*, 1993b) and, in HPV 16- or 18-positive lesions, this post-transcriptional deregulation is related to downregulation of TAP protein (Cromme *et al.*, 1994), but it is unlikely that all class I downregulation is due to this alone. Whatever the mechanism of downregulation is, functionally these changes may be crucial in neoplastic progression. Allele-specific downregulation or the absence of class I would interfere with both NK cell and CTL recognition of targets, whether of viral or cellular origin, disabling the major cytotoxic effector mechanisms.

Cytokines

Both the initiation and the regulation of cell-mediated immune responses are dependent, to a very large degree, on the local cytokine milieu. The production of these molecules is not restricted to immunocytes such as lymphocytes, dendritic cells and macrophages, but the keratinocytes of squamous epithelium themselves are important sources. Pro-inflammatory cytokines such as the type I interferons and TNF-α, when secreted, are potent activators of Langerhans cells.

The type 1 interferons have antiviral, antiproliferative anti-angiogenic and immunostimulatory properties but, crucially, they act as a bridge between innate and adaptive immunity, activating immature dendritic cells (Le Bon *et al.*, 2002). There is relatively little information on the expression of type I interferons in HPV-infected clinical lesions, but good evidence from cervical keratinocyte cell lines that HPV infection deregulates interferon signalling. Microarray studies on cell lines in which HPV 31 is present as the episome show that interferon-inducible genes and the transcriptional regulator Stat-1 are downregulated (Chang *et al.*, 2000), and this seems to be related to E2 expression (Chang *et al.*, 2002). In other work using keratinocytes transfected with HPV 16 E6/E7, expression of IFN-α-inducible genes was inhibited (Nees

et al., 2001). HPV 16 E7 interacts with components of the IFN signalling pathway binding to the p48 component of the interferon-induced transcription complex (Barnard and McMillan 1999), and E6 interacts physically with the JAK kinase tyk-2 (Li *et al.*, 1999). Paradoxically, interferon-inducible gene expression is upregulated in cells in which HPV 16 is integrated compared with cells containing episome only (Alazawi *et al.*, 2002), a phenomenon that may be related to the interferon resistance that appears to accompany neoplastic progression (Bachmann *et al.*, 2002).

In normal cervical epithelium, TNF-α is constitutively expressed by basal and parabasal epithelial cells (Mota *et al.*, 1999), stromal macrophages and endothelial cells (Stanley *et al.*, 2003). A similar pattern of expression is found in most cases of low-grade CIN, but there is an almost complete downregulation of expression by epithelial cells (although not macrophages) in high-grade CIN. This loss of cytokine expression in epithelial cells is also accompanied by loss of TNF receptors (Stanley *et al.*, 2003).

Interleukin 10 (IL-10) is, in contrast to TNF, a cytokine that inhibits Th1 responses, a property partially mediated via its effects on antigen-presenting cells. Keratinocytes can be induced to secrete IL-10, and it is likely that this plays a role in regulating the LC phenotype and function in squamous epithelium. IL-10 is not expressed in normal cervix, but the keratinocytes of high-grade CIN express IL-10 weakly (Mota *et al.*, 1999; Sheu *et al.*, 2001), and infiltrating lymphocytes in CIN3 are IL-10 positive (Stanley *et al.*, 2003). Invasive cervical cancers strongly express IL-10 and another immunosuppressive cytokine, tumour growth factor (TGF) β. IL-10 and TGF-β generate a tumour microenvironment that biases lymphocytes to the Th2/Tc2 phenotype and immunosuppression (Sheu *et al.*, 2001). The role of the TGF-β family of growth factors in growth regulation in cervical epithelium and cervical tumour progression is complex. These molecules inhibit cell cycle progression and the immune response and, in normal cervix, TGF-β 1 and 2 are expressed as intracellular proteins in the intermediate and superficial cells of normal cervical epithelium (Comerci *et al.*, 1996). This epithelial expression is reduced in high-grade CIN and invasive cancer, but extracellular TGF-β 1 secreted by stromal elements is significantly upregulated in invasive cancers. The TGFβ 1 and 2 receptors are mutated or downregulated in invasive cancer cells, the consequence being that the cancer cells are resistant to growth inhibition by the stromally generated TGF-β that contributes at the same time to an immunosuppressive milieu.

SUMMARY AND CONCLUSIONS

The patterns of expression of cell cycle-related molecules, cytoskeletal proteins, cell–cell and cell–matrix adhesion molecules show how exquisitely proliferation and differentiation are regulated and coordinated in normal ecto- and endocervical epithelium. Keratin and cell adhesion molecule expression patterns show that squamous metaplasia is the result of an altered differentiation programme for the reserve cell but not, crucially, a deregulation of proliferation. These studies also provide strong support for the view that among the reserve cells are the stem cells for cervical epithelium. The majority of low-grade CIN are characterised by an increase in the proliferating compartment, but the differentiation programme of the keratinocyte (and hence its eventual death) is completed. These phenomena almost certainly reflect the events of the infectious cycle of the human papillomavirus and reinforce the view that most low-grade CIN are simple viral infections. The switch from low-grade to high-grade CIN is reflected in the deregulation of both proliferation and differentiation, a crucial and irrevocable step in neoplastic progression. This loss of control of the keratinocyte growth and death programme finds its ultimate expression in the progressive autonomy of invasive cancer.

Host defence in the ectocervix is a partnership between the cells of the innate immune system (and this includes the keratinocytes) and the adaptive immune system. The dominant lymphocyte population in the normal cervix is the T cell, with CD4+ cells dominating the immediate subepithelial stroma and both CD4+ and CD8+ cells intraepithelially. The cytokine profile of these cells indicates that they are Th1 biased, and the expression of the CD45RO marker suggests that they are 'antigen experienced'. Langerhans cells are present in the ectocervical epithelium with their cell bodies located in the parabasal layer, and macrophages and stromal dendritic cells constitute the antigen-presenting population of the stroma. B lymphocytes are rare, but plasma cells can frequently be detected in the stroma. The ectocervical keratinocytes express receptors for pro-inflammatory cytokines such as TNF-α and can be induced to secret these cytokines that activate Langerhans cells and bias to a Th1 cell-mediated immune response after wounding or infection. Neoplastic progression results in a change in both the cytokine milieu and the lymphocyte populations. The intraepithelial CD4+ population falls, and CD8+ T cells with a Th2 suppressor-type cytokine profile are recruited to the lesions. The neoplastic keratinocytes upregulate MHC class II protein expression and secrete immunosuppressive cytokines such as IL-10, but they downregulate the expression of pro-inflammatory cytokines such TNF-α and its receptors. Invasive cancers are characterised by this immunosuppressive cytokine milieu and loss or downregulation of key immunological molecules such as MHC class I on the malignant cells. Effective immunotherapies for cervical neoplasia need to reverse this immunosuppressive environment to activate appropriate host effectors.

ACKNOWLEDGEMENTS

I owe all the members of my research laboratory (past* and present) a massive debt of gratitude for their help in preparing the illustrations for this chapter. Special thanks go to Emillie Ikelle, Dawn Ward, Sally Dowen*, Mandy Scott*, Colette Tourlamaine and Mischal Khan* for the cell cycle immunostaining, Nick Coleman* for the immunohistology (and for setting the standards for immunohistology in the laboratory in the long ago days as a graduate student), Tina Rich for advice on microscopy, and Richard Moore for his patient and good-natured explanations and help on the mysteries of jpg and tif files plus other baffling details of electronic imaging. Grateful thanks to Dr Nick Coleman and his graduate student Dr Will Alazawi for the desmosomal protein immunostaining.

REFERENCES

al Saleh W, Delvenne P, van den Brule FA *et al.* (1997) Expression of the 67 KD laminin receptor in human cervical preneoplastic and neoplastic squamous epithelial lesions: an immunohistochemical study. *Journal of Pathology* 181: 287–293.

al Saleh W, Giannini SL, Jacobs N *et al.* (1998) Correlation of T-helper secretory differentiation and types of antigen-presenting cells in squamous intraepithelial lesions of the uterine cervix. *Journal of Pathology* 184: 283–290.

Alazawi W, Pett M, Arch B *et al.* (2002) Changes in cervical keratinocyte gene expression associated with integration of human papillomavirus 16. *Cancer Research* 62: 6959–6965.

Alazawi WO, Morris L, Garrod D *et al.* (2003) Immunohistochemical staining of desmosomal components in cervical intra-epithelial neoplasia. *Virchows Archiv* 443: 51–56.

Bachmann A, Hanke B, Zawatzky S *et al.* (2002) Disturbance of tumor necrosis factor alpha-mediated beta interferon signaling in cervical carcinoma cells. *Journal of Virology* 76: 280–91.

Barnard P, McMillan NA (1999) The human papillomavirus E7 oncoprotein abrogates signaling mediated by interferon-alpha. *Virology* 259: 305–313.

Bartholomew JS, Glenville S, Sarkar S *et al.* (1997) Integration of high-risk human papillomavirus DNA is linked to the down-regulation of class I human leukocyte antigens by steroid hormones in cervical tumor cells. *Cancer Research* 57: 937–942.

Barton SE, Maddox PH, Jenkins D *et al.* (1988) Effect of cigarette smoking on cervical epithelial immunity: a mechanism for neoplastic change? *Lancet* ii: 652–654.

Bell MC, Edwards RP, Partridge EE *et al.* (1995) CD8+ T lymphocytes are recruited to neoplastic cervix. *Journal of Clinical Immunology* 15: 130–136.

Bontkes HJ, de Gruijl TD, Walboomers JM *et al.* (1997) Assessment of cytotoxic T-lymphocyte phenotype using the specific markers granzyme B and TIA-1 in cervical neoplastic lesions. *British Journal of Cancer* 76: 1353–1360.

Bontkes HJ, Walboomers JM, Meijer CJ *et al.* (1998) Specific HLA class I down-regulation is an early event in cervical dysplasia associated with clinical progression. *Lancet* 351: 187–188.

Brown DC, Gatter KC (1990) Monoclonal antibody Ki-67: its use in histopathology. *Histopathology* 17: 489–503.

Chang YE, Laimins LA (2000) Microarray analysis identifies interferon-inducible genes and Stat-1 as major transcriptional targets of human papillomavirus type 31. *Journal of Virology* 74: 4174–4182.

Chang YE, Pena L, Sen GC *et al.* (2002) Long-term effect of interferon on keratinocytes that maintain human papillomavirus type 31. *Journal of Virology* 76: 8864–8874.

Coleman N (1993) The local immune response to human papilloma virus related disease in the female genital tract. PhD Thesis, University of Cambridge, UK.

Coleman N, Stanley MA (1994a) Characterization and functional analysis of the expression of vascular adhesion molecules in human papillomavirus related disease of the cervix. *Cancer* 74: 884–892.

Coleman N, Stanley MA (1994b) Analysis of HLA DR expression on keratinocytes in cervical neoplasia. *International Journal of Cancer* 56: 314–319.

Coleman N, Greenfield IM, Hare J et al. (1993) Characterization and functional analysis of the expression of intercellular adhesion molecule 1 in human papillomavirus related disease of cervical keratinocytes. *American Journal of Pathology* 143: 355–367.

Comerci JT Jr, Runowicz CD, Flanders KC et al. (1996) Altered expression of transforming growth factor-beta 1 in cervical neoplasia as an early biomarker in carcinogenesis of the uterine cervix. *Cancer* 77: 1107–1114.

Cromme FV, Meijer CJ, Snijders PJ et al. (1993a) Analysis of MHC class I and II expression in relation to presence of HPV genotypes in premalignant and malignant cervical lesions. *British Journal of Cancer* 67: 1372–1380.

Cromme FV, Snijders PJ, Van Den Brule AJ et al. (1993b) MHC class I expression in HPV 16 positive cervical carcinomas is post transcriptionally controlled and independent from c myc overexpression. *Oncogene* 8: 2969–2975.

Cromme FV, Airey J, Heemels M-T et al. (1994) Loss of transporter protein encoded by the TAP-1 gene is highly correlated with loss of HLA expression in cervical carcinomas. *Journal of Experimental Medicine* 179: 335–340.

de Boer CJ, van Dorst E, van Krieken H et al. (1999) Changing roles of cadherins and catenins during progression of squamous intraepithelial lesions in the uterine cervix. *American Journal of Pathology* 155: 505–515.

de Gruijl TD, Bontkes HJ, van den Muysenberg AJ et al. (1999) Differences in cytokine mRNA profiles between premalignant and malignant lesions of the uterine cervix. *European Journal of Cancer* 35: 490–497.

Dixon IS, Stanley MA (1984) Immunofluorescent studies of human cervical epithelia in vitro using antibodies against specific keratin components. *Molecular Biology and Medicine* 2: 37–51.

Dowen SE, Scott A, Mukherjee G et al. (2003) Over expression of SKP2 in carcinoma of the cervix does not correlate inversely with p27 expression. *International Journal of Cancer* 22: 2531–2540.

Edwards RP, Kuykendall K, Crowley-Nowick P et al. (1995) T lymphocytes infiltrating advanced grades of cervical neoplasia. CD8-positive cells are recruited to invasion. *Cancer* 76: 1411–1415.

Freeman A, Morris LS, Mills AD et al. (1999) Minichromosome maintenance proteins as biological markers of dysplasia and malignancy. *Clinical Cancer Research* 5: 2121–2132.

Giannini SL, Hubert P, Doyen J et al. (2002) Influence of the mucosal epithelium microenvironment on Langerhans cells: implications for the development of squamous intraepithelial lesions of the cervix. *International Journal of Cancer* 97: 654–659.

Gigi Leitner O, Geiger B, Levy R et al. (1986) Cytokeratin expression in metaplasia of the human cervix. *Differentiation* 31: 191–205.

Glew SS, Connor ME, Snijders PJ et al. (1993) HLA expression in pre invasive cervical neoplasia in relation to human papilloma virus infection. *European Journal of Cancer* 29A: 1963–1970.

Hawthorn RJ, Murdoch JB, MacLean AB et al. (1988) Langerhans' cells and subtypes of human papillomavirus in cervical intraepithelial neoplasia. *British Medical Journal* 297: 643–646.

Hilders CGJM, Houbiers JGA, Krul EJT et al. (1994) The expression of histocompatability-related leukocyte antigens in the pathway to cervical carcinoma. *American Journal of Clinical Pathology* 101: 5–12.

Huang LW, Chao SL, Hwang JL et al. (2002) Down-regulation of p27 is associated with malignant transformation and aggressive phenotype of cervical neoplasms. *Gynecologic Oncology* 85: 524–528.

Hubert P, van den Brule F, Giannini SL et al. (1999) Colonization of in vitro-formed cervical human papillomavirus-associated (pre)neoplastic lesions with dendritic cells: role of granulocyte/macrophage colony-stimulating factor. *American Journal of Pathology* 154: 775–784.

Hughes DE, Rebello G, Al-Nafussi A (1994) Integrin expression in squamous neoplasia of the cervix. *Journal of Pathology* 173: 97–104.

Ivanyi D, Groeneveld E, Van Doornewaard G et al. (1990) Keratin subtypes in carcinomas of the uterine cervix: implications for histogenesis and differential diagnosis. *Cancer Research* 50: 5143–5152.

Johansson EL, Rudin A, Wassen L et al. (1999) Distribution of lymphocytes and adhesion molecules in human cervix and vagina. *Immunology* 96: 272–277.

Kanai M, Shiozawa T, Xin L et al. (1998) Immunohistochemical detection of sex steroid receptors, cyclins, and cyclin-dependent kinases in the normal and neoplastic squamous epithelia of the uterine cervix. *Cancer* 82: 1709–1719.

Klaes R, Friedrich T, Spitkovsky D et al. (2001) Overexpression of p16(INK4A) as a specific marker for dysplastic and neoplastic epithelial cells of the cervix uteri. *International Journal of Cancer* 92: 276–284.

Kobayashi A, Greenblatt RM, Anastos K et al. (2004) Functional attributes of mucosal immunity in cervical intraepithelial neoplasia and effects of HIV infection. *Cancer Research* 64: 6766–6774.

Le Bon A, Tough DF (2002) Links between innate and adaptive immunity via type I interferon. *Current Opinion in Immunology* 14: 432–436.

Levy R, Czernobilsky B, Geiger B (1988) Subtyping of epithelial cells of normal and metaplastic human uterine cervix, using polypeptide specific cytokeratin antibodies. *Differentiation* 39: 185–196.

Li S, Labrecque S, Gauzzi MC et al. (1999) The human papilloma virus (HPV)-18 E6 oncoprotein physically associates with Tyk2 and impairs Jak-STAT activation by interferon-alpha. *Oncogene* 18: 5727–5737.

McKenzie J, King A, Hare J et al. (1991) Immunocytochemical characterization of large granular lymphocytes in normal cervix and HPV associated disease. *Journal of Pathology* 165: 75–80.

Man S (2005) CD8+ T cell responses against oncogenic papillomariruses – are they useful? *Papillomavirus Reports* 16: 1–6.

Matthews K, Leong CM, Baxter L et al. (2003) Depletion of Langerhans cells in human papillomavirus type 16-infected skin is associated with E6-mediated down regulation of E-cadherin. *Journal of Virology* 77: 8378–8385.

Moll R, Franke WW, Schiller DL et al. (1982) The catalog of human cytokeratins: patterns of expression in normal epithelia, tumors and cultured cells. *Cell* 31: 11–24.

Moll R, Levy R, Czernobilsky B et al. (1983) Cytokeratins of normal epithelia and some neoplasms of the female genital tract. *Laboratory Investigation* 49: 599–610.

Mota F, Rayment N, Chong S *et al.* (1999) The antigen-presenting environment in normal and human papillomavirus (HPV)-related premalignant cervical epithelium. *Clinical and Experimental Immunology* 116: 33–40.

Nees M, Geoghegan JM, Hyman T *et al.* (2001) Papillomavirus type 16 oncogenes downregulate expression of interferon-responsive genes and upregulate proliferation-associated and NF-kappaB-responsive genes in cervical keratinocytes. *Journal of Virology* 75: 4283–4296.

Nordstrom B, Einhorn N, Silfersvard C *et al.* (2002) Laminin-5 gamma 2 chain as an invasivity marker for unifocal and multifocal lesions in the lower ano-genital tract. *International Journal of Gynecological Cancer* 12: 105–109.

Poppe WA, Drijkoningen M, Ide PS *et al.* (1998) Lymphocytes and dendritic cells in the normal uterine cervix. An immunohistochemical study. *European Journal of Obstetrics, Gynecology, and Reproductive Biology* 81: 277–282.

Roncalli M, Sideri M, Gie P *et al.* (1988) Immunophenotypic analysis of the transformation zone of human cervix. *Laboratory Investigation* 58: 141–149.

Sano T, Oyama T, Kashiwabara K *et al.* (1998) Expression status of p16 protein is associated with human papillomavirus oncogenic potential in cervical and genital lesions. *American Journal of Pathology* 153: 1741–1748.

Santin AD, Hermonat PL, Ravaggi A *et al.* (2001) Expression of CD56 by human papillomavirus E7-specific CD8+ cytotoxic T lymphocytes correlates with increased intracellular perforin expression and enhanced cytotoxicity against HLA-A2-matched cervical tumor cells. *Clinical Cancer Research* 7: 804s–810s.

Sheu BC, Lin RH, Lien HC *et al.* (2001) Predominant Th2/Tc2 polarity of tumor infiltrating lymphocytes in human cervical cancer. *Journal of Immunology* 167: 2972–2978.

Shiozawa T, Shiohara S, Kanai M *et al.* (2001) Expression of the cell cycle regulator p27(Kip1) in normal squamous epithelium, cervical intraepithelial neoplasia, and invasive squamous cell carcinoma of the uterine cervix. Immunohistochemistry and functional aspects of p27(Kip1). *Cancer* 92: 3005–3011.

Smedts F, Ramaekers F, Robben H *et al.* (1990) Changing patterns of keratin expression during progression of cervical intraepithelial neoplasia. *American Journal of Pathology* 136: 657–668.

Smedts F, Ramaekers F, Troyanovsky S *et al.* (1992) Basal cell keratins in cervical reserve cells and a comparison to their expression in cervical intraepithelial neoplasia. *American Journal of Pathology* 140: 601–612.

Smedts F, Ramaekers F, Leube RE *et al.* (1993) Expression of keratins 1, 6, 15, 16, and 20 in normal cervical epithelium, squamous metaplasia, cervical intraepithelial neoplasia, and cervical carcinoma. *American Journal of Pathology* 142: 403–412.

Stanley MA (2001) Immune responses to human papillomaviruses. In: Sterling JC, Tyring SK (eds) *Human Papillomaviruses. Clinical and Scientific Advances.* London: Arnold, pp. 38–49.

Stanley M, Coleman N, Chambers M (1994) The host response to lesions induced by human papillomavirus. *Ciba Foundation Symposium* 187: 21–32; discussion 32–44.

Stanley MA, Scarpini C, Coleman N (2003) Cell mediated immunity and lower genital tract neoplasia. In: McLean AB, Singer A, Critchley H (eds) *Lower Genital Tract Neoplasia.* London: RCOG Press, pp. 27–44.

Szarewski A, Maddox P, Royston P *et al.* (2001) The effect of stopping smoking on cervical Langerhans' cells and lymphocytes. *British Journal of Obstetrics and Gynaecology* 108: 295–303.

Tay SK, Jenkins D, Maddox P *et al.* (1987) Lymphocyte phenotypes in cervical intraepithelial neoplasia and human papillomavirus infection. *British Journal of Obstetrics and Gynaecology* 94: 16–21.

Vessey CJ, Wilding J, Folarin N *et al.* (1995) Altered expression and function of E-cadherin in cervical intraepithelial neoplasia and invasive squamous cell carcinoma. *Journal of Pathology* 176: 151–159.

Viac J, Guerin Reverchon I, Chardonnet Y *et al.* (1990) Langerhans cells and epithelial cell modifications in cervical intraepithelial neoplasia: correlation with human papillomavirus infection. *Immunobiology* 180: 328–338.

Warhol MJ, Gee B (1989) The expression of histocompatibility antigen HLA DR in cervical squamous epithelium infected with human papilloma virus. *Modern Pathology* 2: 101–104.

PART 2

Physiological and drug-induced alterations within the cervical epithelium

CHAPTER 5

Morphology of the fetal and prepubertal cervicovaginal epithelium

The late Ellis Pixley and Albert Singer

This chapter, dealing with the fetal and prepubertal cervicovaginal epithelium, was written by the late Dr Ellis Pixley of Perth, Western Australia, for the first edition of *The Cervix* in 1974/75. Its contents represented a lifetime of study and observation into the changes occurring in the fetal, young child and adolescent cervix. The material on which he based his observations and conclusions was unique, and no major study on this subject has appeared over the ensuing three decades. We are therefore publishing it in its original form.

When squamous cervical cancer emerges in adult life, it is the epilogue in the play and interplay of perhaps a lifetime of factors which have determined its evolution. The stage is that particular field of cervical epithelial cells within which the initiation and expression of neoplastic potential occurs. The establishment of this and other cell populations of the genital tract during fetal life is an obligatory prologue to the whole play.

The opportunity to study morphology in prepubertal subjects rarely presents in clinical practice, in sharp contrast to the extensive opportunities encountered during reproductive and postmenopausal years. Clinical and histopathological enterprise has quite naturally been focused upon material from age groups relevant to the study of cervical cancer and its precursors, and upon symptomatic gynaecological disorders. In this chapter, the findings made during the study of a large group of fetuses and prepubertal subjects are summarised. Hopefully the summary will provide a prologue to enhance the understanding of the study of material from older age groups.

THE EPITHELIA OF THE LOWER GENITAL TRACT IN THE FETAL AND PREPUBERTAL FEMALE

Materials and methods of study

Observations of prepubertal subjects have of necessity been made largely on necropsy material, which presents certain advantages for detailed study. Substantial portions of the genital tract can be removed *in toto*, preserving the relationships of the various parts to each other. The common causes of perinatal and childhood death are not understood to significantly disturb the epithelial morphology of the lower genital tract. The material may be held to be free of exposure to environmental factors thought to be significant in the evolution of various changes within the cervix and which are characteristic of adolescence and adult life. Providentially, the material has accumulated since 1965 in a medical climate in which administration of diethylstilbestrol (DES) to pregnant females was probably rare. Since epithelial variations of the vagina will be described, the material serves as some form of control for comparison with those changes which occur when intrauterine exposure to DES is known or suspected. Exposure to dietary sources of estrogen cannot be excluded as a cause of variations encountered in the study material.

The material drawn upon for this chapter consists of 330 specimens of sufficient degree of preservation to allow detailed study of epithelial surfaces. The youngest subject was 24 weeks' gestation, the oldest 13 years. The total in each age group was: 24 weeks' gestation to 3 weeks after birth, 170 cases; 4 weeks to 5 years, 104 cases; 5 years to 9 years, 36 cases; 10 years to 13 years, 20 cases.

Observations were made on specimens removed at necropsy so as to include as much of the uterus and vagina as possible. Recently, several specimens have been removed to include the vulva, allowing the epithelial relationships of the whole genital tract to be studied. Histological preparations from blocks taken close to the median sagittal plane have allowed the epithelial continuities, extents and boundaries to be traced (Fig. 5.1). Colpophotographs of the preserved cervix have enabled us to determine the surface configurations (Fig. 5.2). The features pertaining to the lower endocervical canal, ectocervix, vagina and vulva have been the focus of interest. They constitute the area presenting to the clinician for evaluation during clinical examination.

During studies of this nature, the need for a reliable terminology is evident, and the following descriptions will be based upon that need. Terms used are largely compatible with those used in current Anglo-American publications on clinical, colposcopic and histological studies of the adult cervix and vagina (Coppleson *et al.*, 1971).

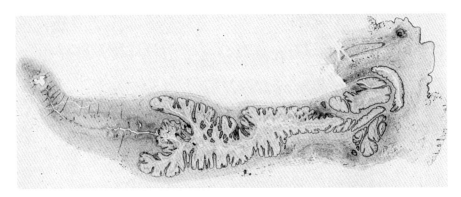

Fig. 5.1 Histological preparation of lower genital tract of fetus at 30 weeks' gestation (×3).

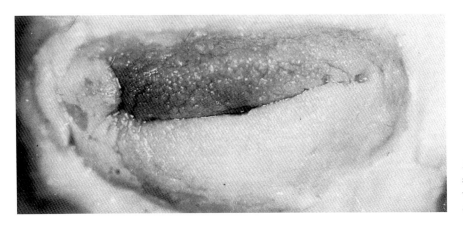

Fig. 5.2 Colpophotograph of preserved specimen from subject aged 3 months. The vagina has been removed to display the cervix (×6).

The original epithelia of the lower genital tract

Present during fetal life, so deserving the application of the term 'original', are three epithelial forms which are conveniently defined at this stage.

The columnar epithelium (see Figs 5.8–5.11) continues cephalad with the endometrium and extends caudad for a variable distance to boundaries with the original metaplastic and original squamous epithelium.

The original metaplastic epithelium (see Figs 5.12–5.15) Present in the majority of subjects before birth, this epithelium is continuous caudad with the original squamous epithelium. It is coextensive with the most caudal expanse of the columnar epithelium and may virtually replace it there. To emphasise its importance to the clinician and colposcopist, the expanse of the metaplastic epithelium in any subject under 1 month of age, whether fetus or neonate, is termed the 'original transformation zone'.

The original squamous epithelium (see Figs 5.16 and 5.17) Proper to the vagina, the usually highly differentiated and stratified original squamous epithelium extends from a junction with vulval epithelium, cephalad to a junction with the columnar epithelium, or with the metaplastic epithelium when present.

It forms part of the integument of vulval structures and usually covers a portion of the cervix, as well as lining the vagina.

Epithelial boundaries of the lower genital tract

The original epithelia are disposed along the lower genital tract in a variable fashion. Where one epithelial form/type meets another is usefully termed a boundary, and an appreciation of these is vital to the understanding of the variations in territories occupied by each form/type.

In histological preparations, as epithelial continuities are traced, the boundary is usually seen as a sharp transition from one epithelial form/type to another, and in histological nomenclature they are usefully termed junctions. In living subjects the boundaries are best observed with the colposcope, when adjacent epithelia may be seen to be separated by a line of abrupt transition of one appearance to another. Junctions of this type can also be observed in the anal canal of fetuses, where the epithelium of the alimentary tract encounters the epithelium of the buttock (Fig. 5.3).

The boundaries to be described, observed as they are in the fetus, prepubertal female and adult, are entities of embryological significance. It seems probable that a boundary may indicate a site at which an epithelial cell population meets another during the organogenetic process by which the surface arrangements are completed. The original squamocolumnar

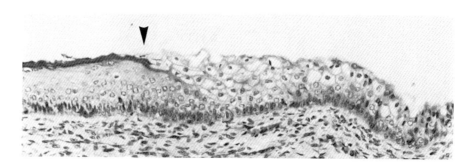

Fig. 5.3 Original epithelial junction. Epithelium of anal canal of newborn. Squamous epithelium of anal cleft on left, separated by oblique line from squamous epithelium evolving with the columnar epithelium of canal (× 160).

junction may well be the line of encounter between cells originating in the Müllerian duct and those of the urogenital sinus. Similarly, when a cell population develops from another, it may well be that the site of that embryological act is marked in adult life by the type of boundary defined as the vulvovaginal line. At that site, presumably, cells destined to form the urogenital sinus originally evolved from ectodermal cells.

In the lower genital tract, four such junctions can be identified:

The vulvovaginal junction When the Schiller's solution is applied to the vaginal introitus of both neonatal and adult subjects, a sharply etched line appears, separating the characteristic mahogany-stained vaginal epithelium cephalad from the non-staining vulval epithelium. The junction circumscribes the introitus from clitoris to fourchette, and passes along the middle of the medial surface of both labia minora (Fig. 5.4). The duct of Bartholin's gland is cephalad to the junction. The line would appear to be homologous with the midline of the ventral portion of the male urethra. Histological examination of the site of the line confirms an abrupt junction between two forms of epithelia (Fig. 5.5).

The original squamocolumnar junction As the original squamous epithelium is traced cephalad, it may be seen to join directly with the columnar epithelium (Fig. 5.6), constituting what is appropriately termed the original squamocolumnar junction. This form of the junction is found in 25% of perinatal material delivered after 36 weeks' gestation. In the remainder of this group (75%), original metaplastic epithelium is present in the most caudal extent of the columnar epithelium, either having replaced it or being coextensive with it. In these subjects, the junction will be observed to separate two multilayered epithelia: caudad will be the original squamous epithelium, and cephalad one of the many and varied appearances of

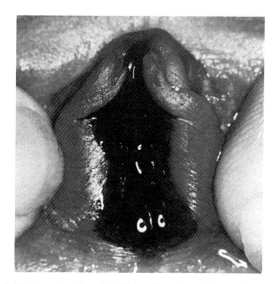

Fig. 5.4 Vulvovaginal junction. Vulva of newborn after application of Schiller's solution. The original squamous (vaginal) epithelium stains deeply and is sharply demarcated from the vulval epithelium.

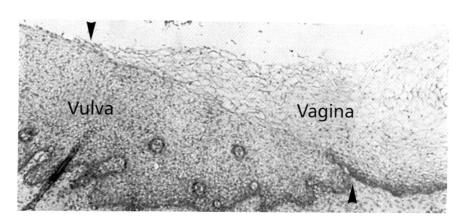

Fig. 5.5 Vulvovaginal junction. Original squamous epithelium of vagina on right, separated by oblique line from vulval epithelium of newborn (× 160).

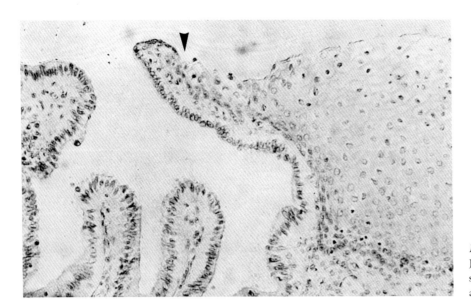

Fig. 5.6 Original squamocolumnar junction. Junction on ectocervix between original squamous and columnar epithelia in neonate aged 8 days (×250).

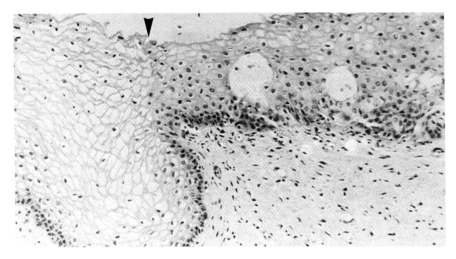

Fig. 5.7 Original squamocolumnar junction. Junction on vaginal wall between original squamous (left) and original metaplastic epithelium (right). Neonate aged 3 days (×160).

the original transformation zone which occurs so frequently at this site (Fig. 5.7). Nevertheless, the site marks the original squamocolumnar junction.

The neosquamocolumnar junction When present, the original metaplastic epithelium extends cephalad to a site beyond which only the columnar epithelium is present. That site deserves definition. The prefix neo- is used in the sense that the junction is established subsequent to the original squamocolumnar junction. In any subject it may be difficult to identify precisely, for the initial phases of metaplasia may affect small isolated areas of columnar epithelium, before becoming confluent to form a plate of epithelium (Fig. 5.12). Nevertheless, at any instant this junction represents the current, cephalic extent of the metaplastic epithelium, and allows the original transformation zone to be defined as that area extending between the two squamocolumnar junctions. During linear studies of living adult subjects, the neosquamocolumnar

junction may be observed to encroach cephalad on the columnar epithelium. Similar studies show that the original squamocolumnar junction does not undergo similar changes, its relationships persisting throughout life largely unchanged. It may be displaced caudad when eversion occurs during pregnancy, following parturition and when the insertion and full opening of a bivalve vaginal speculum distorts its true relationships. Throughout life, as metaplasia brings about a decrease in the amount of columnar epithelium, displacement of the junction cephalad may well occur. This is especially common following the menopause. The original squamocolumnar junction may not be identifiable following electrosurgical and cryosurgical destruction.

The cervico-uterine epithelial junction Traced cephalad, the columnar epithelium merges with the uterine epithelia at the site usually termed the histological internal os. The main object of this study has been to examine the early natural history of those areas which are accessible during clinical and colposcopic examination, and therefore no descriptions of this junction can usefully be offered.

The epithelial forms

The columnar epithelium

At birth, the principal features of the columnar epithelium are already established, and these seem to be similar to the adult arrangements. In specimens less than 30 weeks of gestation, however, the epithelium is usually flat, complicated only by several clefts extending into the stroma (Fig. 5.8). It is evident that in subsequent weeks there is active organogenesis, for in specimens of 34 weeks' gestation onwards numerous papillary and villous surface projections are present, as well as cleft-like structures extending deeply into the stroma (Fig. 5.9). There is extensive interspecimen variation in respect of all features. There is also a tendency for the most cephalic areas to present

the most striking clefts, whereas the caudal, often ectocervical, areas are mainly papillary (Fig. 5.10). In some subjects, however, the columnar epithelium remains largely flat, so that at birth and during childhood the cervix may be covered by a largely uncomplicated epithelium with a few clefts extending into the stroma (Fig. 5.11).

These arrangements no doubt have considerable implications for the functional potential of the cervix as a unit of the reproductive system. However, the principal reason for interest in the surface and stromal configuration is the fashion by which the architecture of the original columnar tissue will be reflected in the morphology of the transformation zone, should this evolve.

Evolution of the transformation zone in the adult has been well described. By the process of metaplasia, columnar epithelium is transformed into squamous epithelium. Portions of the stroma, particularly the original terminal vascular elements, remain as intra- or subepithelial structures, and the imprint of

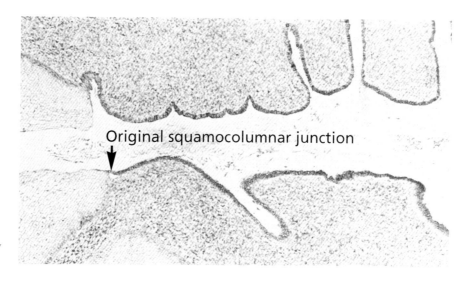

Fig. 5.8 Columnar epithelium. Fetus, 28 weeks' gestation. The original squamocolumnar junction is within the endocervical canal. The columnar epithelium is flat and displays several shallow clefts (×28).

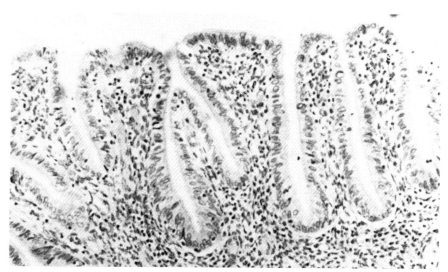

Fig. 5.9 Columnar epithelium. The characteristic surface configuration is evident in a neonate aged 3 weeks (×250).

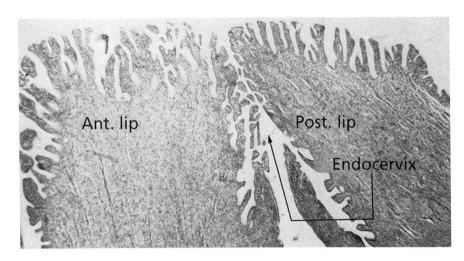

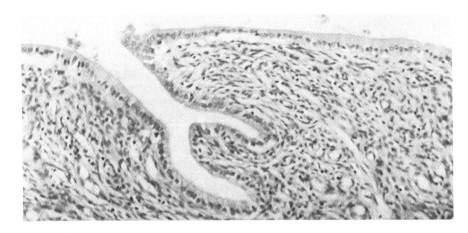

Fig. 5.10 Columnar epithelium. Portion of cervix of infant aged 3 months, showing complex surface configuration (×15).

Fig. 5.11 Columnar epithelium. Flat epithelium with simple clefts on ectocervix and vagina of child aged 1 year (×250).

the original morphology therefore remains, like an archaeological record.

The following description of the original transformation zone needs to be considered with the columnar epithelial variations in mind as a variable scaffold by which the morphological variations of the original transformation zone will be determined.

The original metaplastic epithelium

The metaplastic epithelium is perhaps the most important of the original epithelia to be described. Metaplasia is understood to be an aspect of cellular behaviour which may result in the initiation of neoplastic potential (Coppleson and Reid, 1967). It is the epithelial expanse which forms the transformation zone of the colposcopist and the transition zone of the microscopist. It is surprisingly common and extensive in the fetus and prepubertal female.

Even in preserved specimens the original transformation zone can be identified with the colposcope (Fig. 5.2), but the major portion of this description has been drawn from observations made on the histological preparation from each subject.

The metaplastic epithelium is found most commonly as a multilayered epithelial expanse whose boundaries are the two squamocolumnar junctions previously described, namely the original squamocolumnar junction and the neosquamocolumnar junction. Evolving as it does within the most caudal extent of the original columnar epithelium, the metaplastic epithelium will be coextensive with those glandular elements from the original tissue.

The mixtures of columnar and metaplastic epithelia are infinitely variable; the initial phases of metaplasia may be present in older subjects, whilst mature metaplastic squamous epithelium may be present in the youngest.

Material from youthful subjects is particularly suitable for demonstrating in a single specimen the range of appearances of the complete original transformation zone (Fig. 5.12). Within the zone marked by the junctions, the initial stage of metaplasia is seen affecting several columnar villi at the cephalic limit. Caudad, the process is more complete, and the levelled surface and incorporation of stromal elements is seen. At the original squamocolumnar junction the epithelial change is virtually complete.

Original transformation zone has been identified in speci-

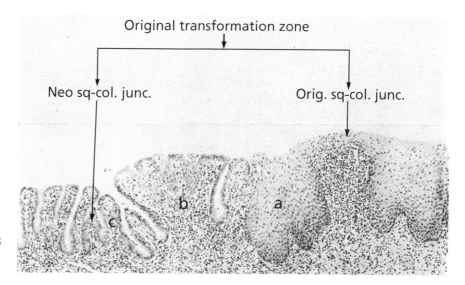

Fig. 5.12 Original transformation zone. The whole extent of the metaplastic epithelium is displayed between the two squamocolumnar junctions in an infant 3 weeks old. (a) Metaplasia virtually completed. (b) Levelling of surface with incorporation of stromal elements, including vascular structures. (c) Initial changes of metaplasia (× 100).

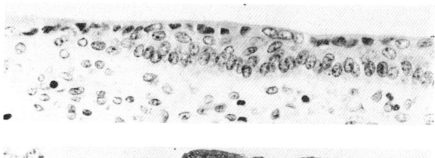

Fig. 5.13 Original transformation zone. Simple flat columnar epithelium, with evolving transformation zone unlikely to develop intraepithelial vascular patterns (× 250).

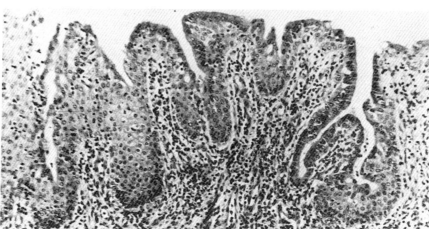

Fig. 5.14 Original transformation zone. Villiform columnar epithelium and evolving transformation zone with incorporation of stromal elements. Persistence as punctation and mosaic is probable (× 160).

mens from fetuses of all gestational ages, metaplasia seeming to be an important feature of epithelial formation during organogenesis. It seems likely that metaplasia occurring *in utero* will result in the evolution of a transformation zone with some characteristics which reflect its fetal origin.

Flat original columnar epithelium with a simple stromal configuration is characteristic of specimens of less than 30 weeks' gestation (Fig. 5.8). Original transformation zone present in these specimens is flat and lacks intraepithelial vascular structures (Fig. 5.13; see also Fig. 5.15). Persisting into adult life, such forms should exhibit vascular patterns of the subepithelial stroma only. It seems likely that metaplasia occurring

later in intrauterine existence will generate a transformation zone with a wider variety of vascular patterns, including punctation and mosaic (Fig. 5.14).

In the adult cervix, the transformation zone adjacent to the original squamocolumnar junction is likely to be of original character. Further studies of the fetal–adult morphological correlation may allow the persisting original transformation zone to be identified as an adult entity.

Original transformation zone

An attempt has been made to assess the frequency and extent of the original transformation zone so that some form of comparison may be made with older age groups. The nature of the study group makes a satisfactory assessment difficult, for the data compiled are from the examination of a single histological section from each of 330 specimens. Such an evaluation must therefore be regarded as cursory. Within the group, there is a great variation in size which does not allow direct measurements of epithelial extents to be compared. The extent of metaplasia has been defined as 'significant' when the distance from the original to the neosquamocolumnar junction is equal to one-half the field of vision provided by a plane 10 objective.

In the 330 specimens constituting the whole group, original transformation zone was present in 219 (66%) and extended to a significant degree in 128 (39%). Among those subjects born alive after 36 weeks of gestation, but dying after less than 1 month of life, a significant original transformation zone was present in 43%. In several of this latter group, the original transformation zone extended cephalad from an original squamocolumnar junction on the vagina, to cover the vagina, vaginal vault, ectocervix and portion of the lower endocervical canal.

It is important to record that such findings are also present in fetuses of 26 weeks' gestation (Fig. 5.15).

The persistence of the original transformation zone through infancy and childhood is evident from the identification of significant extents in 42% of subjects between 1 month of age and 3 years. In a group of 104 subjects aged between 1 month and 4 years, extensive original transformation zone was present in 40% and in 51% of those aged between 5 and 13 years.

During infancy and childhood, metaplastic epithelium may be found within gland clefts, and small glandular dilatations suggestive of early cyst formation have been identified.

The original squamous epithelium

In all subjects the usually well-stratified and highly differentiated original squamous epithelium (Fig. 5.16) can be traced cephalad from the vulvovaginal junction to form the covering of the vestibule, vagina and usually part of the ectocervix. As a result, a portion of the ectocervix is most frequently covered by epithelium which is more vaginal in type and function. This

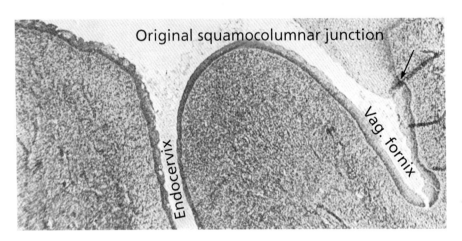

Fig. 5.15 Original transformation zone. Upper vagina and portion of cervix of fetus at 26 weeks. The original squamocolumnar junction is on the vagina, and original transformation zone covers vagina and ectocervix.

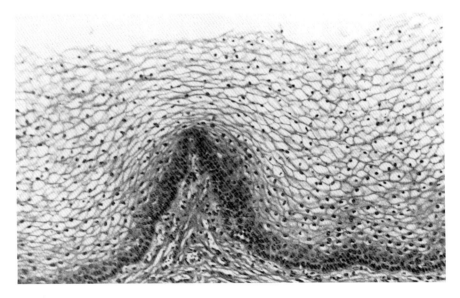

Fig. 5.16 Original squamous epithelium. Highly differentiated, stratified squamous epithelium from neonate aged several days (×160).

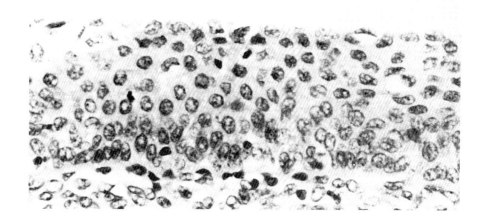

Fig. 5.17 Original squamous epithelium. Appearance of original squamous epithelium from ectocervix of 3-year-old child, showing loss of stratification and differentiation (×250).

aspect is emphasised in some youthful subjects by the presence of a rugose appearance of the cervix.

In subjects dying within several days of birth, this epithelium is thick and very highly differentiated (Fig. 5.16), reflecting the intrauterine hormonal environment. During the years that follow, the absence of hormone stimulation is reflected in loss of the extreme differentiation. Occasionally the apparently normal, youthful vagina and cervix may be covered by an original squamous epithelium which is largely undifferentiated (Fig. 5.17). It seems important to highlight this normal phase of cellular activity and existence in a decade when vaginal biopsy is undertaken on young girls exposed *in utero* to DES.

Variations in epithelial boundaries

The boundaries which separate the various epithelial coverings of the lower genital tract have been of central importance in topographical description. Variations in the disposition of these deserve description.

In histological sections from the sagittal plane it is possible to identify only the junctions between epithelia in that plane; extensive serial sections would therefore be necessary to construct a proper topographical description. Accordingly, the observations in the prepubertal study group have been supplemented by colposcopic observations on the boundaries made previously on adolescent and adult subjects (Coppleson *et al.*, 1971).

The site of the original squamocolumnar junction has been noted in its relationship to three anatomic features: the external os, the vaginal fornix and vaginal walls. The following basic arrangements can be described in mature fetuses.

1 The original squamocolumnar junction occurs at or cephalad to the external os. Present in 30% of subjects at birth, this arrangement ensures that the ectocervix is covered entirely with original squamous epithelium and that the metaplastic and columnar elements are endocervical in situation (Fig. 5.18, line 1).

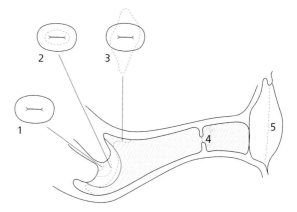

Fig. 5.18 Epithelial boundaries of lower genital tract. 1. The original squamocolumnar junction is at the external os. 2. The original squamocolumnar junction is on the ectocervix. 3. The original squamocolumnar junction is partly on the vagina. 4. Gynatresia; the obstructing membrane separates original squamous epithelium caudad from the Müllerian-derived columnar and metaplastic epithelia found cephalad. 5. The vulvovaginal epithelial junction.

Such an arrangement in the adult is encountered in the cervix and is most commonly termed 'clinically normal' or 'healthy'.

2(a) The original squamocolumnar junction occurs at a site caudad to the external os in 70% of subjects. This arrangement results in the ectocervix being covered by two, or more commonly three, forms of epithelia. Caudad to the junction, the cervix and vagina will be covered by original squamous epithelium. Cephalad, the remainder of the cervix will exhibit a variable mixture of original transformation zone and columnar epithelium. Persisting into adult life, the arrangement constitutes the basis of the appearances of the so-called ectopy, erosion, eversion and ectropion. In their original form, these arrangements form the familiar elliptical area surrounding the external cervical os, which may be quite extensive, at times reaching almost to the vaginal vault (Fig. 5.18, line 2).

2(b) In a small but significant group (3–5%) of subjects, the junction is found at some point caudad to the vaginal fornix. Cephalad to the junction, original transformation zone and columnar epithelium form the covering of the vagina and ectocervix (Fig. 5.15). This variation, persisting into adult life, is presumably the morphological basis for some of the conditions termed vaginal adenosis. In the specimens examined, original transformation zone has been the predominant form in the epithelial mixture covering the vagina and cervix (Fig. 5.18, line 3).

3 There is a further important variation, obviously of congenital origin, not yet encountered in the prepubertal material, which has been observed in five adults. Each had undergone an operation during adolescence for relief of haematocolpos due to atresia. In each subject the vagina above the level of the atresia demonstrated the usual mixture of columnar epithelium and original transformation zone (Fig. 5.18, line 4).

4 In adults, small isolated islands of original transformation zone may be found within the original squamous epithelium, close to the original squamocolumnar junction.

AGE-RELATED TOPOGRAPHICAL ALTERATIONS

During organogenesis, the site of the original squamocolumnar junction undergoes alterations which seem to be restricted to the later weeks of intrauterine existence.

In the subjects of less than 30 weeks' gestation, it is most common for the junction to be at, or cephalad to, the external os (Fig. 5.8). At birth, and subsequently, this arrangement is the least common, indicating a substantial shift caudad during the last 10 weeks of gestation. Presumably rapid proliferation of columnar epithelium and related stroma accounts for this change, causing displacement caudad of the junction.

During the years between birth and puberty, there is apparently no change in relationships that can be described. The characteristic topographic profile persists, for the overall incidence of the second type of arrangement of the original squamocolumnar junction is 67%. The vaginal site of the junction continues to be represented in its usual incidence.

There seems little doubt that the characteristic profiles of the cervicovaginal epithelial variations emerge at birth as a result of the organogenetic processes. They persist through infancy and childhood, in the protected environment of the non-reproductive state, to present at the threshold of reproductive life, awaiting the encounter with the new environmental influences which coitus and its consequences may generate.

DISCUSSION

In clinical practice the appearances of the cervix noted during speculum examination have long been held to be the result of various influences such as infection and trauma. Current practice, inheriting much from tradition, holds that the appearances which allow the diagnosis of erosion, eversion or cervicitis to be made are abnormal. Causal relationships with genitourinary disturbances are drawn, and therapeutic decisions made. The possibility that such appearances result mainly from organogenetic determination with subsequent alterations of environmental and temporal origin is not often considered. The possibility is nevertheless real, and the morphological findings in the study group allow the organogenetic contribution to the adolescent and adult morphology to be defined.

In the adult nulligravida, appearances will no doubt reflect the original topographic profiles, with the alterations superimposed by processes related to environmental factors and to senescence. It seems probable that in every subject the most caudal expanse of the transformation zone may be original. Should that peripheral transformation zone contain histological abnormality, then the interesting possibility of an intrauterine contribution to the neoplastic potential of its cell population emerges. Such a potential appears to be established in some female fetuses exposed by maternal ingestion to DES during pregnancy.

The boundaries that exist between the epithelial types in the lower genital tract of all females would seem to be the persisting evidence of the meeting place of embryonal epithelia. The original squamocolumnar junction may well represent the boundary between the Müllerian epithelia cephalad and the epithelium derived from the urogenital sinus lying caudad. The vulvovaginal junction appears to represent the most caudal extent of epithelium of sinus origin.

Originally the study of fetal and prepubertal subjects by a colposcopically oriented clinician was undertaken to obtain an understanding of early development in the evolution of the adult morphology. The extent to which the youthful epithelial profiles approach those of the adult has been a surprise, emphasising the obligatory nature of the prologue referred to in the opening of this chapter.

ADDENDUM

Professor Albert Singer was fortunate in having the unique experience of studying the material presented in Dr Pixley's chapter under his supervision in 1967. By virtue of a grant from the Royal College of Obstetricians and Gynaecologists (Australian Council), he was able to make his own detailed and unique observations after being given free and unimpeded access to the colposcopic photographs of Dr Pixley and the actual morphological specimens and histological material collected from the specimens. The observations that he made have been published only once before, in a PhD thesis submitted, examined and conferred by the University of Sydney in 1970. It had always been the intention of Dr Pixley and Professor Singer to publish this material but, unfortunately, owing to the untimely death of Dr Pixley, this publication never occurred. It is now presented by Professor Singer as an addendum to Dr Pixley's classic chapter.

FURTHER OBSERVATIONS OF THE FETAL CERVIX

Incorporation of an observational study in conjunction with the histological studies of the fetal cervix as discussed by Dr Pixley would allow a greater appreciation of the evolutionary changes occurring in the fetal and newborn cervix. The unique collection of material, as described in the chapter, was also accompanied by histological records of the actual morphological specimens of the cervix. It has therefore been possible to make further conclusions as to the changes undergone within the fetal cervix as a result of study of this colposcopic material as well as the histological sections that were taken in the form of a single sagittal section from the specimens of each of the 330 cases that he had collected, the youngest being 34 weeks' gestation and the oldest 13 years. The preparations were from blocks taken close to the median sagittal plane and allowed the

epithelial continuities, extent and boundaries within the cervix and its transformation zone to be traced.

Methods of study

Two studies were undertaken on the material as listed above: an observational study and a study of the epithelial composition (histological study).

1 The observational study involved viewing of the colpophotographs in the lateral and planar views (Figs 5.19 and 5.20) so that the position of the original squamocolumnar junction could be determined. Two positions of the junction were noted, and these have been described by Pixley in his chapter and illustrated diagrammatically in Figure 5.18. The two positions were: type I, where the original squamocolumnar junction was situated within the endocervix; and type II, where the original squamocolumnar junction was situated on the ectocervix (Figs 5.19 and 5.20).

2 The histological study was of two types: the first examined the material to determine the histological site of the original squamocolumnar junction, and the classification of this site

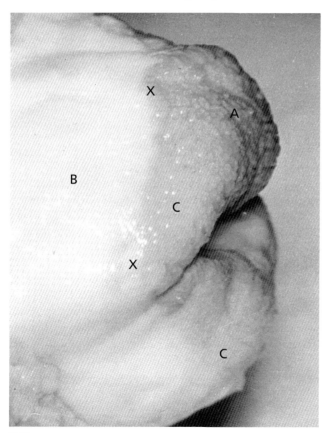

5.19

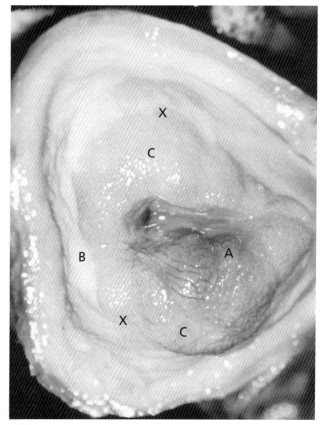

5.20

Figs 5.19 and 5.20 A colpophotograph (× 6) of a preserved post-mortem specimen of a 36-week fetal cervix seen in the lateral (Fig. 5.19) and planar (Fig. 5.20) view. The cervix is classified topographically as type II because the original squamocolumnar junction is situated on the ectocervix (X), which is mainly composed of original (native) columnar epithelium (C), in the form of broad, thick villi (A). Original (native) squamous epithelium exists at (B).

was made according to types I and II as defined above in the observation study; the second study examined the material to assess the epithelial composition of the cervix and its transformation zone components. Exact definition of the position of the original squamocolumnar junction was difficult in a number of cases as a result of post-mortem autolysis and fixation. These were excluded from the analysis. The amount of each epithelial type was assessed semi-quantitatively by measuring their extent within the one sagittal section. A measuring graticule was placed in the eyepiece of the microscope and used to obtain these measurements. The percentage of each type was assessed and a drawing made of each type of epithelium. The epithelial types were defined as follows: (1) original (native) squamous or columnar epithelium; and (2) metaplastic squamous epithelium. The metaplastic squamous epithelium was further graded as to whether it was of an immature or mature nature, the former epithelium usually consisting of one to three layers of recognisable vesicular cells with oval-shaped nuclei and commonly covered with or associated with columnar epithelial remnants. The mature epithelium consisted of distinctly squamous cells, some six to eight cells in thickness. In respect of assessing the upper limit of the transformations and the epithelial constituents of the endocervix, i.e. the original columnar epithelium within the endocervix, the junction with the endometrial epithelium was taken as indicating the most caudal extent of these tissues.

Results

Dr Pixley has already described the extensive morphological variations that occur in the fetal cervix during the last trimester of intrauterine development, and these more detailed results confirm his observations. They allow a more accurate examination to be made of the actual times in intrauterine life at which these changes occur. The highly significant changes that develop in the last 4–5 weeks of development are clearly outlined in Table 5.1 in the colposcopic observational study. Figures 5.19 and 5.20 clearly show examples of a type II cervix

Table 5.1 Topographic aspects of the fetal transformation zone. Observational study of the lateral and planar views as assessed from colpophotographs.

Groups*	n =	Type I (%)	Type II (%)
32–35 weeks' gestation	(21)	14 (67)	7 (33) ***
36 weeks to birth**	(29)	6 (21)	23 (79)

*Two cases were excluded due to post-mortem changes, one case from each group.
**Stillborn or neonatal deaths within 1 week of birth.
***Significant difference.

Table 5.2 Topographic aspects of the fetal transformation zone. Histological study.

Groups	n =	Type I (%)	Type II (%)
18–32 weeks' gestation	17	12 (71)	5 (59)
32–35 weeks' gestation	21	14 (67)	7 (33)
36 weeks to birth*	29	6 (21)	23 (79)

*Stillborn or neonatal deaths within 1 week of birth.

in a 36-week fetus. The histological studies on sagittal sections taken of this group of specimens also clearly confirm the colposcopic observations (Table 5.2).

The observations of Dr Pixley in respect of the epithelial composition of the fetal cervix are further confirmed by the breakdown of the epithelial types. It can be clearly seen from Table 5.3 that the ectocervix becomes progressively more composed of metaplastic squamous epithelium as birth comes closer. However, the endocervix shows very little change in epithelial composition during this time (Table 5.3). The maturity of the epithelium exposed to changing factors within the vagina may well explain the maturity that overtakes the metaplastic epithelium in the last few weeks of uterine life (Table 5.4). Changes on the ectocervix are significant and those alterations within the endocervix are not significant.

Discussion

The results of this detailed observational and histological study confirm those of Dr Pixley. However, explanations have to be given for the changes that have been described.

The gradual increase in the size of the fetal uterus that occurs during the second trimester of pregnancy (Fluhmann, 1960) is replaced by an exceedingly rapid increase in the third trimester, which has been attributed by most authors to the growth that occurs in the size of the cervix at this time (Fluhmann, 1961; Song, 1964). This is due to the hyperplasia of the endocervical glandular elements. Many authors (Epperson *et al.*, 1951; Fluhmann, 1959; Hamperl and Kaufmann, 1959) believe that this increase results from glandular hyperplasia which mirrors that which occurs in the maternal cervix during pregnancy. If a similar process occurs in the fetal cervix, then this would encourage prolapse of the endocervical epithelium into the region of the vaginal vault. Hamperl and Kaufmann (1959), the chief proponents of this theory, also believe that the periphery of the cervix, which is surrounded by a dense elastic sheath, may further encourage downward extension of this epithelium when the cervical volume increases as pregnancy progresses.

Large quantities of estrogen are produced during normal human pregnancy and, after the first 3–4 weeks of gestation, nearly all the estrogen (estradiol and estriol) is produced in the

Table 5.3 Epithelial composition of the fetal cervix (histological assessment).

Groups	n =	Epithelial types (%)		
		Native squamous	Columnar	Metaplastic squamous
Ectocervix				
18–35 weeks' gestation	37	91	5	4 *
36 weeks to birth	32	71	19	10
Endocervix				
18–35 weeks' gestation	37	31	57	12 **
36 weeks to birth	32	17	75	8

*Significant difference.
**No significant difference.

Table 5.4 Degree of squamous metaplastic epithelial maturity (as a percentage of existing squamous metaplastic epithelium).

Groups	n =	Maturity	
		Immature (%)	Mature (%)
Ectocervix			
23–35 weeks' gestation	5	4 (80)	1 (20) *
36 weeks to birth	19	7 (37)	12 (63)
Endocervix			
23–35 weeks' gestation	10	7 (70)	3 (30) **
36 weeks to birth	9	6 (67)	3 (53)

*Significant difference.
**No significant difference.

syncytiotrophoblast of the placenta. The mechanism by which estrogen is produced in the human trophoblast, however, is unique and is described in detail by Casey and MacDonald (1998). Near term, approximately half the estradiol synthesised in the placenta is derived from precursors in the fetal circulation and about half from precursors in the maternal circulation. Progesterone is produced in the human placenta by conversion from cholesterol. More than 90% of estradiol and estriol and 85% of the progesterone formed within the trophoblast are secreted into the maternal circulation, and little of the progesterone in the maternal circulation enters the fetus. Therefore, only a small amount of the steroids in the maternal circulation reaches the fetal compartment; this is due to the rapid clearance of steroids from maternal plasma, which minimises the availability of maternal plasma steroids to the trophoblast, and steroids that do enter the trophoblast re-enter the maternal compartment preferentially, rather than the fetal compartment. However, this still allows a proportionally large amount of the steroids to influence the small fetal tissues.

During its development, the fetus is therefore subjected to these increasing levels of circulating estrogenic and progestogenic hormones. Resultant relatively high fetal tissue levels of these hormones exist, and many of the morphological variations that occur in the fetal cervix and are described above are presumably related to the presence of this hormonal milieu. It is therefore not surprising that the morphological variations undergone by the fetal cervix mirror similar changes that occur in the gravid maternal cervix in relation to adolescence and pregnancy.

The increase in fetal intracervical volume in the third trimester is probably caused by the effect of these hormones. The progestogenic placental hormones have been shown to produce an increased intracervical water concentration, as demonstrated by the decrease in the intracervical collagen concentration (Danforth, 1960). There is also an intense decidual change in the fetal endocervical stroma (Song, 1964). This increase in cervical volume may cause eversional prolapse of the glandular endocervical epithelium as discussed above, with the result that it now occupies an ectocervical position. This leads to the caudal displacement of the original squamocolumnar junction.

The eversion of the endocervical columnar epithelium recognised by many authors and its characteristic appearance have given rise to a veritable glossary of terms, e.g. endocervical prolapse, congenital erosion and pseudo-erosion. However, failure to recognise that the origin of this tissue is from a simple everting process of the endocervical epithelium has led to much confusion. Fischel, in 1880, first described this 'lesion' and regarded it as a congenital anomaly. Robert Mayer (1910) and Rugae (1918) were convinced that this tissue represented a form of erosion associated with a loss of surface epithelium due to an accompanying inflammation. Subsequent studies have shown no evidence of tissue loss, significant histological inflammatory patterns or the presence of major bacterial contamination.

Lack of proper tissue orientation has tended to obscure the real incidence of this everted endocervical tissue, within whose confines lay the foundations for the later development of the transformation zone. Song (1964) quotes figures for its occurrence of 20% at 32 weeks and 16% at full term. In the study of Pixley's material, 80% of fetal cervices examined at birth showed some eversion of endocervical tissue. Subsequent studies (see the main part of this chapter) that examined similar post-mortem material suggest that these changes have persisted into childhood and young adult life. Pixley has made similar observations. The results as presented in this study of the epithelial composition of the cervix support similar evidence obtained from the observational studies that indicated a significant degree of endocervical epithelial eversion in the later stages of intrauterine development, as evidenced by the outward displacement of the original squamocolumnar junction. The decrease in the extent to which the ectocervix was covered by native squamous epithelium at 36 weeks and the increase in the ectocervical area occupied by the native columnar epithelium provide histological evidence of a dynamic change.

Further confirmation of these alterations comes from the studies of Barberini *et al.* (1998a). Although examining material at an early stage in intrauterine life, they have shown that dramatic changes occur in the surface epithelium even in the late first and during the second trimester. From 12 weeks onwards, there is change, especially in the endocervical epi-

thelium. By 21 weeks, the so-called 'plicae palmatae' have developed, and they are covered by cells often showing a smooth area surrounded by microvilli and provided with primary cilia. These ultrastructural changes have been described in relation to the adult cervix (Chapter 2). Using scanning electron microscopy, the differentiation of the human cervix has been shown by Barberini *et al.* (1998b) to occur up to the 31st week. In the 21st week, the first changes in squamous metaplasia have occurred with a number of apoptotic cells also noted. By the 31st week, mature squamous exfoliating cells 'with complex microplicae have covered an hypertrophied portio vaginalis'. They have also shown that squamous cells extend towards the squamocolumnar junction in flat tongue-like projections. In their paper, they show evidence of immature squamous metaplastic cells at this time and suggest that these features are 'similar to those occurring during adult reproductive life', and they have 'hypothesised that during pregnancy the common gestational background may induce somewhat similar morphodynamic processes in the cells and tissues of the fetal reproductive tract'. If this were so, then they would exactly mimic those that occur in the adult.

Study of Pixley's material showed that areas of squamous metaplasia appeared in the region of the native columnar epithelium that had undergone eversion. This metaplastic tissue appearing at 36 weeks' gestation possesses some unique features. It was not confined to the ectocervix (Figs 5.19 and 5.20) but sometimes extended high into the endocervical canal. In the latter situation, it appeared in either of two forms, either as a continuous sheet of metaplastic tissue extending cranially from the external cervical os into the cervical canal (Figs 5.21 and 5.22) or as, isolated islands of metaplastic tissue in a sea of columnar epithelium (Fig. 5.23). In its ectocervical position, it was found in abrupt apposition to the native

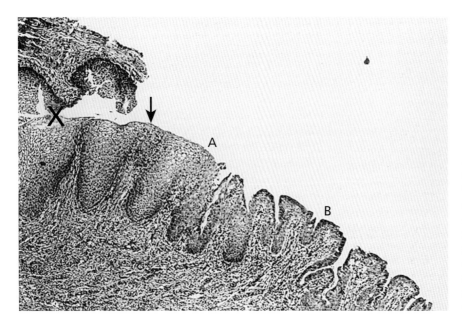

Fig. 5.21 A photomicrograph (× 200) of a section taken from a 37-week fetal cervix. The lateral vaginal fornix and the outer third of the ectocervix is covered by original (native) squamous epithelium (X), while the remainder of the ectocervix is covered by mature metaplastic squamous epithelium (A); immature epithelium exists at (B). The metaplastic epithelium joins the original squamous epithelium at the original squamocolumnar junction marked (↓).

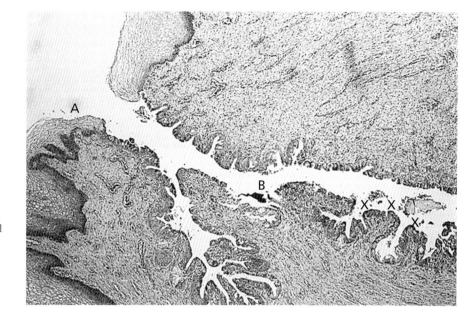

Fig. 5.22 Photogromicrograph (× 100) of a section of a 36-week fetal cervix. The squamocolumnar junction (A) is situated at the level of the external cervical os (topographically type I cervix). Areas of squamous metaplastic epithelium extend a considerable distance into the endocervical canal (B). In some areas, this metaplastic epithelium is six to eight cells thick. Note that the distribution of this metaplastic epithelium is along the crests of the endocervical canal rugae or ridges (X).

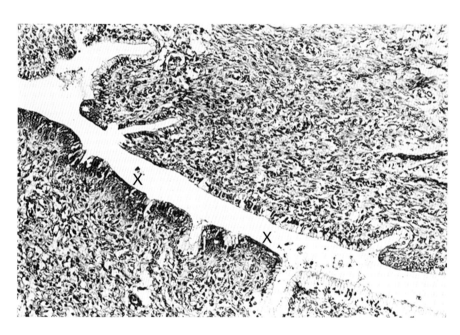

Fig. 5.23 A photomicrograph of a section of a 39-week fetal cervix showing isolated islands of squamous metaplasia existing within a sea of columnar epithelium in the endocervical canal. These areas are situated in the main luminal surface (X), and it is speculated that these positions are likely to be more exposed than other luminal areas to currents of vaginal fluid that enter the endocervical canal and initiate the metaplastic processes.

squamous epithelium in approximately half the specimens examined.

The existence of fetal squamous metaplasia as shown in this study, although recognised by some authors (Fluhmann, 1961; Song, 1964), is disputed by others (Davies and Kasuma, 1962). The latter authors are handicapped by their failure to recognise that the variable histological patterns of squamous metaplasia are essentially variations of one process. Their results are further impaired by their belief that metaplastic epithelium migrates inwards from the native squamous epithelium. Davies and Kasuma (1962), while denying the existence of squamous metaplasia, published photomicrographs of meta-

plastic squamous tissue some six to eight cells thick possessing an abrupt and distinct border with the native squamous epithelium. They are of the opinion that this epithelium is a form of native squamous epithelium that has 'grown in' over the native columnar epithelium.

The characteristic distribution of the metaplastic process provides a clue to its possible initiating stimulus. The prominence of this epithelium on the ectocervix and its distribution in apposition to the native squamous epithelium (the marginal area being the first area of the original native columnar epithelium to be everted) (A in Fig. 5.21) suggest that some factor in the external vaginal environment has contact principally with the ectocervix. This then initiates the metaplastic process. The distribution of the squamous metaplastic epithelium along the crests of the endocervical canal rugae (Figs 5.22 and 5.23) and in isolated islands within the endocervical canal (X in Fig. 5.23) suggests that this external environmental influence has managed to infiltrate the cervical canal and has initiated squamous metaplasia in a similar fashion to that produced on the exposed ectocervix. Many authors (Walz, 1958; Coppleson and Reid, 1967) suggest that the pH of the vaginal fluid is the factor responsible for the initiation of metaplasia. It could be speculated that the vaginal fluids, with their high acidic content, not only bathe the exposed ectocervix, but are able to penetrate the endocervical canal and produce variable streams of current of acidic pH within the canal lumen. The high estrogenic milieu existing in the fetus in the last trimester, as described above, would result in increased vaginal acidity (Lang, 1955) and could possibly accentuate the metaplastic process. The suggestion by some authors (Funck-Brentano *et al.*, 1957) that estrogens per se are the initiators of the metaplastic process is only partly true. It is probable that estrogens contribute indirectly to the induction of squamous metaplasia by their effect in producing increased fetal cervical volume, with resultant endocervical eversion, and by their ability to lower vaginal pH (Lang, 1955).

There was very limited histological evidence from this study to show that an excessive degree of endocervical glandular hyperplasia accounted for the presence of native columnar epithelium in the ectocervical position. The presence of this epithelium at this site was due to an everting process possibly initiated by an increase in the connective tissue and fluid volume of the cervix, rather than an excessive degree of epithelial proliferation.

REFERENCES

Barberini F, Makabe S, Motta PM (1998a) A three-dimensional study of the human fetal endocervix with special reference to its epithelium. *Histology and Histopathology* 13: 635–645.

Barberini F, Makabe S, Corrie S *et al.* (1998b) The fetal development of the human uterine cervix from 12th to the 31st post-menstrual week as revealed by scanning electron microscopy. Anatomical and clinical correlations. *Italian Journal of Anatomy and Embryology* 104(3): 77–87.

Casey ML, MacDonald PC (1998) Endocrine changes in pregnancy. In: Williams RH, Foster DW, Kronenburg HM, Larsen PR (eds) *Williams' Textbook of Endocrinology*, 9th edn. Philadelphia: W.B. Saunders, pp. 1259–1264.

Coppleson M, Reid BL (1967) *Preclinical Carcinoma of the Cervix Uteri. Its Nature, Origin and Management*. Oxford: Pergamon.

Coppleson M, Pixley EC, Reid BL (1971) *Colposcopy. A Scientific and Practical Approach to the Cervix in Health and Disease*. Springfield, IL: Charles C. Thomas.

Danforth D, Buckingham Y, Roddick J (1960) Connective tissue incident to cervical effacement. *American Journal of Obstetrics and Gynecology* 80: 939.

Davis J, Kasuma H (1962) Developmental aspects of the human cervix. *Annals of the New York Academy of Sciences* 97: 534–550.

Epperson JWW, Hillman LM, Galvin GA *et al.* (1951) The morphological changes in the cervix during pregnancy, including intraepithelial carcinoma. *American Journal of Obstetrics and Gynecology* 61: 50–61.

Fischel W (1880) *Archives of Gynaecology* 16: 162.

Fluhmann C (1959) The squamocolumnar transitional zone of the cervix uteri. *Obstetrics and Gynecology* 14: 133.

Fluhmann C (1960) Carcinoma in situ and the transitional zone of the cervix uteri. *Obstetrics and Gynecology* 15: 62.

Fluhmann C (1961) *The Cervix Uteri: Diseases*. Philadelphia: Saunders.

Funck-Brentano P, Moricard R, Robert H (1957) Des modifications de l'endocol après implantation aestrogene chez la femme ménopause; problème du diagnostic differentiel des métaplasies des glandes endo-cervicales (glycogène et mucine) 1. *Bulletin de la Fédération de Gynécologie et d'Obstétrique* 3: 381–387.

Hamperl H, Kaufmann C (1959) The cervix uteri at different ages. *Obstetrics and Gynecology* 14: 621.

Lang W (1955) Vaginal acidity and pH. A review. *Obstetrical and Gynecological Survey* 10: 546–560.

Mayer R (1910) Die Epithelentwicklung der Cervix and Portio vaginalis uteri. *Archiv Gynaekologica* 91: 579–586; 61: 658.

Rugae T (1918) *Archives of Gynaecology* 102: 264.

Song J (1964) *The Human Uterus*, 1st edn. Springfield: Charles Thomas, p. 55.

Walz W (1958) [Über die Genese der sogenannten indirekten Metaplasie im Bereich des Mullerschen-Gang-Systems] Genesis of so-called indirect metaplasia in Mullerian duct systems. *Zeitschrift für Geburtshilfe und Gynäkologie* 151 (1): 1–21.

FURTHER READING

Linhartova A (1970) Congenital ectopy of the uterine cervix. *International Journal of Obstetrics and Gynecology* 8: 653–660.

Song J (1964) *The Human Uterus*. Springfield, IL: Charles C. Thomas.

CHAPTER 6

The cervical epithelium during puberty and adolescence

Anna-Barbara Moscicki and Albert Singer

Adolescence is marked by enormous somatic and visceral changes, as shown by the transformation of the reproductive system. However, adolescence is not an isolated event; rather, it reflects a transitional period between a juvenile state and adulthood with dramatic alterations in hormonal levels resulting from changes in the sensitivity of the hypothalamic–pituitary feedback loop. As one of the major reproductive target organs, the uterus and the uterine cervix are highly influenced by these changes at both the microscopic and the macroscopic level. The uterus and uterine cervix undergo two major landmark events that herald the end of puberty for girls, these being menarche, followed by full reproductive capabilities. Since hormones, particularly estrogen and progesterone, influence the growth and morphology of the cervix, it is important to understand the timing of these hormonal changes.

ENVIRONMENT OF THE ADOLESCENT CERVIX

Hormonal

The hypothalamic–pituitary gonadal axis is fully functional at birth but is tightly controlled with a sensitive negative feedback in place resulting in low levels of circulating estradiol (Grumbach and Kaplan, 1990). At birth, placental sex steroid levels fall, and concentrations of the pituitary luteinising hormone (LH) and follicular-stimulating hormone (FSH) rise to levels found in mid-puberty and remain at that level for several months This rise is probably due to the negative feedback system's response to placental estrogen withdrawal. During this time, serum estradiol levels also rise. By 9–12 months of age, the feedback mechanism once again becomes highly sensitive, resulting in low levels of gonadotrophins and gonadal steroids. The exact mechanism that triggers puberty remains elusive (Fig. 6.1). However, three major changes are noted in girls:

1 Nocturnal pulsatile secretions of the hypothalamic gonadotrophin-releasing hormone (GnRH) and LH occur (Marshall and Kelch, 1986).

2 The sensitivity of the hypothalamus and pituitary to estradiol decreases, resulting in higher and higher levels of LH and FSH; and

3 A positive feedback loop develops so that critical levels of estradiol are reached; these in turn trigger a surge of GnRH agonist, thereby releasing LH to stimulate ovulation.

The first major rise in gonadotrophins occurs prior to sex steroid elevation. FSH secretion is greater than luteinisation hormone secretion in females. The negative feedback loop becomes less sensitive, requiring a greater amount of sex steroids to cause the negative feedback at the hypothalamic level. The positive feedback loop is required for full maturation of the hypothalamic–pituitary–gonadal (HPG) complex. The positive feedback operates when the ovarian follicles are capable of producing a critical level of estrogen. The pituitary responds by releasing a surge of LH that triggers ovulation. This positive feedback loop often does not fully develop until 2–4 years after menarche. Data from Finland (Apter et al., 1993) showed that 55–82% of cycles are anovulatory within the first 2 years after menarche. By 3 years after menarche, 50% of cycles will be anovulatory and, by 5 years, only 10–20% remain anovulatory. Interestingly, this interval appears to be greater if menarche occurs later (Apter and Vikho, 1977).

The variability in the onset of menarche and ovulatory cycles emphasises the enormous changes in hormonal influence that the cervical epithelium is subjected to during adolescence. These data suggest that, early on, the growth of the cervix is primarily influenced by estrogen only and, in some young women, estrogen remains the dominant influence until several years after menarche. On the other hand, progesterone has a significant influence on growth in a proportion of adolescents who ovulate. There are numerous other hormonal changes that affect visceral growth, including increased insulin secretion, growth hormone and insulin-like growth factors (Bloch et al., 1987; Albertsson-Wikland et al., 1994). The influence of androgens, which are similar to estrogen, on cervical development has never been studied. Dramatic changes in androgens due to adrenarche are also seen in adolescents (Apter et al., 1979). The adrenal cortex is responsible for the majority of

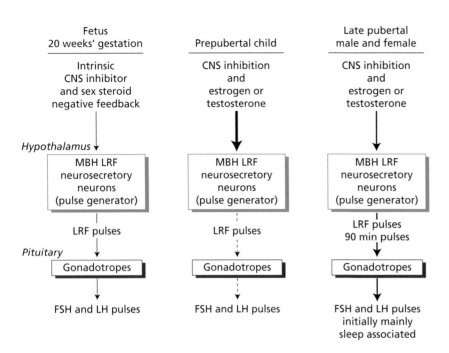

Fig. 6.1 Interaction of sex steroids and gonadotrophic hormones from fetal to late pubertal life. The diagram shows the postulated ontology of the dual mechanism for the inhibition of puberty, highlighting the interaction of sex steroids and gonadotrophic hormones during this time period. Note the action of both components during the juvenile pause (prepuberty). MBH, medial basal hypothalamus; LRF, luteinising hormone-releasing factor. From Grumbach *et al.* (2000), with permission.

circulating androgens in females; however, the ovaries secrete small amounts of androstenedione and testosterone. Polycystic ovarian syndrome, a common disorder found in adolescents, results in anovulatory cycles, excessive androgen secretion and insulin resistance. The role of these changes in cervical development is also completely unknown.

Adolescence is also marked by tremendous changes in cognitive processes. These changes include the development of a sexual identity, achievement of independence and the ability to form intimate relationships (Arnett, 2000). Middle adolescence is often a time when risk-taking behaviours begin to accelerate and sexual activity is initiated (Damon, 1999). With sexual activity, the environment of the cervix also changes with exposure to sperm, sexually transmitted infections and pregnancy-related hormones. The mean age of sexual intercourse for girls in the US is estimated at 16.9 years, 4–5 years after menarche. The effect of sexual intercourse upon the developing cervix of an adolescent is discussed later. Does sexual intercourse have a different influence on the adolescent compared with the adult cervix?

The microenvironment of the adolescent cervix/vagina

The microenvironment of the vagina is considered essential for cervical and vaginal health (Redondo-Lopez *et al.*, 1990). The change in the vaginal/cervical environment from alkaline to acid plays an important role in pubertal changes. Although lactobacilli exist in the prepubertal vagina, the increases in estrogen during puberty appear to foster lactobacillus growth. This creates a more acidic environment because of the secre-

tion of lactate. The effect of chronic alkalinisation on cervical development, such as that found in women with bacterial vaginosis or *Trichomonas vaginalis* infection, is not known. Sperm is also known to create an alkalinising environment (Redondo-Lopez *et al.*, 1990). Adolescents have the highest rates of sexually transmitted infections (STIs) including *Chlamydia trachomatis*, *Neisseria gonorrhoeae*, *T. vaginalis* and human papillomavirus (HPV) (Moscicki *et al.*, 1990, 2000; CDC, 2001). Several studies have suggested that *C. trachomatis* and *N. gonorrhoeae* preferentially adhere and infect columnar cells (Pearce and Buchanan, 1978; Harrison *et al.*, 1985). Observations that rates of 'cervical erosions', 'ectopy' and STIs are highest in adolescent age groups support this notion. Whether the presence of STIs actually affects the development of the cervix or the rates of development of squamous metaplastic transformation is speculative. The influence of STIs is discussed below in further detail.

Summary

The uterine cervix is one of the primary end-organs responsive to pubertal hormonal influences. Unfortunately, most studies of the cervix focus on chronological age and have not included studies of the hormonal variations. Clearly, there is enormous variability in estrogen levels during early to mid-puberty, and many adolescents lack ovulatory cycles and are progesterone deficient. In addition, most studies of premenarchial or perimenarchial populations have small sample sizes because of the difficulty in accessing the cervix in non-sexually active adolescents. Studies that include hormonal changes are necessary in order to complement our understanding of cervical development.

GROWTH CHARACTERISTICS OF THE PREPUBERTAL CERVIX

During the 2–3 years preceding puberty, there is a dramatic increase in the dimensions of the body and cervix of the uterus (Huffman, 1948; O'Rahilly, 1973). Dogma teaches that the cervix dominates the uterus prepubertally with ratios of the body to cervix usually < 1:1 and that uterine body growth dominates the uterus postpubertally. The ratio of the uterine body to cervix is thought to be < 1:1 prepubertally, 1:1 at menarche and > 1:1 postpubertally. Older studies were based on autopsy and consequently included small numbers of children. Using non-invasive ultrasonography, Bridges *et al.* (1996) examined patterns of growth of the uterus and uterine cervix in 358 girls ranging from birth to 16 years of age. This study showed that the uterine body and cervix were very similar with a ratio of 0.95 (0.44–1.75) in the prepubertal child. Growth of the cervix and body increased in parallel with each increasing Tanner stage (2–5). However, uterine growth outpaced cervical growth beginning at Tanner stage 2. The mean ratio for Tanner stage 2 was 1.12 (0.55–2.00); for Tanner stage 3, it was 1.26 (0.77–2.00), for Tanner 4, the ratio was 1.29 (1.0–1.83), and for Tanner 5 the ratio was 1.22 (0.75–2.13). Buzi *et al.* showed similar findings but the girls studied had greater changes in the uterine body with a mean ratio of 1.33 for Tanner stage 2, 1.44 for Tanner stage 3, and 1.45 for Tanner stage 4. Perhaps the most striking observation in both studies was the considerable overlap in dimensions between pubertal stages, in that in some women the cervix continued to predominate even postmenarchially. As the data are cross-sectional, they do not give us insight into individual growth patterns. These data also indicate that the cervical epithelium undergoes a simultaneous change during this increasingly active peripubertal period. However, the exact nature of these morphological alterations is controversial. Some aspects have already been discussed in the preceding chapter and others will be considered below.

EPITHELIAL COMPOSITION OF THE ADOLESCENT CERVIX

Unfortunately, most of the early studies of cervical development available for review are cross-sectional and do not include factors that may influence cervical epithelial change such as STI testing and measures of endogenous hormones; these thereby limit the interpretation of their findings. Notwithstanding these limitations, colposcopic examination of virginal and sexually active adolescents can give us important insight into the changes in the cervical epithelium occupying the transformation zone during adolescence. However, longitudinal studies of large groups of women are needed to elucidate fully these changes during puberty. In addition, understanding the cellular changes within the epithelia and stroma of the cervix is critical as many of the morphological alterations described in adolescents are confusing in terms of their actual histological representation.

Epithelial types within the transformation zone

There has been considerable interest in the epithelial types found within the transformation zone of the cervix as this area has long been identified as vulnerable to the development of neoplastic changes. The four major types of epithelium found in the normal cervix including the transformation zone are:

1 and **2** Original (native) columnar and squamous epithelium.

3 Squamous metaplastic epithelium with all its morphological variations as seen colposcopically, ranging from the earliest stages of development of metaplasia, the so-called immature squamous metaplasia, to more mature stages as seen diagrammatically in Figure 6.2. Intermediate changes are sometimes referred to with the exact title of intermediate squamous metaplastic changes. There are five stages in this process. The first two, (a) and (b), correspond to the single villus of the columnar epithelium which undergoes change whereby, in the exposed apical part of the structure, it adopts a pallor which progresses when the two villi fuse together (c), forming a smooth surface. This stage (c) and the following (d) both signify intermediate stages of metaplasia, and (e) corresponds to the more mature stage. These histological representations can be recognised colposcopically. Reference to Figures 6.3 and 6.4 demonstrates them within adolescent cervices.

4 Atypical epithelium refers to a purely colposcopic description. Within this colposcopic classification (see Chapter 21) are the premalignant and malignant stages of cervical neoplasia as well as those of the benign stages of immature metaplasia, as described above. This last stage would correspond to (c) in Figure 6.2.

The transformation zone (TZ), that area of original (native) columnar epithelium in which the physiological process of metaplasia occurs, is composed of all four epithelial types. It is bounded by the original squamocolumnar junction (Figs 6.3 and 6.4). When there is no atypical epithelium present within its boundaries, it is referred to as a physiological transformation zone; when atypical epithelium occurs within the confines of the TZ, it is referred to as an atypical transformation zone (Fig. 6.5).

When original (native) columnar epithelium is found predominantly on the ectocervix, as seen in Figures 6.3 and 6.4, it is referred to by some authors as 'ectopy'. This has been discussed in Chapter 2. The presentation of original (native) columnar epithelium on the ectocervix is in most cases accompanied by some degree of metaplastic change. However, the original (native) columnar epithelium, when present in this position, is also erroneously referred to as an 'erosion'. This term means loss of superficial tissue, and this rarely occurs physiologically on the cervix; it predominates in pathological lesions, as discussed in Chapter 15.

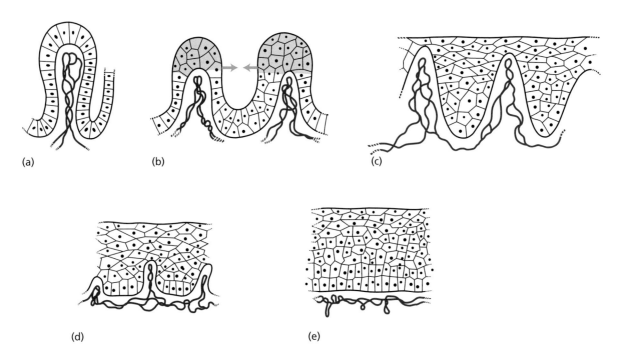

(a)   (b)   (c)

(d)   (e)

Fig. 6.2 (a–e) The process of squamous metaplasia in which the villi of columnar epithelium are replaced by metaplastic epithelium. The capillary structures of the stroma in the villi are compressed and reduced in height, ultimately forming a network. Modified from Kolstad and Stafl, 1982.

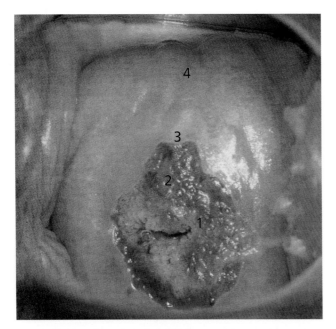

Fig. 6.3 Native columnar epithelium. The squamocolumnar junction (3) is at the mid-distance point between the endocervix and the vaginal fornix. The original columnar epithelium is at (1), with a small island of metaplastic squamous epithelium at (2). Original squamous epithelium is at (4).

Frequency and distribution of epithelial types

Studies have shown conflicting information with regard to the frequency and distribution of these types of epithelium in adolescent cervices. In part, these disparities result from differences in the populations studied. It appears that sexual activity induces or accelerates changes in the cervix. Therefore, it is important to define the epithelial types of the virginal cervix and those in a cervix exposed to sexual intercourse. Further, the composition of the virginal cervix can be divided into premenarchial and postmenarchial types. Sexual activity prior to menarche is rare, and the impact of sexual intercourse during this time is unknown. The embryological development of the cervix up to adolescence is covered in Chapter 1.

In the following sections, the frequency and distribution of epithelial types within cervices of virginal and sexually active adolescents will be discussed.

Within the virginal cervix

Situated on the ectocervix of the peripubertal female is the squamocolumnar junction with large areas of associated original (native) columnar epithelium in the early stages of undergoing squamous metaplastic transformation. These observations are derived from colposcopic studies done by Pixley *et al.* (1967, 1971) and described in the previous chapter and its addendum. They differ from the traditional views long held and derived from the histological studies of Hamperl and Kaufmann (1959) and Fluhman (1961), who

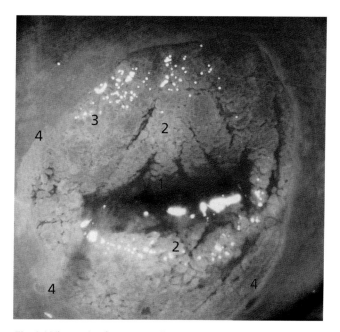

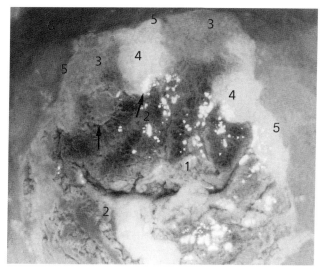

Fig. 6.4 The cervix of a non-sexually active adolescent (16 years) showing all the stages of squamous metaplasia. The endocervix with its original columnar epithelium is at (1). At position (2) is seen stage 2 of squamous metaplasia development with fusion of the villi and, at (3), this has extended to fusion of all the villi. Immature squamous epithelium is present, adjacent and medial to the squamocolumnar junction at (4). Between (2) and (3), it can be seen that the villous structure of the original columnar epithelium has been gradually lost until the surface has become flat with the development of more peripheral immature epithelium. This has developed in an area that is more exposed to the effect of the vaginal pH. The pallor of this immature epithelium (3) contrasts with the redness of the previous columnar epithelium (1). With further maturity, this pallor will be lost as the epithelium becomes thicker.

Fig. 6.5 The transformation zone showing the early metaplastic process in the cervix of a sexually active adolescent (16 years). The original columnar epithelium is at (2) with some opaqueness already developing in the columnar villi at (1). However, at (3), immature metaplastic epithelium has already developed with a typical pallor. It can easily be differentiated from the redness of the original columnar epithelium (2). A line (arrowed) has developed between the metaplastic process and the columnar epithelium, and this represents the new squamocolumnar junction. This signifies the upper extent of the metaplastic process. At (4), there exists a faint micropapillary surface contour that is indicative of the effect of human papillomavirus (HPV). This transformation zone with its abnormal (atypical) epithelium (at 4) would be labelled an atypical transformation zone. The original squamocolumnar junction can be clearly seen at (5), with original (native) squamous epithelium at (6).

stated that the squamocolumnar junction occupied an endocervical position in this premenarchial era. With the appearance of hormonal stimulation at menarche as described above, the epithelium and stroma increase in size within the original (native) squamous epithelium, which correspondingly increases in height from its prepubertal flattened state (Fluhman, 1961). Simultaneously, thickening of the mucosal folds and clefts appears with evidence of secretion present within the glandular epithelium. Retention of fluid within the cervix also occurs as a result of the local action of the newly secreted ovarian hormones, which has been described above. It is therefore not surprising that some degree of eversion of this relatively enlarged endocervical epithelium occurs at this stage. As the point of attachment of the cervix to the vagina is firmly fixed, the only direction in which the enlarged cervix could expand is downwards and outwards by an inverting mechanism, which results in the squamocolumnar junction adopting a more peripheral ectocervical position; the authors refer to this state as an 'ectopic' or 'ectopy' position (Figs 6.3 and 6.4).

Studies describing the frequency of this 'ectopy' are limited because of small sample sizes and the lack of hormonal studies that are related to the time of puberty. In addition, the interpretation of these studies is confusing because colposcopic viewing with a speculum is usually performed, which invariably produces an artificial eversion of the endocervix, the so-called apparent position; with the speculum's closure and removal to the lower and mid-vagina, a position that imitates the normal *in vivo* position becomes apparent, which is referred to as the real position. Exposure of the cervix in the apparent view may reveal large areas of immature and developing metaplasia (stages 2 and 3 in Fig. 6.4) that actually reside within the endocervix and only appear in the ectocervical area in this apparent view. The presence of such 'ectopy' on the ectocervix is important, as this tissue remains vulnerable to infection and changes associated with neoplasia.

There have been very few studies describing the epithelial composition in virginal girls, and these have not been replicated and remain landmark studies which are important to review. Singer's (1975a) study documented planimetric measurements of epithelium within the virginal cervix (Fig. 6.6).

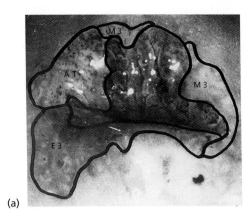

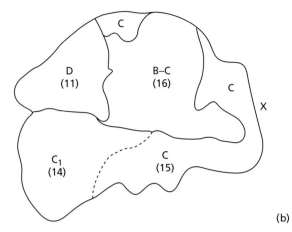

Fig. 6.6 Colpophotograph (×6) with corresponding contour area map of an atypical transformation zone. Planimeter measurement has determined the relative areas of each individual type. (2) represents columnar epithelium with early metaplastic change; E3, recently formed metaplastic squamous epithelium; M3, mature metaplastic squamous epithelium; AT, atypical (abnormal) epithelium. The original squamocolumnar junction is at X.

The results seen in Table 6.1 show that there was four times as much original (native) columnar epithelium present (Fig. 6.3) as in the cervix of a sexually active adolescent. This epithelium constituted 53% of the total area of the virginal transformation zone. However, it appears that it is uncommon to find areas on the ectocervix of the adolescent that are exclusively occupied by columnar epithelium, giving the appearance of an ectopy. Rather, there appears to be a mixed picture within the transformation zone, which includes metaplastic squamous epithelium, an easily recognisable condition colposcopically (Figs 6.3–6.5).

Although the presence of metaplastic squamous epithelium is more common and such epithelium constitutes a larger proportion of the transformation zone in the sexually active adolescents who were studied by Singer (1975b) (Table 6.1), this tissue is also found in the cervix of the virginal transformation zone. Singer reported that 56% of the area of sexually active adolescent cervices contained squamous metaplastic epithelium, usually of the immature to intermediate type; this

compared with only 30% of the area of the virginal transformation zone. In the former group, it was adjacent to areas of atypical epithelium in many cases.

The question remains: 'Do the dramatic hormonal changes seen at puberty and with the onset of sexual behaviour influence the type and distribution of epithelium found within the transformation zone of the adolescent cervix or are these changes preordained at birth?' Traditional wisdom, as described and referenced above, insisted that the transformation zones of the adolescent cervices were predominantly covered with columnar epithelium or the stages of early metaplasia, whereas in the adult they were covered by mature squamous epithelium. This implies that, during late adolescence and early adulthood, the process of squamous metaplastic transformation was accelerated, transforming the original (native) columnar epithelium into a more mature form of metaplastic squamous epithelium. Immunohistochemical studies show that the density of estrogen and progesterone receptors is greatest in areas of immature squamous metaplasia, support-

Table 6.1 Epithelial composition of the adolescent transformation zone as assessed by colposcopy.

		Total area (mm²)	Native columnar	Early squamous metaplasia	Mature squamous metaplasia	Atypical epithelium
Virgins	Mean	170	90	51	27	2
$n = 40$	Range	(112–240)	(45–137)	(32–73)	(10–52)	(0–3)
	Per cent		53	30	16	1
Sexually active girls	Mean	117	14	65	25	13
$n = 170$	Range	(72–132)	(8–26)	(33–84)	(12–32)	(9–27)
	Per cent		12	56	21	11

The differences in the amount of native columnar epithelium and in the amount of early metaplastic epithelium between the two groups was significant ($P < 0.01$).
From Singer (1975b), with kind permission of Blackwell Publishing.

ing the role of hormonal control in accelerating the squamous metaplastic process (Remoue *et al.*, 2003).

However, in clinical practice, it is not unusual to find an adolescent cervix predominantly covered by original (native) squamous epithelium (i.e. stage (e) in Fig. 6.2, Fig. 6.7) and,

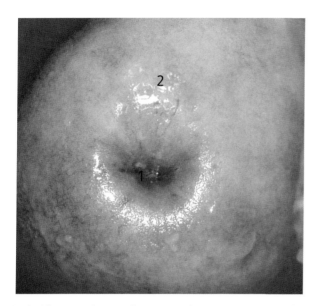

Fig. 6.7 The cervix showing the squamocolumnar junction (1) in the endocervix, with original (native) squamous epithelium (2) covering the ectocervix.

vice versa, to find a cervix in a woman over 40 years of age almost completely covered by columnar epithelium when viewed in the apparent view with the vaginal speculum fully opened. These dichotomies have caused much confusion as to the origin of the composition of cervical epithelium in the adolescent, younger and middle-aged woman.

Within the cervix of sexually active adolescents

Table 6.2 summarises several of the early studies describing the frequency of cervical 'ectopy' in predominantly sexually active adolescents. Unfortunately, comparisons between the studies are limited because factors that may influence cervical epithelial composition were not measured consistently in these older studies. In addition, sexual practices and the composition of hormonal contraceptives have changed dramatically over the last few decades.

Among the early studies, Singer (1975b) and Coppleson (1977) used colposcopic observations to compare the development of the transformation zone in sexually active adolescents with 'high-risk' sexual behaviour and in non-sexually active adolescents. In Coppleson's study, 300 sexually active and nulliparous girls under 17 years of age (mean age 16.4 ± 2.4 years) who were detained in a state institution were obliged by law to undergo cytological and sexually transmitted disease (STD) testing. In a similar study of detained girls in a London prison, Singer (1975a,b) screened 168 nulliparous women aged 21 years and under (mean age 18.8 ± 2.4 years). The mean

Table 6.2 The frequency of epithelial tissue types within the adolescent cervix, as seen colposcopically.

	Virginal adolescents	Sexually active (nulliparous) adolescents		Adolescents (mixed parity)		Adult 'well women' (mixed parity)
	Sydney[1] (14–24 years) n = 40	Sydney[2] (14–17 years) n = 170	London[1] (16–21 years) n = 168	Buenos Aires[3][7] (10–15 years) n = 310	Manchester[4] (15–20 years) n = 100	Sydney[5] (18–55 years) n = 8623
Original (native) columnar epithelium	4 (10%)	–	–	133[8] (43%)	40[9] (40%)	629 (7.3%)
Squamocolumnar junction wholly or nearly within the endocervix	2 (5%)	15[6] (8%)	38 (23%)	47 (15%)	5 (5%)	1365 (15.8%)
Physiological transformation zone	29 (72.5%)	80 (48%)	60 (35%)	100 (32%)	55 (55%)	4908 (56.9%)
Atypical transformation zone	5 (12.5%)	75 (44%)	70 (42%)	30 (10%)	–	1145 (13.2%)
Other						576 (6.8%)

1 Singer (1975b).
2 Coppleson (1977).
3 de Zeiguer (personal communication, 1975).
4 Crompton (1973).
5 Coppleson and Reid (1967).

6 Only includes those with junction completely within endocervix.
7 Early age of coitus.
8 'Ectopy' within transformation zone.
9 'Ectopy'.

age of first coitus was 13.4 (± 2.7) years in the former and 14.9 (± 3.2) years in the latter. Fourteen per cent of the Australian and 10% of the London girls had coitus prior to the menarche. For comparison, Singer (1975b) examined the cervices of 40 virginal girls ranging from 14 to 24 years of age (mean age 19 years) who were admitted to hospital for examination under anaesthesia for such conditions as dysmenorrhoea, rigid hymen or dysfunctional uterine bleeding. All consenting girls were examined using colposcopy and had colpophotographs taken of the cervix after the application of 3% acetic acid with a small self-retaining Cusco speculum fully opened. The extent, distribution and frequency of the individual epithelial types of tissue [i.e. original (native) squamous and columnar, metaplastic squamous and atypical epithelium] from these studies are summarised in Tables 6.1 and 6.2. The method employed (Fig. 6.6) in determining the space occupied by each type involved the projection of a colpophotograph on to graph paper with subsequent planimetric measurement from the contour map of the total area of the transformation zone and of the individual epithelia.

Singer (1975b) and Coppleson (1977) described four distinct patterns in these girls. In the first, the ectocervix medial to the squamocolumnar junction is completely covered by original columnar epithelium (i.e. 'ectopy'). A second pattern is that in which the ectocervix is totally or nearly covered by original squamous epithelium with the squamocolumnar junction wholly (Fig. 6.7) or nearly completely situated within the endocervix. This state has been proposed by some authors as the most common pattern seen in the prepubertal cervix (Hamperl and Kaufmann, 1959; Kaufmann and Ober, 1959; Fluhman, 1961), arising as a result of retraction to within the endocervix by the squamocolumnar junction in the early infancy period. However, the lack of this pattern in the virginal adolescents suggest that subsequent eversion of this junction occurs during adolescence. This mechanism has been supported by many authors (Gruengagel, 1957; Song, 1964; Pixley, 1967, 1971) who have shown the junction to be situated in an ectocervical position in most pre- and postmenarchial girls. The third pattern is that of a typical or normal (physiological) transformation zone, an area comprising both original columnar and metaplastic squamous epithelium (Fig. 6.8).

In the final pattern, these last two epithelial types may be associated with colposcopically recognisable atypical epithelium (atypical transformation zone). This last pattern and its significance to the relationship of neoplasia will be considered later.

Examination of Table 6.2 emphasises the tremendous variability in the frequency and distribution of the different epithelial types within the transformation zone. This suggests that certain factors, in relation to either sexual risk behaviour or developmental stages, are probably operating within these diverse populations. Singer's (1975b) study was the only study to provide information relating to virginal adolescents. Among

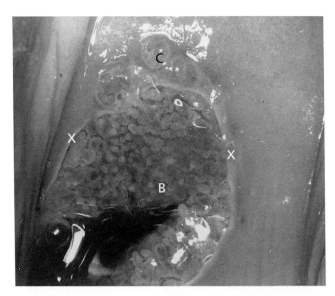

Fig. 6.8 Colpophotograph (× 6) of the transformation zone in a 17-year-old virgin showing large areas of original columnar epithelium (B), with smaller peripheral regions occupied by metaplastic squamous epithelium (C). The squamocolumnar junction is at X.

40 virginal girls examined, only 10% had a predominance of original (native) columnar epithelium visualised on the ectocervix (Fig. 6.4). Although this stage, also referred to as an 'ectopy', is thought to be predominant in nonsexually active girls, this finding may not be surprising as the ages ranged from 14 to 24 years. When other epithelial types were considered, it could be seen that 72% of virginal girls had both columnar and early stages of squamous metaplastic epithelium also present within the transformation zone.

In both Singer's and Coppleson's studies of sexually active adolescents, none of the girls was found to have this pattern of transformation zone completely covered by original (native) columnar epithelium. In contrast to these findings, de Zeiguer (personal communication, 1975) and Crompton (1973) found that in approximately 40% of their sexually active population the transformation zone was predominantly occupied by original (native) columnar epithelium while 32–55% a mixed composition of both columnar and metaplastic epithelium was present. Crompton examined colposcopically 100 girls aged 15–20 years and de Zeiguer examined a younger population aged between 10 and 15 years who were sexually active in Buenos Aires. The higher rates found in these two studies of columnar epithelium predominating within the transformation zone when compared with Singer's study may be explained by the fact that de Zeiguer had a younger population. It may also have been that these last two authors did not discriminate between the various stages of squamous metaplasia as Singer did. However, the studies do agree that completely mature squamous metaplastic epithelium within the transformation zone is not common, occurring in only 5–15% of adolescents.

Moscicki *et al.* (2001a) reported a relatively low rate of 'ectopy' in a group of adolescents who were at relatively high risk sexually (e.g. reporting multiple partners, having a history of sexually transmitted infections). In this population, two-thirds of the adolescents were human immunodeficiency virus (HIV) positive with acquisition through sexual transmission. The mean age of the cohort was 16.8 years. 'Ectopy' in this study was defined as at least 10% of the cervix having evidence of original (native) columnar and early or mid-metaplastic epithelium (Fig. 6.2), as measured on digitised images of the cervix. Ten per cent was used as a cutoff as holding the cervix open with a speculum caused some artificial eversion, and the rate of inter-rater error was 5–10%. 'Ectopy' was noted in 18.5% of the HIV infected and in 29.4% of those who were HIV negative. The difference in rate of 'ectopy' was explained by the fact that the HIV-infected adolescents were more sexually experienced and had a greater number of lifetime partners (Moscicki *et al.*, 2001a). That is, when controlling for number of sexual partners, HIV infection was no longer associated with the presence of 'ectopy'. To examine the distribution of epithelial types more closely, a comparison defining percentage of total cervical area for each epithelial type was performed (Moscicki, personal communication, 2003). As the effect of HIV on cervical development is unknown, the HIV-infected group was excluded. Not surprisingly, the majority of the HIV-uninfected adolescents had a picture of mature metaplastic squamous epithelium consistent with the theory that high-risk sexual behaviour results in enhanced squamous metaplasia and the rapid development of mature squamous metaplastic epithelia. The median percentage area covered by early to midstage metaplasia was 5.5% [interquartile range (IQR) 2.1, 14.3]. Forty-four per cent had some evidence of late-stage squamous metaplasia, but the median area covered by this epithelial type was quite low: 8.7% (IQR 2.8, 14.4). In addition, 8.6% had areas identified as atypical epithelium with the median area constituting 9.8% (IQR 7.5, 12.7).

In a recent ongoing longitudinal study of adolescents and young women started in 1990, Moscicki *et al.* examined the rate of 'ectopy' at entry into the study. The cohort was predominantly defined as HPV positive but included an HPV-negative control cohort, which was selected based on randomisation (Moscicki *et al.*, 1998; Moscicki, personal communication, 2003). Subjects who were younger than 19 years old and had been sexually active for less than 2 years were included in this analysis. Trained nurse practitioners noted the presence of original (native) columnar epithelium and areas of immature to intermediate squamous metaplastic epithelium (Fig. 6.2) and the number of quadrants involved of any particular epithelial type. Examinations were performed at 10× and 16× or 20× magnification using a colposcope after a 3% acetic acid cervical wash. A colpophotograph was also obtained at each examination. All subjects noted to have

Table 6.3 Frequency of early, mid and late squamous metaplasia in adolescents aged 13–18 years with less than 2 years of sexual experience.

Early squamous metaplasia	$n = 45$ (47%)
Mid squamous metaplasia	$n = 31$ (33%)
Late squamous metaplasia	$n = 79$ (83%)
Those with	
early squamous metaplasia only	$n = 2$ (2.1%)
late squamous metaplasia only	$n = 36$ (37.9%)
early *and* mid squamous metaplasia	$n = 6$ (6.3%)
early *and* late squamous metaplasia	$n = 18$ (19.0%)
mid *and* late squamous metaplasia	$n = 6$ (6.3%)
early *and* mid **and** late squamous metaplasia	$n = 19$ (20%)
Of those with early squamous metaplasia	
involvement in two quadrants	$n = 7$ (15.6%)
involvement in four quadrants	$n = 38$ (84.4%)
Of those with mid squamous metaplasia*	
involvement in two quadrants	$n = 1$ (3.5%)
involvement in four quadrants	$n = 28$ (96.5%)
Of those with late squamous metaplasia*	
involvement in one quadrant	$n = 2$ (2.7%)
involvement in two quadrants	$n = 10$ (13.5%)
involvement in three quadrants	$n = 5$ (6.8%)
involvement in four quadrants	$n = 57$ (77%)

original (native) columnar and immature metaplastic epithelium had their colpophotographs reviewed for verification. As the lack of 'ectopy' is less subject to colposcopic error, only 10% of those noted as no 'ectopy' had their colpophotographs reviewed No errors were noted for the 'no ectopy' group and the data are summarised in Table 6.3.

The results showed that approximately half the adolescents had evidence of early squamous metaplasia. Only 2.1% had early squamous metaplasia only. Most adolescents had a mixed picture, with 53% having immature and intermediate stages of metaplasia. Thirty-eight per cent had a relatively mature cervix with some evidence of late squamous metaplasia, and only 8% had completely mature cervices with no evidence of squamous metaplasia. This picture is strikingly different from the high-risk group reported previously by Moscicki *et al.* (2001a). However, the rate of early, middle and late metaplasia in Moscicki's longitudinal group was similar to that reported by Singer and Coppleson several decades ago. In a subset of this group (Moscicki *et al.*, 1999), colpophotographs were digitised, and areas of columnar and early metaplasia were outlined and calculated using a software program and documented as percentage of total transformation zone area. The subjects were selected from the longitudinal study, and a case–control analysis was performed to examine the role of 'ectopy' in the development of low-grade squamous intraepithelial lesions (LGSILs) (Moscicki *et al.*, 1999). Excluding those who developed LGSILs, 21% of the group had evidence of original (native) columnar/immature metaplasia at baseline. The median area of the cervix covered by columnar /early metaplasia was 28.7% (IQR 14.7, 46.6). The area covered by columnar/early metaplasia was greater than the 5.5% found in the higher sexual risk group described earlier (Moscicki *et al.*, 2001a), emphasising the importance of sexual activity and sexual risk in promoting maturation of the epithelial types.

ATYPICAL EPITHELIUM WITHIN THE ADOLESCENT TRANSFORMATION ZONE

The pattern defined by Singer (1975b) and Coppleson (1977) as colposcopically atypical epithelium (Fig. 6.5) occurs in a significant proportion of adolescents. Atypical epithelium is often indistinguishable from dysplastic epithelium and is strongly associated with sexual activity. In Singer's study, only 12.5% of the virginal girls compared with 42% of the sexually active girls were observed to have colposcopically recognisable atypical epithelium. The majority of atypical epithelium cases were found to be composed of immature metaplastic squamous epithelium, with some dysplastic and *in situ* carcinomatous lesions also found. In a study of young adolescents aged 10–15 years of age (de Zeiguer, personal communication, 1975), the rate of atypical epithelium was similar to that of virginal girls, suggesting that pubertal development and risky behaviour are both critical to the development of atypical epithelium. On the other hand, association with infectious agents in these studies was limited because the authors did not test for sexually transmitted infections such as HPV, herpes simplex virus, chlamydia or trichomonas.

Histological appearances

Histological biopsy of the atypical transformation zone under colposcopic vision was taken from some of the sexually experienced Australian patients in Coppleson's study (1977) and from 90% of the young women in the London study (Singer, 1975b). All five virginal cervices with atypical epithelium were biopsied, and all showed a pattern of immature squamous metaplasia. Evidence of some epithelial abnormality existed in 18 of the 63 punch biopsies taken from the London study. Twelve of these contained lesions classified at that time as abnormal epithelium (non-neoplastic) (Fig. 6.9) (as described by Glatthaar, 1950) or benign basal cell hyperplasia (Glatthaar, 1950; Govan *et al.*, 1966). In six patients, the youngest of whom was 16 years of age, dysplastic lesions usually regarded as potentially neoplastic were found. Four of the dysplasias were mild, while one was classified as moderate and another as severe dysplasia with areas of carcinoma *in situ*. The remaining 45 of the 63 punch biopsies showed histological evidence of very active early immature squamous metaplastic epithelium with an associated intense inflammatory and 'round cell' reaction involving the epithelium and subepithelial areas. In view

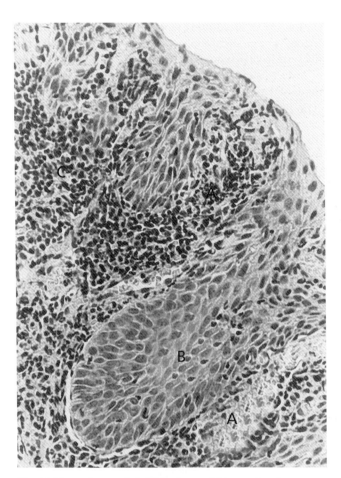

Fig. 6.9 Photomicrograph (× 150) of a punch biopsy taken from colposcopically visible atypical epithelium. The epithelium shows an increase in the basal layers and was classified at the time (1967) as abnormal epithelium (after Glatthaar, 1950). Intraepithelial capillaries (A) extend between the epithelial rete-like pegs (B); the inflammatory infiltrate (C) is composed predominantly of lymphocytes, monocytes and plasma cells.

of the 65% incidence of vaginal infection (cytologically or bacteriologically confirmed), the infiltration of the stroma and epithelium by mononuclear and lymphocytic cells rather than polymorphonuclear leucocytes was puzzling (Fig. 6.10). It has been suggested that this pattern may present an immune reaction to a coitally transmitted mutagen such as HPV (Friedell *et al.*, 1960; Glucksmann *et al.*, 1964; Reid *et al.*, 1971; Rawls and Gardiner, 1972). Interestingly, these speculations were made before HPV testing was broadly available or the role of HPV in the development of cancers was understood.

Correlation between colposcopic and histological appearances

Precise correlation between major colposcopic and histological abnormalities such as dysplasia and carcinoma *in situ* was

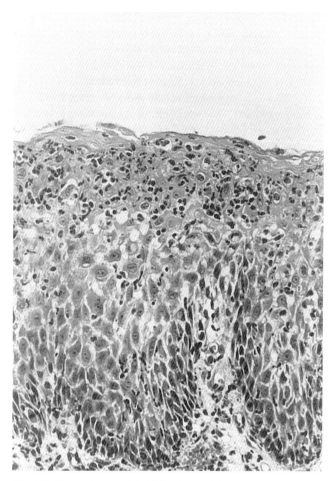

Fig. 6.10 Photomicrograph (× 100) of a punch biopsy taken from colposcopically visible atypical epithelium showing the epithelium and stroma heavily infiltrated by a mixture of inflammatory and 'immune'-type cells. Marked tissue oedema is seen in this benign metaplastic squamous epithelium. The infiltration and oedema have distorted the overlying epithelium so as seriously to impair the passage of reflected light from the subepithelial vascular structures to the surface, thereby allowing the colposcopist to interpret the resulting opaque appearance as atypical.

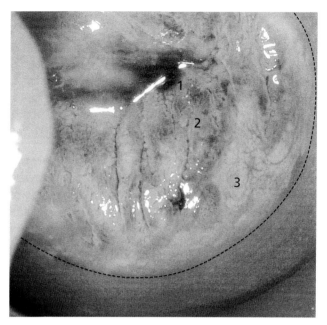

Fig. 6.11 The cervix of a sexually active 15-year-old adolescent. The original columnar epithelium is at (1). Early squamous (immature) metaplasia is seen developing at (2), with fusion of some of the columnar villi. Their original form can still be made out underneath the new metaplastic squamous epithelium. A more advanced stage of squamous metaplasia is seen at (3); again, the form of the original columnar epithelium is just visible as a type of mosaic structure at point (3). The original squamocolumnar junction is marked (dotted line) with a sharp differentiation seen between the two forms of squamous epithelium, i.e. metaplastic and original.

not possible in either Copplesen's or Singer's series. In the latter series, only six (10%) of the 63 biopsied cervices with an atypical transformation zone had a dysplastic lesion. The figure rose to 27% if the 'borderline' lesions of abnormal epithelium (Glatthaar, 1950) and basal cell hyperplasia were included. This seemingly high rate of false-positive colposcopic observations needs some explanation. The answer may lie in the increased thickness of the epithelium caused by the tissue oedema associated with the infiltrative inflammatory process (Figs 6.9 and 6.10), or the relatively excessive cellular proliferation of the recently formed and active metaplastic squamous tissue, or 'borderline lesions' themselves with their marked increase in epithelial dimensions. In all these conditions, the passage of reflected light from the underlying vascular stroma to the colposcopist is impeded. The result is that the overlying epithelium appears opaque, and so will be interpreted as indicative of an atypical transformation zone (Fig. 6.11). An analogous situation was found by Stafl and Mattingly (1975) when observing the cervix and upper vagina of young women exposed to high doses of DES (diethylstilbestrol) *in utero*.

Development of neoplasia: the role of HPV

One of the reasons why the transformation zone and its associated squamous metaplastic epithelium are thought to be important is in its role of sustaining HPV infection, a subject dealt with in Chapter 19. Although the life cycle of HPV is not well understood, it has been suggested that the basal cells of the cervical columnar epithelium are particularly vulnerable to HPV infection because of their accessibility compared with the basal cells of the thick-layered squamous epithelium (Chapter 19). The virus may remain dormant in the basal cells until replication is triggered by factors that are currently unknown. The efficiency of HPV replication appears to be dependent on host cell proliferation and differentiation. Studies have shown that specific viral proteins expressed during the process of viral replication induce cytoskeletal changes in differentiated superficial epithelial cells and lead to basal cell proliferation, resulting in characteristic LGSILs that are also referred to as cervical intraepithelial neoplasia (CIN) I. Moscicki *et al.* (2001b) showed that most adolescents and young girls will acquire HPV within 5 years of the onset of sexual activity. The strongest risk factor for acquiring HPV is having a recent new sexual partner (Moscicki *et al.*, 2001b). These data emphasise the commonness of HPV infections in adolescents and the high rate of transmissibility during sexual activity. Not surprisingly, LGSIL is also common in young women, with 25% of those infected with HPV developing a LGSIL within 3 years of acquiring HPV (Moscicki *et al.*, 2001b). These natural history studies of HPV suggest that there is little risk of significant precancerous lesions going undetected within the first 3–5 years after the onset of sexual activity. The American Cancer Society has recently recommended that screening be initiated within 3 years of the onset of vaginal intercourse but no later than 21 years of age, and Moscicki (2005) has reviewed these new recommendations and concludes that they appear 'to be safe and will decrease the current overreferral and overtreatment of adolescent and young women with HPV infections'.

The association of squamous metaplastic epithelium and HPV

It had long been proposed (Coppleson and Reid, 1975) that the physiological process of squamous metaplasia is intimately related to the development of cervical neoplasia. The studies of Singer (1975a) and Coppleson (1977) indicated that the cervix of the sexually active adolescent has large areas of squamous metaplastic epithelium, the majority of which is in an immature and recently developed stage.

Moscicki *et al.* (1999) examined the risk of developing the earlier stages of premalignancy, the so-called stage LGSIL, in a longitudinal study involving a cohort of women whose cervix was found to have epithelium predominantly showing the stages of immature squamous metaplastic epithelium, i.e. Figure 6.2. This study was a nested case–control design that used subjects from an ongoing prospective study of HPV infection (Moscicki *et al.*, 2001b). As described earlier (Moscicki *et al.*, 1990, 1998, 2001b), the majority of adolescents and young women were selected for participation because they were found to be positive for HPV infection on routine screening. A random group of women who were HPV negative were also asked to participate. Fifty-four sexually active young women who developed LGSIL were matched for age and number of visits with 54 women who never developed LGSIL. The percentage of cervical immaturity was interpreted from colpophotographs obtained at each 4-month visit after the application of 3% acetic acid. The colpophotographs were

computerised using a slide scanner. The computerised copy of the slides was displayed on the computer screen, and areas consistent with the early stages of metaplasia, i.e. Figure 6.2a–c, and original (native) columnar epithelium and the total cervical area were outlined by a single observer blinded to LGSIL or HPV status. Ten per cent of the slides were reviewed by a second observer. This study found no association between baseline measurement of the frequency of 'ectopy' and the risk for the future development of LGSIL. On the other hand, the proclivity of the squamous metaplastic process was strongly associated with LGSIL development. To study further the effect of the propensity for the development of squamous metaplasia and LGSIL, the study measured the alteration in the size of the transformation zone over time. The rate of squamous metaplastic development was defined by the extent of the changes visualised within the area of the transformation zone, especially in relation to the precise stages of the process as described in Figure 6.2, stages 1–3. Obviously, this was between two points in time. The interpretation of this variable was based on the premise that changes from larger areas of immaturity to smaller areas reflect an active process of maturation, resulting in a reduction in the area covered by immature metaplastic epithelium. After correcting for the presence of HPV, the odds ratio (OR) for every 10% change in immaturity was 4.0 [95% confidence interval (CI) 1.45–10.79]. In other words, if a woman had a relatively large area of change, such as 30% reduction in the area of immaturity, she had a 12-fold chance of developing LGSIL. Therefore, it appears that recent active squamous metaplasia development in the face of an HPV infection, and not the original size of the cervical transformation zone, is a risk factor for the development of LGSIL-associated atypical epithelium.

Several questions arise here: 'Does HPV itself stimulate change or vice versa?' The oncoproteins E6 and E7 (Chapter 19) are known to enhance cell proliferation and may lead to enhanced transformation, inducing the process of squamous metaplasia. This might suggest that all women with HPV E6/E7 expression develop LGSIL. However, the greater incidence of HPV infection compared with SIL in young women supports the premise that HPV requires other cofactors for SIL to develop (Moscicki *et al.*, 2001b). In turn, if we believe that women with squamous metaplasia are vulnerable to HPV and LGSIL development, the high rates of HPV and LGSIL in adolescent populations support the notion that rates of squamous metaplasia are also high in this age group. Active squamous metaplasia may support viral replication and protein transcription and, consequently, result in cytological changes consistent with LGSIL. These high rates of LGSIL most probably help to explain the presence of atypical epithelium in adolescents. Whether the metaplastic process was induced by HPV or whether the metaplasia was due to other factors remains unknown. It is certainly feasible

Table 6.4 Univariate and multivariate analysis examining risks for the presence of incidence atypical epithelium* in a cohort with normal cytology†.

Variable	RH	95% CI	P-value
Univariate analysis			
HPV status at visit	2.05	1.29, 3.27	0.003
Presence of HPV 16-like	1.51	1.15, 1.98	0.003
Presence of HPV 18-like	1.48	1.16, 1.90	0.002
Presence of HPV 53/56/66	1.50	1.18, 1.91	0.0008
Bacterial vaginosis	4.5	2.66, 18.36	0.04
History of STI	2.09	1.04, 4.22	0.04
Reid score of 4 at prior visit	1.34	1.17, 1.53	< 0.0001
Number of years sexually active	0.82	0.72, 0.92	0.001
Number of years since menarche	0.88	0.80, 0.96	0.006
Multivariate analysis			
HPV status at visit	1.90	1.19, 3.05	0.006
Bacterial vaginosis at visit	5.10	1.24, 20.95	0.02
History of STI	1.64	0.79, 3.40	0.18
Reid score of 4 at prior visit	1.36	1.18, 1.55	< 0.0001
Number of years sexually active	0.82	0.71, 0.95	0.009
Number of years since menarche	0.95	0.85, 1.06	0.40

*Atypical epithelium was based on colposcopic score (Reid score) of 5 or more. (Moscicki, 1995)
†Subjects with cytological ASCUS or worse at incident event were excluded.
RH, relative hazard.

to conjecture HPV inducing metaplasia in order to support its own replicative process.

To investigate the association between HPV and atypical epithelium more closely, Moscicki *et al.* (1993) examined 84 young sexually active women aged 13–22 years of age who were attending family planning clinics for health care. The majority were seen for annual health examinations. Baseline colposcopic examinations were performed by one of three trained nurse practitioners with the aid of 3% acetic acid and Lugol's solution without knowledge of HPV DNA status. Colposcopic examination noted the presence of atypical epithelium by scoring the presence of vascularity, acetowhiteness, Lugol's staining and the contour of the area of aceto-whiteness, if present. Women with HPV 16/18 were more likely to have an atypical transformation zone identified and were more likely to have higher atypia scores based on the severity of the vasculature, acetowhiteness, Lugol's staining and contour. In the subjects who had atypical epithelium with scores of 6 or more and were biopsied (*n* = 8), three had SIL on biopsy, and three had a stage referred to as 'atypical squamous metaplasia', one had a condyloma acuminatum, and one had acute and chronic inflammation. This study suggested that HPV is associated with atypical epithelium development even in the presence of normal cytology. Unfortunately, this study used a relatively insensitive test for HPV (ViraPap; Digene Diagnostics) and the study was cross-sectional, thus limiting any conclusions.

Other factors

To investigate factors that may also influence the development of atypical epithelium, an analysis was performed to examine risk factors for the incident development of atypical epithelium within the transformation zone of the adolescent cervix (Table 6.4). Using the longitudinal cohort described above (Moscicki, personal communication, 2003), the degree of atypicality within this epithelium was defined colposcopically using a combination of colposcopic criteria (described elsewhere, see above). The so-called Reid colposcopic criteria on which this analysis was performed studied such features of the transformation zone as atypical vasculature (punctation/mosaicism), contour, acetowhiteness and staining in respect of Lugol's iodine (Reid *et al.*, 1984).

Colposcopic examination using acetic acid and Lugol's solution was performed at baseline and at every 4- to 6-month interval visit. Not surprisingly, univariate analysis showed that atypical squamous metaplasia defined by colposcopy was strongly associated with the presence of abnormal cytology including atypical squamous cells of uncertain significance (ASCUS). For analysis, women were excluded who had atypical epithelium at baseline. In addition, all subjects who had abnormal cytology (ASCUS or greater) at the time of the incident atypia were also excluded. Univariate analysis found several factors associated with incident atypical epithelium, which included the presence of HPV infection, the presence of bacterial vaginosis, number of years sexually active, ever having had an STI and number of years since menarche (Table 6.4). However, in multivariate analysis, only HPV as well as the presence of bacterial vaginosis and number of years sexually active continued to have a strong association with atypia (see Table 6.4). The duration of years of sexual activity is interesting as the longer the subject had been sexually active, the less likely she was to have an incident atypia, suggesting that the sexually inexperienced cervix is more vulnerable to the development of atypia. Perhaps rates of squamous metaplasia are greater in this group or immunological factors are more immature. It was also interesting that all HPV types including HPV 16-like, HPV 18-like and low-risk types were also associated with incident atypia. Other risk factors, including age, cigarette use and hormonal contraception, were not associated with atypia.

Summary

In summary, these data suggest that the majority of atypical epithelium in adolescents can be explained by HPV infection with or without the development of abnormal cytology. Changes in the vaginal microenvironment resulting from bacterial vaginosis also appear to play a role in inducing atypical epithelium. Finally, vulnerability to atypical epithelium without evidence of abnormal cytology occurs shortly after the onset of intercourse and the risk decreases with increasing sexual experience. This was supported by the study by Moscicki *et al.* (2001a) described above in which adolescents with more years of sexual experience were less likely to have atypical epithelium than those with fewer years of sexual experience.

FACTORS INFLUENCING THE EPITHELIAL COMPOSITION OF THE ADOLESCENT CERVIX

In reviewing the data presented above, it is clear that both pubertal hormones and sexual activity effect cervical epithelial changes. Premenarchial children have a predominance of original (native) squamous epithelium covering the cervix with subsequent predominance in squamous metaplastic epithelium. As described above, there is an assumption that the process of eversion occurs as a result of endogenous hormonal increases, which in turn results in exposure of the everted original (native) columnar epithelium to the more acidic vaginal environment influencing the process of squamous metaplasia. Consequently, the postmenarchial cervix is predominantly composed of original columnar and mixed squamous metaplastic tissues (early, mid and late). With the onset of sexual activity, tissue composed of the more mature squamous metaplastic epithelium is increasingly prevalent. Whether this process is due to a phenomenon of retraction, a process to be discussed below, or is a result of accelerated metaplastic process is controversial. Some evidence suggests that numerous events may promote the formation of squam-

ous epithelium from the original columnar epithelium by accelerating the squamous metaplastic transformation process. This development has been examined both colposcopically and microscopically. However, conclusions from these studies are limited because of the lack of adequate hormonal level measurements, STD testing and adequate longitudinal follow-up of individuals.

The effect of the menarche

The presence of metaplastic squamous epithelium in the virginal cervix raises the prospect of its formation having occurred as a result of the menarche. Studies have been performed that tend to support this contention. In one of these, the unique post-mortem material from the cervix and upper vagina of some 64 pre- and postmenarchial girls collected by Dr Ellis Pixley in Australia (as described in Chapter 5 and the addendum to that chapter) has been studied. Pixley (1967, 1971) obtained colpophotographic records of the tissue soon after removal. He classified the cervices into two types according to the degree of endocervical eversion, as determined from the colpophotographs taken of cervices in the lateral or planar views (Fig. 6.12). The type 1 position was one in which the squamocolumnar junction was situated within the endocervical canal with original squamous epithelium covering the endocervix. In type 2, the squamocolumnar junction occupied an ectocervical position with variable amounts of original squamous, columnar and metaplastic squamous tissue covering the ectocervix. The colpophotographs taken by Pixley of 36 girls between 10 and 13 years and 28 between 14 and 16 years of age were reviewed by Singer (1972). The age of menarche was known in 26 instances, with the mean being 13.9 years. The whole group for the purpose of this study was divided into two (below and above 14 years of age), which corresponded broadly to the pre- and postmenarchial groups.

The results, as seen in Figure 6.12, show the significant change in frequency of cervical types between the pre- and postmenarchial groups. Twenty-eight per cent of the premenarchial cervices contained type 1 configuration. As a result of the menarche, however, this type accounted for only 12% whereas type 2 cervix increased from a frequency of 72% in the premenarchial era to 88% after the menarche. This suggests that the endocervical tissue becomes everted and adopts an ectocervical position, analogous to the situation occurring during the first pregnancy (Coppleson and Reid, 1967; Coppleson *et al.*, 1971). In this position, the former endocervical tissue, which is usually composed of original columnar epithelium, is subjected to the newly developing vaginal fluid with its acidic pH. It is believed that the contact provides the stimulus for the formation of the metaplastic squamous epithelium (Walz, 1958; Reid *et al.*, 1971). This eversion process is most probably the result of increased intracervical oedema caused by the newly secreted estrogenic and progestogenic hormones. As the

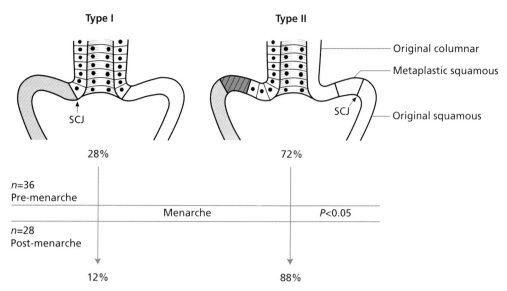

Fig. 6.12 Degree of endocervical epithelial eversion induced by the menarche. SCJ, squamocolumnar junction.

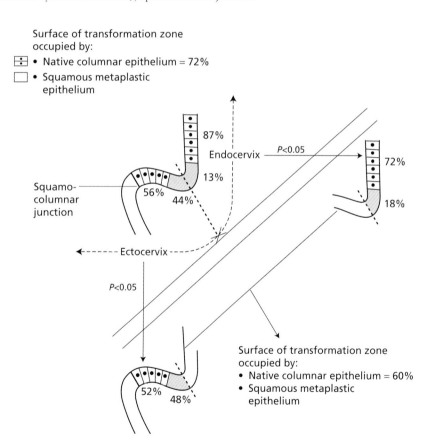

Fig. 6.13 Epithelial surface changes induced
by the menarche.

cervix is attached at a fixed point to the vagina, there is only one direction that this enlarged cervix can expand into, and that is in a caudal and outwards direction by an everting mechanism, as has been described previously (Fig. 6.13).

In further study of Pixley's material of virginal cervices, Singer (1972) calculated semi-quantitatively the area occu-

pied by the different epithelia within the transformation zone using the thick, histological sagittal section of the whole cervix. In Figure 6.13, the effect of the menarche on the composition of epithelial types on both the endo- and the ectocervix is seen. The premenarchial cervix was composed essentially of original columnar epithelium (i.e. 72%), the majority of which was present within the endocervix. After the menarche (simultaneously with the eversion process and the facilitated access of acidic vaginal fluid to the columnar epithelium), the amount of original columnar epithelium decreases (i.e. 72% to 60%) as the development of metaplastic squamous epithelium increases (from 28% to 40%).

The presence of recently formed metaplastic squamous epithelium in the adolescent cervix is to some extent a result of the menarche. However, the excess amount of this tissue found in the transformation zone of the sexually active adolescent, as described previously, has probably arisen as a result of coitus and its accompaniments, i.e. constituents of semen and/or sexually transmitted infections. This factor is the only major variation existing between these two otherwise comparable groups. The stimulus to the formation of the metaplastic squamous epithelium can only be speculated upon. Indeed, it would not have been surprising, in view of the reduction in the area of the transformation zone of the sexually experienced adolescent, to expect a small rather than a large amount of metaplastic squamous epithelium within the transformation zone. It could be that some substance in semen, e.g. prostaglandins, stimulates the development of this tissue in the coitally active girl. Prostaglandins have profound metabolic effects, especially intracellularly, where they stimulate glucose utilisation. The action of cervically or vaginally absorbed prostaglandins (von Euler and Eliasson, 1967; Goshowaki *et al.*, 1988) could be assumed to account for the increase seen in the activity of cervical stromal cells or indeed subepithelial stem-like reserve cells that are evident during the early stages of metaplastic development (Reid *et al.*, 1967, 1971). However, there are no studies to support this assumption. Indeed, Reid *et al.* (1967a,b) and Singer *et al.* (1968) showed that, when examining stages of experimentally induced squamous metaplasia, those cells in the stromal aspects of the new squamous epithelium appeared to be incorporated into this epithelium by the fusion of their periodic acid–Schiff (PAS)-positive capsules with the subsequent disappearance of this capsule around most of the cells other than on its stromal side. These new cells appeared as though they were subepithelial stem-like reserve cells that are described in sections of newly developed metaplastic epithelium. It may be that these stromal cells or, indeed, the later developed epithelial stem-like reserve cells could be the progenitor cells of the new metaplastic epithelium (Coppleson and Reid, 1975), as has also been suggested by other authors (Elson *et al.*, 2000). It could be speculated that these cells may have a role to play in the later development of neoplasia.

Unfortunately, these studies have not been repeated in more recent cohorts with the same detail, thus limiting comparisons. Specifically, recent data on premenarchial or non-sexually active adolescents are lacking. Madile (1976) examined the post-mortem histopathology of 164 girls from birth to 11 years of age. Unfortunately, children from 13 months to 11 years were reported collectively and the hormonal status of the older children was not described. The study found that 'ectopy' was present in 29% of premature infants, whereas 68% of 0- to 1-month-old infants had 'ectopy'. This reversed again after 12 months of age, at which time only one-third of the infants had 'ectopy'. This would suggest that two-thirds of young girls enter puberty with the squamocolumnar junction within the endocervix. There are striking similarities between the transition noted from premature to neonatal infants and the transition from premenarchial to postmenarchial noted in the studies above. The rate of 'ectopy' in premature and premenarchial children is almost identical, and the rate of 'ectopy' (including squamous metaplasia) was similar in the neonates and postmenarchial girls. This study suggested that maternal hormones cause hyperactivity of columnar epithelium and growth of the endocervix, the portio vaginalis and the supravaginal segment of the cervix. These findings are not dissimilar from those described by Pixley in the previous chapter and the addendum to that chapter. The mechanisms that result in adolescent 'ectopy' are unknown. However, similar rises in estrogen in the perimenarchial child may explain the eversion of original columnar epithelium that occurs postmenarchially, a role that may influence cervical epithelial composition. These levels of hormones were not measured consistently in older studies. In addition, sexual practices and the composition of hormonal contraceptives have changed dramatically over the last few decades. Studies described previously for the epithelial composition of the cervix of a virginal girl have not been replicated.

To examine the factors associated with the presence of early squamous metaplasia in a more recent cohort, Moscicki (personal communication, 2003) performed a risk factor analysis in the longitudinal cohort described above. Multivariate analysis showed that the only factor associated with the presence of early squamous metaplasia was an inverse association with years of sexual activity (Table 6.5). That is, the longer a girl had been sexually active, the less likely early squamous metaplasia was identified by colposcopy. This strongly suggests that factors associated with sexual activity such as exposure to semen, trauma and sexually transmitted infections enhance the process of maturation associated with squamous metaplasia.

As the cervix matures, there would be an expectation that the proportion of mature metaplastic squamous epithelium would increase. In Singer's (1975a) study, there was no significant difference in the amount of this epithelium as assessed planimetrically between the virginal and the sexually active girls' cervices. It may be that this tissue has remained from the metaplastic epithelium originally laid down in late intrauterine life. Song (1964), Linhartova (1970) and Pixley in the preceding chapter have all shown its existence in fetal life, and Pixley (1967) believed that its quantity does not change significantly from birth to menarche. Data from

Moscicki's longitudinal cohort show that 83% of cervices from sexually active adolescents had evidence of late squamous metaplasia and 38% of the cervices had only mature squamous metaplasia (Table 6.3). These figures are higher than those reported in Singer's study, where only 25% of the sexually active girls had mature squamous metaplasia (Table 6.1). Moscicki's group may have been sexually active longer than Singer's, which may explain these differences.

The effect of sexual behaviour: sexual partners: oral contraception and infection

Factors associated with sexual risk behaviour have been thought to affect the development of the transformation zone by exposing the cervix to infections, douching practices and the use of hormonal contraceptives (Table 6.5). A recent study by Moscicki *et al.* (2001a) examined factors associated with the presence of 'ectopy', the transformation zone composed of a mixture of original columnar and early/mid-squamous metaplasia in high-risk sexually active girls. Two-thirds of the girls were HIV infected. Univariate analysis showed that 'ectopy' was associated with HIV status, recent oral contraceptive use and number of lifetime partners. However, multivariate logistic regression analysis found that only the number of lifetime sexual partners remained significantly associated with 'ectopy'. This association was inversely related, in that subjects who had more than 10 lifetime sexual partners were less likely to have 'ectopy' [OR =

Table 6.5 Risk factor analysis for presence of 'ectopy' (columnar/early metaplasia) at baseline visit.

Variable	Test used	P-value using esm
Age at baseline	Wilcoxon	0.04
Age at menarche	Wilcoxon	0.57
Years since menarche	Wilcoxon	0.19
Number of lifetime sex partners	Wilcoxon	0.08
Number of recent (new) partners	Wilcoxon	0.28
Years sexually active	Wilcoxon	0.03
Current OC use	χ^2	0.10
Total months of OC use	Wilcoxon	0.08
Daily cigarette smoking	Fisher's exact	0.36
History of Ct or Gc infection	Fisher's exact	0.34
Chlamydia at visit	Fisher's exact	0.59
HPV at visit*	χ^2	0.12
History of HSV†		
Atypia on cytology	Fisher's exact	0.81
LGSIL on cytology	Fisher's exact	1.00

*Twelve observations out of 95 missing.

†None of these women had a history of herpes simplex virus (HSV) infection.

Ct, *Chlamydia trachomatis*; Gc, *Neisseria gonorrhoeae*.

0.47; 95% confidence interval (CI) 0.22–1.00; $P = 0.05$]. This finding is consistent with the finding that exposure to a large number of partners results in a more 'mature' transformation zone. As the multilayered squamous epithelium is less fragile than columnar epithelium, the influence of sexual behaviour on maturation seems logical. The actual cause of the acceleration of metaplasia, however, remains unknown. Schacter *et al.* (1975) showed that chlamydia infection may enhance squamous metaplasia through repeated episodes of cellular repair (Moscicki *et al.*, 1999).

To examine the relationship between the development of squamous metaplasia and oral contraceptive (OC) use and STI, two separate groups were selected from the longitudinal cohort described by Moscicki *et al.* (1999): women who had computerised measurements of the cervix and had (a) an incident STI (chlamydia or gonorrhoea or trichomonas) and (b) began OCs during the study. This allowed us to examine the parallel association between squamous metaplasia and the initiation of OC use and/or STI. Sixteen subjects had photographs of the cervix available for measurement both before and after an incident case of STI. The median percentage change in 'ectopy' was a decrease of 42% between the visit with the infection and the postinfection visit (an average of 4 months later). The interquartile range was −62% to −15%. This suggests that infection with STI may, in fact, induce squamous metaplasia through cellular repair, leading to enhanced maturation of the transformation zone.

We also examined the role of OCs. Examining only women on whom Moscicki *et al.* (1999) had data both before and after initiation, we found no association with OC use and change in 'ectopy', suggesting that the current OCs with low-dose estrogens do not result in eversion. The median percentage change from before to after the initiation of OC was a decrease of 25.89% (ranging from a decrease of 82.45% to an increase of 24.55%). Figures 6.14a–c and 6.15a–c show two young women before and after starting OC use.

Another possible explanation for changes: the retraction theory

Clearly, the presence of congenital 'ectopy' has been established, with at least one-third of neonates displaying 'ectopy'. However, congenital ectopies are also known to disappear. Studies of prepubertal girls have suggested that 'ectopy' reverts with only original (native) squamous epithelium present on the ectocervix. As discussed above, the question remains whether 'ectopy' in puberty is congenital or develops at the time by eversion of the endocervical mucous [i.e. original (native) columnar] epithelium or as a result of shortening of the outer portion of the cervix in comparison with the growth of the inner portions: a form of retraction. Madile's (1976) study showing that 'ectopy' was much more common in the neonate than in the infant older than 12 months

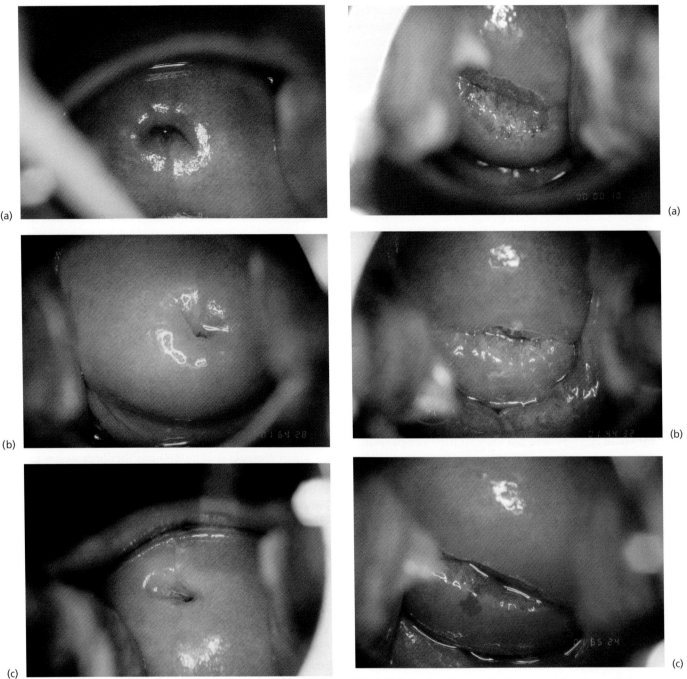

Fig. 6.14 Effect of oral contraception on the cervix. (a) Before starting; (b) 4 months after starting oral contraceptive usage; (c) 4 months after stopping oral contraceptive usage.

Fig. 6.15 Reflection of changes in the cervix with oral contraceptive use. (a) Before starting; (b) 10 months after starting oral contraceptive usage; (c) 8 months after stopping oral contraceptive usage.

strongly suggests that some cervices do undergo such a 'retraction' process.

Only one study (Singer, 1975a) has assessed the area of the adolescent transformation zone in virginal adolescents. In this study, comparison was made between the colpophotographic planimetric measurements of 40 virginal cervices and a ran-domly selected group of 170 out of the 300 sexually active Australian girls from the Coppleson study described above. The results, seen in Table 6.1, showed that the transformation zone of the virginal cervix was about 60% larger in area in vir-ginal adolescents than in sexually active girls. The difference was significant ($P < 0.01$).

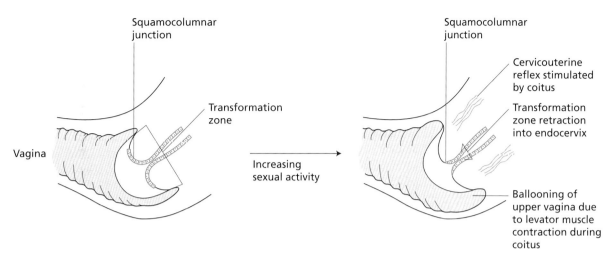

Fig. 6.16 Speculative diagrammatic presentation of the possible effect of coitus upon the position of the transformation zone, induced by retraction of the original squamocolumnar junction to within the endocervix.

The presence of mature squamous epithelium on the adolescent cervix is either due to maturation of columnar epithelium secondary to metaplasia or reflective of the presence of original squamous epithelium at this site. Seventy girls (42%) had an atypical transformation zone, and it was the impression that the majority of the area of this zone was situated within the endocervix. Similarly, of the 156 young prostitutes (mean age 24.5 years) also colposcoped in the same establishment, no fewer than 30 (24%) had evidence of withdrawal of the epithelium to within the endocervix, a condition that may have resulted from a form of retraction of the respective epithelial types. Both these studies support the notion that rapid squamous metaplasia occurred with the development of associated atypical epithelium.

Youssef (1957) reported a similar colposcopic picture with the squamocolumnar junction found completely within the endocervical canal in 12% of cervices (Fig. 6.7). It is therefore possible that this finding in some women results from some form of retractive process, similar to that occurring in the postmenopausal woman, in whom the transformation zone is 'taken back' into the endocervix.

To explain these changes it is necessary to examine the effect of coitus on cervical morphology. Masters and Johnson (1970) provided preliminary evidence that sensory and physiological stimuli, as well as local and reflex actions, may be operating in the genital tract during coitus. It seems as though the sensory signals travel via the sacral segments of the spinal cord through the pudendal nerve and sacral plexus before being transmitted to the cerebrum. These reflexes are also associated with local reflexes that are integrated with the sacral and lumber spinal cord (Janig 1996).

Over the last 14 years Shafik (1993, 1995a–c; Shafik *et al.*, 2005) has suggested no fewer than five reflexes, induced by coitus that may have an effect on the cervix, these acting via stimulation of various pelvic muscles. He has hypothesised that cervical buffeting during coitus effects a reflex pathway that exists between the smooth muscle of the corpus uteri and the cervix. A recent study (Shafik 2005) has shown that there is diminished electrical activity and pressure in the area of the uterine corpus which effects uterine wall relaxation and is associated with a decline in interuterine pressure, aiding possible semen siphonage from the vagina into the uterus. He believes that this reflex is mediated via the cervicouterine inhibitory reflex that is evoked by penile thrusting. Previous studies have demonstrated that this act also evokes reflexes associated with the clitoris and with the lavator pelvic muscles resulting in the upward and lateral retraction of the upper vaginal walls and fornices, and according to Shafik (1995c) and Shafik *et al.* (2005) these events lead to dilatation of the upper vagina, which in turn acts as a receptacle for semen collection. It could be speculated that contraction of these pelvic muscles, be it the puborectalus or the levator can have an effect on the shape of the cervix with a possible resulting retraction of the original squamocolumnar junction to within the endocervix.

In summary, the aetiological factors that could be operating to produce this retractive process, for example in the sexually active population described above, can only be speculated upon at this stage and are summarised diagrammatically in Figure 6.16.

SUMMARY

In summary, it appears that the majority of children enter puberty with cervices covered predominantly with original (native) squamous epithelium. The hormonal influences seen at puberty, which parallel these at birth, result in an eversion with increased exposure of original (native) columnar epithelium. As the majority of cervices seen in adolescents are of mixed epithelial types, hormonal influences most probably cause eversion and squamous metaplasia almost simultaneously.

Exposure of this columnar epithelium to the acidic nature of the vagina or to the vaginal microenvironment may also induce metaplasia. Clearly, sexual activity and exposure to STIs such as *C. trachomatis* also appear to influence the rate of squamous metaplastic activity. The role of HPV in the development of squamous metaplasia remains to be elucidated; HPV may enhance squamous metaplasia in order to support its replicative process. In turn, squamous metaplasia may support HPV replication through its natural processes of proliferations and differentiation. HPV, however, appears to be strongly associated with the development of atypical epithelium.

REFERENCES

Albertsson-Wikland K, Rosberg S, Karlberg J *et al.* (1994) Analysis of 24-hour growth hormone profiles in healthy boys and girls of normal stature: relation to puberty. *Journal of Clinical Endocrinology and Metabolism* 78: 1195–1201.

Apter D, Vihko R (1977) Serum pregnenolone, progesterone, 17-hydroxyprogesterone, testosterone and 5 alpha-dihydrotestosterone during female puberty. *Journal of Clinical Endocrinology and Metabolism* 45: 1039–1048.

Apter D, Pakarinen A, Hammond GL *et al.* (1979) Adrenocortical function in puberty. Serum ACTH, cortisol and dehydroepiandrosterone in girls and boys. *Acta Paediatrica Scandinavica* 68: 599–604.

Apter D, Butzow TL, Laughlin GA *et al.* (1993). Gonadotropin-releasing hormone pulse generator activity during pubertal transition in girls: pulsatile and diurnal patterns of circulating gonadotropins. *Journal of Clinical Endocrinology and Metabolism* 76: 940–949.

Arnett JJ (2000). Emerging adulthood. A theory of development from the late teens through the twenties. *American Psychologist* 55: 469–480.

Bloch CA, Clemons P, Sperling MA (1987). Puberty decreases insulin activity. *Journal of Pediatrics* 11: 481–487.

Bridges NA, Cooke A, Healy MJ *et al.* (1996) Growth of the uterus. *Archives of the Diseases of Childhood* 75: 330–331.

Buzi F, Pilotta A, Dordoni D *et al.* (1998) Pelvic ultrasonography in normal girls and in girls with pubertal precocity. *Acta Paediatrica* 87: 1138–1145.

CDC (2001) *Sexually Transmitted Diseases Surveillance Report, 2001.* Atlanta, GA: Centers for Disease Control, Division of STD Prevention.

Coppleson M (1977) Colposcopy. In: Stallworthy J, Bourne G (eds) *Recent Advances in Obstetrics and Gynaecology.* London: Churchill Livingstone.

Coppleson M, Reid B (1967) *Preclinical Carcinoma of the Cervix Uteri,* Vol. 1. Oxford: Pergamon Press.

Coppleson M, Reid B (1975) The origin of premalignant lesions of the cervix uteri. In: Taymor ML, Green TH (eds) *Progress in Gynecology,* Vol. 6. New York: Grune and Stratton, Ch. 24.

Coppleson M, Pixley E, Reid B (1971) *Colposcopy: A Scientific Approach to the Cervix in Health and Disease,* Vol. 1. Springfield, IL: Charles C. Thomas.

Crompton AC (1973) Quoted in Epithelial abnormalities of the cervix uteri. In: Langley FA, Crompton AC (eds) *Recent Results in Cancer Research,* Vol. 40. Berlin: Springer Verlag, p. 53.

Damon W (1999) The role of peer group stability and change in adolescent social identity. *New Directions in Child and Adolescent Development* 1–8.

Elson DA, Raleigh RR, Lacey A *et al.* (2000) Sensitivity of the cervical transformation zone to oestrogen-induced squamous carcinogenesis. *Cancer Research* 60 (5): 1267–1275.

von Euler V, Eliasson R (1967) *Prostaglandins,* Vol. 1. New York: Academic Press, pp. 125–126.

Fluhmann C (1961) *The Cervix Uteri: Diseases.* Philadelphia: Saunders.

Friedell GH, Hertig AT, Younge PA (1960) *Carcinoma* In Situ *of the Uterine Cervix.* Springfield, IL: Charles C. Thomas.

Glatthaar E (1950). *Studies on the Morphology of the Surface Changes on the Vaginal Portio of the Uterus.* Basle: Karger, pp. 77–79.

Glucksmann A, Cherry C (1964) In: Gary L (ed.) *Dysplasia, Carcinoma In Situ and Microinvasive Carcinoma of the Cervix Uteri.* Springfield, IL: Charles C. Thomas, p. 351.

Goshowaki H, Ito A, Mori Y (1988) Effect of prostaglandins on the production of collagenase by rabbit uterine cervical fibroblasts. *Prostaglandins* 36: 107–114.

Govan AD, Haines RM, Langley F *et al.* (1966) Changes in the epithelium of the cervix uteri. *Journal of Obstetrics and Gynaecology of the British Commonwealth* 73: 886–896.

Grumbach MM, Kaplan SL (1990) The neuroendocrinology of human puberty: an ontogenetic perspective. In: Grumbach MM, Sizonenko PC, Aubert ML (eds) *Control of the Onset of Puberty.* Baltimore: Williams and Wilkins, pp. 1–68.

Grumbach MM, Sizonenko PC, Aubert ML (eds) (2000) *Control of the Onset of Puberty.* Baltimore, MD: Williams and Wilkins.

Gruengagel HH (1957) Die Plattenepithel-Zylinderepithelgrenze an der Portio vaginalis uteri bei unreifen und reifen Neugeorenen, Sauglingen und Kindern bis zu neun Jahren. *Frankfurter Zeitschrift für Pathologie* 68: 465–496.

Hamperl H, Kaufmann C (1959) The cervix uteri at different ages. *Obstetrics and Gynecology* 14: 621.

Harrison HR, Costin M, Meder JB *et al.* (1985) Cervical *Chlamydia trachomatis* infection in university women: relationship to history, contraception, ectopy and cervicitis. *American Journal of Obstetrics and Gynecology* 153: 244–251.

Huffman JW (1948) Mesonephric remnants in the cervix. *American Journal of Obstetrics and Gynecology* 56: 23–40.

Janig W (1996) Behavioural and neurovegetative components of reproductive functions. In: Gregor R, Winhorst U (eds) *Comprehensive Human Physiology: From Cellular Mechanisms to Integration.* Berlin: Springer-Verlag, pp. 2253–2263.

Kaufmann C, Ober K (1959) Morphological changes of the cervix uteri with age and their significance in the early diagnosis of carcinoma. In: Wolstenholme GE, O'Connor M (eds) *Cancer of the Cervix; Diagnosis and Early Forms.* London: Churchill, pp. 61–65.

Kolstad P, Stafl A (1982) *Atlas of Colposcopy,* 3rd edn. Edinburgh: Churchill Livingstone, p. 48.

Linhartova A (1970) Congenital ectopy of the uterine cervix. *International Journal of Gynaecology and Obstetrics* 8: 653–660.

Madile BM (1976) The cervical epithelium from fetal age to adolescence. *Obstetrics and Gynecology* 47: 536–539.

Marshall JC, Kelch RP (1986) Gonadotropin-releasing hormone: role of pulsatile secretion in the regulation of reproduction. *New England Journal of Medicine* 315: 1459.

Masters WA, Johnson VG (1970) *Human Sexual Inadequacy.* Boston, MA: LittleBrown.

Moscicki AB, Palefsky J, Gonzales J *et al.* (1990) Human papillomavirus infection in sexually active adolescent females: prevalence and risk factors. *Pediatric Research* 28: 507–513.

Moscicki AB, Broering J, Powell K *et al.* (1993) Comparison between colposcopic, cytologic, and histologic findings in women positive and negative for human papillomavirus DNA. *Journal of Adolescent Health* 14: 71–79.

Moscicki AB, Shiboski S, Broering J *et al.* (1998) The natural history of human papillomavirus infection as measured by repeated DNA testing in adolescent and young women. *Journal of Pediatrics* 132: 277–284.

Moscicki AB, Grubbs-Burt V, Kanowitz S *et al.* (1999) The significance of squamous metaplasia in the development of low grade squamous intra-epithelial lesions in young women. *Cancer* 85: 1139–1144.

Moscicki AB, Ellenberg JH, Vermund SH *et al.* (2000) Prevalence of and risks for cervical human papillomavirus infection and squamous intraepithelial lesions in adolescent girls: impact of infection with human immunodeficiency virus. *Archives of Pediatric and Adolescent Medicine* 154: 127–134.

Moscicki AB, Ma Y, Holland C *et al.* (2001a) Cervical ectopy in adolescent girls with and without human immunodeficiency virus infection. *Journal of Infectious Diseases* 183: 865–870.

Moscicki AB, Hills N, Shiboski S *et al.* (2001b) Risks for incident human papillomavirus infection and low-grade squamous intraepithelial lesion development in young females. *Journal of the American Medical Association* 285: 2995–3002.

Moscicki AB (2005) Cervical cytology testing in teens. *Current Opinion in Obstetrics and Gynecology* 17: 471–475.

O'Rahilly R (1973) The development of the uterus in late fetal life, infancy, and childhood. In: Norris HJ, Hertig AT, Abell MR (eds) *The Uterus.* Baltimore: Williams and Wilkins.

Pearce WA, Buchanan TM (1978) Attachment role of gonococcal pili: optimum conditions and quantitation of adherence of isolated pili T-human cells in vitro. *Journal of Clinical Investigation* 61: 931.

Pixley E (1967) The cervix during foetal life and the prepubertal era. In: Coppleson M, Reid B (eds) *Preclinical Carcinoma of the Cervix Uteri,* Vol. 1. Oxford: Pergamon, p. 96.

Pixley E (1971) Natural history of squamous metaplasia and the transformation zone. In: Coppleson M, Pixley E, Reid B (eds) *Colposcopy: a Scientific Approach to the Cervix in Health and Disease,* Vol. 1. Springfield, IL: Charles C. Thomas, p. 77.

Rawls WE, Gardiner HL (1972) Herpes genitalis: venereal aspects. *Clinics in Obstetrics and Gynecology* 15: 912–918.

Redondo-Lopez V, Cook RL, Sobel JD (1990) Emerging role of lactobacilli in the control and maintenance of the vaginal bacterial microflora. *Review of Infectious Diseases* 12: 856–872.

Reid BL, Coppleson M (1971) Natural history of the origins of cervical cancer. In: McDonald R (ed.) *Scientific Basis of Obstetrics and Gynecology,* Vol. 1. London: Churchill.

Reid BL, Singer A, Coppleson M (1967a) The process of cervical regeneration after electrocauterisation. Part I. Histological and colposcopic

study. *Australian and New Zealand Journal of Obstetrics and Gynaecology* 7 (3): 125–135.

Reid BL, Singer A, Coppleson M (1967b) The process of cervical regeneration after electrocauterisation. Part II. Histochemical, autoradiographic and pH study. *Australian and New Zealand Journal of Obstetrics and Gynaecology* 7 (3): 136–143.

Reid R, Stanhope C, Herschman B *et al.* (1984) Genital warts and cervical cancer. IV. A colposcopic index for differentiating subclinical papillomaviral infection from cervical intraepithelial neoplasia. *American Journal of Obstetrics and Gynecology* 149: 815–823.

Remoue F, Jacobs N, Miot V *et al.* (2003) High intraepithelial expression of estrogen and progesterone receptors in the transformation zone of the uterine cervix. *American Journal of Obstetrics and Gynecology* 189: 1660–1665.

Schachter J, Hill EC, King EB *et al.* (1975) Chlamydial infection in women with cervical dysplasia. *American Journal of Obstetrics and Gynecology* 123: 753–757.

Shafik A (1993) The cervico-cavernosus reflex: description of the reflex and its role in the sexual act. *International Urogynecological Journal* 4: 70–73.

Shafik A (1995a) Vagino-levator reflex: description of a reflex and its role in sexual performance. *European Journal of Obstetrics, Gynecology and Reproductive Biology* 60: 161–164.

Shafik A (1995b) The clitoromotor reflex. *International Urogynecological Journal* 6: 329–335.

Shafik A (1995c) Vagino-puborectalis reflex: the description of a new reflex and its clinical significance. *International Journal of Gynecology and Obstetrics* 51: 61–63.

Shafik A, Olfat ES, Shafik I *et al.* (2005) Uterine effect of cervical buffeting: role of cervicouterine reflex in coitus. *Journal of Reproductive Medicine* 50: 837–843.

Singer A (1972) The effect of physiological and pathological factors in the cervix uteri. PhD Thesis. University of Sydney, Australia.

Singer A (1975a) Cervical dysplasia in young women. *Proceedings of the Royal Society of Medicine* 68: 14.

Singer A (1975b) The uterine cervix from adolescence to the menopause. *British Journal of Obstetrics and Gynaecology* 82: 81–99.

Singer A, Monaghan J (2000) Diagnosis of cervical precancer: cytology colposcopy and pathology. In: Singer A, Monaghan J (eds) *Lower Genital Tract Precancer.* Oxford: Blackwell Publishing.

Singer A, Reid B, Coppleson M (1968) The role of peritoneal mononuclear cells in the regeneration of the uterine epithelium of the rat. *Australian and New Zealand Journal of Obstetrics and Gynaecology* 8 (4): 163–170.

Song J (1964) *The Human Uterus,* Vol. 1. Springfield, IL: Charles C. Thomas, p. 98.

Stafl A, Mattingly RF (1975). Angiogenesis of cervical neoplasia. *American Journal of Obstetrics and Gynecology* 121: 845–852.

Walz W (1958) Über die Genese der Sogenannten Indirekten Metaplasie im Bereich der Mullerschen Gang Systems. *Zeitschrift fur Geburtshilfe und Gynäkologie* 151: 1–21.

Youssef A (1957) Colposcopy: results in 1000 cases. *Journal of Obstetrics and Gynecology of the British Empire* 64: 801–814.

CHAPTER 7

The cervical epithelium and subepithelium during pregnancy and the puerperium

Albert Singer

Pregnancy and delivery have a profound effect on the cervical epithelium and its subepithelial tissues. The changes occurring during pregnancy prepare the cervix for the enormous physiological task that it must perform during labour when its diameter alone increases 10-fold. There are few organs in the body that exhibit the ability to perform such dramatic changes in so short a span of time. Furthermore, the relative infrequency of long-term damage to the cervix emphasises the physiological propensities of this organ.

The epithelium bears the brunt of the increasing hormonal and metabolic changes that occur in the cervicovaginal region as pregnancy develops. It is therefore not surprising that dynamic alterations occur in its structure, alterations that can easily be monitored by the visual inspection allowed by the colposcope. The subepithelial tissues, comprising smooth muscle, fibrillar and cellular components, ground substance and collagen fibres in their gelatinous matrix, also undergo intense change. These are no less dramatic than those occurring in the epithelium, but are less able to be so efficiently monitored. The biomechanics of the subepithelial tissue during pregnancy and labour will be discussed later (Chapter 13).

As the epithelial and subepithelial tissues are so inexorably linked, primary mechanisms of change in one inevitably affect and involve the other. Although this chapter will deal principally with the epithelium, mention will be made of the role that the subepithelial tissues play in the production of these surface changes.

THE EPITHELIUM

Methods of study

It has been known for some time that pregnancy is the major factor contributing to the variable epithelial patterns present on the adult cervix (Fluhmann, 1948; Nesbitt and Hellman, 1952; Mohler, 1953; McClaren *et al.*, 1961). However, the extent and frequency of these epithelial changes have not been accurately determined because many of the studies have been of an essentially clinical nature employing sequential naked eye observations (Mohler, 1953; McClaren *et al.*, 1961). This form of visual monitoring is unable to detect effectively variations in the morphology of the individual epithelial types that are readily visible colposcopically. The early colposcopic studies (Moricard and Cartier, 1956; Bonham, 1961) presented imprecise conclusions as a result of employing purely descriptive classifications to indicate epithelial alterations, i.e. 'no change', 'better', 'worse', and of not differentiating between different parity states.

Two later colposcopic studies (Coppleson and Reid, 1966; Singer, 1975) followed the epithelial changes occurring on the cervix sequentially throughout pregnancy. By employing colpophotography to record these changes, a more objective assessment of them could be made. In his study, Singer (1975) also used a technique of planimetric measurements to assess the extent of each epithelial type as seen in colpophotographs (see Chapter 6).

Physiological mechanisms operating during pregnancy

Two basic conclusions regarding the physiological mechanisms operating in the cervix and its epithelium during pregnancy were made from the colposcopic observations of Coppleson and Reid (1966) and Singer (1975) (Fig. 7.1). These are:

1 That the endocervical epithelium is subjected to two types of processes which draw it into closer contact with, and exposure to, the vaginal environment. These involve either an *eversion* of the endocervical canal epithelium or a *gaping* of the external cervical os. In both instances, the vaginal environment (or, more precisely, the pH of the vaginal secretions) gains access to this previously protected epithelium which is now exposed.

2 As a result of these two processes, a stimulus is provided to the now *exposed* epithelium, which is usually the original (native) columnar, that induces the development within it of squamous epithelium by the process of metaplastic *transformation*.

The frequency and extent of these changes depend primarily on parity. For example, eversion is more common in the primiparous while gaping predominates in the multiparous cervix. The formation of metaplastic squamous epithelium is more likely to occur in the first pregnancy than in subsequent

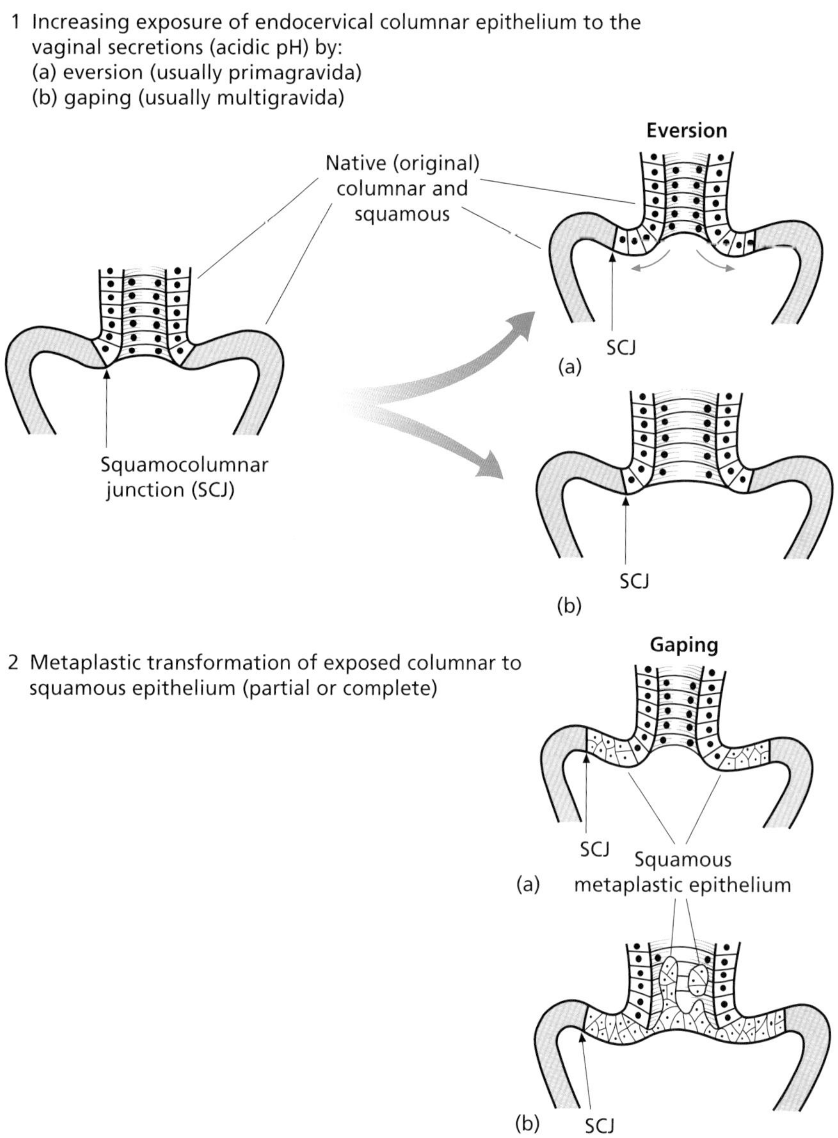

1 Increasing exposure of endocervical columnar epithelium to the vaginal secretions (acidic pH) by:
(a) eversion (usually primagravida)
(b) gaping (usually multigravida)

Eversion

Native (original) columnar and squamous

SCJ
(a)

SCJ
(b)

Squamocolumnar junction (SCJ)

2 Metaplastic transformation of exposed columnar to squamous epithelium (partial or complete)

Gaping

SCJ   Squamous
(a)   metaplastic epithelium

(b)   SCJ

Fig. 7.1 Physiological mechanisms operating in the cervix during pregnancy.

gestations. The method of delivery also influences these changes. In the subsequent analysis, these contributing factors of parity and mode of delivery will be assessed individually.

Epithelial changes as seen colposcopically

Primigravid cervix

In the two major colposcopic studies to date (Coppleson and Reid, 1966; Singer, 1975), a total of 99 primigravidae were colposcoped sequentially during pregnancy. In both studies, colpophotographs were taken with the bivalve vaginal speculum fully opened, thus allowing both ecto- and endocervical epithelia to be seen (called the apparent view), and also with the speculum withdrawn into the lower vagina, enabling the cervix and its epithelia to return to their natural *in vivo* position (called the real view). This allowed an accurate assessment

to be made of the outward movement or eversion of the endocervical epithelium.

Both studies agree on the changes undergone by the epithelia in pregnancy. The primiparous cervix in the early part of the *first trimester* is composed of large areas of columnar epithelium that have not undergone squamous metaplasia (Fig. 7.2). During the later weeks of the first trimester, the metaplastic process commences simultaneously with endocervical eversion and, very rapidly, areas of individual columnar villi fuse and become recognisable as distinct islands of metaplastic squamous epithelium in a sea of columnar epithelium. Biopsy of this new tissue shows it to be composed essentially of immature squamous epithelium.

During the *second trimester*, the metaplastic process becomes more active, and the resultant squamous epithelium appears over larger areas as a smooth opaque covering (Fig. 7.3).

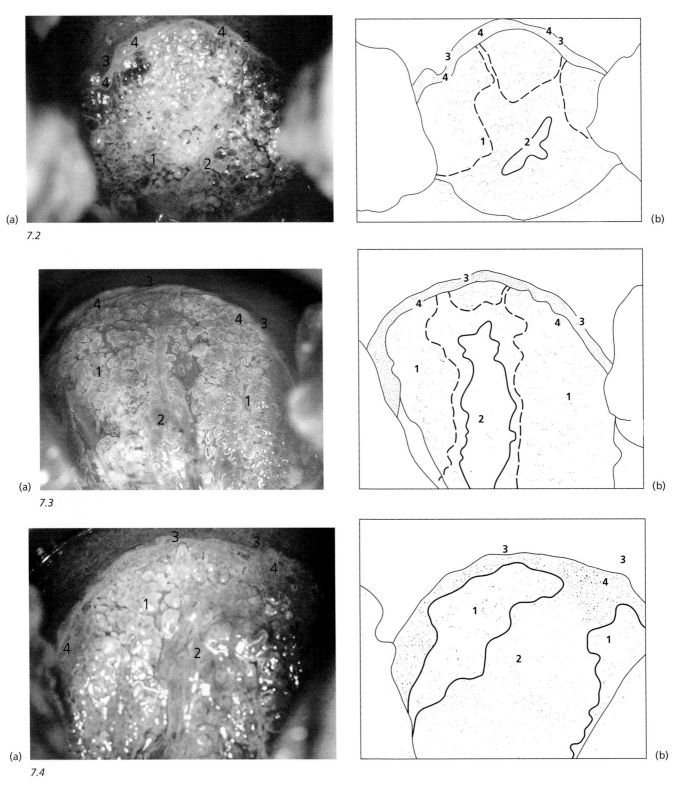

Figs 7.2–7.4 Colpophotographs of a primigravida cervix at 12 (Fig. 7.2), 26 (Fig. 7.3) and 36 (Fig. 7.4) weeks of pregnancy. At 12 weeks, the cervix is mainly composed of original columnar epithelium (1), with a small island of metaplastic squamous epithelium (2). By 26 weeks, this island (2) has enlarged principally by fusion of the adjacent columnar villi. Metaplasia is still developing within the original columnar epithelium at (1), and is in the second stage of the metaplastic process, when there is already fusion between the columnar villi. At 36 weeks, the new metaplastic epithelium (2) has extended to the original squamocolumnar junction (3). Some columnar villi have not undergone complete metaplastic transformation and are seen in an arrested stage at (1). An area of metaplastic squamous epithelium has developed adjacent to the squamocolumnar junction, giving rise to the theory that this epithelium grows inwards and covers the original columnar epithelium. This rim of tissue (4) is already visible by 12 and 26 weeks. The sequence shown here clearly demonstrates the island formation of the new metaplastic epithelium that extends outwards towards the original squamocolumnar junction. The tissue types have the same labels in all three photographs.

During this trimester, a thin rim of squamous metaplastic epithelium appears medial and adjacent to the squamocolumnar junction. This epithelium has usually arisen as a result of *in situ* transformation in the border area (see 4 in Figs 7.3 and 7.4).

In the *third trimester*, squamous metaplasia continues, although fusion of individual metaplastic islands and tongues of tissue has normally ceased by the 34th to 36th weeks (Fig. 7.4). Maturation of this epithelium occurs during this time, as noted by the appearance of a characteristic vascularity within the smooth sheets of epithelium and the development of Nabothian follicles. These appear during the second half of the third trimester and become prominent in the last.

Although the metaplastic squamous epithelium, especially in the third trimester, appears from the study of colpophotographs to have grown in from the original squamous epithelium at the squamocolumnar junction, this is *not* the case as a sharp dividing line can always be seen between this new epithelium and the original squamocolumnar junction (see dotted line in Figs 7.5–7.7). The question of the origin of the metaplastic squamous epithelium is discussed in Chapter 2.

Although the majority of the new metaplastic epithelium develops in areas of columnar epithelium that appear in an ectocervical position as a result of eversion, there is also some metaplastic change occurring within the endocervix. The latter probably occurs as a result of the laxity of the external os and was seen by Singer (1975) in seven (20%) of the 35 primiparous cervices examined. The gaping mechanism involved in this change is described below.

Eversion of endocervical epithelium to occupy an ectocervical position is evident from early in the first trimester and continues throughout pregnancy. It is more marked during the second and early third trimester. Occasionally, however, the degree of initial eversion in the first trimester is not always continued in the later part of pregnancy, as was seen in two cases (6%) in Singer's (1975) study. In three other women (9%), only minimal eversion was evident throughout pregnancy with the formation of minute areas of metaplastic epithelium. All three were delivered by caesarean section, and cervical dystocia was given as the reason for the failure of the

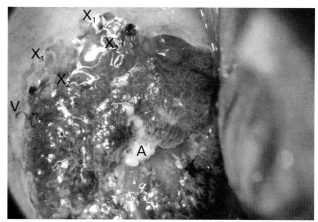

7.5

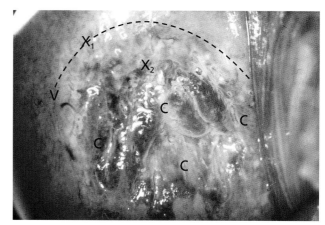

7.6

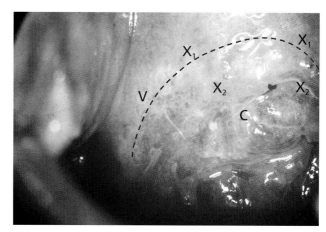

7.7

Figs 7.5–7.7 Colpophotographs (× 6) of a primigravida cervix at 12 (Fig. 7.5), 28 (Fig. 7.6) and 37 (Fig. 7.7) weeks of pregnancy. In Figure 7.5, the transformation zone is composed of original columnar epithelium (A). A small rim of metaplastic squamous tissue already exists between X_1 and X_2. By the 28th week (Fig. 7.6), most of the transformation zone has become occupied by metaplastic squamous epithelium (C). However, the small peripheral area of this epithelium (X_1–X_2) has expanded and seems to be at a more mature stage of development than the more central tissue. A sharp line (– – –) delineates the lateral extension of this area, which is situated at the squamocolumnar junction (X_1). By the 37th week (Fig. 7.7), this rim of metaplastic squamous epithelium has become more pronounced (X_1–X_2), but its sharp border with the original junction still exists

(– – –). Sequential colpophotographs show that the sheet of new metaplastic epithelium (C in Figs 7.6 and 7.7), including the peripheral rim, appears to have grown inwards from the squamocolumnar junction. However, examination of 2 and 3 weekly sequential photographs shows that this new tissue has arisen by the linkage of small islands of metaplastic squamous epithelium and not by any ingrowth from the original squamocolumnar junction. A prominent vessel (V) is 'constant' in all figures.

cervix to dilate in labour. One of the two women with cessation of the eversion process during pregnancy was delivered by caesarean section as a consequence of severe pre-eclampsia and associated retardation of fetal growth developing in the third trimester. Coppleson and Reid (1966) also found a tendency towards absent or minimal eversion in all women they delivered by caesarean section.

The multigravid cervix

The multiparous cervix undergoes to a limited extent during pregnancy most of the epithelial changes that have been described for the primipara. However, there are some differences between the two (Singer, 1975) and these are:

1 The development of metaplastic squamous epithelium occurs predominantly in the last trimester, in contrast to the primipara, in whom it is maximal in the second and early third trimesters.

2 Eversion is most likely to occur in the last trimester.

3 The external os of the multipara tends to open and gape as pregnancy progresses. This occurred in 10 of the 15 (67%) women colposcoped in Singer's series and was evident as early as the 12th week of gestation.

4 Significant areas of metaplastic squamous transformation were noted in 10 out of 15 (67%) cervices seen by Singer. This compares with its nearly universal occurrence, i.e. 32/35 (92%), in the primiparae. Although this new squamous epithelium forms in large sheets or small islands, as in the primiparous cervix, it also has a tendency to develop as distinct furrows within endocervical columnar epithelium (Figs 7.8–7.10). This process usually commences in the second trimester and, by the third trimester, completely covers the sides and ridges of the glandular furrows. Its distribution in these sites is probably caused by the facilitated entry to this area of vaginal fluid (with its acidic pH), passing through the gaping external os.

Coppleson and Reid (1966) did not find significant eversion or squamous metaplasia formation in the 41 multiparae they studied. They argued that the metaplastic squamous epithelium had mainly formed in the first pregnancy.

QUANTITATIVE ASSESSMENT OF EPITHELIAL CHANGES

Singer (1975) measured the total area as well as the region occupied by the four different types of epithelium that constituted the physiological transformation zone. Measurements were made from colpophotographs by the previously published planimetric technique (see Chapter 6); the colposcopic characteristics that allowed recognition of each epithelial type are also described by Coppleson *et al.* (1971). The results are seen in Table 7.1.

The increase in *total* transformation zone area is most marked in the primigravida during the first and second trimester, whereas in the multigravida, this increase occurs

mainly in the third trimester. Each of the epithelial tissue types alters throughout pregnancy, the most dramatic changes being seen in the development of metaplastic squamous epithelium. It is obvious that this new epithelium develops in both primigravid and multigravid cervices. The greatest amount seems to be deposited during the first pregnancy. This is in agreement with the views of most authors (Geschickter and Fernandez, 1962; Coppleson and Reid, 1966). However, the formation of this epithelium in the multiparous cervix as described above is reported infrequently.

FACTORS RESPONSIBLE FOR THE EPITHELIAL ALTERATIONS IN PREGNANCY

Factors producing exposure of columnar epithelium on the ectocervix

Eversion

Studies by Schneppenheim *et al.* (1958), Kaufmann and Ober (1959), Coppleson and Reid (1966) and Singer (1975) confirm that eversion is the major factor in producing exposure of the endocervical columnar epithelium, or uncommonly of small areas of columnar epithelium already exposed on the inner aspects of the ectocervix, to the vaginal environment. The new ectocervical position of this epithelium is produced by a form of protrusion outwards of the glandular portion of the endocervix at the expense of and upon the fibromuscular subepithelial area. This protrusion in turn everts the cervix, and this process progresses during pregnancy. Encouraging this protrusion towards the vagina is the gross hyperplasia undergone by the epithelium (Fluhmann, 1948, 1959; Epperson *et al.*, 1951). The ectocervical position now adopted by this protruded tissue obviously leads to an entire displacement outwards of the squamocolumnar junction (Figs 7.11–7.14).

The absence of eversion or minimal eversion occurs in some primigravidae and is believed by certain authors (Coppleson and Reid, 1967) to be related to an embryonic defect in the cervix, which leads to the glandular cervical tissue becoming unresponsive to the action of estrogens and therefore unable to undergo eversion.

Singer (1975) showed that the multiparous cervix undergoes eversion, but on a much reduced scale to that seen in the primiparae, while Coppleson and Reid (1966) were unable to show any eversion occurring in the multiparous cervix. To explain this process in the multiparae, it must be asked what factor or factors causing eversion act(s) maximally in the primiparae and is/are reduced or even absent in the multiparae. In this regard, the detailed anatomical studies of Hughesden (1952) and Rosa (1965), which deal with the arrangement and action of the two muscular systems (an external and an internal) ensheathing the cervix, are of relevance. Hughesden (1952) believes that the external cervical muscle is composed of fibres that extend from the myometrium caudally and break

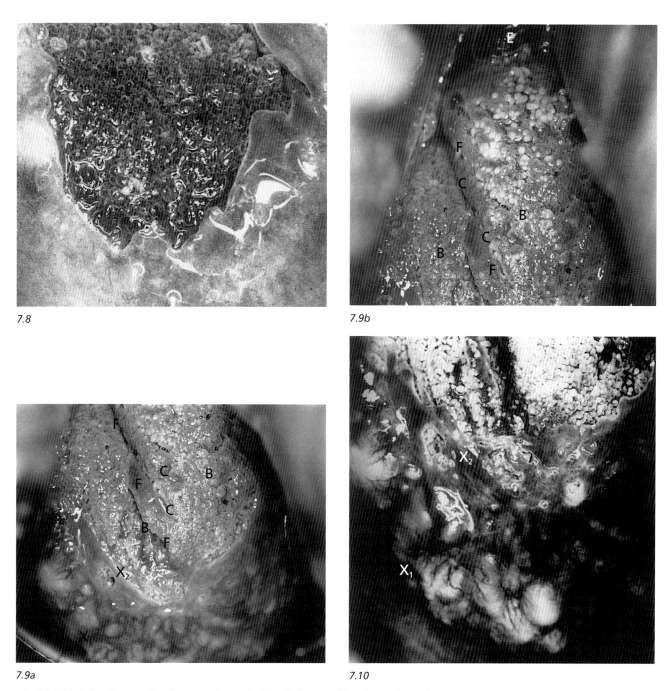

7.8

7.9b

7.9a

7.10

Figs 7.8–7.10 Colpophotographs of the posterior cervical lip of a 26-year-old multigravida at 8 (Fig. 7.8, ×6), 22 (Fig. 7.9a and b, ×10) and 35 (Fig. 7.10, ×20) weeks of pregnancy, showing the gradual development of furrows (F) within the original columnar epithelium (B) and the formation of metaplastic squamous epithelium (C) along the sidewalls of these furrows. Metaplastic squamous tissue at a more advanced stage has developed between X_1 and X_2 in an area exposed by eversion of the endocervical columnar (original) epithelium at the 35-week stage. Figure 7.9b at 22 weeks already shows the endocervix (E) gaping and, because of this 'open' position, facilitating the entry of vaginal secretions.

Table 7.1 The mean areas occupied by different epithelial types within the physiological transformation zone during each trimester of pregnancy as determined by the planimetric measurements of colpophotographs.

	Mean area (mm^2)											
	Primiparae (35 patients)						Multiparae (15 patients)					
	Apparent view*			Real view†			Apparent view			Real view		
Trimester	1	2	3	1	2	3	1	2	3	1	2	3
Total transformation zone area	146	184	176	65	76	110	160	173	220	89	93	125
Columnar epithelium	46	60	16	26	22	18	21	19	15	14	12	15
Columnar epithelium with evidence of metaplastic change	39	42	46	14	12	17	47	39	35	17	15	15
Recently formed metaplastic squamous epithelium	30	54	84	10	25	54	52	63	128	42	48	74
Mature metaplastic squamous epithelium	31	28	32	15	17	21	40	52	42	16	18	21

From Singer (1975) with kind permission of the editor of the *British Journal of Obstetrics and Gynaecology*.
*The apparent view is that view of the cervix obtained when the speculum is fully opened.
†The real view is a view of the cervix obtained when the speculum is withdrawn into the mid- to lower vagina, imitating the cervix in its natural *in vivo* position.

up into further projections that traverse the vaginal fornix and terminate as a sphincter-like ring at the level of the external os. Myometrial contractions during and especially near the end of pregnancy would tend to draw the external os upwards, thereby exposing the endocervical canal contents. The softening of the mucosa and submucosa in pregnancy (Buckingham *et al.*, 1962) allows it to be more readily everted by this contraction mechanism. Obviously, damage to this system during the delivery of the first pregnancy would impair eversion in subsequent pregnancies and therefore reduce the extent of metaplastic epithelial transformation (Hughesden, 1952).

However, there is a second school of thought that believes that changes occurring primarily in the cervix itself account for its dilatational properties and eversion characteristic. For many years, Danforth and colleagues have insisted that the collagen and ground substance composition of the cervix holds the key to the understanding of these mechanisms. They (Danforth *et al.*, 1960, 1974) have shown the striking changes undergone by the connective tissue components of the cervix during pregnancy, particularly the fall in the collagen concentration in the second half of pregnancy, which results in a possible 'loosening up' effect of the cervical interstitium. During late pregnancy, the cervical collagen is actively destroyed, probably as a result of hormonally mediated enzymatic action (collagenases and proteases) (Schubert and Hamerman, 1968; Endo and Yosizawa, 1973; Silbert, 1973). It is possible that the destruction of collagen removes the basic internal support

structure of the cervix and leads in turn to dilatation, gaping and eversion of the endocervical tissues.

Gaping

This feature (Figs 7.8–7.10) is more common in the multiparous than in the primiparous cervix and is explicable on the basis of the muscular damage theory of Hughesden (1952). Damage to the external and internal sphincters, both of which have uterine connections, would make gaping of the external and internal os more liable to occur in the multigravid cervix. Increasing destruction of collagen during pregnancy (Danforth *et al.*, 1974) with resultant loss of internal support in the cervix would also accentuate this phenomenon. Budinska (1972) measured the dilatation of both the internal and the external os in a group of healthy pregnant women of varying parities. Her findings suggest that some dilatation of the cervix normally occurs in pregnancy. She found that 30% of primiparae and 39% of multiparae possessed some dilatation of the external os, enough to admit one finger, by the 24th to 28th week of gestation. In 30% of the former and 36% of the latter, the internal os also admitted one finger at the same time. This figure rose to 61% and 69%, respectively, by the 36th gestational week. Ninety-two per cent of her group of 108 delivered at full term; the 7% who were delivered prior to the 38th week possessed an assortment of obstetrical complications relatively unrelated to a possible incompetence of the cervical os.

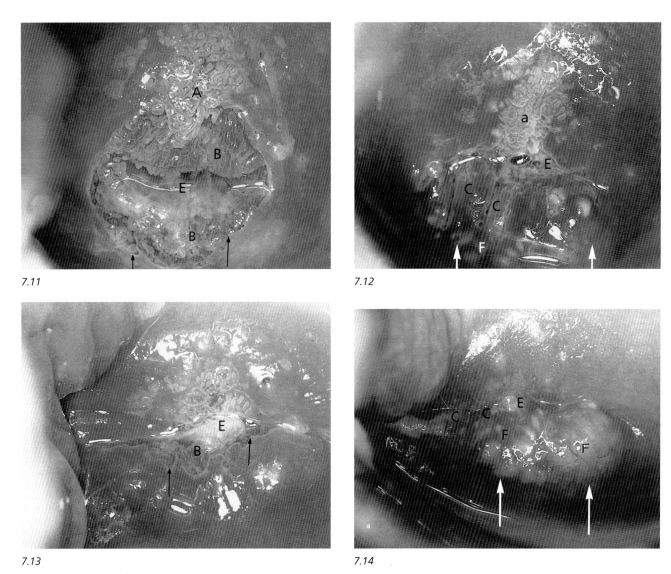

7.11

7.12

7.13

7.14

Figs 7.11–7.14 Colpophotographs (×6) of a primigravida cervix at 12 (Figs 7.11 and 7.12) and 36 (Figs 7.13 and 7.14) weeks of gestation taken in the apparent (Figs 7.11 and 7.13) and real (Figs 7.12–7.14) view. The latter view imitates the normal *in vivo* position of the cervical epithelium and from this the extent of the eversion process can be gauged. The original squamocolumnar junction (↑), as seen in the real views, has extended outwards into an ectocervical position as pregnancy progresses and has resulted in metaplastic squamous transformation (C) of the exposed original columnar epithelium (B) that resides within the endocervix (E) in the non-pregnant state. A Nabothian follicle (F) has developed within the area occupied by the new metaplastic squamous epithelium. A small area of pre-existing low-grade atypical epithelium exists at (a).

Factors inducing metaplastic squamous transformation within the exposed epithelium

The stimulus — vaginal pH

The high incidence of metaplastic squamous epithelial areas in positions exposed to vaginal secretions suggests that a factor or factors exist(s) in these secretions that might be responsible for initiating metaplasia. Evidence presented earlier (Chapter 2) and emanating principally from the work of Reid *et al.* (1967a,b) confirmed earlier suggestions made by Lang (1955) and Walz (1958) that the acid pH of the vaginal secretion initiated the metaplastic transformation within original columnar epithelium.

Singer (1975), employing direct read-out glass microelectrodes (Fig. 7.15), measured the pH on various points across the cervicovaginal portio at different times during pregnancy in 35 women, of whom 26 were primiparae. One hundred and thirty-four measurements were taken, and those obtained from the pregnant cervix were compared with those from 60 non-pregnant women in a study described earlier (Chapter 2).

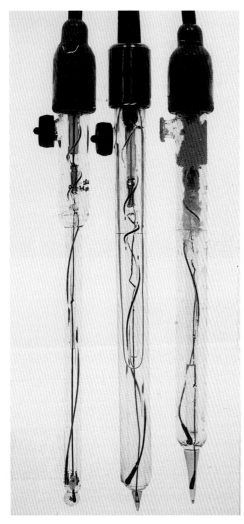

Fig. 7.15 pH combination glass electrodes (Phillips C146A), actual size.

There was a significant drop ($P < 0.01$) in the pH of the vaginal secretions bathing the cervix during early pregnancy (Fig. 7.16), and this drop probably stimulated metaplasia in the everted columnar epithelium when it became exposed to the acidic vaginal secretions.

Further to Singer's (1975) study using direct read-out glass electrodes, no other vaginal pH measuring devices became available until the late 1990s (Roy *et al.*, 2004). Until that time, vaginal and ostensibly cervical pH were measured by the application of a strip of pH paper against the vaginal wall, held in place by either a finger or a forceps placed in the vaginal pool of secretions in the posterior fornix (Rein and Muller, 1990). Studies using this technique confirmed that the normal vaginal wall pH in the reproductive-aged woman is between 3.8 and 4.5 (Smith, 1993).

There seems to be a relationship between vaginal estrogens, the vaginal microflora and their attendant metabolic products

and possibly vaginal and cervical pH. Estrogens encourage proliferation of the vaginal epithelium and, in response to this hormonal stimulation, the glycogen concentration of the vaginal cells increases. When these cells are subsequently released (desquamated) into the vagina, they may encourage or contribute to the growth of various strains of bacteria that produce hydrogen peroxide and lactic acid (lactobacilli), each contributing to the acidic pH of the vagina (Gregoire *et al.*, 1971; Boskey *et al.*, 1999). It would seem obvious that the increased amount of estrogen occurring during pregnancy would have a significant effect on this process. It is well known that certain forms of vaginitis also increase the vaginal pH (to over 4.5), with infectious agents such as *Trichomonas vaginalis* and group B streptococcus as well as other pathogenic organisms and bacterial vaginosis being prominent in this respect (Caillouette *et al.*, 1997).

There have been no studies to assess the effects of extreme variations in vaginal pH on the cervical epithelium and surrounding tissues except for those studies in relation to bacterial vaginosis, where a link has been suggested between the presence of this condition and the causation of premature labour (Klein and Gibbs, 2004; Romero *et al.*, 2004). It may be that a prolonged elevated pH in association with gestation may induce changes within the cervical epithelium and subepithelial tissues that may in some way stimulate uterine contractions. What effect these extreme changes in pH have in the premenopausal and postmenopausal woman are unknown. It may be that the development of metaplasia in the premenopausal patient could be influenced by these extremes in the physiological environment or, for that matter, in the postmenopausal woman, in whom the pH dramatically rises over 4.5 as a result of the low estradiol levels that exist at that time (Nilsson *et al.*, 1995; Garcia-Closas *et al.*, 1999). The introduction of estrogen replacement treatment for many of these postmenopausal women results in the vaginal pH returning to under 4.5, which is usually indicative of an estradiol level above 40 pg/mL and with an increase in vaginal epithelial proliferation and glycogenation (Caillouette *et al.*, 1997).

THE EFFECT OF VAGINAL DELIVERY ON THE CERVICAL EPITHELIUM

The passage of the fetus through the dilated cervix produces gross and easily recognisable injury to the epithelial and subepithelial areas. However, there have been only a few observational studies of these injuries and the subsequent repair process. In three colposcopic studies of the cervix in the immediate postpartum period (Zimskind and Lang, 1958; Coppleson and Reid, 1966; Wilbanks and Richart, 1966, 1967), the presence of specific injuries related to delivery was recognised, but their reported extent and distribution differed from study to study. The findings in these colposcopic studies

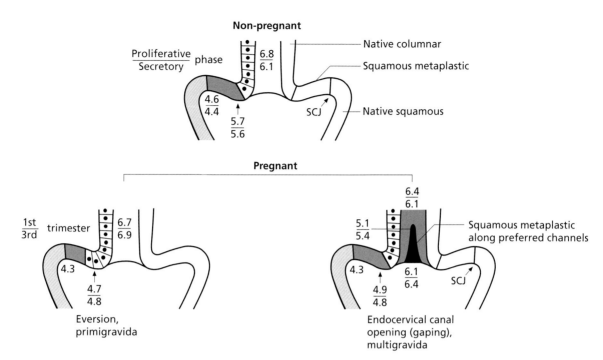

Fig. 7.16 Diagrammatic representation of pH changes across the cervicovaginal portio as found in the pregnant and non-pregnant state. Redrawn from Singer (1975). SCJ, squamocolumnar junction.

differed from results obtained from the less precise naked eye observations of Johnson *et al.* (1959). In none of the studies were sequential observations made with colpophotographic recording of the cervix during late pregnancy and in the immediate puerperium. It could be argued that it is only by observing the cervix before and after delivery that an accurate assessment can be made of the effect of delivery on the cervix. Singer (1975), however, overcame this objection when he observed the cervices of 50 women with colposcopy and colpophotography regularly during pregnancy and into the puerperium. In addition, a further 125 selected women were examined by colposcopy within 2–5 days of delivery, of whom about half were multiparous.

Types of epithelial injuries caused by delivery

In three of the four colposcopic studies mentioned above, an attempt was made to classify certain distinctive tissue injuries resulting from delivery. Zimskind and Lang (1958) found a 'true erosion' (where loss of surface epithelium existed) to be present in 56% of 81 multiparous women colposcoped soon after delivery. Lacerations occurred in 31% and bruising in 4%. They concluded, after colposcopy at the sixth to eighth week post partum, 'that one may consider the epithelial pattern of the immediate post partum cervix as being practically identical with the prenatal cervix'.

Singer (1975) used a classification to describe four specific types of lesion that occurred immediately post partum

(Figs 7.17–7.19) based on the suggestions of Wilbanks and Richart (1966, 1967). The lesions were: *ulceration* (an area recognised colposcopically and histologically by the absence of the original overlying cervical epithelium); *laceration* (an area defined by a linear separation or tear within the epithelium and which extended into the stroma); *bruising* (an area of subepithelial haemorrhagic discoloration which ranged from a small petechial haemorrhage to an area of gross contusion); and *yellow areas* (distinctly coloured tissue regions usually associated with the edges of deep laceration and composed histologically of structureless necrotic tissue with inflammatory cell infiltration).

Using this classification, he found that the cervix was involved by traumatic lesions in 72% of primiparae and 52% of multiparae. This difference was significant ($P < 0.01$). The anterior lip of the cervix tended to be damaged more often than the posterior lip, being involved in 78% of primiparae and in 61% of multiparae compared with a respective involvement of the posterior lip of 66% and 42%. These differences were significant ($P < 0.05$). Ulcerations of the cervix were seen in 83% of primiparae and in 72% of multiparae who had a traumatised cervix. They were significantly ($P < 0.01$) more common than lacerations, which were the next most frequent lesions. Wilbanks and Richart (1967) reported similar findings with 97% of primiparous and 58% of multiparous cervices traumatised.

When Singer (1975) examined the cervices showing lacerations or ulcerations 6–12 weeks later, he found it uncommon

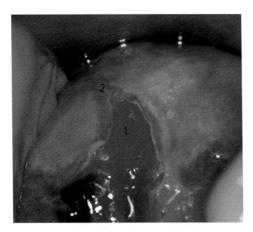

Fig. 7.17 Colpophotograph (× 18) of the anterior lip of the cervix in a primipara at 36 hours after a normal delivery. The epithelium is missing over a large area (1). Healing by metaplastic squamous epithelium (confirmed on biopsy) has already occurred over the upper part of this lesion (2), which is classed as an ulceration.

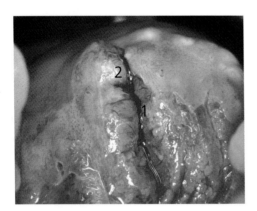

Fig. 7.18 Colpophotograph (× 20) of the anterior lip of the cervix in a primipara at 24 hours after a normal delivery. A large laceration (1), extending into the cervical stroma, radiates from the cervical canal. In the laceration, small Nabothian follicles (2) are visible. Six weeks post partum healing has occurred and, where the laceration had previously been, squamous metaplastic epithelium has appeared.

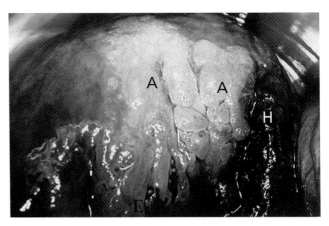

Fig. 7.19 Colpophotograph (× 10) of an atypical transformation zone 48 hours after delivery with a haematoma (H) occupying its lateral area. Biopsy of the atypical epithelium (A) prior to pregnancy showed it to contain histological evidence of carcinoma *in situ*. The endocervix is at E.

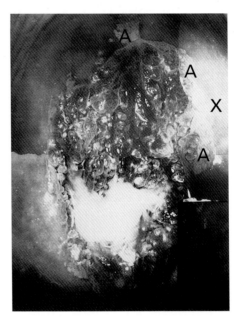

Fig. 7.20 Colpophotographic montage (× 9) of the same cervix as in Figure 7.19, now at 8 weeks post partum. Only a few small areas of atypical epithelium (A) are visible, and no cytological or histological evidence could be obtained to confirm a continuing presence of any epithelium with carcinoma *in situ*. The original squamocolumnar junction is at (X).

to see any residual evidence of the lesion (Figs 7.19–7.22). The cervix at this stage rarely bore any resemblance to its predelivery appearance. This is different from the colposcopic findings of some authors such as Coppleson and Reid (1966), and from the naked eye findings under similar conditions of Johnson *et al.* (1959), who insisted that 'pregnancy and/or delivery has very little effect on the appearance of the cervix'. Wilbanks and Richart (1967), even though finding a high rate of traumatic lesions after delivery, could find only 10% of cervices showing residual traumatic damage or alteration in overall shape when seen 6 weeks post partum. They did not,

however, perform any observations prior to delivery. It is also difficult to reconcile the findings of Coppleson and Reid's (1966) study, in which they concluded that 'minimal physical trauma is suffered by the cervix during delivery'.

The high frequency of traumatic change to the cervix suggests that this event is physiological. The ease with which they heal so rapidly would tend to support this contention.

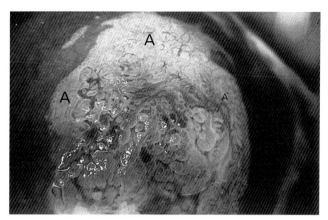

7.21

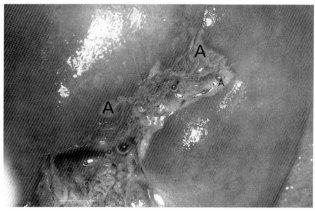

7.22

Figs 7. 21 and 7.22 Two colpophotographs of the cervix of a primigravida during pregnancy and the puerperium. In Figure 7.21, taken at 12 weeks' gestation, an area of atypical epithelium (A) involving the anterior lip exists. Punch biopsy has shown this to be composed of mild/moderate dysplasia. In Figure 7.22, taken 6 weeks after delivery, the overall contour of the cervix has been extensively altered with large segments of a colposcopically atypical area (A) having disappeared and been replaced by normal squamous metaplastic epithelium.

The proclivity of the anterior cervical lip to traumatic damage is most likely to be related to the anterior-directed expulsive pressure of the fetal head on this area during delivery. This anterior lip usually retracts behind the fetal head and out of the path of the oncoming fetal head. However, it is not unusual for delivery to occur in the presence of a small rim of undilated cervix, the rigid nature of which in the primipara makes it more vulnerable to compression and probably accounts for the higher frequency of damage in this group. In the Wilbanks and Richart (1967) study, there seemed to be no aetiological factor other than primiparity which predisposed the cervix to the occurrence of these lesions. In some earlier studies (Peckham, 1934; Gainy *et al.*, 1953), the length of labour seemed to be correlated with a likelihood of developing cervical laceration.

However, this observation has not been confirmed in subsequent investigations.

The rapid healing process of the traumatic epithelial lesions

Colposcopic studies attest to the rapid epithelial covering of traumatic injuries caused by delivery (Figs 7.19–7.22). However, there have been few studies of the cellular dynamics of the healing process. Singer (1973) took biopsies under colposcopic vision from the lesions that he classed as erosions, and in which the surface layer had been avulsed. Biopsies were taken within 48 hours of delivery. He subsequently biopsied at 24-hour intervals the area adjacent to the initial biopsy. Histological and autoradiographic studies were performed on these biopsies; the latter procedure used culture with tritiated thymidine from 1 to 4 hours, and exposure with liquid emulsion for 2 weeks (Figs 7.23 and 7.24).

He found that, within 48 hours of delivery, there was histological evidence of some cellular invasion of the denuded and essentially amorphous necrotic tissue of the erosion (Fig. 7.23) by what appeared to be mononuclear cells. Multiple biopsies over the subsequent 2 days suggested that these cells migrated along tissue spaces towards the free surface. At 5 days, cylindrical collections of these cells spread upwards and laterally towards the surface from the tissue depths and, by day 6, had covered the free surface. Thereafter, they rapidly formed a multilayered epithelium some six to eight cells thick (Fig. 7.24). The transition from collections of mononuclear cells to multilayered epithelium was apparently quite rapid because free mononuclear cells and well-defined squamous epithelium co-existed.

A high rate of cellular proliferation and differentiation within the mononuclear cells in the necrotic tissue was evident and, as the cells formed an epithelium, the rate and capacity for isotopic incorporation increased (Figs 7.23 and 7.24). These autoradiographic and histological findings of postpartum epithelial regeneration are similar to those obtained from a study of the repair process that follows cervical electrocauterisation (Reid *et al.*, 1967b). The significance of these findings has been discussed in Chapter 2.

DEVELOPMENT OF THE ATYPICAL TRANSFORMATION ZONE DURING PREGNANCY

Histological studies of the cervical epithelium and stroma during pregnancy attest to the dynamic nature of the development of squamous metaplasia (Carrow and Greene, 1951; Nesbitt and Hellman, 1952; Moricard and Cartier, 1956). It is surprising in view of these histological studies and some of a colposcopic nature (Coupez, 1965; Coppleson and Reid,

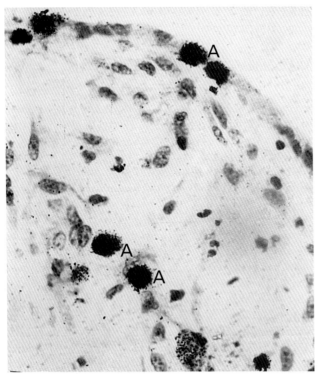
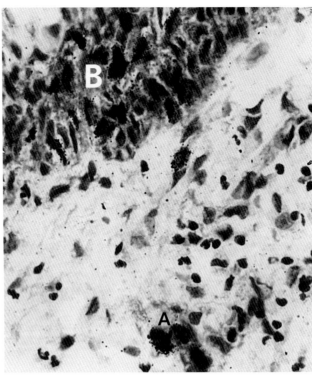

7.23   7.24

Figs 7.23 and 7.24 Photomicrographs of autoradiographic sections (× 200) taken from adjacent areas of a traumatic cervical ulcer at 56 (Fig. 7.23) and 84 hours (Fig. 7.24) after delivery. Heavily labelled mononuclear-type cells (A) appear in the amorphous and necrotic stroma (Fig. 7.23) and most probably contribute to the new monolayered epithelium at this stage (Coppleson and Reid, 1967a,b). Subsequently, the radioisotopic label (tritiated thymidine) was found in the multilayered epithelium (B) (Fig. 7.24), which rapidly covered the denuded area.

1966) that no precise explanation can be given for the insistence by the epidemiologist that pregnancy, usually in conjunction with an associated HPV infection, is a major aetiological factor in the development of cervical carcinoma (Maliphant, 1949; Boyd and Doll, 1964; Muñoz *et al.*, 2002b; Sheilds *et al.*, 2004). It is well known that women who have had seven or more full-term pregnancies are at increased risk of cervical cancer. Those women who are HPV positive had a fourfold increased risk of cervical cancer compared with similar HPV-positive women who were nulliparous (OR 3.8%; 95% CI 2.7–5.5). There was still a twofold increased risk when women reported seven or more pregnancies compared with HPV-positive women who reported one or two full-term pregnancies (Bosch *et al.*, 2002). Indeed, there have been other authors, especially pathologists, who have contended that pregnancy per se is unrelated to cervical carcinogenesis and that its only relevance to the latter is because 'histological changes within the cervix during pregnancy could be easily confused with malignancy' (Moore and Taylor, 1965). Some also believe that 'pregnancy is only a complication of the epithelial reaction rather than a cause of it' (Rutledge and Christopherson, 1962).

Parity seems to play a distinct role in the development of cervical carcinoma. Parous rather than non-parous women may be more prone (Wynder *et al.*, 1954; Rotkin, 1962). It is possible that other behavioural factors associated with pregnancy also contribute to this increased risk. For example, high and early parity is usually associated with an early age of first coitus and multiple sexual partners, which are common aetiological denominators for cervical cancer (Rotkin, 1973; Hildesheim *et al.*, 2001; Muñoz *et al.*, 2002a). Smoking, sexually transmitted diseases and use of oral contraception are also risk factors linked, in many cases, to high parity and, in all cases, HPV infectivity is a common denominator (de Sanjose *et al.*, 1994; Kjaer *et al.*, 1998; Bosch *et al.*, 2002).

There is, however, evidence dating to the 1950s–1970s that supports the premise that pregnancy is directly involved in the origin of cervical neoplasia. Many authors contend that dysplasia and carcinoma *in situ* are abnormal forms of squamous metaplasia (Kaufmann and Ober, 1959; de Brux and Dupre-Fremont, 1960; Reagan and Patten, 1962; Johnson *et al.*, 1964). It is possible that a mutagenic or carcinogenic agent gains entry to the epithelium during this process and, indeed, Coppleson and Reid (1967a, 1992) have shown the absorptive capacity of the metaplastic epithelium to one such potential agent (i.e. spermatozoa).

Table 7.2 Development of the atypical transformation zone during pregnancy.

Case no.	Time of first antenatal visit (weeks)	Time of appearance of atypical transformation zone (weeks)	Histological diagnosis (ex biopsy)
1	16	32	Carcinoma *in situ*, moderate dysplasia
2	12	34	Severe dysplasia (Figs 7.25–7.28)
3	18	Post partum	Severe dysplasia
4	20	26	Mild dysplasia (Figs 7.29–7.31)
5	8	Post partum	Abnormal epithelium, basal cell hyperplasia
6	18	Post partum	Abnormal epithelium
7	16	Post partum	Abnormal epithelium, basal cell hyperplasia

Colposcopic studies

There have been only three major colposcopic studies of the cervix during pregnancy in which the development of an atypical transformation zone was observed (Coupez, 1965; Coppleson and Reid, 1966; Kolstad and Stafl, 1972), a feature believed to have neoplastic potential. Coppleson and Reid (1966) noted the presence of three such zones in their study of 105 primi- and multiparous women examined in pregnancy. No sequential colposcopic observations of their development were made either in that study or in those of Coupez (1965) or Kolstad and Stafl (1972). Singer (1975) was able to make such observations during a study of 35 unselected primigravidae during pregnancy. In seven instances, an atypical transformation zone developed. None developed in the 15 multigravidae also studied. Details of these cases are listed in Table 7.2.

Histological evidence was obtained via punch biopsy from these atypical areas in all women after the 16th postpartum week. One biopsy showed the presence of carcinoma *in situ*, and two showed severe dysplasia, as was the classification of intraepithelial neoplasia at that time, i.e. 1968/9. In a further one, mild dysplasia was demonstrated and, in the remaining three, basal cell hyperplasia or abnormal epithelium (Glatthaar, 1950) was noted. Cervical cytology in each of the three major lesions was negative at the first antenatal visit but had changed to doubtful (Papanicolaou class III) in two patients and positive in one patient by the third month after delivery. All four of the minor type of lesions possessed negative cytology both before and shortly after delivery. Two of these patients were colposcoped again 2 years later, and the atypical transformation zone was still present; one patient now had a doubtful smear (Papanicolaou class III). The other two were lost to follow-up. Three of the women in Singer's (1975) series first developed atypical epithelium at 26, 32 and 34 weeks of pregnancy. In the others, it was first seen in the puerperium. He delayed punch biopsy until the fourth month in case spontaneous regression occurred. The series of colpophotographs (Figs 7.25–7.31) shows the development of two such lesions

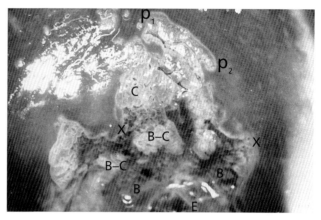

Fig. 7.25 Colpophotograph (×9) of the anterior lip of the cervix in a 19-year-old primipara at 12 weeks' gestation showing columnar epithelium at point B and columnar epithelium with very early metaplastic transformation at point B–C. Early metaplastic squamous epithelium is at C and between p_1 and p_2. The endocervical canal is at E. The squamocolumnar junction is at x. From Singer (1975) with kind permission of the editor of the *British Journal of Obstetrics and Gynaecology*.

in a 19-year-old (Figs 7.25–7.28) and the other in a 22-year-old primigravida (Figs 7.29–7.31).

In all four colposcopic studies (Coupez, 1965; Coppleson and Reid, 1966; Kolstad and Stafl, 1972; Singer, 1975), no obvious difference was observed between the formation of the new metaplastic squamous and atypical epithelium, as regards their topographical distribution within the transformation zone and the time of development. It would appear that the 'former commences insidiously within and probably at the time of occurrence of the latter' (Coppleson and Reid, 1966). A similar process may well operate in the adolescent cervix in which the development of these two forms of epithelium seems to occur simultaneously. It is difficult to avoid the conclusion that a neoplastic potential is endowed on some cervical epithelia during the formation of metaplastic squamous

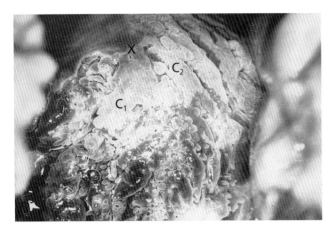

Fig. 7.26 Colpophotograph (× 15) of the anterior lip of the cervix shown in Figure 7.25 at 24 weeks' gestation showing eversion of the anterior cervical lip. The previous islands of columnar epithelium (B–C in Fig. 7.25) have undergone metaplastic transformation to squamous epithelium (C_1/C_2) and have joined the original squamocolumnar junction at X. The whiteness between points C_1 and C_2 is artificial and caused by flashlight reflection. From Singer (1975) with kind permission of the editor of the *British Journal of Obstetrics and Gynaecology.*

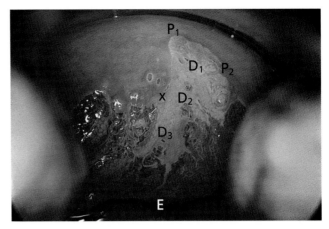

Fig. 7.28 Colpophotograph (× 9) of the anterior lip of the cervix, as shown in Figures 7.25–7.27, 6 weeks after delivery. Atypical epithelium D_1–D_3 extends longitudinally towards the endocervix. This epithelium exists in an area that was originally occupied by columnar (Fig. 7.25) and then by metaplastic squamous epithelium (Figs 7.26 and 7.27). Biopsy at multiple points along this longitudinal atypical area (D_1–D_2) showed severe dysplasia. Points x, P_1 and P_2 correspond to the similarly labelled points in Figure 7.27. From Singer (1975) with kind permission of the editor of the *British Journal of Obstetrics and Gynaecology.*

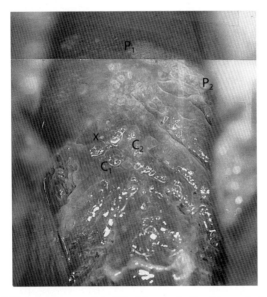

Fig. 7.27 Colpophotograph (× 12) of the anterior lip of the cervix shown in Figures 7.25 and 7.26 at 34 weeks' gestation. Complete metaplastic transformation has occurred. A very faint abnormal vascular pattern exists between points P_1 and P_2. Points x, C_1 and C_2 are at the same points as in Figure 7.26. From Singer (1975) with kind permission of the editor of the *British Journal of Obstetrics and Gynaecology.*

epithelium in pregnancy. A possible relationship between estrogenic hormone stimulation of the cervical epithelium and neoplasia has been discussed in relation to the oral contraceptive steroids (Chapter 9).

ALTERATION AND REGRESSION OF THE ATYPICAL TRANSFORMATION ZONE AS A RESULT OF DELIVERY

Regression of intraepithelial lesions within the cervical epithelium has been suggested by many authors (Kottmeier, 1953; Simon and Sheehan, 1961; Koss *et al.*, 1963; Reagan, 1964; Richart, 1967), with regression rates of between 13% and 70% being quoted. It is further suggested by some (Koss *et al.*, 1963) that these epithelial lesions are so poorly established and fragile that a number of minor procedures such as small biopsies or curettage, or even drugs (for example, locally applied tetracyclines), can induce regression. The physiological effect of trauma associated with delivery has been incriminated as the cause of the decrease in the prevalence of atypical cytology (ranging between 20% and 75%) that is noted during and after pregnancy (Marsh, 1956; Rawson and Knoblick, 1957; McKay *et al.*, 1959). It is presumed that the actual epithelial lesions causing this abnormal cytology have been altered by this trauma (Slate and Merrith, 1961; Bret and Coupez, 1961; Koss *et al.*, 1963; Singer, 1975).

de Brux and Brechet (1979) reviewed 12 300 pregnant women over a 10-year period and showed that 180 of them had cervical atypia, as assessed cytologically. However, only 106 were able to be followed up but, on this number, the authors concluded that 58% showed cytological 'improvement' and 41% remained 'unchanged'. For comparison, they studied a group of 11 090 sexually active women who were taking a high-dose estrogen/progestogen pill and, within this group,

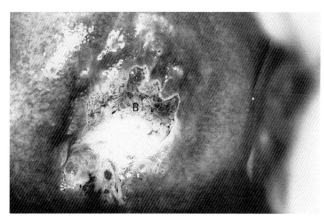

7.29

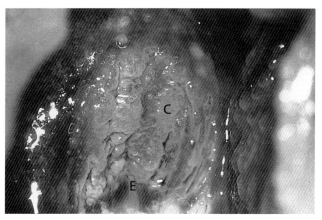

7.30

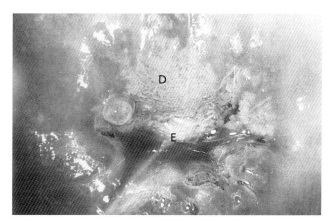

7.31

Figs 7.29–7.31 Colpophotographs of a 22-year-old primigravida at 8 (Fig. 7.29, × 4) and 22 (Fig. 7.30, × 9) weeks during pregnancy and at the eight postpartum week (Fig. 7.31, × 4). The development of atypical epithelium (D) as seen in Figure 7.31 has occurred in an area initially occupied by native columnar epithelium (B in Fig. 7.29), followed by what appeared colposcopically to be metaplastic squamous epithelium (C in Fig. 7.30). Biopsy of the atypical epithelium (D in Fig. 7.31) revealed histological evidence of mild dysplasia. The endocervical canal is at E.

1.27% had cytological abnormalities, ranging as in the former group from invasive cancer to borderline lesions. In this group, they showed that 44% 'improved' cytologically and 55% remained 'unchanged'. Two further studies supported the contention that regression occurs in abnormal cytological findings during pregnancy. Strinic *et al.* (2002) showed that, of 107 pregnant women diagnosed with abnormal cytology in the immediate antepartum period, 50 of them (46.7%) returned 6 months after delivery with a normal smear while in a further 11 (12%), there was some regression of the cytological findings. This was in comparison with 43 of the original group (40%) in whom persistence of the cytological abnormality was noted, and the antenatal findings progressed after delivery in only three (3%). The authors suggested that 'desquamation of the cervical epithelium or enhancement of the localised reparative immunological response after vaginal delivery could be an important role in the spontaneous regression of cervical dysplasia in the postpartum period'.

In the second recent study by Paraskevaidis *et al.* (2002), 98 women with antenatal cytological or colposcopic impression of cervical intraepithelial neoplasia (CIN) were followed during pregnancy with cytology and colposcopy being performed. When examined 2 months post partum, a large loop excision of the transformation zone was performed. In 14 of the 39 (35.9%) women who had antenatal impression of CIN1 and 25 of the 51 (48.1%) in whom a CIN2 or 3 lesion was suspected, there was regression when the cervices of these women were examined in the postpartum period. In seven women, there had been a suspicion of microinvasion on colposcopy, and so a small loop biopsy had been procured during the actual pregnancy. One more case was diagnosed postnatally. In total, it was assessed that 84.6% of women who subsequently had evidence of regression, as found by the absence of CIN in the resultant excised specimen, and 67.3% of women who continued to have CIN, or indeed had evidence of progression of the disease, had been delivered vaginally. The authors concluded that there was a considerable rate of regression of CIN associated with pregnancy and delivery, and they attributed this to loss of the abnormal cervical epithelium that occurred in relation to cervical ripening and the vaginal delivery.

However, other authors such as Johnson (1973) challenge these views and, after an extensive review of the literature at that time, they concluded that dysplasia and carcinoma *in situ* are not altered in any way by pregnancy or delivery. Indirect evidence as to the status of the atypical epithelium during pregnancy, as derived from extensive cytological or random punch biopsy studies (as quoted by Johnson, 1973), cannot accurately determine the effect of pregnancy or delivery on this epithelium. Sequential colposcopic monitoring, as undertaken in the Paraskevaidis *et al.* (2002) study, allows a more direct and efficient avenue by which to observe these dynamic epithelial alterations.

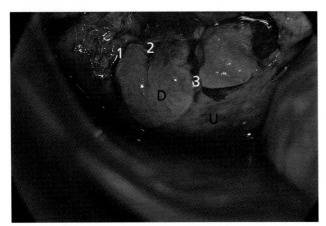
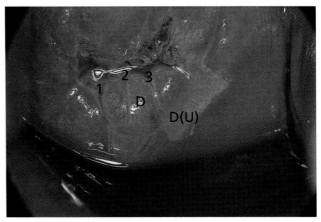

Figs 7.32 and 7.33 Colpophotograph of an atypical transformation zone at 36 hours (Fig. 7.32, × 10), and 8 weeks (Fig. 7.33, × 6) after delivery. Biopsy of the atypical epithelium (D) during pregnancy revealed histological evidence of moderate dysplasia. In Figure 7.32, this epithelium has been removed from over a large area of the posterior cervical lip by a traumatic ulcerative lesion (U). There is some residual atypical epithelium remaining (D). When seen 8 weeks later (Fig. 7.33), fresh atypical epithelium (D) had regenerated in this previously traumatic area D(U), and biopsy again revealed moderate dysplasia. Points 1, 2 and 3 are on identical areas in both figures.

Colposcopic studies

Three colposcopic and colpomicroscopic studies have evaluated the effect of pregnancy and delivery on the atypical transformation zone (Richart, 1963; Coppleson and Reid, 1967b; Singer, 1975). In his study, Singer (1975) has shown both colposcopic and histological evidence of variable regressive alterations occurring in atypical epithelium as a result of parturition, while Richart (1963) and Coppleson and Reid (1967) hold opposite views and insist that minimal changes occur in such tissue during gestation. Richart (1963) followed with the colpomicroscope 40 women with dysplasia and carcinoma *in situ* during pregnancy and after delivery without finding obvious morphological change in them. Coppleson and Reid (1967b) state that they 'have never witnessed the disappearance of an atypical appearance associated with dysplasia', although they admit that regression is theoretically possible.

Singer (1975) showed that the atypical and physiological transformation zones sustain similar traumatic injuries at delivery. He followed 12 women with an atypical transformation zone throughout pregnancy and delivery. When colposcoped 6–8 weeks post partum, he observed that, in six cases, a marked and, in four cases, a minor reduction had occurred in the area occupied by the atypical epithelium. Some type of traumatic lesion induced by delivery had involved all these cervices in the immediate postpartum period (Figs 7.19–7.22). In 10 of these 12 cases, the atypical area that had been removed was replaced by immature metaplastic squamous epithelium as confirmed histologically from punch biopsy material. In two further cases, however, the removed atypical area was again replaced by dysplastic epithelium at the eighth postpartum week (Figs 7.32 and 7.33). In these cases, it could be specu-

lated that the subepithelial cells, believed by Reid (1964) and Reid *et al.* (1967a,b) to be the progenitor cell of regenerating squamous epithelium, contained a neoplastic potential that became re-expressed in the formation of atypical epithelium. Either that or the more common HPV virus, present in the lower genital tract, reinfected the regenerating tissue.

It is possible that the epithelium of the atypical transformation zone can be affected in three ways as a result of delivery.

1 Partial or complete removal may occur with resulting regression of the lesion.

2 Partial removal or damage may induce some alteration in its neoplastic potential.

3 The lesion may remain unaltered or recur after temporary removal in its previous form with subsequent expression of its preneoplastic or neoplastic potential.

Pregnancy and delivery have effects upon the atypical transformation zone, the assessment of which may help to clarify the presently controversial topic of the natural history of cervical dysplasia and carcinoma *in situ*.

THE SUBEPITHELIAL TISSUES

Ultrastructure and biomechanical properties of subepithelial tissues

The subepithelial tissues, composed predominantly of elastic tissue with a small amount of smooth muscle, have undergone intense study (Leppert and Yu, 1991). When examined under scanning electron microscopy (SEM), the elastic tissue, composed of collagen and elastin, has been shown to be composed of two distinct structures: fibrils and thin sheets of elastic membranes. The fibrils are arranged into fishnet-like structures, while within the thin elastic membranes there are fenestrations and pits with diameters of some 3–5 μm. In the Leppert and Yu (1991) study, the concentration of the insoluble elastin was found to be approximately 1.4% of the dry, defatted tissues of the cervix, while the total collagen was estimated to be between 64% and 72%. The orientation of the elastic tissues within the cervix has been described in detail by Leppert *et al.* (1986), who have shown that they are orientated from the external os to the periphery and from there in a band upwards towards the internal os, where they become sparse in that area of the cervix which contains the greatest amount of smooth muscle, just below the internal os.

Rotten *et al.* (1988) studied the elastic fibres with a specific polyphenolic compound stain which enabled automatic image analysis. They showed that the elastic fibre network is composed of two types: first, fibres that run parallel to the basement lamina of the epithelium and, second, thinner perpendicular fibres. With their sophisticated image analysis, they were able to show a decline in the cervical elastin content during pregnancy. This constant decline is associated with disorganisation and dissociation of the fibres as pregnancy progresses, so much so that, by the fifth to seventh week post partum, the elastic fibre network appeared almost completely restructured. These changes support a role for elastin in the process of cervical maturation and reconstruction during delivery and in the postpartum period.

The tensile strength and firmness of the cervix is derived from the collagen which is the predominant protein of the extracellular matrix. Minamoto *et al.* (1987) have described four types of collagen within the dense fibrous tissue of the cervix which, at term, is broken down by the enzyme collagenase. It would seem that the cells involved in this degeneration during the process of dilatation are not resident fibroblasts, as had previously been assumed, but rather polymorphonuclear leucocytes that migrate from blood vessels within the cervix (Osmers *et al.*, 1992). Not surprisingly, there is an elevation in serum collagenase levels during the ripening process at term and, in active labour, it increases further.

Assessment of the biochemical and muscular contractile ability of the cervix has shown no significant difference in these physical properties (Petersen *et al.*, 1991) between tissues taken from the distal and proximal parts of the elastic tissues. Petersen *et al.* (1991) concluded that the passive biomechanical strength of the cervix markedly exceeds the active muscular contractile ability, and this is explained by a high collagen concentration and a low content of smooth muscle within the cervical tissues (this subject is further discussed in Chapter 13).

REFERENCES

Bonham D (1961) The cervix ante and postpartum. *Proceedings of the Royal Society of Medicine* 54: 717–719.

Bosch FX, Lorincz A, Muñoz N *et al.* (2002) The causal relation between human papillomavirus and cervical cancer. *Journal of Clinical Pathology* 55: 244–265.

Boskey ER, Telsch KM, Whaley KJ *et al.* (1999) Acid production of vaginal flora in vitro is consistent with the rate and extent of vaginal acidification. *Infection and Immunity* 67: 5170–5175.

Boyd JT, Doll R (1964) A study of the aetiology of carcinoma of the cervix uteri. *British Journal of Cancer* 18: 419–434.

Bret AJ, Coupez F (1961) Reserve cell hyperplasia, basal cell hyperplasia and dysplasia. *Acta Cytologica* 5: 259–261.

Buckingham JC, Selden R, Danforth DN (1962) Connective tissue changes in the cervix during pregnancy and labour. *Annals of the New York Academy of Sciences* 97: 733–742.

Budinska MB (1972) The changes in the cervix uteri in pregnancy. *Acta Europaea Fertilitatis* 3: 79–82.

Caillouette JC, Sharp CF, Zimmerman GJ *et al.* (1997) Vaginal pH as a marker for bacterial pathogens and menopausal status. *American Journal of Obstetrics and Gynecology* 176: 1270–1277.

Carrow L, Greene R (1951) The epithelia of the pregnant cervix. *American Journal of Obstetrics and Gynecology* 61: 237–252.

Coppleson M, Reid B (1966) A colposcopic study of the cervix during pregnancy and the puerperium. *Journal of Obstetrics and Gynaecology of the British Commonwealth* 73: 575–585.

Coppleson M, Reid B (1967a) *Preclinical Carcinoma of the Cervix Uteri*. Oxford: Pergamon Press, p. 274.

Coppleson M, Reid B (1967b) *Preclinical Carcinoma of the Cervix Uteri*, 1st edn. Oxford: Pergamon Press, p. 130.

Coppleson M, Pixley E, Reid B (1971) *Colposcopy, a Scientific and Practical Approach to the Cervix in Health and Disease*, 1st edn. Springfield, IL: Charles C. Thomas, pp. 155–193.

Coupez F (1965) Les dysplasies du cot uterin. *Revue Française de Gynécologie et d'Obstétrique* 60: 579–586.

Danforth DN, Buckingham JC, Roddick JW (1960) Connective tissue changes incident to cervical effacement. *American Journal of Obstetrics and Gynecology* 89: 939–945.

Danforth DN, Veis A, Breen M *et al.* (1974) The effect of pregnancy and labour on the human cervix: changes in collagen, glycoproteins and glycosaminoglycans. *American Journal of Obstetrics and Gynecology* 120: 641–651.

de Brux J, Brechet M (1979) Epithelial dysplasias of the uterine cervix during pregnancy and its evolution (author's translation from French). *Bulletin du Cancer* 66: 147–153.

de Brux JA, Dupre-Fremont J (1960) Differentiation of endocervical glandular and metaplastic cells. *Acta Cytologica* 4: 299–303.

de Sanjose S, Muñoz N, Bosch FX (1994) Sexually transmitted agents and cervical neoplasia in Colombia and Spain. *International Journal of Cancer* 56: 358–363.

Endo M, Yosizawa Z (1973) Hormonal effect on glycoproteins and glycosaminoglycans in rabbit uteri. *Archives of Biochemistry and Biophysics* 156: 397–403.

Epperson JW, Hellman LM, Galvin GA *et al.* (1951) The morphological changes in the cervix during pregnancy including intraepithelial carcinoma. *American Journal of Obstetrics and Gynecology* 61: 50–61.

Fluhmann CF (1948) A clinical and histopathological study of lesions of the cervix uteri in pregnancy. *American Journal of Obstetrics and Gynecology* 55: 133–150.

Fluhmann CF (1959) The glandular structures of the cervix uteri during pregnancy. *American Journal of Obstetrics and Gynecology* 78: 990–1003.

Gainy HL, Keeler JE, Nicolay KS (1953) Cervical damage in obstetrics. Part I. Cervical lacerations in primiparas. *Obstetrics and Gynecology* 1: 333–338.

Garcia-Closas M, Herrero R, Bratti C *et al.* (1999) Epidemiologic determinants of vaginal pH. *American Journal of Obstetrics and Gynecology* 180: 1060–1066.

Geschickter CF, Fernandez F (1962) Epidermization of the cervix. *Annals of the New York Academy of Sciences* 97: 638–652.

Glatthaar E (1950) *Studien über die Morphogenese des Plattenepithelcarcinomas der Portio vaginalis uteri*. Basle: Karger.

Gregoire AT, Kandil O, Ledger WJ (1971) The glycogen content of human vaginal epithelial tissue. *Fertility and Sterility* 22: 64–68.

Hildesheim A, Herrero R, Castle PE (2001) HPV cofactors related to the development of cervical cancer; results from a population-based study in Costa Rica. *British Journal of Cancer* 84: 1219–1226.

Hughesden PE (1952) The fibromuscular structure of the cervix and its changes during pregnancy and labour. *Journal of Obstetrics and Gynaecology of the British Empire* 59: 763–776.

Johnson LD (1973) Dysplasia and carcinoma in situ in pregnancy. In: Norris HJ, Hertig A, Abell MR (eds) *The Uterus*, Vol. 1, Ch. 18. Baltimore: Williams and Wilkins.

Johnson LD, Sheps MC, Esterday CL (1959) The cervix in the pregnant and postpartum period. *Obstetrics and Gynecology* 14: 452–460.

Johnson LD, Esterday CL, Gore H *et al.* (1964) The histogenesis of carcinoma in situ of the uterine cervix. A preliminary report of the origin of carcinoma in situ in subcylindrical cell anaplasia. *Cancer* 17: 213–229.

Kaufmann C, Ober KG (1959) The morphological changes in the cervix uteri with age and their significance in the early diagnosis of carcinoma. In: Wolstenholme GEW, O'Connor M (eds) *Cancer of the Cervix, Diagnosis and Early Forms*. London: Churchill, pp. 61–65.

Kjaer SK, Van den Brull AJC, Svare E (1998) Different risk factor patterns for high grade and low grade intraepithelial lesions on the cervix amongst HPV-positive and HPV-negative women. *International Journal of Cancer* 76: 613–619.

Klein L, Gibbs R (2004) Use of microbial cultures and antibiotics in the prevention of infection-associated pre-term births. *American Journal of Obstetrics and Gynecology* 190: 1493–1502.

Kolstad P, Stafl A (1972) *Atlas of Colposcopy*, 1st edn. Oslo: Universitetsforlaget, p. 75.

Koss LG, Stewart FW, Foote FW *et al.* (1963) Some histological aspects of the behaviour of in situ epidermoid carcinoma and related lesions of the uterine cervix. *Cancer* 16: 1160–1211.

Kottmeier HL (1953) *Carcinoma of the Female Genitalia*. The Abraham Flexner Lecture Series, Number 11. Baltimore: Williams and Wilkins.

Lang WR (1955) Vaginal acidity and pH. *Obstetrical and Gynaecological Survey* 10: 546–560.

Leppert PC, Yu SY (1991) Three-dimensional structures of uterine elastic fibers: scanning electron microscopic studies. *Connective Tissue Research* 27: 15.

Leppert PC, Cerreta JM, Mandl I (1986) Orientation of elastic fibers in the human cervix. *American Journal of Obstetrics and Gynecology* 155: 219.

McClaren H, Attwood M, Nixon W *et al.* (1961) The cervix ante and postpartum. *Proceedings of the Royal Society of Medicine* 54: 712–720.

McKay D, Terjaman B, Younge P *et al.* (1959) Clinical and pathological significance of atypical hyperplasia of the cervix. *Obstetrics and Gynecology* 13: 2–21.

Maliphant R (1949) The incidence of cancer of the cervix. *British Medical Journal* 1: 978–982.

Marsh M (1956) The original site of cervical carcinoma. *Obstetrics and Gynecology* 7: 444–452.

Minamoto T, Arai K, Hirakawa S *et al.* (1987) Immunohistochemical studies on collagen types in the uterine cervix in pregnant and non-pregnant states. *American Journal of Obstetrics and Gynecology* 156: 138.

Mohler R (1953) The clinical significance of misplaced endocervical tissue. *American Journal of Obstetrics and Gynecology* 65: 748–757.

Moore D, Taylor H (1965) In: Gray L (ed.) *Dysplasia, Carcinoma In Situ and Microinvasive Carcinoma*, Vol. 1. Springfield, IL: Charles C. Thomas, p. 386.

Moricard R, Cartier R (1956) Topographic orificielle des dystrophies et de l'epithelioma intraepithelial du col utérin. *Bulletin de la Fédération des Sociétés de Gynécologie et d'Obstétrique de Langue Française* 8: 314–339.

Muñoz N, Franceschi S, Bosch FX *et al.* (2002a) The influence of reproductive and menstrual factors on cervical cancer in HPV positive women. *Lancet* 359: 1093–1101.

Muñoz N, Franceschi S, Bosett C *et al.* (2002b) Role of parity and human papillomavirus in cervical cancer: the IARC multicentre case–control study. *Lancet* 359: 1093–1101.

Nesbitt R, Hellman L (1952) Histopathology of the cervix during pregnancy. *Surgery, Gynecology and Obstetrics* 94: 10–20.

Nilsson K, Risberg B, Heimer G (1995) The vaginal epithelium in the postmenopause—cytology, histology and pH as methods of assessment. *Maturitas* 21: 51–56.

Osmers WD, Raff MW, Alderman-Grill BG (1992) Origin of cervical collagenase during parturition. *American Journal of Obstetrics and Gynecology* 166: 1455.

Paraskevaidis E, Koliopoulos G, Kalantaridou S *et al.* (2002) Management and evolution of cervical intraepithelial neoplasia during pregnancy and postpartum. *European Journal of Obstetrics, Gynecology and Reproductive Biology* 104: 67–69.

Peckham CH (1934) An investigation of some effects of pregnancy noted six weeks and one year after delivery. *Bulletin of the Johns Hopkins Hospital* 54: 186.

Petersen LK, Oxlund H, Uldbjerg N *et al.* (1991) *In vitro* analysis of muscular contractile ability and passive biomechanical properties of uterine cervical samples from non-pregnant women. *Obstetrics and Gynecology* 77: 772.

Rawson AJ, Knoblick R (1957) Clinicopathological study of cervical atypical epithelium. *American Journal of Obstetrics and Gynecology* 73: 120–126.

Reagan JW (1964) In: Gray L (ed.) *Dysplasia, Carcinoma In Situ and Microinvasive Carcinoma*, Vol. 1. Springfield, IL: Charles C. Thomas, p. 294.

Reagan JW, Patten SF (1962) Dysplasia, a basic reaction to injury of the uterine cervix. *Annals of the New York Academy of Sciences* 97: 662–682.

Reid BL (1964) The behaviour of human sperm towards cultured fragments of human cervix uteri. *Lancet* i: 21–22.

Reid B, Singer A, Coppleson M (1967a) The process of cervical regeneration after electrocauterization. Part I. Histological and colposcopic study. *Australian and New Zealand Journal of Obstetrics and Gynaecology* 7: 125–135.

Reid B, Singer A, Coppleson M (1967b) The process of cervical regeneration after electrocauterization. Part II. Histochemical, autoradiographic and pH study. *Australian and New Zealand Journal of Obstetrics and Gynaecology* 7: 136–143.

Rein MF, Muller M (1990) *Trichomonas vaginalis* and trichomoniasis. In: Holmes KK, Mardh P-A, Sparling PF *et al.* (eds) *Sexually Transmitted Diseases*, 2nd edn. New York: McGraw-Hill, pp. 481–492.

Richart RM (1963) Cervical neoplasia and pregnancy. *American Journal of Obstetrics and Gynecology* 87: 474–477.

Richart RM (1967) The natural history of cervical intraepithelial neoplasia. *Clinical Obstetrics and Gynaecology* 10: 748–784.

Romero R, Chaiworapongsa T, Kuipaniemi H *et al.* (2004) Bacterial vaginosis, the inflammatory response and the risk of pre-term births; a role for genetic epidemiology in the prevention of pre-term birth. *American Journal of Obstetrics and Gynecology* 190: 1509–1519.

Rosa P (1965) La structure du myomètre humain et la signification fonctionelle. *Bulletin de la Fédération des Sociétés de Gynécologie et d'Obstétrique de Langue Française* 17: 5–78.

Rotkin ID (1962) Relation of adolescent coitus to cervical cancer risk. *Journal of the American Medical Association* 179: 486–491.

Rotkin ID (1973) A comparison of key epidemiological studies in cervical cancer related to current searches for transmissible agents. *Cancer Research* 33: 1353–1367.

Rotten D, Gavignet C, Colin MC *et al.* (1988) Evolution of the elastic fibre network of the human uterine cervix before, during and after pregnancy. A quantitative evolution by automated image analysis. *Clinics in Physiology and Biochemistry* 6: 285–292.

Roy S, Caillouette J, Faden J (2004) Vaginal pH is similar to follicle-stimulating hormone for menopause diagnosis. *American Journal of Obstetrics and Gynecology* 190: 1272–1277.

Rutledge CE, Christopherson WM (1962) Cervical dysplasia and carcinoma in pregnancy. *Obstetrics and Gynecology* 19: 351–354.

Schneppenheim P, Hamper H, Kaufmann C *et al.* (1958) Die Beziehungen des Schleimepithels zum plattenepithel an der Cervix Uteri in Lebenslauf der Frau. *Archiv für Gynäkologie* 190: 303–345.

Schubert J, Hamerman D (1968) *A Primer of Connective Tissue Biochemistry*, Vol. 1. Philadelphia: Lea and Febiger, p. 228.

Sheilds TS, Brinton LA, Burk RD *et al.* (2004) A case–control study of risk factors for invasive cervical cancer among US women exposed to oncogenic human papillomavirus. *Cancer Epidemiology Biomarkers and Prevention* 13: 1574–1582.

Silbert JE (1973) In: Pereo-Tamayo R, Rojkind M (eds) *Molecular Pathology of Connective Tissue*, Vol. 1. New York: Marcel Dekker, p. 391.

Simon TR, Sheehan JF (1961) The behaviour of cervical atypia and carcinoma in situ in pregnancy, a study of 120 patients. *Proceedings of the 1st International Congress of Exfoliative Cytology*. Philadelphia: Lippincott, pp. 116–120.

Singer A (1973) *The Effect of Physiological and Pathological Factors on the Cervix Uteri*. PhD thesis, University of Sydney, Australia.

Singer A (1975) The uterine cervix from adolescence to the menopause. *British Journal of Obstetrics and Gynaecology* 82: 81–99.

Slate TA, Merrith JW (1961) The behaviour of cervical atypia and carcinoma in situ in pregnancy, a study of 120 patients. *Proceedings of the 1st International Congress of Exfoliative Cytology*. Philadelphia: Lippincott, pp. 128–132.

Smith KPB (1993) Estrogens and the urogenital tract: studies on steroid hormone receptors and a clinical study on a new estradiol releasing vaginal ring. *Acta Obstetrica et Gynecologica Scandinavica* 72 (suppl.): S1–26.

Strinic T, Bukovic D, Karelovic D *et al.* (2002) The effect of delivery on regression of abnormal cervical cytologic findings. *Colloques de Anthropologie* 26: 577–582.

Walz W (1958) Über die genese der Sogenannten indirekten Metaplasie in bereich des Müllerschen Gang-Systems. *Zeitschrift für Geburtshilfe and Gynäkologie* 151: 1–21.

Wilbanks GD, Richart RM (1966) The postpartum cervix and its relationship to cervical neoplasia, a colposcopic study. *Cancer*, 19: 273–276.

Wilbanks GD, Richart RM (1967) The puerperal cervix, injuries and healing, a colposcopic study. *American Journal of Obstetrics and Gynecology* 97: 1105–1110.

Wynder EL, Cornfield J, Schroff PD *et al.* (1954) A study of environmental factors in carcinoma of the cervix. *American Journal of Obstetrics and Gynecology* 68: 1016–1052.

Zimskind PD, Lang WR (1958) The immediate effect of delivery on the portio of the uterine cervix, a colposcopic study. *Fertility and Sterility* 9: 426–434.

CHAPTER 8

Decidual ectopy of the uterine cervix

Antoni Basta

Decidual transformation occurs in endometrial tissue. However, in pregnancy, the decidual foci can occur outside the uterine cavity or in other areas of the female reproductive tract (ovaries, fallopian tubes, cervix, vagina) and within the general pelvic and abdominal cavities (Bayer, 1885; Lapan, 1949; Kwan and Pong, 1964; Herr *et al.*, 1978; Suster and Moran, 1990).

FREQUENCY

Initially, most reported cases of ectopic localisation of decidual transformation were isolated case reports, diagnosed by histological examination. However, decidual ectopy involving the pregnant cervix was originally described by Bayer in 1885 and, at that time, it was thought to be a rare occurrence. Link (1971) and Schneider and Barnes (1981) examined hysterectomy specimens removed for either benign or neoplastic disease in pregnancy and found decidual changes in 30.8% and 61.4% respectively.

Decidual ectopy detected by colposcopy was reported for the first time by Hinselmann (1929): he believed this change to be rare. Madej *et al.* (1965) also described the changes and also thought them to be rare. However, routine colposcopic assessment of the cervix in pregnant women reveals that decidual changes within the cervix are much more common, affecting 3–34% of women (Schneider and Barnes, 1981; Basta *et al.*, 1984). At the University Department of Krakow, Poland, colposcopy is performed routinely in pregnant women, and the frequency of decidual ectopic changes is 6.2% (Basta *et al.*, 1984; Madej *et al.*, 1989).

Decidual transformation has never been reported in the cervix of women with an ectopic pregnancy. It can, however, be seen in the cervix of non-pregnant women, albeit rarely.

AETIOLOGY

In pregnancy

There are two possible explanations for the presence of decidual cervical tissue. The first is that of decidual transformation of foci of endometriosis within the cervix which, in pregnancy, may be influenced by the same progesterone stimulation as endometrial tissue (Cartier 1984). The second is the decidualisation of connective tissue cells, especially fibrocytes in pregnancy (Weller 1935). Mayer (1913) suggested that the inflammatory process that may change the connective tissue cells of the stroma could be important in the decidualisation process. These cells may act as receptors for hormones produced by the corpus luteum and placenta. In addition to progesterone and human chorionic gonadotrophin, human placental lactogen, prolactin, prostaglandins and other proteins may also be involved in inducing the ectopic decidual changes (Basta *et al.*, 1984; Madej *et al.*, 1989; Kularbkaew *et al.*, 1998; Gornall *et al.*, 2000).

In the non-pregnant cervix

Although the aetiology of decidual ectopy in the cervix of the non-pregnant woman is not clear, the author suggests from his own observations that it may result from the so-called superluteal status, the result of prolonged activity of the corpus luteum.

Hormonal, neurohormonal and inflammatory agents have been proposed as producing decidual ectopic transformation within the cervix and within the abdominal cavity, but these processes do not seem to be enough to explain all the occurrences of ectopic decidual change.

Three questions need to be asked in respect of decidual change:
1 Why does decidual change not develop in every pregnancy?
2 Why is decidual ectopy not seen in ectopic pregnancy?
3 Why, in some pregnant women, is the decidual cervical tissue diagnosed only microscopically while in others it is observed macroscopically?

However, certain factors are known such as:
1 Decidual tissue develops within the stroma underlying original squamous, columnar and metaplastic squamous epithelium and within the transformation zone.
2 Decidual changes most commonly occur within the cervix in women aged 20–35 years of age (Basta *et al.*, 1984; Madej *et al.*, 1989; Basta, 1988).

3 Over 70% of foci of cervical decidual change are diagnosed between the fifth and 12th weeks of pregnancy.

4 In early pregnancy, ectopic cervical decidual tissue may bleed spontaneously, thus raising the suspicion of a threatened abortion; the lesions are usually multiple and often multi-coloured (white, yellow, pink or brown), and the surface may be ulcerated. Such lesions may raise the suspicion of malignancy, especially sarcoma. The less experienced colposcopist will always need to take a biopsy to confirm and to exclude malignancy.

COLPOSCOPIC APPEARANCES

Colposcopy is the optimum way to diagnose decidual changes. The colposcopic classification of decidual ectopy is based on their localisation within the cervix, their degree of proliferation and their shape. The classification is as follows:

1 decidual ectopy of the cervix:
infiltrative form
ulcerative form
polypoidal form
papillary form
2 decidual polyps of the endocervical canal.

Decidual ectopy of the cervix

In primagravidae, the ectopic changes are seen most frequently on the ectocervix but, in multigravidae, the ectopic changes are seen with equal frequency on the ectocervix and in the endocervical canal (Table 8.1).

Infiltrative and ulcerative forms occur in the stroma of squamous epithelium. The polypoid form occurs in the stroma of squamous, columnar and transformation zone epithelium. The papillary form is localised exclusively to areas of columnar epithelium. (Note: the papillary form is different from the decidual polyps which are located in the endocervical canal.)

Table 8.1 Localisation of cervical decidual ectopy: an assessment of 459 cases.

	Primigravidae	*Multigravidae*
Decidual ectopy of the ectocervix	114 (78.6%)	161 (51.3%)
Decidual endocervical polyps	31 (21.4%)	153 (48.7%)
Total	145	314

Infiltrative form

Colposcopically, the infiltrative form appears as a smooth or coarse protrusion or swelling covered by squamous epithelium within which a cavity, dimple or depression may be observed. In some cases, capillaries are seen on the surface (similar to the capillaries seen on Nabothian follicles). Following the application of acetic acid, the smooth transparent appearance of the surface diminishes and, in areas that are not covered with epithelium, there is a dense acetowhite appearance. The areas stain with iodine, but some small areas are non-staining with iodine (Fig. 8.1a–c).

Ulcerative form

Colposcopically, the ulcerative form is seen as areas that have been denuded of the superficial squamous epithelium – the areas have sharp borders and an irregular friable surface. Following the application of acetic acid, the ulcerated areas appear to have a dense acetowhite appearance: these areas are non-staining with iodine (Figs 8.2 and 8.3).

Polypoidal form

The polypoidal form is seen macroscopically as polyp-shaped lesions arising from the ectocervix and having a yellow–brown colour. Colposcopically recognisable blood vessels are usual

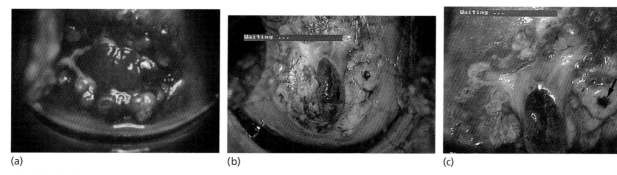

(a)   (b)   (c)

Fig. 8.1 (a) Infiltrative nodular decidual ectopy. (b) Colpophotograph showing the bizarre changes associated with decidual ectopy: decidualisation in pregnancy. An endocervical polyp is seen at (1) with squamous metaplasia apparent at its tip (arrowed). (c) A higher magnification of the view seen in (b) showing gland openings becoming large and prominent, giving the appearance of a raised lesion with a central cavity, which may appear, as in this photograph, as a central dimple or depression (arrowed). This is a characteristic finding of the infiltrative form of deciduosis.

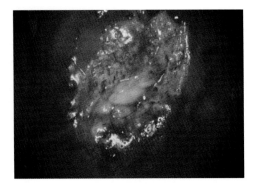

Fig. 8.2 Mixed, i.e. ulcerative and papillary, decidual ectopy.

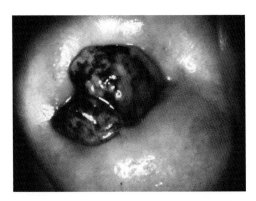

Fig. 8.3 Ulcerative infiltrative decidual ectopy on posterior cervix. A necrotic decidual polyp with blood in the external os.

on the surface and areas are densely acetowhite. The polyps are non-staining with iodine (Figs 8.3, 8. 4a–c and 8.5).

Papillary form

The papillary form occurs only in columnar epithelium. The grape-like columnar epithelial villi become larger and have a pale, white colour. These changes are most pronounced following the application of acetic acid (Fig. 8.2).

Decidual polyps of the cervical canal

Decidual changes may occur in columnar epithelial polyps that had been present before pregnancy but, more often in pregnancy, the decidual transformation begins in the stroma of the endocervical canal. Colposcopically, the polyps are single

(Figs 8.1b, 8.6, 8.7) or multiple and tend to be grain-shaped or bean-shaped; sometimes, they have a hedgehog shape (usually being multicoloured, yellow, pink, brown or white). This multicoloration is related to changes in the blood vessel and represents small haematomas or necrosis. In some instances, two types of blood vessels may be seen – linear/spiral vessels or asymmetric looped vessels (Madej 1982). Polyps are densely acetowhite but, interestingly, the blood vessels do not disappear. The polyps are non-staining with iodine.

CYTOLOGICAL AND PATHOLOGICAL DIAGNOSIS

The role of cytology in the diagnosis of decidual ectopy has improved (Schneider and Barnes, 1981; Basta *et al.*, 1984) but,

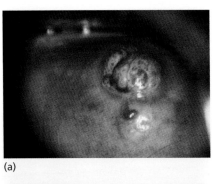

(a)

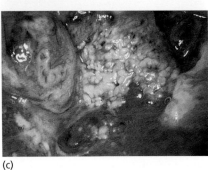

(c)

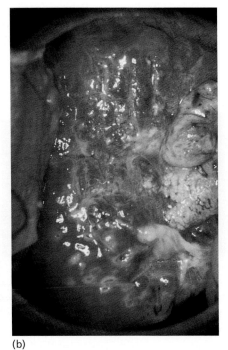

(b)

Fig. 8.4 (a) Polypoid decidual ectopy. (b) Polypoidal form of deciduosis in a woman of 14 weeks' gestation showing the oedematous nature of the polyp-shaped lesions arising from the ectocervix. The oedematous epithelium in this photograph is of both squamous and columnar tissues. At low power. (c) A higher magnification of the view seen in (b).

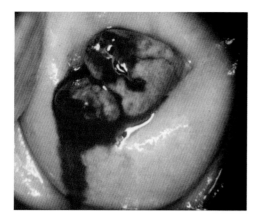

Fig. 8.5 Polypoid form of decidual ectopy. Secondary transparency and bleeding.

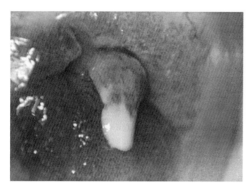

Fig. 8.6 Decidual polyp of the cervical canal. Spiral blood vessels and whitening of the top of the polyp. Mosaic changes are present in the posterior lip of the epithelium.

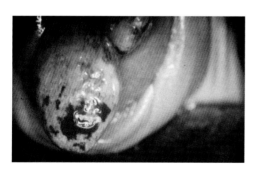

Fig. 8.7 Decidual polyp of the cervical canal with linear/spiral blood vessels. Necrosis with bleeding.

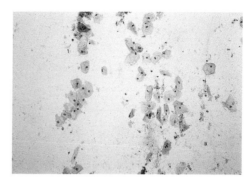

Fig. 8.8 Characteristic cytological changes. The cells are essentially superficial squames and are oedematous and abnormal in appearance. Necrosis is apparent with contact bleeding.

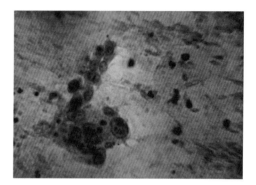

Fig. 8.9 Pap smear of a pregnant woman with decidual ectopy. The nucleocytoplasmic ratio is changed, with nuclear enlargement and hyperchromasia. Changes are similar to those seen in sarcoma.

Characteristic histological changes show widely expanded cells that underlie a superficial single layer of cuboidal cells that are present on the upper surface of the elevated protrusions. These features are seen in Figures 8.10 (low power) and 8.11 (high power).

CLINICAL SIGNIFICANCE

The clinical significance of decidual ectopy resides in the fact that many of its features, i.e. macroscopic, colposcopic and microscopic, can be confused with identical characteristics existing in both carcinomatous and sarcomatous lesions of the cervix. For example, the irregular surface of these lesions, the reduced transparency of the epithelium and the fact that there is no staining with iodine may be mistaken by the inexperienced colposcopist as changes suggestive of malignancy. The colposcopic features that help to differentiate between decidual ectopy and cancer are:

1 Decidual foci are localised within areas of original or metaplastic squamous or columnar epithelium and have a sharp line of demarcation with original squamous epithelium. Cancer, on the other hand, is localised within the atypical transformation

even so, the accuracy of colposcopy is higher than the accuracy of cytology. There are characteristic cytological changes: the cells are essentially superficial squames and are oedematous and abnormal in appearance (Fig. 8.8). They also contain a considerable amount of fluid. In about one-third of cases with decidual ectopy, cytology is negative. Furthermore, in some cases, it is difficult for the Pap test to differentiate between decidual cells and cells suggestive of carcinoma, especially sarcoma (Fig. 8.9) (Krupiński and Madej, 1981).

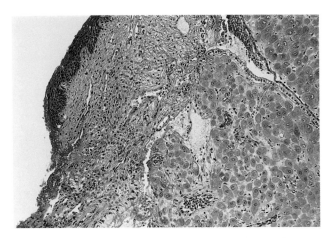

Fig. 8.10 View under low power of characteristic histological changes showing widely expanded cells that underlie a superficial single layer of cuboidal cells present on the upper surface of the elevated protrusions.

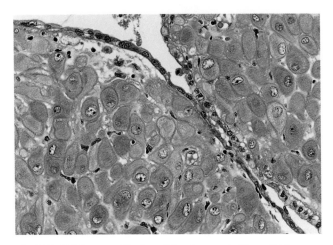

Fig. 8.11 A higher magnification of the view seen in Figure 8.10.

zone and is often surrounded by foci of lower pathology (CIN).

2 Decidual ectopy is usually multifocal and of small size, whereas cancer is usually a solitary tumour with an irregular papillary surface.

3 The capillary pattern in the decidual foci may mimic the atypical vessels of cancer but, in decidual foci, the vessels are of small calibre, the intercapillary distance is small and, following the application of acetic acid, the vessels of decidual ectopy do not disappear whereas those of cancer often do.

4 The multicoloration of decidual changes, the younger age of the woman, the presence of pregnancy and bleeding or necrosis all favour a diagnosis of decidual foci. However, if the colposcopist is unsure of the diagnosis, a punch biopsy should always be taken.

5 Sometimes, decidual changes and CIN or cancer may occur simultaneously.

The decidual changes of the cervix may easily become infected by vaginal bacteria, and this may result in excessive vaginal discharge in the pregnant woman.

It should be remembered that areas of decidual change in early pregnancy can bleed spontaneously and may mimic a miscarriage. Colposcopy will allow the source of such bleeding to be identified (Figs 8.5 and 8.7) and, when coupled with a normal ultrasound, the pregnant woman can be reassured that her bleeding is due not to miscarriage, but rather to decidual change.

In Krakow, Poland, it is felt that colposcopy should be an integrated part of antenatal assessment. The colposcopist should remember that decidual changes within the endocervical canal may not be visible to colposcopy but may nevertheless be the source of bleeding in early pregnancy. Colposcopic observation shows that ectopic decidual changes in the cervix are found most commonly before the 16th week of gestation but, in a small percentage of cases, the changes can appear for the first time up to 25 weeks. After 25 weeks, the decidual lesions regress. Regression particularly occurs in the decidual polyps of the endocervical canal and occurs as a result of compression of the blood vessels in the pedicle of the endocervical polyps, which results in necrosis and shedding of the polyp. Most of the decidual changes (60–70%) have regressed by the 38th week of pregnancy while the remainder regress shortly after delivery, which is why the decidual changes in the cervix do not need to be treated surgically.

ACKNOWLEDGEMENT

The author wishes to thank Professor A. Singer and Mr J.M. Monaghan for allowing him to reproduce Figures 8.1b, 8.1c, 8.2, 8.4b, 8.4c, 8.8, 8.10 and 8.11 from their text, *Lower Genital Tract Precancer, Colposcopy, Pathology and Treatment*. Oxford: Blackwell Science, 2nd edn, 2000, pp. 312–313.

REFERENCES

Basta A (1988) The course of pregnancy and labour and the condition of the newborn in women with decidual ectopy of the cervix. *Wiadomości Lekarskie* 41: 925–929.

Basta A, Krzysiek J, Ciocheń G *et al.* (1984) The importance of colposcopic diagnosis of decidual ectopy in the cervix in early pregnancy. *Ginekologia Polska* 55: 351–358.

Bayer H (Red.) (1885) *Zur physiologischen un pathologischen Morphologie der Gebärmutter W: Gynäkologische Klinik*. Strasburg: W.A. Frennd, pp. 369–662.

Cartier R (1984) Practical colposcopy. *Laboratoire Cartier* 274.

Gornall AS, Naftalin NJ, Brown LJR *et al.* (2000) Massive necrosis of cervical ectopic decidua presenting in labour. *British Journal of Obstetrics and Gynecology* 107: 573–575.

Heer JC, Heidger PM Jr, Scott JR (1978) Decidual cells in the human ovary at term. Incidence, gross anatomy and ultrastructural features of endocrine secretion. *American Journal of Anatomy* 152: 7–22.

Hinselmann H (1929) Deziduaknötchen in der Umwandlungszone der Portio bei einer Gravida Mens III. *Zeitschrift für Geburtshilfe und Gynäkologie* 95: 1121.

Krupiñski L, Madej J (1981) Zytologische und kolposkopische Diagnose der dezidualen Ektopie der Zervix. *Geburtshilfe und Frauenheilkeit* 41: 474–477.

Kularbkaew Ch, Jutanaviboonchai W, Pairojkul Ch (1998) Molar pregnancy I. Associated ectopic decidua; Report of a case and review of the literature. *Journal of the Medical Association of Thailand* 81: 918–923.

Kwan D, Pong LS (1964) Deciduosis peritonei. *Journal of Obstetrics and Gynaecology of the British Commonwealth* 7: 804–806.

Lapan B (1949) Deciduosis of the cervix and vagina simulating carcinoma. *American Journal of Obstetrics and Gynecology* 58: 743–747.

Link M (1971) Über die deziduale Reaktion der Zervixschleimhaustroma im Verlauf der Gravidität. *Zenterblatt Gynäkologie* 93: 1481–1488.

Madej J (1982) *Kolposkopia*. Warszawa: PZWL.

Madej J, Matuszewski H, Cielecki J *et al.* (1965) Ectopic decidual growth on the uterine vaginal portion. *Ginekologia Polska* 36: 569–575.

Madej J, Krzysiek J, Basta A *et al.* (1989) Decidual ectopy on the uterine cervix. The diagnostic and clinical consideration. *Materia Medica Polonia* 1 (69): 20–26.

Mayer R (1913) Die Entzundung als Enstehungsursache ektopischer Dezidua oder Paradezidua. *Zeitschrift für Geburtshilfe und Gynäkologie* 74: 250.

Schneider V, Barnes LA (1981) Ectopic decidual reaction of the uterine cervix. *Acta Cytologica* 25: 616–621.

Suster S, Moran CA (1990) Deciduosis of the appendix. *American Journal of Gastroenterology* 85: 841–845.

Weller CV (1935) The ectopic decidual reaction and its significance in endometriosis. *American Journal of Pathology* 1: 287–290.

CHAPTER 9

The effects of oral contraceptive steroids, menopause and hormone replacement therapy on the cervical epithelium

Sun Kuie Tay and Albert Singer

INTRODUCTION

Cervical epithelium changes throughout the lifespan of a woman, most notably at puberty, during pregnancy and menopause and under the influence of exogenous female sex steroid hormones. The dynamics of cervical epithelium is further modified by the microenvironment and the pH milieu of the endocervix and vagina (see Chapter 7). Cervical squamous epithelium has a rapid cell turnover rate during the reproductive ages of women. Proliferation of the basal cells of the epithelium produces new cells, which enter the end-stage differentiation and maturation as they pass through the process of stratification to become the superficial cells. On average, the mature squamous epithelium of the cervix has a thickness of between 20 and 30 cell layers.

In contrast, the endocervical epithelium is composed of a single layer of columnar cells. The epithelium forms clefts with architectural organisation of glands. These cells demonstrate both proliferative and secretory functions. Under the influence of a surge in circulating blood levels of estrogen and progesterone, the cervix everts and exposes the caudal portion of the endocervical columnar epithelium to the relatively more acidic microenvironment of the vagina. The exposed columnar epithelium undergoes a process of squamous metaplasia. A matured metaplastic squamous epithelium is indistinguishable from the native squamous epithelium. The true nature of its metaplastic origin is revealed only by the presence of glands under the epithelium on histological examination (see Chapter 2).

THE ROLE OF SEX STEROID RECEPTORS IN TARGET TISSUES

These characteristics of cervical epithelia are the consequence of intricate interactions between the female sex steroids and their receptors on the target tissues. In this respect, estrogen and progesterone receptors are the most essential. Using an autoradiographic method, Gould *et al.* (1983) reported the presence of estrogen binding sites in squamous and stromal cells of the human cervix. More recent immunohistochemical staining studies (Remoue, 2003) also showed that only estrogen but not progesterone receptors are present in the human ectocervical epithelium. These receptors are localised mainly in the basal cells, with only weak expression in occasional parabasal cells. Estrogen receptor expression vanishes as the cells mature progressively towards the superficial strata of the epithelium. Estrogen receptor expression, however, does not display any discernible change throughout the menstrual cycle (Scharl *et al.*, 1988; Cano *et al.*, 1990). In the endocervical epithelium, both estrogen and progesterone receptors can be demonstrated. Estrogen receptor expression is reduced during the secretory phase of the menstrual cycle, but progesterone receptor expression is not affected by fluctuation of the endogenous hormones. Estrogen is the physiological inducer of progesterone receptors *in vivo* (Lin, 1984). Strong estrogen receptor expression is also seen in metaplastic epithelial cells (Ciocca *et al.*, 1986).

Recently, Remoue (2003) has shown that the expression of estrogen receptors and progesterone receptors is significantly higher in the transformation zone than in the ectocervix, particularly in the hormone receptor-positive cells which are seen to be located in parabasal and intermediate cell layers in the transformation zone, and also in the ectocervical epithelium. It seems as though the cells of immature squamous metaplasia show a significantly high density of hormone receptor-positive cells in them compared with those in the ectocervical epithelium, which are predominantly original (native) epithelial cells.

Experiments with rats show that estrogen receptors and retinoid receptors play a critical role in squamous cell differentiation and maturation. During the oestrous cycle, estrogen induces proliferation and squamous differentiation of the cervical epithelium, while progesterone and retinoids maintain the simple columnar epithelium of the endocervix (Celli *et al.*, 1996). In humans, the regulatory roles of estrogen may be mediated via the two distinct alpha and beta estrogen receptors (Wang *et al.*, 2001). Although the exact roles of the two estrogen receptors are yet to be ascertained, the available evidence suggests that low levels of alpha estrogen receptor and high levels of progesterone receptor are associated with an increased apoptosis index in the epithelial cells (Ramos *et al.*, 2002). On the other hand, low levels of estrogen and the presence of oncogenic human papillomavirus (HPV) may facilitate the metaplastic transformation of the subepithelial stem-like reserve cells towards squamous rather than columnar cells and eventual development of neoplasia (Elson *et al.*, 2000).

The specific distribution of estrogen and progesterone receptors and their interactions with female sex steroids determine the dynamic state of the cervical epithelium in physiological conditions and also determine the response of this tissue to exogenous sex steroid therapies.

THE EFFECTS OF ORAL CONTRACEPTIVE STEROIDS

Oral contraceptive pills (OCPs) are a combination of synthetic estrogens and progestogens. They have emerged as a major method of contraceptive practice among women for the last four decades. Annually, 100 million women worldwide, including 10 million women in the USA, take oral contraceptive pills (Abma *et al.*, 1997). Recent progress in the development of OCPs has brought about a steady decline in the dosage of ethinylestradiol within these preparations from 100 μg daily in the 1960s to 30 μg in the 1980s and 20 μg in the 1990s. The progestogens have also undergone changes over this time including the development of levonorgestrel in the 1980s from the original norethisterone. Gestodene, desogestrel and norgestimate were later developments in the 1990s. The newer or the third-generation progestogens are less androgenic and carry lesser adverse effects on the metabolism of carbohydrates and lipids than the progestogens of earlier generations (Kuhl, 1996). Their potent progestogenic property in respect of the stability of endometrium permits progressive lowering of estrogen dosage in the newer OCPs. These advances have resulted in a lowering of cardiovascular, hypertensive and thromboembolic diseases associated with the use of OCPs (WHO Collaborative Study of Cardiovascular Disease and Steroid Hormone Contraception, 1995, 1997; Carr and Ory, 1997; Suissa *et al.*, 1997; Chasen-Taber and Stampfer, 1998; Hatcher *et al.*, 1998).

These synthetic female sex steroids are potent ligands of estrogen and progesterone receptors on cervical epithelium (Gould *et al.*, 1983; Cunha *et al.*, 1982). Their effects on cervical epithelium and the development of cervical neoplasia are of great importance to clinicians, researchers and public health policy-makers. Of great concern is the high prevalence of *Chlamydia trachomatis*, a very common sexually transmitted infection which in most cases is asymptomatic or mildly symptomatic, in women using oral contraceptives. It would

seem as though *C. trachomatis* preferentially infects the columnar cells that are the major epithelial target of this condition. The increased exposure of the susceptible cells aids the infection and its passage through the cervix into the uterine and pelvic cavity, inducing pelvic inflammatory disease with significant reproductive sequelae. It has also been suggested that oral contraceptives have a direct effect on the genital tract's immune system, as well as increasing the susceptibility of the host cells within the cervical ectropion, induced by the oral contraceptive steroids, to infection (Jacobson *et al.*, 2000a).

Clinical features of OCP effects on the cervix

The effect of OCPs on the cervix varies according to the content of estrogen and progestogen and the duration of their use. In a major proportion of pill users, the cervix is gradually seen to enlarge and soften as a result of oedema within the stroma. These changes result in the bulky vaginal portion of the cervix everting to a variable degree, a process seen in pregnancy (see Chapter 7). The well-estrogenised native squamous epithelium seems to be unaffected by the OCPs and remains smooth and pink. The most prominent changes occur in the transformation zone and the endocervical columnar epithelium, again similar to those seen in pregnancy. There is an obvious extension of endocervical columnar epithelium onto the ectocervix, producing the classical appearance of what is clinically referred to as an ectopy or ectropion (Critchlow *et al.*, 1985; Jacobson *et al.*, 2000b). There is usually an associated area of erythema and oedema at the periphery (Fig. 9.1a and b).

As a result of estrogen stimulation, the exposed endocervical columnar cells increase their intracellular mucus synthesis. Under the influence of progestogen, the biochemical composition of the mucus changes to become thick and viscous, with loss of cyclic variations seen with ovulatory menstrual cycles (Mohsenian *et al.*, 1981; Gaton *et al.*, 1982; Hull and Moghissi, 1986). The endocervical crypts also increase in dimension, and these changes may be related to the biological potency of the synthetic progestogens. In this respect, the third-generation OCPs containing gestodene, desogestrel and norgestimate, which contain potent progestogens, may show a higher cellular activity than the older pills containing weaker progestogens (Dallenbach-Hellweg and Fenzel, 1985; Kuhl, 1996). Clinically, a thick and viscous plaque of mucoid secretion can be seen to cover the cervix (Fig. 9.2a).

Colposcopic features of OCP effects on the cervix

The cervical ectopy or ectropion described above, commonly seen in women taking OCPs, is associated with exposure of the transformation zone components, namely the original columnar epithelium. After the application of acetic acid,

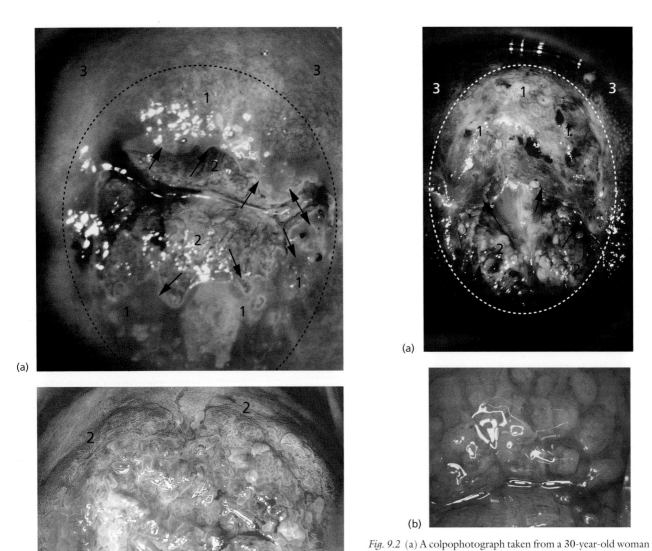

(a)

(b)

Fig. 9.1 (a) A colpophotograph from a 26-year-old woman on oral contraceptive pills for 12 months. The overall appearance is commonly referred to as an ectropion or as ectopy. There is surrounding erythema, and the transformation zone is clearly demarcated by the new (→→) and original (– – –) squamocolumnar junctions. The epithelium within the transformation zone represents areas of squamous metaplasia (1). Original columnar epithelium is prominent and extends from the anatomical os to the ectocervix (2). The peripheral native squamous epithelium shows the typical fine reticular vascular network (3). (b) The development of ectopy or ectropion, with the columnar epithelium situated on the ectocervix in a young woman taking oral contraceptive steroids. The endocervix is at

(a)

(b)

Fig. 9.2 (a) A colpophotograph taken from a 30-year-old woman who had been on oral contraceptives for 5 years. There is a large transformation zone with prominent squamous metaplasia (1). The exposed endocervical columnar epithelium shows florid proliferative activity with enlarged globular and grape-like surface appearance (2). The mucus is viscous and opaque. The original (native) squamous epithelium assumes a bluish hue (3). The overall impression of the cervix is similar to pregnancy-induced changes. The new squamocolumnar junction is marked by arrows (→) and the original junction is also shown (– – –). (b) Colpophotograph of the cervix of a young woman who has been taking a high estrogen dosage oral contraceptive for 15 years. The individual columnar villi are grossly enlarged and fused, giving a polypoid appearance. There is an apparent eversion of these columnar villi, which protrude from the endocervical canal; this results in an ectropion or ectopy.

---

(1) and the original squamocolumnar junction at (2). In between, there are columnar villi that are clumped and present as irregular but small polypoid structures. These look quite abnormal to the naked eye and imitate the appearance of malignancy. Colposcopy allows the benign nature of this lesion to be confirmed.

metaplastic squamous epithelium of the transformation zone displays a pearly white appearance on the ectocervix (1 in Fig. 9.1), with a well-demarcated new squamocolumnar junction (see Fig. 9.1). There may be intermingling areas of squamous metaplasia at different stages of maturation. The columnar epithelium may show a prominent globular topographic appearance, which reflects the high cellular proliferation and mucin production rates of the endocervical cells. Under the influence of a prolonged period of OCP use, the globular columnar epithelium may enlarge and elongate to assume an appearance of short villi (Fig. 9.2a and b).

It is also possible to have clumping of the villi, which produces an irregular polypoidal mass (Fig. 9.2b). With some of the high-dose oral contraceptives (50 μg of ethinylestradiol), there develops gross oedema and hyperaemia of the columnar epithelium in association with the irregular polypoidal masses seen in Figure 9.2b.

All types of progestogens used in OCPs exert a direct angiogenesis effect on blood vessels (Hague *et al.*, 2002) (see also Chapter 20). This may explain the faint bluish hue of the cervix in some women using OCPs for a long period (3 in Fig 9.2a). The increased vascularity is manifested within the columnar epithelium by the ease with which bleeding occurs on contact during examination.

The native or original squamous epithelium demonstrates a strong iodine reaction on the application of Schiller's iodine. The area of dark iodine staining on the cervix increases with the duration of use of low-dose OCPs.

Cytological features of OCP effects on the cervical epithelium

The cellular components of a satisfactory cervical smear taken from women not taking OCPs shows a cyclic variation relating to the hormonal state of the physiological menstrual cycle. It includes a mixture of squamous cells at different stages of maturation and endocervical cells. The cyclic variation in the proportion of different cell types is lost in women consuming OCPs steadily. There is a reduction in the number of superficial cells and an increase in the number of endometrial cells in the smears from these women (Liu *et al.*, 1967). Typically, the karyopyknotic index is low. There may be some navicular cells, with marked curling and folding of cells, and occasional cells showing large cellular nuclei beyond 5 μm (Katira and Dayal, 1987).

Quantitative measurement shows a statistically significant difference in the nuclear–cytoplasmic ratio on the visually normal intermediate cells between the patients and normal control subjects among women in natural ovulatory cycles. This difference is masked by the use of OCPs for three cycles (Kwikkel *et al.*, 1986). These OCP effects may sometimes confuse the cytological interpretation of neoplasia in the intermediate cells.

Histological features of OCP effect on the cervical epithelium

In women on long-term OCPs, interactions between sex steroids and estrogen and progesterone receptors on different cell types within the cervical epithelium can lead to a number of histological changes. The most noteworthy histological variations occur in the endocervical columnar epithelium, resulting in specific histological changes described as endocervical cribriform adenomatous hyperplasia or microglandular endocervical hyperplasia (MEH) (Fig. 9.3a and b).

Moltz and Becker (1977) examined the histology of punch biopsies of the cervix from 79 women taking OCPs, nine women taking progestogen-only pills and 14 control women with natural menstrual cycles. There was a tendency for a higher prevalence of cribriform adenomatous hyperplasia of the endocervical glands among women on hormones, than in the control group. However, the difference between the groups was not statistically significant.

Microglandular hyperplasia is seen clinically as polypoidal lesions in the endocervical canal (Fig. 9.3c). The classical histological features show closely packed glands of variable sizes and shapes interspersed by infiltration of acute and chronic inflammatory cells. The cells lining these glands are flattened or cuboid, with eosinophilic cytoplasm containing a small quantity of mucin. The nucleus may be hyperchromic and occasionally pleomorphic (Wright and Holinka, 2002). The mitotic index is low (Fig. 9.3a and b).

The pathogenesis of microglandular hyperplasia has long been thought to be associated with pregnancy and exogenous hormones, particularly OCPs (Gondos, 1976). However, Chumas *et al.* (1985) reported that more than half the 43 women with microglandular hyperplasia in their series had no history of OCP use. In a blinded case–control study, Greeley *et al.* (1995) reported that a documented pregnancy or OCP use in the preceding 6 months was found in 57.9% (22 of 38) of patients with microglandular hyperplasia and in 47.4% (18 of 38) of control subjects. There was no statistically significant difference in the prevalence of pregnancy or OCP use between the patients with microglandular hyperplasia and the control subjects. Comparing 18 patients with endocervical adenocarcinoma and adenosquamous carcinoma with age-matched subjects with squamous cell carcinoma, Jones and Silverberg (1989) reported a positive OCP history in 28% of cases and 39% of control subjects. Microglandular hyperplasia was seen in five cases of adenocarcinoma and one case of squamous cell carcinoma. There was no statistical association between microglandular hyperplasia and endocervical carcinoma.

Nonetheless, microglandular hyperplasia is an important entity, in that it can give rise to confusion in cytological inaccuracies and histological diagnosis of malignancy. Alvarez-Santin *et al.* (1999) reported the cytological features of 54 cases of microglandular hyperplasia: the glandular cells form

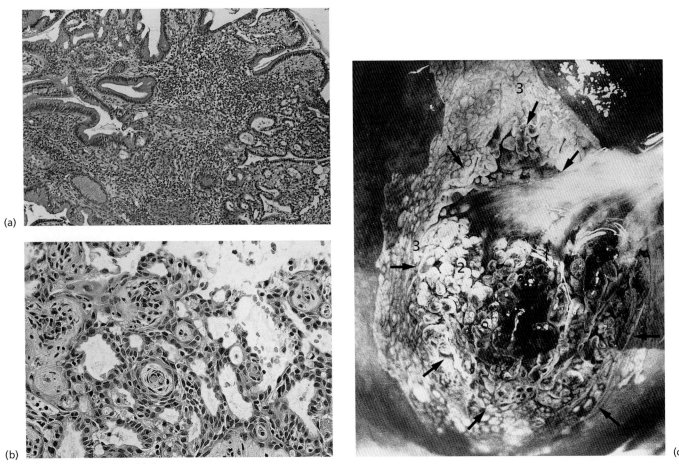

Fig. 9.3 Biopsy taken from a woman with a history of long-term oral contraceptive use; microglandular endocervical hyperplasia (MEH) is evident. (a) A low-power view. (b) Part of this view at higher magnification. Multiple, and apparently complex, superficial cervical crypts are present, and numerous small glandular spaces are lined by regular cuboidal cells. The nuclei are uniform and vesicular, with occasional nucleoli. Mitotic figures are not present here, but can sometimes be found. Vacuoles also appear in an extracellular position. The stromal cells are present between the glandular elements, and these have the appearance of reserve cells. Two important features of MEH are the presence of irregular nuclei and the virtual absence of mitotic figures. These should be kept in mind when this condition is to be differentiated from invasive carcinoma. (c) Typical colposcopic findings of oral contraceptive use; the columnar villi are enlarged and have adopted a small capillary loop pattern at (1). Squamous metaplastic epithelium appears at (2) and the original squamocolumnar junction is arrowed. Biopsy of the area around (1) showed the pattern characteristic of microglandular hyperplasia. The epithelium at (3) is characteristic of that found in the congenital transformation zone (see Chapter 2).

clusters and may be cuboid or cylindrical, with vacuolated or dense cytoplasm, or with basaloid appearances. The cells may sometimes demonstrate various degrees of atypia, which leads to misdiagnosis of malignancy or high-grade squamous epithelial neoplasia (Yahr and Lee, 1991; Young and Scully, 1992; Valente and Schantz, 1994).

Mucosal immunity and predisposition to infection

Cervical epithelium harbours a significant population of immune-reactive cells which constitutes the mucosal cellular and humoral immune systems. B lymphocytes are located predominantly in the subepithelial compartment. In women of reproductive age, the main types of immunoglobulins are IgA

and IgG. The levels of these immunoglobulins show a cyclic fluctuation corresponding to endogenous estradiol levels. In contrast, IgA is the predominant immunoglobulin in women taking OCPs. Its level was higher than the peak level seen in the ovulatory phase of a normal menstrual cycle (Franklin and Kutteh, 1999). The impact of these changes in producing a protective effect in respect of OCP-associated cases of sexually transmissible diseases is unclear (Montes *et al.*, 2000).

The cellular immune system is represented by the antigen-presenting cells (Langerhans cells), monocytes, T-helper and T-cytotoxic cells (Tay *et al.*, 1987a–c). These dendritic Langerhans cells form a mesh of fine network in the cervical epithelium, strategically placed to detect any invading viruses and microbes. There is a dense population of helper and killer

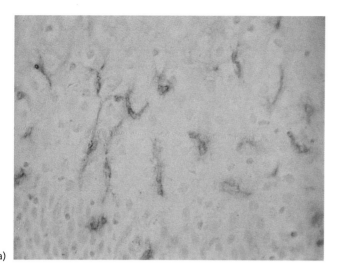
(a)

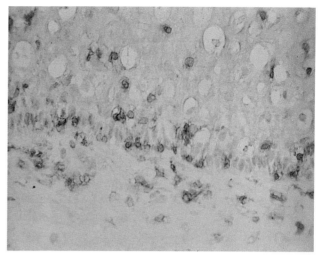
(b)

Fig. 9.4 Microphotographs of the cervical epithelial cellular immune system. (a) Immunohistochemical staining with CD6 monoclonal antibody to demonstrate the distribution of antigen-presenting Langerhans cells within the squamous epithelium of a normal cervix. These dendritic cells form an intricate network for antigen detection within the epithelium. (b) Immunohistochemical staining with CD8 monoclonal antibody. Abundance of cytotoxic T lymphocytes can be seen at the basal layers of the epithelium in close proximity to Langerhans cells.

T lymphocytes at the basal compartment of the epithelium to effect the antiviral activities (Fig. 9.4a and b). The use of OCPs does not cause any discernible changes in the cellular immune system in cervical epithelium (Tay, unpublished data), although Remoue *et al.* (2003) have recently proposed an effect of sex hormones on the regulation of these cells, particularly Langerhans/dendritic cells, by influencing the production of cytokines/chemokines.

The role of OCP in cervical carcinogenesis

Squamous neoplasia

An excess prevalence of cervical neoplasia among women on long-term OCPs was first reported in large cohort studies. Meisels *et al.* (1977) studied 84 540 women with no cytological abnormality and 2017 patients with mild and moderate dysplasia, and reported a highly significant correlation between the use of contraceptive pills and mild and moderate dysplasia. Vessey *et al.* (1983) reported a rising trend of incidence of cervical neoplasia in women using OCPs in a 10-year follow-up surveillance for the Oxford Family Planning Association. Compared with the incidence of 1.0 per 1000 women–years among intrauterine device (IUD) users, the incidence of cervical neoplasia rose from 0.9 per 1000 women–years among women with less than 2 years' OCP use to 2.2 per 1000 women–years among women with more than 8 years' use. However, in a similar set-up, the New Zealand Contraception and Health Study Group (1994) reported that no discernible difference in the incidence of cervical intraepithelial neoplasia (CIN) was observed between pill users and IUD users.

In a prospective follow-up study of 6622 women, Gram *et al.* (1992) found that, after adjusting for age, marital status, smoking and frequency of alcohol intoxication, the relative rate for current pill users was 1.5 (95% CI 1.1–2.1), and the relative rate for past users was 1.4 (95% CI 1.0–1.8), compared with those who had never used oral contraceptives. Similarly, some case–control studies with adjustment for confounding factors did not show a consistent association of OCP usage and CIN (Clarke *et al.*, 1985; Molina *et al.*, 1988; Coker *et al.*, 1992; de Vet *et al.*, 1993; Zondervan *et al.*, 1996; Ylitalo *et al.*, 1999).

Zondervan *et al.* (1996) suggested that the observed excess prevalence of CIN in some studies may result from confounding HPV infection. Indeed, in a case–control study adjusted for HPV infection, Coker *et al.* (2001) reported no association of OCP use and CIN development. These studies contradict the findings of Ylitalo *et al.* (1999), who reported a fourfold increase among current pill users compared with non-users, after adjustment for HPV types 16 and 18.

Brinton *et al.* (1990) studied 759 invasive cervical cancer patients and 1430 control subjects in Panama, Costa Rica, Colombia and Mexico and reported that, after adjustment for confounding factors and history of cervical smear, there was no observable effect on OCP use and squamous cell carcinoma of the cervix [odds ratio (OR) 1.1].

In a study to assess the effect of use of oral contraceptives on the risk of cervical cancer in women who tested positive for HPV DNA, Moreno *et al.* (2002) reported that, compared with never-users, patients who had used oral contraceptives for less than 5 years did not have an increased risk of cervical cancer (OR 0.66; 95% CI 0.45–0.98). The OR for use of oral

Table 9.1 Impact of different strategies of HPV adjustment on associations between cofactors and risk of cervical cancer (from the IARC case–control studies).

	All women			HPV-positive women	
Cofactor	Cases/controls	Not HPV-adjusted OR (95% CI)	HPV-adjusted OR (95% CI)	Cases/controls	OR (95% CI)
Full-term pregnancies (status and number)					
Never	95/164	1	1	57/24	1
Ever	2183/2209	1.08 (0.80–1.47)	1.32 (0.88–1.98)	1616/229	2.45 (1.33–4.51)
1 or 2	444/747	0.82 (0.60–1.12)	0.99 (0.65–1.50)	279/59	1.79 (0.94–3.40)
3 or 4	644/677	1.33 (0.97–1.83)	1.68 (1.09–2.57)	450/70	2.61 (1.37–5.00)
5	1095/785	1.73 (1.24–2.41)	2.03 (1.30–3.16)	887/100	3.88 (1.99–7.55)
OC use (status and years)					
Never	1419/1508	1	1	1071/163	1
Ever	864/886	1.09 (0.94–1.27)	0.97 (0.79–1.19)	605/92	1.13 (0.80–1.59)
1–4 years	351/445	0.90 (0.75–1.09)	0.75 (0.58–0.97)	274/64	0.66 (0.45–0.98)
5+ years	510/427	1.33 (1.11–1.59)	1.17 (0.92–1.49)	331/28	2.35 (1.44–3.85)
Smoking (status and amount)					
Never	1645/1905	1	1	1265/218	1
Ever	636/488	1.30 (1.11–1.52)	1.68 (1.36–2.08)	409/36	1.99 (1.29–3.07)
1–5 cigarettes per day	251/200	1.21 (0.98–1.51)	1.46 (1.09–1.97)	181/17	1.72 (0.98–3.01)
6+ cigarettes per day	320/216	1.79 (1.45–2.22)	2.07 (1.56–2.75)	211/18	2.16 (1.18–3.97)

Odds ratios (ORs) adjusted for centre, age (< 37, 37–45, 46–55, ≥56 years), educational level (none, primary, secondary or higher), smoking amount (never, 1–5 cigarettes per day, ≥6 cigarettes per day), age at first sexual intercourse (< 17, 17–18, 19–22, ≥23), lifetime number of sexual partners (1, 2–3, ≥4), OC use (never, 1–4 years, 5–9 years, ≥10 years), lifetime number of Pap smears (0, 1–5, ≥6) and parity (0; 1 or 2; 3 or 4; 5 or 6; ≥7). Table adapted from Castellsague and Muñoz (2003), with permission of Oxford University Press and the National Cancer Institute.

contraceptives was 2.32 (95% CI 1.44–3.85) for 5–9 years, and 4.03 (2.09–8.02) for use for 10 years or longer (see also Chapter 18). In Table 9.1 from Castellsague and Muñoz (2003), two other risk factors, namely full-term pregnancy and smoking, are shown in relation to HPV positivity and the adjustments that have been made for HPV. Both parity and smoking increase the risk in HPV-positive women after 5 years. Castellsague and Muñoz (2003) have summarised a number of studies and, again, the role of oral contraceptives as a cofactor in cervical carcinogenesis among HPV DNA-positive women can be seen (Table 9.2). It is remarkable that the findings in both these studies are strongly dependent on the background prevalence of the exposure of interest and of the practice of screening. In Table 9.2, the impact of oral contraceptives on cervical cancer (in some countries on cervical precancer lesions) is more evident in countries that do not have proper screening programmes. This strongly suggests that there is an association between screening and oral contraceptive use in many populations. It may be that women who receive oral contraceptive prescriptions have Pap smears more often than other women. Interpretation of many of these studies is therefore questionable.

One of the largest reviews of the literature in respect of cervical cancer and hormone contraception was a systematic analysis performed by Smith *et al.* (2003), in which 28 eligible studies that included 12 551 women with cervical cancer were examined. Compared with never-users of oral contraceptives, the relative risk of cervical cancer increased with increasing duration of use; 5-, 5–9 and 10-year periods were examined, and the relative risks were broadly similar for invasive and *in situ* cervical cancers as well as for squamous and adenocancers. Adjustment for HPV status, sexual partners, the impact of cervical screening, smoking and the use of barrier contraception was made and, with the limited data available, it was suggested that the relative risk of cervical cancer may decrease after oral contraceptive use cessation, but this fact, at the moment, cannot be evaluated properly from the 'published data'.

Finally, Green *et al.* (2003) have investigated infection by HPV in relation to the use of oral contraceptives. They conducted a systematic review of 19 epidemiological studies concerning the risk of genital HPV infection and oral contraceptive use, and the results showed that there was no evidence for a strong negative or positive association between HPV positivity and the ever-use or long duration of use of oral

Table 9.2 Summary results of studies assessing the role of OC use as a cofactor in cervical carcinogenesis among HPV DNA-positive women.

Exposure measures	Study (study outcome)					
	Denmark (HSIL)	USA, Eastern (CIS and CC)	Manchester (CIN3)	Costa Rica (HSIL and CC)	USA, Portland (CIN3 and CC)	IARC (CIS and CC)
OC use status						
Ever vs. never	NR	5.4 (0.7–43.4)	NR	NR	NR	1.4 (1.0–2.0)
Former vs. never	NR	3.1 (0.4–27.5)	1.2 (0.6–2.1)	0.9 (0.6–1.6)	NR	NR
Current vs. never	NR	17.1 (1.5–188.2)	1.3 (0.7–2.5)	1.5 (0.8–2.8)	0.8 (0.5–1.5)	NR
OC use duration						
[Years] vs. never	Decreasing risk	[–2] 4.0 (0.4–44.3)	[–3] 1.2 (0.6–2.4)	[–4] 1.8 (0.6–4.9)	NR	[1] 0.7 (0.4–1.1)
	with increasing	[–6] 4.8 (0.4–51.9)	[–8] 0.8 (0.4–1.5)	[≥5] 3.1 (1.1–9.1)		[–4] 0.8 (0.5–1.2)
	duration	[≥7] 6.2 (0.7–52.7)	[>8] 1.5 (0.8–2.9)			[–9] 2.8 (1.5–5.4)
						[≥10] 4.0 (2.1–7.8)
P for trend	NR	0.12	NR	NR	NR	<0.001
Comments	ORs not reported	For adenocarcinoma *in situ*		Duration estimates computed among women with fewer than three pregnancies pregnancies	Relative risk refers to current vs. not current OC use at enrolment	For both squamous cell and adenocarcinoma

NR, not reported; NS, not significant. Bold figures denote statistical significance. CIN, cervical intraepithelial neoplasia; HSIL, high-grade squamous intraepithelial lesion; CIS, carcinoma *in situ*; CC, cervical cancer.
Table adapted from Castellsague and Muñoz (2003), with permission of Oxford University Press and the National Cancer Institute.

contraceptives. They felt that more research was needed into the role played by oral contraceptives in the persistence and detectability of cervical HPV infections.

Recently, IARC (2006) published a report on the subject of 'Combined (oestrogen–progestogen) contraceptives and combined oestrogen–progesterone menopausal therapy'. This is a consensus document compiled by experts who, when considering the risk of cervical cancer in women using combined estrogen–progestogen contraceptives, were of the opinion that the risk of cervical cancer increased with the duration of use of the combined oral contraceptives. In the report, they stated that studies that investigated HPV infection suggested that the prevalence of infection was not increased in women who used the combined contraceptives, but that the increased risk of cervical cancer was recorded in analyses of data from women who were already positive for HPV. It also detailed *in vitro* and animal studies that suggested that estrogens and progestogens enhanced the expression of certain HPV genes and stimulated cell proliferation in the cervix through hormone response elements in the viral genome and through receptor-mediated mechanisms, although other mechanisms, they stated, could also be involved.

Adenocarcinoma

Dallenbach-Hellweg (1984) reported that 82% of women who developed endocervical adenocarcinoma under the age

of 50 years used OCPs. Similar carcinoma was produced experimentally in Rhesus monkeys exposed to high-dose medroxyprogesterone. However, earlier reports from case–control studies were contradictory (Valente and Hanjani, 1986; Honore *et al.*, 1991). In a well-conducted, hospital-based, case–control study adjusted for confounding epidemiological risk factors, Thomas and Ray (1996) reported that the risk of developing adenocarcinoma of the cervix increased with duration of oral contraceptive use and was highest among current pill users. The trends in these risks were strongest for cancers that occurred in young women below the age of 35 years. A twofold increase in the risk of adenocarcinoma of the cervix was also reported by Brinton *et al.* (1990) among pill users, after adjustment for HPV infection and other epidemiological risk factors for cervical cancers. Other reports reached a similar conclusion (Persson *et al.*, 1987; Hildesheim *et al.*, 1990; Honore *et al.*, 1991; Ursin *et al.*, 1994; Thomas and Ray, 1996).

Possible mechanism involved in carcinogenesis

Cervical carcinogenesis seems to be influenced by sex hormones. It has been shown that sex hormones induce HPV gene expression directly or indirectly through steroid response elements in the viral genotypes (Monsonego *et al.*, 1991; Yuan *et al.*, 1999). Likewise, HPV oncogenes and the expression of estrogen receptors have been seen in some basal cells

(Arbeit *et al.*, 1996), and it has been suggested that these receptors in some way signal pathways that 'may synergise with the cellular effects of the HPV 16 oncoproteins' (Elson *et al.*, 2000). It has also been suggested by a number of authors (Remoue *et al.*, 2003) that hormones sensitise the transformation zone to neoplastic change by altering the local immune microenvironment via Langerhans/dendritic cells, which particularly are involved with immunosurveillance (al Saleh, 1995). Furthermore, sex hormones have been shown to be directly involved in the production of cytokines/chemokines which influence the migration and function of Langerhans/dendritic cells (Wira *et al.*, 2000).

Progesterone has been shown to be a potent factor for transcription of upstream E6 and E7 promoters of the oncogenic HPV genome through a glucocorticoid-dependent pathway (Pater *et al.*, 1988; Chan *et al.*, 1989). Indeed, progesterone enhances the ability of the viral DNA to transform cells (Pater *et al.*, 1990). Estrogen may increase the risk of cervical cancer development by inducing progesterone receptor synthesis (Monsonego *et al.*, 1991).

Recently, a review by Moodley *et al.* (2003) emphasised the important role played by high-risk HPV in the carcinogenic mechanisms of women on oral contraceptives. They point out that steroid contraception has been postulated to be one mechanism whereby HPV exerts a tumorigenic effect on cervical tissue. They emphasise the role played by steroids in binding specific DNA sequences within transcriptional regulatory regions on the HPV DNA, which can either increase or suppress the transcription of various genes; this process is seemingly further enhanced by the discovery of hormone receptors in cervical tissue (as described by Remoue *et al.*, 2003). They emphasise, as well, the role of the upstream regulatory region (URR) of HPV 16 DNA, which mediates transcriptional control of the HPV genome and is thought to contain enhancer elements that are activated by steroid hormones (Von Knebel Doeberitz *et al.*, 1991), highlighting the fact that steroid hormones bind to specific glucocorticoid response elements within HPV DNA (Strahle *et al.*, 1987).

Experimental evidence has revealed that high-risk HPV 16 is able to stimulate the development of vaginal and cervical squamous cell carcinomas in transgenic mice. Arbeit *et al.* (1996) showed that these mice, when subjected to slow-release pellets of 17β-estradiol in the presence of human keratin 14 promoters, were able to be diverted to a neoplastic course. They also showed that squamous cell cancers developed in a multistage pathway only in these transgenic mice and not in non-transgenic mice. Elson *et al.* (2000) also treated transgenic mice with estrogens. They found that, as they lowered the estrogen dose, they were able to induce squamous carcinogenesis solely at the cervical transformation zone compared with other reproductive tract sites. In further studies, they were able to delineate the stages of the transformation zone carcinogenesis, including the formation of hyperplastic

lower uterine glands and the emergence of multiple foci of metaplasia from individual stem-like glandular reserve cells followed by neoplastic progression of metaplasia to dysplasia and squamous cancer. They postulated that the combination of low-dose estrogens and low-level HPV oncogenes had an effect on the glandular reserve cells, programming them towards squamous rather than columnar epithelial differentiation. They summarised their results by concluding that 'synergistic activation of proliferation by viral oncoprotein cell cycle dysregulation and estrogen receptor signalling together with altered paracrine stromal–epithelial interactions may conspire to support and promote neoplastic progression and cancer formation'.

A number of authors have shown that the E16 oncoprotein of HPV 16 will bind to the p53 tumour-suppressor gene and, in so doing, will stimulate its degradation by ubiquitin-dependent protease systems (Zimmermann *et al.*, 1999; Duensing *et al.*, 2000; Sherr, 2000). It is thought that these E6 and E7 HPV 16 oncogenes, whose expression is increased by steroid hormones, bind to and subsequently degrade the p53 product, leading to cell death (apoptotic failure and eventual carcinogenesis) (Hubbert *et al.*, 1992; Kessis *et al.*, 1993; Galloway and McDougall, 1996).

Remoue *et al.* (2003) showed that estrogen and progestogen receptors are highly expressed in the immature squamous metaplastic epithelium of the transformation zone in comparison with the original (native) squamous epithelium. The 'immune characteristics' of the transformation zone could, according to Remoue *et al.* (2003), explain in part the high susceptibility of this region to HPV infection and carcinogenesis.

EFFECTS OF MENOPAUSE ON CERVICAL EPITHELIUM

Menopause leads to atrophy of the entire female reproductive system. The rate of atrophy varies greatly between individuals. Clinically, progressive atrophy associated with increasing duration of menopause steadily reduces the volume and length of the vaginal portion of the cervix. In extreme cases, the cervix is seen flush with the vaginal fornix.

Atrophic cervical squamous epithelium is thin and dry consequent to the reduced proliferative activity of the basal cells because of the marked diminution of estrogen receptors after menopause (Cano *et al.*, 1990; Bulten *et al.*, 2000a). In an experimental model of cultured human ectocervical epithelium, Gorodeski (2000) elegantly demonstrated that estrogen deficiency from menopause increases the resistance to water permeability at the tight junctions between the epithelial cells, leading to the characteristic clinical state of dryness of the cervical epithelium (Fig. 9.5a and b). Other studies have shown that significant breakdown of collagen occurs as the menopause progresses. Gill *et al.* (2003), using autofluorescence to examine collagen, were able to show changes in the

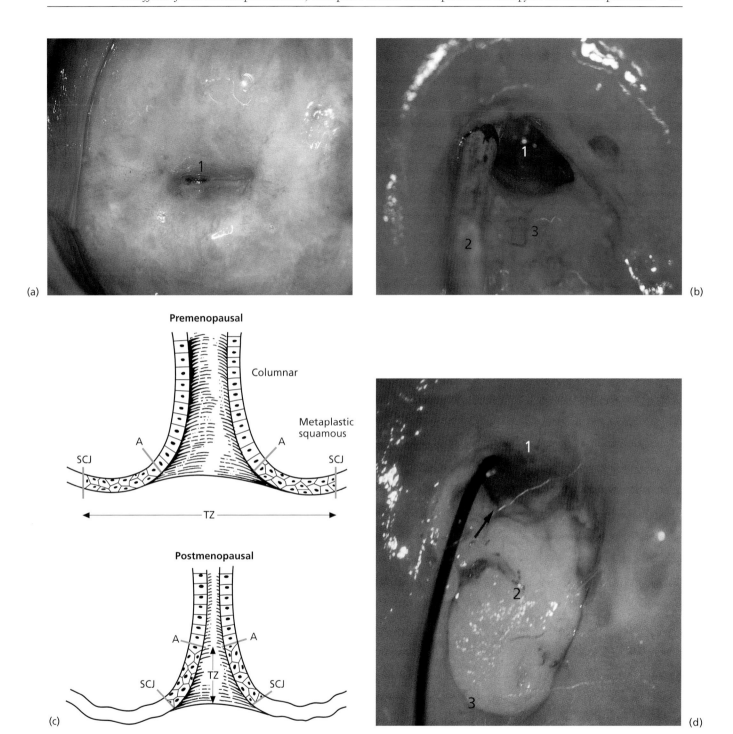

Fig. 9.5 (a) The cervix of a 58-year-old woman, 10 years postmenopausal. A large area of the transformation zone has retracted within the endocervical canal (1). The ectocervix is covered with atrophic epithelium, and it is difficult to differentiate original squamous from metaplastic squamous epithelium. (b) In this colpophotograph, the transformation zone extends into the endocervical canal (1). A probe (2) is shown opening up the canal, and the mature squamous metaplastic epithelium with normal branching vessels is seen at (3). The new squamocolumnar junction, indicating the upper extent of the transformation zone, is high in the cervical canal and cannot be seen. (c) Diagrammatic representation showing the retraction of the transformation zone into the endocervix with the development of the menopause. The transformation zone (T2) is situated between point A and the squamocolumnar junction (SCJ). (d) A colpophotograph showing an atypical transformation zone in a postmenopausal woman. Acetowhite epithelium is seen extending from the anterior (1) but mainly from the posterior lip (2) of the cervix to within the endocervical canal. The direction of the new squamocolumnar junction (arrowed) cannot be seen as it has retracted to within the endocervix, making the colposcopic examination unsatisfactory. The original junction is at (3).

Continued on following page

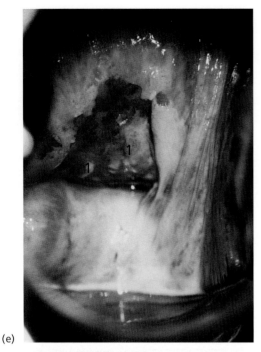

(e)

Fig. 9.5 (cont'd) (e) High-grade lesion (1) extending into the endocervix of a 56-year-old woman. Retraction has caused the new squamocolumnar junction to be invisible, and therefore this colposcopy is unsatisfactory.

collagen cross-linking within the tissues as the menopause developed. This may account for some of the 'retraction' seen within the epithelium as the menopause progresses, which is discussed below.

Endocervical atrophy as a result of the menopause causes the ectocervix to invert and retract to within the endocervical canal (Fig. 9.5c). This results in the squamous metaplastic epithelium of the transformation zone being withdrawn within the endocervical canal (Singer, 1975). Megevand *et al.* (1996) reported that a significant degree of extension of the transformation zone into the endocervical canal was present in a large proportion of menopausal women among 461 patients undergoing loop electro-excision procedure for CIN. Kirkup and Singer (1979) showed that the number of women with unsatisfactory colposcopic examinations increased in relation to their age. Among women in the fifth decade of life the incidence of unsatisfactory examinations was at least 40%; in contrast, the incidence among those in the second decade was only 3%. This was because of retraction of the new squamocolumnar junction to within the endocervix as a result of menopausal atrophy. Likewise, Toplis *et al.* (1986) also showed that more than half the colposcopic examinations conducted in the postpartum period were unsatisfactory (Fig. 9.5d and e).

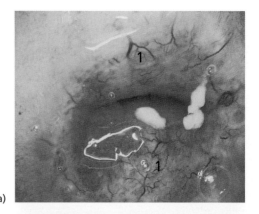

(a)

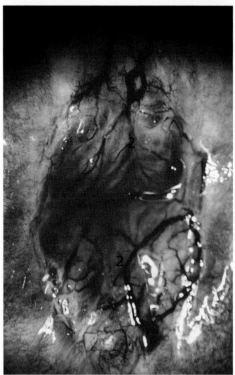

(b)

Fig. 9.6 (a,b) Colpophotographs of postmenopausal cervices with prominent vessels. The candelabra appearance of the vessels results from the thin atrophic nature of the metaplastic squamous epithelium in (1) and of the columnar epithelium in (2). The larger terminal vessels have irregular branching patterns, with the branches decreasing in size (diameter) so as to terminate in a fine meshwork capillary network. There is no suggestion of abnormal vascularity.

Colposcopic features of menopausal epithelium

In the early phase of menopause, the squamous epithelium loses its usual moist, shiny and pearly appearance. There is a prominent display of the fine reticular pattern of the epithelial and subepithelial capillaries (Fig. 9.6a and b). The endocervical columnar cells diminish in their tallness. The loss of globular surface of the endocervix results in displays of prominent vessels across the epithelium. The apparent translucency with obvious vessel morphology can be so prominent that it may occasionally be mistaken for malignant change (Fig. 9.6b).

The size of the transformation zone does not change significantly with the advent of the menopause. However, the metaplastic squamous epithelium that has matured within the transformation zone is sometimes difficult to differentiate from the original (native) squamous epithelium (Fig. 9.5a). In late menopausal women, the cervical epithelium assumes a uniform opacity without reticular vascular pattern. The epithelial cells lack cytoplasmic glycogen, and the epithelium stains light yellow on Schiller's test. Three-dimensional ultra-structural studies of the ectocervix and vaginal squamous cell surface show a reduction in the number of microridges that are typical of these tissues, and changes are also obvious in the typical structural organisation of these cells. These findings are the result of the decline in estrogens (Makabe *et al.*, 1998).

As the menopause progresses, the process of atrophy continues at different rates across the squamous epithelium. The atrophic opaque epithelial surface is interrupted by islands of less atrophic pink epithelium, giving rise to the characteristic 'strawberry' appearance (Fig. 9.7).

Atrophic changes in cervical epithelial cells pose a challenge to colposcopists in assessing the severity of intraepithelial neoplasia and HPV-associated epithelial changes (Fig. 9.8).

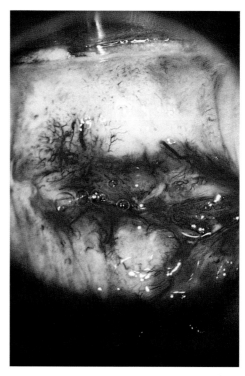

Fig. 9.8 A colpophotograph from a 62-year-old woman who has been menopausal for 12 years. The cervix is covered by atrophic opaque epithelium, which accentuates the very prominent vessels that may sometimes be confused with an underlying neoplasia. In this case, some of the vessels possess the characteristic features associated with malignant vessels, as has been described in Chapter 24. There is no neoplasia present in these tissues.

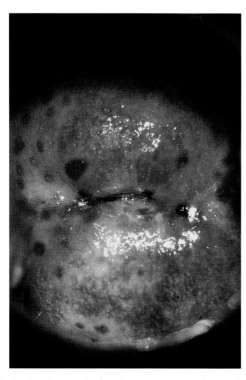

Fig. 9.7 A colpophotograph showing postmenopausal cervical atrophy with typical 'strawberry' appearance.

Cytology effect of menopause on cervical epithelium

Postmenopausal atrophic epithelium is thin and prone to infection. Not surprisingly, Papanicolaou smears are persistently inflammatory in 43% of these women (Toplis *et al.*, 1986). Cytology of atrophic squamous epithelium is dominated by the basal and parabasal squamous cells, which are characterised by uniform nuclear enlargement (Abati *et al.*, 1998). There may be other atypical features such as various degrees of prominent perinuclear halos, nuclear hyperchromasia, variation in nuclear size and multinucleation. These atypical features may mimic koilocytosis of HPV infection or high-grade CIN (Jovanovic *et al.*, 1995; Bulten *et al.*, 2000b).

Mucosal immune system

Judging by the cellular densities of CD3+ and CD4+ T cells and dendritic cells, the cervical mucosal immune system is not affected by the menopause (White *et al.*, 1997).

EFFECTS OF HORMONE REPLACEMENT THERAPY ON CERVICAL EPITHELIUM

The physical effects of the menopause are the sequelae of estrogen deficiency resulting from ovarian failure and are reversible upon estrogen replacement. Yasui *et al.* (2001) demonstrated that the minimum concentration of estradiol required varies with the different target tissue responses. Hormone replacement therapy (HRT) with estrogen has been well established as an important preventative health measure for postmenopausal women since the 1970s (Wren 1985; Daly *et al.*, 1992). Later, the role of unopposed estrogen treatment in the development of endometrial hyperplasia and neoplasia became clear, and progestogen is included in the HRT regimen for postmenopausal women with an intact uterus (Williams and Moley, 1994). The most commonly administered estrogens are either the natural conjugated equine estrogens or synthetic estradiol, whereas the most commonly employed progestogen is medroxyprogesterone acetate.

It has been estimated that approximately 15% of women between the ages of 40 and 60 years in the United Kingdom are on HRT (Barlow *et al.*, 1991; Wilkes and Meades, 1991). With the rapidly increasing population of postmenopausal women worldwide, any adverse reactions from HRT are likely to have a profound impact on public health (Beral *et al.*, 2002).

Clinical features of HRT on the cervix

Estrogen replacement restores the intercellular permeability to water in the cervical epithelium (Gorodeski, 2000). A thin layer of moisture appears on the cervix. The increased basal cell proliferation and maturation of the epithelial cells return the pink lustre to the cervical epithelium. However, only a small degree of cervical eversion occurs, and cervical ectopy is uncommon, even after a prolonged period of HRT.

Colposcopic features of HRT on the cervix

After 6 or more weeks of HRT, the squamous epithelium of the cervix resumes the premenopausal features in terms of its thickness and the fine reticular vascular morphology. Maturation of the surface epithelial cells is seen by the increase in the cytoplasmic glycogen content, which can be illustrated by the dark-brown discoloration on staining with Lugol's iodine solution. The transformation zone is predominantly represented by mature squamous metaplastic epithelium and may still encroach onto the endocervical canal. Nonetheless, the post-HRT change is sufficient to expose the new squamocolumnar junction to allow satisfactory colposcopy to be performed in 70% of postmenopausal women (Paterson *et al.*, 1982; Toplis *et al.*, 1986) (Fig. 9.9).

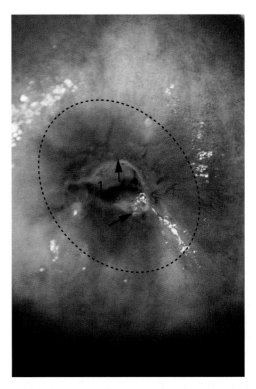

Fig. 9.9 A colpophotograph of a postmenopausal woman who has been treated with hormone replacement therapy for 14 months. The atrophic epithelium has shown satisfactory estrogenisation. A small transformation zone is seen within the line of the original squamocolumnar junction (– – –), as is the new squamocolumnar junction (→). It would seem as though partial eversion of the transformation zone has occurred as a result of therapy, as there is now original (native) columnar epithelium present in an ectocervical position. This epithelium would previously have been hidden within the endocervix but, as a result of HRT and estrogenisation, is now everted and exposed.

HRT and cervical carcinogenesis

Several studies examining the potential role of HRT in cervical carcinogenesis have been the subject of interest, especially those investigating the interaction between sex steroids and oncogenic HPV. There is a positive correlation between serum levels of progesterone and HPV DNA detection rates in cervical scrapes in women between the ages of 40 and 62 years (Kedzia *et al.*, 2000). Kutza *et al.* (2000) demonstrated that the presence of HPV DNA, in HRT users when compared with never-users of HRT, produced an odds ratio adjusted for age, reproductive and sexual history, and cigarette smoking of 1.50 (95% CI 0.55–4.07) for current HRT users and 1.96 (CI 0.56–6.86) for past HRT users. The observed trend of higher relative risk for HPV DNA detection among HRT users was not statistically significant. More importantly, it is noteworthy that the prevalence of oncogenic HPV was very low at 2.8%.

A similarly low prevalence was reported by Ferenczy *et al.* (1997). In a randomised clinical trial of estrogen–progestogen interventions in 105 postmenopausal women between the ages of 45 and 64 years over a 2-year period, no association between the detection rate of oncogenic HPV and duration of HRT use was found (Smith *et al.*, 1997).

Sawaya *et al.* (2000) reported in a prospective cohort study and randomised, double-blind, placebo-controlled trial of hormone therapy that there was no significant difference in the incidence of cytological abnormalities between HRT users and non-users.

In a case–control study involving 645 women aged 40–75 years with cervical cancer and 749 women aged 40–75 years as control subjects, Parazzini *et al.* (1997) found that, compared with non-users, the overall odds ratio for cervical cancer among the HRT users was 0.5 (95% CI 0.3–0.8). The protection against cervical cancer among HRT users increases with the duration of hormone use. Long-term cohort studies also confirmed that the use of HRT is not associated with a higher incidence of cervical cancers (Hunt *et al.*, 1987; Adami *et al.*, 1989). Even the use of a combined contraceptive vaginal ring for up to 12 months, during which a silastic ring that released a small amount of ethinylestradiol daily was left in the upper vagina in close proximity to the cervix, did not induce any increase in the number of cervical neoplastic lesions (Roumen *et al.*, 1996).

Although HRT reverses many characteristics of the epithelial atrophy from estrogen deficiency, it does not play a significant role in cervical carcinogenesis. It is unclear whether this observation is related to the low proliferative state of menopausal cervical epithelium or the low prevalence of oncogenic HPV infection among postmenopausal women.

REFERENCES

Abati A, Jaffurs W, Wilder AM (1998) Squamous atypia in the atrophic cervical vaginal smear: a new look at an old problem. *Cancer* 84: 218–225.

Abma JC, Chandra A, Musher WD *et al.* (1997) Fertility, family planning and women's health: new data from the 1995 national survey of family growth. *Vital Health Statistics* 19: 1–114.

Adami H-O, Persson I, Hoover R *et al.* (1989) Risk of cancer in women receiving hormone replacement therapy. *International Journal of Cancer* 44: 833–839.

al Saleh W, Delvenne P, Greimers R *et al.* (1995) Assessment of Ki-67 antigen immunostaining in squamous intraepithelial lesions in the uterine cervix. Correlation with histological grades of human papillomavirus. *American Journal of Clinical Pathology* 104: 154–160.

Alvarez-Santin C, Sica A, Rodriguez M *et al.* (1999) Microglandular hyperplasia of the uterine cervix. Cytologic diagnosis in cervical smears. *Acta Cytologica* 43: 110–113.

Arbeit JM, Howley PM, Hanahan D (1996) Chronic estrogen-induced cervical and vaginal squamous carcinogenesis in human papillomavirus type 16 transgenic mice. *Proceedings of the National Academy of Sciences of the USA* 93: 2930–2935.

Barlow DH, Brockie JA, Rees CMP (1991) Study of general practice consultation and menopausal problems. *British Medical Journal* 302: 274–276.

Beral V, Banks E, Reeves G (2002) Evidence from randomised trials on the long-term effects of hormone replacement therapy. *Lancet* 360: 942–944.

Brinton LA, Reeves WC, Brenes MM *et al.* (1990) Oral contraceptive use and risk of invasive cervical cancer. *International Journal of Epidemiology* 19: 4–11.

Bulten J, de Wilde PC, Schijf C *et al.* (2000a) Decreased expression of Ki-67 in atrophic cervical epithelium of post-menopausal women. *Journal of Pathology* 190: 545–553.

Bulten J, de Wilde PC, Boonstra H *et al.* (2000b) Proliferation in 'atypical' atrophic pap smears. *Gynecology and Oncology* 79: 225–229.

Cano A, Serra V, Rivera J *et al.* (1990) Expression of estrogen receptors, progesterone receptors, and an estrogen receptor-associated protein in the human cervix during the menstrual cycle and menopause. *Fertility and Sterility* 54: 1058–1064.

Carr BR, Ory H (1997) Estrogen and progestin components of oral contraceptives: relationship to vascular disease. *Contraception* 55: 267–272.

Castellsague X, Muñoz N (2003) Causal relation between cofactors and cervical cancer, global evaluation: review. *Journal of the National Cancer Institute Monograph* 31: 20–28.

Celli G, Darwiche N, De Luca LM (1996) Estrogen induces retinoid receptor expression in mouse cervical epithelia. *Experiments in Cell Research* 226: 273–282.

Ciocca DR, Puy LA, Lo Castro G (1986) Localization of an estrogen-responsive protein in the human cervix during menstrual cycle, pregnancy, and menopause and in abnormal cervical epithelia without atypia. *American Journal of Obstetrics and Gynecology* 155: 1090–1096.

Chan WK, Klock G, Bernard HV (1989) Progesterone and glucocorticoid response elements occur in the long control regions of several human papillomaviruses involved in anogenital neoplasia. *Journal of Virology* 63: 3261–3269.

Chasen-Taber L, Stampfer MJ (1998) Epidemiology of oral contraceptives and cardiovascular disease. *Annals of Internal Medicine* 128: 476–477.

Chumas JC, Nelson B, Mann WJ *et al.* (1985) Microglandular hyperplasia of the uterine cervix. *Obstetrics and Gynecology* 66: 406–409.

Clarke EA, Hatcher J, McKeown-Eyssen GE *et al.* (1985) Cervical dysplasia: association with sexual behavior, smoking, and oral contraceptive use? *American Journal of Obstetrics and Gynecology* 151: 612–616.

Coker AL, McCann MF, Hulka BS *et al.* (1992) Oral contraceptive use and cervical intraepithelial neoplasia. *Journal of Clinical Epidemiology* 45: 1111–1118.

Coker AL, Sanders LC, Bond SM *et al.* (2001) Hormonal and barrier methods of contraception, oncogenic human papillomaviruses, and cervical squamous intraepithelial lesion development. *Journal of Women's Health and Gender Based Medicine* 10: 441–449.

Critchlow CW, Wolner-Hanssen P, Eschenbach DA *et al.* (1995) Determinants of cervical ectopia and of cervicitis: age, oral contraception, specific cervical infection, smoking, and douching. *American Journal of Obstetrics and Gynecology* 173: 534–543.

Cunha GR, Shannon JM, Vanderslice KD *et al.* (1982) Autoradiographic analysis of nuclear estrogen binding sites during postnatal development of the genital tract of female mice. *Journal of Steroid Biochemistry* 17: 281–286.

Dallenbach-Hellweg G (1985) On the origin and histological structure of adenocarcinoma of the endocervix in women under 50 years of age. *Pathology in Research and Practice* 179: 38–50.

Dallenbach-Hellweg G, Fenzel J (1985) Dependence of morphologic changes in portio, cervix and endometrium on dosage or potency of synthetic gestagens *Geburtshilfe und Frauenheilkunde* 45: 238–243.

Daly E, Roche M, Barlow D *et al.* (1992) HRT: an analysis of benefits, risks and costs. *British Medical Bulletin* 48: 368–400.

de Vet HC, Knipschild PG, Sturmans F (1993) The role of sexual factors in the aetiology of cervical dysplasia. *International Journal of Epidemiology* 22: 798–803.

Duensing S, Lee LY, Duensing A *et al.* (2000) The human papillomavirus type 16, E6 and E7 oncoproteins co-operate to induce mitotic defects and genomic instability by uncoupling centrosome duplication from the cell division cycle. *Proceedings of the National Academy of Sciences of the USA* 97: 10002–10007.

Elson DA, Riley RR, Lacey A *et al.* (2000) Sensitivity of the cervical transformation zone to estrogen-induced squamous carcinogenesis. *Cancer Research* 60: 1267–1275.

Ferenczy A, Gelfand MM, Franco E *et al.* (1997) Human papillomavirus infection in postmenopausal women with and without hormone therapy. *Obstetrics and Gynecology* 90: 7–11.

Franklin RD, Kutteh WH (1999) Characterization of immunoglobulins and cytokines in human cervical mucus: influence of exogenous and endogenous hormones. *Journal of Reproductive Immunology* 42: 93–106.

Galloway DA, McDougall JK (1996). The disruption of cell-cycle checkpoints by papillomavirus oncoproteins contributes to anogenital neoplasia. *Cancer Biology* 7: 309–15.

Gaton E, Zejdel L, Bernstein D *et al.* (1982) The effect of estrogen and gestagen on the mucus production of human endocervical cells: a histochemical study. *Fertility and Sterility* 38: 580–585.

Gill EM, Malpica A, Alford RE *et al.* (2003) Relationship between collagen autofluorescence of the human cervix and menopausal status. *Photochemistry and Photobiology* 77: 653–658.

Gondos B (1976) Histologic changes associated with oral contraceptive usage. *Annals of Clinical and Laboratory Science* 6: 291–299.

Gorodeski GI (2000) Effects of menopause and estrogen on cervical epithelial permeability. *Journal of Clinical and Endocrinology and Metabolism* 85: 2584–2595.

Gould SF, Shannon JM, Cunha GR (1983) The autoradiographic demonstration of estrogen binding in normal human cervix and vagina during the menstrual cycle, pregnancy, and the menopause. *American Journal of Anatomy* 168: 229–238.

Gram IT, Macaluso M, Stalsberg H (1992) Oral contraceptive use and the incidence of cervical intraepithelial neoplasia. *American Journal of Obstetrics and Gynecology* 167: 40–44.

Greeley C, Schroeder S, Silverberg SG (1995) Microglandular hyperplasia of the cervix: a true 'pill' lesion? *International Journal of Gynecology and Pathology* 14: 50–54.

Green J, Berrington de Gonzalez A, Smith JS *et al.* (2003) Human papillomavirus infection and use of oral contraceptives. *British Journal of Cancer* 88: 1713–1720.

Hague S, MacKenzie IZ, Bicknell R *et al.* (2002) In-vivo angiogenesis and progestogens. *Human Reproduction* 17: 786–793.

Hatcher RA, Trussel J, Stewart F *et al.* (1998) *Contraceptive Technology*, 17th rev. edn. New York: Ardent Media.

Hildesheim A, Reeves WC, Brinton LA *et al.* (1990) Association of oral contraceptive use and human papillomaviruses in invasive cervical cancers. *International Journal of Cancer* 45: 860–864.

Honore LH, Koch M, Brown LB (1991) Comparison of oral contraceptive use in women with adenocarcinoma and squamous cell carcinoma of the uterine cervix. *Gynecological and Obstetric Investigation* 32: 98–101.

Hubbert NL, Sedman SA, Schiller JT (1992) Human papillomavirus type 16, E6 increases the degradation rate of p53 in human keratinocytes. *Journal of Virology* 66: 6237–6241.

Hull ME, Moghissi KS (1986) Effects of norgestimate (0.250 mg) in combination with ethinyl estradiol (0.035 mg) on cervical mucus. *Advances in Contraception* 2: 71–77.

Hunt K, Vessey M, McPherson K *et al.* (1987) Long-term surveillance of mortality and cancer incidence in women receiving hormone replacement therapy. *British Journal of Obstetrics and Gynaecology* 94: 620–635.

IARC (2006) *Monograph on the Evaluation of Carcinogenic Risk to Humans.* Vol. 91. Combined oestrogen–progestogen contraceptives and combined oestrogen–progestogen menopausal therapy. Lyon: International Agency for Research on Cancer (in press).

Jacobson DL, Peralta L, Farmer M *et al.* (2000a) Relationship of hormonal contraception and cervical ectopy as measured by computerized planimetry to chlamydial infection in adolescents. *Sexually Transmitted Diseases* 27: 313–319.

Jacobson DL, Peralta L, Graham NM *et al.* (2000b) Histologic development of cervical ectopy: relationship to reproductive hormones. *Sexually Transmitted Diseases* 27: 252–258.

Jones MW, Silverberg SG (1989) Cervical adenocarcinoma in young women: possible relationship to microglandular hyperplasia and use of oral contraceptives. *Obstetrics and Gynecology* 73: 984–989.

Jovanovic AS, McLachlin CM, Shen L *et al.* (1995) Postmenopausal squamous atypia: a spectrum including 'pseudo-koilocytosis'. *Modern Pathology* 8: 408–412.

Katira V, Dayal SS (1987) Vaginal cytology in women using oral contraceptives. *Journal of the Anatomical Society of India* 36: 94–100.

Kedzia W, Gozdzicka-Jozefiak A, Kwasniewska A *et al.* (2000) Relationship between HPV infection of the cervix and blood serum levels of steroid hormones among pre- and postmenopausal women. *European Journal of Gynaecological Oncology* 21: 177–179.

Kessis TD, Slebos RJ, Nelson WG *et al.* (1993) Human papillomavirus 16, E6 expression disrupts the p53-mediated cellular response to DNA damage. *Proceedings of the National Academy of Sciences of the USA* 90: 3988–3992.

Kirknp W, Singer A (1980) Colposcopy in the management of women with abnormal smears. *British Journal of Obstetrics and Gynaecology* 87: 322–325.

Kuhl H (1996) Comparative pharmacology of newer progestogens. *Drugs,* 51: 188–215.

Kutza J, Smith E, Levy B *et al.* (2000) Use of hormone replacement therapy (Hrt) and detection of human papillomavirus (HPV) DNA in postmenopausal women. *Annals of Epidemiology* 10: 465–466.

Kwikkel HJ, Boon ME, van Rijswijk MM *et al.* (1986) Masking effect of hormonal contraceptives on discriminating quantitative features of visually normal intermediate cells in positive and negative cervical smears. *Analysis and Quantification of Cytology and Histology* 8: 227–232.

Lin TT (1984) Progesterone receptor in the human uterine cervix. *Acta Medica Okayama* 38: 41–48.

Liu W, Koebel L, Shipp J *et al.* (1967) Cytologic changes following the use of oral contraceptives. *Obstetrics and Gynecology* 30: 228–232.

Makabe S, Motta PM, Naguro T *et al.* (1998) Microanatomy of the female reproductive organs in postmenopause by scanning electron microscopy. *Climacteric* 1: 63–71.

Megevand E, Denny LA, Soeters R *et al.* (1996) The influence of hormonal status on excision margins after large loop excision of the transformation zone (LLETZ). *European Journal of Gynaecological Oncology* 17: 223–227.

Meisels A, Begin R, Schneider V (1977) Dysplasias of uterine cervix: epidemiological aspects: role of age at first coitus and use of oral contraceptives. *Cancer* 40: 3076–3081.

Mohsenian M, Moghissi KS, Borin K (1981) Effects of norgestimate in combination with ethinyl estradiol on cervical mucus. *Contraception* 24: 173–181.

Molina R, Thomas DB, Dabancens A *et al.* (1988) Oral contraceptives and cervical carcinoma in situ in Chile. *Cancer Research* 48: 1011–1015.

Moltz L, Becker K (1977) Cribriform polypoid adenomatous (atypical) hyperplasia of the endocervical glands of the uterus under hormonal contraception. *European Journal of Obstetric Gynecology and Reproductive Biology* 7: 331–336.

Monsonego J, Magdelena H, Catalan F *et al.* (1991) Estrogen and progesterone receptors in cervical human papillomavirus related lesions. *International Journal of Cancer* 48: 533–539.

Montes MB, Ferreira AC, Fenolio JC *et al.* (2000) Effects of oral contraceptives in vaginal cytology. *Pathologica* 92: 185–188.

Moodley M, Moodley J, Chetty R *et al.* (2003) The role of steroid contraceptive hormones in the pathogenesis of invasive cervical cancer: a review. *International Journal of Gynecology and Cancer* 13: 103–110.

Moreno V, Bosch FX, Muñoz N *et al.* (2002) International Agency for Research on Cancer. Multicentric Cervical Cancer Study Group. Effect of oral contraceptives on risk of cervical cancer in women with human papillomavirus infection: the IARC multicentric case–control study. *Lancet* 359: 1085–1092.

New Zealand Contraception and Health Study Group (1994) Risk of cervical dysplasia in users of oral contraceptives, intrauterine devices or depot-medroxyprogesterone acetate. *Contraception* 50: 431–441.

Parazzini F, La Vecchia C, Negri E *et al.* (1997) Case–control study of oestrogen replacement therapy and risk of cervical cancer. *British Medical Journal* 315: 85–88.

Pater MM, Hughes GA, Hyslop DE *et al.* (1988) Glucocorticoid-dependent oncogenic transformation by type 16 but not type 11 human papilloma virus DNA. *Nature* 335: 832–835.

Pater A, Bayatpour M, Pater MM (1990) Oncogenic transformation by human papillomavirus type 16 deoxyribonucleic acid in the presence of progesterone or progestins from oral contraceptives. *American Journal of Obstetrics and Gynecology* 162: 1099–1103.

Paterson ME, Allen J, Jordan JA (1982) Effects of the climacteric and sequential mestranol and norethisterone on the cervix and genital tract. *British Journal of Obstetrics and Gynaecology* 89: 657–664.

Persson E, Einhorn N, Pettersson F (1987) A case–control study of oral contraceptive use in women with adenocarcinoma of the uterine cervix. *European Journal of Obstetric Gynecology and Reproductive Biology* 26: 85–90.

Ramos JG, Varayoud J, Bosquiazzo VL *et al.* (2002) Cellular turnover in the rat uterine cervix and its relationship to estrogen and progesterone receptor dynamics. *Biology of Reproduction* 67: 735–742.

Remoue F, Jacobs N, Miot V *et al.* (2003) High intraepithelial expression of estrogen and progesterone receptors in the transformation zone of the uterine cervix. *American Journal of Obstetrics and Gynecology* 189: 1660–1665.

Roumen F J, Boon M E, van Velzen D *et al.* (1996) The cervico-vaginal epithelium during 20 cycles' use of a combined contraceptive vaginal ring. *Human Reproduction* 11: 2443–2448.

Sawaya GF, Grady D, Kerlikowske K *et al.* (2000) The positive predictive value of cervical smears in previously screened postmenopausal women: the Heart and Estrogen/progestin Replacement Study (HERS). *Annals of Internal Medicine* 133: 942–950.

Scharl A, Vierbuchen M, Graupner J *et al.* (1988) Immunohistochemical study of distribution of estrogen receptors in corpus and cervix uteri. *Archives of Gynecology and Obstetrics* 241: 221–233.

Sherr CJ (2000) The Pezcoller lecture: cancer cell cycles revisited. *Cancer Research* 60: 3689–3695.

Singer A (1975) The uterine cervix from adolescence to the menopause. *British Journal of Obstetrics and Gynaecology* 82: 81–99.

Smith EM, Johnson SR, Figuerres EJ *et al.* (1997) The frequency of human papillomavirus detection in postmenopausal women on hormone replacement therapy. *Gynecology and Oncology* 65: 441–446.

Smith JS, Green J, Berrington de Gonzalez A *et al.* (2003) Cervical cancer and use of hormonal contraceptives: a systematic review. *Lancet* 361: 1915.

Stamm WE, Holmes KK (1997) *Chlamydia trachomatis* of the adult. In: Holmes KK (ed.) *Sexually Transmitted Diseases*. New York: McGraw Hill.

Strahle U, Klock G, Schutz G (1987) A DNA sequence of 15 base pairs is sufficient to mediate both glucocorticoid and progesterone induction of gene expression. *Proceedings of the National Academy of Sciences of the USA* 84: 7871–7875.

Suissa S, Blais L, Spitzer WO *et al.* (1997) First time use of newer oral contraceptives and the risk of venous thromboembolism. *Contraception* 56: 141–146.

Tay SK, Jenkins D, Maddox P *et al.* (1987a) Subpopulations of Langerhans cells in cervical neoplasia. *British Journal of Obstetrics and Gynaecology* 94: 10–15.

Tay SK, Jenkins D, Maddox P *et al.* (1987b) Lymphocyte phenotypes in cervical intraepithelial neoplasia and human papillomavirus infection. *British Journal of Obstetrics and Gynaecology* 94: 16–21.

Tay SK, Jenkins D, Maddox P *et al.* (1987c) Tissue macrophage response in human papillomavirus infection and cervical intraepithelial neoplasia. *British Journal of Obstetrics and Gynaecology* 94: 1094–1097.

Thomas DB, Ray RM (1996) Oral contraceptives and invasive adenocarcinomas and adenosquamous carcinomas of the uterine cervix. The World Health Organization Collaborative Study of Neoplasia and Steroid Contraceptives. *American Journal of Epidemiology* 144: 281–289.

Toplis PJ, Casemore V, Hallam N *et al.* (1986) Evaluation of colposcopy in the postmenopausal woman. *British Journal of Obstetrics* 93: 843–851.

Ursin G, Peters RK, Henderson BE *et al.* (1994) Oral contraceptive use and adenocarcinoma of cervix. *Lancet* 344: 1390–1394.

Valente PT, Hanjani P (1986) Endocervical neoplasia in long-term users of oral contraceptives: clinical and pathologic observations. *Obstetrics and Gynecology* 67: 695–704.

Valente PT, Schantz HD, Schultz M (1994) Microglandular hyperplasia of the uterine cervix. Cytologic diagnosis in cervical smears. Cytologic atypia associated with microglandular hyperplasia. *Diagnostic Cytopathology* 10: 326–331.

Vessey MP, Lawless M, McPherson K *et al.* (1983) Neoplasia of the cervix uteri and contraception: a possible adverse effect of the pill. *Lancet* 2: 930–934.

Von Knebel Doeberitz M, Bankrecht T, Bartsch D *et al.* (1991) Influence of chromosomal integration on glucocorticoid-regulated transcription of growth stimulating papillomavirus genes E6 and E7 in cervical carcinoma cells. *Proceedings of the National Academy of Sciences of the USA* 88: 1411–1415.

Wang H, Stjernholm Y, Ekman G *et al.* (2001) Different regulation of oestrogen receptors alpha and beta in the human cervix at term pregnancy. *Molecular Human Reproduction* 7: 293–300.

White HD, Yeaman GR, Givan AL *et al.* (1997) Mucosal immunity in the human female reproductive tract: cytotoxic T lymphocyte function in the cervix and vagina of premenopausal and postmenopausal women. *American Journal of Reproductive Immunology* 37: 30–38.

WHO Collaborative Study of Cardiovascular Disease and Steroid Hormone Contraception (1995) Venous thromboembolic disease and combined oral contraceptives: results of an international, multicentre, case-controlled study. *Lancet* 346: 1575–1582.

WHO Collaborative Study of Cardiovascular Disease and Steroid Hormone Contraception (1997) Acute myocardial infarction and combined oral contraceptives: results of an international, multicentre, case-controlled study. *Lancet* 349: 1202–1209.

Wilkes HC, Meades TW (1991) Hormone replacement therapy in general practice; a survey of doctors in the MRC's general practice framework. *British Medical Journal* 302: 1317–1320.

Williams DB, Moley KH (1994) Progestin replacement in the menopause: effects on the endometrium and serum lipids. *Current Opinion in Obstetrics and Gynecology* 6: 284–292.

Wira CR, Rossoth RM, Kavshic C (2003) Antigen-presenting cells in the female reproductive tract: influence of estradiol on antigen presentation of vaginal cells. *Epidemiology* 141: 2877–2885.

Wren BG (1985) Estrogen replacement therapy in the management of an endocrine deficiency disease. *Medical Journal of Australia* 142 (Suppl.): S1–S5.

Wright TC, Holinka CF, Ferenczy A (2002) Estriol-induced hyperplasia in endometrial biopsies from women on hormone replacement therapy. *American Journal of Surgical Pathology* 10: 1269–1275.

Yahr LJ, Lee KR (1991) Cytologic findings in microglandular hyperplasia of the cervix. *Diagnostic Cytopathology* 7: 248–251.

Yasui T, Uemura H, Tezuka M *et al.* (2001) Biological effects of hormone replacement therapy in relation to serum estradiol levels. *Hormone Research* 56: 38–44.

Ylitalo N, Sorensen P, Josefsson A *et al.* (1999) Smoking and oral contraceptives as risk factors for cervical carcinoma in situ. *International Journal of Cancer* 81: 357–365.

Young RH, Scully RE (1992) Uterine carcinomas simulating microglandular hyperplasia. A report of six cases. *American Journal of Surgical Pathology* 16: 1092–1097.

Yuan F, Auborn K, James C (1999) Altered growth and viral gene expression in HPV-16 containing cancer lines treated with progesterone. *Cancer Investigations* 17: 19–29.

Zimmermann H, Degenkolbe R, Bernard HU *et al.* (1999) The human papillomavirus type 16, E6 oncoprotein can down-regulate p53 activity by targeting the transcriptional co-activator CBP/p300. *Journal of Virology* 73: 6209–6219.

Zondervan KT, Carpenter LM, Painter R *et al.* (1996) Oral contraceptives and cervical cancer—further findings from the Oxford Family Planning Association contraceptive study. *British Journal of Cancer* 73: 1291–1297.

CHAPTER 10

Diethylstilbestrol (DES) and the cervicovaginal epithelium

J. Michael Emens

INTRODUCTION

Tragic mistakes caused by administration of drugs during pregnancy are usually recognised at the time of delivery, as in the case of thalidomide, but sometimes the adverse effects of the drug are recognised only after many years. The story of stilbestrol is a classic example.

In 1948, Smith reported the results of the use of diethylstilbestrol (DES) in pregnant patients to prevent miscarriage. Stilbestrol, synthesised by Sir Charles Dodds in 1936, was the first inexpensive, orally effective synthetic estrogen. The drug proved to be efficacious as a replacement therapy in estrogen-deficient postmenopausal women, in the management of dysfunctional uterine bleeding, in the treatment of inoperative prostate cancer and for the relief and prevention of postpartum breast engorgement. However, the evidence to support the use of the drug to prevent miscarriages was not conclusive (Goldziecher and Benigno, 1958).

Diethylstilbestrol was given to pregnant women in the belief that it would provide luteal support in situations such as threatened miscarriage or poor reproductive performance and particularly that associated with maternal diabetes (White and Hunt, 1943). It was widely used for this purpose in the USA but less frequently in the UK and Europe from about 1940 onwards. Two randomised controlled trials (RCT) were conducted in the 1950s, one in the USA involving 2000 non-diabetic pregnant women (Dieckmann *et al.*, 1953) and one in the UK between 1950 and 1953 (Reid, 1955). In the latter, 80 diabetic patients received DES and ethisterone and were compared with 76 non-hormone-treated control subjects. Neither trial showed any benefit for the treated group. Nevertheless, the use of DES was still being described in a 1971 reprint of the third edition of Jeffcoate's textbook *Principles of Gynaecology*.

DES AND VAGINAL CARCINOMA

In May 1966, Dr Howard Ulfelder in Boston (Herbst *et al.*, 1971) examined a teenage patient whose complaint was abnormal vaginal bleeding, thought to be anovulatory dysfunctional bleeding; however, the examination revealed a malignant growth in the vagina which histologically was adenocarcinoma. The finding of vaginal adenocarcinoma in such a young girl was quite unusual (Fig. 10.1a and b).

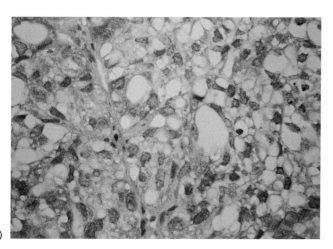
(a)

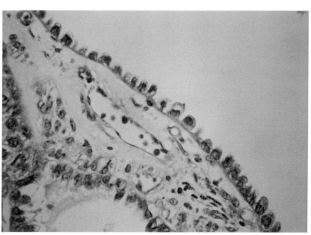
(b)

Fig. 10.1 (a) Clear cell tumour of the vagina (H&E × 120). (b) Higher power of the same tumour as above showing cystic margins (H&E × 300).

Links between hormones and vaginal and vulval cancer

Primary carcinoma of the vagina represents less than 2% of all gynaecological malignancies, and its relative rarity is exaggerated by its definition, which excludes tumours of the vagina which also invade either the cervix or the vulva. Squamous cell carcinoma of the vagina represents approximately 85% of all histological types, followed by adenocarcinoma (8%), sarcoma and melanoma (3%) and, more rarely, undifferentiated small cell and endodermal sinus tumour (Helm and Chan, 1996).

The mean age at presentation is the seventh decade of life, but it occurs in younger women, and many series report its occurrence in the third decade. Most commonly, it involves the upper third of the vagina. A case–control study showed limited education, low family income and a history of genital warts and abnormal cervical smears as risk factors: smoking and sexual behaviour, which are strongly associated with cervical carcinoma, were not implicated (Brinton *et al.*, 1990).

THE HISTORY OF DES

Following Ulfelder's findings, Herbst and Skully (1970) reported seven cases of clear cell adenocarcinoma (CCA) of the vagina in adolescent girls in the Boston area of the USA. An eighth case was added in 1971 in a retrospective study that linked these cases with the maternal ingestion of DES during pregnancy (Herbst *et al.*, 1971). Since then, there have been an enormous number of papers, mainly from the USA but increasingly from Europe, where the drug was used up to almost 10 years later than in the USA. Over 500 cases of CCA of the vagina and cervix have been registered, 25% having no history of exposure to DES. Despite the fact that the majority of cases occurred in the 1970s and 1980s, new cases of the disease continue to appear. Recently, it has been estimated that as many as 20 new cases and 10–15 recurrent cases occur in the USA every year (Herbst and Anderson, 1990). In about one-third of cases, there is no history of exposure to DES or any other non-steroidal estrogen.

Waggoner *et al.* (1994) hypothesised that the natural history of DES-exposed vaginal CCA and DES-unexposed vaginal CCA may differ. His cases were taken from the US Registry for Research on Hormonal Transplacental Carcinogenesis, which maintains information on cases of CCA of the lower genital tract occurring in women born after 1940. Four hundred and thirty-one cases satisfied FIGO criteria for primary vaginal carcinoma, of which 318 had hospital or pharmacy records available for review. Eighty per cent of these cases (255 of 318) had well-documented evidence of DES exposure and 20% (63 of 318) were without DES exposure. Waggoner found that survival of patients with vaginal CCA was significantly influenced by DES exposure, with a greater proportion of DES-exposed patients being alive 5 and 10 years after diagnosis. Thus, the prognosis and metastatic behaviour of CCA of the vagina appear to be influenced by DES exposure.

The DES-negative cases have a worse prognosis and a higher rate of distant metastasis than cases associated with exposure to DES. These observations do not appear to result from differences in clinical prognostic factors, such as tumour stage or diameter, but instead suggest differences in tumour behaviour, for as yet undetermined reasons.

The risk of developing CCA, calculated from birth to the age of 34 years, is estimated to be about one for every 1000 women exposed *in utero*. Melnick *et al.* (1987) and Herbst *et al.* (1986) also reported that women whose mothers were given DES before 12 weeks' gestation had a relative risk of developing CCA of the vagina and cervix three times higher than the relative risk for women whose mothers were given the drug during week 13 of gestation or later. The youngest patient diagnosed as having CCA was 7 years old and the oldest exposed patient in the USA was 42 years old at the time of diagnosis. Among DES-exposed daughters, 91 cases were diagnosed when the patients were aged 15–17 years and more than half these cases were diagnosed between 17 and 23 years of age. The incidence rate among those over 44 years of age is as yet unknown, because the first cohort is now just entering this age range. At present, it is not known whether a secondary rise in the age incidence will occur for patients beyond the fifth or sixth decade of life, the time when CCA occurs more commonly in the DES-unexposed population. However, this possibility emphasises the importance of long-term follow-up of the DES-exposed population. Hanselaar *et al.* (1996) reported his data from the Central Netherlands Registry showing twin age-incident peaks of CCA of the vagina and cervix. These were first at a mean age of 26 years and secondly at a mean age of 76 years.

This is reinforced by the most recent data from the DES Registry where some patients were over the age of 50 years at the time of diagnosis. A.L. Herbst (personal communication, 2002) states that these cancers will continue to develop rarely among the exposed and 'There clearly is no safe period'. Why CCA develops in only a small proportion of the exposed population is unknown. A steep rise in the age incidence curve occurs after the age of 14 years, suggesting that the events of the menarche may be important in promoting CCA. However, current data only imply, but do not prove, that increased endogenous secretion of steroid hormones in puberty is associated with the occurrence of these cancers. Both the shape of the age incidence curves and the rarity of this tumour among the exposed suggest that DES is an initiator of a carcinogenic process that is facilitated by the later action of promoters.

DES AND SQUAMOUS CELL CANCER

Some authors have suggested that DES-exposed females are at an increased risk of developing squamous cell neoplasia because of the extensive transformation zone and greater surface area of immature metaplastic epithelium exposed to a possible carcinogen (Robboy *et al.*, 1984). An early prevalence study of 744 closely matched pairs of DES-exposed and unexposed daughters from the National Co-operative Diethylstilboestrol Adenosis Project (DESAD) found 26 cases of cervical intraepithelial squamous neoplasia (CIN) and vaginal intraepithelial neoplasia (VIN) among DES-exposed daughters and 35 cases among unexposed control subjects. However, incidence data from the first 10 years of the DESAD project reported twice the incidence of high-grade CIN in the exposed daughters (15.7 vs. 7.9 cases per 1000 person–years of follow-up). The exposed and control groups were similar with respect to many variables, including the number of sexual partners and the frequency of several sexually transmitted diseases. Examination followed a uniform protocol, which included pelvic examination, colposcopy, vaginal and cervical cytology, and biopsy when colposcopic abnormalities were detected. The data suggest that the risk of lower genital tract neoplasia may be twice as high among DES-exposed daughters. However, there are insufficient data to assess the magnitude of the risk or trends in the risk of squamous carcinoma of the cervix and vagina upon ageing of this cohort. Bornstein *et al.* (1988) claimed that Robboy's findings were confounded by an increased prevalence of herpes simplex virus and human papillomavirus.

BENIGN LESIONS ASSOCIATED WITH DES EXPOSURE

Fosberg (1966), in a series of elegant experiments, showed that ovarian injections of 5 mg of estradiol resulted in large regions of untransformed pseudostratified epithelium in the upper two-thirds of the developing mouse vagina and, moreover, that this untransformed epithelium persisted into the adult stage, at which time it formed glandular-like downgrowths into the stroma. In the most pronounced cases, the normal structure of the whole uterine cervix was hidden. Stilbestrol injected in the same dose and according to an identical time schedule as estradiol resulted in the same type of changes (Fosberg, 1972).

It is now well established that the intake of stilbestrol during human pregnancy is associated with the development of vaginal adenosis and, in a small number of cases, with clear cell adenocarcinoma (Herbst *et al.*, 1971). It is now generally agreed that these changes occur in Müllerian-derived epithelium. Thus, stilbestrol inhibits mitotic activity in the human pseudostratified Müllerian epithelium, and also inhibits transformation of the human Müllerian epithelium into a stratified one, which is important in the expansion of the vaginal plate. The large transformation zone extending into the vagina of girls exposed to DES shows persistent columnar Müllerian epithelium, which develops into adenosis. A scheme of the extension of the transformation zone can be seen in Figure 10.2a and b.

Although the principal effect of DES on the development of the vagina has been the production of ectopic columnar epithelium, there are a number of macroscopic changes that are typical and clearly evident on examination. Figure 10.3a–e shows the typical gross findings.

Figure 10.3d and e shows a cervix with a transverse vaginal septum, which can be either partial, as in Figure 10.3d, or virtually complete like a collar, necessitating division in some cases for adequate visualisation of the cervix. With all these findings,

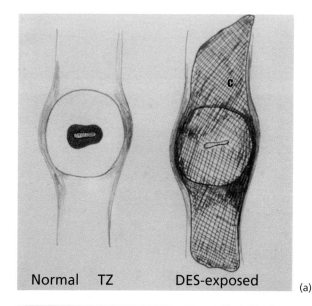

Normal TZ   DES-exposed   (a)

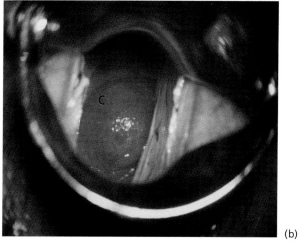

(b)

Fig. 10.2 (a) Schema of the extension of the transformation zone (TZ) in DES-exposed girls (right) and unexposed girls (left). In unexposed girls, the transformation zone encircles the external os while in DES-exposed girls, the transformation zone sometimes extends from across the cervix to cover the entire vagina. C = columnar epithelium. From Stafl *et al.* (1974), with kind permission of the editors of the *American Journal of Obstetrics and Gynecology*. (b) Colposcopic appearance of the transformation zone in a DES-exposed girl. C = columnar epithelium (×6).

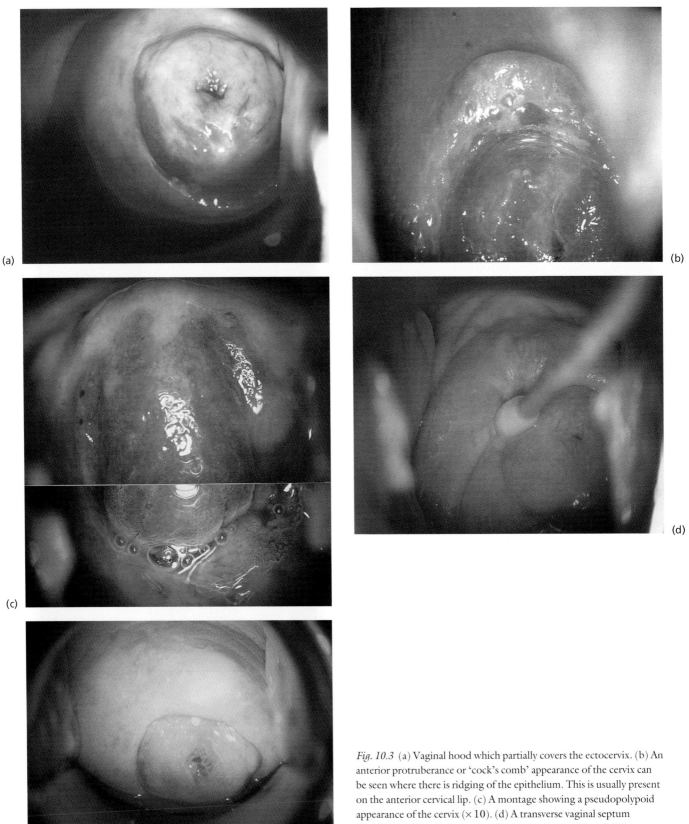

Fig. 10.3 (a) Vaginal hood which partially covers the ectocervix. (b) An anterior protruberance or 'cock's comb' appearance of the cervix can be seen where there is ridging of the epithelium. This is usually present on the anterior cervical lip. (c) A montage showing a pseudopolypoid appearance of the cervix (× 10). (d) A transverse vaginal septum partially covering the cervix (× 10). (e) Cervical hood partially covering the cervix post acetic acid (× 16).

Table 10.1 Macroscopic benign findings in Birmingham series.

	Number	Percentage
Vaginal hood	15	14
Cock's comb	13	12
Columnar epithelium	43	40
Transverse septum	11	10
No changes visible	26	24

J.M. Emens, personal series, 2001.

there is also obliteration of the fornices and the finding of the ectocervix almost flush with the vault. Table 10.1 shows the typical findings in the Birmingham series.

VAGINAL ADENOSIS

By definition, vaginal adenosis is the presence of glandular columnar epithelium in the vagina. Stafl *et al.* (1974) demonstrated that columnar epithelium in the vagina is colposcopically and histologically identical to the endocervical type of columnar epithelium, and that the terminal vascular network of columnar epithelium is identical to that which is found in the cervix. Vaginal adenosis in the non-DES-exposed female does occur, albeit rarely, and Sandberg and his co-workers (1968) were able to identify 45 reported cases. It was not until 1971 when Herbst and his co-workers first drew attention to the relationship of intrauterine DES exposure and the subsequent development of clear cell adenocarcinoma that columnar epithelium in the vagina once again become an important clinical finding. Stafl's series in 1974 drew attention to the importance of colposcopic examination in recognising this condition. Undoubtedly, accurate recognition of vaginal adenosis can be achieved only with clear visualisation with the colposcope (Fig. 10.4a and b).

The main objective is to identify the location of the original squamocolumnar junction. This is established by the identification of the extent of the colposcopic transformation zone, the presence of gland openings and Nabothian cysts and by the differences in the vascular pattern in the transformation zone and the original squamous epithelium. The location of the original squamocolumnar junction is shown in Table 10.2a and b.

CLINICAL ASSESSMENT AND MANAGEMENT OF DES-EXPOSED DAUGHTERS

DES-exposed daughters need meticulous examinations of the vagina and the ectocervix and should be examined as soon as possible after the menarche. They rarely need examination under anaesthesia, but should be advised to use tampons 3–6 months before their first examination to facilitate colposcopic

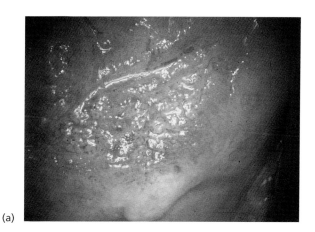

(a)

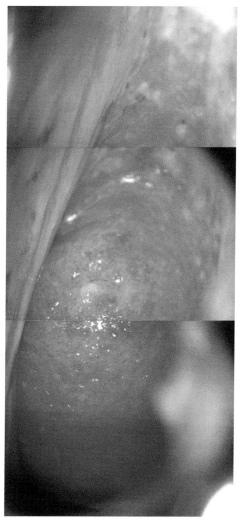

(b)

Fig. 10.4 (a) An area of vaginal adenosis (× 10).
(b) Colpophotomontage showing extensive ectopic columnar epithelium (adenosis) in the vagina of a virginal DES-exposed patient (× 16).

Table 10.2a Extension of columnar epithelium.

	Number	Percentage
Lower third of vagina	17	6
Middle third of vagina	57	20
Upper third of vagina	74	26
Vaginal fornices	83	30
Cervix, portio	49	18

After Stafl *et al.* (1974).

Table 10.2b Extension of columnar epithelium: Birmingham series.

	Number	Percentage
Lower third of vagina	17	16
Middle third of vagina	17	16
Upper third of vagina	34	32
Vaginal fornices	11	10
Cervix, portio	28	26

J.M. Emens, personal series, 2001.

examination. They should be referred to the appropriate referral centre. Careful digital examination of the vagina should first be carried out to exclude any nodular areas that may be suggestive of CCA. After digital palpation, an appropriate-sized speculum is placed in the vagina and gently rotated to allow visualisation of the anterior and posterior vaginal walls. Samples for cytology should be taken from the cervix and the endocervical canal and all four vaginal walls. After the application of 5% acetic acid, the extent of the transformation zone should be noted and any abnormal colposcopic vascular patterns recorded. The transformation zone is often striking for not staining with iodine and is clearly outlined. Careful recording of these findings, including photography, is desirable. Biopsies are rarely necessary unless there is a suspicion of a carcinoma or if there is persistent abnormal cytology needing evaluation (Anderson *et al.*, 1992).

The colposcopic findings are often of acetowhite epithelium with fine mosaicism and punctation (Fig. 10.5a–f). Previous investigation of this epithelium, including scanning electron microscopy, has shown that these abnormalities consist of active squamous metaplasia rather than neoplasia (McDonnell *et al.*, 1984). These areas usually revert to normal over a period of 2 or 3 years and gradually become glycogenated, and treatment is rarely necessary (Emens, 1980).

Figure 10.6a–h shows the gradual regression of this epithelium to normal. Annual follow-up is advisable. As CCA can occur at any time, lifelong follow-up is advisable.

FERTILITY AND PREGNANCY

A number of case–control studies have evaluated fertility in DES daughters and have found no differences in fertility between exposed and unexposed daughters. An *in vitro* fertilisation (IVF) study shows that DES exposure has no influence on oocyte quality and fertilisation (Kerjean *et al.*, 1999). Adverse outcomes of pregnancy, including preterm birth, ectopic pregnancies and intrauterine deaths, have been reported more commonly among DES daughters than among DES-exposed women. Despite this, more than 80% of DES daughters who desire pregnancy or who have become pregnant have been delivered of at least one liveborn infant. However, the risk of ectopic pregnancy would appear to be increased 10-fold while the risk of spontaneous miscarriage is doubled, as is the incidence of preterm labour. In a meta-analysis by Goldberg and Falcone (1999), 59% of DES-exposed women delivered at term, with a 76% live birth rate, compared with 83% and 92%, respectively, in non-exposed control subjects. Pregnant women who know that they were exposed to DES *in utero* should inform their obstetrician and be aware of the increased risks of ectopic pregnancy and preterm labour. Vaginal ultrasound in early pregnancy should be performed to confirm an intrauterine pregnancy.

DES AND BREAST CANCER

It has been hypothesised that *in utero* estrogen exposure may influence later breast cancer risk (Trichopoulous, 1990). Studies designed to evaluate this hypothesis have assessed several different prenatal factors related to pregnancy estrogen levels: pre-eclampsia, eclampsia, twin pregnancy, maternal age at the time of pregnancy, preterm birth and birthweight (Potischman and Troisi, 1999). In the case of prenatal DES exposure, DES was prescribed at the first trimester and continued daily for several months or until the end of pregnancy. Thus, the offspring of these women are likely to have had *in utero* exposure to very high levels of estrogen. Do these women therefore have an increased risk of breast cancer in later life?

Julie Palmer and her associates (2002) evaluated a cohort of 4821 exposed women and 2095 unexposed women, most of whom were first identified in the mid-1970s. Their results showed that DES was not associated with increased risk of breast cancer in women under 40 years but, among women aged 40 and older, the rate ratio was 2.5 [95% confidence interval (CI) 1.0–6.3]. The rate ratio for the association of DES exposure with estrogen receptor-positive tumours was 1.9 (95% CI 0.8–4.5); while not statistically significant, the overall 40% excess risk arising exclusively from the subset of estrogen receptor-positive cases raises a concern calling for continued investigation. This is supported by another study (Titus-Ernstoff *et al.*, 2001), which indicated that

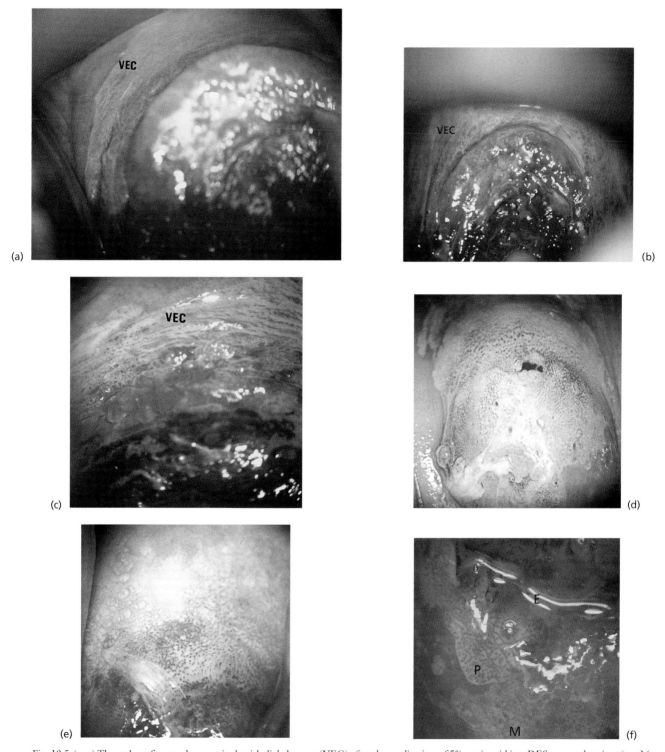

Fig. 10.5 (a–c) These three figures show vaginal epithelial changes (VEC) after the application of 5% acetic acid in a DES-exposed patient (a × 16; b × 6; c × 25). (d and e) In these two figures, the acetowhite epithelium in DES-exposed patients is seen, showing the marked punctation on the anterior lip extending into the anterior vaginal fornix (× 16). (f) High-powered view (× 25) of the acetowhite epithelial changes on the posterior cervical lip just outside the boundary of the endo- and ectocervix (E). An area to the left shows typical fine punctation (P); that to the right and lower has a suggestion of fine mosaic epithelium (M).

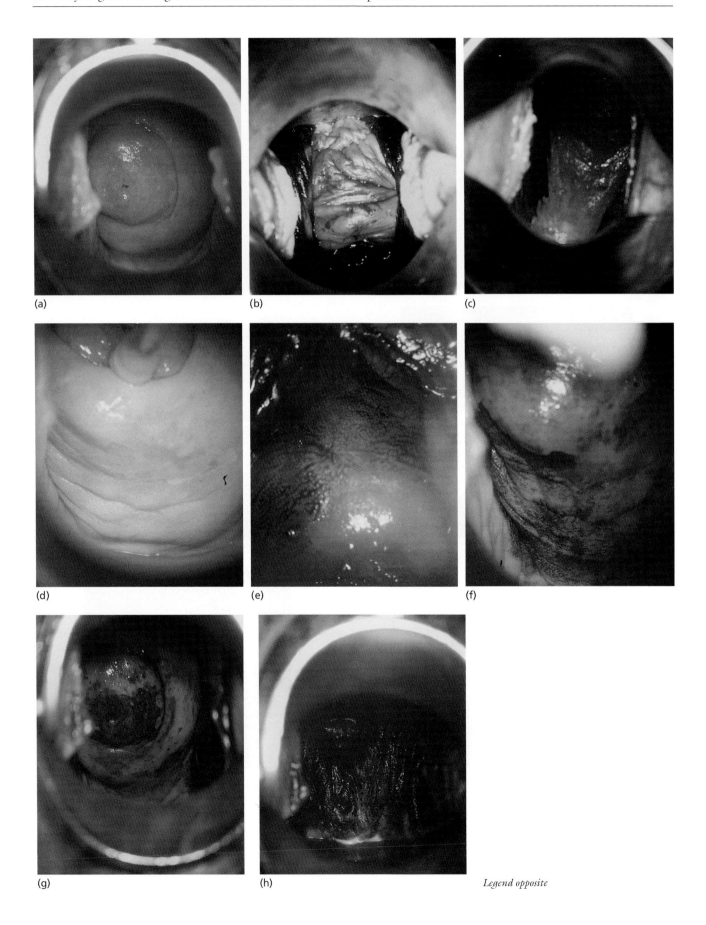

(a)

(b)

(c)

(d)

(e)

(f)

(g)

(h)

Legend opposite

approximately 16% of women who were prescribed DES while pregnant developed breast cancer. In comparison, approximately 13% of women who were not prescribed DES while pregnant are likely to develop breast cancer. The increased risk of breast cancer did not appear to be interactive with other risk factors [such as use of hormone replacement therapy (HRT), use of birth control pills or family history of breast cancer]. That means that DES exposure, in addition to HRT or family history, did not increase the risk of breast cancer higher than that caused by DES exposure alone.

Further follow-up of DES-exposed women is imperative in order to establish whether there is a causal association with breast cancer risk and to assess the hypothesis raised by their data. A cohort of USA women exposed to DES in the 1950s and 1960s have now reached the age at which breast cancer incidence is appreciable. The receptor testing currently occurs more routinely, and it should be possible to determine the receptor status for almost all new cases. DES-exposed women should follow the advice given to all women aged 40 years and over in the USA and 50 years and over in the UK and undergo screening mammography and regular breast examinations.

CONCLUSIONS

It would be prudent for those females who believe that they may have been exposed to DES *in utero* and who are anxious about the risks of vaginal and cervical cancer to be carefully monitored by annual colposcopic examinations in specialist centres. These examinations should be commenced as soon as possible after the menarche and be repeated indefinitely for the reasons outlined below. There is a need to be aware of the biphasic peaks of incidence of vaginal CCA, especially as exposed females will now be approaching their fifth decade. Evidence for an increased risk of other cancers in both them-

selves and their mothers is less convincing, but they would be sensible to participate in the National Breast Screening Programme. Pregnant women who know that they were exposed to DES *in utero* should inform their obstetrician and be aware of the increased risks of ectopic pregnancy and preterm labour. Notwithstanding these risk factors, only a small minority of DES-exposed individuals will experience serious problems, and a proper perspective should be maintained.

REFERENCES

Anderson M, Jordan JA, Morse A *et al.* (1992) *Text and Atlas of Integrated Colposcopy.* London: Chapman & Hall Medical, Ch. 19, pp. 211–212.

Bornstein J, Adam E, Adler-Storhz K *et al.* (1988) Development of cervical and vaginal squamous cell neoplasia as a late consequence of in utero exposure to diethylstilboestrol. *Obstetric and Gynaecology Surveys* 43: 1521.

Brinton LA, Nasca PC, Mallin K *et al.* (1990) Case control study of in-situ and invasive carcinoma of the vagina. *Gynaecologic Oncology* 38: 49–54.

Dieckmann WJ, Davis HE, Rynknewicz LM *et al.* (1953) Does the administration of diethylstilboestrol during pregnancy have therapeutic value? *American Journal of Obstetrics and Gynecology* 66: 1062–1081.

Emens JM (1980) The significance of white epithelium on the vagina and cervix of diethylstilboestrol (DES) exposed and non-exposed sexually active teenage girls. MD Thesis, University of Birmingham.

Fosberg JG (1966) Effect of estradiol 17 beta on the epithelium in the mouse vaginal anlage. *Acta Anatomica* 63: 71–88.

Fosberg JG (1972) Estrogen, vaginal cancer and vaginal development. *American Journal of Obstetrics and Gynecology* 113: 80–87.

Goldberg JM, Falcone T (1999) Effect of DES on reproductive function. *Fertility and Sterility* 72: 1–7.

Goldziecher JW, Benigno BB (1958) The treatment of threatened and recurrent abortion. A critical review. *American Journal of Obstetrics and Gynecology* 75: 1202–1214.

Hanselaar A, van Loosbroek M, Schuurbiers O *et al.* (1996) Clear cell adenocarcinoma of the vagina and cervix. *Cancer* 79: 2229–2236.

Helm CW, Chan KK (1996) Vaginal cancer. In: Shingleton HM, Jordan JA, Fowler WC (eds) *Gynaecological Oncology.* Philadelphia: W.B. Saunders, pp. 109–119.

Herbst AL, Anderson D (1990) Clear cell adenocarcinoma of the vagina and cervix secondary to intrauterine exposure to diethylstilboestrol. *Seminars in Surgical Oncology* 6: 343–346.

Herbst AL, Skully RE (1970) Adenocarcinoma of the vagina: a report of seven cases including six clear cell carcinomas (so called mesonephromas). *Cancer* 25: 745–757.

Herbst AL, Ulfelder H, Poskanzer DC (1971) Adenocarcinoma of the vagina: an association of maternal stilboestrol therapy with tumour appearance in young women. *New England Journal of Medicine* 284: 878–881.

Herbst AL, Anderson D, Hubby MM *et al.* (1986) Risk factors for the development of diethylstilboestrol-associated clear cell adenocarcinoma: a case–control study. *American Journal of Obstetrics and Gynecology* 154: 814–822.

Fig. 10.6 (opposite) (a) The cervix of a DES patient stained with saline . This colpophotograph was taken in April 1976 (× 6). (b) The same colpophotograph of the same cervix as in (a) after the application of Schiller's iodine. The anterior vaginal fornix is stained positive (× 6). (c) The same cervix as in (a) and (b), again with Schiller's iodine applied, but this time to the posterior vaginal fornix (× 6). (d) View of the same cervix as in (a) to (c), now photographed in February 1978. The view of the posterior vagina after the application of acetic acid shows a very faint white staining. This view can be interpreted as a virtually normal colposcopic appearance (× 10). (e) A view of the anterior vagina of the same cervix as in (d), showing partial glycogenation after the application of Schiller's iodine. (f) The same cervix as in (d) and (e), again after the application of Schiller's iodine, showing partial glycogenation (× 10). (g) Colpophotograph of the same cervix as in (a) to (f), now in February 1979, showing glycogenation of the cervix after the application of Schiller's iodine (× 6). (h) The same cervix as in (g) with complete glycogenation having taken place over the anterior vaginal vault.

Jeffcoate TNA (1971) *Principles of Gynaecology*, 3rd edn. London: Butterworth.

Kerjean A, Poiro C, Epelboin S *et al.* (1999) Effect of in-utero DES exposure on human oocyte quality and fertilization in a programme of in-utero fertilization 1999. Laboratoire de Biologie de la Reproduction, Universitie Paris V–Hospital Cochin, Paris, France.

McDonnell JM, Emens JM, Jordan JA (1984) The congenital cervico-vaginal transformation zone in young women exposed to DES in-utero. *British Journal of Obstetrics and Gynaecology* 91: 580–584.

Melnick S, Cole PA, Atherson D *et al.* (1987) Rates and risks of diethyl-stilboestrol related to clear-cell adenocarcinoma of the vagina and cervix. *New England Journal of Medicine* 316: 514–516.

Palmer JR, Hatch EE, Rosenberg CL *et al.* (2002) Risk of breast cancer in women exposed to diethystilboestrol in-utero: preliminary results (United States). *Cancer Causes and Control* 13: 753–758.

Potischman N, Troisi R (1999) In-utero and early life exposures in relation of risk of breast cancer. *Cancer Causes and Control* 10: 561–573.

Reid DD (1955) The use of hormones in the management of pregnancy in diabetes: report to the Medical Research Council by their Conference on Diabetes and Pregnancy. *Lancet* 6895: 833–836.

Robboy SJ, Nollar KL, O'Brian P *et al.* (1984) Increased incidence of cervical and vaginal dyplasia in 3980 diethylstilboestrol exposed young women. *Journal of the American Medical Association* 252: 2979–2983.

Sandberg EC (1968) The incidence and distribution of occult vaginal adenosis. *American Journal of Obstetrics and Gynecology* 101: 322–334.

Smith OW (1948) Diethylstilboestrol in the prevention and treatment of complications of pregnancy. *American Journal of Obstetrics and Gynecology* 56: 821–831.

Stafl A, Mattingley RF, Foley DV *et al.* (1974) Clinical diagnosis of vaginal adenosis. *Obstetrics and Gynaecology* 43: 118–128.

Titus-Ernstoff L, Hatch EE, Hoover RN *et al.* (2001) Long term cancer risk in women given diethylstilboestrol (DES) during pregnancy. *British Journal of Cancer* 84: 125–133.

Trichopoulos D (1990) Does breast cancer originate in utero? *Lancet* 335: 939–940.

Waggoner MD, Millendorf R, Nana Biney PH *et al.* (1994) Influence of in-utero diethystilboestrol exposure on the prognosis and biologic behaviour of vaginal clear-cell adenocarcinoma. *Gynaecological Oncology* 55: 238–244.

White P, Hunt H (1943) Pregnancy complicating diabetes. *Journal of Clinical Endocrinology* 3: 500–511.

PART 3

The cervix and fertility and infertility

CHAPTER 11

The structure, chemistry and physics of human cervical mucus

Khaldoun Sharif and Olufemi Olufowobi

The main product of the uterine cervix is the mucus. Understanding its physical and chemical structure is helpful in discerning its function and malfunction.

STRUCTURE OF HUMAN CERVICAL MUCUS

The endocervical glands are deep slit-like invaginations of the surface epithelium with blind-ending tubules arising from the clefts. The epithelial cells that line these glands produce mucus. There are several hundred mucus-secreting units in the cervical canal. The daily production varies in relation to the cyclical changes of the menstrual cycle, varying from 600 mg during midcycle to 20–60 mg during other periods of the cycle.

Cervical mucus is a heterogeneous mixture of secretions whose rate of production depends on several factors. These include the number of mucus-secretory units in the cervical canal, the percentage of mucus-secreting cells per unit and the secretory activity and the response of the cells to circulating hormones (Stevens and Lowe, 1997).

Based on nuclear magnetic resonance studies, Odeblad (1968a) (Fig. 11.1) proposed a theoretical model for the spatial organisation of cervical mucus infrastructure. He reported that the glycoprotein solid phase is organised as a network of fibrils linked together by oblique or transverse bonds, in a 'tricot-like macromolecular arrangement'. At midcycle, the glucoprotein chains that constitute the framework of the mucoid hydrogel organise themselves into fibrils forming a meshwork, approximately 3 μm, large enough to allow spermatozoa to pass through. The low-viscosity aqueous phase or cervical plasma occupies the interspaces of the micelle structure. However, outside the midcycle, the fibrillar micelles are rare, and thus the arrangement is a much denser network, approximately 0.3 μm, presenting a most effective barrier to

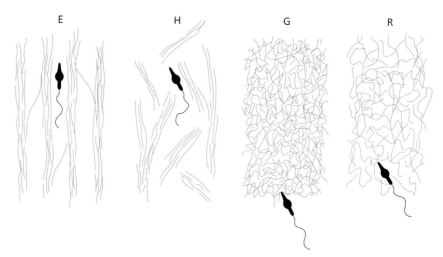

Fig. 11.1 Schematic picture of the gel structure for some types of cervical mucus. In type E, the thread-formed macromolecules lie together in long parallel bundles, or micelles, with spaces between them filled with cervical plasma. The spermatozoa can easily swim in these spaces. In type H, the micelles are shorter, and the connections between them are broken so that the parallel arrangement is lost. In type G, no micelle formation occurs, but the long macromolecules form a large, three-dimensional, irregular, dense network (average size 0.3 μm) that does not allow spermatozoa to enter. In type R, there is also an irregular network but with somewhat larger mesh size (average size 0.5 μm) that, however, is sufficiently narrow to prevent effective sperm migration. From Odeblad and Rudolfsson-Åsberg (1973), with kind permission of the editor (Professor R.A. Blandau) and the publisher (University of Chicago Press).

spermatozoa, as the diameter of a sperm head is approximately 2.5 μm. This model was corroborated by several investigators using either scanning electron microscopy or rheological techniques (Singer and Reid, 1970; Chrétien and Psychoyos, 1975; Chrétien *et al.*, 1976; Chrétien and David, 1978; Takano *et al.*, 1979). The cyclical nature of these changes suggests that they are under hormonal influence, and appear to be responsible for the receptivity, and hostility, of the mucus to sperms at various phases of the menstrual cycle.

On the other hand, Lee *et al.* (1977) refuted the above model based on studies on cervical mucus using laser light scattering techniques. The authors proposed a cervical mucus model composed of 'an ensemble of tangled random-coiled macromolecules' rather than a fibrillar macromolecular network. Additionally, the authors queried the validity of the data generated by either nuclear magnetic resonance or scanning electron microscopy, which was deemed to be 'largely artifactitious'. Their data contradicted the actual results gained with hydrogels and entangled macromolecules (De Gennes, 1976; Gould *et al.*, 1976; Adam and Delsanti, 1977a,b). These inconsistencies prompted a systematic study of human cervical mucus by Volochine *et al.* (1988). Using laser light scattering proton correlation and spectral analysis, it was shown that cervical mucus is a non-Newtonian hydrogel with large meshes (~ 5 μm), thus corroborating the model of hydrogel structure. They also agreed with earlier extensive mechanical studies carried out on cervical mucus by other investigators (Meyer *et al.*, 1975; Litt *et al.*, 1976).

Some of the inconsistencies above have been attributed to the changes that mucin undergoes during the course of an experiment. Beeson *et al.* (1982) demonstrated that the changes were dependent on the technique and nature of the experiment. In their experiment, human cervical mucus samples were frozen as described by Parish *et al.* (1981) and later studied by the scanning electron microscope (SEM). The authors reported that the observed 'pored' structure (crystal voids) was inversely proportional to the freezing rate. Their observation corroborated the findings and conclusion of Parish *et al.* (1982) that the porous structure seen in frozen specimens is a product of the freezing procedure used prior to examination in the SEM and does not represent a structure present in the natural state. In spite of this, they speculated that the observed change in the artefact in one specimen (and its similarity to that which can be induced by calcium ions) suggests that alterations in the SEM appearances may still parallel *in vivo* modifications in mucus composition, which may in turn be relevant to fertility.

Branching and cross-linking between micelles occur and aid the formation of network gel structure. Intermicellar spaces play a key role in sperm migration. The channels or spaces have been classified into three types. They are: (1) DT, direct, sperm-transmitting spaces, 2–5 μm wide (mainly E_s type mucus; see below); (2) DN, directed but not sperm-transmitting space, 1–2 μm wide (mainly E_1 type mucus); and (3) NO, non-oriented spaces with no sperm-transmitting capacity, spaces 0.3–1 μm wide (mucus type G). It is worth mentioning that the molecular assemblies such as micelles are dynamic structures, vibrating and of varying shapes. Consequently, the intermicellar spaces also vary in size.

Secretions in human cervical mucus

Odeblad (1969) characterised the two main types of secretions in normal cervical mucus. He designated them as type E (estrogenic) and type G (progestogenic) (Table 11.1). During the menstrual cycle, both types are always mixed together in different proportions. Type E is under estrogen dominance and is characterised by thin, watery mucus in pure form (Fig. 11.2). Type G, under progestogenic dominance, corresponds to the thick, sticky mucus. Thus, type E predominates at the time of ovulation (about 97% E and 3% of type G). Type G dominates during the normal luteal phase or when the combined oral contraceptive pill is used (Fig. 11.3).

Two types of fibrous structures have been demonstrated in midcycle cervical mucus: (1) long, thick fibres that vary in diameter from 0.5 to 5 μm and run parallel to each other; and (2) microfibrils that range from 500 to 1500 Å in diameter (Zeneveld *et al.*, 1975). These investigators speculated that the fibres most probably represented the micelles that give spermatozoa their directional approach through the cervix. Using nuclear magnetic resonance (NMR) analysis of the contents of a single crypt and comparing this with sperm migration on well-preserved mucus explants, Odeblad (1976) established the biological functions of two types of estrogen type E cervical mucus secretions, labelled as E_s and E_1 (s for string, l for loaf).

NMR implies radiofrequency absorption in atomic nuclei in a homogeneous field. It permits a non-destructive study of cervical mucus. The E_s mucus conveys the spermatozoa from the vaginal pool, but the E_1 type has a very limited role in this respect. The E_s–E_1 system is very dynamic. Ovulatory mucus contains 20–25% type E_s, 72–77% type E_1 and 3% type G. Furthermore, E_s and E_1 differ in their protein content. Protein is low in the intermicellar spaces of E_s mucus. The very low viscosity of E_s intermicellar fluid permits very rapid sperm migration. The E types of secretions have characteristic molecular architecture. The mucins contain macromolecules, which are peptides with carbohydrate and other side groups attached at certain points to the peptide chain. The mucin macromolecules are thread-like and occur in assemblies in which they lie almost in parallel. The assembly, which varies in diameter and arrangement, is called a micelle.

Other types of cervical mucus secretions have been identified. Odeblad (1969) labelled the secretion associated with chronic cervicitis type Q. Cervical mucus compositions vary depending on the type, degree and duration of the inflammatory

Table 11.1 Biological properties of some types of cervical mucus.

Type	Condition	Molecular structure of gel channels	Dry substance (%)	Cell contents	Main cell types*	Cell arrangements	Macro+ viscosity (poise)	R_1 (s^{-1})
E	Estrogenic	Micelles, ordered DT channels	1.5–3	Low	Eo	Scattered	1–19	0.5–2
G	Estrogenic	Dense network NO spaces	5–12	High	Ep, Le	Dense, scattered	10–1000	5–20
H_1	Hyper-estrogenic	Micelles, disordered	1–3	Low	Ep	Scattered	0.1–3	0.1–0.3
H_2								
H_3								
Q	Chronic inflammation	Unknown	5–15	Very high	Ep, Le, Ly	Dense	100–1000	10–100
L	Acute inflammation	Unknown	–	Varying	Varying	Dense	–	–
N	Retained mucus	Mixed	Varying	Varying	Varying	–	–	–
R	Retrosteroid	Loose DN channels	2–4	High	Ep, Le	Dense, scattered	1–10	1–3
B	Mechanical stimulation	–	2–3	–	–	–	0.03–0.1	0.1–0.3
DE	Iso-E glands		Similar to type E					
DG	Iso-D glands		Similar to type G					

*Ep, epithelial cells; Le, leucocytes; Ly, lymphocytes.

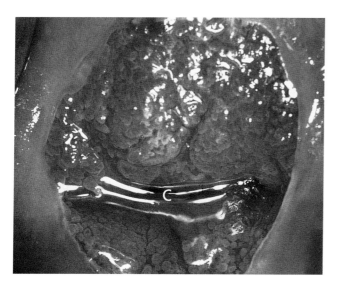

Fig. 11.2 Within the cervical canal (C), there is typical estrogenic mucus which is thin, watery and clear.

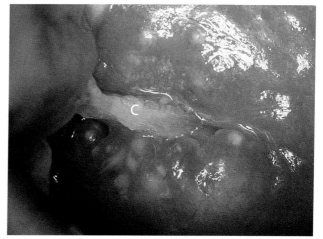

Fig. 11.3 Within the endocervix (C), opaque mucus is seen, typical of that visualised during the normal luteal phase or in women who are taking the oral contraceptive steroid.

condition. The crypts (Fig. 11.4) releasing this type of secretion have a limited response to hormonal stimulation. Odeblad (1966a) also described single glands within the transformation zone with these characteristics. Such secretory units have been designated isomucorrhoeic glands, isoglands or isounits (Odeblad, 1966b). Isounits also occur in acute inflammatory conditions and produce a serous type of secretion of low viscosity and high leucocyte content, the V type. The secretions in most cases of inflammation are of mixed type, containing all types, E, G, Q and V, in different proportions varying from

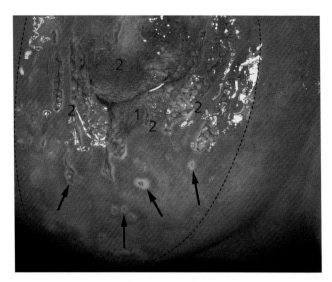

Fig. 11.4 Colpophotograph showing a transformation zone with single glands (arrowed), proposed by Odeblad (1966a) to secrete mucus only autonomically with very little or no response at all to steroid stimulation. Its glands are called isomucorrhoeic or isoglands, and Odeblad referred to this mucus as isosecretions and denoted it type D (D for destroyed normal response). Within this photograph, original columnar epithelium is at (1), the new squamocolumnar junction at (2) and, between it and the original junction (dotted line), is metaplastic squamous epithelium.

case to case and during the course of the disease. Thus, the cervical mucus is a heterogeneous mixture with one or other secretory type predominating. This gives the mucus complex rheological (flow and deformation) and biological properties.

In conclusion, the changing functions of cervical mucus in different endocrine states are compatible with their molecular and biological concepts. The cervical mucus consists of the mucoid hydrogel and the cervical plasma. The mucoid hydrogel (a glycoprotein solid phase) is organised as a network of fibrils linked together by oblique or transverse bonds. This meshwork is interspaced by cervical plasma. The fibrillar micelles vary in density during the different phases of the menstrual cycle, suggesting hormonal influence, and this appears to regulate sperm migration through the cervical mucus. Two types of secretions in normal cervical mucus are under hormonal control. Type E, mainly produced under estrogenic dominance, is watery and thin. Its microfibrils give spermatozoa the directional approach through the cervix. The type G secretion that is thick and sticky is produced under progesterone dominance. It is unfavourable to sperm migration. Other types of cervical secretion are produced under pathological conditions. In general, the cervical mucus is a heterogeneous mixture with one or more secretory types predominating; this gives the mucus its complex rheological and biological properties.

THE CHEMISTRY OF HUMAN CERVICAL MUCUS

The chemistry of cervical mucus is closely associated with its functions. Similarly, abnormalities are associated with infertility and impairment of local immunity of the female genital tract.

Cervical mucus constituents

Cervical mucus is a hydrogel composed of a low-molecular-weight component (cervical plasma) and a high-molecular-weight component (gel phase). The low-viscosity component consists mainly of electrolytes, organic components of low molecular weight such as glucose and amino acids, and soluble proteins (Schumacher, 1970; Gibbons and Selwood, 1973). The gel phase consists of a network of macromolecular glycoproteins called mucin. The extremely large mucins with high carbohydrate content are responsible for the high viscosity of cervical mucus (Schumacher, 1977).

Cervical mucus contains approximately 90% water. In the pre- and postovulatory phases, cervical mucus normally contains approximately 93%, while in the midcycle it may rise as high as 98% (Pommerenke, 1946). Depending on the viscosity and water content, it functions as a barrier or a transport medium for spermatozoa. Abnormality in the properties of the mucus may cause subfertility (the so-called 'cervical factor').

Mucin

In the study of human cervical mucus composition and properties using agar gel electrophoresis, Moghissi *et al.* (1962) were able to identify protein bands and a non-migrating zone. The non-migrating zone amounted to approximately 43% of the total stainable material. The authors suggested that this area, which was intensely periodic acid–Schiff (PAS) positive, might be the carbohydrate-rich factor, mucin, which gives the cervical mucus its unique characteristics. Furthermore, Neuhaus and Moghissi (1962), in their preliminary study of the mucoid component of the cervical mucus, observed the effect of trypsin and chemotrypsin on the whole cervical mucus and on the PAS-positive electrophoretically non-migrating material. Proteolysis caused the formation of PAS-positive electrophoretically migrating components, the disappearance of spinnbarkeit (elasticity) and viscidity and the elimination of precipitability with cetyltrimethylammonium bromide. Comparisons were made with saliva, purified salivary mucoid, orosomucoid, synovial fluid and chondroitin sulphates. The authors concluded that the carbohydrate-rich component, later called mucin, of the cervical mucus is a glycoprotein, or mucoid, and not a mucopolysaccharide. The same was suggested earlier by Werner (1953), who also proposed that the glycoproteins were of fucose and sialic acid type and are responsible for the specific characteristics.

The constituents and biochemical properties of mucin

It is widely believed that the biological and rheological properties of the cervical mucus gel depend on the cervical mucus glycoprotein, mucin (Moghissi *et al.*, 1960; Wolf *et al.*, 1977). Variations in mucus rheology observed during the normal menstrual cycle reflect, in part, the response of the cervix to steroid hormones. Estrogen stimulates the production of thin, isotonic mucus containing increased amounts of high-molecular-weight glycoproteins (highest at midcycle), whereas progesterone dominance leads to a relatively dry, viscous mucus (Moghissi, 1966a,b, 1972; Moghissi *et al.*, 1960). Thus, the physical and physiological properties of cervical mucus reflect alterations in the macromolecular composition or concentration of its components during the menstrual cycle. Various investigators have suggested that the mucin network is maintained by a peptide of ~ 30 kDa. This peptide connects mucin molecules through disulphide bridges (S–S), thus forming mucin micelles of 100 to 1000 glycoprotein chains (Schumacher, 1970; Sheehan and Carlstedt, 1982). This association of micro- ppears to be a relatively fragile one because it is capable of being readily disrupted by physical means, rendering it less viscous. The filamentous structure of mucin is said to be exhibited in physical properties such as spinnbarkeit and birefringence when the cervical mucus is stretched. Between the mucin network lies the cervical plasma, which consists of organic compounds and soluble proteins. The distance between the glycoproteins varies according to the phase of the menstrual cycle.

The presence of highly charged negative groups on the oligosaccharide side-chains of the glycoprotein molecules, such as terminal sialic acid(s), may be involved in the structural integrity of the mucin. Daunter *et al.* (1977) showed that 90% of the copper present in the cervical mucus is associated with mucin. Pigman and Horton (1970) reported that the sialic acid(s) moieties of the glycoproteins might bind copper in a way similar to that of calcium by the sialic acid moieties in salivary mucin. Thus, the process may link individual glycoproteins to each other via the carboxylic acid groups of the sialic acid(s) (COO^-–Cu^{2+}–^-OOC) to form 'fibres', which then associate by hydrogen bonding to form the mucin.

Mucin quantification

Analysis of monkey mucin demonstrated changes in the oligosaccharide structure depending on the phase of the menstrual cycle (Hatcher *et al.*, 1977). For decades, the sialic acid content of human cervical mucin was widely studied. The reports concerning the variation in sialic acid or other carbohydrate moieties during the menstrual cycle are sometimes contradictory (Van Kooji *et al.*, 1980; Meyer *et al.*, 1975; Moghissi and Syner, 1976; Guslandi, 1981; Chantler, 1982). Fleetwood *et al.* (1986) suggested that the variation in results might be due to the absence of calculations of concentration changes as well as of total amounts. In an analysis that involved the quantification of human cervical mucin during consecutive days and hourly on 1 day at midcycle, Fleetwood and co-investigators (1986) showed that the concentration of mucin varies significantly during midcycle. The decrease correlated with the luteinising hormone (LH) peak followed by an increase in late midcycle. The decrease in mucin was attributed possibly to: (1) increase in water content; (2) decrease mucin content; or (3) increase in both water and mucin contents with a relatively more pronounced water increase. Thus, the correlation between serum estradiol level and the amount of mucin secreted on cycle day LH-1 (the day of peak LH) is in agreement with the concept that estradiol stimulates the secretion of mucin. In the same study, it was shown that repeated mucus sampling resulted in a significant decrease in the total amount of mucin recovered during repeated sample collections. The concentration of mucin was not affected, as mucin and water were removed to the same extent.

Cervical plasma

The low-molecular-weight component (cervical plasma) constitutes the soluble component of cervical mucus. It consists of inorganic salts, trace elements, low-molecular-weight organic compounds and soluble proteins.

Soluble proteins

Cervical mucus protein content is estimated to be between 0.5% and 3%, with a total nitrogen content of approximately 12%. Soluble proteins make up about 30% of the non-dialysable material that is dispersed in the aqueous phase of the cervical mucus gel. Local tissue production and derivation from the serum are the sources of soluble proteins.

Serum proteins are present in the cervical mucus probably as a result of capillary permeability (Von Kaulla *et al.*, 1957). In a paper on the electrophoretic examination of cervical mucus from normal, pregnant and carcinomatous patients, Spencer and colleagues (1957) found two main bands, one non-migratory and the other diffuse. The non-migratory band was composed of insoluble polysaccharides and cell debris, and albumin accompanied by globulins was identified. No peaks were identifiable with the usual serum proteins. The authors suggested that the presence of an albumin peak could be indicative of some pathological state in the genital tract. However, the highly viscous character of cervical mucus makes paper electrophoretic studies of mucus open to highly significant questions. A subsequent paper by Moghissi and colleagues (1962), using agar gel electrophoresis, showed the presence of albumin and other electrophoretically identifiable protein areas as well. Following this, Moghissi and Neuhaus (1962) used immunoelectrophoretic studies to show the presence of albumin, gamma-globulins, a migrating zone (similar to the alpha- and beta-globulins) and a non-migrating zone. The non-migrating zone constituted approximately 43% of the total stainable material. There was no high concentration of immunologically active material coinciding with the so-called non-migrating fraction. Therefore, it was suggested that the non-migrating fraction was not a protein fraction of serum origin. Furthermore, the fact that the non-migrating fraction was intensely PAS positive suggested that it might be the carbohydrate-containing factor, mucin, that makes the cervical mucus characteristically unique (Moghissi *et al.*, 1962).

The proteins of human cervical mucus

Rohr and co-workers (1992) first performed an initial comprehensive evaluation of smaller molecules of mucus in their native state using high-resolution nuclear magnetic resonance spectroscopy. It proved to be a valuable new method for differentiated biochemical analysis of human cervical mucus. Recently, Sahrbacher and co-workers (2002) used high-resolution proton magnetic resonance spectroscopy to study late follicular phase cervical mucus from a group of infertile women who were pretreated with oral estrogen to standardise the hormonal influence on mucus properties. Of the 20 proteogenic amino acids, 13 were regularly observed. It was supposed that the remaining amino acids probably occur at concentrations below the limit of detection of about 10 µmol. Morales and colleagues (1993) have studied the concentration of protein in the mucus and its ability to sustain sperm migration. The peri-ovulatory and 60 days post partum mucus exhibited low protein concentrations as revealed by sodium dodecyl sulphate polyacrylamide gel electrophoresis (SDS-PAGE). The data showed a statistically significant inverse relationship between protein concentration in the mucus and its ability to sustain sperm migration. Many of the soluble proteins showed their lowest concentration during the fertile period of the cycle, when cervical mucus is most receptive to sperm penetration. An earlier study by Moghissi and Neuhaus (1966) on cervical proteins employed separation electrophoretically by dilute agar to demonstrate the cyclical changes during menstrual cycles. Albumin, globulin and non-migrating mucoid were determined in the cervical mucus of four healthy fertile women throughout one menstrual cycle. A decrease in albumin and an increase in the amount of mucoid component prior to and at ovulation were shown, and these changes were reversed shortly after ovulation. Globulin concentration did not change remarkably during the menstrual cycle. These findings were put forward as a possible means of detecting ovulation. They also suggested that the reciprocal changes in the albumin and mucoid components are apparently the result of normal cyclic release of estrogen and progesterone (Moghissi and Neuhaus, 1966). Human spermatozoa invariably live longer in ovulation cervical mucus than in their own seminal fluid. This can be observed in slide cover glass or capillary tube preparations. The cervical mucus components have been shown to have nutritional capacity for a growing embryo. Shettles (1971) fertilised an oocyte in ovulation cervical mucus and incubated the mixture. After 5 days, the oocytes had become a blastocyst.

Cervical immunoglobulins

Cervical mucus contains immunoglobulins that constitute part of the local immune defence mechanism. Cervical immunoglobulins (Ig) are a combination of transudate and local tissue production (Behrman, 1973). IgA is the principal immunoglobulin present within external secretions. Secretory IgA is the product of two distinct cells: plasma cells and epithelial cells. Epithelial cells produce secretory component (SC), which acts as a regulatory transport protein. Labelled amino acids have been incorporated into IgA and IgG in cultured human cervical tissue. More commonly, more IgA than IgG has been found in the culture fluids. Also, IgA- and IgG-producing plasma cells have been demonstrated in biopsied cervical tissue, although the number has varied from one biopsy site to another. Masson and Ferin (1969) showed a relatively higher number of IgA-producing cells. Ovorectomised rats showed that the sex steroids influence total levels of IgA, IgG and SC in the reproductive tract secretions. Administration of estradiol resulted in a decline in the cervical and vaginal content of IgA, IgG and SC. In contrast, estradiol stimulated an increased tissue content of IgA in the uterus and induced an increased production of SC. The addition of progesterone blocked these responses. The opposing effect of estrogen on the secretion of immunoglobulins by the uterus and cervix demonstrates a different response of each compartment of the female reproductive tract to hormonal stimulus.

The levels of IgA and IgG in cervical mucus vary markedly throughout the cycle; the early proliferative phase is markedly characterised by high levels of IgG (100–300 mg/dL) and IgA (20–70 mg/dL). These concentrations decrease markedly at midcycle to approximately 4 mg/dL for IgA and 10 mg/dL for IgG (Schumacher, 1980). Specific antibodies against several microorganisms have been identified in human cervical mucus. Cyclical changes in specific antibody titre in cervical secretions were noted in monkeys experimentally immunised with T4 coliphage (Yang and Schumacher, 1979). The cervix is an organ with a prominent role in local immunity of the female reproductive tract because of its numerous immunoglobulin-producing cells (Brandtzaeg, 1997). The female reproductive tract has multiple defence mechanisms against invading pathogens, including non-specific epithelial and mucosal barriers. Protection at this site involves a unique interaction of secretory IgA, cytokines and reproductive hormones.

As noted above, the female reproductive tract immunity varies with the phase of the reproductive cycle. Both estrogen and progesterone regulate genital tract immunity and potentially affect susceptibility to infection in the female reproductive tract. The presence and stimulatory effects of cytokines on the mucosal immune system have been reported in both human subjects and rodents (Prabhala and Wira, 1991, 1995; Kutteh *et al.*, 1998). Finkelman *et al.* (1990) reported the multiregulatory effects of cytokines such as interleukin 1β (IL-1β), IL-6 and IL-10 in the maturation of B lymphocytes to immunoglobulin-producing plasma cells.

Quantification of immunoglobulins

Kutteh and Franklin (2001), using enzyme-linked immuno-sorbent assay (ELISA), quantified the immunoglobulins and cytokines in human cervical mucus during each trimester of pregnancy. The authors demonstrated that levels of IgG in cervical mucus were greater than levels of IgA during each trimester. Levels of IgA in cervical mucus remained high and constant throughout pregnancy. Peak levels of IgA and IgG during all trimesters of pregnancy significantly exceeded the ovulatory and postovulatory phases of menstrual cycles. They suggested that the enhancement of IgA and IgG in women during pregnancy might be the result of the increased levels of estrogens and progesterones that are produced in large quantities and contribute to the maintenance of the pregnancy. The increased production of these immunological factors may provide for enhanced immunity and improve protection against invading pathogens. An earlier report by the same group (Franklin and Kutteh, 1999) showed that an increase in the concentrations of cervical mucus IgA and IgG correlated with an increase in the progestin component of oral contraceptives. Peak levels of IgA and IgG in cervical mucus from women taking oral contraceptives significantly exceeded the levels in cervical mucus obtained from women during the ovulatory and postovulatory phases of the menstrual cycle. These hormone-dependent changes in immunoglobulin or cytokine levels were attributed to the progestin component of the pills. They proposed that there might be a complex regulatory effect of both estrogens and progestogens on the expression of immunoglobulins in cervical mucus. Increases in IL-1β corresponded in general with increases in IgA. When IL-1β levels were low (< 500 pg/mL), IgG and IgA levels were < 10 mg/dL. As IL-1β levels increased, a correlation was observed with increased levels IgG and IgA levels in cervical mucus during pregnancy and during oral contraceptive use. Additionally, amounts of IL-1β in cervical mucus during pregnancy and oral contraceptive use were approximately 10-fold greater than in the cervical mucus of normally cycling women.

Increased levels of cervical mucus IgA and IgG have been reported in women with gonorrhoea, trichomoniasis, candidosis and herpes genitalis in comparison with a control group of uninfected women (Chipperfield and Evans, 1975). Coughlan and Skinner (1977) reported a similar finding in a similar study. The data indicate a marked enhancement of immune factors in the presence of local disease and suggest the induction of a local immune response.

Other antimicrobial components of cervical mucus

Ascending lower tract infection is well documented as a cause of intrauterine infection with consequences such as preterm labour and delivery and its associated problems of neonatal infection, neonatal death, neurological impairment and developmental delay (Minkoff, 1983; Goldenberg *et al.*, 2000).

Hein and colleagues (2002) analysed the composition and the antimicrobial activity of cervical mucus plugs of pregnant women using Western blot and immunostaining. The cervical mucus plug proved to be a rich source of antimicrobial proteins and peptides, including secretory leucocyte protease inhibitor (SLPI), lysozyme, calprotectin, lactoferrin, the neutrophil defensins (human neutophil peptides 1 to 3; HNP1–3) and the epithelial beta-defensin (human beta-defensin; HBD-1). The same group and Ganz (2001) earlier reported similar findings and antimicrobial activities. The observation by Hein and colleagues of very high concentrations of SLPI in cervical mucus confirmed an earlier report (Helmig *et al.*, 1995) and raised the possibility that SPLI in host defence secretion may protect antimicrobial polypeptides from excessive proteolysis and inactivation by inflammatory proteases. The antimicrobial activity of SLPI has been attributed to lysozymes (Chimura *et al.*, 1993). The concentrations of lysozyme in cervical mucus plugs are about twice as high as in cervical mucus and well within the range of antimicrobial activity (Ellison and Giehl, 1991). Furthermore, Thompson *et al.* (1991) suggested that the leucocytes, mainly neutrophils, play a role in both the cellular defence line of the cervix and the 'selective' mechanisms (phagocytosis of abnormal spermatozoa) of spermatozoa transport through the cervix. Their result corroborates an earlier report by Pandya and Cohen (1985). The authors concluded that seminal leucocytes were not a significant contributor to the elevated levels of leucocytes detected in postinsemination cervical mucus samples and that the leucocytic reaction is a cervical response to semen samples.

Calprotectin is a complex protein with fungistatic activity (Murthy *et al.*, 1993). In general, the constituent antimicrobial polypeptides in cervical mucus plugs are remarkably similar to those of nasal secretion (Cole *et al.*, 1999) except that the concentrations of SLPI and HBD-1 are higher in plugs. This is no surprise if one considers that both cervical mucus plugs and nasal fluid fill spaces that separate the microbe-rich external environment from the sterile interior (the lungs or the uterine cavity). Previous investigators have shown that the substances that are present in nasal fluid interact additively and synergistically to kill microbes (Travis *et al.*, 1999). Therefore, given the similarity of composition, the same would be expected of the cervical mucus plug.

Hein and colleagues (2002) suggested that the physical and biochemical differences between cervical plugs and cervical mucus might reflect an evolutionary requirement for sperm penetration through cervical mucus, a constraint that does not apply to the plugs. The higher concentration of lysozymes in cervical plugs compared with cervical mucus may be due to a higher concentration of one or more antimicrobial proteins in the former material and/or a hormonally induced alteration of the secretions of cervical glands in pregnancy.

Trace elements of cervical mucus

Zinc, copper, iron, manganese and selenium are trace elements that have been identified in the cervical mucus. Their hormone-dependent cyclical variation during different phases of the menstrual cycle has been demonstrated (Hagenfeldt *et al.*, 1973; Pandey *et al.*, 1986). Low levels of copper and iron have been associated with ovulatory cervical mucus (Chowdhury *et al.*, 1981). Zipper and colleagues in 1969 reported excess of copper or ferric ions in ovulatory mucus to be unfavourable for sperm penetration.

Pandey *et al.* (1986) estimated trace elements in cervical mucus of infertile and fertile subjects and reported the concentrations of zinc, copper and iron in the mucus of both groups in the preovulatory, ovulatory and postovulatory phases. The authors found the concentration of these trace elements to be significantly higher than that of manganese and selenium. In both groups, iron ions recorded a marked fall from preovulatory to ovulatory to postovulatory phases, while copper levels at ovulatory and postovulatory phases were either higher or lower than in the preovulatory phase. In contrast, manganese levels exhibited a rise from preovulatory to ovulatory and postovulatory phases. In both primary and secondary infertility, copper, iron and selenium levels in the cervical mucus were elevated compared with levels in fertile women. Zinc content was reduced, while the manganese level remained unaltered. The authors surmised that a certain concentration of these essential elements in cervical mucus was critical for normal fertility. The spermatotoxic effect and altered cervical mucus receptivity of copper have been shown by various investigators (Elstein and Ferrer, 1973; Randic *et al.*, 1973).

Cyclical hormonal variations in concentrations of sodium and chloride ions have been shown, reaching peak level at the immediate preovulatory period. The level of sodium decreased in the presence of progestogen. Potassium ions did not show this cyclical variation (Lieberman, 1966; Kopito *et al.*, 1973).

Other constituents of human cervical mucus

Human cervical mucus lipids contain 10.5% free fatty acids in an entire pooled cycle. Cyclical variation in amount has been a notable observation resulting from hormonal influence at different phases of the cycle. The levels rise in the estrogenic phase and fall in the progestogenic phase. The most abundant fatty acids are myristic, palmitic, stearic, oleic and linoleic. The use of the oral contraceptive pill alters the composition of free fatty acids, which become more saturated, but the change in total amount is minimal (Singh and Swartwout, 1973).

Cervical mucus contains prostaglandins (PGE_1, PGE_2, PGD_2, $PGF_{1\alpha}$ and $PGF_{2\alpha}$). The prostaglandin content increases in the preovulatory mucus. The source of the PG is thought to be the secretory cells of the crypts. The biological importance of cervical mucus PG has been attributed to an increase in motility, drive and spermatozoa penetration, the maintenance of a continued milieu of a PG-rich environment, the seminal plasma, leading to another PG-rich environment, the cervical mucus. These are all effects that could provide better fertility (Charbonnel *et al.*, 1982).

Various enzymes have been identified in human cervical mucus, while cervical amylase has been shown to be elevated in the secretory phase (Gregoire *et al.*, 1967). The acid and alkaline phosphatase activities do not exhibit cyclic changes in natural cycles, but administration of progestogen significantly increases enzyme activity (Gregoire *et al.*, 1972). Also, peroxidase profiles have been suggested as markers for a woman's fertile period (Tsibris *et al.*, 1989).

Beller and Weiss (1966) revealed a fibrinolytic enzyme system in human cervical mucus. The activator of the system appeared to have an inverse relationship to the activity of endogenous estrogen, being lowest at midcycle and highest before and after menstruation.

In conclusion, cervical mucus contains approximately 90% water. Depending on the water content, which varies during the menstrual cycle, the mucus functions as a barrier or a transport medium to spermatozoa. The macromolecular glycoprotein component (mucin) that is responsible for its unique characteristics varies in concentration during the phases of the menstrual cycle, being lowest at the fertile period (the midcycle). The disulphide bridges of the mucin network are fragile, rendering the cervical mucus less viscous. The presence of highly charged negative groups on the oligosaccharide sidechains of the glycoprotein molecules has been linked with the structural integrity of cervical mucin. The levels of cervical proteins vary during the menstrual cycle, being lowest at ovulation. There is an inverse relationship between protein concentration in the mucus and its ability to support sperm migration. Cervical mucus provides local immunity through a unique interaction of the immunoglobulins, cytokines and reproductive hormones. The prostaglandins and the trace elements also show hormone-dependent cyclical variations. Raised levels of copper, iron and selenium have been associated with primary and secondary infertility.

THE PHYSICS OF HUMAN CERVICAL MUCUS

The physics of cervical mucus relates to the forces within the structural framework and their relationship to sperm migration and infertility.

Cervical mucus intermolecular forces

In mammals, if a spermatozoon is to fertilise an ovum, it must leave the semen and enter into the cervical mucus. The force that separates two different fluids is an interfacial one, known as the surface tension. The surface tension of human cervical mucus was found by Lippes and Hurwitz (1965) to change with the phases of the menstrual cycle. In their study of 70 cervical specimens from healthy volunteers, they demonstrated that the lowest surface tension index (STI) value occurred prior to ovulation. A steep rise in STI occurred with or immediately after ovulation, coincidentally with the progesterone-induced thermogenic shift. Also, in women of high parity, STI rose to higher values post ovulation than were seen in the general series. This suggests that these cyclical variations in surface tension are under hormonal influence. Their biological significance is probably to favour (or deter) sperm migrations at different times of the menstrual cycle.

As mentioned earlier, cervical mucus is a hydrogel composed of a high-molecular-weight component (gel phase) and a low-molecular-weight component (cervical plasma). NMR has been used extensively to investigate the protons of the aqueous phase of cervical mucus. Investigations by Odeblad spanned over a decade (1959a–c, 1963, 1966a,b, 1968a–d, 1969, 1972; Odeblad and Rudolfsson-Asberg, 1973). In these studies, NMR permitted the study of proton mobility, bonding in water and binding of water molecules to the macromolecular system in cervical mucus. NMR implies radiofrequency (RF) absorption in atomic nuclei (here protons) in a homogeneous magnetic field. The magnetic fields used were 6900, 11 000 or 37 000 G, corresponding to frequencies 28.9, 47.1 or 157 MHz, supplied to a detector coil surrounding the sample. In these studies, the proton relaxation rate R (the inverse of T1, i.e. the interaction time for proton spins with the molecular surroundings or lattice) was determined among other variables. Highly mobile protons are present in free water and, as a result, the interaction between spin and lattice is small and R is small (about 0.33 per second). Water tied up by macromolecules had reduced average proton mobility, which implied that each proton was exposed to the surrounding for a longer time, the interaction became stronger and R became larger (30 per second for albumin, 40 per second for estrogenic cervical mucin and 85 per second for gestagenic mucin. On average, type E (estrogenic) mucus has a proton NMR relaxation rate of 1.1 per second and contains 97% water. The water contributes approximately $0.97 \times 0.3 = 0.3$ per second to the relaxation rate. The water bound to albumin (0.5%) contributes $30 \times 0.005 = 0.15$ per second to the relaxation rate. As hydrated water or NaCl (sodium chloride) does not differ significantly from free water as regards relaxation rate, the remaining 0.55 per second must be due to water hydrated on mucins. This typically has a relaxation rate of 40 per second for bound protons. Thus, approxim-

ately 0.014 or 1.4% of the water is hydrated to a mucin (1.3%). The gel therefore binds 1.4/1.3 = 108%, mainly by hydrogen bonding, as indicated by the negative shift of the proton NMR signal.

In the viscous type G mucus, characteristic of the progestational phase, there is much more organic material capable of binding water, and the micelles are split into a dense network with an extensive surface exposed to and tying up water molecules. On average, the type G mucus has a relaxation rate of 12 per second and contains 89% water, contributing $0.89 \times 0.2 = 0.27$ per second to relaxation rate. Albumin (2.5%) contributes $30 \times 0.025 = 0.75$ per second. The remainder, 10.98 per second, must be contributed to the mucin mainly by water. This typically has a relaxation time of 85 per second for absorbed water. Thus, 13% is hydrated, or the degree of hydration is 13/7.5 = 185%, and is bound mainly by dipole bonding, as indicated by the positive NMR shift. The intermesh spaces are of the non-oriented type. The proton spin can be either parallel or antiparallel to the magnetic field, and there is normally a small excess of protons with parallel spins. The proton magnetic signal is due to this small excess. The excess (and thus the NMR signal) can be removed if a strong pulse of RF radiation is imposed on the samples (saturation). After saturation, the excess gradually reappears, and the signal grows with rate R. The study of signal regrowth after saturation therefore allows direct visualisation of proton relaxation. Different cervical mucus types would have different relaxation rates when subjected to this experiment. A less laborious and more rapid method of relaxation devised later required the use of simple equipment called a marginal oscillator to determine the average proton relaxation rate. This average rate permits approximate evaluation of the relative proportions of type E and type G secretions in the cervical mucus.

The biologically significant information comes from the fact that the measured R is a sum of partial rates:

$$R = \Sigma_n \, p_n R_n$$

where p_n is the fraction of water of the inherent relaxation rate R_n.

Sheehan and Carlstedt (1982) studied the speed-dependent sedimentation velocity of human cervical mucus in the analytical ultracentrifuge. This was an attempt to study the size heterogeneity and polydispersity (the sedimentation behaviour) of large mucin molecules at different rotor speeds of an analytical ultracentrifuge. The following were the three observations from the experimental results: (1) boundary broadening occurred to such a degree that the boundary could not be monitored for more than 80–90 minutes; (2) a perturbed baseline appeared behind the sedimenting boundary; and (3) there was a loss of material that could not be accounted for by radial dilution. The boundary broadening did not appear to be consistent with the high molecular weight of the molecules. Similar findings have been reported for very large DNA molecules (Aten and Cohen, 1965; Schumaker and Zimm, 1973), and this prompted the investigation of the sedimentation rate as a function of rotor speed. Sheehan and Carlstedt (1982) concluded that the experimental observations might be explained by speed-dependent aggregation as noted for DNA (i.e. clusters of molecules sediment ahead of the boundary) and a rate-dependent sticking of the mucin molecules to the surface of the centrifuge cell. They also suggested that the transition from a slow to a fast sedimentation rate depended on the velocity of the boundary.

In conclusion, the cervical mucus surface tension index shows hormone-dependent cyclical variation, being lowest during the fertile period (at ovulation) when cervical mucus is most receptive to sperm migration through the cervix. Proton relaxation rate as determined by the NMR method permits approximate evaluation of the relative proportions of type E and type G secretions in the cervical mucus. Also, the sedimentation behaviour of cervical mucus correlates with the rate of aggregation of the molecules and the rate-dependent sticking of the mucin molecules on the surface of the centrifuge cell.

ACKNOWLEDGEMENT

Figures 11.2, 11.3 and 11.4 are from Singer A., Monaghan J.M. (2000) *Lower Genital Tract Precancer*, 2nd edn, Oxford: Blackwell Science, with thanks.

REFERENCES

Adam M, Delsanti M (1977a) Photon beat study of internal modes in large polymer coils. *Journal of Physical Letters* 38: 271–277.

Adam M, Delsanti M (1977b) Dynamic properties of polymer solutions in good solvent by Rayleigh scattering experiments. *Macromolecules* 10: 1229–1232.

Aten JBT, Cohen JA (1965) Sedimentation viscosity studies of high molecular weight DNA. *Journal of Molecular Biology* 12: 537–548.

Beeson MF, Parish GR, James SL *et al.* (1982) A scanning electron microscopic study of human cervical mucus. *Advances in Experimental Medicine and Biology* 144: 293–296.

Behrman SJ (1973). Biosynthesis of immunoglobulins by the cervix. In: Blandau RJ, Moghissi KS (eds) *The Biology of the Cervix*. Chicago: University of Chicago Press, Ch. 12, pp. 237–249.

Beller FK, Weiss G (1966) The fibrinolytic enzyme system in cervical mucus. *Fertility and Sterility* 17: 655–662.

Brandtzaeg P (1997) Mucosal immunity in the female genital tract. *Journal of Reproductive Immunology* 36: 23–50.

Charbonnel B, Kremer M, Gerozissis K *et al.* (1982) Human cervical mucus contains a large amount of prostaglandins. *Fertility and Sterility* 38: 109–111.

Chantler E (1982) Structure and function of cervical mucus. In: Chantler E, Elder JB, Elstein M (eds) *Mucus in Health and Disease*, Vol. 144. New York: Plenum, pp. 251–263.

Chimura T, Hirayama T, Takase M (1993) Lysozymes in cervical mucus of patients with chorioamnionitis. *Japanese Journal of Antibiotics* 46: 726–729.

Chipperfield EJ, Evans BA (1975) Effects of local infection and oral contraceptives on immunoglobulin levels in cervical mucus. *Infection and Immunity* 11: 215–221.

Chowdhury AR, Singh S, Kutty D *et al.* (1981) Metallic ions in cervical mucus. *Indian Journal of Medical Research* 73: 277–279.

Chrétien FC, David G (1978) The ultrastructure of human cervical mucus under scanning electron microscopy study. *European Journal of Obstetrics, Gynecology and Reproductive Biology* 816: 307–316.

Chrétien FC, Psychoyos A (1975) Temporary obstructive effect of human cervical mucus on spermatozoa throughout reproductive life: a scanning electron microscopy study. *Proceedings of the Polish Gynecology Society*.

Chrétien FC, Cohen J, Psychoyos A (1976) Préparation du mucus cervical à l'observation au microscope électronique à balayage. *Journal of Gynecology, Obstetrics and the Biology of Reproduction* 5: 313–330.

Cole AM, Dewan P, Ganz T (1999) Innate antimicrobial activity of nasal secretions. *Infection and Immunity* 67: 3267–3275.

Coughlan BM, Skinner GA (1977) Immunoglobulin concentrations in cervical mucus in patients with normal and abnormal cervical cytology. *British Journal of Obstetrics and Gynaecology* 84: 129–134.

Daunter B, Chantler EN, Elstein M (1977) Trace metals (Cu, Mn, Zn, Fe), sulphydryl and disulphide groups of cervical mucus. *Contraception* 15: 543–552.

De Gennes PG (1976) Dynamics of single polymer chain. *Macromolecules* 9: 587–596.

Ellison RT, Giehl TJ (1991) Killing of gram-negative bacteria by lactoferrin and lysozyme. *Journal of Clinical Investigation* 88: 1080–1091.

Elstein M, Ferrer K (1973) The effect of a copper-releasing intrauterine device on sperm penetration in human cervical mucus in vitro. *Journal of Reproductive Fertility* 32: 1109–1111.

Finkelman FD, Holmes J, Katona IM *et al.* (1990). Lymphokine control of in vivo immunoglobulin isotype selection. *Annual Review of Immunology* 8: 3030–3033.

Fleetwood L, Landgren B, Eneroth P (1986) Quantification of human cervical mucin during consecutive days and hourly during one day at mid-cycle. *Gynecological and Obstetric Investigations* 22: 145–152.

Franklin RD, Kutteh WH (1999) Characterisation of immunoglobulins and cytokines in human cervical mucus: influence of exogenous and endogenous hormones. *Journal of Reproductive Immunology* 42: 93–106.

Ganz T (2001) Antimicrobial proteins and peptides in host defense. *Seminars in Respiratory Infection* 16: 4–10.

Gibbons RA, Selwood R (1973) The macromolecular biochemistry of cervical secretions. In: Blandau RJ, Moghissi KS (eds) *The Biology of the Cervix*. Chicago: University of Chicago Press.

Goldenberg RL, Hauth JC, Andrews WW (2000) Intrauterine infection and preterm delivery. *New England Journal of Medicine* 342: 1500–1507.

Gould KG, Martin DE, Graham CE (1976) *Scanning Electron Microscope of Human Cervical Mucus*. Proceedings of a Workshop on Scanning Electron Microscopy in Reproductive Biology. Chicago, IL: ITT Research Institute.

Gregoire AT, Rankin J, Johnson W *et al.* (1967) Alpha-amylase content in cervical mucus of females receiving sequential, nonsequential, or no contraceptive therapy. *Fertility and Sterility* 18: 836.

Gregoire AT, Kandil O, Beyers G (1972) The acid and alkaline phosphatase activity in human cervical mucus of females using either a coil or combined hormone contraceptive therapy. *Fertility and Sterility* 23 (1): 15–17.

Guslandi M (1981) Sialic acid and mucus rheology. *Clinica et Chemica Acta* 117: 3–5.

Hagenfeldt K, Plantin LO, Diczfalusy E (1973) Trace elements in the human endometrium: zinc, copper and manganese levels in the endometrium, cervical mucus and plasma. *Acta Endocrinologia* 72: 115–126.

Hatcher VB, Schwarzmann OH, Jeanloz RW *et al.* (1977) Purification, properties and partial structure elucidation of a high-molecular-weight glycoprotein from cervical mucus of the bonnet monkey (*Macaca radiata*). *Biochemistry* 16: 1515–1524.

Hein M, Helmig RB, Schonheyder HC *et al.* (2001) An in vivo study of antibacterial properties of cervical mucus plug in pregnancy. *American Journal of Obstetrics and Gynecology* 185: 586–592.

Helmig R, Uldbjerg N, Ohlsson K (1995) Secretory leucocyte protease inhibitor in the cervical mucus and fetal membranes. *European Journal of Obstetrics, Gynecology and Reproductive Biology* 58: 95–101.

Kopito LE, Kosasky HJ, Sturgis SH *et al.*(1973) Effect of chlormadione acetate on water and sodium in cervical mucus. *International Journal of Fertility* 18: 174–176.

Kutteh WH, Moldoveanu Z, Mesteckky J (1998) Mucosa immunity in the female reproductive tract: correlations of immunoglobulins, cytokines, and reproductive hormones in human cervical mucus around the time of ovulation. *AIDS Research in Human Retroviruses* 14 (Suppl. 1): S51–5.

Kutteh WH, Franklin RD (2001) Quantification of immunoglobulins and cytokines in human cervical mucus during each trimester of pregnancy. *American Journal of Obstetrics and Gynecology* 5: 865–874.

Lee WI, Verdugo P, Blandan RJ *et al.*(1997) Molecular arrangement of cervical mucus: a re-evaluation based on laser light-scattering spectroscopy. *Gynecological Investigations* 8: 154–166.

Lieberman BL (1966) Quantitative determinations of anions and cations in cervical mucus. *Surgical Forum* 17: 395–396.

Lippes J, Hurwitz L (1965) The dilution effect on surface tension of cervical mucus and its variability with the menstrual cycle. *Fertility and Sterility* 16: 722–726.

Litt M, Khan MA, Wolf DP (1976) Mucus rheology: relation to structure and function. *Biorheology* 13: 37–48.

Masson PL, Ferin J (1969) Protein constituents of cervical mucus. *Gynecologie et Obstetrique* 68: 419–432.

Meyer FA, King M, Gelman R (1975) On the role of sialic acid in the rheological properties of mucus. *Biochimica et Biophysica Acta* 392: 223–232.

Minkoff H (1983) Prematurity: infection as an etiologic factor. *Obstetrics and Gynecology* 62: 137–144.

Moghissi KS (1966a) Cyclic changes in cervical mucus in normal and progestin-treated women. *Fertility and Sterility* 17: 663–675.

Moghissi KS (1966b) Cyclic changes of cervical mucus proteins. *International Journal of Fertility* 11: 284–286.

Moghissi KS (1972) The function of the cervix in fertility. *Fertility and Sterility* 23: 295–306.

Moghissi KS, Neuhaus OW, Stevenson CS (1960) Composition and properties of human cervical mucus: electrophoretic separation and identification of proteins. *Journal of Clinical Investigation* 39: 1358–1363.

Moghissi K, Neuhaus OW (1962) Composition and properties of human cervical mucus. Immunoelectrophoretic studies of the proteins. *American Journal of Obstetrics and Gynecology* 83: 149.

Moghissi K, Neuhaus OW (1966) Cyclical changes of cervical mucus proteins. *American Journal of Obstetrics and Gynecology* 9: 91–95.

Moghissi KS, Syner FN (1976) Cyclic changes in the amount and sialic acid of cervical mucus. *International Journal of Fertility* 21: 246–250.

Moghissi K, Neuhaus OW, Stevenson CS (1962) Composition and properties of human cervical mucus. Electrophoretic separation and identification of proteins. *American Journal of Obstetrics and Gynecology* 89: 1358.

Morales P, Roco M, Vigil P (1993) Human cervical mucus: relationship between biochemical characteristics and ability to allow migration of spermatozoa. *Human Reproduction* 8: 78–83.

Murthy AR, Lehrer RI, Harwig ST *et al.* (1993) In vitro candidastic properties of the human neutrophil calprotectin complex. *Journal of Immunology* 151: 6291–6301.

Neuhaus OW, Moghissi KS (1962) Composition and properties of cervical mucus. A preliminary study of the mucus component. *Fertility and Sterility* 13: 550.

Odeblad E. (1959a) The physics of cervical mucus. *Acta Obstetrica et Gynecologica Scandinavica* 38 (Suppl. 1): 44–58.

Odeblad E (1959b) In general discussion to conference on the cervix. *Acta Obstetrica et Gynecologica Scandinavica* 38 (Suppl. 1): 126–127.

Odeblad E (1959c) Research in obstetrics and gynaecology with nuclear magnetic resonance. *Acta Obstetrica et Gynecologica Scandinavica* 38: 599–617.

Odeblad E (1963) Studies of the molecular structure and function of human cervical mucus. *Journal of the Japanese Obstetrical and Gynaecological Society* 10: 273.

Odeblad E (1966a) Micro-NMR in high permanent magnetic fields. Theoretical and experimental investigations with application to the secretions from single glandular units in the human uterus cervix. *Acta Obstetrica et Gynecologica Scandinavica* 45 (Suppl. 2).

Odeblad E (1966b) Micro-NMR in high permanent magnetic fields. *Acta Obstetrica et Gynecologica Scandinavica* 45: 139–154.

Odeblad E (1968a) The functional structure of human cervical mucus. *Acta Obstetrica et Gynecologica Scandinavica* 47 (Suppl. 1): 59–79.

Odeblad E (1968b) An NMR method for the determination of ovulation. *Acta Obstetrica et Gynecologica Scandinavica* 47 (Suppl. 1): 39–47.

Odeblad E (1968c) Biophysical composition of cervical mucus and sperm migration during treatment with Conluten and Conlunett. *Acta Obstetrica et Gynecologica Scandinavica* 47: 7–19.

Odeblad E (1969) Types of human cervical secretions. *Acta Europea Fertilitatis* 1: 99–116.

Odeblad E (1972) Biophysical techniques of assessing cervical mucus and microstructure of cervical epithelium. In: *Cervical Mucus in Human Reproduction*. Geneva: World Health Organization Colloquium, pp. 58–74. Copenhagen: Scriptor.

Odeblad E (1976) The biophysical aspects of cervical mucus. In: Jordan J, Singer A (eds) *The Cervix*, 1st edn. London: Saunders, pp. 156–163.

Odeblad E, Rudolfsson-Asberg C (1973) Types of cervical secretions: biophysical characteristics. In: Blandau RA (ed.) *The Biology of the Cervix*. Chicago: University of Chicago Press, pp. 267–283.

Pandey S, Chuwdhury AR, Tewari SR *et al.* (1986) Trace elements in cervical mucus of infertile women. *Indian Journal of Medical Research* 84: 163–166.

Pandya IJ, Cohen J (1985) The leucocytic reaction of the human uterine cervix. *Journal of Reproductive Fertility* Abstract series 5: No. 12.

Parish GR, Beeson MF, Brown DT *et al.* (1982) A freezing artefact associated with the preparation of mucin for examination using the scanning electron microscope. *Advances in Experimental Medicine and Biology* 144: 297–300.

Pigman W, Horton D (1970) *The Carbohydrates*, Vol. 2B. London: Academic Press.

Pommerenke WT (1946) Cyclic changes in the physical and chemical properties of cervical mucus. *American Journal of Obstetrics and Gynecology* 52: 1023.

Prabhala RH, Wira CR (1991) Cytokine regulation of the mucosal immune system: in vivo stimulation by gamma-interferon of secretory component and immunoglobulin A in uterine secretions and proliferation of lymphocytes from spleen. *Endocrinology* 129: 15–23.

Prabhala RH, Wira CR (1995) Sex hormone and IL-6 regulation or antigen presentation in the female reproductive tract mucosal tissues. *Journal of Immunology* 155: 56–73.

Randic L, Musacchio I, Epstein JA (1973) Copper level in cervical mucus of women with copper-bearing and non-copper-bearing intrauterine devices. *Biology of Reproduction* 8: 499–503.

Rohr G, Eggert-Kruise W, Pehlke A *et al.* (1992) Biochemical analysis of cervical mucus by nuclear magnetic resonance spectroscopy. *Human Reproduction* 7: 915–917.

Sahrbacher U, Pehlke-Rimpf A, Rohr G *et al.* (2002) High resolution proton magnetic resonance spectroscopy of human cervical mucus. *Journal of Pharmacology and Biomedical Analysis* 28: 827–840.

Schumacher GFB (1970) Biochemistry of cervical mucus. *Fertility and Sterility* 21: 697–705.

Schumacher GFB (1977) The uterine cervix. In: *Reproduction*. Stuttgart: Georg Thieme, pp. 101–107.

Schumacher GFB (1980) Humoral immune factors in the female reproductive tract and their changes during the cycle. In: Dhindsa D, Schumacher GFB (eds) *Immunological Aspects of Infertility and Fertility Regulation*. New York: Elsevier, pp. 903–912.

Schumaker VN, Zimm BH (1973) Anomalies in sedimentation II. Testing the enlargement hypothesis. *Biopolymers* 12: 869–876.

Sheehan J, Carlstedt I (1982) Speed-dependent sedimentation-velocity of human cervical mucus in the analytical ultracentrifuge. *Advances in Experimental Medicine and Biology* 144: 277–279.

Shettles LB (1971) Human blastocyst grown in vitro in ovulation cervical mucus. *Nature* 229: 343.

Singer A, Reid BL (1970) The ultrastructure of cervical mucus. *Journal of Reproductive Fertility* 21: 377.

Singh EJ, Swartwout JR (1973) Effects of oral contraceptives on free fatty acids of human cervical mucus. *Obstetrics and Gynaecology* 41 (5): 743–747.

Spencer B, Sunseri LZ, Sunseri SG (1957) Electrophoretic examination of human cervical mucus from normal, pregnant and carcinomatous patients. *Clinica et Chimica Acta* 2: 485.

Stevens A, Lowe J (1997) *Human Histology*, 2nd edn. London: Mosby.

Takano N, Maekawa I, Takamizawa H (1979) The ultrastructure of human cervical mucus observed by cryo-scanning electron microscopy. *Fertlility and Sterility* 32 (5): 604–607.

Thompson LA, Tomlinson MJ, Barratt CLR *et al.* (1991) Positive immunoselection. A method of isolating leucocytes from leukocytic reacted human cervical mucus samples. *American Journal of Reproductive Immunology* 26: 58–61.

Travis SM, Conway BA, Zabner J *et al.* (1999) Activity of abundant antimicrobials of the human airway. *American Journal of Respiratory Cell and Molecular Biology* 20: 872–879.

Tsibris JCM, Lewis V, Langenberg PW *et al.* (1989) Cervical mucus enzymes as markers for the woman's fertile period. *International Journal of Gynecology and Obstetrics* Suppl. 1: 73–82.

Van Kooij RJ, Roelofs HJ, Kathmann GA *et al.* (1980) Human cervical mucus and its mucous glycoproteins during the menstrual cycle. *Fertility and Sterility* 34: 226–233.

Volochine B, Cazabat AM, Chretien FC *et al.* (1988) Structure of human cervical mucus from light scattering measurements. *Human Reproduction* 3: 577–582.

Von Kaulla KN, Aikawa JK, Burns PD *et al.* (1957) Secretory function of the human uterine cervix; studies with radioisotopes. *Fertility and Sterility* 8: 444–454.

Werner I (1953) Studies on glycoproteins from mucus epithelium and epithelia secretions. *Acta Societa Medica Upsaliensis* 58: 1.

Wolf DP, Blasco L, Khan MA (1977) Human cervical mucus: changes in viscoelasticity during the ovulatory menstrual cycle. *Fertility and Sterility* 28: 47–52.

Yang SL, Schumacher GFB (1979) Immune response after vaginal application of antigens in the rhesus monkeys. *Fertility and Sterility* 32: 588–598.

Zeneveld DVM, Tauber RF, Port C *et al.* (1975) Structural aspects of human cervical mucus. *American Journal of Obstetrics and Gynecology* 122: 650–654.

CHAPTER 12

Sperm transport in the human and mammalian cervix and genital tract: its relation to fertility

Anne M. Jequier

The cervix is the first organ to meet the sperm after ejaculation and thus plays an important role in fertility. It is the port of entry for the sperm into the female genital tract and thus can be the site of problems that result in infertility.

The cervix is situated high in the vagina and is angled on the anteverted uterus so that the external os faces downwards and forwards and indents the anterior wall of the vagina. During intercourse, however, the vagina is distended by the penis and loses contact with the anterior vaginal wall. This will ensure that the external os achieves maximal possible contact with the external penile meatus and the ejaculate that issues from it. When the uterus is retroverted, the cervix lies up in the anterior fornix while the semen will be deposited in the posterior fornix. Thus, marked retroversion, particularly when also associated with severe retroflexion, can occasionally result in infertility.

In the following review, it has been necessary to incorporate some concepts not directly related to the cervix, especially those in respect of seminal fluid, passage of sperm through the uterus and fallopian tube and the actual process of fertilisation and the mechanisms immediately preceding this event. However, the cervix plays a critical role in fertility, especially in respect of capacitation and, in order to understand this pivotal function in fertility, it is important to understand the concepts and mechanisms than are indirectly responsible for maintaining fertility.

THE SECRETIONS THAT MAKE UP THE EJACULATE

Seminal fluid is a grey opalescent and somewhat turbid fluid. The turbidity is largely due to the presence of the spermatozoa and other cellular components in the fluid, and the opalescence results from its high protein content. The protein in the semen acts as a buffer that helps to protect the spermatozoa from the acidity of the vagina as the pH of the vaginal secretions can be as low as 3.5 or 4 around the time of ovulation.

The seminal fluid that makes up the ejaculate arises from five different sources (Lundquist, 1949), and their volumetric

Table 12.1 The percentage contributions that make up seminal fluid.

Sources of semen	Percentage of ejaculate
Testes and their excurrent ducts	5
Seminal vesicles	46–80
Prostate gland	13–33
Bulbo-urethral and urethral glands	2–5

Source: Lundquist (1949).

contribution to the ejaculate as well as their chemical content vary greatly (Table 12.1).

The testicular contribution

The testes are made up of the seminiferous tubules around which lie the Leydig cells. The seminiferous tubules are lined by an epithelium formed by Sertoli cells between which lie the developing sperm. Close to the base are the spermatogonia that form firstly primary and then secondary spermatocytes. Meiotic division and spermatogenesis are completed with the formation of the spermatids. These haploid cells then develop into spermatozoa in a process called spermiogenesis, and these leave the epithelium to enter the lumen of the seminiferous tubule in a process known as spermiation. Around each tubule are clusters of Leydig cells that are the main source of testosterone that is essential for normal testicular function. The contents of each testis are contained within a thick, non-distensible fibrous sac known as the tunica albuginea (Fig. 12.1).

While still within the testes, the spermatozoa pass out of the seminiferous tubule into a network of channels known as the rete testis and then exit the testis by means of 10–15 efferent ductules. These ductules then join together to form the epididymal duct, which is convoluted and is some 6 metres in length.

The testicular component of the ejaculate is the most important when considering fertility as it is this component that contains the spermatozoa. However, the testicular secretions

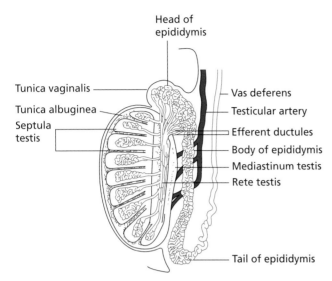

Fig. 12.1 A diagrammatic representation of the testis and its excurrent ducts.

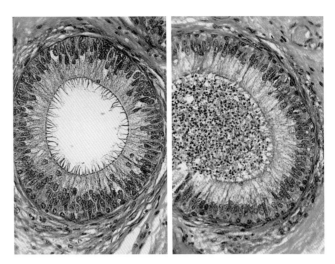

Fig. 12.2 Histological sections of the epididymal duct in the caput (left) and cauda (right) of the epididymis. Owing to the spontaneous activity of the myocytes in the wall of the duct, few sperm are seen in the caput. In the cauda, there is storage of sperm as the contractile activity of this section of the duct is confined to emission and ejaculation.

make up only around 5% of the total ejaculatory volume. Thus, men who have undergone a vasectomy notice no change in their semen volume.

The fluid that emerges from the testis is known as rete testis fluid and contains the spermatozoa. In its passage through the efferent ductules, water is absorbed from this fluid and, thus, the sperm suspension becomes concentrated. In their passage down the epididymal duct, the sperm acquire motility. On their arrival in the epididymal cauda, the sperm are stored in the cauda of the epididymis until ejaculation (Fig. 12.2).

The sperm bring with them a number of different substances that are important to their function and which can be used diagnostically. The three main substances that are produced by the testes are inhibin B, testosterone and transferrin.

Inhibin B is produced by the Sertoli cells and is the main negative feedback for follicle-stimulating hormone (FSH). It is present in semen, where it falls to undetectable levels in men with obstructive lesions of the excurrent ducts or in whom there is testicular atrophy (Anderson, 2001).

Testosterone is present in semen in both the free and the bound form and is the source of testosterone for the normal function of the excurrent ducts.

The iron-carrying protein, transferrin, is also produced by the Sertoli cells. Its function in semen is unclear, but it is thought to be important in maintaining the integrity of the sperm cell membrane (Fuse *et al.*, 1994). Similarly, the copper-carrying protein, ceruloplasmin, is also produced by the Sertoli cells, but its function in semen remains unclear.

The sugar inositol is concentrated by the epididymal duct and its function is unknown. Both L-carnitine and glycerophosphorylcholine are also found in epididymal secretions and are probably an energy source for the spermatozoa.

The secretions of the seminal vesicles

After leaving the epididymal duct, this component of the semen passes into the vasa deferentia and is propelled up each vas by muscular contraction to be stored in the ampulla of each vas. The ampulla of each vas joins with the duct of the seminal vesical to form the ejaculatory ducts (Fig. 12.3).

The seminal vesicles are situated at the back of the bladder and lie inferiorly to the ampulla of the vasa deferentia (Fig. 12.3). Volumetrically, this is the largest of the contributions that make up the seminal fluid as these secretions form around 60% of the total ejaculatory volume. The seminal vesicular secretions contain the sugar fructose, which is an important energy source for the spermatozoa.

The seminal vesicles are also a major source of prostaglandins, which are mainly of the PGE and 19-OH PGE groups. The role of these prostaglandins is uncertain: they were at one time thought to enhance sperm motility but this has recently been disproved (Hellstrom *et al.*, 1998). They are now believed to promote the calcium influx that triggers the acrosome reaction (Shimizu *et al.*, 1998).

The seminal vesicles also secrete a substance that has been called semengelin or Sg1 (Roberts and Gagnon, 1999), which is acted upon by the prostatic enzyme vesiculase to induce the clotting of the semen that occurs at ejaculation.

The prostatic secretion

The prostatic contribution to the semen makes up some 30% of the total ejaculate and is biochemically very active. This emerges into the urethra by a series of ducts that drain each area of the prostate gland (Fig. 12.4).

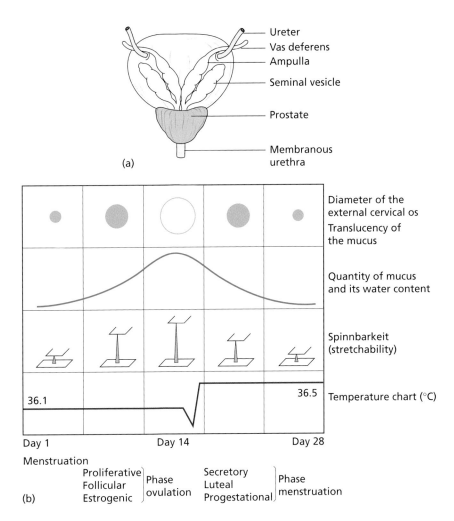

Fig. 12.3 (a) Diagrammatic representation of the seminal vesicles at the back of the bladder. (b) Changes in the cervix and its mucus during the menstrual cycle.

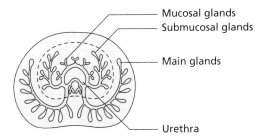

Fig. 12.4 Diagram showing the arrangement of the ducts that drain the secretions of the prostate gland into the prostatic urethra.

The contribution from the prostate also contains the enzyme prostatic acid phosphatase (PAP) as well as prostate-specific antigen (PSA), both of which are used in forensic science for the identification of seminal fluid.

Citric acid is also present in this contribution to the semen and reduces the pH of the semen to within the acid range. The role of the citric acid in semen is unclear, but it may act by chelating calcium ions and thus inhibiting any premature triggering of the acrosome reaction (Ford and Harrison, 1984).

The prostatic fluid also contains a large number of proteases and peptidases that break down the clot induced by vesiculase. Thus, the seminal vesicular secretions induce clotting, and the prostatic secretions lyse the clotted semen. The prostatic secretions also contain a bacteristatic amine called spermine, which can precipitate out in semen as crystals of spermine phosphate. This part of the ejaculate also contains substances such as acid phosphatase and citrates.

Zinc and magnesium are also present in reasonable concentrations, but their exact function is not known although zinc is believed to act by stabilising the condensed chromatin in the sperm head (Kvist *et al.*, 1990).

Bulbo-urethral and urethral glands

These secretions form a very small proportion of the ejaculate and are made up almost solely of mucus. The bulbo-urethral glands open into the membranous urethra and the urethral glands into the lacuna close to the external meatus of the penis. These secretions are merely lubricants and usually have no real pathological significance. However, they can at times be the source of anti-sperm antibodies in the semen.

ERECTION: EJACULATION AND EMISSION

Erection

The penis is made up of two parts, namely the root of the penis, which is contained within the perineum, and the main body of the penis, which is free from the perineum and is entirely covered by skin.

The penis is made up of three bodies of erectile tissue. Within the root of the penis, the two lateral erectile bodies known as the crura are firmly adherent to the ischiopubic ramus of the pelvis while, between them, on the undersurface of the perineal triangle lies the third erectile body known as the bulb of the penis (Fig. 12.5). Each crus is covered by the ischiocavernosus muscle while the bulbocavernosus muscle covers the bulb.

The two crura pass forwards into the main body of the penis as the corpora cavernosa. The bulb also extends forwards to become the corpus spongiosum and expands at the end of the penis into the glans penis. The erectile bodies are held together by a dense fibrous tunica albuginea, the corpus spongiosum lying in the groove beneath the two corpora cavernosa

(Fig. 12.5). The urethra perforates the corpus spongiosum and is contained within it down the main body of the penis.

Each erectile body is made up of smooth muscle arranged to surround the cavernous spaces and lined by a flat epithelium. When the penis is in a flaccid state, this smooth muscle is contracted and the cavernous spaces are relatively small.

The blood supply of the penis is by means of the dorsal arteries of the penis, which arise from the pudendal arteries within the pelvis. Branches of these arteries perforate the erectile tissue down its length. The venous drainage of the erectile tissue is by means of small veins that emerge tangentially through the tunica albuginea to drain into the deep and the superficial veins of the penis.

The nerve supply of the penis involves the sacral segments S2, S3 and S4 by means of the pudendal nerve and the sacral plexus. They contain a large parasympathetic element, and it is these nerves that are important in the generation of an erection (Fig. 12.6).

The initiation of erection occurs as the result of visual, tactile and also probably olfactory stimuli. As the result of these stimuli, there is a massive increase in the arterial blood flow into the erectile tissue by means of the dorsal arteries to the penis. At the same time, the smooth muscle in the erectile tissue undergoes relaxation and the now large cavernous spaces fill with blood. Venous drainage of the erectile tissue is greatly impeded by the tangential exit of the veins through the tunica albuginea. Thus, the penile erection is maintained.

During erection, the penis becomes distended and increases in both length and diameter. Contraction of the ischiocavernosus and bulbocavernosus muscles forces the now rigid penis into an almost vertical position.

Ejaculation and emission

Ejaculation is a complex process. It is controlled by the

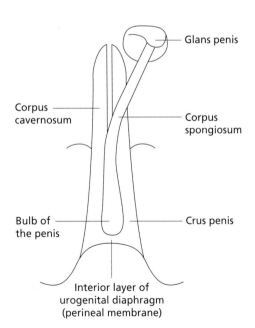

Fig. 12.5 Diagram showing the erectile bodies of the human penis.

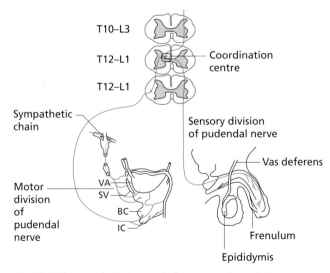

Fig. 12.6 The neurological control of erection and ejaculation.

Table 12.2 The order of emission into the urethra of the components that make up seminal fluid.

i) The urethral and the bulbo-urethral secretions
ii) The testicular and epididymal secretions
iii) The prostatic secretions
iv) The seminal vesicular secretions

sympathetic system, but both these processes require cerebral input as well and are thus frequently absent in men with spinal injury. It must not be forgotten that the brain is a major sexual organ (Fabbri *et al.*, 1997). The process of ejaculation is thought to be controlled by a coordinating centre in the spinal cord around the level of T12 (Truitt and Coolen, 2002). Damage to the cord in this region will always result in loss of the ability to ejaculate. The nervous control of erection and ejaculation is depicted diagrammatically in Figure 12.6.

The secretions that make up the ejaculate enter the posterior urethra in a set order in a process known as emission, which is under the control of the thoracolumbar outflow (T12–L3). The first secretions are those of the bulbo-urethral and the urethral glands, and they may be in the urethra early during intercourse.

As climax approaches, the circular muscle that surrounds the bladder neck in the male contracts strongly, thus preventing reflux of the semen into the bladder. The first major secretion that arrives in the posterior urethra is that from the testes and the epididymal ducts. This is followed by the prostatic secretions and lastly by the secretions of the seminal vesicles (Table 12.2).

Rhythmic contractions of the bulbocavernosus and the ischiocavernosus muscles now occur, and the seminal fluid is rapidly and forcefully milked down the urethra and out through the penile meatus in the process of ejaculation. Thus, the components of the ejaculate do not in fact come together until they reach the vagina.

THE RELEVANCE OF THE CLOTTING MECHANISM

The clotting of semen occurs straight after ejaculation and is commonly seen in many mammals. In rodents, the coagulum is very firm and is known as the 'plug'. However, in the bull and the ram, the semen remains liquid after ejaculation.

The coagulation of the semen is advantageous to fertility as it protects the spermatozoa from the midcycle acidity of the vagina. It may also hold the ejaculate close to the cervical os where the clot mixes with the cervical mucus, ensuring that the sperm, on lysis of the coagulum, are able to enter the cervical mucus with some ease. The clot usually lyses within 5–20 minutes of ejaculation when the sperm are slowly released and can enter the cervical mucus. There can be abnormalities of liquefaction where the sperm are unable to escape the clot, and this can result in infertility.

THE CERVIX AT MIDCYCLE

The cervix undergoes important changes as the menstrual cycle approaches ovulation (Fig. 12.3b). The rise in estrogen also increases the vascularity of the cervix, which becomes soft, allowing the external os to gape somewhat. This may help to accommodate the entry of the spermatozoa into the cervical canal. The cervical mucus increases its water and ion content, thus allowing easier penetration of the polymeric mucus by the spermatozoa. Both the quantity and the quality of the cervical mucus are controlled by estrogen, and increase as ovulation approaches. Progesterone, however, reverses these effects on the cervical mucus and reduces its water and ionic content dramatically. It is important to remember that this rise in progesterone often precedes ovulation. Thus, even before ovulation and actual follicular rupture, the postcoital test may become negative.

Close to ovulation, the estrogen level is maximal and the progesterone level is very low. As a consequence, the mucus increases in quantity, and its water and ionic contents are also greatly increased. The mucus can also be stretched in a phenomenon known as spinnbarkeit (Fig. 12.7). The mucus polymers thus become separated, giving easy access by the sperm to the cervical canal. On contact with the cervical mucus, the sperm enter the mucus in phalanxes. The sperm then induce a massive influx of white blood cells into the area. The exact function of these white cells is not known, but this

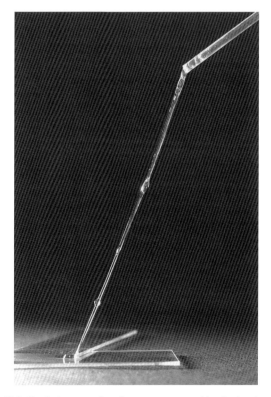

Fig. 12.7 Cervical mucus taken from a woman at midcycle showing marked spinnbarkeit.

could be a means of removing dead or dying sperm from the mucus. The white cells could also be a means of producing an immunological response and thus inducing tolerance to paternal antigens (Head and Billingham, 1986). The sperm pass up into the uterus through the cervical mucus but also invade all areas of the cervix including the cervical glands.

THE SCORING OF THE CERVIX AND THE CERVICAL MUCUS

A scoring system that involves the examination of the cervix as well as the cervical mucus has been devised and is known as the Insler score. This scoring system (Table 12.3) involves the assessment of four features of the cervix, namely degree of gaping of the external cervical os, the amount of mucus present at the os, its spinnbarkeit and the presence or absence of ferning.

To test spinnbarkeit, the cervical mucus is aspirated from the cervix, and one end of the mucus is placed on a clean glass slide and anchored by a coverslip. The mucus is now put on the stretch and, at midcycle, should elongate to around 5–10 centimetres.

Also at midcycle, the ionic content of the cervical mucus is greatly increased and can be precipitated out on drying to form branch-like crystals that resemble the branches of a fern (Fig. 12.8). This phenomenon is known as ferning. Its presence is induced by estrogen, and it is thus absent when the estrogen levels are low, as occurs early in the cycle. It is also suppressed by progesterone, and thus ferning is seen only around ovulation in the middle of the cycle. To demonstrate ferning, a small amount of cervical mucus is placed on a glass slide, and a drop of distilled water is added to the mucus. The preparation is then allowed to dry out, after which the ferning pattern can easily be seen using low-power microscopy.

This test of course also suffers from a great degree of subjectivity, particularly in relation to the degree of gaping of the os and the estimation of the amount of mucus present, but it gives the clinician a rough idea of the response of the cervix to estrogen stimulation and, indeed, the level of estrogen stimulation present. Each assessment scores up to three points

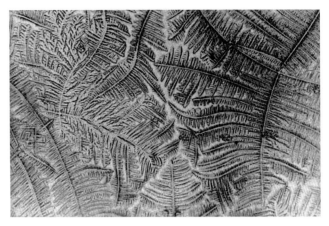

Fig. 12.8 The ferning pattern seen in midcycle mucus that has been allowed to dry out on a slide.

for each evaluation, giving a maximum score of 12 (Table 12.3). A score of 10 indicates good-quality cervical mucus and a receptive cervix. The presence of a positive postcoital test adds to the validity of the cervical response.

THE POSTCOITAL TEST AND OTHER TESTS OF SPERM PENETRATION OF CERVICAL MUCUS

There are several ways in which the ability of the sperm to penetrate cervical mucus can be tested.

The *in vivo* postcoital test

This is a commonly used method for testing the ability of sperm to enter the cervical mucus (Glazener *et al.*, 2001). The cervical mucus is at its most copious and its penetrability is maximal when the estrogen level is high and the progesterone is low. Thus, the time to perform this test is close to but not at or past ovulation. The timing of the postcoital test is thus essential for its correct interpretation. Indeed, the most common reason for a negative postcoital test is that it is performed at the wrong time of the cycle. Thus, the level of both estrogen and progesterone on the day of the test must be known in order to interpret the test correctly. If the estrogen level is not maximal (below some 500 pmol/L) and the progesterone is high (at or above 5 pmol/L), then the test is likely to be negative, and a false conclusion can be made as to the cause of a patient's infertility. Thus, the interpretation of this test, especially when it is negative, can be difficult (Oei *et al.*, 2000).

For this test, the couple are asked to have intercourse after 2 days of abstinence. The mucus is then examined for the presence of spermatozoa some 9–24 hours later. The problem with this test is that, for practical reasons, it is very difficult to standardise the time at which the mucus is examined as well as

Table 12.3 The Insler score and the method of scoring the cervix and the cervical mucus contained within it (the subjectivity of this test is clearly very great).

	Poor	*Moderate*	*Good*
The gaping of the external os	1	2	3
Amount of mucus	1	2	3
Spinnbarkeit	1	2	3
Ferning	1	2	3

Total possible score = 12.

to standardise the effects of the estrogen on the mucus itself. Its interpretation is thus very difficult, and it should be used only as a rough guide to sperm penetration of the mucus. It must also be remembered that the quality of the semen sample may determine the numbers of sperm in the mucus, and this test cannot be used as an alternative to a semen analysis. Sometimes, when men are asked to have intercourse to order, the patient will have difficulty in ejaculation or ejaculation may even be totally absent. This phenomenon will of course also give rise to a negative postcoital test but may also have the advantage that it can indicate the presence of coital difficulties in a couple. The difficulty in the interpretation of this test, however, cannot be overemphasised.

To carry out the mucus examination, an unlubricated speculum is inserted into the vagina, and the cervix and posterior fornix are viewed. Using a syringe attached to a quill, the semen in the posterior fornix is aspirated. Using another syringe and quill, the mucus that is protruding through the cervical os is also aspirated. Both samples are now placed separately on glass slides and examined microscopically at a magnification of around × 400, preferably using a phase-contrast system.

In the sample taken from the posterior fornix, all the sperm will be immotile as they will have come in contact with the highly acidic secretions of the midcycle vagina. However, the presence of sperm in the vagina will at least indicate that ejaculation has occurred and will give a very rough idea of the sperm count, but this should already be known. In the sample of cervical mucus, the test is deemed to be positive if there are five or more sperm per high-power field and at least one of these sperm is motile.

A positive postcoital test gives a good prognosis for pregnancy, whereas a negative postcoital test may be caused by an abnormality of sperm function or an abnormality of the cervical mucus. However, the difficulties in standardising this test must always be borne in mind. Badly timed postcoital tests will frequently give a negative result. Postcoital tests will also usually be negative in anovulatory women.

Sperm–cervical mucus interaction tests

In this test, the sperm–cervical mucus interaction is carried out not in the patient but in the laboratory. It is sometimes known as the Kurzrok–Miller test. Some midcycle cervical mucus is taken from the cervix, placed on a glass slide and covered with a coverslip. Some fresh semen is placed at the edge of the coverslip, and the preparation is incubated for some 30 minutes at 37°C. The cervical mucus is observed microscopically using phase contrast. A good result is reported where many sperm penetrate the mucus and show forward progression (Fig. 12.9).

Another way to examine sperm–cervical mucus interaction *in vitro* is known as the Kremer test. This test was initially

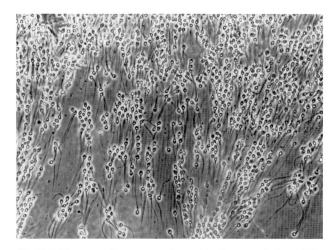

Fig. 12.9 The entry of spermatozoa into midcycle mucus during a slide test for mucus penetration.

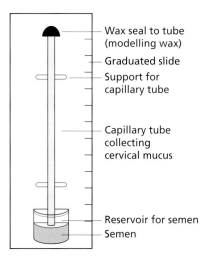

Fig. 12.10 Diagram of the apparatus used in the Kremer test that examines sperm–mucus interaction.

designed to detect the presence of anti-sperm antibodies in both semen and cervical mucus (Kremer and Jager, 1976). In this procedure, the mucus is aspirated into a capillary tube, and the end of the tube is placed into a pool of semen. This preparation is also incubated at 37°C for 30 minutes (Fig. 12.10). The contents of the tube are then examined microscopically at 10, 40 and 70 millimetres from the end of the capillary tube, and the number of sperm seen per high-power field are counted. The more sperm there are at a distance from the end of the tube, the more satisfactory the test. This is again a very subjective test with little or no attempt at any standardisation.

Hyaluronate migration test

This is a useful test as it examines the ability of the sperm to migrate into an artificial mucus (Mortimer, 1997). It is thus a test only of the migratory ability of the sperm and not any aspect of the patient's cervical mucus itself. In this test, a solution of the polysaccharide sodium hyaluronate contained in a tube (Select Medical Systems, VT, USA) is used. The capillary tube containing the solution is upended into an aliquot of the solution, and the preparation is then incubated at 37°C for 60 minutes. The advance of the sperm into the solution is then examined microscopically, and the number of sperm seen at 10, 20, 30 and 40 millimetres are counted. This test correlates very well with the ability of the sperm to penetrate cervical mucus and has the advantage of a certain degree of standardisation. It does not of course take into account any existing abnormality of the female partner's cervical mucus.

CERVICAL ABNORMALITIES THAT CAUSE INFERTILITY

Abnormalities of the cervical mucus can also be a cause of infertility, and these very commonly relate to poor estrogen rises in relation to defective ovulation or premature progesterone rises. Thus, it is unwise clinically to make an assessment of mucus quality without knowing the level of estrogen and progesterone in the serum. Surgical or ablative removal of the cervical canal, as occurs during a cone biopsy (Fig. 12.11), or treatment of cervical precancer causes cervical constriction or even stenosis (Figs 12.12 and 12.13) and can also at times cause infertility by removing the glands that secrete the mucus but, interestingly, this form of infertility is uncommon (Buller

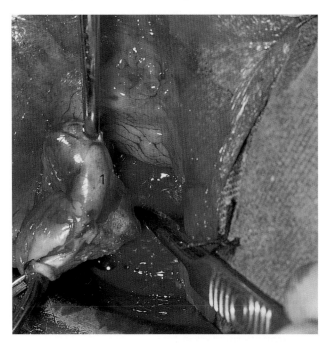

Fig. 12.11 Surgical cone biopsy (1) being undertaken for an extensive cervical precancer, showing the removal of both the ecto- and much of the endocervix.

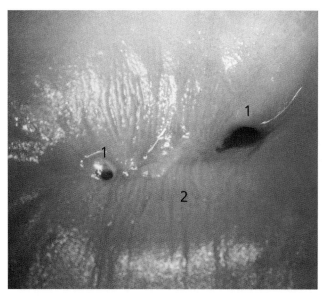

Fig. 12.12 Superficial twin ora (1) produced by the centre of the cervix (2) healing over following ablative treatment (cryosurgery). The cervical canals have been reduced to virtual pinhead openings.

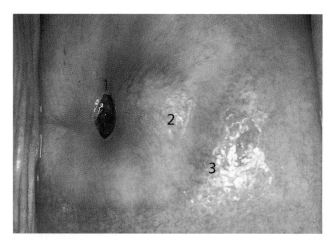

Fig. 12.13 Severe constriction of the ectocervix following previous large cone biopsy. The constricted endocervix is seen at (1), the scarred treatment area at (2) and the remaining cervix at (3).

and Jones, 1982). Anti-sperm antibodies can also be found in the mucus (Kremer and Jager, 1988), and these antibodies may both immobilise the sperm as well as coat the sperm with immunoglobulins.

THE CAPACITATION OF SPERM

This phenomenon was first described by Austin (1952) and Chang (1951). Capacitation confers on the sperm the ability to fertilise an intact oocyte. The process of capacitation consists of a variety of functional and structural changes in the sperm, many of which are poorly understood. The discovery of

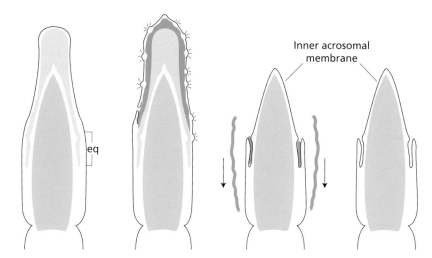

Fig. 12.14 Diagrammatic representation of the acrosome reaction.

capacitation was extremely important, as it is the first of the steps that allows the *in vitro* fertilisation of a human oocyte.

The process of capacitation starts when the sperm enters the cervical mucus. There are several changes that are recognised as being part of the process known as capacitation.

Hyperactivation

The most obvious of these is the change in sperm movement now known as hyperactivation. This has been accurately defined by Mortimer (1997). Sperm showing hyperactivation demonstrate a great increase in the bending of the sperm tail so that it resembles a whiplash movement. At the same time, there is a major increase in the lateral movement of the sperm head. Such sperm therefore have limited forward progression but have a greatly increased thrust. Such hyperactivated movement may thus aid the passage of sperm through the pinnae of the endometrium, and this type of movement would be of particular advantage for its negotiation of the folds formed by the tubal epithelium. The increased thrust will also enhance the ability of the sperm to penetrate the zona pellucida.

However, the premature occurrence of hyperactivation would considerably impede the passage of the sperm through the cervical mucus and could be a cause of infertility. However, it is now known that cervical mucus in fact suppresses hyperactivated sperm movement (Eriksen *et al.*, 1998).

Human sperm are also able to change from hyperactivated to non-capacitated sperm movement, but the mechanism that controls these changes is unclear.

The acrosome reaction

Capacitated sperm also undergo a process known as the acrosome reaction. This phenomenon is the result of an influx of calcium into the sperm. This influx can be induced by proges-

terone, by follicular fluid and by a protein that forms part of the zona pellucida that is known as zona pellucida protein 3 (ZP3) (Primakoff and Myles, 2002). The acrosome reaction can also be triggered by a calcium ionophore, and this has been used in the past to test the ability of the sperm to undergo the acrosome reaction (Cummins *et al.*, 1990). A disordered or deficient acrosome reaction can be a reason for infertility of unknown cause and for fertilisation failure in *in vitro* fertilisation (IVF) (Liu and Baker, 2003).

The acrosome reaction is a fairly complex procedure that results in major structural changes to the sperm head. It takes place prior to the penetration of the cumulus by the sperm and is essential for natural fertilisation. The first change that takes place is a fusion by the plasma membrane of the sperm head with the outer acrosomal membrane. Vesiculation now occurs between these two membranes, after which they break down to release the enzymes of the acrosome (Fig. 12.14). These enzymes consist of hyaluronidase as well as proteases and peptidases that break down protein and may assist in the separation of the cumulus cells (Fig. 12.15) and thus facilitate access of the sperm to the oocyte. Equally, they may also help in the penetration of the zona pellucida by the sperm head.

A proportion of the sperm, usually around 10%, undergoes the acrosome reaction spontaneously, but such sperm are never able to fertilise an oocyte.

THE PASSAGE OF THE SPERM THROUGH THE UTERUS AND INTO THE FALLOPIAN TUBE

Upon entering the uterus, the spermatozoa are now suspended in the small amount of fluid secreted by the endometrium. Their presence in the uterus may again induce a local leucocytosis. How the sperm pass up the uterus and into the fallopian tube continues to be unclear, but their propulsion probably

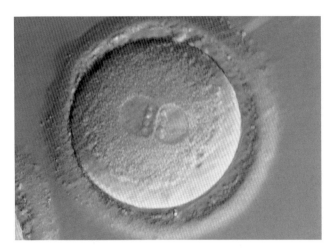

Fig. 12.15 A fertilised human egg showing the pronuclei and the prominent nucleoli within them.

relates to myometrial contractions, to the movement of the endometrial pinnae and to the motility of the spermatozoa themselves (Kunz *et al.*, 1996).

On entering the cornu of the fallopian tubes, the passage down to the ampulla where fertilisation will take place is likely to result from the contractions of the tubal wall itself.

How many sperm arrive in the fallopian tube is still uncertain, but it is thought to be only several thousand. However, many sperm can be found in the peritoneal fluid in the pouch of Douglas after intercourse at midcycle (Templeton and Mortimer, 1982). The absence of sperm from the peritoneal fluid has in fact been cited as a cause of infertility. There is in fact no evidence to support the presence of any chemotactic influence on the sperm by the oocyte.

How many sperm are needed to achieve reliable fertilisation is again uncertain, but this of course will also depend upon the presence of the acrosome reaction and will probably relate to the number of sperm that arrive in the tube having undergone capacitation.

Although the lifespan of the egg after ovulation is only some 12–18 hours, the life of the spermatozoa in the tube is probably very much longer; indeed, there are anecdotal reports of pregnancy occurring from intercourse that took place in the previous menstrual cycle.

SPERM BINDING AND THEIR PENETRATION OF THE ZONA PELLUCIDA

The zona pellucida surrounds the whole oocyte and is basically made up of three proteins supported by a zona matrix. These proteins are known as ZP1, ZP2 and ZP3. These proteins induce the acrosome reaction, induce hyperactivated sperm movement and enhance binding of the sperm to the zona pellucida.

The binding of the sperm to the zona pellucida takes place between the zona and the postacrosomal region of the sperm head that is close to the equatorial ring. The hyperactivated sperm movement that now occurs is providing the sperm with maximal thrust and an enhanced ability to penetrate the zona pellucida.

THE BINDING OF THE SPERM TO THE OOLEMA

After the sperm has penetrated the zona to enter the perivitelline space, the sperm head fuses with the plasma membrane of the oocyte. In the experimental animal, this fusion seems to be dependant upon a glycoprotein known as PH-20 (Primakoff and Myles, 2002), but its presence in the human has not been confirmed. This substance consists of two subunits known as α and β subunits. The α subunit is markedly hydrophilic and assists fusion between the sperm head and the plasma membrane of the oocyte. Another substance, the metalloprotease known as 'fertilin' (or a substance like it) that is found on the postequatorial segment of the sperm, may also play a role in sperm–membrane fusion (Bronson *et al.*, 1999).

As soon as the fusion between the egg and the sperm has taken place, there occur oscillations in calcium concentrations over the egg surface that cause the release of secretory granules into the egg cytoplasm just beneath the oolemma in a process that is known as the cortical granule reaction. These small vesicles contain enzymes such as hyaluronidase that are released into the perivitelline space. The cortical granule reaction is thought to be induced by the oscillations of the calcium ions on the surface of the oolemma. Within seconds, this phenomenon induces a block to any further penetration of the space by other spermatozoa and thus prevents polyspermic fertilisation.

Interestingly, the cortical reaction is also seen after intracytoplasmic sperm injection (ICSI) (Ghetler *et al.*, 1998). It has also been suggested that a deficiency in the cortical reaction may be a cause of repeated polyspermic fertilisation in IVF (Schalkoff *et al.*, 1996).

THE FERTILISATION OF THE HUMAN EGG

This begins as soon as the sperm enters the oocyte. After fusion with the oolemma, the sperm including its tail is engulfed by the oocyte and, at this point, all sperm movement ceases. On its arrival within the cytoplasm of the oocyte, the sperm head undergoes decondensation. A new membrane is formed around the DNA in the sperm head to form the male pronucleus. While this is taking place, the oocyte is activated and the second reduction division takes place, resulting in the formation of the female pronucleus and the extrusion of the second polar body.

The male and female pronuclei are initially apart within the oocyte but, some 20 hours after fertilisation, they migrate to

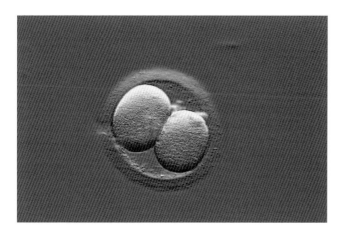

Fig. 12.16 A two-cell human embryo.

the centre of the oocyte to lie alongside each other. Prominent nucleoli may be seen, and the arrangement of these nucleoli (Fig. 12.15) within the pronuclei may be important in the prognosis for IVF (Boiso *et al.*, 2002). The membranes of both pronuclei then break down, and the contents of the pronuclei fuse together in a process known as syngamy. Syngamy completes the process of fertilisation. The zygote then undergoes its first cleavage division (Fig. 12.16).

PROBLEMS FACING THE SPERMATOZOA IN THEIR JOURNEY THROUGH THE FEMALE GENITAL TRACT

The sperm first have a major task in protecting themselves from the acidity of the female genital tract at midcycle. The journey facing the sperm as they enter the cervical mucus is a long one; indeed, it has been estimated to be the equivalent, in human terms, of a journey of 100 miles. Each sperm must then find its way through the thick layers of cumulus cells that surround each newly ovulated oocyte, after which it must penetrate the relatively dense protein covering of the egg known as the zona pellucida.

The journey to the oocyte by the sperm is thus an arduous one, at which only relatively few succeed. However, the great advantage that the sperm have over the egg is longevity: it is probable that the spermatozoa can survive many days or even weeks in the fallopian tube while the life of the egg is extremely limited.

The whole process of fertilisation begins at the interaction between the ejaculate and the cervix and, as such, the cervix is one of the most important organs involved in fertilisation and the generation of the conceptus.

ACKNOWLEDGEMENT

Figures 12.11, 12.12 and 12.13 are from Singer A., Monaghan J.M. (2000) *Lower Genital Tract Precancer*, 2nd edn, Oxford: Blackwell, with thanks.

REFERENCES

Anderson RA (2001) Clinical studies: inhibin in the adult male. *Molecular and Cellular Endocrinology* 180: 109–116.

Austin CR (1952) The capacitation of the mammalian spermatozoa. *Nature* 170: 326.

Boiso I, Veiga A, Edwards RG (2002) Fundamentals of human embryonic growth in vitro and the selection of high-quality embryos for transfer. *Reproduction Online* 5: 328–350.

Bronson RA, Fusi FM, Calzi F *et al.* (1999) Evidence that a functional fertilin-like ADAM plays a role in human sperm–oolemmal interactions. *Molecular Human Reproduction* 5: 433–440.

Buller RE, Jones HW III (1982) Pregnancy following conisation. *American Journal of Obstetrics and Gynecology* 142: 506–512.

Chang MC (1951) The fertilising capacity of spermatozoa deposited in the Fallopian tubes. *Nature* 168: 697–698.

Cummins JM, Pember SM, Jequier AM *et al.* (1990) A test for the human acrosome reaction following ionophore challenge. Relationship to fertility and other seminal parameters. *International Journal of Andrology* 12: 98–103.

Eriksen GV, Carlsedt I, Uldbjerg N *et al.* (1998) Cervical mucins affect the motility of human spermatozoa in vitro. *Fertility and Sterility* 70: 350–354.

Fabbri A, Aversa A, Isodori A (1997) Erectile dysfunction: an overview. *Human Reproduction Update* 3: 455–466.

Ford WC, Harrison A (1984) The role of citrate in determining the activity of calcium ions in human semen. *International Journal of Andrology* 7: 198–202.

Fuse H, Satomi S, Okumura M *et al.* (1994) Seminal plasma transferrin concentration: relationship with seminal parameters and plasma hormone levels. *Urology International* 49: 158–162.

Ghetler Y, Raz T, Ben Nun I *et al.* (1998) Cortical granules reaction after intracytoplasmic injection. *Molecular Human Reproduction* 4: 289–294.

Glazener CM, Ford WC, Hull MG (2001) The prognostic power of the post-coital test for natural conception depends on duration of infertility. *Human Reproduction* 16: 1051–1053.

Head JR, Billingham RE (1986) Concerning the immunology of the uterus. *American Journal of Immunology and Microbiology* 10: 76–81.

Hellstrom WJ, Wang R, Petersen CA *et al.* (1998) Effects of alprostadil and prazosin on motility, viability and membrane integrity of human sperm. *Journal of Urology* 159: 1559–1562.

Kremer J, Jager S (1988) Sperm–cervical mucus interaction, in particular in the presence of anti-sperm antibodies. *Human Reproduction* 3: 69–73.

Kunz G, Beil D, Deininger H *et al.* (1996) The dynamics of rapid sperm transport through the female genital tract: evidence from vaginal sonography of uterine peristalsis and hysterosalpingoscintigraphy. *Human Reproduction* 11: 627–632.

Kvist U, Kjellberg S, Bjorndahl L *et al.* (1990) Seminal fluid from men with agenesis of the Wolffian ducts: zinc binding properties and effects on sperm chromatin stability. *International Journal of Andrology* 13: 245–252.

Liu D, Baker HW (2003) Disordered zona pellucida-induced acrosome reaction and failure of in vitro fertilisation in patients with unexplained infertility. *Fertility and Sterility* 79: 74–80.

Lundquist F (1949) Aspects of the biochemistry of semen. *Acta Physiologica Scandinavica* 19 (Suppl. 66): 7–105.

Mortimer D, Mortimer ST, Shu MA *et al.* (1990) A simplified approach to sperm cervical mucus interaction testing using a hyaluronate migration test. *Human Reproduction* 5: 835–841.

Mortimer S. (1997) A critical review of the physiological importance and analysis of sperm movement in mammals. *Human Reproduction Update* 5: 835–841.

Oei SG, Helmerhorst FM, Keirse MJ (2001) When is the post-coital test normal? A critical appraisal. *Human Reproduction* 10: 1711–1714.

Primakoff P, Myles DD (2002) Penetration, adhesion and fusion in mammalian sperm–egg interaction. *Science* 296: 2182–2185.

Roberts M, Gagnon C (1999) Semengelin 1: a coagulum forming multifunctional seminal vesicle protein. *Cellular and Molecular Life Sciences* 55: 944–960.

Schalkoff ME, Powers RD, Oskowitz SP (1996) An ultrastructural analysis of an oocyte from an in vitro fertilization patient with repeated polyspermic fertilization. *Journal of Assisted Reproduction and Genetics* 13: 477–484.

Shimizu Y, Jorimitsu A, Maruyama Y *et al.* (1998) Prostaglandins induce calcium influx in human spermatozoa. *Molecular Human Reproduction* 4: 555–561.

Templeton AA, Mortimer D (1982) Laparoscopic sperm recovery in infertile women. *British Journal of Obstetrics and Gynaecology* 87: 1128–1131.

Truitt WA, Coolen LM (2002) Identification of a potential ejaculation generator in the spinal cord. *Science* 297: 1460–1461.

PART 4

The cervix in pregnancy and labour

CHAPTER 13

Mechanics, biochemistry and pharmacology of the cervix and labour

Harold Gee

INTRODUCTION

The uterus maintains the pregnancy and delivers it at parturition. The two parts of the uterus, cervix and corpus, have to complement each other at every stage. Premature delivery or delayed progress in spontaneous labour may be described in terms of mismatches between these functions.

The myometrium, almost certainly because of its overt activity, has captured most attention. The cervix, in contrast, has been considered passive, responding only to myometrial activity. However, despite clinicians having the means to control myometrial function, problems continue to plague practice and paradoxes go unexplained (Olah and Gee, 1992, 1996). It is the thesis of this chapter that solutions lie in the hidden subtlety and complexity of the cervix.

Clinical paradoxes and justification for a paradigm shift

The paradigm that the cervix is 'passive' and the myometrium 'active' has driven the clinical management of labour for over 40 years (Danforth, 1954; O'Driscoll et al., 1969). If this is correct, suppression of myometrial activity or augmentation should prevent premature delivery and correct delay in labour respectively. However, tocolysis does not delay premature delivery for more than 48–72 hours (Goldenberg, 2002; Coomarasamy et al., 2002), and oxytocin augmentation has not reduced the need for caesarean section in labour (Frigoletto et al., 1995; Thornton and Lilford, 1994).

A paradox presents itself in normal, spontaneous labour: the rate of cervical dilatation in the first stage of labour is greater in multiparous women than it is in nulliparous ones. Classically, this is explained by more efficient or greater myometrial activity. However, this is not the case. Multiparous women dilate their cervixes faster but with *less* uterine activity (Al-Shawaf et al., 1987), i.e. resistance is lower.

The ability to augment uterine activity in labour offered the prospect of eliminating poor progress in labour, excluding cephalo-pelvic disproportion. However, failure to progress in labour continues to be a major indication for caesarean section (Kiwanuka and Moore, 1987). Cephalo-pelvic disproportion may be more common than expected, but there is little evidence for this (Gee, 1994a). The paradox that presents itself is that two out of three women who have caesarean sections for failure to progress go on to deliver successfully when they attempt vaginal delivery in subsequent pregnancies (Rosen and Dickinson, 1990). This is not much different from the rate among women who have had caesarean sections for non-recurrent indications.

Lastly, concepts accepted in one part of practice are not transferred to another. Cervical ripeness is an important factor for the successful induction of labour. However, cervical influence on intrapartum events is rarely considered, and only the forces of labour are manipulated.

MECHANICS

Functional anatomy in pregnancy and parturition

The cervix is tubular with a central canal having external and internal openings. The 'internal os' has been considered critical for competence. It may be defined as the constriction in the uterine lumen between corpus and cervix that coincides with the fibromuscular junction between the muscular myometrium and the fibrous cervix. Great play used to be made of the 'isthmic' portion of the cervix, which was said to lie between the 'anatomical' internal os, as just defined, and the 'histological' internal os, the transition between the endometrial and endocervical epithelia. The isthmus was said to form the lower segment. This may be so in other primates but not in the human. Functionally, it is better and simpler to consider the cervix as a single functional entity without subdividing it, on little evidence, into parts that do not exist.

Pregnancy

The cervix is predominantly a connective tissue structure (Danforth, 1947), with collagen and its associated ground substance accounting for 80% of its dry weight. There is also a small amount of smooth muscle (15%) (Danforth, 1947,

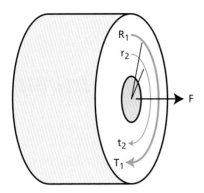

Fig. 13.1 Schematic representation of a cross-section of the cervix to demonstrate the Laplace equation. The radial force (F) induces greater tension in the outer fibres (T_1) compared with the inner ones (t_2) because of the differences in their radii of curvature (R_1, r_2).

1954) and, paradoxically, a relatively extensive capillary bed, given its low metabolic requirements.

The collagen that forms the cervix is similar to that in other load-bearing connective tissues such as tendons. It is mainly composed of type I and III collagen fibres (Kleissl *et al.*, 1978). Like other collagens, cervical collagen is inelastic with a steep stress–strain relationship (Stevens, 1977). It is, therefore, an ideal fibre to resist passive load.

In the non-pregnant state and in early pregnancy, the cervix is between 30 and 50 mm long and in the later part of pregnancy it is 20–30 mm long (Cook and Ellwood, 2000; Rozenberg *et al.*, 2002). The clinical importance of cervical length, as evaluated by ultrasound imaging, has increased with its predictive value for premature labour. The collagen fibres are tightly wound around the canal with a small radius of curvature (Fig. 13.1).

The Laplace relationship

This relates radial force (F) [pressure (P) in a closed vessel] with circumferential tension (T) and radius of curvature (R) in the wall:

$$P(F) \propto 2(T/R)$$

It is why balloons get easier to inflate as they get bigger and why aneurysms rupture according to their size. It is, however, simplistic *in vitro*, because it does not take account of visco-elasticity, but it is useful to illustrate and explain certain functions and paradoxes regarding the cervix and its interaction with the corpus.

Perhaps the amount of force required to dilate such a system can be illustrated by an everyday surgical procedure. The radial force imparted to cervical tissue by a Hegar's dilator, used to dilate the cervix prior to instrumentation of the uterine cavity, is 40 times the operator's effort!

Thus, the form of the cervix is ideally suited to its pregnancy function. Closure can be maintained with minimal tension in

its inelastic collagen fibres and no energy expenditure. The problem lies with reconciling this with its function in labour, when it has to yield. Furthermore, it has to be able to perform these functions repeatedly in subsequent pregnancies. The cervix does not lose its competence with parity.

Parturition

In labour, myometrial contractions impart tension to the wall of the uterus and to the cervix, subjecting it to a dilating force (Gee *et al.*, 1988). The amount of dilatation will be the resultant of the contraction strength and cervical resistance/ compliance.

According to the Laplace equation, intra-uterine pressure is directly proportional to wall tension, assuming constant size. Intra-uterine pressure (IUP) has been used to quantify contraction amplitude and derive uterine activity (Steer *et al.*, 1975). However, in this system, the cervix is in series with the myometrium. Its compliance modulates (reduces) wall tension (Gee *et al.*, 1988). Thus, the 'passive' cervix, as well as the active myometrium, determines both uterine wall tension (and thus IUP/uterine activity) *and* cervical dilatation. Simultaneous recordings of cervical dilatation and IUP during contraction cycles demonstrate a fall in IUP as cervical response improves, the so-called CAP (cervical augmentation/attenuation of pressure) effect (Gee, 1994b). Thus, one of the paradoxes given above, regarding nulliparous and multiparous labours, can be explained in terms of cervical behaviour. The more compliant cervix of the multiparous woman reduces contraction amplitude/uterine activity *and* permits a better rate of dilatation. Furthermore, limitation of the amplitude of contractions (Gee, 1983) protects placental perfusion and fetal oxygenation. This may not occur when contractions are augmented in the presence of a non-compliant cervix.

The small amount of smooth muscle in the cervix has already been noted. Condensations occur circumferentially around the upper part of the cervical canal and longitudinally along its lateral aspects in continuity with the vagina (Hughesdon, 1952). These muscles have been shown to act during labour (Pajntar *et al.*, 1987), but histological estimation of the amount led to the belief that they were not strong enough to have a functional effect (Danforth, 1954). However, examination of cervical response to myometrial contractions using a cervimeter has shown that the cervix can constrict simultaneously with myometrial contractions (Olah *et al.*, 1993). Electromyographic studies demonstrate (Pajntar *et al.*, 2001) smooth muscle activity. This occurs only under specific conditions, namely when the cervix is uneffaced and undilated. Returning, again, to the Laplace equation, even 'weak' muscle fibres will generate significant tension when they act with small radius of curvature at low cervical dilatation. Cervical contractions have been associated with prolonged latent phase, which in turn is associated with poor fetal outcome (Chelmow *et al.*, 1993).

Effacement, formation of the lower segment and dilatation

These are all familiar concepts to the clinician, but precise definition of the underlying processes is not easy.

Effacement is thinning of the cervix, changing it from the 25–30 mm thickness it has in later pregnancy to almost nothing at the time of labour. Removal of tissue reduces cervical resistance but which bit of tissue moves, and to where, is unclear.

Possibly, tissue is removed like peeling back the skins of an onion from the outside (Fig. 13.2).

This would obey the Laplace relationship whereby outer parts of the uterine wall and cervix are at greater tension as a result of greater radius of curvature. In the cervix and lower segment, this would amount to about 5% difference across the thickness of the wall. This is significant over repetitive contraction cycles.

The lower segment has many definitions according to clinical circumstance. The ultrasonographer looking for a low-lying placenta will recognise it differently from the surgeon performing a caesarean section. Almost certainly, the tissues redeployed from the cervix contribute to the lower segment.

Its fibres run more horizontally and circumferentially like those in the cervix, and it is thinner than the upper segment. However, its anatomical boundaries are notional and its component parts ill-defined.

Dilatation would seem more obvious. Contractions simply stretch the cervix over the head, using it as a dilator. However, measurement of head–cervix forces shows that, in progressing labour, these forces are not distributed evenly (Lindgren, 1961; Gee, 1982; Gough *et al.*, 1990; Allman *et al.*, 1996a,b), as would be expected by this concept. On the contrary, it is poorly progressing labour that demonstrates an even distribution of resistive forces (Gee, 1982). The force distribution between head and cervix in normal, efficient labour remains to be fully explained. Cervical dilatation is not a simple, mechanical process.

The cervix in labour — the clinical aspects

Friedman meticulously documented the behaviour of the cervix in labour (Friedman, 1954, 1967). Friedman's work is still the most objective documentation of labour and is the foundation of current cervicography, the plotting of cervical dilatation with time to monitor progress in labour. He divided the first stage of labour into two parts according to the rate of cervical dilatation, the latent and active phases (Fig. 13.3).

The latent phase

The onset of labour and, hence, the start of these graphical representations of progress has always been problematic and always will be. Friedman took the establishment of regular, painful contractions as his start point. Other researchers (Hendricks *et al.*, 1970; Studd, 1973; Cardozo *et al.*, 1982) have chosen more precise but totally arbitrary points, such as the time of admission to the delivery suite, as their start of labour. This has led to confusion over findings and definitions. Furthermore, if labour is diagnosed only in terms of evidence of active dilatation of the cervix, i.e. the active phase of labour,

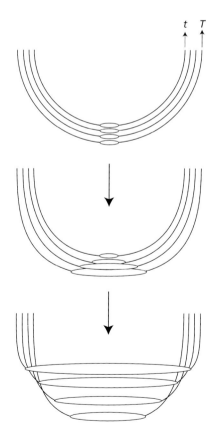

Fig. 13.2 Diagrammatic representation of the way effacement and dilatation could be produced by differential tensions (T, t) across tissue 'layers' of the lower segment and cervix as a result of the Laplace equation.

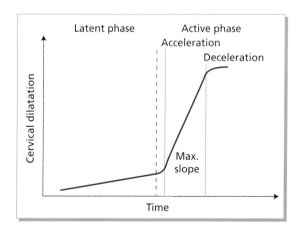

Fig. 13.3 Friedman's graphical representation of cervical dilatation in the first stage of labour.

then the latent phase is not labour at all but 'prelabour'. This is important clinically. Detection of slow dilatation and interventions to accelerate it should be confined to the active phase. Diagnosis of labour only in terms of the active phase facilitates good pragmatic clinical management but ignores an important physiological part of labour.

During the latent phase, the cervix is transforming from 'pregnancy' mode (no cervical change) into 'labour' mode (active dilatation). The presence of uterine activity means that the myometrium is already in 'labour' mode. Primarily, effacement is taking place in preparation for dilatation in the active phase. The two processes are more distinct and sequential in first than in subsequent labours when dilatation is often evident before effacement is complete.

Prolonged latent phase. The latent phase can last up to 20 hours (mean 8.6 hours) in first labours and 14 hours (mean 5.3 hours) in subsequent ones. True prolongation is associated with increased maternal and neonatal morbidity (Cardozo *et al.*, 1982; Chelmow *et al.*, 1993). Caesarean section is 10 times more likely and one-third of neonates will have poor Apgar scores. Response to augmentation of the powers is poor. All else being well, pain relief and waiting until the active phase has been entered is a better option. With time, the biochemical and physical properties of the cervix can improve to facilitate effacement and subsequent dilatation.

Prospective monitoring of the latent phase is not easy. The inductograph (Beazley and Alderman, 1976), which plots Bishop score against time in the latent phase of induced labour, is analogous to the cervicograph in the active phase. It has not, however, found widespread acceptance.

The end of the latent phase occurs at about 3 cm dilatation when active dilatation begins. Retrospective identification is easy but, prospectively, it can be difficult. As a rule of thumb, if in doubt, assume that the latent phase has not reached active phase. This avoids inappropriate application of cervimetric standards and acceleration.

Active phase

Friedman identified 200 primigravidae (Friedman, 1955) retrospectively from a larger heterogeneous group of patients [a second paper followed the same practice for multiparae (Friedman, 1956)] to identify 'ideal' labour, i.e. no iatrogenic interventions (apart from 'prophylactic low forceps'), vaginal deliveries and average-sized, healthy neonates. These patients' labour curves were analysed to identify statistical limits. Means and standard deviations were used, although this could be questioned given that the data were not evenly distributed with a tail towards longer labour.

A lower limit of maximum slope dilatation of 1.2 cm/h for nulliparae and 1.5 cm/h for multiparae was produced. Similar values were found in other populations, and a lower limit of progress of 1 cm/h has now become almost universally accepted for clinical practice (Philpott and Castle, 1972a,b). However, using a 1 cm/h 'alert' line and an 'action' line set 2 hours behind, the likelihood of needing an operative delivery is only 50:50 (Studd, 1973).

Primary dysfunctional labour The active phase progress rate is less than 1 cm/h (Friedman *et al.*, 1969). This is the commonest pattern of aberrance, affecting 26% of spontaneous nulliparous and 8% of multiparous labours. The underlying pathology has never been specified. Hypotonic uterine activity is a major contributor and should be looked for. Some 80% of nulliparae and 90% of multiparae respond to oxytocin augmentation, and this is a logical and specific treatment for hypotonic uterine activity. However, the empirical use of oxytocin to manage any aberrant pattern has been found wanting in clinical trials (Frigoletto *et al.*, 1995; Cammu and Van Eeckhout, 1996). Other pathologies should be considered if there is delay with normal uterine activity. Cervical resistance has not conventionally been considered, but poor biochemical preparation has been associated (Granstrom *et al.*, 1991).

Secondary arrest Cervical dilatation ceases after a normal portion of active phase dilatation (Friedman and Kroll, 1971). This pattern has been associated with cephalo-pelvic disproportion and abnormalities with the mechanisms of labour.

CERVICOGRAPHY

The cervicograph is a fundamental component of the partogram or partograph (Studd, 1973), a chart that records observations on mother and fetus with time during labour. It is an aid to the management of labour (Beazley, 1972; Beazley and Kurjak, 1972), representing graphically a clinical sign. It is *not* a diagnosis in itself. When progress is within limits, little more needs be done (a good negative predictive value). However, poor progress requires a proper evaluation of the patient, her labour and the fetus to determine a diagnosis. Unfortunately, this is often impossible with current knowledge. Because of this, clinicians have had to rely on try-it-and-see interventions designed to augment the powers that, when subjected to scientific scrutiny, have failed to live up to expectations (Thornton and Lilford, 1994; UK Amniotomy Group, 1994; Frigoletto *et al.*, 1995; Cammu and Van Eeckhout, 1996). Only research and a better understanding of the pathophysiology of labour will resolve these frustrations.

BIOCHEMISTRY

Cervical collagen

Collagen molecules are synthesised as single polypeptide chains (Fietzek and Kuhn, 1976) in fibroblasts and, possibly, smooth muscle cells. Each peptide chain carries an N-terminal peptide extension, the procollagen peptide. Proline and lysine amino acids are hydroxylated and carbohydrate moieties attached, allowing condensation of the chains into a triple helical conformation. The triple helical procollagen molecule is secreted into the extracellular space (Rechberger, 1993), where the procollagen peptide is enzymatically cleaved, permitting the peptide to polymerise into fibrils. These fibrils are stabilised by electrostatic bonding between peptide side-chains and by hydrogen bonding between the carbohydrate moieties and glycoprotein in the ground substance.

Ehlers–Danlos syndrome (EDS) is a heterogeneous group of inherited connective tissue disorders with at least 10 distinct types, all demonstrating decreased processing of procollagen to collagen (Minor *et al.*, 1986). The effect on pregnancy is varied but, in particular, cervical dysfunction is reflected in a high preterm delivery rate (23%) and spontaneous abortion (29%) (Kulkarni and LaGrenade, 1992; Sorokin *et al.*, 1994; Lind and Wallenburg, 2002).

In animals, collagen accounts for 8% by weight of the non-pregnant cervix, falling to 4% at the end of pregnancy (Harkness and Harkness, 1959), and human studies have shown a fall in collagen concentration of 40–60% over the same period (Granstrom *et al.*, 1989). Two processes could account for these changes. First, dispersion of the collagen fibres resulting from changes in cross-bonding and increased hydration of ground substance and, secondly, degradation of the collagen fibres themselves due to the action of collagenases and elastases secreted from macrophages and, possibly, fibroblasts (Junqueira *et al.*, 1980).

Ground substance

Ground substance is the material between the collagen fibrils and other structural components of the cervix. Its most important component is glycoprotein. Glycoproteins (Ruoslahti, 1988) are complex molecules containing a long protein 'spine' with covalently attached side-chains of unbranched polysaccharides, the glycosaminoglycans (GAGs). GAGs are composed of repeating disaccharide units with an amino sugar. The carbohydrate portion of the glycoprotein molecule may account for 90% of their mass.

Glycoproteins have two important functions: first, they impart 'texture' to the tissue and, secondly, they are labile molecules, whose physical properties can be changed dramatically and rapidly.

The 'texture' of the connective tissue, i.e. its stiffness, can be determined by the constituent GAGs (Osmers *et al.*, 1993). The cervix has been shown to contain hyaluronic acid, chondroitin-4- and chondroitin-6-sulphates, dermatan sulphate, heparan sulphate and keratan sulphate. Dermatan sulphate has a high affinity for collagen, which it stabilises, and it binds fibronectin, another structural glycoprotein that has high affinity for collagen (Rath *et al.*, 1994; Winkler and Rath,

1999). It is, therefore, important structurally and it stiffens connective tissue. Hyaluronic acid and chondroitin sulphate have weak affinities for collagen. In addition, hyaluronic acid increases tissue hydration (Fujimoto *et al.*, 1995) because of a high water-binding capacity.

Hydrogen bonding between GAG amino sugars and polar side-chains in collagen peptides can be altered by temperature, hydration, pH and calcium ion concentration among others. An example of the lability of glycoproteins can be demonstrated by jelly. Edible jelly is traditionally made from gelatine — glycoprotein derived from animal connective tissues. Simply by increasing its hydration, the solid block can be changed to a gel — still solid but with markedly different stress–strain properties.

Cervical ripening

Cervical ripening is easily recognised as softening leading to effacement and dilatation. However, the underlying mechanisms are poorly understood. It has been likened to an inflammatory reaction with tissue oedema, infiltration of inflammatory cells and involvement of inflammatory mediators (Winkler and Rath, 2001; Young *et al.*, 2002) such as prostaglandins (Calder, 1994), cytokines (Denison *et al.*, 1999; Fujimoto *et al.*, 1995; Sennstrom *et al.*, 2000) and vascular permeability factors (Sisi *et al.*, 1995; Sugano *et al.*, 2001).

Inflammatory cascade
In the latent phase, a peak in hyaluronic acid concentration can be demonstrated (Osmers *et al.*, 1993) (Fig. 13.4).

Rising concentrations of hyaluronic acid can be a potent inducer of IL-8 synthesis (Belayet *et al.*, 1999) by various leucocyte populations, and an increase in IL-6 (Hebisch *et al.*, 2001) synthesis stimulates prostaglandin and leukotriene production, causing dilatation of cervical vessels and further promoting the extravasation of leucocytes. Degranulation of these cells is triggered by an increased concentration of IL-8. Degranulation releases proteases that encounter an already destabilised collagenous fibre network. As a sustained action of proteases may lead to severe tissue damage, this process is strictly limited in time and is controlled by increasing concentrations of tissue inhibitors in the lower uterine segment immediately after delivery.

Increased vascular permeability and leucocyte infiltration
An infiltration of leucocytes (Winkler and Rath, 1999), including eosinophils (Luque *et al.*, 1998; Ramos *et al.*, 2000), macrophages and mast cells (Radestad *et al.*, 1993), has been demonstrated. It is highly likely that cell types and fibroblasts interchange morphologically and functionally. They almost certainly come from the capillary circulation, facilitated by increased vascular permeability resulting from agents such as

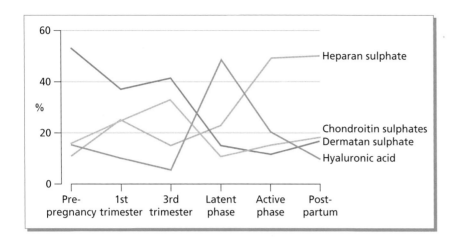

Fig. 13.4 Changes in the GAG composition of the cervix.

vascular endothelial growth factor (VEGF). The difference between the nulliparous and multiparous cervix (and thus performance in labour) may be due to the development and response of the capillary bed as a result of neovascularisation at the time of the first labour. Functionally, these cells remodel glycoproteins and collagen through synthesis of enzymes such as collagenases, elastases and metalloproteins. Estrogen receptors have been demonstrated on their cell membranes (Wang *et al.*, 2001), and they are chemotactically attracted by cytokines and interleukins.

Increased hydration

In the human, the increased hydration amounts to about 5% and can be demonstrated *in vivo* (Olah, 1994). This occurs as part of the normal hormonal milieu towards the end of pregnancy, but the peak in concentration of hyaluronic acid has already alluded been to. This GAG carries with it water. Increased hydration alters the physical characteristics of structural GAGs, resulting in dispersion of the collagen fibres and fibrils. The fluid ground substance allows the collagen lattice to open and fibres to slip apart from each other.

Changes in glycoproteins (see Fig. 13.4)

There is a marked fall in the main structural GAG, dermatan sulphate, and a rise in heparan sulphate, a 'packing' GAG with little collagen affinity. This is in keeping with the observed dispersion of the collagen fibres. Abnormalities in these glycoprotein changes have been associated with poor cervical dilatation (Granstrom *et al.*, 1991).

Collagen remodelling

Changes in glycoprotein and increased hydration produce disaggregation of collagen fibrils and fibres. In addition, there is evidence of increased collagen turnover (Maillot and Zimmermann, 1976; Kleissl *et al.*, 1978; Junqueira *et al.*, 1980; Ekman *et al.*, 1986; Granstrom *et al.*, 1992; Osmers *et al.*, 1995). The overall result is a reduction in collagen density,

although it must be emphasised that the collagen skeleton remains.

Thus, the cervix is anything but passive at parturition. The end-result of these changes is an alteration in the visco-elastic properties of the cervix. Theoretical calculation of the change in stiffness of the connective tissue from the observed reduction in collagen concentration, disorganisation of collagen fibre orientation and increased hydration would amount to a 12-fold reduction (Aspden, 1988). This is consistent with measured reductions on tissue testing that range between five- and 20-fold. A more 'fluid' tissue can 'flow' in response to applied forces. The resultant deformation allows tissue to be redistributed from the cervix to the 'lower segment'.

Visco-elasticity implies that deformation depends not only on the force applied but also on the rate of application. The same force applied more gradually will produce more deformation than if the same force were to be applied suddenly. This is important. It explains why labour is a gradual process and should question why clinicians are so obsessed with interventions that simply augment applied forces.

PHARMACOLOGY OF CERVICAL RIPENING AND INDUCTION OF LABOUR

Progesterone and mifepristone

As the name implies, progesterone promotes gestation and is the pregnancy hormone. Mifepristone is a steroid that binds to progesterone receptors and acts as an antagonist. It was developed to induce early abortion. Subsequently, it has been found to have ripening effects on the cervix. Treatment with mifepristone increases neovascularisation followed by infiltration of polymorphs, macrophages and mast cells due to the production of IL-8, IL-1β and monocyte chemotactic (MCP-1) protein (Denison *et al.*, 2000). These effects are independent of prostaglandins. An increase in enzyme activity can also be demonstrated, namely increases in neutrophil elastase and matrix metalloproteins (-1, -8 and -9) while metalloprotein inhibitors are not affected.

Although mifepristone has been shown to increase myometrial responsiveness to prostaglandins and oxytocin, its main effect is to produce cervical ripening without necessarily inducing labour (Wing *et al.*, 2000). It is, therefore, ideal for preparation of the cervix for surgical dilatation and sequential use with prostaglandins.

Estrogens

Women with placental sulphatase deficiency — low circulating estrogens — do not ripen their cervices (Rajabi *et al.*, 1991). The presence of estrogen receptors on cervical leucocytes (Stygar *et al.*, 2001) suggests that estrogen may directly regulate leucocyte functions in the cervix. Estrogen can be shown to trigger eosinophil invasion (Ramos *et al.*, 2000). This is affected by the estrogen receptor antagonist tamoxifen and by the mRNA synthesis blocker actinomycin D, suggesting a genomic action of estrogens. Furthermore, the estrogen effect is blocked by progesterone, and this inhibition is reversed by mifepristone. Further data suggest that estrogens may be involved in cervical ripening through the enhancement of collagenase activity (Rajabi *et al.*, 1991; Yoshida *et al.*, 1993).

Estrogens have been tried clinically to induce ripening, usually by local application (Tromans, 1981). Ripening does occur, but they appear to be less effective than prostaglandins for inducing labour and delivery. However, there are insufficient data to draw any conclusions (Thomas *et al.*, 2001).

Prostaglandins

It is not clear how prostaglandins (PGs) produce cervical ripening, but the mechanism does not depend on myometrial activity as was once proposed. Prostaglandin receptors have been demonstrated (Smith *et al.*, 2000), and the cervix can produce a variety of prostaglandins (Ellwood *et al.*, 1980). Production increases towards term (Allport *et al.*, 2001). Prostaglandins may affect fibroblast activity through their production of glycoproteins. They have been shown to influence the production of hyaluronic acid. Prostaglandins are chemotactic agents, increasing the numbers of leucocytes and macrophages in connective tissues.

PGE_2

PGE_2 is usually administered vaginally or intracervically. It is efficient in producing both ripening and labour induction (Witter, 2000). In many clinical settings, it has become the standard method for inducing labour.

Prostaglandins PGE_2 and $PGF_{2\alpha}$ can be administered orally and intravenously but produce significant gastrointestinal side-effects.

Misoprostol

Misoprostol is a PGE_1 analogue, originally developed for the treatment of gastric ulcers. It is finding a widening range of applications in obstetrics and gynaecology. In contrast to other prostaglandins, misoprostol is cheap, insensitive to heat and light and appears to cause fewer maternal side-effects. It appears to have a greater effect on the cervix than PGE_2 (Hofmeyr and Gulmezoglu, 2000). Because of this, misoprostol has been used prior to transcervical interventions in gynaecology and for curettage in the cases of silent miscarriage (missed abortion). Mifepristone-induced termination of pregnancy is routinely and effectively complemented by misoprostol.

Misoprostol appears to be more effective in inducing labour than conventional methods of cervical ripening and labour induction, particularly so in cases of an unripe cervix or preterm rupture of membranes (Hofmeyr and Gulmezoglu, 2001). However, there is an apparent increase in uterine hyperstimulation and tachysystole, although the studies so far are not large enough to be conclusive about the risks. Care should be exercised if uteroplacental insufficiency is suspected (Lukoschus *et al.*, 2002) and, after uterine surgery such as caesarean section or myomectomy, there is a significant risk of uterine rupture (Hill *et al.*, 2000), to the point where these conditions act as contraindications.

Oral and vaginal routes of administration have been tried without clear benefits of one above the other. Vaginal administration results in slower absorption compared with oral and longer activity (up to 4 hours). This has theoretical attractions, giving a more gradual and constant process but, in practice, oral administration (50 µg every 3 hours) is effective and without statistically significant differences with respect to intrapartum complications, tachysystole, uterine hyperstimulation or adverse neonatal outcomes. Buccal misoprostol, however, results in a higher incidence of tachysystole than does intravaginal administration.

Vaginally applied 50 µg of misoprostol, compared with a regime using 25 µg, gives shorter induction–delivery intervals with less need for labour augmentation but increased risks of uterine contractile abnormalities and postpartum haemorrhage (El-Sherbiny *et al.*, 2001; Sanchez-Ramos *et al.*, 2002). The lower dose, given every 4 hours, can induce labour safely and effectively.

Mechanical stimulation and other endogenous releasers of ripening agents

Mechanical methods were the first methods developed to ripen the cervix or to induce labour. Tents made from dried seaweed that would swell as a result of absorption of tissue fluid were used in the eighteenth century. Balloon catheters, introduced into the cervical canal to permit the extra-amniotic instillation of estrogens and prostaglandins, were found to be effective without the pharmacological agent. Potential advantages of mechanical methods, compared with pharmacological methods, may include simplicity of preservation, lower cost and reduction in the side-effects. However, there are drawbacks and contraindications, for example risk of infection and maternal discomfort.

A meta-analysis (Boulvain *et al.*, 2001) of 45 studies comparing mechanical methods with placebo/no treatment, usually in women with unfavourable cervices and intact membranes, shows that the risk of caesarean section is similar between groups; hyperstimulation with fetal heart rate changes is not reported. There are no reported cases of severe neonatal and maternal morbidity.

Compared with PGE_2 and misoprostol, the effectiveness of mechanical methods appears to be similar. There is no difference in the risk of caesarean section between mechanical methods and prostaglandins.

Relaxin

Relaxin is a 6-kDa peptide of the insulin family that is present at increased levels in the circulation during pregnancy. The protein promotes connective tissue remodelling (Mushayandebvu and Rajabi, 1995), which allows cervical ripening and separation of the pelvic symphysis in various mammalian species. In the rat, PGE_2 stimulates eosinophilic invasion, and relaxin promotes a widespread reorganisation of collagen fibres (Too *et al.*, 1986). There is evidence for action on monocytic cells (Parsell *et al.*, 1996), THP-1. Relaxin triggered intracellular signalling events. Other members of the insulin-like family of proteins (insulin, insulin-like growth factors I and II and relaxin-like factor) were unable to displace the binding of relaxin to THP-1 cells, suggesting that a distinct receptor for relaxin exists on this monocyte/macrophage cell line.

Nitric oxide (NO) donors

There is evidence for the existence of a NO system within the human uterine cervix and a role for NO in the control of cervical function and relaxation of cervical smooth muscle (Ekerhovd *et al.*, 2000). NO causes morphological changes similar to those seen during spontaneous cervical ripening. Increased expression of NO synthase isoforms (Ali *et al.*, 1997) in late pregnancy supports the hypothesis that NO is involved in the process of cervical ripening. Ripening due to NO may be mediated in part via increased (Selvemini *et al.*, 1993; Ledingham *et al.*, 1999) $PGF_{2\alpha}$ synthesis, PGE_2 and cyclic guanosine monophosphate (Ekerhovd *et al.*, 2002). NO enhances matrix metalloprotein (MMP-1) production by cervical fibroblasts (Yoshida *et al.*, 2001).

NO donors may provide an alternative to prostaglandins for cervical ripening. Sodium nitroprusside applied into the cervical canal induces a rapid and significant softening of the cervix (Facchinetti *et al.*, 2000), and isosorbide mononitrate and glyceryl trinitrate can effect cervical ripening like the prostaglandin analogue gemeprost. However, no advantage has been demonstrated by combining isosorbide mononitrate with misoprostol compared with misoprostol alone for preoperative cervical ripening in the first trimester (Ledingham *et al.*, 2001).

COX inhibitors

Cervical application of the cyclo-oxygenase (COX) 2 inhibitor nimesulide prevents the physiological process of cervical ripening in late pregnancy (Bukowski *et al.*, 2001). The inhibition is not the result of changes in cross-linked collagen content. Inhibition of cervical ripening with locally administered COX 2 inhibitors may be a potentially valuable treatment for patients at risk of preterm delivery. Indomethacin compares favourably with tocolytics. Side-effects on the fetal ductus arteriosus and kidney are the main concerns regarding their wider use (Butler-O'Hara and D'Angio, 2002; Suarez *et al.*, 2002).

CONCLUSION

In everyday practice, paradoxes present themselves that indicate the importance of the cervix and provide clues to future research. An understanding of the molecular physiology of cervical ripening can provide the means to manipulate cervical resistance as required, to increase it to delay premature delivery and to reduce it to facilitate delivery. Although efficient ripening agents are available, they tend to stimulate myometrial activity. While this may be desirable for inducing labour, it may be a drawback when the fetus is compromised or when the myometrium is already active but the cervix is unresponsive. Control over the powers that drive labour has not provided the answers to common clinical problems. To solve these, perhaps a similar degree of control has to be achieved over resistance to delivery. The cervix is the key.

REFERENCES

Ali M, Buhimschi I, Chwalisz K *et al.* (1997) Changes in expression of the nitric oxide synthase isoforms in rat uterus and cervix during pregnancy and parturition. *Molecular Human Reproduction* 3: 995–1003.

Allman AC, Genevier ES, Johnson MR *et al.* (1996a) Head-to-cervix force: an important physiological variable in labour. 1. The temporal relation between head-to-cervix force and intrauterine pressure during labour. *British Journal of Obstetrics and Gynaecology* 103: 763–768.

Allman, AC, Genevier, ES, Johnson, MR *et al.* (1996b) Head-to-cervix force: an important physiological variable in labour. 2. Peak active force, peak active pressure and mode of delivery. *British Journal of Obstetrics & Gynaecology* 103: 769–775.

Allport VC, Pieber D, Slater DM *et al.* (2001) Human labour is associated with nuclear factor-kappaB activity which mediates cyclo-oxygenase-2 expression and is involved with the 'functional progesterone withdrawal'. *Molecular Human Reproduction* 7: 581–586.

Al-Shawaf T, Moghraby SA, Al-Meshari AA (1987) Normal levels of uterine activity in primigravidae and mothers of high parity in spontaneous labour. *Journal of Obstetrics and Gynecology* 8: 18–23.

Aspden RM (1988) The theory of fibre-reinforced composite materials applied to changes in the mechanical properties of the cervix during pregnancy. *Journal of Theoretical Biology* 130: 213–221.

Beazley JM (1972) Use of partograms in labor. *Proceedings of the Royal Society of Medicine* 65: 700.

Beazley JM, Alderman B (1976) The 'inductograph' – a graph describing the limits of the latent phase of labour. *British Journal of Obstetrics and Gynaecology* 83: 513–517.

Beazley JM, Kurjak A (1972) Influence of a partograph on the active management of labour. *Lancet* 2: 348–351.

Belayet HM, Kanayama N, Khatun S *et al.* (1999) Dehydroepiandrosterone sulphate promotes hyaluronic acid-induced cervical ripening in rabbits. *Human Reproduction* 14: 1361–1367.

Boulvain M, Kelly A, Lohse C *et al.* (2001) Mechanical methods for induction of labour. *Cochrane Database of Systematic Reviews* 4.

Bukowski R, Mackay L, Fittkow C *et al.* (2001) Inhibition of cervical ripening by local application of cyclooxygenase 2 inhibitor. *American Journal of Obstetrics and Gynecology* 184: 1374–1378; discussion 1378–1379.

Butler-O'Hara M, D'Angio CT (2002) Risk of persistent renal insufficiency in premature infants following the use of indomethacin for suppression of preterm labor. *Journal of Perinatology* 22: 541–546.

Calder AA (1994) Prostaglandins and biological control of cervical function. *Australian and New Zealand Journal of Obstetrics and Gynaecology* 34: 347–351.

Cammu H, Van Eeckhout E (1996) A randomised controlled trial of early versus delayed use of amniotomy and oxytocin infusion in nulliparous labour. *British Journal of Obstetrics and Gynaecology* 103: 313–318.

Cardozo LD, Gibb DM, Studd JW *et al.* (1982) Predictive value of cervimetric labour patterns in primigravidae. *British Journal of Obstetrics and Gynaecology* 89: 33–38.

Chelmow D, Kilpatrick SJ, Laros RK (1993) Maternal and neonatal outcomes after prolonged latent phase. *Obstetrics and Gynecology* 81: 486–491.

Cook CM, Ellwood DA (2000) The cervix as a predictor of preterm delivery in 'at-risk' women. *Ultrasound in Obstetrics and Gynecology* 15: 109–113.

Coomarasamy A, Knox EM, Gee H *et al.* (2002) Oxytocin antagonists for tocolysis in preterm labour — a systematic review. *Medical Science Monitoring* 8: 269–273.

Danforth DN (1947) The fibrous nature of the human cervix and its relation to the isthmic segment in gravid and nongravid uteri. *American Journal of Obstetrics and Gynecology* 53: 541–557.

Danforth DN (1954) The distribution and functional activity of the cervical musculature. *American Journal of Obstetrics and Gynecology* 68: 1261–1271.

Denison FC, Calder AA, Kelly RW (1999) The effect of mifepristone administration on leukocyte populations, matrix metalloproteinases and inflammatory mediators in the first trimester cervix. *American Journal of Obstetrics and Gynecology* 180: 614–620.

Denison FC, Riley SC, Elliott CL *et al.* (2000) The action of prostaglandin E2 on the human cervix: stimulation of interleukin 8 and inhibition of secretory leukocyte protease inhibitor. The distribution and functional activity of the cervical musculature. *Molecular Human Reproduction* 6: 541–548.

Ekerhovd E, Brannstrom M, Weijdegard B *et al.* (2000) Nitric oxide synthases in the human cervix at term pregnancy and effects of nitric oxide on cervical smooth muscle contractility. *American Journal of Obstetrics and Gynecology* 183: 610–616.

Ekerhovd E, Weijdegard B, Brannstrom M *et al.* (2002) Nitric oxide induced cervical ripening in the human: Involvement of cyclic guanosine monophosphate, prostaglandin F(2α), and prostaglandin E(2). *American Journal of Obstetrics and Gynecology* 186: 745–750.

Ekman G, Malmstrom A, Uldbjerg N *et al.* (1986) Cervical collagen: an important regulator of cervical function in term labor. *Obstetrics and Gynecology* 67: 633–636.

Ellwood DA, Mitchell MD, Anderson ABM *et al.* (1980) The in vitro production of prostanoids by the human cervix during pregnancy: Preliminary observations. *British Journal of Obstetrics and Gynaecology* 87: 210–214.

El-Sherbiny MT, El-Gharieb IH and Gewely HA (2001) Vaginal misoprostol for induction of labor: 25 vs. 50 microg dose regimen. *International Journal of Gynaecology and Obstetrics* 72: 25–30.

Facchinetti F, Piccinini F, Volpe A (2000) Chemical ripening of the cervix with intracervical application of sodium nitroprusside: a randomized controlled trial. *Human Reproduction* 15: 2224–2227.

Fietzek PP, Kuhn K (1976) The primary structure of collagen. *International Review of Connective Tissue* 7: 1–60.

Friedman EA (1954) The graphic analysis of labor. *American Journal of Obstetrics and Gynecology* 68: 1568–1575.

Friedman EA (1955) Labor in multiparas. *Obstetrics and Gynecology* 6: 567–589.

Friedman E (1956) Primigravid labor. *Obstetrics and Gynecology* 8: 691–703.

Friedman EA (1967) *Labor Clinical Evaluation and Management.* New York: Meredith.

Friedman EA, Kroll BH (1971) Computer analysis of labor progression. IV. Diagnosis of secondary arrest of dilatation. *Journal of Reproductive Medicine* 7: 176–178.

Friedman EA, Niswander KR, Sachtleben MR *et al.* (1969) Dysfunctional labor. 8. Relative accuracy of clinical and graphic diagnostic methods. *Obstetrics and Gynecology* 33: 145–152.

Frigoletto, FDJ, Lieberman E, JM L *et al.* (1995) A clinical trial of active management of labor. *New England Journal of Medicine* 333: 745–750.

Fujimoto T, Savani RC, Watari M *et al.* (1995) Induction of the hyaluronic acid-binding protein, tumor necrosis factor-stimulated gene-6, in cervical smooth muscle cells by tumor necrosis factor-[alpha] and prostaglandin E2. *American Journal of Pathology* 160: 1495–1502.

Gee H (1982) Uterine activity and cervical resistance determining cervical change in labour. Unpublished MD thesis. Liverpool: University of Liverpool.

Gee H (1983) The interaction between cervix and corpus uteri in the generation of intra-amniotic pressure in labour. *European Journal of Obstetrics, Gynecology and Reproductive Biology* 16: 243–252.

Gee H (1994a) Trials of labor. *Contemporary Review of Obstetrics and Gynaecology* 6: 31–35.

Gee H (1994b) The cervix in labour. *Contemporary Review of Obstetrics and Gynaecology* 6: 84–88.

Gee H, Taylor EW, Hancox R (1988) A model for the generation of intra-uterine pressure in the human parturient uterus which demonstrates the critical role of the cervix. *Journal of Theoretical Biology* 133: 281–291.

Goldenberg RL (2002) The management of preterm labor. *Obstetrics and Gynecology* 100: 1020–1037.

Gough GW, Randall NJ, Genevier ES *et al.* (1990) Head-to-cervix forces and their relationship to the outcome of labor. *Obstetrics and Gynecology* 75: 613–618.

Granstrom L, Ekman G, Ulmsten U *et al.* (1989) Changes in the connective tissue of corpus and cervix uteri during ripening and labour in term pregnancy. *British Journal of Obstetrics and Gynaecology* 96: 1198–1202.

Granstrom L, Ekman G, Malmstrom A (1991) Insufficient remodelling of the uterine connective tissue in women with protracted labour. *British Journal of Obstetrics and Gynaecology* 98: 1212–1216.

Granstrom LM, Ekman GE, Malmstrom A *et al.* (1992) Serum collagenase levels in relation to the state of the human cervix during pregnancy and labor. *American Journal of Obstetrics and Gynecology* 167: 1284–1288.

Harkness MLR, Harkness RD (1959) Changes in the physical properties of the uterine cervix of the rat during pregnancy. *Journal of Physiology* 148: 524–547.

Hebisch G, Grauaug AA, Neumaier-Wagner PM *et al.* (2001) The relationship between cervical dilatation, interleukin-6 and interleukin-8 during term labor. *Acta Obstetrica et Gynecologica Scandinavica* 80: 840–848.

Hendricks CH, Brenner WE, Kraus G (1970) Normal cervical dilatation pattern in late pregnancy and labor. *American Journal of Obstetrics and Gynecology* 106: 1065–1082.

Hill DA, Chez RA, Quinlan J *et al.* (2000) Uterine rupture and dehiscence associated with intravaginal misoprostol cervical ripening. *Journal of Reproductive Medicine* 45: 823–826.

Hofmeyr GJ, Gulmezoglu AM (2001) Vaginal misoprostol for cervical ripening and induction of labour. *Cochrane Database of Systematic Reviews* 2.

Hofmeyr GJ, Gulmezoglu AM (2002) Vaginal misoprostol for cervical ripening and labour induction in late pregnancy. *Cochrane Database of Systematic Reviews* 3.

Hughesdon PE (1952) The fibromuscular structure of the cervix and its changes during pregnancy and labour. *Journal of Obstetrics and Gynaecology of the British Empire* 59: 763–776.

Junqueira LCU, Zugaib M, Montes GS *et al.* (1980) Morphological and histochemical evidence for the occurrence of collagenolysis and for the role of neutrophilic polymorphonuclear leukocytes during cervical dilation. *American Journal of Obstetrics and Gynecology* 138: 273–281.

Kiwanuka AI, Moore WMO (1987) The changing incidence of caesarean section in the Health District of Central Manchester. *British Journal of Obstetrics and Gynaecology* 94: 440–444.

Kleissl HP, van der Rest M, Naftolin F *et al.* (1978) Collagen changes in the human uterine cervix at parturition. *American Journal of Obstetrics and Gynecology* 130: 748–753.

Kulkarni S, LaGrenade L (1992) Ehlers–Danlos syndrome in pregnancy. *West Indian Medical Journal* 41: 86–87.

Ledingham MA, Denison FC, Kelly RW *et al.* (1999) Nitric oxide donors stimulate prostaglandin F(2α) and inhibit thromboxane B(2) production in the human cervix during the first trimester of pregnancy. *Molecular Human Reproduction* 5: 973–982.

Ledingham MA, Thomson AJ, Lunan CB *et al.* (2001) A comparison of isosorbide mononitrate, misoprostol and combination therapy for first trimester pre-operative cervical ripening: a randomised controlled trial. *British Journal of Obstetrics and Gynaecology* 108: 276–280.

Lind J, Wallenburg HC (2002) Pregnancy and the Ehlers–Danlos syndrome: a retrospective study in a Dutch population. *Acta Obstetrica et Gynecologica Scandinavica* 81: 293–300.

Lindgren CLS (1961) Measurement and interpretation of the pressures upon the cervix during normal and abnormal labour. *Journal of Obstetrics and Gynaecology of the British Commonwealth* 68: 901–915.

Lukoschus H, Nierhaus M, Vetter K (2002) Misoprostol in gynaecology and obstetrics. *Gynakologische Praxis* 26: 9–21.

Luque EH, Muñoz de Toro MM, Ramos JG *et al.* (1998) Role of relaxin and estrogen in the control of eosinophilic invasion and collagen remodeling in rat cervical tissue at term. *Biology of Reproduction* 59: 795–800.

Maillot KV, Zimmermann BK (1976) The solubility of collagen of the uterine cervix during pregnancy and labour. *Archiv fur Gynakologie* 220: 275–280.

Minor RR, Sippola-Thiele M, McKeon J *et al.* (1986) Defects in the processing of procollagen to collagen are demonstrable in cultured fibroblasts from patients with the Ehlers–Danlos and osteogenesis imperfecta syndromes. *Journal of Biological Chemistry* 261: 10006–10014.

Mushayandebvu TI, Rajabi MR (1995) Relaxin stimulates interstitial collagenase activity in cultured uterine cervical cells from nonpregnant and pregnant but not immature guinea pigs; estradiol-17β restores relaxin's effect in immature cervical cells. *Biology of Reproduction* 53: 1030–1037.

O'Driscoll K, Jackson JA, Gallagher JT (1969) Prevention of prolonged labour. *British Medical Journal* 2: 447–480.

Olah KS (1994) The use of magnetic resonance imaging in the assessment of the cervical hydration state. *British Journal of Obstetrics and Gynaecology* 101: 255–257.

Olah KS, Gee H (1992) The prevention of pre-term delivery: Can we afford to continue to ignore the cervix? *British Journal of Obstetrics and Gynaecology* 99: 278–280.

Olah KS, Gee H (1996) The active mismanagement of labour. *British Journal of Obstetrics and Gynaecology* 103: 729–731.

Olah KS, Gee H, Brown JS (1993) Cervical contractions: the response of the cervix to oxytocic stimulation in the latent phase of labour. *British Journal of Obstetrics and Gynaecology* 100: 635–640.

Osmers R, Rath W, Pflanz MA *et al.* (1993) Glycosaminoglycans in cervical connective tissue during pregnancy and parturition. *Obstetrics and Gynecology* 81: 88–92.

Osmers R, Rath W, Adelmann-Grill BC *et al.* (1995) Origin of cervical collagenase during parturition. *American Journal of Obstetrics & Gynecology* 166: 1455–1460.

Pajntar M, Roskar E, Rudel, D (1987) Electromyographic observations on the human cervix during labor. *American Journal of Obstetrics and Gynecology* 156: 691–697.

Pajntar M, Leskosek B, Rudel D *et al.* (2001) Contribution of cervical smooth muscle activity to the duration of latent and active phases of labour. *British Journal of Obstetrics and Gynaecology* 108: 533–538.

Parsell DA, Mak JY, Amento EP *et al.* (1996) Relaxin binds to and elicits a response from cells of the human monocytic cell line, THP-1. *Journal of Biological Chemistry* 271: 27936–27941.

Philpott RH, Castle WM (1972a) Cervicographs in the management of labour in primigravidae. I. The alert line for detecting abnormal labour. *Journal of Obstetrics and Gynaecology of the British Commonwealth* 79: 599–602.

Philpott RH, Castle WM (1972b) Cervicographs in the management of labour in primigravidae. II. The action line and treatment of abnormal labour. *Journal of Obstetrics and Gynaecology of the British Empire* 79: 592–598.

Radestad A, Thyberg J, Christensen NJ (1993) Cervical ripening with mifepristone (RU 486) in first trimester abortion. An electron microscope study. *Human Reproduction* 8: 1136–1142.

Rajabi MR, Dodge GR, Solomon S *et al.* (1991) Immunochemical and immunohistochemical evidence of estrogen-mediated collagenolysis as a mechanism of cervical dilatation in the guinea pig at parturition. *Endocrinology* 128: 371–378.

Ramos JG, Varayoud J, Kass L *et al.* (2000) Estrogen and progesterone modulation of eosinophilic infiltration of the rat uterine cervix. *Steroids* 65: 409–414.

Rath W, Osmers R, Stuhlsatz HW *et al.* (1994) Biochemical fundamentals of cervical ripending and dilatation. *Zeitschrift fur Geburtshilfe und Perinatologie* 198: 186–195.

Rechberger TWJF (1993) Collagenase, its inhibitors, and decorin in the lower uterine segment in pregnant women. *American Journal of Obstetrics and Gynecology* 168: 1598–1603.

Rosen MG, Dickinson JC (1990) Vaginal birth after cesarean: a meta-analysis of indicators for success. *Obstetrics and Gynecology* 76: 865–869.

Rozenberg P, Gillet A, Ville Y (2002) Transvaginal sonographic examination of the cervix in asymptomatic pregnant women: review of the literature. *Ultrasound in Obstetrics and Gynecology* 19: 302–311.

Ruoslahti E (1988) Structure and biology of proteoglycans. *Annual Review of Cell Biology* 4: 29–55.

Sanchez-Ramos L, Kaunitz AM, Delke I (2002) Labor induction with 25 microg versus 50 microg intravaginal misoprostol: a systematic review. *Obstetrics and Gynecology* 99: 145–151.

Selvemini D, Misko TP, Masferrer JL *et al.* (1993) Nitric oxide activates cyclooxygenase enzymes. *Proceedings of the National Academy of Science USA* 90: 7240–7244.

Sennstrom MB, Ekman G, Westergren-Thorsson G *et al.* (2000) Human cervical ripening, an inflammatory process mediated by cytokines. *Molecular Human Reproduction* 6: 375–381.

Sisi P, Li F, Gee H *et al.* (1995) In: Cervical ripening mediated by vascular endothelial growth factor. *Meeting of the Growth Factor Group.* London.

Smith GCS, Wu WX, Nathanielsz PW (2000) Effects of gestational age and labor on the expression of prostanoid receptor genes in the pregnant baboon cervix. *Prostaglandins* 63: 153–163.

Sorokin Y, Johnson MP, Rogowski N *et al.* (1994) Obstetric and gynecologic dysfunction in the Ehlers–Danlos syndrome. *Journal of Reproductive Medicine* 39: 281–284.

Steer PJ, Little DJ, Lewis NL *et al.* (1975) Uterine activity in induced labour. *British Journal of Obstetrics and Gynaecology* 82: 433–441.

Stevens J (1977) In: Black MM, English MJ (eds) Uniaxial tensile testing of cervical tissue in vitro in relation to dilatation of the cervix. *Physical Science Techniques in Obstetrics and Gynaecology.* London: Pitman Press, p. 47.

Studd J (1973) Partograms and nomograms of cervical dilatation in management of primigravid labour. *British Medical Journal* 4: 451–455.

Stygar D, Wang H, Vladic YS *et al.* (2001) Co-localization of oestrogen receptor [β] and leukocyte markers in the human cervix. *Molecular Human Reproduction* 7: 881–886.

Suarez VR, Thompson LL, Jain V *et al.* (2002) The effect of in utero exposure to indomethacin on the need for surgical closure of a patent ductus arteriosus in the neonate. *American Journal of Obstetrics and Gynaecology* 187: 886–888.

Sugano T, Narahara H, Nasu K *et al.* (2001) Effects of platelet-activating factor on cytokine production by human uterine cervical fibroblasts. *Molecular Human Reproduction* 7: 475–481.

Thomas J, Kelly AJ, Kavanagh J (2001) Oestrogens alone or with amniotomy for cervical ripening or induction of labour. *Cochrane Database of Systematic Reviews* 4.

Thornton, JG and Lilford, RJ (1994) Active management of labour: current knowledge and research issues. *British Medical Journal* 309: 366–369.

Too CKL, Kong JK, Greenwood FC *et al.* (1986) The effect of oestrogen and relaxin on uterine and cervical enzymes: collagenase, proteoglycanase and beta-glycuronidase. *Acta Endocrinologica* 111: 394–403.

Tromans PM (1981) A comparative study of oestradiol and prostaglandin E2 vaginal gel for ripening the unfavourable cervix before induction of labour. *British Medical Journal* 282: 679.

UK Amniotomy Group (1994) A multicentre randomised trial of amniotomy in spontaneous first labour at term. *British Journal of Obstetrics and Gynaecology* 101: 307–309.

Wang H, Stjernholm Y, Ekman G *et al.* (2001) Different regulation of oestrogen receptors [alpha] and [beta] in the human cervix at term pregnancy. *Molecular Human Reproduction* 7: 293–300.

Wing DA, Fassett MJ, Mishell DR (2000) Mifepristone for preinduction cervical ripening beyond 41 weeks' gestation: a randomized controlled trial. *Obstetrics & Gynecology* 96: 543–548.

Winkler M, Rath W (1999) Changes in the cervical extracellular matrix during pregnancy and parturition. *Journal of Perinatal Medicine* 27: 45–60.

Winkler M, Rath W (2001) Cervical ripening and dilatation as a molecular process. *Gynakologie* 34: 510–520.

Witter FR (2000) Prostaglandin E2 preparations for preinduction cervical ripening. *Clinical Obstetrics and Gynecology* 43: 469–474.

Yoshida K, Tahara R, Nakayama T *et al.* (1993) Effect of dehydroepiandrosterone sulphate, oestrogens and prostaglandins on collagen metabolism in human cervical tissue in relation to cervical ripening. *Journal of International Medical Research* 21: 26–35.

Yoshida M, Sagawa N, Itoh H *et al.* (2001) Nitric oxide increases matrix metalloproteinase-1 production in human uterine cervical fibroblast cells. *Molecular Human Reproduction* 7: 979–985.

Young A, Thomson AJ, Ledingham M *et al.* (2002) Immunolocalization of proinflammatory cytokines in myometrium, cervix, and fetal membranes during human parturition at term. *Biology of Reproduction* 66: 445–449.

CHAPTER 14

The incompetent cervix

Roy G. Farquharson

INTRODUCTION

The clinical entity of cervical incompetence represents an enigma of medical understanding. Wherever there is a dearth of fact and knowledge within clinical practice, the vacuum is filled by unsubstantiated opinion and emotional debate. When reproducible and verifiable evidence is produced, clarity and calm can appear. The area of cervical incompetence remains a vacuum with a poorly reproducible basis for methodological diagnosis, treatment interventions based on quasi-randomised, small-scale studies and a complex case mix of clinical presentation.

From this beginning, the chapter will attempt to describe the historical path of diagnosis, assessment of recent surgical treatments and the emerging importance of multiple pathology that causes the late loss of pregnancy between 12 and 24 weeks associated with cervical incompetence.

The historical recognition of cervical incompetence has an undoubted pedigree as well as being an overdiagnosed condition. In 1658, Grant gave a tentative description of possible cause and effect:

> . . . The orifice of the womb is so slack that it cannot rightly contract itself to keep in the seed; which is chiefly caused by abortion or hard labour or childbirth, whereby the fibres of the womb are broken in pieces from one another and they, and the inner orifice of the womb overmuch slackened.

For the purposes of this chapter, a representative sample of the literature has been culled to reflect the changing views during the past four decades. An extensive and critical review (Romero *et al.*, 2006) assesses the new techniques which can be used to identify those patients who will benefit from cervical cerclage.

DIAGNOSIS

The classical description of cervical incompetence is alleged to cause midtrimester loss (MTL) or premature labour which, in turn, is precipitated by rupture of the membranes and which proceeds painlessly. As questioned by Jeffcoate (1975), 'this classical description is not supported by the facts'. For

example, there may be no history of prior pregnancy, trauma or operation. Those women with 'a gaping cervix' do not necessarily miscarry and, when midtrimester loss does occur, the process can be associated with pain and bleeding. This fulsome clinical description attracted the idea of a functional or inherent defect, which still carries weight more than 25 years later. Perhaps it is time to rename the condition cervical weakness rather than incompetence in view of the variable functional element of clinical appearance rather than an absolute physical entity, which fails to be measured accurately by investigative assessment. In addition, the word incompetence carries non-politically correct associations and holds aspects of personal denigration for the patient concerned. Following critical appraisal, these features have recently been highlighted and supported as well as endorsing the need for change in nomenclature (Harger, 2002).

Gestation of pregnancy loss

Early (< 12 weeks)

Cervical incompetence has been considered aetiological in early pregnancy loss (Edmonds, 1988), leading to a treatment intervention trial in early pregnancy with cerclage insertion before 7 weeks' gestation. Although this small study found a high cure rate, the absence of preconceptual investigation and treatment randomisation weakens the case for use in early pregnancy loss with non-verifiable effectiveness.

The recognition of cervical incompetence as the primary cause of preterm labour and delivery has had firm believers. The recent use of transvaginal ultrasound (TVU) in the assessment of cervical length, dilatation or shortening has been described when compared against the known physiological shortening process of advancing gestation (Fig. 14.1). During pregnancy, several authors, with a view to early detection of signs and treatment intervention, have studied this area intensively (Rozenberg *et al.*, 2002). The consensus seems to suggest that cervical length measurement (CLM) is best reserved for those high-risk groups with a significant MTL history and that CLM should be performed at 20–24 weeks. There is an inverse correlation between CLM and preterm

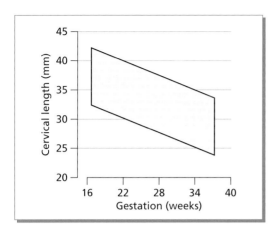

Fig. 14.1 Cervical length changes during pregnancy using TVU (Murakawa *et al.*, 1993).

delivery (Iams *et al.*, 1996). However, there is a high negative predictive value if CLM is applied as a screening tool.

In addition, screening is worthwhile only if an effective therapy is available. A retrospective study of observation versus intervention in the same unit showed a similar preterm delivery (< 33 weeks) rate of 21% vs. 26% and no significant difference in mean gestational age at delivery (34.6 vs. 34.4 weeks) between both groups, totalling 177 patients (Berghella *et al.*, 2002). A recent review by the same author states that transvaginal ultrasound is an effective way to predict preterm birth, especially when a cervical length of below 25 mm is found between 16 and 24 weeks' gestation (Berghella, 2004). In addition, transabdominal pressure over the midtrimester uterine fundus for 15 seconds may reveal evidence of funnelling as well as a shortened cervical length (Fig. 14.2).

In a prospective study of 64 women, Airoldi *et al.* (2005) have shown that in women with uterine anomalies, a cervical length of less than 25 mm, as shown by ultrasound scan, carries a risk of preterm birth that is 13 times greater than normal. The sensitivity, specificity, and positive and negative predictive values of a short cervical length were 71%, 91%, 50%, and 96% respectively (RR 13.5, 95% CI 3.49–54.74).

Investigation of midtrimester loss (12–24 weeks)

In modern practice, the diagnosis of cervical incompetence involves adherence to a strict investigation protocol (Fig. 14.3) to exclude conditions and diseases that are known to contribute to second trimester miscarriage (Fig. 14.4). An important consideration is that an underlying cause for late pregnancy loss may be present in isolation (40%) or combined (10%) or absent in 50% despite intensive investigation. Women undergoing investigation of MTL represent a heterogeneous group, displaying widely varying presentation and aetiology. In addition, the ascertainment of possible multiple pathologies must always be considered in a woman with repeated second trimester miscarriage (Drakeley *et al.*, 1998).

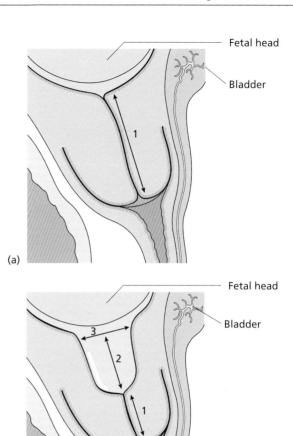

(a)

(b)

Fig. 14.2 Illustration showing the normal cervix (a) and a short cervix (b) with significant funnelling. The latter is associated with cervical weakness. Ultrasonic characteristics of these cervices assesses (1) cervical length; (2) funnel length; (3) funnel width.

To determine the presence of cervical incompetence, a careful history and detailed assessment of the sequence of events leading up to late pregnancy loss becomes absolutely essential. Clear description and accurate history will provide a powerful analysis of potential cause and help in counselling as well as planned pregnancy management in the future (Table 14.1).

Cervical weakness (incompetence)

As stated by the Euro-Team Early Pregnancy protocol (Berry *et al.*, 1995), there is no agreed definition of cervical weakness by absolute measurable and reproducible criteria. It is important that, before cervical weakness is confirmed, certain diagnostic criteria are applied and other causes excluded, as resultant management is invasive and carries a recurrence risk of an adverse outcome.

A consensus definition that is frequently used includes painless dilatation of the cervix (Fig. 14.5) followed by ruptured

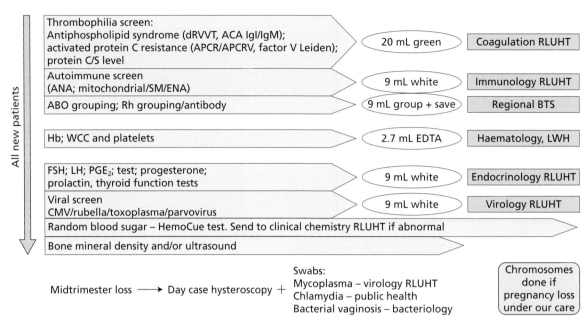

Fig. 14.3 List of investigations performed in miscarriage clinic. ACA, anticardiolipin antibody; ANA, antinuclear antibody; CMV, cytomegalovirus; dRVVT, dilute Russel viper venom time; ENA, extractable nuclear antibody; FSH, follicle-stimulating hormone, LH, luteinising hormone; WCC, white cell count; BTS, blood transfusion service; RLUHT, Royal Liverpool University Hospitals Trust.

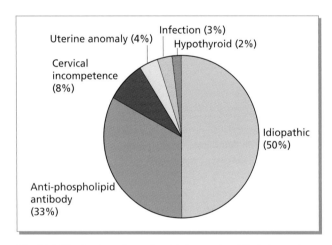

Fig. 14.4 Distribution of cause in midtrimester loss (Drakeley *et al.*, 1998).

Table 14.1 Analysis of causes of midtrimester loss.

History questions
Time order of event sequence *essential*, e.g. bleeding, pain, ruptured
  membranes, cervical dilatation
Detail each miscarriage in chronological order
Gestation at time of miscarriage
Was a fetal heart observed on ultrasound scan and until what gestation?
Was the miscarriage painful (like labour pains) or painless?
Was evacuation of the uterus required or repeated?
Was cytogenetic placental/fetal testing ever done to investigate the cause?
Is there a family history of thrombophilia, e.g. mother or sister?
Previous history of thromboembolic event?

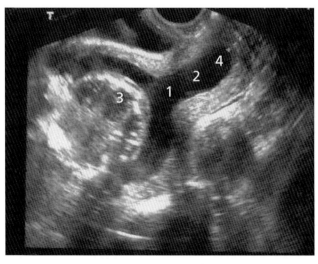

Fig. 14.5 Transvaginal scan at 16 weeks' gestation demonstrating open internal os (1) and full cervical length dilatation (2) due to cervical weakness with fetal head above (3). Salvage cerclage revealed bulging membranes (4) on speculum examination prior to suture insertion. The patient delivered eventually at 26 weeks, resulting in a live birth.

membranes, resulting in second trimester miscarriage or extreme preterm delivery. An example of such a case is illustrated in Figure 14.5.

In the non-pregnant state, the passage, without resistance, of a size 9 Hegar dilator through the cervix acts as a surrogate measure. A recent definition for entry into a controlled treatment trial includes the initial painless, progressive dilatation of the uterine cervix, where preterm delivery seems inevitable without interference. The diagnosis is made in the absence of other causes of preterm delivery such as uterine anomaly, fibroids or infection (*vide infra*) and where only singleton pregnancies are included (Althuisius *et al.*, 2001). As has been written recently as the premise for another randomised controlled trial, 'the overuse of prophylactic cerclage is a manifestation of our inability to diagnose cervical incompetence with any degree of reliability on the basis of historical criteria alone' (Rust *et al.*, 2000).

Uterine anomalies

The urogenital system develops from a common mesodermal ridge (intermediate mesoderm) along the posterior wall of the abdominal cavity and, initially, the excretory ducts of both systems enter a common cavity, the cloaca. Duplication of the uterus results from a lack of fusion of the paramesonephric ducts, in a localised area or throughout the length of the ducts. In its extreme form, the uterus is entirely double (uterus didelphys); in the least severe form, it is only slightly indented in the middle (uterus arcuatus). One of the more common anomalies is the uterus bicornis, in which the uterus has two horns entering a common vagina. This condition is normal in many mammals below the primates. The uterine septum should normally disappear by the end of the third month of embryonic life (Sadler, 1995).

In 1931, Smith reported one case of double uterus for every 7040 consecutive obstetric patients in New York from 1899 to 1924. Having taken an interest in the finding, Smith's detection rate for the years 1925 to 1930 increased the reported incidence by five times. Harger *et al.* (1993) reported an incidence of 27% of uterine anomalies in their data set of late miscarriage patients. Miscarriage can occur where there is only limited uterine space available, at a point when the semi-uterus is unable to expand further (Strassman, 1966) or when implantation occurs into an avascular septum (DeCherney *et al.*, 1986).

The mode of diagnosis for uterine anomalies has evolved with time. In the past, hysterosalpingography was the mainstay of investigation, but it is painful and is limited by a two-dimensional image. Pelvic ultrasound is highly specific for uterine anomaly, is non-invasive and may be suitable for screening purposes (Clifford *et al.*, 1993). Magnetic resonance imaging (MRI) has been proposed for the same reason, although it is much more expensive (Kirk *et al.*, 1993). Hysteroscopy is now widely used for directly visualising septal defects and intra-uterine synechiae, which can be combined with laparoscopy to assess fundal dimpling.

Fibroids

The role of leiomyomata in MTL is also unclear. Proposed theories suggest that fibroids in pregnancy can show rapid growth and undergo red degeneration, causing the uterus to become irritable, and that they alter the oxytocinase activity, endometrial stroma or vasculature (Buttram and Reiter, 1981). Large submucous and intramural fibroids can compromise placental implantation, especially midtrimester second-wave trophoblast invasion, leading to late miscarriage associated with cervical incompetence.

Infection

The role of infection in the aetiology of miscarriage appears to be in the second trimester rather than the first (Oakeshott *et al.*, 2002). Bacterial vaginosis (BV) is known to contribute to late fetal loss (Llahi-Camp *et al.*, 1996). The most sensitive and specific method of diagnosing BV is by examining a Gram stain of a vaginal smear for clue cells. Ideally, this should be done in the first quarter of the menstrual cycle when levels are highest. A positive diagnosis should be treated with intravaginal clindamycin or, alternatively, with a combination of oral erythromycin and metronidazole (Adinkra and Lamont, 2002). Infrequently, other pathogens, such as *Chlamydia* or *Mycoplasma*, can be detected with cervical swabs.

Recently, a study (Gomez *et al.*, 2005) has shown that there is a relationship between ultrasonically determined cervical length and the presence of culture-proven microbial invasion of the amniotic cavity in women who develop preterm labour and who have intact membranes. A total of 401 patients were admitted in preterm labour between 22 and 35 weeks, and the cervix was dilated as assessed at digital examination to be less than 3 cm. Cervical length was assessed by transvaginal ultrasound on admission and the outcome variables with the presence of microbial invasion of the amniotic cavity as defined by the presence of a positive amniotic culture and the occurrence of preterm delivery before 35 weeks. It was shown that the prevalence of microbial invasion of the amniotic cavity was 7% and spontaneous preterm delivery, i.e. under 35 weeks, occurred in 21.4% of the patients. When an ROC (receiver–operator characteristic) curve was analysed, it showed that there was a significant relationship between the frequency of microbial invasion of the amniotic cavity and the length of the uterine cervix. Patients who had a length of the cervix < 15 mm had a higher rate of positive amniotic fluid culture than those with a cervical length of > 15 mm. The difference was significant. Moreover, patients with a cervix under 15 mm, and this was defined as a short cervix, were more likely to deliver before 32 weeks. Forty per cent of patients who had a cervix > 30 mm long had a number of factors in their favour, which included a low risk of spontaneous delivery under 35 weeks. A low risk of microbial invasion of the amniotic cavity also existed in this group.

Recently, the prognostic role of endocervical inflammation has been recognised, with Sakai *et al.* (2006) showing that cerclage reduced preterm labour in women with a short cervix (< 25 mm) and associated low levels of interleukin 8 in cervical mucus between 20 and 24 weeks' gestation. It may increase the likelihood of preterm labour in those cerclaged women with short cervices and elevated interleukin 8 concentrations.

TREATMENT INTERVENTION

Future implications following a second midtrimester loss (MTL)

Subsequent pregnancy outcome after a second trimester miscarriage remains largely unknown, as few studies have generated large numbers of adequately investigated groups for logistic regression analysis and success prediction. Unpublished data from Liverpool following 200 women with recurrent MTL (≥ 1 loss after 12 weeks) would suggest that this is related to the number of associated pathologies identified (Drakeley and Farquharson, 2002). Patients with multiple pathologies are less frequent and, as a result, patient numbers are too small to reach statistical significance (Table 14.2). Nonetheless, a distinct trend for increasing failure is seen with increasing number of pathologies.

Cervical cerclage

Surgical treatment of cervical weakness is aimed at strengthening the internal os in order to maintain the pregnancy. Emmett described the first elective reconstruction of the non-pregnant cervix in 1874 (Emmett, 1874). This technique involved a V-shaped incision to remove the scar from a cervix damaged by obstetric trauma. The surfaces were then apposed with silver wire sutures.

In the twentieth century, Shirodkar (1955) (Fig. 14.6) and McDonald (1957) (Fig. 14.7) described the two classical techniques of vaginal cervical cerclage. In Shirodkar's technique (Fig. 14.6), the bladder is reflected to enable a suture to be placed as close to the internal cervical os as possible per vaginam. Bladder reflection is not required for McDonald's description (Fig. 14.7).

Results

Although there are no comparative studies, the success rate for both types of vaginal suture is similar. The MRC/RCOG trial on cervical cerclage (1993) studied more than 1200 patients and concluded that cerclage is beneficial to patients with three or more pregnancies ending before 37 weeks' gestation (midtrimester losses). Cerclage was also associated with a higher rate of medical intervention, puerperal pyrexia, use of β sympathomimetics, hospital admissions, induction of labour and caesarean section. More recently, a treatment intervention trial randomly assigned 61 women to either cervical cerclage or no cerclage on presentation with ultrasonographically detected second trimester preterm dilatation of the internal os. The study was unable to demonstrate an improved perinatal outcome with cerclage (Rust *et al.*, 2000). The authors proposed a hypothesis that ultrasonographically detectable dilatation of the internal os, prolapse of the membranes into the endocervical canal and shortening of the distal cervix during the second trimester represent a final common pathway of multiple pathophysiological processes, such as infection, immunologically mediated inflammatory stimuli and subclinical abruptio placentae.

At a similar time, the preliminary results of the Dutch CIPRACT treatment trial (Cervical Incompetence Prevention

Table 14.2 Subsequent pregnancy outcome and diagnostic group.

Group	Success rate (%)	Subsequent MTL rate (%)	Early embryo loss rate (%)
Idiopathic ($n = 82$)	78	5	17
Single factor ($n = 59$)	66	12	22
Multiple factor ($n = 13$)	62	23	15

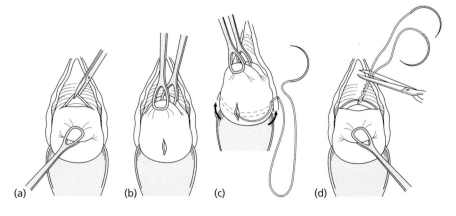

(a)　(b)　(c)　(d)

Fig. 14.6 The technique for repair of an incompetent cervix as described by Shirodkar (1955).

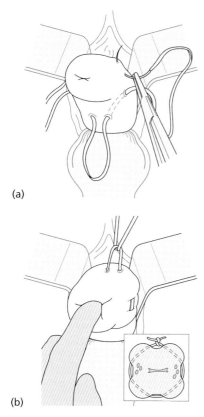

(a)

(b)

Fig. 14.7 Technique used with a McDonald cerclage. (a) A purse-string suture is placed around the cervix and no dissection of the vaginal mucosa is performed. (b) The stitch is tied anteriorly. The operator can place a finger into the external os to assess closure. Transverse section through the cervix is illustrated in an insert, and the location of the cervical vessels as mentioned in the text is seen in the 3 o'clock and 9 o'clock positions.

Randomised Cerclage Trial) showed no significant differences between the prophylactic cerclage group and the observational group in terms of preterm delivery rate at < 34 weeks' gestation and the neonatal survival rate. In this study, patients were initially randomised to cerclage or no cerclage using ultrasound determination of cervical length measurement. In the no cerclage arm, if the cervical length decreased to < 25 mm, the 35 eligible women underwent a second randomisation to either cerclage and bed rest or simply bed rest. Interim results indicated that transvaginal ultrasonographic follow-up examination of the cervix can save the majority of women from unnecessary intervention (Althuisius *et al.*, 2000). The final results showed that therapeutic cerclage with bed rest reduces preterm delivery before 34 weeks' gestation and compound neonatal morbidity, but showed no statistically significant difference in neonatal survival between the two groups (Althuisius *et al.*, 2001). In contrast, screening for short cervical length (< 15 mm, *n* = 470) in a low-risk population (*n* = 47 123) followed by observation or cervical cerclage failed to reduce

the preterm delivery rate before 34 weeks (22% in cerclage vs. 26% in observation group, RR = 0.84, 95% CI 0.54–1.31, *P* = 0.44) (To *et al.*, 2004).

Transabdominal cervical cerclage

In developing an abdominal approach, Benson and Durfee (1965) uniquely reasoned that: 'If cervical cerclage during gestation is indicated but the vaginal approach is impossible, why not accomplish constriction from above?'

When cervical cerclage became widely used for the prevention of MTL, it became apparent that there was a small subgroup of patients for whom the vaginal approach was inappropriate. This group included those patients in whom the cervix was extremely short or absent secondary to a surgical procedure such as cone biopsy, or congenitally deformed as a result of exposure to stilbestrol *in utero*. In addition, those patients whose cervices were markedly scarred or lacerated as a consequence of obstetric trauma or as a result of previously failed vaginal cerclage also fell within this group.

Protocol and technique

The first abdominal procedures, as described by Benson and Durfee in 1965, were performed between 14 and 24 weeks' gestation. At this gestation, a midline incision was used to improve access to the cervical region. Dissection involved opening the broad ligament and mobilisation of the uterine vessels to identify an avascular space through which to pass a 5-mm Mersilene tape. Several series have been published since 1965 (Table 14.3), and modifications in timing of the operation, surgical technique, postoperative management and patient selection have been reported to decrease the morbidity (especially haemorrhage) reported with earlier series and, secondly, to avoid the necessity for a midline scar. The protocol at Liverpool Women's Hospital is described in this chapter, and the first 30 consecutive cases performed from 1994 are reported.

Patient selection

Following a second trimester miscarriage, a detailed history and investigation was undertaken as described above (Fig. 14.3). Following analysis and counselling, those patients with diagnosed cervical weakness were offered transabdominal cerclage when they had a failed elective vaginal cerclage history or where the cervix was so severely damaged that vaginal cerclage was considered impossible. Preconceptual counselling required careful handling and considerable explanation regarding risks of failure, complications of insertion following previous surgery, e.g. classical caesarean section delivery, hourglass constriction of cervix and adjacent major vessels, bowel or bladder damage and the need for two major operations. All factors need to be addressed so that the patient has all relevant information before conception in the knowledge that abdominal cerclage should be seen as a last resort.

Table 14.3 Pregnancy outcome studies following TAC.

Authors	Year	No. of patients	No. of pregnancies	Indications for cerclage	Fetal survival before cerclage (%)	Fetal survival after cerclage (%)
Benson and Durfee	1965	10	13	Shape of cervix, cervicitis	11	82
Mahran	1978	10	10	Shape of cervix and history of failed transvaginal cerclage	10	70
Novy	1982	16	22	Shape of cervix	24	95
Olsen and Tobiassen	1982	17	17	Past obstetric history and shape of cervix	12	88
Herron and Parer	1988	8	13	Shape of cervix and failed cerclage	15	85
Gibb and Salaria	1995	50	61	Shape of cervix or previous failed vaginal cerclage	6.1	85
Cammarano *et al.*	1995	23	29	Shape of cervix or history of failed vaginal cerclage	18	93
Craig and Fleigner	1997	12	14	History and failed vaginal cerclage	17.8	69
Anthony *et al.*	1997	13	13	Previous failed cerclage or shape of cervix	16	86.6
Turnquest *et al.*	1999	11	12	Previous failed vaginal cerclage or anatomical defect	NA	83
Davis *et al.*	2000	82	96	Previous failed vaginal cerclage	NA	82

The procedure

Laparotomy for insertion of a transabdominal cerclage is usually performed by ultrasound between 9 and 13 weeks. Fetal viability is confirmed the day before the procedure.

The procedure is performed under general anaesthesia. The bladder is emptied and the catheter left *in situ* during the procedure. In our experience, we have found that packing the vagina before laparotomy can elevate the uterus with improved access to the cervico-isthmic region.

The patient is placed in the Trendelenburg position. A low transverse abdominal incision is made, and packs are used to keep the bowel away from the operative field. The peritoneum of the vesicocervical fold is incised transversely in the midline. Often it is not necessary to reflect the bladder inferiorly as the bladder reflection lies at the level of the isthmus. The uterine vessels and isthmus are identified digitally.

Double-stranded 2-gauge nylon suture (Ethicon, UK) is mounted on to a loose 40-mm round-bodied Mayo needle. The isthmus is grasped between the thumb and forefinger to stabilise the uterus. The suture is inserted postero-anteriorly through the substance of the cervix lateral to the canal but medial to the uterine vessels, at the level of the uterine isthmus above the insertion of the uterosacral ligaments (Fig. 14.8).

The needle is remounted and the procedure repeated again postero-anteriorly on the opposite side (Fig. 14.8). The knot is tied anteriorly and covered by a loose peritoneal fold and the abdomen closed (Figs 14.9 and 14.10).

There were no cases of severe haemorrhage in our series although several cases required the knot to be tightly closed to achieve adequate haemostasis.

A single dose of intra-operative antibiotics is given. Non-steroidal anti-inflammatory agents (diclofenac sodium suppositories 100 mg) are given for pain relief and uterine quiescence over the following 72 hours. Preoperative thromboprophylaxis was recommenced on the first postoperative day using dalteparin 5000 units subcutaneously daily and low-dose aspirin 75 mg per os daily.

Women remained in hospital for 5–7 days until removal of the skin sutures; fetal viability was confirmed on scan prior to discharge.

Follow-up included fetal anatomy scan at 20 weeks and serial fetal growth scans. Adjuvant treatment was continued for co-existing pathologies, e.g. low-molecular-weight heparin and low-dose aspirin for antiphospholipid syndrome (APS); clindamycin cream for bacterial vaginosis.

Prophylactic antenatal steroid treatment was prescribed once only at 24 weeks' gestation where dual pathology was present and the mother consented to the administration. Transvaginal ultrasound measurement of cervical length in several cases has shown little change compared with that expected with physiological shortening seen with advancing gestation. Prophylactic

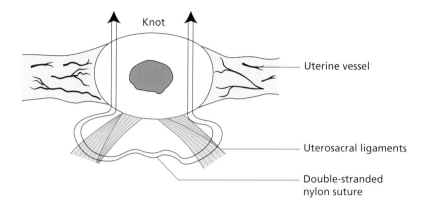

Fig. 14.8 Transabdominal cerclage technique, showing the double-strand nylon suture being inserted through the uterosacral ligaments.

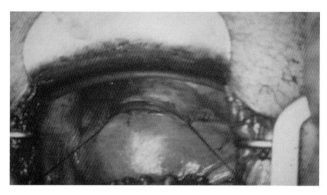

Fig. 14.9 Transabdominal cerclage showing the preconceptual suture insertion.

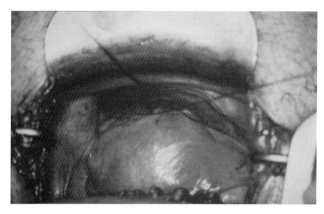

Fig. 14.10 Transabdominal cerclage showing the tying of the suture anteriorly. For clarity, this is a non-pregnant woman.

bed rest was not used. Pregnancies progressing beyond viability were delivered by caesarean section; the suture was left in place if the woman wished to consider another pregnancy.

Results of transabdominal cerclage (TAC)

Of 30 patients who underwent transabdominal cervical cerclage, 27 had a successful outcome (defined as a live birth with no ensuing neonatal death), and three experienced midtrimester loss or extreme preterm delivery and neonatal death. The success rate was 88%.

Five pregnancies ended prior to 30 weeks' gestation (Fig. 14.11). The three recorded failures showed a mixed pattern of presentation. One patient aborted at 12 weeks' gestation associated with APS. A second had spontaneous rupture of the membranes at 17 weeks followed by chorioamnionitis and intra-uterine death, necessitating hysterotomy. The third pregnancy failure was delivered by caesarean section at 25 weeks following preterm rupture of the membranes and labour. The infant died at 3 days of age from acute pulmonary haemorrhage and extreme prematurity. Two further deliveries occurred before 30 weeks, progressing to 27 and 29 weeks, respectively, and both infants subsequently did well. Eight babies were delivered at a gestation of 30–36 weeks. This was for a variety of reasons including preterm rupture of the membranes, preterm

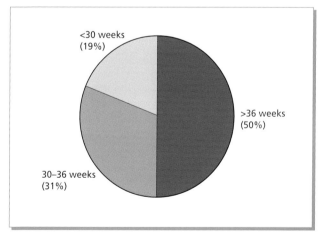

Fig. 14.11 Gestation at delivery following transabdominal cerclage.

labour and intra-uterine growth restriction. All infants are now doing well.

As 50% of pregnancies progressed to near term, we looked at the presence of other pathologies found on initial screening at the miscarriage clinic (Table 14.4). This demonstrated that

Pathology	Delivery at < 30 weeks	Delivery at 30–36 weeks	Delivery > 36 weeks	Total
Cervical weakness alone	0	3	7	10
Cervical weakness and one other pathology	2	5	5	12
Cervical weakness with two other pathologies	3	0	1	4
Total	5	7	12	26

Table 14.4 Gestation at subsequent delivery following TAC in relation to pathology identified during screening (*n* = 26 patients).

Preterm delivery rate (< 36 weeks) is 30% (3/10) for cervical weakness alone but rises to 62% (10/16) when another pathology is present.

62% (16/26) of delivered patients had another pathology in conjunction with the cervical weakness and that the presence of more than one pathology increased the risk of preterm delivery. Of the four patients with two pathologies as well as cervical weakness, three delivered prior to 30 weeks and only one of the infants survived, which emphasises the importance of co-existing pathology and its detrimental effect.

The role of transabdominal cerclage

There is little doubt that transabdominal cervical cerclage is an effective surgical technique in reducing fetal loss in a highly selective group of patients with true cervical weakness and/or a past history of failed vaginal cerclage (Novy, 1991).

Examination of published series fails to highlight the co-existence of further pathology, especially the presence of thrombophilia. The data from Liverpool suggest that the presence of co-existing pathology increases the risk of preterm delivery to 45% (12/26), which increases to 75% when there are two or more co-existing pathologies. It is important that women are aware of this confounding variable, as the patient will require laparotomy to insert the suture and abdominal delivery irrespective of gestation, both of which require continued thromboprophylaxis.

The presence of co-existing pathology in 60% of patients stresses the need for a full preconceptual screen in all patients with cervical weakness to look for dual pathology that can be treated. The commonest cofactor was APS, found in 33% of cases. All were treated with low-dose aspirin and low-molecular-weight heparin. Bacterial vaginosis was treated with oral erythromycin throughout pregnancy (14–32 weeks) combined with a week-long course of clindamycin cream per vaginam every month. Two cases of uterine anomaly were untreated by surgery, and both had a successful outcome.

There is no study comparing the insertion of transabdominal cervical cerclage during pregnancy with insertion prepregnancy. In the non-pregnant state, more manipulation of the tissues is possible as well as improved access (Figs 14.9 and 14.10). To counterbalance this advantage, there is the problem of early pregnancy loss before 10 weeks' gestation, when spontaneous miscarriage may allow the suture to tear through the substance of the pregnant cervix. In addition, fetal loss rates are higher in the presence of the commonest thrombophilia, APS, where suction evacuation may pose a considerable threat to the integrity of a preconceptual abdominal cerclage. Furthermore, in the non-pregnant state, the uterine vessels are not as easily identified, and it is more difficult to ensure that they are not caught within the suture. Also, cervical tissue is not as soft and it is difficult to pass the round-bodied needle through the substance of the cervix.

Preconceptual transabdominal cerclage was performed in two of 30 cases. One patient was homozygous for factor V Leiden and at high risk of thrombosis, having suffered two previous episodes of venous thromboembolic disease. The second patient had laboured at 25 weeks after insertion of her first transabdominal cerclage, and had an emergency classical caesarean section when the suture was removed and subsequent access to the lower segment was poor.

There are case reports describing insertion and removal of transabdominal cerclage laparoscopically (Scibetta *et al.*, 1997; Lesser *et al.*, 1998); there is at yet no series published using the laparoscopic approach.

Clinical experience with transabdominal cerclage is limited in the United Kingdom to a few centres (Gibb and Salaria, 1995; Topping and Farquharson, 1995, 2002; Anthony *et al.*, 1997). Selection criteria vary between centres and often include patients with preterm delivery histories and bad outcome as well as classical MTL due to true cervical weakness. Our series contains only MTL patients.

There are as yet no randomised trials comparing the use of transabdominal cerclage with the transvaginal approach. A highly selective retrospective study (Davis *et al.*, 2000) looked at the outcome of a group of patients with previous failed vaginal cerclage who were assigned either repeat vaginal cerclage or TAC. Assignment to either group was at the discretion of the authors and no randomisation occurred. They found that delivery at < 35 weeks occurred significantly less frequently in the transabdominal group (18% vs. 42%) and that preterm premature rupture of the membranes also occurred less commonly (8% vs. 29%). Extrapolation from these data should be viewed with caution as no prospective analysis has been made available, and a considerable number of performed cases were excluded from the report.

It is unlikely that a randomised controlled trial will be feasible, because women referred for this procedure often perceive it as their last chance and are unlikely to accept randomisation. We are also looking at a small number of patients, and the possibility of recruiting sufficient numbers to satisfy a credible power calculation is unlikely.

Adjuvant treatment intervention

Antiphospholipid syndrome and thrombophilias

The antiphospholipid antibody syndrome comprises lupus anticoagulant (LA) and anticardiolipin antibodies (aCL) that are known to bind to negatively charged phospholipids and are regarded as markers of thrombosis (Birdsall and Pattison, 1993). Various theories exist as to how they cause miscarriage: binding to platelet membrane activating release of thromboxane and subsequent platelet aggregation and thrombosis; binding to endothelial cells, inhibiting prostacyclin production or involvement with other clotting factors. It is likely that APS is a family of autoantibodies. A high index of suspicion is needed in any patient with an unexplained intra-uterine death (Lubbe *et al.*, 1984), especially if associated with thrombocytopenia and arterial or venous thromboses.

APS is associated with miscarriage in any trimester. Fetal loss commonly occurs in the first trimester (Rai *et al.*, 1995), while others have found that their patients with APS mostly miscarried in the second or early third trimester (Branch *et al.*, 1985). Prevalence rates for APS of up to 42% have been recorded in an MTL group (Unander *et al.*, 1987). As placental thrombosis has been presumed to be the historical cause, the mainstay of treatment has been the use of anticoagulants to provide thromboprophylaxis in the form of either low-dose aspirin and/or unfractionated/low-molecular-weight heparin. Recent evidence supports the use of low-dose aspirin alone (Pattison *et al.*, 2000; Farquharson *et al.*, 2002), whereas others support the use of combined aspirin/heparin (Kutteh, 1996; Rai *et al.*, 1997).

Uterine surgery

Results from metroplasty studies have claimed good success rates ranging from 73% to 85% (Strassman, 1966; DeCherney *et al.*, 1986; Kirk *et al.*, 1993); however, invasive intervention is beneficial only in highly selected patients. Successful hysteroscopic myomectomy for submucous fibroids up to 2 cm in diameter has been described (Buttram and Reiter, 1981).

The majority of women with uterine abnormality will successfully achieve a pregnancy without intervention, although the incidence of miscarriage, malpresentation and caesarean section is increased (Heinonen *et al.*, 1982; Acien, 1993). As recommended by the authors, these pregnancies should always be treated as high risk and supervised accordingly with regular ultrasound surveillance of fetal growth and cervical length.

Evidence of benefit from hysteroscopic metroplasty surgery in recurrent miscarriage is of poor quality and should be interpreted with caution. This is because there are no reported randomised trials, and eligible groups are heterogeneous and follow-up is incomplete. In women with second trimester loss and preterm labour, metroplasty may improve pregnancy outcome, but they remain at increased risk of preterm delivery, although the data are again of poor quality (Matts *et al.*, 2000). Furthermore, hysteroscopic metroplasty does not improve outcome or 'cure' unexplained infertility.

ACKNOWLEDGEMENTS

The author would like to thank AnnMaria Hughes, Kath Moore, Joanne Topping and Siobhan Quenby of the Miscarriage Clinic, Liverpool Women's Hospital, for their generous help over the years, and all patients who helped with our research.

REFERENCES

Acien P (1993) Reproductive performance in women with uterine malformations. *Human Reproduction* 8: 122–126.

Adinkra PE, Lamont RF (2002) Abnormal genital tract flora and pregnancy loss. In: Farquharson RG (ed.) *Miscarriage*. Dinton, Wilts: Quay Books Division, Mark Allen Publishing, pp. 108–130.

Airoldi J, Berghella V, Sehdeu H (2005) Transvaginal ultrasonography of the cervix to predict preterm birth in women with uterine anomalies. *Obstetrics and Gynecology* 106: 553–556.

Althuisius SM, Dekker GA, van Geijn HP *et al.* (2000) Cervical Incompetence Prevention Randomized Cerclage Trial (CIPRACT): study design and preliminary results. *American Journal of Obstetrics and Gynecology* 183: 823–829.

Althuisius SM, Dekker GA, Hummel P *et al.* (2001) Final results of the Cervical Incompetence Prevention Cerclage Trial (CIPRACT): therapeutic cerclage with bed rest versus bed rest alone. *American Journal of Obstetrics and Gynecology* 185: 1106–1112.

Anthony GS, Walker RG, Cameron AD *et al.* (1997) Transabdominal cervico-isthmic cerclage in the management of cervical incompetence. *European Journal of Obstetrics, Gynaecology and Reproductive Biology* 72: 127–130.

Benson RC, Durfee RB (1965) Transabdominal cervico-uterine cerclage during pregnancy for the treatment of cervical incompetence. *Obstetrics and Gynecology* 25: 145–155.

Berghella V (2004) The short and funneled cervix: what do I do now? *Contemporary Obstetrics and Gynaecology* April: 26–34.

Berghella V, Haas S, Chervoneva I *et al.* (2002) Patients with second trimester loss: prophylactic cerclage or serial transvaginal sonograms? *American Journal of Obstetrics and Gynecology* 187: 747–751.

Berry CW, Brambati B, Eskes TKAB *et al.* (1995) The Euro-Team Early Pregnancy (ETEP) protocol for recurrent miscarriage. *Human Reproduction* 10 (6): 1516–1520.

Birdsall MA, Pattison NS (1993) Antiphospholipid antibodies in pregnancy: clinical associations. *British Journal of Hospital Medicine* 50 (5): 251–260.

Branch DW, Scott JR, Kochenour NK *et al.* (1985) Obstetric complications associated with the lupus anticoagulant. *New England Journal of Medicine* 313 (21): 1322–1326.

Buttram VC, Reiter RC (1981) Uterine leiomyomata: etiology, symptomatology and management. *Fertility and Sterility* 36: 433–445.

Cammarano CL, Herron MA, Parer JT (1995) Validity of transabdominal cervicoisthmic cerclage for cervical incompetence. *American Journal of Obstetrics and Gynecology* 172: 1871–1875.

Clifford K, Rai R, Watson H *et al.* (1994) An informative protocol for the investigation of recurring miscarriage: preliminary experience of 500 consecutive cases. *Human Reproduction* 9: 1328–1332.

Craig S, Fleigner JRH (1997) Treatment of cervical incompetence by transabdominal cervicoisthmic cerclage. *Australian and New Zealand Journal of Obstetrics and Gynecology* 37: 407–411.

Davis G, Berghella V, Talucci M *et al.* (2000) Patients with a prior failed transvaginal cerclage: a comparison of obstetric outcomes either transabdominal or transvaginal cerclage. *American Journal of Obstetrics and Gynecology* 183: 836–839.

DeCherney AH, Russell JB, Graebe RA *et al.* (1986) Resectoscopic management of mullerian fusion defects. *Fertility and Sterility* 45: 726–728.

Drakeley AJ, Farquharson RG (2002) Midtrimester loss. In: Farquharson RG (ed.) *Miscarriage*. Dinton, Wilts: Quay Books Division, Mark Allen Publishing, pp. 191–200.

Drakeley AJ, Quenby S, Farquharson RG (1998) Mid-trimester loss — appraisal of a screening protocol. *Human Reproduction* 13 (7): 1975–1980.

Edmonds DK (1988) Use of cervical cerclage in patients with recurrent first trimester abortion. In: *Early Pregnancy Loss Mechanisms and Treatment*. London: RCOG Press, pp. 411–415.

Emmett TA (1874) Laceration of the cervix uteri as a frequent and unrecognised cause of disease. *American Journal of Obstetrics and Gynecology* 7: 44–46.

Farquharson RG, Quenby SM, Greaves M (2002) Antiphospholipid syndrome in pregnancy: a randomised controlled trial of treatment. *Obstetrics and Gynecology* 100: 418–424.

Gibb DMF, Salaria DA (1995) Trans-abdominal cervico-isthmic cerclage in the management of recurrent second trimester miscarriage and pre-term delivery. *British Journal of Obstetrics and Gynaecology* 102: 802–806.

Gomez R, Romero R, Nien JK *et al.* (2005) A short cervix in women with pre-term labour and intact membranes: a risk factor for microbial invasion of the amniotic cavity. *American Journal of Obstetrics and Gynecology* 192: 678–689.

Harger JH (2002) Cerclage and cervical insufficiency: an evidence-based analysis. *Obstetrics and Gynecology* 100: 1313–1327.

Harger JH, Archer DF, Marchese SG *et al.* (1983) Etiology of recurrent pregnancy losses and outcome of subsequent pregnancies. *Obstetrics and Gynaecology* 62: 574–581.

Heinonen PK, Saarikoski S, Pysteynen P (1982) Reproductive performance of women with uterine anomalies: an evaluation of 182 cases. *Acta Obstetrica et Gynecologica* 62: 157–162.

Herron MA, Parer JT (1988) Transabdominal cerclage for fetal wastage due to cervical incompetence. *Obstetrics and Gynecology* 71: 865–868.

Iams JD, Goldenberg RL, Meis PJ *et al.* (1996) The length of the cervix and the risk of spontaneous preterm delivery. *New England Journal of Medicine* 334: 567–572.

Jeffcoate TNM (1975) *Principles of Gynaecology*. London: Butterworth Publishing Group, pp. 192–193.

Kirk EP, Chuong CJ, Coulam CB *et al.* (1993) Pregnancy after metroplasty for uterine anomalies. *Fertility and Sterility* 59: 1164–1168.

Kutteh WH (1996) Antiphospholipid antibody-associated recurrent pregnancy loss: treatment with heparin and low dose aspirin is superior to low dose aspirin alone. *American Journal of Obstetrics and Gynecology* 174: 1584–1589.

Lesser KB, Childers JM, Surwit EA (1998) Transabdominal cerclage a laparoscopic approach. *Obstetrics and Gynaecology* 91: 855–856.

Llahi-Camp JM, Rai R, Ison CR *et al.* (1996) Association of bacterial vaginosis with a history of second trimester miscarriage. *Human Reproduction* 11: 1575–1578.

Lubbe WF, Butler WS, Palmer SJ *et al.* (1984) Lupus anticoagulant in pregnancy. *British Journal of Obstetrics and Gynaecology* 91: 357–363.

McDonald IA (1957) Suture of the cervix for inevitable miscarriage. *Journal of Obstetrics and Gynaecology of the British Empire* 64: 346–350.

Mahran M (1978) Transabdominal cerclage during pregnancy, a modified technique. *Obstetrics and Gynecology* 52: 502–506.

Matts SJF, Clark TJ, Khan KS *et al.* (2000) Surgical correction of congenital uterine anomalies. *Hospital Medicine* 61: 246–249.

MRC/RCOG Working Party on Cervical Cerclage (1993) Final Report of the Medical Research Council/Royal College of Obstetricians and Gynaecologists multicentre randomised trial of cervical cerclage. *British Journal of Obstetrics and Gynaecology* 100: 516–523.

Murakawa H, Utumi T, Hasegawa I *et al.* (1993) Evaluation of threatened preterm delivery by transvaginal ultrasonographic measurement of cervical length. *Obstetrics and Gynecology* 82: 829–832.

Novy MJ (1982) Transabdominal cervicoisthmic cerclage for the management of repetitive abortion and preterm delivery. *American Journal of Obstetrics and Gynecology* 143: 44–54.

Novy JJ (1991) Transabdominal cervivoisthmic cerclage. A reappraisal 25 years after its introduction. *American Journal of Obstetrics and Gynecology* 164: 1635–1642.

Oakeshott P, Hay P, Hay S *et al.* (2002) Association between bacterial vaginosis or chlamydial infection and miscarriage before 16 weeks gestation: prospective community based cohort study. *British Medical Journal* 325: 1334–1336.

Olsen S, Tobiassen T (1982) Transabdominal isthmic cerclage for the treatment of incompetent cervix. *Acta Obstetrica et Gynecologica Scandinavica* 61: 473–475.

Pattison NS, Chamley LW, Birdsall MA *et al.* (2000) Does aspirin have a role in improving pregnancy outcome for women with the antiphospholipid syndrome? A randomised controlled trial. *American Journal of Obstetrics and Gynecology* 183: 1008–1012.

Rai RS, Clifford K, Cohen H *et al.* (1995) High prospective fetal loss rate in untreated pregnancies of women with recurrent miscarriages and antiphospholipid antibodies. *Human Reproduction* 10: 3301–3304.

Rai R, Cohen H, Dave M *et al.* (1997) Randomised controlled trial of aspirin and aspirin plus heparin in pregnant women with recurrent miscarriage associated with phospholipid antibodies. *British Medical Journal* 314: 253–257.

Romero R, Espinoza J, Hassan S (2006) The role of cervical cerclage in obstetric practice. Can the patient who could benefit from this procedure be identified. *American Journal of Obstetrics and Gynecology* 194: 1–9.

Rozenberg P, Gillet A, Ville Y (2002) Transvaginal sonographic examination of the cervix in asymptomatic pregnant women: review of the literature. *Ultrasound in Obstetrics and Gynaecology* 19: 302–311.

Rust OA, Atlas RO, Jones KJ *et al.* (2000) A randomized trial of cerclage versus no cerclage among patients with ultrasonographically detected second-trimester preterm dilatation of the internal os. *American Journal of Obstetrics and Gynecology* 183: 830–835.

Sadler TW (1995) In: Sadler TW (ed.) *Langman's Medical Embryology*, 7th edn. Philadelphia: Williams & Wilkins, pp. 272, 296–297.

Sakai M, Shiozaki A, Tabata M *et al.* (2006) Evaluation of effectiveness of prophylactic cerclage of a short cervix according to interleukin-8 in cervical mucus. *American Journal of Obstetrics and Gynecology* 194: 14–19.

Scibetta JJ, Sanko SR, Phipps WR (1997) Laparoscopic transabdominal cervicoisthmic cerclage. *Fertility and Sterility* 69: 161–163.

Shirodkar VN (1955) A new method of operative treatment for habitual abortion in the second trimester. *Antiseptic* 52: 299–300.

Smith FR (1931) The significance of incomplete fusion of the Mullerian ducts in pregnancy and parturition, with a report on 35 cases. *American Journal of Obstetrics and Gynecology* 22: 714–728.

Strassmann EO (1966) Fertility and unification of double uterus. *Fertility and Sterility* 17: 165–176.

To MS, Alfirevic Z, Heath VCF *et al.* (2004) Cervical cerclage for prevention of preterm delivery in women with short cervix: randomised controlled trial. *Lancet* 363: 1849–1853.

Topping J, Farquharson RG (2002) Transabdominal cervical cerclage. In: *The Yearbook of Obstetrics and Gynaecology*, Vol. 10. London: RCOG Press, pp. 254–261.

Topping J, Farquharson RG (1995) Transabdominal cervical cerclage. *British Journal of Hosp Med*, 54: 510–512.

Turnquest MA, Britton KA, Brown HL (1999) Outcome of patients undergoing transabdominal cerclage: a descriptive study. *Journal of Maternal and Fetal Medicine* 8: 225–227.

Unander AM, Norberg R, Hahn L *et al.* (1987) Anticardiolipin antibodies and complement in ninety-nine women with habitual abortion. *American Journal of Obstetrics and Gynecology* 156: 114–119.

PART 5

Cervical infections

CHAPTER 15

Pathology of inflammatory diseases of the cervix

Kasturi Das, Michele Burday and Debra S. Heller

INTRODUCTION

This chapter will describe the pathology of inflammatory diseases of the cervix. Pathogenesis, clinical manifestations, diagnosis and treatment will be covered in the two subsequent chapters.

The aetiology of cervicitis can be divided into infectious and associated with specific aetiologies and non-infectious (non-specific). The agents causing infectious cervicitis can be further divided into bacterial, viral, fungal, protozoan and parasitic; all will be discussed later. Non-infectious causes include local causes of inflammation such as repair of epithelial damage, intra-uterine device (IUD), chemotherapy, radiation therapy, localised lesions such as cervical endometriosis, and inflammation associated with neoplasia (Table 15.1). Systemic inflammatory diseases such as polyarteritis nodosa and Behçet's syndrome may also manifest as cervical inflammation.

The pathological changes associated with inflammatory diseases of the cervix are predominantly non-specific tissue responses to the non-infectious and infectious aetiologies. Frequently, the presence of normal stromal inflammatory cells of the cervix leads to a misdiagnosis of cervicitis (Winkler and Richart, 1985) (Figs 15.1–15.3), and inflammatory cells are frequent in Papanicolaou smears (Fig. 15.4).

The inflammatory responses to specific aetiologies may be variable and range from the acute to the chronic. They may be

Table 15.1 Cervicitis: aetiological agents.

Inflammatory disease with specific aetiology	
A. Infections	
1. Bacteria	Gonorrhoea
	Chlamydia
	Syphilis
	Tuberculosis
	Donovanosis (granuloma inguinale)
	Actinomycosis
	Lymphogranuloma venereum
2. Viral	Herpes simplex
3. Fungal	Moniliasis
4. Protozoan and parasitic	Trichomonas
	Schistosomiasis
	Amoebiasis
	Oxyuriasis
	Hydatid disease
B. Inflammation associated with systemic inflammatory disease	
	Polyarteritis nodosa
	Asymptomatic arteritis of cervix
	Behçet's syndrome
C. Inflammation associated with neoplasia	
	Reaction to primary tumour
	Postirradiation inflammation
Non-specific inflammations	
A. Associated with mechanical, physical and chemical trauma	
B. Associated with non-specific infections.	

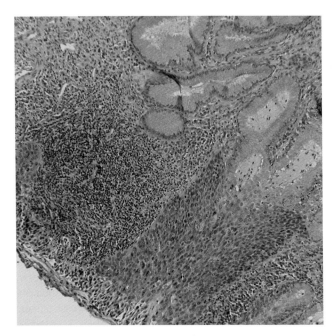

Fig. 15.1 Acute inflammatory reaction of the cervix.

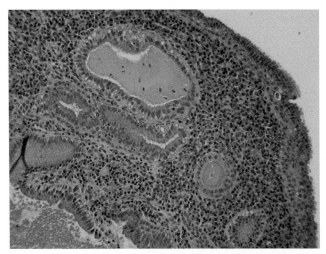

(a)

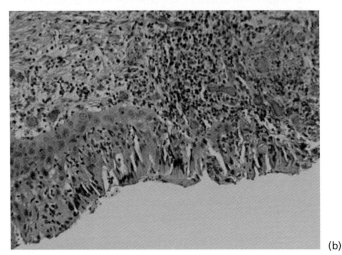

(b)

Fig. 15.2 (a) Non-specific chronic inflammation of the endocervix. (b) Reparative changes are seen in this area of inflammation and squamous metaplasia. Note prominent nucleoli.

of an acute inflammatory type, characterised by marked neutrophilic infiltration of cervical stroma and epithelium. These changes are commonly seen associated with bacterial infections (mucopurulent cervicitis). Chronic inflammatory changes with intense lymphoplasmacytic infiltration with germinal centre formation are seen in infection due to *Chlamydia*. Granulomatous inflammation is associated with necrotising granuloma formation as in syphilitic gummas or tuberculous infection, while necrotising cervicitis is seen associated with herpes viral infection with destruction of glands and stroma. Infiltration of both neutrophils and plasma cells and foreign body giant cells may be a response associated with IUD use. Some of these morphological changes in the clinically 'inflamed' cervix are documented in Table 15.2.

Cytological changes associated with cervical inflammation in cervical Pap smears, irrespective of aetiology, are characterised by minimal nuclear enlargement, bi- or multinucleation, mild nuclear hyperchromasia, karyopyknosis, karyorrhexis, smooth nuclear contours, the presence of prominent nucleoli, cytoplasmic vacuolisation, polychromasia and perinuclear halos (Fig. 15.5a). In addition to the inflammatory response, there are reparative epithelial changes seen in the ecto- and endocervix, which may mimic intraepithelial neoplasia histologically and cytologically. Features that help to distinguish reactive atypia from cervical intraepithelial neoplasia (CIN) are lack of nuclear pleomorphism, well-defined cytoplasmic membranes, orderly maturation of the squamous epithelium, maintenance of polarity, confinement of mitotic figures to the basal and parabasal layers and the presence of inflammatory cells within the epithelium (Wright and Ferenczy, 1994).

Ulcerations lead to granulation tissue formation, and persistence of the inciting agent may result in stromal fibrosis and scarring with distortion of endocervical glands as seen in chronic gonorrhoeal cervicitis (Winkler and Richart, 1985).

Ulceration and necrosis, features of invasive cancer, produce within the resultant smear the presence of what is called an 'ulcerative diathesis'. Within the smear can be found the presence of pleomorphic, keratinised and parabasal squamous cells that often have pale, degenerate nuclei. Not surprisingly, inflammatory cell exudate with attendant necrotic tumour cells (ghost) and resultant blood can be found. Sometimes, these changes can be mimicked by the lesser comedo-like crypt CIN3 lesions. The finding of 'fibre' cells suggests early invasion and reflects either surface flattening in large cell, keratinising CIN3 (carcinoma *in situ*) or marginal areas of focal differentiation that accompany microinvasion or high-grade squamous intraepithelial lesions (Fig. 15.5b and c).

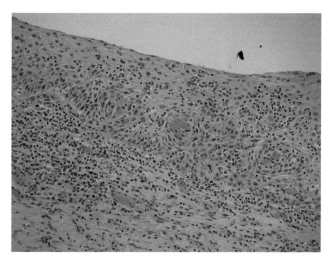

Fig. 15.3 Non-specific acute and chronic inflammation of the ectocervix.

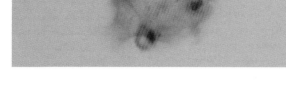

Fig. 15.4 Non-specific inflammation on Pap smear. There are neutrophils with the squamous cells showing reactive changes.

BACTERIAL INFECTIONS

Gonorrhoea

One of the oldest known human diseases is gonorrhoea. Ancient Chinese writings and the Old Testament have references to it. The term gonorrhoea, 'flow of seed', was given by Galen (130 AD). Neisser described the causative organism in 1879, and in 1882 Leistikow and Loeffler first cultured it. Effective therapy against gonorrhoea was available with the advent of sulphonamides in the 1930s and penicillin in 1943. An estimated 600 000 new cases occur each year occur in the United States (Workowski and Levine, 2002). The highest incidence in the US is in the 20- to 24-year-old age range. Risk factors for gonorrhoea in the US are low socioeconomic and educational status, urban residence, early onset of sexual activity, large number and variety of sexual partners and a past history of gonorrhoea (Fitzgerald, 1984). Gonorrhoea is the most commonly reported infectious disease in the US (Fitzgerald, 1984).

Pathology

The aetiological agent of gonorrhoea is *Neisseria gonorrhoeae*, which is a non-motile, non-spore-forming Gram-negative diplococcus transmitted by contact with the mucosal surfaces of an infected host (usually a sexual partner). The columnar epithelial cells of the endocervix are most susceptible to *N. gonorrhoeae* infection. The bacteria attach to the cells mediated by pili and other surface proteins. (This process is discussed in detail in the following chapter.) In the next 24–48 hours, the organism is transported into the cell by pinocytosis followed by intracellular replication and egestion of the gonococci into submucosal tissue, usually by the third day (Zenilman and Wiesner, 1991). An intense local polymorphonuclear

Table 15.2 Morphological changes in the clinically 'inflamed' cervix.

Inflammatory reaction	Connective tissue response	Associated epithelial changes
Acute e.g. gonorrhoea	Cellular phenomena: polymorphonuclear leucocytes, lymphocytes, histiocytes, epithelioid cells, giant cells	Cell degeneration and necrosis, proliferation, hyperplasia, metaplasia, cellular atypia
Chronic e.g. non-specific cervicitis	Vascular changes: capillary dilatation, capillary proliferation, endarteritis	Cysts and Nabothian follicles

Granulomatous
  e.g. tuberculosis,
    schistosomiasis
	Stroma, repair:
	fibroblast proliferation,
	granulation tissue, fibrosis	

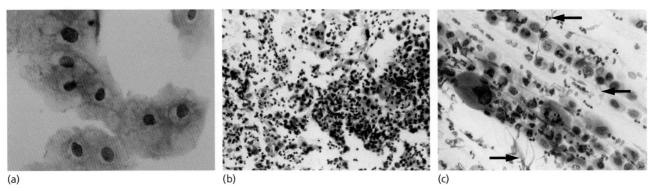

(a)   (b)   (c)

Fig. 15.5 (a) Pseudokoilocytes, associated with non-specific inflammation, as seen on a Pap smear. (b) A background ulcerative diathesis typical of early invasive cancer, showing pleomorphic and keratinised parabasal cells, some with pale, degenerate nuclei in association with inflammatory cell exudate, necrotic tumour cells and keratinising cells. (c) A higher power of an ulcerative diathesis, typical of invasive cancer, showing pleomorphic, keratinising parabasal cells associated with fibre cells (arrowed).

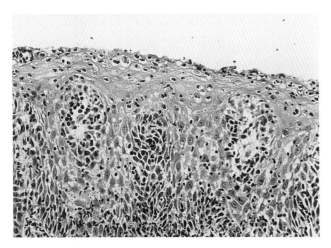

Fig. 15.6 Biopsy of the ectocervix in a woman with acute gonococcal infection, showing marked degeneration of the superficial epithelium and an acute inflammatory infiltrate. Intercellular oedema is prominent and there is some basal cell hyperactivity.

inflammatory response ensues with surface epithelial sloughing, the formation of submucosal microabcesses and exudation of purulent material (Fig. 15.6). A Gram stain of the exudate reveals large numbers of Gram-negative diplococci within few neutrophils. If left untreated, this is followed by lymphoplasmacytic and histiocytic infiltration, which persists for weeks to months, after which gonococci can no longer be isolated.

Chlamydia

The most prevalent bacterial sexually transmitted disease in the world is chlamydial infection. In women, the most important complication of sexually transmitted chlamydial infection is pelvic inflammatory disease, which has a major impact on

fertility as a result of tubal damage and may lead to ectopic pregnancy and infant pneumonia. The Centers for Disease Control and Prevention (CDC) estimates that there are approximately 4 million new *Chlamydia trachomatis* infections per year in the US. According to the World Health Organization, 50–70 million chlamydial infections are detected annually worldwide. On the other hand, a rapid decline in the incidence of gonococcal infections has been noted in many western countries. This has not been observed with chlamydial infections, suggesting that epidemiological control measures against chlamydia are not as effective as those against gonorrhoea.

Pathology

Chlamydia trachomatis infects the epithelial cells of the cervix uteri, with the endocervical cells being more susceptible (Wright and Ferenczy, 1994). Hence, patients with columnar ectropion, such as pregnant women or younger women, are more susceptible to chlamydial infection. Chlamydial infection of the cervix is not common in older postmenopausal women or before menarche.

Colposcopically, the cervix may be completely normal or exhibit oedema, erythema and hypertrophy with mucopurulent discharge. Closer examination will reveal typical follicles across the ectocervix, and there will occasionally be loss of superficial epithelium within the endocervix, which will appear eroded (Fig. 15.7a).

Histologically, an initial acute inflammatory response is seen at the squamocolumnar junction predominantly in the endocervical epithelium, which may be eroded. There is diffuse infiltration of endocervical glands (Fig. 15.7b) and stroma by plasma cells, lymphocytes and histiocytes with plasma cells predominating. Lymphocytic follicular cervicitis, seen in tissue and cytological samples (Fig. 15.8a–c), is strongly correlated with chlamydial infection, and *Chlamydia* has been reported to be a

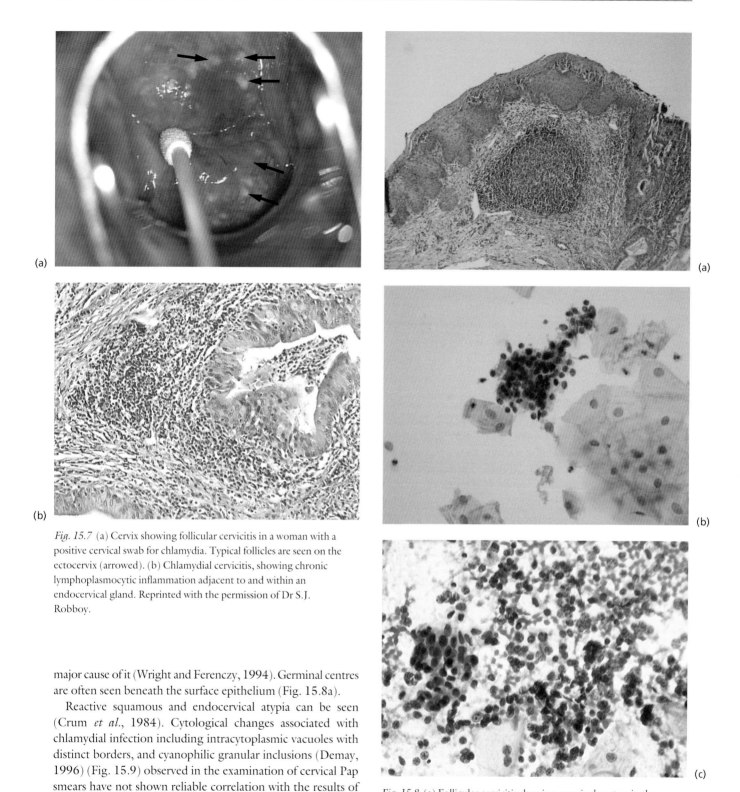

Fig. 15.7 (a) Cervix showing follicular cervicitis in a woman with a positive cervical swab for chlamydia. Typical follicles are seen on the ectocervix (arrowed). (b) Chlamydial cervicitis, showing chronic lymphoplasmocytic inflammation adjacent to and within an endocervical gland. Reprinted with the permission of Dr S.J. Robboy.

Fig. 15.8 (a) Follicular cervicitis showing germinal centres in the cervical stroma. (b) and (c) Follicular cervicitis as seen in a Pap smear.

major cause of it (Wright and Ferenczy, 1994). Germinal centres are often seen beneath the surface epithelium (Fig. 15.8a).

Reactive squamous and endocervical atypia can be seen (Crum *et al.*, 1984). Cytological changes associated with chlamydial infection including intracytoplasmic vacuoles with distinct borders, and cyanophilic granular inclusions (Demay, 1996) (Fig. 15.9) observed in the examination of cervical Pap smears have not shown reliable correlation with the results of culture and immunocytochemical antibody studies (Bonfiglio, 1997). The sensitivity and specificity of Pap smears for making a diagnosis is low (Giampaolo *et al.*, 1983). As chronic follicular cervicitis has been associated with chlamydial infections,

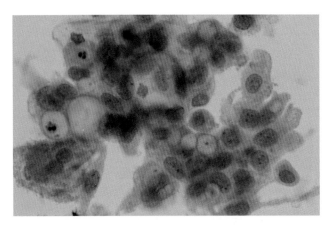

Fig. 15.9 Although not a reliable marker, cytological changes that may reflect chlamydial infection include intracytoplasmic vacuoles with distinct borders and granular inclusions.

the presence of mature lymphocytes and germinal centre cells in a Pap smear raises the possibility of chlamydial infection.

Syphilis

Syphilis is a chronic venereal infection with systemic involvement caused by the spirochaete *Treponema pallidum*. About 134 000 cases were reported to the US Public Health Service in 1990 (Ross, 1997a). The highest case rates in women are seen between the ages of 15 and 30 years (Lossick and Kraus, 1991). Syphilis is transmitted by direct contact of infected epithelium with abraded skin and mucosa of the lower genital tract. Some 10–40% of women with syphilis have primary chancres, usually on the vulva, but these may also be found on the cervix (Anderson *et al.*, 2002). The cervix can also be involved by the mucous patch of secondary syphilis and the gumma of tertiary syphilis (Wright and Ferenczy, 1994; Sweet, 1998; Tramont, 2000).

Pathology

The histological features of a chancre are non-specific, but the diagnosis is favoured when there is an intense plasma cell infiltration and scattered histiocytes and lymphocytes beneath the epithelium (Fig. 15.10). The plasma cells are often perivascular in distribution. Endothelial cell hyperplasia, lymphoplasmacytic infiltration and fibroblastic proliferation of small vessel walls eventually result in endarteritis obliterans. Treponemes can be demonstrated by silver stain or immunofluorescence techniques (direct fluorescent antibody tests) at the surface of the ulcer. The histological features of secondary syphilis are similar to those of primary syphilis with less intense inflammation. The gumma of tertiary syphilis is characterised by central coagulative necrosis surrounded by palisading histiocytes, fibroblasts, lymphocytes and marked plasma cell infiltrate at the periphery. Gummas may be single or multiple and

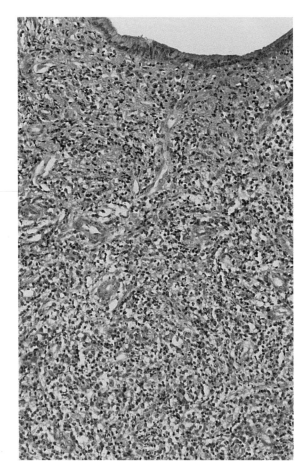

Fig. 15.10 Syphilis of the cervix. There is vasculitis and a plasma cell infiltrate. Reprinted with the permission of Dr S.J. Robboy.

vary in size from microscopic lesions to tumour-like masses. Treponemes are difficult to demonstrate within these gummas (Samuelson, 1999). Concomitant infection with syphilis is seen in one-fifth of women with human immunodeficiency virus (HIV) (Sweet, 1998; Tramont, 2000).

Tuberculosis

Over the last decade, there has been an increase in tuberculosis (TB) in the US; however, genital tract tuberculosis remains uncommon. Primary genital tuberculosis is rare (Schaeffer, 1970) and has been reported in women with male partners with tuberculous epididymitis or genitourinary tuberculosis. Based on a series of clinical, laboratory, roentgenological and laparoscopic procedures in 965 cases, genital tuberculosis is found as primary in only 0.2% (Schaeffer, 1970), as haematogenous in 59.2% and as descending via the lymphatics from the lungs to intestinal lymph nodes and thence to the fallopian tubes in 40.6%. Tuberculosis of the cervix is almost always secondarily acquired by direct spread from the endosalpinx or

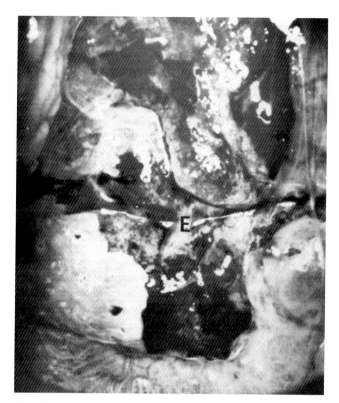

Fig. 15.11 Colpophotograph (×9) showing tuberculous ulceration of endo- and ectocervix. The endocervical canal is at (E). Courtesy of the late Dr Renée Cartier, Paris.

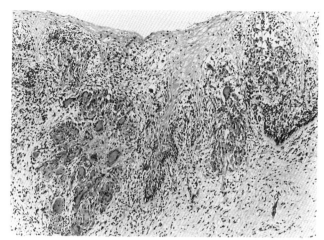

Fig. 15.12 Biopsy of ectocervix showing florid granulomatous reaction beneath the epithelium with many Langerhans-type giant cells. The epithelium is thinned and ulcerated in adjacent sections. Culture for tubercle bacilli was positive. Courtesy of Dr D. Lovell, London.

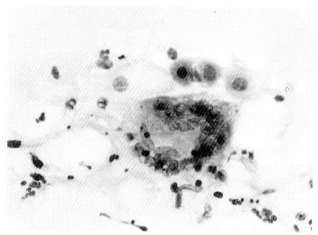

Fig. 15.13 Langerhans-type multinuclear giant cell found in the cervical smear of patient with tuberculous endocervicitis. Courtesy of Dr A. Smithies, London.

endometrium, and is often associated with pulmonary TB. The incidence of cervical involvement in genital TB is 5–15% (Samuelson, 1999). In 57% of cases of cervical TB, there has been simultaneous infection of the endometrium (Chakraborty *et al.*, 1995).

On gross examination, the cervix may be normal, inflamed, hypertrophied or ulcerated with cervical erosions. The most common type is ulcerative (Schaeffer, 1970) (Fig. 15.11), which may mimic squamous cell carcinoma. Histological examination of the hypertrophied lesions shows hyperkeratosis and pseudoepitheliomatous hyperplasia of the squamous epithelium, with sparse epithelioid histiocytes, rare giant cells and absence of caseation (Chakraborty *et al.*, 1995). The ulcerative lesion shows histological findings (Fig. 15.12) characteristic of tuberculous infection seen anywhere in the body, which is the presence of multiple tubercles or granulomas. These are characterised by central caseous necrosis, epithelioid histiocytes and Langerhans giant cells with a dense lymphoplasmacytic infiltrate at the periphery (Wright and Ferenczy, 1994). Necrotising granulomatous inflammation of the cervix may also be due to a non-tuberculous aetiology such as lymphogranuloma venereum, granuloma inguinale, sarcoidosis or schistosomiasis. To establish an unequivocal diagnosis of tuberculous cervicitis, the organisms must be identified.

Some interest has arisen in the recognition of cervical tuberculosis in cytological preparations (Meisels and Fortin, 1995). Epithelioid cells may be recognised among the normal epithelial content of an inflammatory cervical smear as a second population of pale cells with eosinophilic cytoplasm and indistinct borders, sometimes forming syncytia (Fig. 15.13). Langerhans-type giant cells also appear, but these must be distinguished from histiocytic-type giant cells which may be noted in postmenopausal smears, especially after irradiation and in *Trichomonas* infection. Moreover, these cytological appearances are not diagnostic of tuberculosis, but purely reflect the granulomatous nature of the lesion. Tissue biopsy is still necessary to confirm the diagnosis.

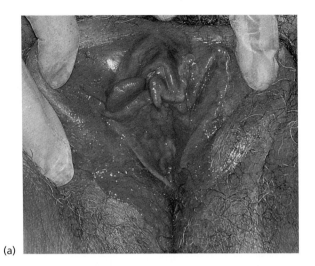

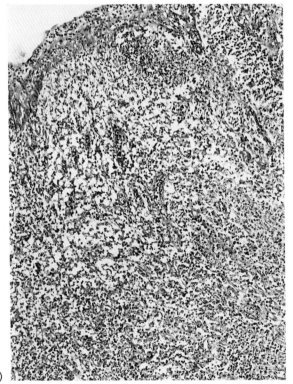

Fig. 15.14 (a) Initially presenting as a papular or nodular lesion, after a 7- to 10-day incubation period, tissue breakdown in the labia minora and fourchette area has occurred, resulting in a soft granulating ulcer that spreads progressively and may eventually involve large areas of perineum and anus and is typical of Donovanosis. (b) Biopsy from the cervix of a woman who had a clinical diagnosis of carcinoma of the cervix but in whom the diagnosis was of Donovanosis. There was marked inflammatory infiltrate in the stroma, with lymphocytes and histocytes prominent and a large contribution from plasma cells. The supra-adjacent epithelium consists of large macrophages with lymphocytes and acute inflammatory cells, but there is no histological evidence of neoplasia. Courtesy of Professor M. Hutt, London.

Presumptive identification can be made based on the detection of acid-fast bacilli by Ziehl–Neelsen stain on histological sections. As other mycobacterium stain similarly, other more specific methods such as culture or direct nucleic acid amplification (Haas, 2000) are required for definitive identification. It should be noted that histological identification of *Mycobacterium tuberculosis* in tissue specimens is very insensitive, as the organisms are scarce.

Donovanosis (granuloma inguinale)

Donovanosis, also known as granuloma inguinale, is rare in developed countries. Fewer than 50 cases a year are reported in the US (Ross, 1997b). It is a major cause of genital ulcers in south India, New Guinea, the Caribbean, parts of South America, Africa, South-East Asia and Australia (Ballard, 2000). It is caused by an encapsulated pleomorphic Gram-negative bacillus, *Calymmatobacterium granulomatis*. The primary lesion starts as a small painless papule or induration that ulcerates to form an exuberant granulomatous ulcer with rolled edges with a friable surface which bleeds easily on contact (Ballard, 2000). The labia and the fourchette are the most frequent sites of the primary lesion (Fig. 15.14a). The cervix may be involved more commonly by spread from the external genitalia, but may occasionally present as a primary lesion (Sengupta and Das, 1984), leading to vaginal bleeding or mimicking cervical cancer. In a study by Cooper *et al.* (Hoosen *et al.*, 1990), 50% of their patients with Donovanosis had a clinical diagnosis of carcinoma of the cervix. Other conditions that may mimic cervical cancer are syphilis, lymphogranuloma venereum and chancroid (Wright and Ferenczy, 1994).

Microscopically, all these conditions produce granulomatous inflammation (Fig. 15.14b). Ulcers of granuloma inguinale are associated with a mixed infiltrate of polymorphonuclear leucocytes, histiocytes and plasma cells.

Typical Donovan bodies (Fig. 15.15) shaped like small safety pins can be demonstrated within histiocytes by staining histological sections or touch preparations with Warthin–Starry silver or Giemsa stains. Papanicolaou-stained smears have also been used to detect Donovan bodies in women with cervical lesions (Ballard, 2000).

Actinomycosis

Actinomycosis infection of the cervix is most commonly caused by *Actinomyces israelii*, a Gram-positive, non-spore-forming anaerobe. Pelvic actinomycosis is most commonly associated with an intra-uterine contraceptive device: it is usually asymptomatic and detected on routine cervical cytology. Actinomycosis should always be treated even if asymptomatic. Reports of actinomycosis infection have been described in cases associated with pessaries, clinical abortion, surgical instrumentation and as a consequence of appendicitis or rectal disease (Samuelson,

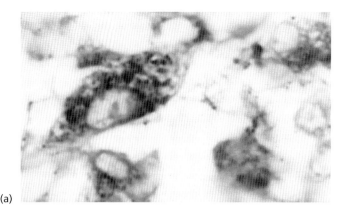

(a)

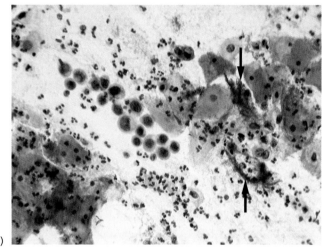

(b)

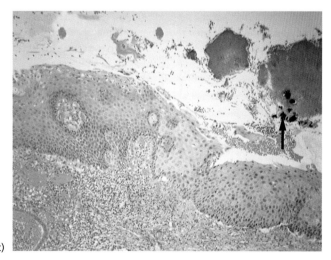

(c)

Fig. 15.15 (a) Silver staining showing numerous intracellular Donovan bodies included in macrophages and characteristic of Donovanosis (granuloma inguinale) (Grocott × 990 approximately). Courtesy of Professor M. Hutt, London. (b) Papanicolaou smear showing a pattern of severe dyskaryosis (high-grade squamous intraepithelial lesion, HSIL) with typical actinomycosis organisms that present as a clump of dark basophilic and filamentous organisms (arrowed). There is a background representing an acute inflammatory infiltrate. (c) CIN2 epithelial lesion with associated actinomycosis seen as dark sulphur granules in the space above the cervical epithelium (arrowed).

1999). Clinically, patients may be asymptomatic or present with fever, weight loss, foul-smelling vaginal discharge, abnormal uterine bleeding, lower abdominal/pelvic pain and, if undetected or left untreated, 'frozen pelvis' mimicking malignancy or endometriosis. The lesions have a yellow granular appearance, often described as 'sulphur granules'. Actinomycetes in routine cervicovaginal Papanicolaou-stained smears appear as clumps of dark, basophilic, filamentous organisms arranged radially at the periphery, associated with an acute inflammatory infiltrate (Bonfiglio, 1997) (Fig. 15.15b and c).

Histological sections reveal large abscesses with occasional granuloma formation. The organisms can be detected in the centres of these abscesses. Direct immunofluorescence techniques to detect actinomycetes in cervical smears have been reported to have a high sensitivity and specificity (Russo, 2000). Significant fibrosis and scarring may result from chronic actinomycosis infection of the cervix. Treatment of actinomycosis has changed significantly with the use of penicillin or tetracycline.

VIRAL INFECTIONS

Herpes simplex virus (see also Chapter 17)

Genital herpes affects an estimated 30 million Americans. Some 500 000 new cases are believed to occur each year (Ross, 1997c). However, an accurate estimation of the prevalence of genital herpes is difficult to make as 70% of HSV 2 infections appear to be asymptomatic (Corey and Holmes, 1983a), leading to a discrepancy between antibody prevalence and clinical infection (Corey and Holmes, 1983b). The reported trends in incidence of genital herpes have shown an increase in the US between 1966 and 1981 and in Great Britain between 1977 and 1981 (Corey and Holmes, 1983a). Seroprevalence of antibody to HSV 2 is higher in prostitutes, women with multiple sexual partners and individuals of low socioeconomic status. Antibodies to HSV 2 do not appear until the early teens and peak by age 35 (Corey and Holmes, 1983a).

Primary genital herpes infection manifests as painful vesicular lesions on an erythematous base accompanied by vaginal discharge. The vesicles rapidly ulcerate, and the cervix is diffusely friable. Often extensive ulcerative lesions of the ectocervix or severe necrotic cervicitis result (Corey and Holmes, 1983a,b). There have been reports of fungating necrotic masses developing on the ectocervix as a result of the extensive ulcerative and necrotic process mimicking carcinoma (Wright and Ferenczy, 1994). Symptoms of recurrent infection are less severe than those of primary disease. Papanicolaou-stained cervical smears reveal characteristic multinucleated giant cells (Fig. 15.16) with nuclear moulding, margination of chromatin, intranuclear eosinophilic inclusions (Cowdry type A inclusions; Fig. 15.17), and a ground glass appearance of infected nuclei (not cells) may also be seen. There may be

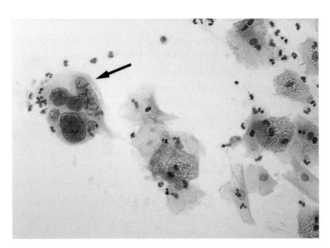

Fig. 15.16 Cytological changes of HSV, as seen characterised by large multiple nuclei that are moulded together (arrowed) and show margination of chromatin and generally empty nuclei. It is important to differentiate these cells from the binuclear cells that are commonly found in association with HPV infection and, from their bizarre appearance, they may be mistaken for those exfoliated from an invasive cancer. These changes may also be generated following radiotherapeutic treatment of cervical cancer.

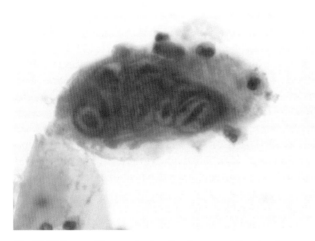

Fig. 15.17 A case of herpes simplex showing several Cowdry A inclusions seen in an infected cell on Pap smear.

associated reparative and regenerative changes in background squamous cells. Histological sections of herpetic vesicles reveal suprabasal intraepidermal vesicles with degenerated epidermal cells and the characteristic multinucleated giant cells with intranuclear inclusions with a perinuclear halo (Wright and Ferenczy, 1994). As the disease progresses, an acute necrotising cervicitis evolves with extensive necrosis, destruction of stroma, glands and vessels, and dense stromal infiltration with acute and chronic inflammatory cells (Fig. 15.18).

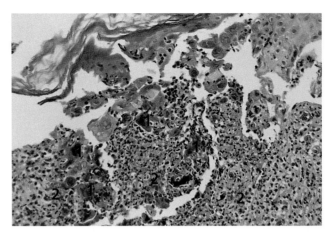

Fig. 15.18 Biopsy taken from a herpetic cervix approximately 36 hours after symptoms commenced. At this stage, vesicle formation and ulceration are present on the cervix. Examination of the former shows it to be composed of giant cells at the edge (1) and in the base; polymorphonuclear leucocytes (2) are present in the surrounding epithelium. There may be some basal cell hyperplasia in the surrounding epithelium.

Human papillomavirus (HPV)

The subject of the human papillomavirus has been discussed in many places in this text. However, in this section, a résumé of the histology and pathology that accompanies this infection in the cervix will be discussed.

Case–control studies, case series and prevalence surveys have unequivocally shown that HPV DNA can be detected in adequate specimens of cervical cancer and precancer in 100% of cases compared with a prevalence of 5–20% in cervical specimens from women identified as suitable as epidemiological control subjects (Bosch *et al.*, 2002; Bohmer *et al.*, 2003).

HPV produces two types of lesions on the cervix. These are: (1) clinical condyloma, various forms; and (2) a subclinical non-condylomatous type that is obvious only after the application of acetic acid.

The condylomatous lesions have been described histologically by Burghardt (1991), and their colposcopic representations are as follows. The so-called primary condyloma is the most common and is composed of thickened epithelium that forms excrescences on the cervix. Scaffolds of delicate stromal stalks rich in blood vessels give rise to its classical clinical appearance (Fig. 15.19). Histologically, the epithelium is squamous with a predominant basal layer as well as a thick layer of prickle cells that are in turn overlain by a zone of cells of clear cytoplasm reminiscent of normal cervical squamous epithelium (Fig. 15.20). The clear cytoplasm is due to a large perinuclear halo that is offset by rather dense cytoplasm. These cells are often binucleated or multinucleated and are referred to as koilocytes. Nuclear atypia and not just a perinuclear halo

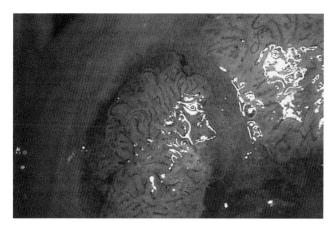

Fig. 15.19 Condylomata accuminata on the cervix with typical blood vessel appearance.

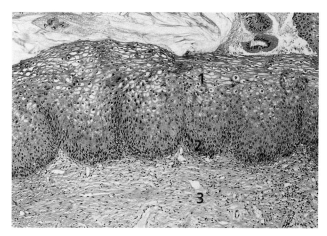

Fig. 15.21 Squamous epithelium showing the features of wart virus infection; the surface (1) displays prominent koilocytic changes in the cells immediately beneath the surface. The basal cells (2) show some nuclear atypia, and the lesion is classified as a flat condyloma.

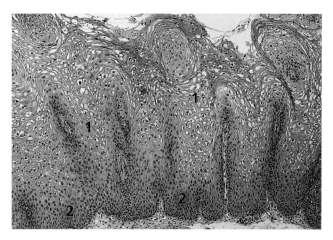

Fig. 15.20 A condyloma with a papillary surface configuration. There are widespread areas of koilocytosis at (1); normal stroma is present at (2).

are essential for a diagnosis of koilocytosis. These koilocytes, characteristic of HPV infection, have a wrinkled nuclear membrane and various degrees of hyperchromasia ('raisin' nuclei).

Four other types of lesions are described, and these include the second type, or spiked condyloma. The flat condyloma makes up the third type, and their pathology is characterised by the presence of the HPV antigen with koilocytes with perinuclear halos being present and also cells that have nuclear pleomorphism with dense cytoplasm, especially in the middle superficial layers of the epithelium (Fig. 15.21). Other authors consider this type of lesion to be synonymous with the subclinical papillomavirus infections to be described below (Coppleson and Pixley, 1992).

The fourth and an uncommon type of condyloma is the so-called inverted condyloma, which is characteristically present within the areas of endocervical crypts. It is impossible to distinguish histologically between the flat condyloma and

low-grade squamous intraepithelial lesions (CIN1), and many pathologists consider these to be one and the same lesion. In the US, these five types of HPV infection described above have all been classified as low-grade squamous intraepithelial lesions (CIN1). However, colposcopically, it would seem as though differentiation into these five types may be of benefit in trying to correlate colposcopic and histological/ pathological images.

The final type is the subclinical non-condylomatous papillomavirus infections that are clinically unapparent minor-grade lesions which show a number of features that differentiate them from more significant CIN or high-grade lesions. These subclinical lesions contain many of the histological features of the condylomatous type described above. Typical examples histologically are seen in Figures 15.21, 15.22 and 15.23, and Figures 21.2 and 21.4 in Chapter 21.

The cytological changes that are readily revealed by Papanicolaou staining show the characteristic koilocytes (1) as seen in Figure 15.24. There is nuclear enlargement, some hyperchromasia, binucleation and clearing or 'cavitation' of the central part of the cell. This produces a characteristic koilocytotic appearance. The nuclear changes are indistinguishable from so-called mild dyskaryosis [low-grade squamous intraepithelial lesions (LSIL)/CIN1] (Fig. 15.24).

The mucosal epithelial microenvironment plays a part in the initiation and progression of these HPV-associated changes within the cervix. The immune surveillance of the epithelium is undertaken in part by Langerhans cells that are present within the endo- and ectocervix. Giannini *et al.* (2002) have recently investigated the influence of the local microenvironment existing within the transformation zone on the function and density of the Langerhans cells. They noted that there was a significant reduction in the density of immature Langerhans

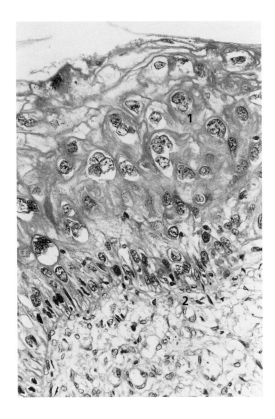

Fig. 15.22 Biopsy from a lesion that showed signs of subclinical papillomavirus infection (SPI); classical features of koilocytosis and multinucleation (1) are present, especially within the middle and superficial layers. There is pleomorphism and hyperchromasia in the basal layer and in increase in cellular proliferation. The stroma can be seen at (2).

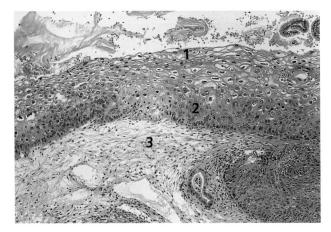

Fig. 15.23 Biopsy from the cervix of a 24-year-old woman who presented cytological evidence of typical koilocytes and mild dyskaryosis (LSIL/CIN1). Punch biopsy shows that koilocytes (1) are present in the superficial layer, whereas there is some basal cell proliferation with very mild nuclear atypia and multinucleation at (2). The stroma (3) is normal.

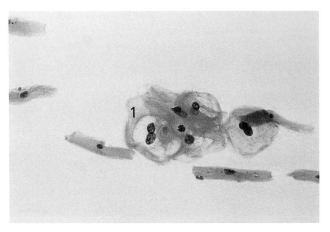

Fig. 15.24 The cytological changes that are readily revealed by Papanicolaou staining show the characteristic koilocytes (1). There is nuclear enlargement, some hyperchromasia, binucleation and clearing or 'cavitation' of the central part of the cell. This produces a characteristic koilocytotic appearance. The nuclear changes are indistinguishable from so-called mild dyskaryosis (LSIL/CIN1).

cells (CD1a–/Lag) within the transformation zone compared with the density of those existing on the ectocervix, which is composed of original (native) squamous epithelium. They found that, when intraepithelial neoplasia develops in relation to HPV, there seems to be a relative increase in the density of the immature Langerhans cells within the transformation zone. They showed that the variation in Langerhans cells was correlated with a differential expression of tumour necrosis factor (TNF) α, macrophage inflammatory protein (MIP) 3α and in interleukin (IL) 10 production within the microenvironment of the transformation zone and the intraepithelial neoplastic areas. They concluded that the immunosurveillance within the epithelium of the transformation zone was intrinsically altered as a result of changes in the expression of chemokines/cytokines and the simultaneous diminished density of Langerhans cells. They also concluded that, following HPV infection and the development of intraepithelial neoplasia, the function of Langerhans cells was further incapacitated by some viral-associated mechanisms (Giannini *et al.*, 2002).

Cytomegalovirus

Cytomegalovirus (CMV) infection is widespread in the general population, but it is usually asymptomatic. In the US, 85% of the population may be infected by adulthood (Smiley and Huang, 1990). CMV is a double-stranded DNA virus and morphologically resembles other herpesviruses. Prevalence of CMV infection in the adult population varies from 40% in Europe to 100% in Africa. The virus can be isolated from the cervix, semen and saliva, and sexual transmission is thought to be a major mode of spread. CMV can be isolated from the

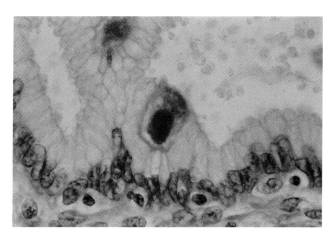

Fig. 15.25 CMV cervicitis, showing characteristic intranuclear inclusion. Reprinted with the permission of Dr S.J. Robboy.

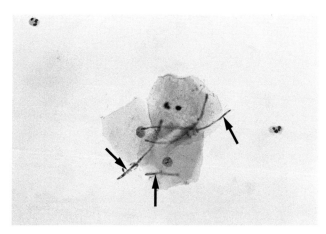

Fig. 15.26 Cervical smear with spores and hyphae of *Candida albicans* presenting as thin, red lines in the cervical smear (arrowed).

cervix of approximately 8% of women (Pereira *et al.*, 1990). Cytomegalovirus infection of the cervix has been reported to be present concurrently with other organisms such as *N. gonorrhoeae* (Pereira *et al.*, 1990), and women with another genital infection are at a higher risk of having CMV. CMV appears to be tropic for the glandular cells of the endocervix rather than the squamous cells of the ectocervix and also infects endothelial cells. The infected cell is enlarged, with a single large round to oval, red to purple, intranuclear inclusion surrounded by a halo (Fig. 15.25). Small basophilic cytoplasmic inclusions may also be seen. Clinical suspicion of CMV infection must be confirmed by available laboratory tests such as viral isolation, serology, electron microscopy, histological evaluation, immunohistochemical staining of tissue or nucleic acid hybridisation techniques.

MYCOTIC INFECTIONS

Candida

The cervix may be involved in vulvovaginal candidiasis. Some 80–95% of fungal vaginitis is attributed to *Candida albicans* and 3–16% to *Torulopsis glabrata* (Clark and Rosenfeld, 1989). The majority of genital fungal infections are not sexually acquired. Predisposing factors for candidiasis include pregnancy, oral contraceptive pills, antibiotics that disrupt the normal flora, menstruation, diabetes mellitus, immunosuppressive agents and poor hygiene. The most common presenting symptom is pruritus. There may be a cottage cheese-like vaginal discharge. On examination, the ectocervix may appear normal or erythematous. Papanicolaou-stained cervical smears show eosinophilic to grey-brown budding yeasts and filamentous forms of the fungus with pseudohyphae (Fig. 15.26) associated with an intense polymorphonuclear leucocytic infiltrate. Non-specific reactive changes may be seen in the

squamous cells such as nuclear enlargement, indistinct perinuclear halos and nuclear debris (Bonfiglio, 1997). Diagnosis of candidiasis can be confirmed by microscopic examination of a wet mount preparation of the vaginal discharge, Gram stain smears, Papanicolaou-stained cervicovaginal smears or culture. Occasionally, organisms can be identified histologically. A variety of antifungal agents are available for therapy.

The vaginal discharge of candidiasis varies from paltry to thick and white with plaques of this discharge adherent to the ectocervical mucosa. Histological examination of the mucosa below these plaques shows the underlying tissue to be markedly erythematous with tiny punctate ulcers. As the condition progresses and in more severe cases, the organism even penetrates and proliferates between and within the basal and parabasal cells of the ectocervix, with disruption of the normal architecture. The latter is partly due to the infiltration of the epithelium by inflammatory cells, the principal ones being the polymorphonuclear leucocytes. This would appear to be a tissue reaction to try to eliminate the *C. albicans* infection as well as a response to the release of the associated cytolytic enzymes by the yeast. It has been suggested by Garcia-Temaio *et al.* (1982) that this intracellular growth may be protected against humoral and cellular attack and a way of resisting antimycotic therapy.

PARASITIC INFECTIONS

Trichomoniasis

Trichomoniasis affects approximately 3 million American women annually. It is a common sexually transmitted disease caused by a flagellated protozoon, *Trichomonas vaginalis*. There is often concurrent infection with other sexually transmitted diseases such as gonorrhoea and *C. trachomatis* infection. The incubation period ranges between 5 and 28 days. Trichomoniasis

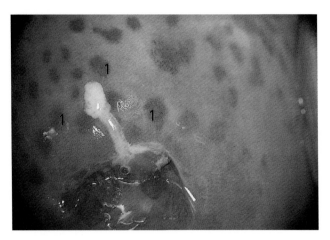

Fig. 15.27 A typical 'strawberry' cervix of a woman with severe trichomonal cervicitis.

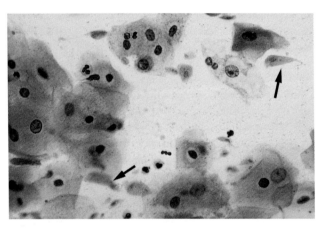

Fig. 15.28 A cervical smear showing the protozoon infection of *Trichomonas vaginalis.* The characteristic appearance is of a small, blue-grey, ill-defined body within elongated nuclei (arrowed).

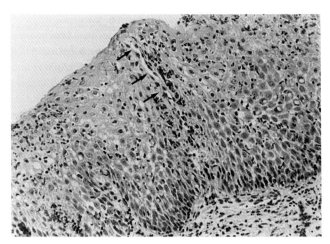

Fig. 15.29 Biopsy from an ectocervix infected with *Trichomonas vaginalis.* There is much epithelial degeneration and inflammatory infiltrate. Note the capillary cut longitudinally and arrowed, which runs almost to the surface, giving rise to the typical 'strawberry' cervicitis.

can be asymptomatic in women. An estimated 10–50% of women attending sexually transmitted disease clinics are asymptomatic carriers (Rein, 2000). The vaginal microenvironment, including the presence of menstrual blood, pH and hormone levels, has been observed to affect the pathogenicity of *T. vaginalis* (Rein and Muller, 1990). Symptoms of trichomoniasis include a yellow-green bubbly vaginal discharge and irritation. The vaginal walls and ectocervix are acutely inflamed. The endocervix is uninvolved. On colposcopic examination, punctate haemorrhages are observed on the cervix, giving it a strawberry appearance (Fig. 15.27).

These strawberry patches of cervicitis or vaginitis are characterised by a multitude of tiny red dots, each of which is the tip of a subepithelial capillary that reaches almost to the surface (Fig. 15.28). Wet mount preparations of vaginal secretions are used to identify typical flagellated, motile, ovoid parasites in a

background of polymorphonuclear leucocytes. The organisms appear in Papanicolaou-stained smears as small oval to round structures with a pale grey-blue cytoplasm with red granules and an eccentric nucleus (Fig. 15.29). There is associated acute inflammation, and reactive cytological changes such as nuclear enlargement and perinuclear halos are seen in the squamous cells. Squamous epithelium of the trichomonally infected cervix shows degenerative changes that are more marked in the superficial layers, suggesting that the parasite has a direct effect. In about 25% of cases, there is a marked degeneration of the surface epithelium and partial replacement by a purulent exudate or pseudomembrane (Fig. 15.30). Deep ulceration and full-thickness necrosis of the epithelium is uncommon, but the adjacent epithelium shows various abnormalities such as nuclear enlargement, binucleate forms and much variability in cell size in association with a diffuse permeation by acute inflammatory cells. Intercellular oedema is marked, and many of these squamous cells also show a perinuclear halo at all levels of the epithelium caused by intracellular oedema. Tests more sensitive than the wet mount are available, such as direct fluorescent antibody staining, latex agglutination and enzyme-linked immunosorbent assay techniques. However, culture remains the most sensitive of all the techniques. Metronidazole remains the drug of choice for the treatment of trichomoniasis.

Schistosomiasis

Schistosomiasis of the female genital tract is a well-known clinical entity in parts of Africa, South America and some Asian countries. Cervical schistosomiasis is the most common of all genital schistosomiasis (Schwartz, 1984; Kjetland *et al.*, 1996)

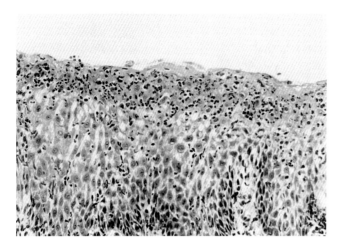

Fig. 15.30 Cervical tissue adjacent to that in Figure 15.29, showing marked superficial inflammation and degeneration with the formation of a pyogenic membrane in the upper portion of the epithelium. Note the well-marked intercellular oedema and the diffuse infiltration with acute inflammatory cells.

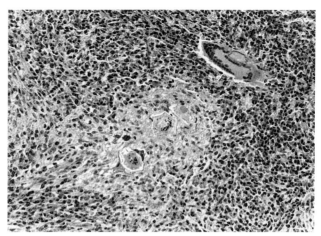

Fig. 15.31 Cervical biopsy in a 49-year-old Tanzanian woman, showing florid granulomatous reaction about fragmented schistosome ova. A multinucleate giant cell is seen, but the inflammatory component is mainly lymphohistiocytic, with numerous eosinophils.

and is chiefly associated with *Schistosoma hematobium* infection. The vesical venous plexus is preferentially parasitised by *S. hematobium*, and its proximity to the uterovaginal plexus and female genital organs is the source of the increased frequency of *S. hematobium* genital infection compared with genital infection by the intestinal form of the disease caused by *Schistosoma mansoni*. Clinical manifestations of cervical schistosomiasis include irregular vaginal bleeding (Schwartz, 1984), dyspareunia, infertility, a friable cervix, dysmenorrhoea and backache, and recent reports suggest a possible increased risk of cervical neoplasia (Moubayed *et al.*, 1995; North *et al.*, 2003). The predominant colposcopic findings are reported to be sandy patches (Helling-Giese *et al.*, 1996) on the cervix. Other findings described are papillomatous growths, nodules, cauliflower-like masses, friable areas and ulcers (Schwartz, 1984; Helling-Giese *et al.*, 1996). Eggs are most commonly deposited in the endocervical subepithelial tissue close to the transformation zone (Berry, 1996). The ova of *S. hematobium* are oval shaped with a chitinous shell varying in length from 80 μm to 186 μm and in breadth from 30 μm to 93 μm with a terminal spine (Berry, 1996) (Fig. 15.32b and c). On microscopic examination of the cervix, a wide range of histopathological changes have been noted, which include no change to chronic cervicitis with lymphoplasmacytic and histiocytic infiltration in subepithelial connective tissue, eosinophilic abscesses, ulceration, acanthosis of squamous epithelium with pseudoepitheliomatous hyperplasia and foreign body granuloma formation progressing to fibrosis and calcification (Berry, 1996) (Fig. 15.31). Ova may be seen as single or numerous, mature and viable or degenerated forms within granulomas or in the subepithelial connective tissue beneath the hyperplastic surface epithelium (Figs 15.32a and 15.33).

Schistosomiasis as a cause of cervical cancer is a topic of debate, and there are conflicting reports as to the role of *S. hematobium* in the genesis of cervical cancer (Schwartz, 1984; Moubayed *et al.*, 1995; North *et al.*, 2003).

Entamoeba histolytica and other parasites

Amoebiasis is of widespread occurrence in tropical and subtropical countries, usually producing syndromes of intestinal and hepatic involvement (Spencer, 1973). Mucocutaneous amoebiasis with destructive ulceration may occur with spread from anus to perineum and subsequent involvement of the pudenda (Cohen, 1973), but direct venereal infection may also occur (Mylius and Ten Seldam, 1962). There is extensive destruction of the tissues with shallow ulcers covered by necrotic yellow slough, friable granulation tissue and accompanied by a profuse serosanguinous discharge. Cervical ulceration is frequently eccentric, sparing the external os, but, in cases coming to autopsy, the infection may extend to the body of the uterus (Weinstein and Weed, 1948).

Amoebic ulceration may simulate cervical carcinoma (Braga and Teoh, 1964). Numerous trophozoite forms of the parasite may be found in wet vaginal smears, but biopsy is necessary to establish the diagnosis for, occasionally, amoebiasis and carcinoma occur simultaneously (Carter *et al.*, 1954).

Other parasitic infections of the cervix are rare. Threadworms (*Oxyuris vermicularis*) may infect the genital tract, spreading from the bowel and producing a necrotising granulomatous inflammation in the vagina, cervix and fallopian tubes with numerous eosinophils (Symmers, 1950). Hydatid disease may sometimes affect pelvic organs with involvement of the uterus and cervix (Langley, 1973).

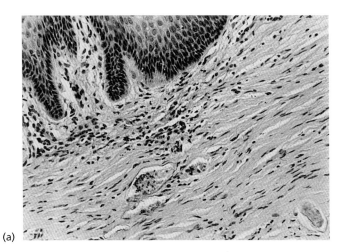

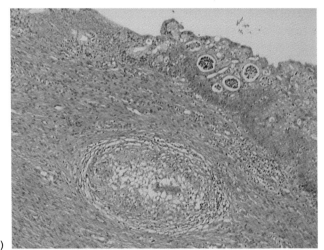

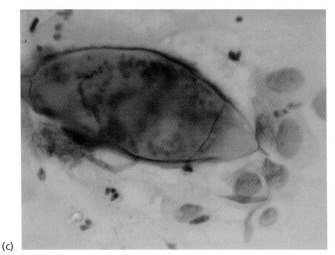

Fig. 15.32 (a) A biopsy from a hard, craggy cervix in a 48-year-old Nigerian woman clinically diagnosed as having cancer. Schistosome ova are seen in the dense fibrotic stroma, with relatively minor inflammation beneath an acanthotic but non-neoplastic epithelium. (b) Schistosome ova clearly visible within the epithelium of a fibrotic stroma with a central granuloma. (c) A classic schistosome ovum as seen on a Pap smear.

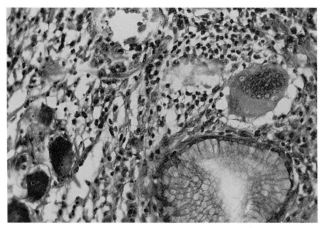

Fig. 15.33 Schistosomiasis. Inflammatory reaction with a multinucleated giant cell is seen adjacent to ova. Reprinted with the permission of Dr S.J. Robboy.

INFLAMMATORY DISEASE ASSOCIATED WITH THE CERVIX

Polyarteritis nodosa and isolated arteritis

Polyarteritis nodosa is occasionally found in the genital tract with the cervix being involved as part of a generalised lesion and overshadowed in a severe systemic illness. Patalano and Sommers (1961) found isolated uterine arteritis in six out of 17 necropsied cases, while Ansell *et al.* (1974) demonstrated a similar localised necrotising arteritis as an incidental finding in surgically resected cervices. The medium-sized muscular arteries are affected with occasional arteriolar involvement. Subintimal hyaline deposition and fibrinoid necrosis also occur, but there is a relative paucity of neutrophil and eosinophil polymorphonuclear leucocytes (Figs 15.34 and 15.35).

Thrombosis and aneurysm formation are not seen, and the appearances thus differ from classical polyarteritis nodosa. Nevertheless, the histological differences are not sufficiently specific to exclude polyarteritis in an individual case. The significance of these isolated changes is uncertain. No evidence can be elicited to incriminate in the aetiology an immune or drug reaction, trauma or a secondary result of superficial inflammation. The lesion appears to be benign, and the subsequent development of systemic polyarteritis has not been reported. Isolated uterine and cervical arteritis has been reported as a chance finding in cone biopsy specimens and in hysterectomy specimens, but its significance is uncertain (Crowe and McWhinney, 1979). The outcome of cases that resemble closely isolated arteritis of the appendix or gall bladder appears to be generally excellent but, as in individual cases, prediction is uncertain. For that reason, simple exclusion of systemic arteritis by haematological and renal screening would seem

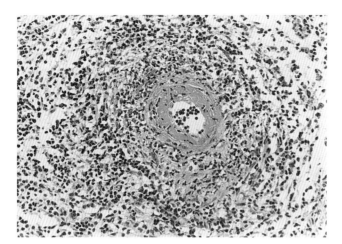

Fig. 15.34 Isolated arteritis of the cervix resected as part of a Manchester repair. Note the marked perivascular inflammatory component, consisting mainly of round cells but with a minor acute cell component. Inflammatory cells permeate the vessel wall, which is eosinophilic but does not show fibrinoid necrosis (H&E × 170).

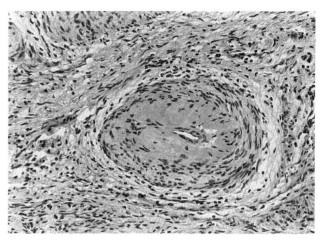

Fig. 15.35 Adjacent artery showing minor arteritic lesion with well-marked subintimal hyalinisation (H&E × 170).

sensible. Sometimes, it is difficult to find an aetiological agent such as a drug or immune reaction, or a secondary response to some pre-existing inflammation, either locally or in another part of the body, or trauma. The lesions usually run a benign course, and the subsequent development of systemic disease has only rarely been reported (Ganesan *et al.*, 2000).

Behçet's syndrome

Behçet (1940) described a chronic relapsing syndrome characterised by oral and genital ulceration and ocular inflammation. Since the original description, the syndrome has been widened to include other lesions: encephalitis (McMenemy and Lawrence, 1957), cutaneous ulceration, colitis (Bøe *et al.*, 1958) and thrombophlebitis. There is a variable course with remissions and exacerbation; fulminant cases with death from encephalitis or colitis may occur. The definition of the syndrome is imprecise, and separation from both simple aphthosis and chronic ulcerative colitis with systemic lesions may be difficult. The diagnosis of Behçet's syndrome is based only on clinical grounds, and there are no pathognomonic laboratory or histological features. However, in 1990 at an international study group on Behçet's syndrome, Wechsler and Piette (1992) recommended diagnostic criteria that are usually associated with Behçet's syndrome.

1 Recurrent oral ulceration is an obligatory finding.
2 No. (1) must be accompanied by two of the following symptoms or signs:
   a recurrent genital ulceration;
   b eye lesions;
   c cutaneous lesions.

The causative agent may be viral and the pathogenesis of the lesion is probably vascular. An association with HLA-B5 has been described, but immunogenetic factors may vary in different parts of the world.

The genital ulceration usually occurs on the vulva as a very painful acute lesion 2–3 cm in diameter with associated painless vaginal and cervical lesions (O'Duffy *et al.*, 1971) (Fig. 15.36). Biopsy of the ulcers shows a non-specific chronic or subacute inflammation. Some reports (O'Duffy *et al.*, 1971; Chajek and Fainaru, 1975) stress that there may be a vasculitis of submucosal venules, capillaries and arterioles with vascular infiltration by lymphocytes and plasma cells. These appearances seem to be variable (Bøe *et al.*, 1958), although perivascular cuffing with lymphocytes is a constant finding (Strouth and Dyker, 1964; Lehner, 1969; Hurt *et al.*, 1979). Decreased plasma fibrinolytic activity in patients with active Behçet's syndrome has been noted, suggesting possible defects in the blood coagulation mechanisms (Chajek and Fainaru, 1975). 'Autoantibodies' to human mucous membrane occur in the sera of patients with Behçet's syndrome, but these are variable and show poor correlation with disease activity (Lehner, 1969). Immunological studies have not provided any clear definition of Behçet's syndrome or any indication of aetiology, which remains obscure. A virus is considered to be involved in its causation, although it has been suggested that it may be an immunopathological response to an HSV type 1 infection (Elgin *et al.*, 1982) as circulating immune complexes have been found in blood.

Behçet's syndrome is a rare disease and vaginal/cervical ulceration an uncommon manifestation. Nevertheless, it is important because of the serious sequelae of the syndrome. It is also imperative to exclude invasive squamous cancer. Recurrent herpes and recurrent untreated syphilis have to be

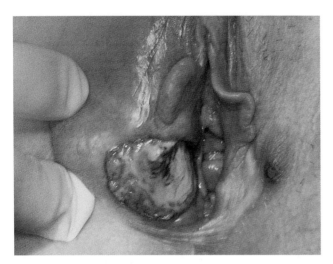

Fig. 15.36 A patient with extensive Behçet's syndrome showing labia minora involved with a typical lesion encompassing all the features common to a Behçet's ulcer. The genital lesion is highly destructive, which has resulted in fenestration and scarring, with progressive loss of the vulval tissue, extending outwards from the labia minora. Notice the depth of involvement of the lesion. In this woman, viral and bacterial cultures were negative, as was the darkfield examination. Serological tests for syphilis were non-reactive, but biopsy showed a non-specific chronic inflammatory process with associated vasculitis. This patient also had lesions on her lips, tongue, buccal mucosa and palate.

considered and tested for their presence, as does pemphigus, which may cause lesions of both the genitalia and the mouth. Pemphigus, which is described below, can be excluded by using specific immunofluorescent stains on fresh tissue samples.

Megaloblastic disease

Vitamin B12 and folate deficiencies interfere with the metabolism of the epithelium. Van Nierker (1966) and Whitehead *et al.* (1973) also presented evidence that may be related to the oral contraceptive steroids. Megaloblasts are formed in the squamous epithelium of the cervix, and these mirror similar forms found in bone marrow and epithelium elsewhere. The epithelial changes involve both the basal and the parabasal layers, and there is enlargement of the nuclei and cytoplasm and the formation of multinucleate cell forms (Van Nierker, 1962). The chromatin is finely dispersed in the nucleus, resembling that of bone marrow and megaloblasts. Atypical cells, multinucleation and hyperchromatism can more often be associated with B12 deficiency than with folate deficiency and, as Koss (1974) emphasised, these atypical epithelial megaloblasts are found in cervical smears but the appearances are seldom diagnostic. The presence of neoplasia needs to be excluded.

Pemphigus vulgaris

Changes on the cervix where ulceration is common in this very rare condition mirror those found in the skin (Friedman *et al.*, 1971). The cervix, being so fragile, is easily traumatised during examination, giving rise to the so-called positive Nikolsky sign (Segher *et al.*, 1974).

INFLAMMATION ASSOCIATED WITH NEOPLASIA

Inflammatory reaction to primary tumour

Many types of primary malignant tumours are associated with an inflammatory reaction both within the tumour and in the adjacent stroma. There is a lymphoreticular reaction with invasion of the tumour by lymphocytes, plasma cells and macrophages (Carr and Underwood, 1974). This may be associated with sinus histiocytosis in the regional lymph nodes. These reactions are characteristic of an immune response and the degree of lymphoid infiltrates in neuroblastoma (Lauder and Aherne, 1972), choriocarcinoma (Elston, 1969) and breast carcinoma (Hamlin, 1968). These reactions have been positively correlated by certain authors with the clinical course of the malignancy. However, Turner and Berry (1972) were unable to confirm such a correlation in carcinoma of the breast. Carter (1975) described the local tumour infiltrates as typical neither of a homograft reaction nor of delayed hypersensitivity and concluded that, although the lymphoplasmacytic infiltrate represents an immunological response, its mode of action is not clear (Fig. 15.37). Similar lymphocytic and plasma cell infiltrates in the epithelium and stroma of preinvasive and invasive carcinomas of the cervix are common (Friedell *et al.*, 1960; Lowe *et al.*, 1981). Reid and Coppleson (1971), in an extensive review, suggested that the reaction in the cervix develops as a reaction to potentially malignant lesions with a particular role in limiting mutagenic changes in the epithelium. There is a frequent and acute associated inflammatory reaction with invasion of the lesion by neutrophil and eosinophil polymorphonuclear leucocytes. This acute reaction appears to be related primarily to necrosis and secondary infection (Lowe *et al.*, 1981; Lowe and Fletcher, 1984). The vascular reaction in the stroma may be increased in part as a result of the normal inflammatory processes.

Inflammatory reaction after irradiation

Irradiation of cervical carcinoma produces its effects by direct action on the tumour cells and indirectly by changes in the tumour bed (Haines and Taylor, 1975). When the response is favourable, the tumour shrinks in bulk and necrosis may be a major feature. In the stroma, vascular dilatation and ectasia is seen but endarteritis is often marked. Associated with this,

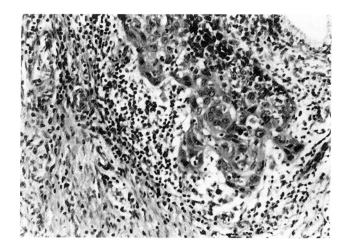

Fig. 15.37 Invasive cords of squamous carcinoma are surrounded by inflammatory cells, mainly plasma cells and lymphocytes. Note that there is a close relationship with inflammatory cells infiltrating into the tumour tissue.

there is an inflammatory cellular infiltrate including both acute and chronic cells. Plasma cells and giant cells may predominate. In the later stages, the associated reparative reaction may produce a diffuse marked fibrosis and this, in association with giant cells, can provide bizarre histological appearances (Pawson, 1981).

NON-SPECIFIC CERVICITIS

Acute non-specific cervicitis may result from direct trauma such as the laceration of childbirth (Chapter 7). Florid bacterial inflammations may also follow the complications of puerperal endometritis and septic abortion. Acute cervicitis (Fig. 15.38a and b) may result from the use of douches and ointments or from abortifacients in common usage prior to legally available abortion. In previous times, the use of potassium permanganate was associated with such changes (Philipp, 1953). All these agents may produce ulceration and bleeding from the vagina and cervix. Genital ulceration may rarely complicate drug hypersensitivity.

The range of organisms isolated from cervices showing histological evidence of chronic inflammation is wide: coliforms and commensal vaginal organisms may be grown as well as chlamydia (Gutman *et al.*, 1972), mycoplasma (Dunlop, 1974) and *Haemophilus vaginalis* (Langley, 1973). This does not necessarily indicate that they play a primary infective role, and their presence may only be secondary to alteration in the cervical milieu. Vaginal and cervical infections with severe ulceration are very uncommon but, in debilitated and marasmic patients, may follow infection with anaerobic coliforms, streptococci and organisms of Vincent's angina.

Chronic non-specific cervicitis is a common gynaecological disorder, which may be due in part to low-grade infection in

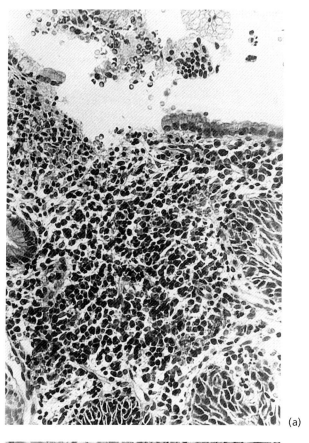

(a)

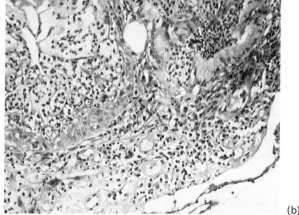

(b)

Fig. 15.38 (a) and (b) An acute inflammatory cervicitis, showing the infiltration of inflammatory cells throughout the stroma with some surface ulceration.

a locally altered cervical environment (Fig. 15.38a and b). In the cervix distorted by minor lacerations, exposure of the cervical canal to the lowered pH of vaginal secretions and altered bacterial flora provides a nidus and an opportunity for chronic infection. Moreover, established inflammation in endocervical glands produces structural changes (oedema and reparative fibrosis) which impair drainage from the mucous glands and help to perpetuate optimal conditions for continuing infection.

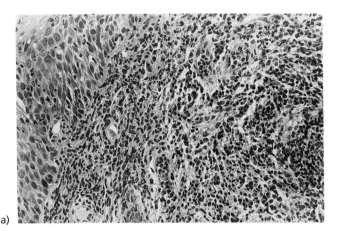

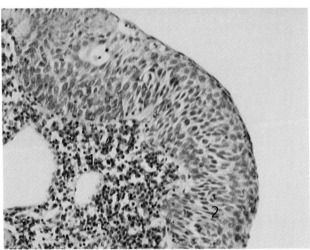

(a)

(b)

Fig. 15.39 (a) and (b) An intense chronic inflammatory/immune reaction (1) underlines an area of intraepithelial neoplasia (2).

Some chronic inflammatory infiltrates in the cervix may represent immune reactions to local alterations in the cervical epithelium (Fig. 15.39a and b). The cervix is exposed to a wide range of insults including potentially coitally transmitted mutants. The inflammatory changes induced by the absorption of such new antigens into the epithelium and stroma may represent a form of host defence mechanism, and these changes, when noted in the malignant cervical epithelium and stroma, may indicate a further and active extension of this defence mechanism.

ACKNOWLEDGEMENTS

The authors wish to thank Professor A. Singer for the kind provision of Figures 15.5b, 15.5c, 15.7a, 15.14a, 15.16, 15.18, 15.19, 15.20–15.24, 15.26–15.28 and 15.36. A number of figures appeared in the original first edition of *The Cervix*, and these are designated in the legend. Dr A.R.S. Deery of St George's Hospital, London, contributed Figures 15.15b, 15.32b, 15.32c, 15.38b and 15.39b.

REFERENCES

Anderson MC, Robboy SJ, Russell P *et al.* (2002) The cervix — benign and non-neoplastic conditions. In: Robboy S, Anderson M, Russell P (eds) *Pathology of the Female Reproductive Tract.* London: Churchill Livingstone, pp. 105–135.

Ansell ID, Evans DJ, Wight DGD (1974) Asymptomatic arteritis of the uterine cervix. *Journal of Clinical Pathology* 27: 664–668.

Ballard RC (2000) Calymmatobacterium granulomatis (donovanosis, granuloma inguinale) In: Mandell GL, Bennett JE, Dolin R (eds) *Principles and Practice of Infectious Diseases.* New York: Churchill Livingstone, pp. 2457–2459.

Behçet H (1940) Some observations of the clinical picture of the so called triple symptoms complex. *Dermatologica* 81: 73–77.

Berry A (1996) A cytopathological and histopathological study of bilharziasis of the female genital tract. *Journal of Pathology and Bacteriology* 9: 325.

Bøe J, Dalgaard JB, Scott D (1958) Mucocutaneous ocular syndrome with intestinal involvements. *American Journal of Medicine* 25: 857–867.

Bohmer G, Van den Brule AJ, Brummer O *et al.* (2003) No confirmed case of human papillomavirus DNA-negative cervical intraepithelial neoplasia grade 3 or invasive primary cancer of the uterine cervix among 511 patients. *American Journal of Obstetrics and Gynecology* 189: 118–120.

Bonfiglio TA (1997) Benign cellular changes. In: Bonfiglio TA, Erozan YS (eds) *Gynecologic Cytopathology.* Philadelphia: Lippincott-Raven, pp. 33–50.

Bosch FX, Lorincz A, Monoz N *et al.* (2002) The causal relation between human papillomavirus and cervical cancer. *Journal of Clinical Pathology* 55: 244–265.

Braga CA, Teoh TB (1964) Amoebiasis of the cervix and vagina. *Journal of Obstetrics and Gynaecology of the British Commonwealth* 71: 299–301.

Burghardt E (1991) *Colposcopy, Cervical Pathology, Textbook and Atlas,* 2nd edn. Stuttgart: George Thieme Verlag.

Carr I, Underwood JCE (1974) The ultrastructure of the local cellular reaction to neoplasia. In: Bourne EGH, Denielli JF (eds) *International Review of Cytology.* New York: Academic Press.

Carter B, Jones CP, Thomas WL (1954) Invasion of squamous cell carcinoma of the cervix uteri by *Entamoeba histolytica. American Journal of Obstetrics and Gynecology* 68: 1607–1610.

Carter RL (1975) Immunological control of metastatic growth. In: Stoll BA (ed.) *Host Defence in Breast Cancer.* London: Heinemann.

Chajek T, Fainaru M (1975) Behçet's disease. Report of 41 cases and review of the literature. *Medicine* 53: 179–196.

Chakraborty P, Roy A, Bhattacharya S *et al.* (1995) Tuberculous cervicitis: a clinicopathological and bacteriological study. *Journal of the Indian Medical Association* 93: 167–168.

Clark J, Rosenfeld WD (1989) Vulvovaginitis and cervicitis. *Pediatric Clinics of North America* 36: 489–511.

Cohen C (1973) Three cases of amoebiasis of the cervix uteri. *Journal of Obstetrics and Gynaecology of the British Commonwealth* 80: 476–479.

Coppleson M, Pixley E (1992) Effect of human papillomavirus infections. In: Coppleson M (ed.) *Gynaecological Oncology*, Vol. 1, 2nd edn. Edinburgh: Churchill Livingstone, p. 303.

Corey L, Holmes KK (1983a) Genital herpes simplex virus infection:

current concepts in diagnosis, therapy and prevention. *Annals of Internal Medicine* 98: 973–983.

Corey L, Holmes KK (1983b) Genital herpes simplex virus infection: clinical manifestations, course, and complications. *Annals of Internal Medicine* 98: 958–972.

Crowe J, McWhinney N (1979) Isolated arteritis of the cervix uteri. *British Journal of Obstetrics and Gynaecology* 86: 393–398.

Crum CP, Mitao M, Winkler B *et al.* (1984) Localizing chlamydial infection in cervical biopsies with the immunoperoxidase technique. *International Journal of Gynecological Pathology* 3: 191–197.

Demay R (1996) A micromiscellany of microbiology. In: *The Art and Science of Cytopathology Exfoliative Cytology.* Chicago: ASCP Press, pp. 55.

Dunlop EMC (1974) Non specific genital infection — laboratory aspects. In: Morton RS, Harris JWR (eds) *Recent Advances in Sexually Transmitted Diseases,* No. 1. Edinburgh: Churchill Livingstone.

Elgin RP, Lehner T, Subak-Sharpe JH (1982) Detection of RNA complementary to Herpes simplex virus in mononuclear cells from patients with Behçet's syndrome and recurrent oral ulcers. *Lancet* 2: 1356.

Elston CW (1969) Cellular reaction to choriocarcinoma. *Journal of Pathology* 97: 261–267.

Fitzgerald FT (1984) The classic venereal diseases syphilis and gonorrhea in the 80s. *Postgraduate Medicine* 75 (8): 91–101.

Friedell GH, Hertig AT, Younge PA (1960) *Carcinoma in situ of the Uterine Cervix.* Springfield: Charles C. Thomas.

Friedman D, Haim S, Pal DE (1971) Refractory involvement of the cervix uteri in a case of pemphigus vulgaris. *American Journal of Obstetrics and Gynecology* 110: 1023–1024.

Ganesan R, Ferryman SR, Meier L *et al.* (2000) Vasculitis of the female genital tract with clinico-pathological correlation: a study of 46 cases with follow-up. *International Journal of Gynecological Pathology* 19: 258–265.

Garcia-Temaio J, Castillo G, Martinez AJ (1982) Human genital candidiasis; histochemistry, scanning and transmission electromicroscopy. *Acta Cytologica* 26: 7–14.

Giampaolo C, Murphy J, Benes S *et al.* (1983) How sensitive is the papanicolaou smear in the diagnosis of infections with chlamydia trachomatis? *American Journal of Clinical Pathology* 80: 844–849.

Giannini SL, Hubert P, Doyen J *et al.* (2002) Influence of the mucosal epithelium microenvironment on Langerhans cells: implications for the development of squamous intraepithelial lesions of the cervix. *International Journal of Cancer* 97: 654–659.

Gutman LT, Wiesner PJ, Holmes KK *et al.* (1972) Microbiologic correlates of cervicitis. *Clinical Research* 20: 529.

Haas DW (2000) *Mycobacterium tuberculosis.* In: Mandell GL, Bennett JE, Dolin R (eds) *Principles and Practice of Infectious Diseases.* New York: Churchill Livingstone, pp. 2576–2604.

Haines M, Taylor CW (1975) *Gynaecological Pathology,* 2nd edn. Edinburgh: Churchill Livingstone.

Hamlin IME (1968) Host resistance in breast cancer. *British Journal of Cancer* 22: 383–401.

Helling-Giese G, Feldmeier H *et al.* (1996) Female genital schistosomiasis (FGS): relationship between gynecological and histopathological findings. *Acta Tropica* 62: 257–267.

Hoosen AA, Draper G, Moodley J *et al.* (1990) Granuloma inguinale of the cervix: a carcinoma look-alike. *Genitourinary Medicine* 66: 380–382.

Hurt WG, Cooke CL, Jordan WP *et al.* (1979) Behçet's syndrome associated with pregnancy. *Obstetrics and Gynaecology* 53: 319.

Kjetland EF, Feldmeier H *et al.* (1996) Female genital schistosomiasis due to *Schistosoma haematobium.* Clinical and parasitological findings in women in rural Malawi. *Acta Tropica* 62: 239–255.

Koss LG (1974) Megaloblastic changes in the cervical epithelium. *Journal of the American Medical Association* 227: 1263.

Langley FA (1973) The pathology of the vagina. In: Fox H, Langley FA (eds) *Postgraduate Obstetrical and Gynaecological Pathology.* Oxford: Pergamon.

Lauder I, Aherne W (1972) The significance of lymphocytic infiltration in neuroblastoma. *British Journal of Cancer* 26: 321–330.

Lehner T (1969) Pathology of recurrent oral ulceration in Behçet's syndrome. *Journal of Pathology* 97: 481–494.

Lossick JG, Kraus SJ (1991) Syphilis. In: Evans AS, Brachman AS (eds) *Bacterial Infections of Humans: Epidemiology and Control.* New York, Plenum Publishing Corporation, pp. 675–693.

Lowe D, Fletcher CDM (1984) Eosinophilia in squamous cell carcinoma of the oral cavity, external genitalia and anus; clinical correlations. *Histopathology* 8:627–632.

Lowe D, Jorizzo J, Hutt M (1981) Tumour-associated eosinophilia: a review. *Journal of Clinical Pathology* 34: 1343–1348.

McMenemy WH, Lawrence BJ (1957) Encephalomyopathy in Behçet's disease. *Lancet* ii: 353–358.

Meisels A, Fortin R (1975) Genital tuberculosis: cytological detection. *Acta Cytologica* 19: 79–81.

Moubayed P, Ziehe A, Peters J *et al.* (1995) Carcinoma of the uterine cervix associated with schistosomiasis and induced by human papillomavirus. *International Journal of Obstetrics and Gynaecology* 49: 175–179.

Mylius RE, Ten Seldam REJ (1962) Venereal infection by Entamoeba histolytica in a New Guinea native couple. *Tropical and Geographical Medicine* 14: 20–27.

North M, Dubinchik I, Hamid A *et al.* (2003) Association between cervical schistosomiasis and cervical cancer; report of two cases. *Journal of Reproductive Medicine* 48 (12): 995–998.

O'Duffy JD, Carney JA, Deodhar S (1971) Behçet's disease. *Annals of Internal Medicine* 74: 561–570.

Patalano VJ, Sommers SC (1961) Biopsy diagnosis of polyarteritis nodosa. *Archives of Pathology* 72: 1–7.

Pawson ME (1981) Cervicitis. In: Fischer AM, Gordon G (eds) *Clinics in Obstetrics and Gynaecology* 8:1. London: Saunders, pp. 201–207.

Pereira LH, Embil JA, Haase DA *et al.* (1990) Cytomegalovirus infection among women attending a sexually transmitted disease clinic: association with clinical symptoms and other sexually transmitted diseases. *American Journal of Epidemiology* 131: 683–692.

Philipp EE (1953) Vaginal bleeding due to potassium permanganate. *Lancet* ii: 1278–1279.

Reid BL, Coppleson M (1971) Natural history of the origins of cervical cancer. In: McDonald R (ed.) *Scientific Basis of Obstetrics and Gynaecology,* Vol. 1. Oxford: Churchill.

Rein MF (2000) *Trichomonas vaginalis.* In: Mandell GL, Bennett JE, Dolin R (eds) *Principles and Practice of Infectious Diseases.* New York: Churchill Livingstone, pp. 2943–2945.

Rein MF, Müller M (1990) *Trichomonas vaginalis* and trichomoniasis. In: Holmes KK, Mardh P, Sparling PF *et al.* (eds) *Sexually Transmitted Diseases.* New York: McGraw-Hill, pp. 481–492.

Ross LM (1997a) General information on syphilis. In: *Sexually Transmitted Diseases Sourcebook*, Health reference series, Vol. 26. Detroit: Omnigraphics, p. 413.

Ross LM (1997b) Donovanosis. In: *Sexually Transmitted Diseases Sourcebook*, Health reference series, Vol. 26. Detroit: Omnigraphics, pp. 466–468.

Ross LM (1997c) Genital herpes. In: *Sexually Transmitted Diseases Sourcebook*, Health reference series, vol. 26. Detroit: Omnigraphics, pp. 210–215.

Russo TA (2000) Agents of actinomycosis. In: Mandell GL, Bennett JE, Dolin R (eds) *Principles and Practice of Infectious Diseases*. New York: Churchill Livingstone, pp. 2645–2646.

Samuelson J (1999) Infectious diseases. In: Cotran RS, Kumar V, Collins T (eds) *Robbins Pathologic Basis of Disease*, 6th edn, Philadelphia: WB Saunders, pp. 362–364.

Schaeffer G (1970) Tuberculosis of female genital tract. *Clinics in Obstetrics and Gynecology* 13: 965–998.

Schwartz DA (1984) Carcinoma of the uterine cervix and schistosomiasis in West Africa. *Gynecological Oncology* 19: 365–370.

Segher F, Bercovici B, Romem R (1974) Nikolsky sign on cervix uteri in pemphigus. *British Journal of Dermatology* 90: 407–409.

Sengupta SK, Das N (1984) Donovanosis affecting cervix, uterus, and adenexae. *American Journal of Tropical Medicine and Hygiene* 33: 632–636.

Smiley L, Huang E (1990) Cytomegalovirus as a sexually transmitted infection. In: Holmes KK, Mardh P, Sparling PF *et al.* (eds) *Sexually Transmitted Diseases*. New York: McGraw-Hill, pp. 415–423.

Spencer H (1973) Amoebiasis. In: Spencer H (ed) *Tropical Pathology*. Berlin: Springer-Verlag.

Strouth JC, Dyker M (1964) Encephalopathy of Behçet's disease. *Neurology* 14: 794–805.

Sweet RL (1998) The enigmatic cervix. *Dermatologic Clinics* 16: 739–745.

Symmers CW (1950) Pathology of oxyuriasis. *Archives of Pathology* 50: 475–560.

Tramont EC (2000) *Treponema pallidum* (syphilis). In: Mandell GL, Bennett JE, Dolin R (eds) *Principles and Practice of Infectious Diseases*. New York: Churchill Livingstone, pp. 2474–2489.

Turner DR, Berry CL (1972) A comparison of two methods of prognostic typing in breast cancer. *Journal of Clinical Pathology* 25: 1053–1055.

Van Nierker WA (1962) Cervical cells and megaloblastic anaemia of the puerperium. *Lancet* 1: 1277–1279.

Van Nierker WA (1966) Cervical cytological abnormalities caused by folate acid deficiency. *Acta Cytologica* 10: 67–73.

Wechsler B, Piette JC (1992) Behçet's disease. *British Medical Journal* 304: 1199–1200.

Weinstein BB, Weed JC (1948) Amoebic vaginitis. *American Journal of Obstetrics and Gynecology* 56: 180–183.

Whitehead N, Reyner F, Lindenbaum J (1973) Megaloblastic changes in the cervical epithelium. *Journal of the American Medical Association* 226: 1421.

Winkler B, Richart RM (1985) Cervical/uterine pathologic considerations in pelvic infection. In: Zatuchni GI, Goldsmith A, Sciarra JJ (eds) *Intrauterine Contraception: Advances and Future Prospects*. New York: Harper & Row, pp. 438–449.

Workowski KA, Levine WC (2002) Sexually transmitted diseases treatment guidelines 2002. In: *CDC MMWR Morbidity and Mortality Weekly Report*, May 10, 2002. Vol. 51, No. RR-6, p. 36.

Wright TC, Ferenczy A (1994) Benign diseases of the cervix. In: Kurman RJ (ed.) *Blaustein's Pathology of the Female Genital Tract*. New York: Springer-Verlag, pp. 203–227.

Zenilman J, Wiesner PJ (1991) Gonococcal infections. In: Evans AS, Brachman AS (eds) *Bacterial Infections of Humans: Epidemiology and Control*. New York: Plenum Publishing Corporation, pp. 264–265.

CHAPTER 16

Common non-viral infections of the cervix: clinical features and management

Sebastian Faro

INTRODUCTION

This chapter will examine the clinical features and management of four common non-viral infections that affect the cervix, namely those involving *Neisseria gonorrhoeae*, *Chlamydia trachomatis*, *Trichomonas vaginalis* and *Treponema pallidum*. The pathology of other bacterial and viral, fungal, protozoal and parasitic infections as they infect the cervix is described in the preceding chapter.

WHY IS THE CERVIX SO VULNERABLE?

The cervix presents a significant surface area for the colonisation, attachment and invasion of sexually transmitted microorganisms. Key factors in the acquisition of sexually transmitted microorganisms capable of causing infection are: a surface area of tissue that permits the organisms to adhere; an inoculum size that is sufficient to overcome the host defensive mechanism to ward off infection; and an environmental milieu that permits growth and reproduction of the infecting organism. Conditions that could be present and favour the acquisition of sexually transmitted microorganisms are inflammatory vaginal conditions such as bacterial vaginitis, which can result in inflammatory changes in the cervix. Such conditions, in turn, create a cervical inflammation that facilitates acquisition of the sexually transmitted microorganisms. Bacterial vaginosis has been implicated in the acquisition of the human immunodeficiency virus (HIV). The patient's sexual behaviour practices are the most important factor in determining whether or not she places herself at risk of contracting a sexually transmitted disease (STD).

Cervical anatomy: role of the transformation zone

A detailed discussion of the development and anatomy of the cervix is presented in Chapters 1 and 2. The important anatomical areas of the cervix with regard to the acquisition of STDs are the portio and the endocervix. The portio is covered by squamous epithelial cells and is relatively resistant to bacterial colonisation and infection, unless it has been traumatised,

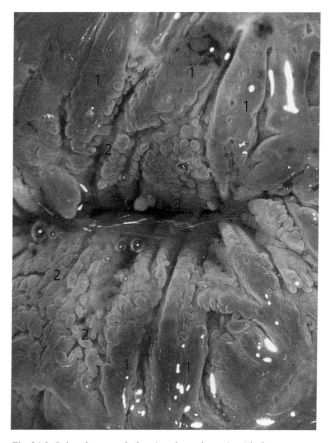

Fig. 16.1 Colpophotograph showing the endocervix with the development of squamous metaplasia (1) associated with areas of original columnar epithelium (2) emanating from the endocervix (3).

thus creating breaks in the epithelial lining, which will permit bacteria and viruses to attach to invade into the deeper tissues. The endocervix is a canal lined by columnar epithelial cells and has a rather rich blood supply (Fig. 16.1). The endocervix consist of folds of columnar epithelium forming numerous branches (Fig. 16.2) that result in crypts (Fig. 16.3), thus creating a large surface area of receptive cells to which microorganisms adhere. In many individuals, the endocervical epithelium turns outwards creating a large area of columnar

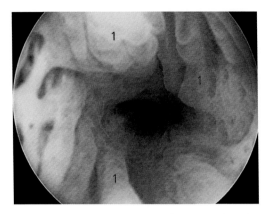

Fig. 16.2 Further view into the endocervix showing the branching effect of the original columnar epithelium (1).

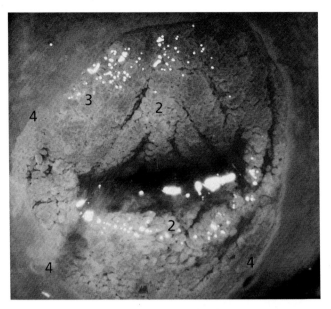

Fig. 16.4 A colpophotograph of what is referred to as an erosion or ectropion, showing the endocervix at (1), original columnar epithelium at (2), early stages of immature squamous metaplasia at (3) and the original squamocolumnar junction at (4). The area medial to the original squamocolumnar junction is correctly termed the transformation zone, but this clinical appearance can also be known as an ectropion and erosion.

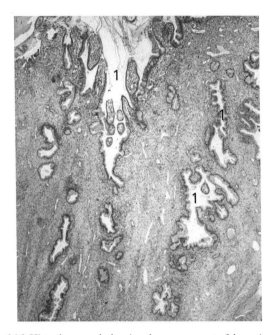

Fig. 16.3 Histophotograph showing the arrangement of the native (original) columnar epithelium into crypts within the cervix (1), thereby creating a large surface area of receptive cells to which microorganisms can adhere.

epithelium that is present on the ectocervix, which is referred to as an eversion, ectopy or ectropion, or sometimes described erroneously as an erosion (Fig. 16.4). During the reproductive years, the squamocolumnar junction, the line where the original (native) columnar epithelium abuts the original (native) squamous epithelium, lies external or close to the external cervical os (Fig. 16.4). The location of the transformation zone, the area situated medial to and bounded by the original

squamocolumnar junctions, in which metaplastic transformation occurs, is affected by the endogenous or exogenous hormones, the age of menarche, coitus, and pregnancy (see Chapters 2, 4 and 6). The transformation zone lies within the endocervical canal in approximately 28% of prepubertal adolescents (Singer, 1976). Following menarche, it is situated on the ectocervix in 88% of women. This is the result of a process of eversion of the endocervical epithelium, occurring in relation to puberty (Singer, 1976). In sexually active women, the composition of the transformation zone's epithelial tissues is different from that in virgins (Chapter 6).

It would seem as though the oral contraceptive steroids induce cervical ectopy and that this, in turn, is associated with an increased risk of chlamydial infection (Stamm and Holmes, 1997; Jacobson *et al.*, 2000). The organism *Chlamydia trachomatis* preferentially infects the columnar cells that are the major epithelial component of this area. Ectopy therefore increases the exposure of these susceptible cells to the infection.

Protective role of cervical mucus (see Chapter 11)

The cervix secretes mucus that covers the endocervical canal as well as the mucus that covers the vaginal epithelium (Elstein, 1978). Mucus production is controlled by hormones, with the amount and viscosity changing as the concentrations of estrogen and progesterone change (Gibbons, 1978). It is believed that mucus acts in a variety of ways to prevent microorganisms from colonising and infecting the cervix (Hein *et al.*, 2002). One way is by the tenacity of mucus in preventing penetration by microorganisms into the endocervical canal, thus protecting the exposed columnar epithelium from being colonised and infected. Mucus contains a variety of carbohydrates and the sugar moieties (Fleetwood *et al.*, 1986) that provide sites for microorganism to bind to, thus preventing them from gaining contact and adherence to the endocervical epithelium (Elstein, 1978; Gibbons, 1978). The carbohydrates in the mucus may also attract endogenous bacteria and thereby prevent the pathogenic bacteria from invading the upper genital tract. The endocervical mucus also contains other protective substances such as defensin, lactoferrin, lysozyme and antibodies. The mucus also provides the environment necessary to enable phagocytic cells to engulf bacteria and kill them once absorbed within the phagocytic cell. Another protective mechanism involves the lysozyme-hydrolysed β-1,4 linkages in the bacterial cell wall, which results in the bacterial cell taking in more water and causing osmotic lysis of the cell (Strominger and Ghuysen, 1967). Lactoferrin is a protein that binds iron and can also interfere with bacterial growth by competing for the iron available in the environment (Oram and Reiter, 1968). The lactoferrin concentration is at its greatest immediately after menstruation, and it is known that women on combination oral contraceptive pills have persistently low levels of lactoferrin (Cohen *et al.*, 1990).

There is evidence from animal experiments that the hormonal environment at the time of infection has a profound effect on the outcome of microbial infections in the cervix and uterus. Kaushic *et al.* (2000) used oophorectomised rats which were administered either estradiol or progesterone or a combination of both and then infected with *Chlamydia* via the intrauterine route and sacrificed 5 days later. They showed that progesterone increased and estradiol decreased the susceptibility to intrauterine chlamydial infection in this model.

Antibody production (see Chapter 4)

Antibody production in the lower genital tract is derived mainly from plasma cells found in the submucosal tissue of the cervix and vagina (Braantzaeg, 1997), and appears to be predominantly of IgA. The concentration of IgA appears to exceed the concentration of IgM and IgG (Waldman *et al.*, 1972; Chipperfield and Evans, 1975). Colonisation of the cervix with certain organisms such as group B *Streptococcus* results in increased production of specific IgA and IgG antibodies in cervical secretions (Hordnes *et al.*, 1996).

Natural antimicrobials/immunoglobulins

The cervix responds to bacterial colonisation and infection by producing a variety of antimicrobial substances and immuno-

globulins (Kutteh *et al.*, 1998, Kutteh and Franklin, 2001). The bacteria, in turn, produce substances that can interfere with the function of the host cell by inhibiting or blocking the mechanisms in the host cell. The result is initiation of infection with the possibility that it will advance to the upper genital tract, especially in pregnancy (Goldenberg *et al.*, 2000; Keelan *et al.*, 2003; Klein and Gibbs, 2004; Romero *et al.*, 2004). Lower genital tract bacteria may also act locally by the production of enzymes such as sialidase or mucinase, which in turn may weaken and destroy the protective effect of cervical mucus, thereby also promoting bacterial invasion of the upper genital tract (McGregor *et al.*, 1994).

Mucosal immunity in the lower genital tract is very well developed, with cytotoxic T lymphocytes functioning in both the cervix and the vagina in pre- and postmenopausal women. White *et al.* (1997) investigated the mucosal immune system in terms of the immune cells present and the cytolytic capacity of mucosal CD3+ T cells in the lower reproductive tract. They showed that the area is certainly immunocompetent as judged by the presence of such cells as CD3, CD4, CD8, as well as macrophages and the immune-presenting cells in the form of dendritic cells that were particularly present in both the endo- and the ectocervix. All these cells were likewise present in the vagina in both pre- and postmenopausal women. They also showed that CD3+ T cells with cytolytic activity were present in both these organs during both phases of the menstrual cycle (proliferative/secretory) and also postmenopausally.

Infection also initiates a cytokine response that, along with the immunological response, can result in elimination of the infection by the host. However, if the infection is not resolved either with or without antimicrobial therapy, then progression to the upper genital tract can occur (Eckert *et al.*, 2004; Klein and Gibbs, 2004). Progressive infection without downregulation of the cytokine response can cause significant tissue damage to the fallopian tubes, which may result in infertility or ectopic pregnancy. Therefore, infection of the cervix should be viewed as the early stages of pelvic inflammatory disease.

THE INFECTING ORGANISM

Neisseria gonorrhoeae

Neisseria gonorrhoeae is an obligate human pathogen and is a fastidious Gram-negative diplococcus. In a Gram-stained preparation, *N. gonorrhoeae* is often found within white blood cells and appears kidney shaped with concave opposed surfaces. This bacterium is acquired through sexual intercourse with an infected male partner. It is exquisitely sensitive to drying, heat, soapy water, other cleansing agents and antiseptic solutions.

Epidemiology

The Centers for Disease Control and Prevention (CDC) in the United States estimated that, in 1999, there were approximately

150–175 cases of gonorrhoea/100 000 women (Centers for Disease Control and Prevention, 2001). This represents a decrease from approximately 300 cases/100 000 women in 1984. There was a steady decrease until 1996 when the prevalence of gonorrhoea seemed to remain at approximately 150–170 cases/100 000 women. The rate varies in different regions of the country (Centers for Disease Control and Prevention, 2001).

It would seem as though women are more vulnerable to acquiring this infection, with the risk of 'catching' *N. gonorrhoeae* being greater for a woman who has sex with an infected male partner than for a man who has sex with an infected female partner. The bacterium is able to achieve infection quite easily. It is estimated that an uninfected female who has sexual intercourse with an infected male has a 60–90% chance of acquiring the infection (Holmes *et al.*, 1970; Barlow *et al.*, 1976; Evans, 1976; Hooper *et al.*, 1978). However, an uninfected male who has sex with an infected female has only a 20–50% chance of becoming infected (Holmes *et al.*, 1970; Hooper *et al.*, 1978). This is most likely because the cervix presents a larger surface for the gonococcus to adhere to than the male urethra, especially if there is an eversion of the columnar epithelium, i.e. an ectopy is present (Fig. 16.4). It has been shown that an estimated 5×10^3 to 8×10^6 gonococci/mL exist in infected cervical mucus (mean 1.0×10^6 bacteria/mL) and, in the vaginal fluid, there are 1.0×10^3 to 1.0×10^6 with a mean of 8.4×10^4 bacteria/mL (Young *et al.* 1983).

Pathogenesis

Approximately 60–70% of gonococcal cervicitis is asymptomatic and, in women who become symptomatic, the symptoms begin within 9–10 days of acquiring infection (Wallin, 1975). In women, sites of infection are the endocervix, urethra, Skene's glands, Bartholin's glands, anus and pharynx. Vaginal infection can occur in prepubertal girls and postmenopausal women and is more common in women who are not on estrogen replacement therapy. Urethral infection occurs in up to 90% of women with cervical gonococcal infection (Barlow and Phillips, 1978). Concomitant cervical and anal infection occurs in up to 50% of women, and the anus is the sole site of infection in approximately 5% of women (Curran *et al.*, 1976). Symptoms associated with rectal gonococcal infection are pruritus, mucoid discharge and, in some cases, severe proctitis.

Infected patients who develop symptoms usually do so within 10 days of acquiring the infection and, if the cervix is infected, then they are more likely to develop pelvic inflammatory disease, especially at the time of menstruation. Although the patient may have asymptomatic gonococcal cervicitis, examination can reveal an inflamed cervical erosion (Fig. 16.5). The endocervical canal may contain mucopus.

Specific gonococcal types are able to infect the columnar epithelium of the cervix, and those types that can infect

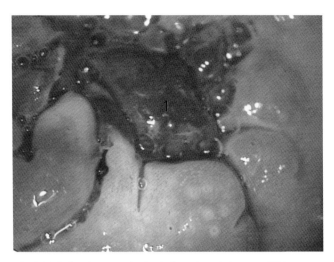

Fig. 16.5 Colpophotograph of an inflamed cervical ectopy (1) in a woman with proven gonorrhoeal cervicitis. Some contact bleeding had occurred when an endocervical swab was taken.

humans possess pili on their surface, in contrast to gonococci that do not posses pili and therefore, cannot cause infection (Kellogg *et al.*, 1963). The pili facilitate adherence of the bacterium to the epithelium, which is a prelude to endocytosis of the bacterium; this is the initial step in the infectious process. Endocytosis allows the bacterium to gain exposure to the necessary nutrients, which allows the bacterium to grow and propagate. Once inside the phagocyte, the bacterium becomes vulnerable to host defensive mechanisms, but the bacterium is able to protect itself, e.g. from lysozyme, by surrounding itself with a sialated lipopolysaccharide capsule (Meyer, 1999). Additional proteins that facilitate endocytosis of the gonococcus by epithelial cells have been identified, e.g. Pori (prion protein), which is located on the outer membrane (Meyer, 1999). Bacterial adhesion to the host epithelium is also enhanced by a group protein designated as Opa proteins (James and Swanson, 1978; Makino *et al.*, 1991). The pathogenic *N. gonorrhoeae* possesses Opa proteins and gives the colonies, when grown on culture medium, an opaque colour, whereas gonococci lacking the genes to synthesise Opa proteins appear translucent. It is the Opa-negative gonococci that have been isolated from the fallopian tubes of patients with pelvic inflammatory disease (PID) (Draper *et al.*, 1980). There appear to be a number of Opa proteins and most function to enhance and facilitate adhesion of the bacterium to epithelial and phagocytic cells. Opa_{59} plays a significant role in endocytosis of the bacterium. All pathogenic strains of *N. gonorrhoeae* possess a protein that blocks IgM antibodies and prevents bacterial killing. This protein is known as reduction modifiable protein (RMP) (Rice *et al.*, 1994).

Neisseria gonorrhoeae produces the following additional virulence factors:

1 lipopolysaccharide or endotoxin, which causes the cytotoxic effects in infected tissue, i.e. cervix and fallopian tubes; endotoxin is also responsible for the systemic effect associated with infection, fever and sepsis;

2 IgA protease, which destroys secretory IgA;

3 iron-repressible protein, which enables the gonococcus to take up iron that is necessary for bacterial growth; and

4 peptidoglycan, which is a tissue toxin (Mulks and Plaut, 1978; Hook and Holmes, 1985).

Experimental studies by Edwards *et al.* (2000) using clinically derived cervical specimens have shown that the gonococcus is capable of infecting and invading both the endo- and the ectocervix. Their electron microscopy studies using tissue culture control systems showed that invasion was found to occur primarily in an 'actin-dependent manner and does not appear to require *de novo* protein synthesis by either the bacterium or the host cervical cell'. They noted a unique morphological observation in that membrane ruffling of the cervical cells seems to appear in response to the gonococcal infection. The gonococcus was found residing within macropinosomes, and a concentrated accumulation in actin-associated proteins was also observed occurring in response to this infection. Membrane ruffling was also associated with lamellipodia formation and cytoskeletal changes. These changes also seem to occur in the cervical epithelium of women with naturally acquired gonococcal cervicitis. This study clearly demonstrates the ability of this organism to invade both the endo- and the ectocervix.

Clinical presentation

The clinical presentation of gonococcal cervicitis varies from truly asymptomatic, with no visibly detectable signs or patient-recognised abnormalities, to subtle changes in the morphology of the cervix, to the symptomatic. The patient with symptomatic cervicitis typically presents with a purulent vaginal discharge, dysuria, endocervical mucopus, recent onset of postcoital bleeding and abnormal vaginal bleeding. The patient with a truly asymptomatic infection has no symptoms, and examination of the cervix does not reveal any abnormalities. The patient with subtle symptoms and signs of cervical infection may notice postcoital spotting, dysuria, hypertrophy of the endocervical columnar epithelium and the presence of endocervical mucopus. The cervix also bleeds briskly when gently palpated with a cotton- or Dacron-tipped applicator or when obtaining a pap smear (Fig. 16.6).

Confirmation of diagnosis

There is no rapid test available for the diagnosis of gonococcal infection of the cervix. Most clinicians now rely on non-culture methods for detecting *N. gonorrhoeae* in specimens obtained from the endocervix. Amplified DNA probes are used routinely in the US (Hook and Handsfield, 1998). This test is based on hybridising a single strand of DNA to ribosomal RNA of *N. gonorrhoeae*. The specificity of this non-amplified nucleic

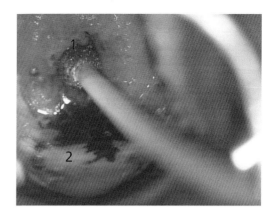

Fig. 16.6 Colpophotograph showing contact bleeding from a woman with proven gonococcal cervicitis during the application of a Dacron-tipped swab within the endocervix (1). There is mucopus present at (2) which has been displaced from the endocervix when the swab was taken.

acid test is 99% with a sensitivity of 89–97%, and it is comparable to culture using selective media (Panke *et al.*, 1991). DNA amplification is available for the detection of *N. gonorrhoeae*, e.g. polymerase chain reaction (PCR) test and the ligase chain reaction (LCR) test. These tests have a sensitivity of 99% and a specificity of 100%. The LCR assay can be used to detect *N. gonorrhoeae* DNA in urine, therefore eliminating the need to do a pelvic examination for the sole purpose of obtaining a specimen from the cervix. This LCR test would be appropriate for screening large numbers of both women and men. The PCR and LCR assays can also be performed on specimens obtained via a swab of the vagina (Hook *et al.*, 1997). However, these methods for obtaining specimens should only be used for screening a large number of patients and should not replace the pelvic examination.

Treatment (Table 16.1)

When treating gonococcal cervicitis, the antibiotic chosen should also provide activity against *Chlamydia trachomatis*. It is estimated that 10–30% of women with gonococcal cervicitis will also be infected with *C. trachomatis* (Centers for Disease Control and Prevention, 2002). The treatment regimens listed in Table 16.1 (CDC recommendation 2002) will also effectively treat urethral and rectal infection.

None of the cephalosporins have activity against *C. trachomatis*. Therefore, if *C. trachomatis* cannot be ruled out, an antimicrobial with activity against *C. trachomatis* must be added to the cephalosporin administered to treat the gonococcal infection. If the patient is suspected of having a pharyngeal infection or one has been documented, ceftriaxone 125 mg, administered in a single dose intramuscularly, or ciprofloxacin 500 mg, administered in a single oral dose, is effective. The quinolone and tetracycline regimens are contraindicated if the patient is pregnant or breastfeeding. It is not necessary to obtain a test-of-cure specimen when following

Table 16.1 Treatment regimens for gonococcal cervicitis.

Antibiotic choices if *Chlamydia trachomatis* is not present:
    Single oral dose regimens:
        Cefixime 400 mg
        Ciprofloxacin 500 mg
        Ofloxacin 400 mg
        Levofloxacin 250 mg
    Intramuscular regimen:
        Ceftriaxone 125 mg
If *Chlamydia trachomatis* is suspected, one of the following should be added to one of the above regimens:
        Azithromycin 1 g orally
        Doxycycline 100 mg orally twice a day for 7 days
    Alternative regimens:
        Spectinomycin 2 g in a single intramuscular (IM) dose
        Ceftizoxime 500 mg IM
        Cefoxitin 2 g IM plus probenecid 1 g orally
        Cefotaxime 500 mg IM
        Gatifloxacin 400 mg orally
        Norfloxacin 800 mg orally
        Lomefloxacin 400 mg orally

the CDC guidelines for treating cervical infection caused by *N. gonorrhoeae* or *C. trachomatis* (Centers for Disease Control and Prevention, 1999).

Chlamydia trachomatis

Chlamydia trachomatis is a true intracellular bacterial parasite and the only known host is the human. It is considered the most common sexually transmitted bacteria, and it frequently causes asymptomatic infection that may be present for long periods without being detected. *C. trachomatis* causes a significant number of PID cases that are also asymptomatic. A delay in the detection of an asymptomatic upper genital tract infection, especially salpingitis, can result in significant damage to the fallopian tubes. This can result in the development of ectopic pregnancy or infertility.

Epidemiology
It is estimated that there are 3 million new cases of *C. trachomatis* annually in the US (Groseclose *et al.*, 1999). The serotypes responsible for cervicitis, endometritis and salpingitis are D, E, F, G, H, I, J and K. These same serotypes are responsible for inclusion conjunctivitis, non-gonococcal urethritis, proctitis, epididymitis and neonatal pneumonia. Unmarried sexually active women between the ages of 15 and 25 years are at the greatest risk of contracting cervical infection caused by *N. gonorrhoeae* and/or *C. trachomatis*. Individuals experiencing their first chlamydial infection before the age of 15 years have an eightfold increased risk of having a recurrent infection, while individuals between 15 and 19 years of age have a fivefold increased risk. Women between the ages of 20

Table 16.2 Risks factors for contracting *Chlamydia trachomatis*.

Young age
Socioeconomic status
African-American
Number of sexual partners
Not living with current sexual partner
Use of oral contraceptive pills

and 29 years have a twofold increased risk compared with women between 30 and 44 years old (Hillis *et al.*, 1994). The risk factors associated with the acquisition of *C. trachomatis* are similar to those for contracting any sexually transmitted disease (Table 16.2). The cervical carriage rate of *C. trachomatis* in sexually active women not in a truly monogamous relationship is 3–5%. The actual prevalence of infection depends upon the population being screened (Thompson and Washington, 1983; Chacko and Lovchik, 1984; Cates and Wasserheit, 1991; Mangione-Smith *et al.*, 1999). In summary, *C. trachomatis* infection of the cervix is easily acquired, tends to be asymptomatic, can progress to upper genital tract infection causing significant morbidity and can easily be transferred to the male partner.

Pathogenesis
Chlamydia trachomatis is unique among bacteria because it is a true bacterial parasite requiring the host to supply adenosine triphosphate (ATP) in order to complete its life cycle. It is similar to other bacteria in that it possesses DNA and RNA, reproduces by binary fission, has a rigid cell wall similar to that found in Gram-negative bacteria and is susceptible to certain antibiotics. The organism can exist in one of two forms — the elementary body, which is also referred to as the infection particle, and the reticulate body or metabolic form. The elementary body initiates infection by stimulating receptive epithelial cells to phagocytose the elementary body. The bacterium remains in the phagosome throughout the life cycle (Friis, 1972; Byrne and Moulder, 1978; Zhang and Stephens, 1992). The phagosome containing the chlamydial organism appears to be protected from the intracellular lysosome via phagolysosomal fusion by the presence of antigens on the surface of the bacterium (Friis, 1972). The entire life cycle takes between 48 and 72 hours and has been divided into stages:
1 attachment of the infectious particle or elementary body to the host cell;
2 endocytosis or phagocytosis of the bacterium;
3 once inside the host cell and within the phagosome, metamorphosis to become a reticulate body;
4 metabolism and reproduction;
5 metamorphosis back to elementary bodies; and
6 lysis of the host cell to release elementary bodies (Schachter, 1999a).

Table 16.3 Chlamydial genital infection: sites of infection.

Skene's glands
Urethra
Bartholin's glands
Cervix
Uterus
Fallopian tubes
Ovaries

Clinical presentation

Chlamydia trachomatis, like *N. gonorrhoeae*, can infect a variety of anatomical sites within the genital tract (Table 16.3). Infection of the cervix is typically asymptomatic. However, the astute clinician can gain insight to the possible existence of infection by assessing the patient's potential risk for contracting a STD by taking a detailed history. Meticulous inspection of the cervix can reveal signs of infection, thus increasing the examiner's suspicion that the patient may have a cervical infection. The typical appearance of chronic follicular cervicitis may be seen in Fig. 16.7. However, it is estimated that two-thirds of women with chlamydial cervicitis do not have any signs of infection (Friis, 1972; Zhang and Stephens, 1992). However, signs of cervicitis attributed to infection are hypertrophy and intense erythema of the endocervical epithelium. Endocervical mucopus is present and the cervix bleeds easily when gently palpated with a cotton- or Dacron-tipped applicator (Fig. 16.8). In some cases, pain can be elicited on palpation of the cervix. The patient may also give a history of the recent onset of dyspareunia. The CDC has published guidelines regarding who should be screened for *C. trachomatis* (Table 16.4).

Confirmation of diagnosis

The diagnosis is established by obtaining a specimen from the endocervix for detection of *C. trachomatis* (Fig. 16.8). Traditional tissue culture methods are no longer employed except for research purposes. The tests commonly used are fluorescein-labelled specific antibodies (DFA), immunohistochemical detection of antigen (EIA) and detection of DNA (Harrison *et al.*, 1985; Schachter, 1999b). The DNA detection tests can be divided into two basic methods: the DNA probe (Gen Probe) and DNA amplification accomplished via the PCR. The DNA probe detection system has both high sensitivity (85%) and specificity (99%) (Yang *et al.*, 1991; Hosein *et al.*, 1992; Blanding *et al.*, 1993; Black, 1997). This is a good test for screening large numbers of patients and good to employ in a private practice setting because it does not require elaborate specimen collection or storage under special conditions. An advantage of this test is that it can also be used to test for the presence of *N. gonorrhoeae*.

DNA amplification is an extremely sensitive testing system for detecting the presence of a bacterial pathogen. This testing is commonly referred to as PCR; it can detect a single copy and

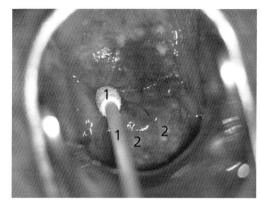

Fig. 16.7 Swab (1) being taken from the endocervix of a woman with chlamydial cervicitis, showing typical follicles across the ectocervix (2). This is an appearance of chronic follicular cervicitis.

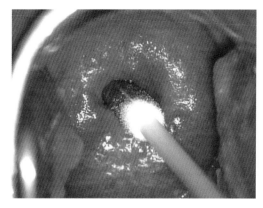

Fig. 16.8 Colpophotograph showing contact bleeding from the endocervix in a previously asymptomatic woman subsequently proven to have chlamydial cervicitis.

Table 16.4 CDC recommendations for prevention and treatment of chlamydial infection in women.*

Screen all sexually active women ≤ 25 years old
Screen women > 25 years old if at increased risk
Women with mucopurulent cervicitis, or inconsistent use of barrier contraception, or new sexual partner in the past 3 months having a prior history of a sexually transmitted disease
Screen pregnant women in the first trimester
Rescreen high-risk women in the third trimester

*CDC (2002) Screening tests to detect *Chlamydia trachomatis* and *Neisseria gonorrhoeae* infection. *Morbidity and Mortality Weekly Report* 51: 37.

is highly sensitive. This has become the gold standard for many diagnostic tests in a variety of diseases. Another significant attribute of PCR and DNA amplification is that specimens can be obtained from non-invasive and minimally invasive specimen acquisition, e.g. urine and vaginal swabs

(Lee *et al.*, 1995; Black, 1997; Stary *et al.*, 1998; Schachter, 1999b). PCR and LCR are the two most widely used nucleic acid amplification tests. Comparing the available non-culture chlamydial detection tests, the EIA test's lower limit of detection is 10 000 elementary bodies, the DNA probe test detects as little as 1000 elementary bodies, culture detects 10–100 elementary bodies, and the PCR and LCR detect a single gene copy.

Treatment

The treatment of *C. trachomatis* should always include treatment for *N. gonorrhoeae* unless the latter has been proven not to be present. Treatment should also include the patient's sexual partner. Pregnant patients should be treated and rescreened in both second and third trimesters because treating the pregnant patient prevents transmission of *C. trachomatis* to the newborn. Treatment regimens recommended by the CDC are presented in Table 16.5. Of note is that doxycycline, ofloxacin and levofloxacin are contraindicated for use in pregnancy and women who are breastfeeding.

Trichomonas vaginalis

Trichomonas vaginalis is a protozoan belonging to the order Trichomonadidae; there are four species found in humans. The most common species known to gynaecologists and obstetricians is *Trichomonas vaginalis*; the other species are *T. tenax* (found in the oral cavity), *T. faecalis* (found in only one patient) and *Pentrichomonas hominis* (Honigberg, 1990).

Epidemiology

Trichomonas vaginalis is believed to be the only trichomonad pathogenic for humans. *T. vaginalis* is a common cause of vaginitis and has been found to cause infection, although rarely, at other anatomical locations, e.g. renal disease, perinephric abscess, cutaneous lesions, acute and subacute arthritis, gastritis, ascites and hepatomegaly (Csonka, 1974; Suriyanon *et al.*, 1975). *T. vaginalis* has also been found to cause pneumonia in newborn infants (McLaren *et al.*, 1983; Hiemstra *et al.*, 1984).

Table 16.5 Treatment regimens for *Chlamydia trachomatis* cervicitis.*

Azithromycin 1 g orally in a single dose, or
Doxycycline 100 mg orally twice a day for 7 days, or
Erythromycin base 500 mg orally four times a day for 7 days, or
Erythromycin ethylsuccinate 800 ng orally four times a day for 7 days, or
Ofloxacin 300 mg orally twice a day for 7 days, or
Levofloxacin 500 mg orally once a day for 7 days.

---

*Centers for Disease Control and Prevention (2002).

Vaginitis is probably one of the most common reasons that women seek gynaecological care for symptomatic problems. The incidence of *T. vaginalis* vaginitis seen in the private practice of a gynaecologist/obstetrician is not known. However, *T. vaginalis* vaginitis accounts for approximately one-third of the cases of vaginitis seen in public health clinics (Rein, 1990). In 1999, the CDC in the US reported that out of 900 000 office visits in 1998 approximately 10 000 were for *T. vaginalis* vaginitis (Division of STD Prevention 1999). The presence of *T. vaginalis* vaginitis should initiate investigation for the presence of other sexually transmitted diseases.

Clinical presentation

Although *T. vaginalis* is most frequently found to cause vaginitis, the cervix is also equally infected. Up to 75% of patients with *T. vaginalis* vaginitis reports a profuse discharge. The discharge is typically a dirty grey colour but, in 5–20% of cases, the discharge is yellow or green. The classically described frothy discharge is actually present in only about 10% of cases (Ronnike, 1964) (Fig. 16.9a).

Odour is not a common finding unless there is a significant number of anaerobic bacteria, such as occurs in the case of concomitant presence of bacterial vaginosis (BV). Approximately 25–50% of patients report one or more of the following symptoms: dysuria, dyspareunia, vaginal irritation and itching. The vaginal epithelium often becomes erythematous or may contain local areas of erythema or petechiae, often referred to as the 'strawberry' cervix, which is seen in 5–25% of patients infected with *T. vaginalis* (Figs 16.9a and b and 16.10).

Biopsy from the ectocervix infected with this organism shows much epithelial degeneration and inflammatory infiltrate. In Fig. 16.10b, marked superficial inflammation and degeneration are seen with a distinct pyogenic membrane having been formed in the upper part of the epithelium.

There is marked intracellular oedema and diffuse infiltration with the acute inflammatory cells not only in the stroma but also in the endothelium.

Confirmation of diagnosis

The diagnosis of *T. vaginalis* vaginitis and cervicitis is accomplished by examining the discharge from the vagina and the endocervix under ×40 magnification. Microscopic examination of the discharge (wet prep) (Fig. 16.11) has a sensitivity of 60–80% (Whittington, 1957; Clark and Solomons, 1959; Fouts and Kraus, 1980). In patients whose vaginal discharge contains many white blood cells (WBCs), but no pathogenesis is observed in the wet preparation, a specimen should be obtained from the endocervix for the detection of *N. gonorrhoeae* and *C. trachomatis*. Additionally, a specimen should be obtained from the vagina and used to inoculate Diamond's medium for the culture and identification of *T. vaginalis*.

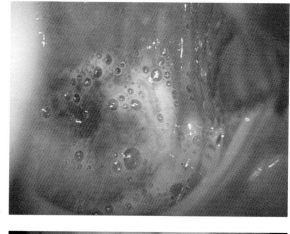

(a)

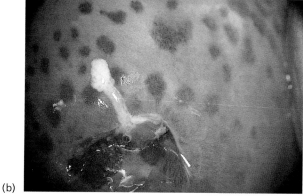

(b)

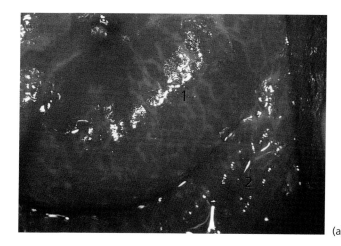

(a)

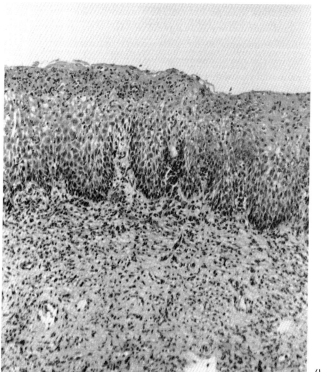

(b)

Fig. 16.9 (a) Colpophotograph showing the typical frothy discharge of a woman with *T. vaginalis*. (b) Typical appearance of a cervix in a woman with trichomonal vaginitis. This clinical appearance is termed a 'strawberry' cervix.

Treatment

In the US, treatment of *T. vaginalis* vaginitis is limited to metronidazole. There are two regimens currently recommended by the CDC: metronidazole 2 g administered in a single oral dose and metronidazole 500 mg administered orally twice daily for 7 days. The patient's sexual partner should be treated simultaneously. The patient should also insist that her sexual partner wear a condom during sexual intercourse. Patients failing to respond to either treatment should receive metronidazole 500 mg orally twice a day for 7 days. If the patient fails therapy again, the following procedure should be followed: (1) ensure that the patient understands that the infection is transmitted via sexual intercourse; (2) have the patient abstain from sexual intercourse until it can be documented that the infection has resolved; (3) impress on the patient that she and her sexual partner must complete a full course of therapy within the same time period; and (4) the patient should be treated with a single 2-g dose of metronidazole and the dose should be repeated once a day for 3–5 days.

Fig. 16.10 A photograph of a cervix and upper vagina showing the intense inflammatory process present in trichomonal vaginitis and cervicitis. The cervix shows the typical pattern of a 'strawberry' appearance (1). The upper vagina shows marked erythema and localised nodular swelling (2). (b) Biopsy from the ectocervix infected with this organism shows much epithelial degeneration and inflammatory infiltrate. There is also marked superficial inflammation and degeneration with a distinct pyogenic membrane having formed in the upper part of the epithelium.

Treponema pallidum

Treponema pallidum is a spirochaete that causes syphilis. In women, the disease almost always goes undetected, especially if the initial infection occurs in the vulva, vagina or perianal

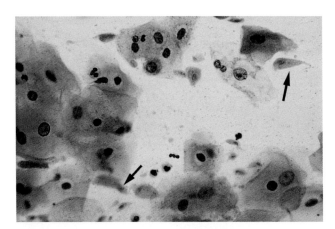

Fig. 16.11 Wet stain preparation with arrows pointing out the active *Trichomonas*.

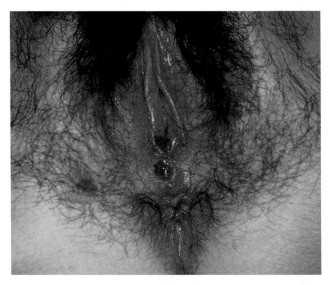

Fig. 16.12 A photograph of the vulva of a woman with primary syphilis. Two small ulcerated areas with a dull red base form the classical presentation of a chancre (1).

area. The primary infection is undetected because the initial ulcer or chancre is painless and women infrequently examine their own genitalia. The diagnosis of syphilis is typically established by serological testing, i.e. non-specific testing, and confirmed by specific treponemal antigen antibody testing.

Epidemiology

The incidence of syphilis appears to have cyclic increases and decreases. In the US in 1982, there were approximately 23 cases of primary and secondary syphilis/100 000 population and, in 1985, there were approximately 16 cases/100 000 population (Division of STD Prevention, 1999). In 1990, there were approximately 23 cases/100 000 population followed by a substantial decrease in 1998 with approximately three cases/100 000 population (Division of STD Prevention, 1999). The increase in 1990 was attributed to an increase in infection among African-Americans (approximately 142 cases/100 000 population) and the fact that 10–12% of the cases occurred in adolescents (Rolfs *et al.*, 1990; Singh and Romanowski, 1999). The majority of these cases were attributed to the use of crack cocaine, the exchange of sex for drugs and the use of spectinomycin for the treatment of gonorrhoea (Rolfs *et al.*, 1990). Although the overall incidence of syphilis has decreased, it continues to remain high in African-Americans (30 cases/100 000 population) (Singh and Romanowski, 1999).

Clinical presentation

Syphilis consists of three stages: primary, secondary and tertiary. Secondary syphilis is divided into two stages: disease of less than 1 year duration (early latent syphilis) and late latent syphilis. Syphilis is acquired through sexual contact, perinatal transmission (congenital syphilis) and non-venereal transmission, e.g. via blood.

Primary syphilis of the cervix or the associated vagina will go unnoticed because the chancre or ulcer is painless. The labia majora seem to be a very common site for a primary chancre (Fig. 16.12); in Fournier's original (1906) series, some 46% occurred in this site: 22% on the labia minora and only 5% on the cervix (Fig. 16.11). A diagnosis of syphilis is established when the patient has a positive, non-specific antibody test, either the rapid plasma reagin (RPR) test or the Venereal Disease Research Laboratory (VDRL) test. Once a patient has a positive RPR or VDRL, the presence of syphilis is confirmed by a positive, treponeme-specific antibody antigen test. The cervical lesion of primary syphilis is a painless cervical ulcer (Fig. 16.13). Lesions may be single or multiple and usually begin as an indurated papule which erodes to form an ulcer. The resultant primary chancre has a typical indurated base with firm rolled edges and is irregularly shaped. It may resemble a traumatic ulcer or indeed a squamous carcinoma as in Figure 16.13. The base is usually level with the surrounding skin, and there may be no associated induration. In this situation, they are invariably painless unless they become secondarily infected. The iliac lymph nodes can become enlarged and, if left untreated, the ulcer will resolve within 3–9 weeks after it appears (Lynch, 1978). Secondary and tertiary syphilis does not manifest signs in the cervix and a complete discussion of syphilis is beyond this book. Suffice it to state that the lesions of early latent syphilis are skin lesions such as macular rash (roseola), papular and papulosquamous lesions that are commonly found all over the body including the scalp, face, palms and soles, and condylomata lata on the genitalia.

Confirmation of diagnosis

Syphilis is typically diagnosed by serological testing. The non-specific tests are screening tests, VDRL and RPR. These tests

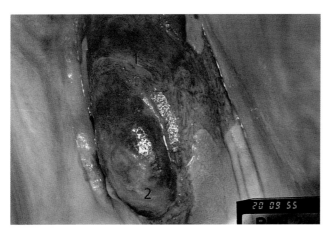

Fig. 16.13 A 52-year-old woman presenting with an ulcerative, painless lesion extending across the anterior vaginal fornix (1) and extending to involve the anterior lip of the ectocervix (2). The base of this lesion is indurated and firm with rolled edges and is level with the surrounding skin. This lesion was initially diagnosed as a primary syphilitic chancre; subsequent biopsy and serological tests excluded primary syphilis and confirmed the presence of a poorly differentiated squamous cell carcinoma of the vagina.

Table 16.6 Treatment regimens for the treatment of syphilis.

Primary and early latent syphilis:
    Benzathine penicillin G 2.4 million units intramuscularly in a single dose
Late latent syphilis or latent syphilis of unknown duration
    Benzathine penicillin G 2.4 million units intramuscularly weekly for 3 weeks

ACKNOWLEDGEMENT

The author wishes to thank Professor A. Singer and Mr J.M. Monaghan for the contribution of Figures 16.1 to 16.13, all of which originally appeared in *Lower Genital Tract Precancer*, 2nd edn, Oxford: Blackwell Publishing, 2000.

are based on the presence of cardiolipin antibodies that appear 7–10 days after the chancre appears or within 3–5 weeks following infection. A positive RPR or VDRL must be confirmed by a specific treponemal test (FTA-ABS, the fluorescent treponemal antibody absorbed; or TP-PA, pallidum particle agglutination test). False-positive results can occur with the non-treponemal tests, RPR and VDRL, whereas false-positive results with the treponemal-specific tests are rare.

Not all patients who have been successfully treated for syphilis will revert to being seronegative when retested using the non-treponemal test. Some individuals will remain serofast for life, usually with a titre of 1:4 or 1:2. Individuals with a positive FTA-ABS or TP-PA will remain positive for life. However, 10–15% of individuals successfully treated for primary syphilis will convert to being FTA-ABS or TP-PA negative (Centers for Disease Control and Prevention, 2002).

Patients with a positive RPR or VDRL with titres of 1:1 or 1:2 and a negative FTA-ABS or TP-PA do not have syphilis and can be considered to have a false-positive non-specific test. This can be seen in a variety of conditions with the most common being lupus.

Treatment
In the treatment of syphilis, the antibiotic of choice is penicillin, especially in the pregnant patient (Table 16.6). In the non-pregnant patient, tetracycline can be used in place of penicillin if the patient has an allergy to penicillin. The pregnant patient allergic to penicillin must be desensitised in order to treat her successfully and prevent congenital syphilis.

REFERENCES

Barlow D, Phillips I (1978) Gonorrhea in women. Diagnostic, clinical, and laboratory aspects. *Lancet* 1: 761–764.

Barlow D, Nayyar K, Phillips I *et al.* (1976) Diagnosis of gonorrhea in women. *British Journal of Venereal Disease* 52: 326–328.

Black CM (1997) Current methods of laboratory diagnosis of *Chlamydia trachomatis* infections. *Clinical Microbiology Review* 10: 160–184.

Blanding J, Hirsch L, Stranton N *et al.* (1993) Comparison of Clearview Chlamydia, the PACE 2 assay, and culture for detection of *Chlamydia trachomatis* from cervical specimens in a low-prevalence population. *Journal of Clinical Microbiology* 31: 1622–1625.

Braantzaeg P (1997) Mucosal immunity in the female genital tract. *Journal of Reproductive Immunology* 36: 23–50.

Byrne GI, Moulder JW (1978) Parasite-specified phagocytosis of *Chlamydia psittaci* and *Chlamydia trachomatis* by L and HeLa cells. *Infection and Immunity* 19: 598–606.

Cates W Jr, Wasserheit JN (1991) Genital chlamydial infections: epidemiology and reproductive sequelae. *American Journal of Obstetrics and Gynecology* 164: 1771–1781.

Centers for Disease Control and Prevention (1999) Summary of notifiable diseases – United States 1998. *Morbidity and Mortality Weekly Report* 47: 3.

Centers for Disease Control and Prevention (2001) Sexually transmitted disease – United States 1999. *Morbidity and Mortality Weekly Report* 49: 29–39.

Centers for Disease Control and Prevention (2002) Sexually transmitted diseases treatment guidelines. *Morbidity and Mortality Weekly Report* 51: 1–80.

Chacko MR, Lovchik JC (1984) *Chlamydia trachomatis* infection in sexually active adolescents: prevalence and risk factors. *Pediatrics* 73: 836–840.

Chipperfield EJ, Evans BA (1975) Effect of local infection and oral contraception on immunoglobulin levels in cervical mucus. *Infection and Immunity* 11: 215–221.

Clark DH, Solomons E (1959). An evaluation of routine culture examinations for *Trichomonas vaginalis* and *Candida*. *American Journal of Obstetrics and Gynecology* 78: 1314–1319.

Cohen MS, Weber RD, Märdh P-A (1990) Genitourinary mucosal defenses. In: Holmes KK, Märdh P-A. Sparling PF *et al.* (eds) *Sexually Transmitted Diseases.* New York: McGraw-Hill, pp. 117–127.

Csonka GW (1974) Trichomoniasis and the dermatologist. *British Journal of Dermatology* 90: 713–714.

Curran JW, Rendtorff RC, Chandler RW *et al.* (1976) Female gonorrhea: its relation to abnormal uterine bleeding, urinary tract symptoms, and cervicitis. *Obstetrics and Gynecology* 45: 195–198.

Division of STD Prevention (1999) *Sexually Transmitted Disease Surveillance, 1998.* Department of Health and Human Services. Atlanta: Centers for Disease Control and Prevention (CDC), pp. 26–29 and 36.

Draper DL, James JF, Brooks GE *et al.* (1980) Comparison of virulence markers of peritoneal and fallopian tube isolates with endocervical *Neisseria gonorrhoeae* isolates from women with acute salpingitis. *Infection and Immunity* 27: 882–888.

Eckert LO, Thwin S, Hillyer SL *et al.* (2004) The antimicrobial treatment of subacute endometritis; a proof of concept study. *American Journal of Obstetrics and Gynecology* 190: 305–313.

Edwards JL, Shao JQ, Ault KA *et al.* (2000) *Neisseria gonorrhoeae* elicits membrane ruffling and cytoskeletal arrangements upon infection of primary human endo- and ectocervical cells. *Infection and Immunity* 68 (9): 5354–5363.

Elstein M (1978) Functions and physical properties of mucus in the female genital tract. *British Medical Bulletin* 34: 83–88.

Evans BA (1976) Detection of gonorrhea in women. *British Journal of Venereal Disease* 52: 40–42.

Fleetwood L, Landgren B, Eneroin P (1986) Quantification of human cervical mucin during consecutive days and hours during one day at mid-cycle. *Gynecological and Obstetric Investigation* 22: 145–152.

Fournier J (1906) Quoted by Stokes JH (1994) *Modern Clinical Syphilogy.* Philadelphia: WB Saunders.

Fouts AC, Kraus SJ (1980). *Trichomonas vaginalis*: reevaluation of its clinical presentation and laboratory diagnosis. *Journal of Infectious Diseases* 141: 137–143.

Friis RR (1972) Interaction of L cells and *Chlamydia psittaci*: entry of the parasite and host responses to its development. *Journal of Bacteriology* 110: 706–721.

Gibbons RA (1978) Mucus of the mammalian genital tract. *British Medical Bulletin* 34: 34–38.

Goldenberg RL, Hauth JC, Andrews WW (2000) Intrauterine infection and preterm delivery. *New England Journal of Medicine* 342: 1500–1507.

Groseclose SL, Zaidi AA, DeLisle SJ *et al.* (1999) Estimated incidence and prevalence of genital *Chlamydia trachomatis* infections in the United States 1996. *Sexually Transmitted Diseases* 26: 339–344.

Harrison HR, Costin M, Meder JB *et al.* (1985) Cervical *Chlamydia trachomatis* infection in university women: relationship to history, contraception, ectopy and cervicitis. *American Journal of Obstetrics and Gynecology* 153: 244–251.

Hein M, Valore VE, Helmik AB *et al.* (2002) Antimicrobial factors in the cervical mucus plug. *American Journal of Obstetrics and Gynecology* 187: 137–144.

Hiemstra I, Van Bel F, Berger HM (1984) Can *Trichomonas vaginalis* cause pneumonia in newborn babies? *British Medical Journal* 289: 355–356.

Hillis SD, Nakashima A, Marchbanks PA *et al.* (1994) Risk factors for recurrent *Chlamydia trachomatis* infections in women. *American Journal of Obstetrics and Gynecology* 170: 801–806.

Holmes KK, Johnson DW, Trostle HJ (1970) An estimate of the risk of men acquiring gonorrhea by sexual contact with infected females. *American Journal of Epidemiology* 91: 170–174.

Honigberg BM (1990) Taxonomy and nomenclature. In: Honigberg BM (ed.) *Trichomonads Parasitic in Humans.* New York: Springer-Verlag, pp. 3–4.

Hook EW, Ching SF, Stephens J *et al.* (1997) Diagnosis of *Neisseria gonorrhoeae* infections in women by using the ligase chain reaction on patient-obtained vaginal swabs. *Journal of Clinical Microbiology* 35: 2129–2132.

Hook EW, Handsfield HH (1998) Gonococcal infection in adults. In: Holmes KK, Sparling PF, Mardh P-A (eds) *Sexually Transmitted Diseases*, 3rd edn. New York: McGraw-Hill, pp. 421–466.

Hook EW, Holmes KK (1985) Gonococcal infections. *Annals of Internal Medicine* 102: 229–243.

Hooper RR, Reynolds GH, Jones OG *et al.* (1978) Cohort study of venereal disease. I. The risk of gonorrhea transmission from infected women to men. *American Journal of Epidemiology* 108: 136–144.

Hordnes K, Tynning T, Kvam AI *et al.* (1996). Colonization in the rectum and uterine cervix with group B streptococci may induce specific antibody responses in cervical secretions of pregnant women. *Infection and Immunity* 64: 1643–52.

Hosein IK, Kaunitz AM, Craft SJ (1992). Detection of cervical *Chlamydia trachomatis* and *Neisseria gonorrhoeae* with deoxyribonucleic acid probe assays in obstetric patients. *American Journal of Obstetrics and Gynecology* 167: 588–91.

Jacobson DL, Piralta L, Graham NM *et al.* (2000) Histological development of cervical ectopy; relationship to reproductive hormones. *Sexually Transmitted Diseases.* 27 (5): 252–258.

James JF, Swanson J (1978) Studies on gonococcus infection. XIII. Occurrence of color/opacity colonial variants in clinical cultures. *Infection and Immunity* 19: 332–40.

Kaushic C, Zhou F, Murdin AD *et al.* (2000) Effect of Estradiol and progesterone on susceptibility and immune responses to *Chlamydia trachomatis* infection in the female reproductive tract. *Infection and Immunity* 68: 4207–4216.

Keelan JA, Blumenstein M, Helliwell RJA *et al.* (2003) Cytokines, prostaglandins and parturition: a review. *Placenta* 17: S33–46.

Kellogg DS Jr, Peacock WL Jr, Deacon WE *et al.* (1963) *Neisseria gonorrhoeae.* I. Virulence genetically linked to clonal variation. *Journal of Bacteriology* 85: 1274–1279.

Klein L, Gibbs RS (2004) Use of microbial cultures and antibiotics in the prevention of infection-associated pre-term birth. *American Journal of Obstetrics and Gynecology* 190: 1493–1502.

Kutteh WH, Franklin RD (2001) Quantification of immunoglobulins and cytokines in human cervical mucus during each trimester of pregnancy. *American Journal of Obstetrics and Gynecology* 184: 865–874.

Kutteh WH, Moldoveanu Z, Mesteckky J (1998). Mucosa immunity in the female reproductive tract: correlations of immunoglobulins, cytokines, and reproductive hormones in human cervical mucus around the time of ovulation. *AIDS Research and Human Retroviruses* 14 (Suppl. 1): S51–5.

Lee HH, Chernesky MA, Schachter J *et al.* (1995) Diagnosis of *Chlamydia trachomatis* genitourinary infection in women by ligase chain reaction assay of urine. *Lancet* 245: 213–216.

Lynch PJ (1978). Sexually transmitted diseases: granuloma inguinale, lymphogranuloma venereum, chancroid, and infectious syphilis. *Clinics in Obstetrics and Gynecology* 21: 1041–1052.

McGregor JA, French JI, Jones W *et al.* (1994) Bacterial vaginosis is associated with pre-maturity and vaginal fluid mucinase and sialidase: results of a controlled trial of topical clindamycin cream. *American Journal of Obstetrics and Gynecology* 170: 1048–1060.

McLaren LC, Davis LE, Healy GR *et al.* (1983) Isolation of *Trichomonas vaginalis* from the respiratory tract of infants with respiratory disease. *Pediatrics* 71: 888–890.

Makino S, van Putten JP, Meyer TF (1991) Phase variation of the opacity outer membrane protein controls invasion by *Neisseria gonorrhoeae* into human epithelial cells. *EMBO Journal* 10: 1307–1315.

Mangione-Smith R, O'Leary J, McGlynn EA (1999) Health and cost-benefits of chlamydia screening in young women. *Sexually Transmitted Diseases* 26: 309–316.

Meyer TF (1999) Pathogenic neisseriae: complexity of pathogen–host interplay. *Clinical Infections Diseases* 28: 433–441.

Mulks MH, Plaut AG (1978) IgA protease production as a characteristic distinguishing pathogenic from harmless Neisseriaceae. *New England Journal of Medicine* 299: 973–976.

Oram JD, Reiter B (1968) Inhibition of bacteria by lactoferrin and other iron-chelating agents. *Biochimica et Biophysica Acta* 170: 351–365.

Panke ES, Yang LI, Leist PA *et al.* (1991) Comparison of Gen-Probe DNA probe test and culture for the detection of *N. gonorrhoeae* in endocervical specimens. *Journal of Clinical Microbiology* 29: 883–888.

Rein MF (1990) Clinical manifestations of urogenital trichomoniasis in women. In: Honigberg BM (ed.) *Trichomonads parasitic in humans.* New York: Springer-Verlag, pp. 225–234.

Rice PA, McQuillen DP, Gulati S *et al.* (1994) Serum resistance of *Neisseria gonorrhoeae.* Does it thwart the inflammatory response and facilitate the transmission of infection? *Annals of the New York Academy of Sciences* 730: 7–14.

Rolfs RT, Goldberg M, Sharrar RG (1990) Risk factors for syphilis: cocaine use and prostitution. *American Journal of Public Health* 80: 853–857.

Romero R, Chaiworapongsa T, Kuivaniemi H *et al.* (2004) Bacterial vaginosis, the inflammatory response and the risk of pre-term birth; a role for genetic epidemiology in the prevention of pre-term birth. *American Journal of Obstetrics and Gynecology* 190: 1509–1519.

Ronnike F (1964) Discharge symptomatology in 1000 gynaecological cases examined with a view to *Trichomonas vaginalis.* Results of metronidazole (Flagyl) treatment. *Acta Obstetrica et Gynecologica Scandinavica* 42 (Suppl. 6): 63–70.

Schachter J (1999a) Biology of *Chlamydia trachomatis.* In: Holmes KK, Sparling PF, Mardh P-A. *et al.* eds. *Sexually Transmitted Diseases.* New York: McGraw Hill, pp. 391–400.

Schachter J. (1999b) Infection and disease epidemiology. In: Stephens RS (ed.) Chlamydia trachomatis *Biology Pathogenesis and Immunology.* Washington, DC: American Society for Microbiology, pp. 139–169.

Singer A (1976) The cervical epithelium during pregnancy and the puerperium. In: Jordan JA, Singer A (eds) *The Cervix.* London: WB Saunders, p. 105.

Singh AE, Romanowski B (1999) Syphilis: review with emphasis on clinical, epidemiologic, and some biologic features. *Clinical Microbiology Review* 12: 187–209.

Stamm WE, Holmes KK (1997) Chlamydial trachomatis of the adult. In: Holmes KK (ed.) *Sexually Transmitted Diseases.* New York: McGraw-Hill.

Stary A, Schuh E, Kerschbaumer M (1998) Performance of transcription-mediated amplification and ligase chain reaction assays for detection of chlamydial infection in urogenital samples obtained by invasive and non-invasive methods. *Journal of Clinical Microbiology* 36: 2666–2670.

Strominger JL, Ghuysen JM (1967) Mechanisms of enzymatic bacteriolysis. Cell walls of bacteria are solubilized by action of either specific carbohydrates or specific peptidases. *Science* 156: 213–221.

Suriyanon V, Nelson KE, Choomsai NA *et al.* (1975) *Trichomonas vaginalis* in a perinephric abscess. A case report. *American Journal of Tropical Medicine and Hygiene* 24: 776–780.

Thompson SE, Washington AE (1983) Epidemiology of sexually transmitted *Chlamydia trachomatis* infections. *Epidemiological Reviews* 5: 96–123.

Waldman RH, Cruz JM, Rowe DS (1972) Immunoglobulin levels and antibody to *Candida albicans* in human cervicovaginal secretions. *Clinics in Experimental Immunology* 10: 427–434.

Wallin J (1975) Gonorrhoea in 1972. A 1-year study of patients attending the VD Unit in Uppsala. *British Journal of Venereal Disease* 51: 41–47.

White HD, Yeaman GR, Givan AL *et al.* (1997) Mucosal immunity in the human female reproductive tract: cytotoxic T-lymphocyte function in the cervix and vagina of pre-menopausal and post-menopausal women. *American Journal of Reproductive Immunology* 37: 30–38.

Whittington MJ (1957) Epidemiology of infections with *Trichomonas vaginalis* in the light of improved diagnostic methods. *British Journal of Venereal Disease* 33: 80–91.

Yang LI, Panke ES, Leist PA *et al.* (1991). Detection of *Chlamydia trachomatis* endocervical infection in asymptomatic and symptomatic women: comparison of deoxyribonucleic acid probe test with tissue culture. *American Journal of Obstetrics and Gynecology* 165: 1444–1453.

Young H, Sarafian SK, Harris AB *et al.* (1983) Non-cultural detection of *Neisseria gonorrhoeae* in cervical and vaginal washings. *Journal of Medical Microbiology* 16: 183–91.

Zhang JR, Stephens RS (1992) Mechanisms of *Chlamydia trachomatis* attachment to eukaryotic host cells. *Cell* 69: 861–865.

CHAPTER 17

Common viral infections of the cervix (excluding human papillomavirus): clinical features and management

Raymond H. Kaufman and Ervin Adam

A variety of common viral infections involve the human cervix. However, very few of them manifest clinical evidence of infection in the cervix. The viral infections that involve the lower genital tract include the following:

1 human papillomavirus (discussed in Chapter 15);
2 herpes simplex, types 1, 2, 6, 7 and 8;
3 cytomegalovirus.

The pathology of these lesions and their effect on the cervix and lower genital tract has been described in Chapter 16.

Other viruses can affect the lower genital tract, including molluscum contagiosum, herpes zoster and vaccinia. However, no good evidence has been demonstrated to suggest that these viruses specifically involve the cervix.

HERPES SIMPLEX VIRUS INFECTIONS OF THE CERVIX

Table 17.1 lists the human herpesviruses and their disease associations. A variety of herpes simplex viruses (HSV) can infect the human cervix. These include HSV 1, 2, 6, 7 and 8. Apparently, HSV 2 is the most significant of these herpesviruses to infect the cervix. However, a number of studies have been conducted investigating the presence of HSV 6, 7 and 8 in the cervix. This chapter will therefore consider these types in two sections: the first considers types (HSV) 6, 7 and 8 and the second the clinically more common types 1 and 2.

Types

Herpes virus 6 (HSV 6)

Herpes virus 6 (HSV 6) is a highly prevalent virus. There are two HSV 6 subtypes, A and B, with subtype A causing the majority of HSV 6 infections. Maeda *et al.* (1997) found human herpes virus 6 (HHV 6) DNA in 25.5% of vaginal swabs taken from 110 pregnant women collected between 4 and 8 weeks of gestation. The virus itself, however, could not be isolated from any vaginal sample. The presence of HSV 6

DNA within the genital tract of the pregnant women did not affect the health of the infants and, thus, it was felt that the virus was not transmitted to infants through the genital tract. Baillargon *et al.* (2000) studied 569 pregnant and non-pregnant women attending a family planning clinic and 345 women attending two obstetric clinics in San Antonio, Texas. They studied blood for HSV 6 IgG antibodies and vaginal swabs for the presence of HSV 6 DNA. They found that all women studied were HSV 6 antibody positive. The antibody titres in non-pregnant women were significantly higher than those seen in the pregnant women. HSV 6 shedding in the genital tract was observed in 2% of the pregnant women and 3.7% of the non-pregnant women. Okuno *et al.* (1995) obtained cervical swabs from women late in pregnancy and found that 19.4% of 72 samples contained detectable HSV 6. It does not appear that infection with HHV 6 has any impact upon the fetus nor does its presence in the cervix appear to contribute to the development of cervical carcinoma. However, Chen *et al.* (1994) found sequences of HSV 6 in six of 72 cases of cervical carcinoma and cervical intraepithelial neoplasia (CIN). Human papillomavirus (HPV) 16 was found in four of the HSV 6-positive cases. None of the 30 normal cervices and biopsies of patients with cervicitis were positive for HHV 6 DNA. Their study raised the possibility of an association between HHV 6 and cervical neoplasia. This, however, has never been confirmed. HHV 6 infection is purported to be involved in a variety of neurological disorders as well as lymphoproliferative diseases. HSV 6 and HPV can interact to transactivate HPV in cervical epithelial cells. Beyond this, no direct relationship between the virus and cervical carcinoma has been established. For a review of human herpesvirus infections, Clark has presented a comprehensive review of human herpes virus 6 (2000).

Herpes virus 8 (HSV 8)

Whitley *et al.* (1999) investigated the seroprevalence of HSV 8 in a population of women attending a sexually transmitted disease clinic and human immunodeficiency virus

Table 17.1 The human herpes viruses and their disease associations.

Subfamily and virus	Disease association
Alphaherpesviruses	
Herpes simplex virus type 1 (HSV 1)	Oral lesions, encephalitis, keratitis
Herpes simplex virus type 2 (HSV 2)	Genital lesions, meningitis
Varicella zoster virus (VZV)	Chicken pox, herpes zoster
Betaherpesviruses	
Human cytomegalovirus (HCMV)	Congenital infection, mononucleosis, post-transplant, CMV disease, retinitis
Human herpes virus 6A (HHV 6A)	Exanthem subitum (rarely)
Human herpes virus 6B (HHV 6B)	Exanthem subitum, febrile convulsions, transplant complications
Human herpes virus 7 (HHV 7)	Exanthem subitum, pityriasis rosea, CMV disease
Gammaherpesviruses	
Epstein–Barr virus (EBV)	Mononucleosis, B-cell lymphomas, oral leucoplakia, nasopharyngeal carcinoma
Human herpes virus 8 (HHV 8)	Kaposi's sarcoma, primary effusion lymphoma, multicentric Castleman's disease

From Black and Pellet (1999).

(HIV) clinic in London. The seroprevalence of HSV 8 was 18.3%, with the highest prevalence seen in women from Africa. The presence of antibodies appeared to be independent of the HIV serostatus. They suggested that there was a low prevalence of HSV-8 in the general heterosexual population in the US and UK. Embom *et al.* (2001) investigated the presence of Epstein–Barr virus (EBV) and HSV 8 DNA from the cervical secretions of Swedish women using polymerase chain reaction (PCR). They concluded that there was a possible sexual route of transmission of EBV but not HSV 8. They found EBV DNA in 10 cervical secretion samples from 112 women.

Herpes simplex virus 8 may well be an aetiological factor leading to the development of Kaposi's sarcoma. Martin *et al.* (1998) evaluated 400 men who were infected with HIV and a sample of 400 uninfected men. Serum samples were assayed for antibodies to HSV 8 at the start of the study. They found anti-HSV 8 antibodies in 37.6% of homosexual men who reported any homosexual activity in the previous 5 years and in none of 195 heterosexual men. The antibody positivity correlated with the history of sexually transmitted diseases and was directly related to the number of male sexual intercourse partners. The 10-year probability of Kaposi's sarcoma was 49.6% among the men who were infected with both HIV and HSV 8 at baseline. They observed that the presence of HHV 8 infection was associated with the development of Kaposi's sarcoma and felt that there may well be an aetiological role of this virus in the development of Kaposi's sarcoma. Boivin *et al.* (2000) studied 195 samples from HIV-seropositive women and 89 from HIV-seronegative women. HHV 8 DNA was not detected in any of the genital samples, including two from women with Kaposi's sarcoma. All these women were sexually active. They concluded that Canadian women, even though

exposed to men who were themselves at risk of HHV 8 infection, are unlikely to acquire this infection. Their findings suggest the possibility that heterosexual transmission of HHV 8 is not an effective means of viral transmission. Their findings also correlate with the low prevalence of Kaposi's sarcoma in HIV-infected women in contrast to HIV-infected men who have sexual contact with men. Whitley *et al.* (1999) studied a group of women attending a sexually transmitted disease clinic and an HIV clinic at a London hospital as well as a group of women attending a colposcopy clinic. They concluded that there is a low prevalence of HSV-8 in the general heterosexual population in the US and the UK.

Herpes virus 7 (HSV 7)

Human herpes virus 7 (HHV 7) is a lymphotrophic member of the betaherpesvirus subfamily of herpesviruses. Its prevalence in the general population is extremely high, with primary infection usually occurring during childhood. It has been associated, as noted in Table 17.1, with a variety of clinical symptoms, but its impact in lower genital tract disease is insignificant. Okuno *et al.* (1995) obtained cervical swabs from 72 women in late pregnancy. They recovered HHV 7 genomes in two (2.7%) of the 72 women studied. The significance of this finding is unknown. Rather than being sexually transmitted, this virus is usually transmitted through the saliva. It is believed that, once primary infection occurs, the virus may enter a latent state in T cells. It is also thought that salivary glands are a likely site of persistent viral infection and the source of infectious transmission. Despite the high prevalence of this infection and the many clinical manifestations associated with it, it does not appear to affect the lower genital tract significantly.

HERPES SIMPLEX VIRUSES 1 AND 2: COMMON (CLINICAL) TYPES

Lower genital tract infection with herpes genitalis has traditionally been thought to be related primarily to infection with HSV 2. However, more recent studies have demonstrated that a significant number of infections of the lower genitalia are related to HSV 1. Most recently, Lafferty *et al.* (2000) observed that HSV 1 was identified in over 20% of initial genital HSV infections. They recovered HSV 1 virus in 27% of initial infections and 16% of recurrent infections in heterosexual women. White race and oral sex had a positive association with HSV 1 genital tract infection. The prevalence of HSV 2 infection has risen steadily over the past decades. The third National Health and Nutrition Examination survey (Fleming *et al.*, 1997) demonstrated a prevalence of HSV 2 antibodies of 21.9% among 13 094 individuals surveyed. In the female population, the prevalence was 25.6%. There was an overall increase in HSV 2 antibodies of 30% in both sexes between the years 1976–1980 and 1988–1994.

Characteristics of infection

Natural history

It is well established that genital tract infection with the HSV is sexually transmitted. Genital HSV infection is frequently associated with the presence of other sexually transmitted diseases. Most primary infections are seen in teenage and unmarried women. Infection is transmitted by direct sexual contact, often when an active virus-secreting lesion is present, but it can also be transmitted through asymptomatic shedding of the virus. Multiple studies have now demonstrated the recovery of HSV in the cervices of asymptomatic women (Adam *et al.*, 1980; Barton *et al.*, 1986; Brock *et al.*, 1990; Wald *et al.*, 1995). Wald *et al.* (1995) followed 110 women with a clinical history of genital herpes infection. Subclinical shedding of HSV 2 was observed in 55% of the women; 52% demonstrated subclinical shedding of both HSV 1 and HSV 2, and 29% of the women were found to be shedding HSV 1. Wald *et al.* (2000) also observed that the frequency of subclinical shedding of HSV 2 in women with no history of genital herpes was similar to that in the subjects with a history of infection. After a primary infection, the herpes simplex virus remains latent in the sensory sacral ganglia that supply the segments of the genitalia where the infection was clinically seen. Recurrence of infection is likely to develop within 6 months in approximately 60% of individuals with a primary infection. Most women infected with HSV never develop clinical manifestations of a primary infection. Many with unrecognised latent infections do develop subsequent symptomatic recurrences (Langenberg *et al.*, 1989; Wald *et al.*, 2000). Recurrent episodes occur at sporadic intervals, and the exact mechanism that results in recurrence is unknown. However, Cohen *et al.*

(1999) reported that persistent significant stress predicted genital herpes recurrences. The effect of stress on asymptomatic shedding, however, has not been adequately studied yet. Primary genital HSV infection is one that occurs in an individual without antibodies to either HSV 1 or HSV 2. Initial non-primary infections are the first clinically found episodes that occur in an individual with the presence of antibodies to either HSV 1 or HSV 2. Antibodies to HSV 1 appear to have a modifying effect upon the initial infection with HSV 2.

Symptoms

Symptoms of primary infection usually develop within 3–7 days after exposure to the virus. An initial infection can be relatively mild or completely asymptomatic. However, the individual with a primary infection may develop significant debilitating symptoms. Mild paraesthesia and burning is often experienced before lesions become visible. Often patients complain of pain radiating to the back or hips or down the legs. After development of the lesions, patients report severe pain and tenderness in the affected tissues. Inguinal and pelvic pain may be seen and is related to inflammation of the lymph nodes and associated lymphadenopathy. Often the individual will have systemic symptoms consisting of headache, generalised aching and malaise and fever. Significant dysuria and even urinary retention may occur and result from infection of the urethra and bladder mucosa, rather than from discomfort caused by voiding over the infected vulva. When the cervix is involved, as it usually is in primary disease, a severe herpes cervicitis may develop with an associated profuse watery discharge.

Clinical manifestations

The clinical manifestations of primary infection are often quite severe with the individual developing extensive involvement of the labia majora, labia minora, perianal skin and vestibule of the vulva as well as the ectocervical mucosa (Figs 17.1–17.4). Soon after the onset of symptoms, multiple vesicles may be seen scattered over the above areas, but they rapidly rupture leaving shallow, ulcerated areas.

Indurated papules with vesiculation and ulceration are also seen. Superficial ulcers may arise on the ectocervix (Figs 17.5 and 17.6) and even within the vagina. Occasionally, a fungating necrotic mass visibly covers the ectocervix, and this is often clinically confused with invasive cervical carcinoma (Figs 17.7 and 17.8).

The cervix may be exquisitely tender, bleed easily and, when it is manipulated, provoke severe pelvic pain. Inguinal lymphadenopathy is frequently present. Primary lesions may persist for 2–6 weeks but, after healing, there is no residual scarring or induration (Figs 17.9–17.11). Uncommonly, meningitis and encephalitis may be seen in association with the primary infection. The prognosis for a patient with meningitis

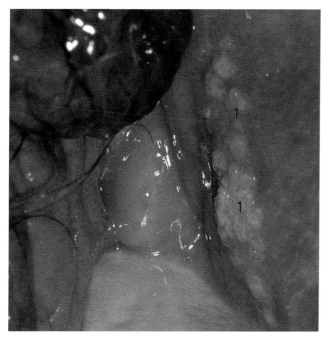

Fig. 17.1 The vulva, showing characteristic small vesicles (1) that are typical of the initial stages of HSV infection.

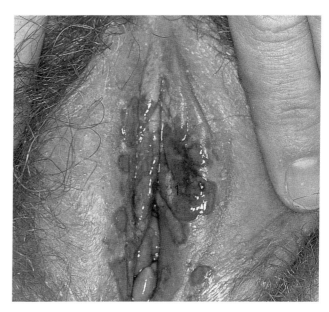

Fig. 17.3 Occasionally, there may be less symptomatic lesions that appear more localised (1) than the usual types of lesions, and these are frequently seen when recurrent attacks occur.

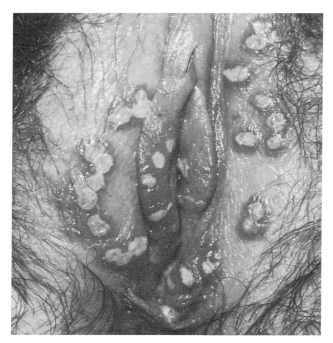

Fig. 17.2 The vulva, showing the vesicles as seen in Figure 17.1, enlarging quickly and surrounded by an erythematous skin reaction. They subsequently rupture and develop into shallow ulcerative lesions that are multiple, painful and may coalesce and develop serpiginous red borders and pale yellow centres.

Fig. 17.4 (right) In this photograph of the vulva, the vesicles have enlarged and again are surrounded by an erythematous skin reaction. These lesions will subsequently rupture and develop into the classical shallow ulcerative lesions seen in Figures 17.2 and 17.3. Some ulcers may be present within the urethra, and those that are within the vestibule may cause such distress that urinary retention is not uncommon.

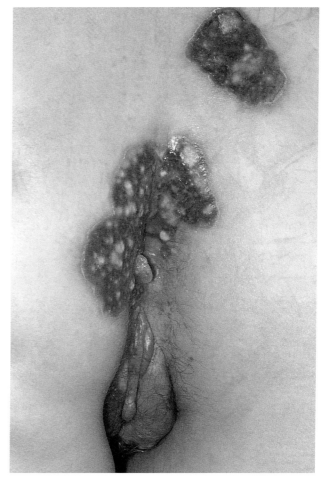

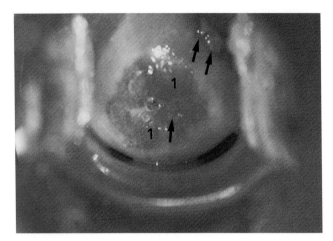

Fig. 17.5 Colposcopic changes of early infection with vesicles arrowed and epithelial congestion (1) caused by cellular infiltration that occurs just before ulceration.

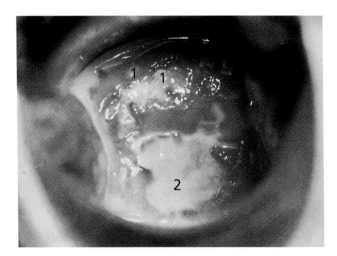

Fig. 17.6 The epithelial congestion (1) associated with the cellular infiltration has now led to ulceration (2), which is usually associated with some secondary infection. In Figures 17.6 to 17.8, the ulceration that has been associated with the secondary infection leads to an appearance designated as non-specific acute necrotising cervicitis.

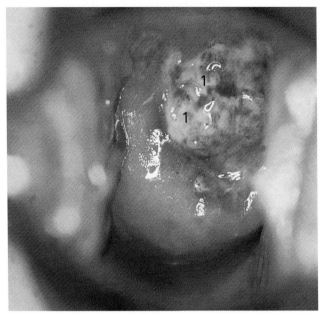

Fig. 17.7 The ulceration is clearly seen at (1) where it is localised.

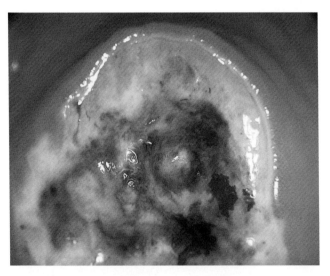

Fig. 17.8 The whole anterior lip of the cervix has been involved in the process of ulceration.

is excellent; however, mortality is high in patients developing HSV 2 encephalitis.

Symptoms seen in association with a recurrent infection are considerably milder than those seen with a primary infection. Recurrent infection usually reaches its peak within 48 hours of the onset of symptoms with maximal pain, size of lesions and virus titre and excretion occurring within this time period. The recurrence pattern after a primary infection differs significantly between HSV 2 and HSV 1. Lafferty *et al.* (1987) observed that genital recurrences develop significantly more often following HSV 2 primary infection than following HSV 1 primary infection. The frequency of symptomatic recurrences appears to decrease over time in many but not all patients

(Benedetti *et al.*, 1999). Cervical shedding of the virus in individuals with recurrent disease has been reported to occur in varying frequencies by different authors. Guinan *et al.* (1981) found cervical cultures to be positive in 30% of individuals studied on the first day of clinical manifestations. However, Kawana *et al.* (1982) reported that only two of 12 women with recurrence of disease shed virus from the cervix. The clinical manifestations of recurrent disease consist of the development of single vesicles or multiple clusters on an erythematous base. These vesicles may vary from 1 to 5 mm in diameter and rapidly rupture on the mucoid surfaces, leaving

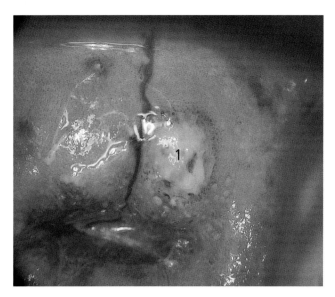

Fig. 17.9 The tiny vesicles seen in the initial infection do not last as long on the cervix as in the vulva, and they rapidly coalesce, producing the appearance of a single, small herpetic ulcer in the process of healing as seen at (1).

shallow painful ulcers. On the skin surface, vesicles last longer and are followed by crusting that persists until complete healing takes place. Healing occurs within 7–10 days after the onset of symptoms. Patients will usually complain of vulvar burning and pain that lasts from 5 to 7 days. Superficial ulcerations of the cervix and vagina are also noted and are similar to those seen in primary disease (Figs 17.7 and 17.8).

Histopathology

The histopathology associated with herpesvirus infections is quite characteristic. An intraepithelial vesicle caused by degeneration of the epithelium with acantholysis and accumulation of fluid beneath the stratum corneum is noted (Fig. 17.12). There is an intense leucocytic infiltration within the epidermis and dermis. The ballooning degeneration of epithelial cells is characteristic, and these cells frequently enlarge, become multinucleated and give rise to viral-type giant cells. These giant cells are most prominent at the edges of the lesion. An eosinophilic inclusion body is often seen within the nucleus and surrounded by a clear halo. These microscopic changes are reflected in those noted on cytology. The latter findings are characteristic of HSV infections. These changes consist of intranuclear vacuoles with irregularly arranged small basophilic intranuclear particles. The nuclei often have a homogeneous 'ground glass' appearance. Discrete eosinophilic intranuclear occlusions are also frequently seen (Fig. 17.13).

Differential diagnosis

The characteristic clinical history of herpes genitalis should usually help distinguish it from other vesiculo-ulcerative diseases of the vulva. Herpes zoster is usually easy to distinguish because of its unilateral distribution and failure to recur in the same site, longer duration and larger more persistent lesions. Viral culture and PCR will distinguish the two. Other disease processes to eliminate are other ulcerative lesions that could be confused with a herpetic infection. These include multiple chancres occasionally seen with syphilis, chancroid, Behçet's syndrome and vaccinia. Occasionally, excoriations associated with candidiasis may be confused with a herpetic infection.

Prevention and treatment

The herpes virus may either cause symptomatic infection or assume a latent existence within the sensory dorsal ganglia

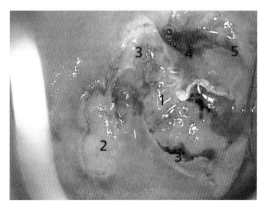

Fig. 17.10 A herpetic ulceration involving the posterior cervical lip (1). Remnants of the acute non-specific necrotising cervicitis are seen at (2). The rolled margins of the ulcer could be confused with the edges of an invasive cervical cancer, as seen at (3). Points (4) and (5) mark the external os.

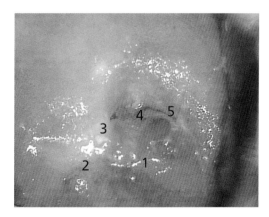

Fig. 17.11 The same cervix as photographed in Figure 17.10, seen some 35 days later. There has been complete healing of the ulcer that had previously been present at (1) by squamous epithelium. Necrotising cervicitis seen at position (2) has completely disappeared, as have the rolled edges of the ulcer that were previously at position (3). Points (4) and (5) are in exactly the same position as in Figure 17.10 and define points on the external os.

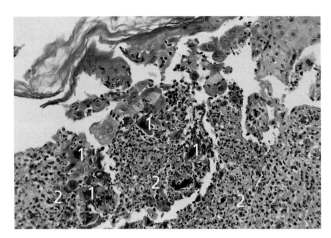

Fig. 17.12 Histophotograph showing the histological representation of vesicle formation and ulceration. The infection commences in the parabasal cells of the squamous epithelium, where there is nuclear enlargement and development of multinucleated cells. Vesicle formation and ulceration follow within 36 hours. The histological examination of the vesicle is then composed of giant cells at the edge (1) and in the base; polymorphonuclear leucocytes (2) are present in the surrounding epithelium.

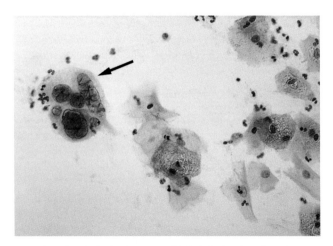

Fig. 17.13 Cytological appearance of HSV infection is easily recognisable with the cytological changes characterised by large multiple nuclei that are moulded together (arrowed) and show margination of chromatin and generally empty nuclei. Large intranuclear inclusions are also commonly seen.

neurons. Methods of managing this infection have included the use of antiviral agents to treat acute infection or suppress the development of recurrent infection, and vaccination. Recently, Stanberry *et al.* (2002), utilising a glycoprotein D-2 vaccine along with adjuvant, found that individual women who were seronegative for both HSV 1 and HSV 2 were protected from both diseases. However, they were unable to demonstrate any significant effect in males. This raises some interesting questions as to why it should be effective in women and not in males. However, further study is certainly necessary to clarify the efficacy of this vaccine.

Three effective drugs for the management of genital herpes virus infection are clinically available. These are acyclovir, valacyclovir and famcyclovir. They are all effective in shortening the duration of the clinical symptoms and viral shedding in both initial and recurrent infections. They are also effective as suppressant therapy in decreasing the frequency of recurrences. The Centers for Disease Control and Prevention (Workowski *et al.*, 2002) have published treatment guidelines for individuals with herpesvirus infections. These recommendations are noted in Tables 17.2–17.4. In individuals with primary disease, if healing is not complete within the 10-day course of therapy, the medication can be continued for a longer period of time. If the individual is unresponsive to the recommended dose, the dose can be increased. Gilbert *et al.* (2001) have reported that, in those individuals who are totally unresponsive to management with these drugs, especially if the patient is immunodeficient, the topical application of imiquimod may be effective in speeding up healing of the ulcers. They report one case demonstrating an excellent result utilising the 5% imiquimod cream three times a week. Active treatment of both primary and non-primary first-episode genital herpes has no effect on the subsequent rate of recurrences.

The Centers for Disease Control (Workowski *et al.*, 2002) recommended treatment for individuals with recurrent disease is outlined in Table 17.3. Treatment is effective in reducing the duration of viral shedding and in shortening the healing time when compared with patients treated with placebo. Treatment of recurrent infection should begin as soon after the onset of symptoms as possible, preferably even during the prodromal period that precedes many outbreaks.

In women with frequent recurrences, suppressive therapy utilising any of the three antiviral drugs has proved to be

Condition or need	Recommended treatments
Genital herpes	
First clinical episode	Oral acyclovir, 400 mg 3 times daily for 7–10 days or
	Oral acyclovir, 200 mg 5 times daily for 7–10 days or
	Oral famcyclovir, 250 mg 3 times daily for 7–10 days or
	Oral valacyclovir, 1 g twice daily for 7–10 days

Table 17.2 Recommendation from the Centers for Disease Control and Prevention 2002 Guidelines for the Treatment of Sexually Transmitted Diseases.

Table 17.3 Recommendation from the Centers for Disease Control and Prevention 2002 Guidelines for the Treatment of Sexually Transmitted Diseases.

Condition or need	Recommended treatments
Genital herpes	
Episodic recurrences	Oral acyclovir, 400 mg 3 times daily for 5 days or Oral acyclovir, 200 mg 5 times daily for 5 days or Oral acyclovir, 800 mg twice daily for 5 days or Oral famcyclovir, 125 mg twice daily for 5 days or Oral valacyclovir, 500 mg twice daily for 3–5 days or Oral valacyclovir, 1 g twice daily for 5 days

Table 17.4 Recommendation from the Centers for Disease Control and Prevention 2002 Guidelines for the Treatment of Sexually Transmitted Diseases.

Condition or need	Recommended treatments
Genital herpes	
Suppression	Oral acyclovir, 400 mg twice daily or Oral famcyclovir, 250 mg twice daily or Oral valacyclovir, 500 mg once daily or Oral valacyclovir, 1 g once daily

effective in reducing the frequency of recurrence. There is a decrease in frequency of recurrences of 70–80% when patients are maintained on continuous therapy. Acyclovir has been used continuously for well over 6 years, and it has continued to be effective and has been demonstrated to be safe over this prolonged period of time. It appears as if the longer the patient is maintained on suppressive therapy, the less frequent are the recurrences observed. This was observed by Goldberg *et al.* (1993). Despite the effectiveness of suppressive therapy in reducing the frequency of recurrences, patients may still occasionally demonstrate asymptomatic viral shedding. This has been demonstrated by Wald *et al.* (1996), who demonstrated over 90% reduction in viral shedding rate in individuals on suppressive acyclovir therapy compared with those receiving placebo. Even though these antiviral drugs are effective in preventing recurrences and apparently in decreasing the frequency of viral shedding, it is still possible for individuals to transmit the disease to a sexual partner in the absence of lesions. There is no good evidence as yet to demonstrate the development of resistance of the virus to the antiviral drugs currently being used. The recommended regimes for suppressive management are presented in Table 17.4.

Antiviral treatment reduces symptomatic and asymptomatic shedding of HSV from genital mucosa. Until recently, it has been difficult to acquire evidence to say whether this translates into a real, clinically important reduction in the transmission of genital herpes to an uninfected partner. Corey *et al.* (2004) have recently published a study of 1484 heterosexual, immunocompetent couples to determine whether daily vala-

cyclovir could reduce the sexual transmission of genital herpes. One partner from each couple had clinically diagnosed genital HSV 2 infection and the other was HSV 2 seronegative; the infected partner was randomised to 500 mg of the drug once daily or placebo for 8 months. The couple were followed for symptoms of genital HSV. It was found that symptomatic genital herpes was observed in 2.2% of partners of individuals treated with placebo but in only 0.5% of those treated with valacyclovir. This represented a 75% reduction in relative risk. The couples had been offered condoms at each visit, and it was found that genital herpes was transmitted less often in those couples using barrier contraception, but the benefit of using valacyclovir was in addition to the protective effect of condoms. Of the 141 individuals who took the drug and used condoms, none transmitted symptomatic genital herpes to their partners, especially when condoms were used for 90% of sexual encounters. The study showed that the rate of transmission in these monogamous HSV 2 discordant couples was very low, at under 5% over an 8-month period. The Food and Drug Administration (FDA) has recently accepted the results of this study and has approved a new indication for valacyclovir, i.e. the prevention of sexual transmission of HSV infection.

Recently, Barton (2005) has emphasised that these data were obtained in immunocompetent, heterosexual couples who were motivated to participate in this trial, and he feels that the benefits may be altered when used 'in pregnancy, across same sex relationships or among individuals with HIV infection'. He also questions whether a notable reduction in transmission provided by valacyclovir is mirrored by other antiviral drugs such as acyclovir or famcyclovir. Other studies would need to be performed to resolve this question. However, Barton also points out that part of the positive aspect of this study was that no evidence of viral resistance was detected in those individuals who became infected in the study. It is important to note that some susceptible individuals did become infected, and this reinforces the message that 'valacyclovir reduced the frequency of HSV reactivation, subclinical shedding, and transmission of genital herpes, but it did not eliminate it'.

There is no effective vaccine at the present time to prevent recurrences of genital lesions. Resiquimod gel 0.01% has been utilised two to three times weekly for up to a period of 3 weeks and has been observed to delay the median days to first recurrence compared with a control group of women. Spruance *et al.* (2001) studied 52 patients with frequently recurrent genital herpes and applied resiquimod gel 0.01% two or three times a week or 0.05% once or twice a week to herpes lesions for a period of 3 weeks. The median days to first recurrence in the resiquimod-treated group was significantly less than that observed in the placebo group. They suggested that the 0.01% gel is more satisfactory than the 0.05% gel as the latter often produced significant inflammation at the lesion sites.

Herpesvirus infections in pregnancy

One of the most serious complications of HSV infections is that associated with activation of the infection at the time of delivery. This often results in infection of the neonate with subsequent severe complications. About 50% of the infants who are infected who are not treated die and those who survive frequently suffer from severe neurological sequelae. Neonatal herpetic infection is relatively rare, seen in approximately 1 in 3000 to 1 in 30 000 live births. Prevention of infection is extremely difficult because approximately 70% of the infants delivered who develop neonatal herpes are born to mothers who have neither signs nor symptoms of disease at or around the time of delivery. Approximately 35–50% of mothers delivering newborn infants who develop HSV infections have no history of prior infection or even exposure to the infection. Theoretically, routine screening for HSV 2 antibodies would identify those women at highest risk for recurrent shedding of the virus at the time of delivery. However, at the present time, this is relatively impractical as most commercial laboratories do not as yet perform antibody studies that clearly distinguish between prior infection with HSV 1 and HSV 2. Rouse and Stringer (2000) created a decision analysis model to assess the cost-effectiveness of herpes simplex antibody screening during pregnancy and concluded that screening for type-specific HSV antibodies in the pregnant mother could not be recommended at the present time to prevent neonatal herpes. Obtaining a history of prior infection in the mother is certainly of some help in identifying the woman at risk of viral shedding; however, as already indicated, the majority of women who have had prior infection have no history of this. Another aspect to consider is the history of genital herpesvirus infection in the male partner of the woman who is pregnant. In addition, a history should be elicited regarding oral herpes infection in the patient and her sexual partner. If there is such a history, all cunnilingus during the third trimester of pregnancy should be avoided.

Primary infection and delivery

Of great significance is the acquisition of a primary infection at or near the time of delivery. Under these circumstances, the risk of transmission of virus to the infant is exceedingly high.

As indicated above, the likelihood of transmission of HSV to the neonate is as high as 50% among women who acquire an initial genital herpes infection near the time of delivery. Furthermore, Brown *et al.* (1996) noted that the asymptomatic genital shedding of HSV at the onset of labour with subclinical primary genital infection is associated with preterm delivery.

However, in women with a history of recurrent herpes who are actively shedding virus at term, the likelihood of transmission of infection to the infant is extremely low, varying between 1% and 5%. Despite this relatively low risk of transmission of infection to the infant, reactivation of maternal HSV infection still accounts for more than 50% of neonatal exposure. The presence of neutralising antibodies to HSV 2 acquired in the infant from the mother appears to be protective against the development of neonatal disease. In 1987, Brown *et al.* followed 29 women who had acquired genital herpes during pregnancy. Fifteen of these women had a primary first episode of genital HSV 2, and 14 had a non-primary first episode. Six of the 15 women with primary genital herpes but none of the 14 with non-primary first episodes had infants with serious perinatal morbidity. Among five women developing primary HSV infection in the third trimester, four of the deliveries were associated with significant perinatal morbidity such as prematurity, intra-uterine growth retardation and neonatal infection. In a study conducted in 1997, Brown *et al.* evaluated seroconversion of women during pregnancy and observed that, of women who were seronegative for HSV 1 and HSV 2, seroconversion occurred in 3.7% of the cases. Acquisition of genital herpes virus infection was known in 60 of 94 women who converted. Three per cent occurred in the first trimester, 30% in the second trimester and 40% in the third trimester. Nine women converted shortly before labour and, of these, there were four neonatal infections and one neonatal death.

Recently, Williams *et al.* (2006) published a study that estimated the efficacy of valacyclovir-suppressive therapy in pregnant women with recurrent genital herpes. Results showed that administration of this drug to these women beginning at 36 weeks' gestation reduced the number of them having subsequent clinical HSV recurrences.

Protocol for monitoring during pregnancy

When the neonate does develop an HSV infection, it appears that the presence or absence of antibodies to HSV 2 is not related to the severity of the neonatal infection (Whitley *et al.*, 1980). On the basis of the extensive accumulation of data related to genital herpesvirus infection during pregnancy, we have established a protocol for following pregnant women. It is extremely difficult to distinguish primary and recurrent infections clinically during pregnancy (Hensleigh *et al.*, 1997). Thus, it is important when a patient with no history of prior herpesvirus infection develops symptoms suggestive of a primary infection that appropriate viral cultures and antibody studies be performed to evaluate whether or not one is dealing with a true primary infection or a recurrent infection. This will have a significant impact for the prognosis of the infant. The protocol we currently recommend is:

1 At the initial visit, each pregnant patient should have a careful history taken that will elicit evidence of a prior genital HSV infection. A history of a similar infection in the male partner should also be elicited. Ideally, blood specimens should be obtained from both the pregnant woman and the prospective father for the detection of antibodies to HSV 1 and HSV 2 but, as already mentioned, this appears not to be practical at the present time.

2 If symptoms develop that are suggestive of an HSV infection, the patient should be seen as soon as possible after the onset of symptoms so that a culture can be taken from the lesions or sites of prodromal symptoms. At the same time, blood should be drawn to detect the presence or absence of antibodies to HSV 1 and HSV 2. If antibodies analogous to those recovered on the culture are detected, this can be assumed to be a recurrent infection.

3 In the woman with a prior history of genital HSV infection or one who develops herpetic lesions during pregnancy that are culture positive, no further cultures need be taken during the pregnancy until the patient enters the hospital in labour. At that time, careful inspection of the vulva, vagina and cervix should be carried out looking for lesions of genital herpes. If none is found, cultures should be taken from the sites of prior lesions and from the cervix. In the absence of clinical evidence of disease, vaginal delivery should be permitted.

4 Any woman in labour with active genital lesions should be delivered by caesarean section regardless of the length of time the membranes have been ruptured. The presence of intact membranes does not guarantee that a neonatal infection will not develop (Stone *et al.*, 1989).

5 Women with non-genital active lesions of the buttocks or lower trunk in labour should be considered for caesarean section as shedding of the virus from the cervix has been documented in these individuals.

6 Information regarding a positive culture that is obtained from the mother after delivery should be rapidly communicated to the paediatrician. Current thinking as to the advisability of treating the infants is, as yet, not clear. A cord blood sample obtained from all such infants tested for the presence of neutralising antibodies may be of some predictive value in indicating which infants are more likely to develop infection. If the infant is exposed to the virus of a primary infection, cultures should be taken from the urine, stool, cerebrospinal fluid, eyes and throat. If a positive culture is obtained beyond 48 hours of neonatal age or if the cerebrospinal fluid is abnormal, treatment with acyclovir should be started (Prober *et al.*, 1992). If the infant is exposed to a recurrent infection, the parents should be instructed to report lethargy, poor feeding, fever or the development of lesions. Weekly cultures from the eyes, nose, mouth and skin should be obtained for a period of 4–6 weeks despite the fact that no clear evidence shows that weekly cultures from these areas are worthwhile (Prober *et al.*, 1992).

7 A woman who develops a primary infection in the third trimester of pregnancy is at risk of preterm delivery. Such an individual should have a culture performed on a weekly basis until a negative culture has been obtained. Once this occurs, the patient should be managed as outlined previously. If active viral shedding is present at the time of the last culture prior to onset of labour, consideration should be given to performing a caesarean section. Although the occurrence of intra-uterine HSV infection is uncommon, it is most likely to occur in the presence of a primary infection. Thus, even if the maternal culture is negative at the time of delivery, infants born to mothers developing primary infection, especially late in pregnancy, should be very carefully monitored for the presence HSV infection. A fetal scalp electrode should not be used on the patient with a history of HSV infection or in the presence of active maternal infection at the time of labour because of the increased risk of transmitting the virus to the neonate.

8 A woman without a known history of genital herpes who has a sexual partner with such a history should avoid intercourse during the third trimester of pregnancy. Prior to this, during pregnancy, intercourse with condoms is advisable. Furthermore, if the pregnant woman has no known history of oral labial herpes but her partner does, she should avoid cunnilingus, especially during the third trimester of pregnancy. Ideally, antibody studies should be done on the pregnant woman to see if she does have antibodies to HSV 1 and/or HSV 2. Likewise, the blood from her partner should be studied. Certainly, if both have already been infected with the same virus, the likelihood of serious consequences decreases significantly.

9 There are those who advocate the use of prophylactic acyclovir late in pregnancy for individuals with a history of recurrent genital herpes late in pregnancy. They suggest starting suppressive acyclovir therapy at approximately 36 weeks of pregnancy and continuing the medication until delivery. Published results have been conflicting. Quite possibly, this acyclovir prophylaxis in late pregnancy may be effective in preventing recurrent genital infection and decreasing the likelihood of viral shedding and will be associated with a decreased frequency of caesarean section (Braig *et al.*, 2001). However, Brown (2002) questioned whether we should use acyclovir to suppress genital herpes in late pregnancy. He raised an obvious question as to what the long-term outcome of prolonged fetal exposure to acyclovir in late pregnancy would be. There are no available data that can answer this question. The acyclovir registry has information on 1246 women exposed to acyclovir during their pregnancies. The majority of these were exposed in the first trimester of pregnancy. There was no increase in malformations in infants born to these women compared with the general population. Likewise, exposure in the second and third trimesters did not result in any adverse outcomes that could be related to drug exposure. However, there have been no follow-up studies to evaluate the long-term effect on the infant.

Relation of herpes simplex virus type 2 to cervical carcinoma

There is a growing body of evidence suggesting a relationship between HSV 2 infection and the development of cervical carcinoma. However, studies by Vonka *et al.* (1984) and Adam *et al.* (1985) have raised questions about this concept. Vonka prospectively followed more than 10 000 women for at least 4 years after initial serum samples had been obtained. They could not demonstrate any relationship between the presence of antibodies to HSV 2 and the subsequent development of cervical intraepithelial neoplasia or invasive carcinoma. Adam *et al.* (1985) prospectively followed for more than 7 years more than 900 women who had been exposed *in utero* to diethylstilbestrol. Twenty-three women developed varying degrees of cervical intraepithelial neoplasia. They could find no relationship between the presence of antibodies to HSV 2 and the development of cervical neoplasia compared with a control population of women.

CYTOMEGALOVIRUS INFECTION

Characteristics of infection

Natural history
Another common herpesvirus that may infect the lower genital tract is cytomegalovirus (CMV). The significance of infection with CMV is the potential for transmission of infection to the fetus. Gaytan *et al.* (2002) reviewed data on 19 studies between 1977 and 1997. They found that the incidence of congenital CMV infection varied from 0.15% to 2% and was related to the level of pre-existing immunity in the population in general. Pre-existing maternal immunity significantly reduced transmission to the infant. However, the severity of congenital CMV infection was not significantly greater when neonatal infection occurred as a result of a primary infection compared with a recurrent or reinfection in the mother. CMV is the largest member of the human herpesvirus family. Based on variation in glycoprotein B in the viral capsule, CMV may be subdivided into four subtypes. Primary CMV infection is a systemic infection following which the virus enters a latent state and can be reactivated. In most instances, in healthy individuals, this infection is not clinically obvious. However, in about 10% of primary infections, patients develop a clinical syndrome similar to infectious mononucleosis. Primary infection during pregnancy will result in a congenital infection in 30–40% of cases. Ninety per cent of congenitally infected infants have no signs or symptoms at birth, but about 10% will ultimately develop long-term sequelae such as hearing loss, delay of psychomotor development and blindness. Ten per cent of congenitally infected infants have symptoms at birth, and approximately 25% of these infants will die. In women with recurrent infections during pregnancy, congenital infection will be found in less than 1% of infants and, of these, 99% will be asymptomatic at birth. Late sequelae will develop in approximately 5–10% of these asymptomatic infants.

CMV infections and the cervix
As with most other herpesviruses briefly discussed above, there are no obvious clinical manifestations identified in association with CMV infections involving the cervix. However, there is evidence of shedding of CMV virus from the cervix. Embil *et al.* (1985) investigated the association of CMV with HSV of the cervix in four different clinic populations. They found CMV infection of the cervix to be 2.5 times more prevalent than HSV in each of the populations studied. The overall infection rate for CMV was 4.1% and for HSV 1.7%. In a sexually transmitted disease clinic, the prevalence was even higher at 12.5% for CMV and 5.6% for HSV. Considering the fact that this virus can be shed from the cervix, several investigators have looked into the possible role of CMV in the genesis of intraepithelial and invasive carcinoma of the cervix. Mostad *et al.* (2000) observed that asymptomatic cervical shedding of both HSV and CMV occurred often in women infected with the HIV type 1. No association between CMV of the cervix and intraepithelial neoplasia or invasive cervical carcinoma has been found (Neill *et al.*, 1985; Schon *et al.*, 1992).

CMV and cervical neoplasia
In a recent study, Daxnerova *et al.* (2003) evaluated the prevalence of CMV DNA in cervical smears in almost 1000 women seen in a colposcopy clinic. CMV DNA was found in 8% of the specimens. Of interest is the fact that, in 58% of these women, koilocytosis was noted in the cervical vaginal smear. Despite these findings, there was no evidence to suggest that CMV plays a significant role in the development of cervical carcinoma. However, what it does emphasise is that the finding of what is often interpreted as koilocytosis may not always reflect infection with human papillomavirus.

Treatment
There is no effective treatment for CMV infection. Gancyclovir has been used to treat symptomatic congenital infections, but its effectiveness is limited and it can cause bone marrow suppression and gonadal toxicity. There is no available CMV vaccine to prevent infection; however, active studies are being conducted in the hope of developing such a vaccine. It is questionable whether such a vaccine will be effective in preventing transmission of CMV to the fetus.

ACKNOWLEDGEMENT

The authors wish to thank Professor A. Singer for the contribution of Figures 17.9, 17.10, 17.11 and 17.18.

REFERENCES

Adam E, Kaufman RH, Mirkovic R *et al.* (1980) Persistence of virus shedding in asymptomatic women after recovery from herpes genitalis. *Obstetrics and Gynecology* 154: 171–173.

Adam E, Kaufman RH, Adler-Storthz K *et al.* (1985) A prospective study of association of herpes simplex virus and human papillomavirus infection with cervical neoplasia in women exposed to diethylstilbestrol in utero. *International Journal of Cancer* 35: 19–26.

Baillargon J, Piper J, Leach CT (2000) Epidemiology of human herpes virus V6 (HHV-6) infection in pregnant and unpregnant women. *Journal of Clinical Virology* 16: 149–157.

Barton SE (2005) Reducing the transmission of genital herpes; antiviral therapy is effective but should be used with safer sex practices and counselling. *British Medical Journal* 330: 157–158.

Barton SE, Wright LK, Link CM *et al.* (1986) Screening to detect asymptomatic shedding of herpes simplex virus (HSV) in women with recurrent genital HSV infection. *Genitourinary Medicine* 62: 181–185.

Benedetti JK, Zeh J, Corey L (1999) Clinical reactivation of genital herpes simplex virus infection diseases in frequency over time. *Annals of Internal Medicine* 131: 14–20.

Black JB, Pellet PE (1999) Human herpesvirus 7. *Review of Medical Virology* 9: 245–262.

Boivin G, Hankins C, Lapointe N *et al.* (2000) Human herpesvirus 8 infection of the genital tract of HIV-seropositive and HIV-seronegative women at risk of sexually transmitted diseases. Canadian Women's HIV Study Group. *AIDS* 14: 1073–1075.

Braig S, Luton D, Sibony O *et al.* (2001) Acyclovir prophylaxis in late pregnancy prevents recurrent genital herpes and viral shedding. *European Journal of Obstetrics Gynecology and Reproductive Biology* 96: 55–58.

Brock BV, Selke S, Benedetti J *et al.* (1990) Frequency of asymptomatic shedding of herpes simplex virus in women with genital herpes. *Journal of the American Medical Association* 263: 418–420.

Brown ZA (2000) Should we use acyclovir to suppress genital herpes in late pregnancy? *Contemporary Obstetrics and Gynecology* 5: 67–70.

Brown ZA, Bontver LA, Benedetti J *et al.* (1987) Effects on infants with a first episode of genital herpes during pregnancy. *New England Journal of Medicine* 317: 1246–1251.

Brown ZA, Benedetti JK, Selke S *et al.* (1996) Asymptomatic maternal shedding of herpes simplex virus at the onset of labor; relationship to preterm labor. *Obstetrics and Gynecology* 87: 483–488.

Brown ZA, Selke S, Zea J *et al.* (1997) The acquisition of herpes simplex virus shedding during pregnancy. *New England Journal of Medicine* 337: 509–515.

Chen M, Wang H, Woodworth CD *et al.* (1994) Detection of human herpes virus 6 and human papillomavirus 16 in cervical carcinoma. *American Journal of Pathology* 145: 1509–1516.

Clark DA (2000) Human herpes virus 6. *Review of Medical Virology* 10: 155–173.

Cohen F, Kemeny ME, Kearney KA *et al.* (1999) Persistent stress as a predictor of genital herpes recurrence. *Archives of Internal Medicine* 159: 2430–2436.

Corey L, Wald A, Patel R *et al.* for the Valacyclovir HSV Transmission Study Group (2004) Once-daily valacyclovir to reduce the risk of transmission of genital herpes. *New England Journal of Medicine* 350: 11–20.

Daxnerova Z, Berkova Z, Kaufman FH *et al.* (2003) Detection of human cytomegalovirus DNA on 986 women studied for human pappilomavirus associated cervical neoplasia. *Journal of Lower Genital Tract Disease* 7: 187–193.

Embil JA, Garner JB, Pereira LH *et al.* (1985) Association of cytomegalovirus and herpes simplex virus infection of the cervix in four clinic populations. *Sexually Transmitted Disease* 12: 224–228.

Embom M, Strand A, Fark KI *et al.* (2001) Detection of Epstein–Barr virus, but not human herpes virus 8 DNA from cervical secretions from Swedish women by realtime polymerase chain reaction. *Sexually Transmitted Disease* 28: 306.

Fleming DT, McQuillan GM, Johnson RE *et al.* (1997) Herpes simplex virus type-2 in the United States 1976 to1994. *New England Journal of Medicine* 337: 1105–1111.

Gaytan MA, Steegers EA, Semmekrotb A *et al.* (2002) Congenital cytomegalovirus infection: review of the epidemiology and outcome. *Obstetrics and Gynecology Survey* 57: 245–256.

Gilbert J, Drehs MM, Weinberg JM (2001) Topical imiquimod for acyclovir–unresponsive herpes simplex virus 2 infection. *Archives of Dermatology* 137: 1015–1017.

Goldberg LH, Kaufman R, Kurtz TO *et al.* (1993) Long term suppression of recurrent genital herpes with acyclovir. A 5-year benchmark. Acyclovir study group. *Archives of Dermatology* 129: 582–587.

Guinan ME, MacCalman J, Kern ER *et al.* (1981) The course of untreated recurrent persistent herpes simplex infection in 17 women. *New England Journal of Medicine* 304: 759–763.

Hensleigh PA, Andrews WW, Brown V *et al.* (1997) Genital herpes during pregnancy: inability to distinguish primary and recurrent infections clinically. *Obstetrics and Gynecology* 89: 891–895.

Kawana T, Kawagoe K, Takizawa K *et al.* (1982) Clinical and virologic studies on female genital herpes. *Obstetrics and Gynecology* 60: 456–461.

Lafferty WE, Downey L, Celum C *et al.* (2000) Herpes simplex virus type-1 as a cause of genital herpes: impact on surveillance and presentation. *Journal of Infectious Disease* 181: 1454–1457.

Langenberg A, Benedetti J, Jenkins J *et al.* (1989) Development of clinically recognizable lesions among women previously identified as having asymptomatic herpes simplex virus type-2 infection. *Annals of Internal Medicine* 110: 882–887.

Maeda T, Okuno T, Eon T *et al.* (1997) Outcomes of infants whose mothers were positive for human herpes virus-6 DNA within the genital tract in early gestation. *Acta Paediatrica Japonica* 39: 653–657.

Martin JN, Ganem DE, Osmond DH *et al.* (1998) Sexual transmission and the natural history of human herpes virus VIII infection. *New England Journal of Medicine* 338: 948–954.

Mostad, SB, Kreiss JK, Ryncar ZA *et al.* (2000) Cervical shedding of herpes simplex virus and cytomegalovirus throughout the menstrual cycle in women infected with human immunodeficiency virus type 1. *American Journal of Obstetrics and Gynecology* 183: 948–955.

Neill WA, Norval M (1985) Cell mediated immune responses to cytomegalovirus in patients with dysplasia of the uterine cervix. *Gynecological and Obstetric Investigations* 20: 96–102.

Okuno T, Oishi H, Hayashi K *et al.* (1995) Human herpes viruses 6 and 7 in cervices of pregnant women. *Journal of Clinical Microbiology* 33: 1968–1970.

Prober EG, Corey L, Brown ZA *et al.* (1992) The management of pregnancies complicated by genital infection with herpes simplex virus. *Clinics in Infectious Diseases* 5: 1031–1038.

Rouse BJ, Stringer JS (2000) An appraisal of screening for maternal type-specific herpes simplex virus antibodies to prevent neonatal herpes. *American Journal of Obstetrics and Gynecology* 183: 400–406.

Schon HJ, Schurz B, Marz R *et al.* (1992) Screening for Epstein–Barr and cytomegalovirus in normal and abnormal smears by fluorescent in situ cytohybridization. *Archives of Virology* 125: 205–214.

Spruance SL, Tyring SK, Smith MH *et al.* (2001) Application of a topical immune response modifier, resiquimod gel, to modify the recurrence rate of recurrent genital herpes: a pilot study. *Journal of Infectious Diseases* 184 (2): 196–200.

Stanberry LR, Spruance SL, Cunningham AL (2002) Glycoprotein-D adjuvant vaccine to prevent genital herpes. *New England Journal of Medicine* 347: 1652–1661.

Stone KM, Brooks CA, Guinan ME *et al.* (1989) National surveillance for neonatal herpes simplex virus infections. *Sexually Transmitted Disease* 16: 152–156.

Vonka V, Kanka J, Hirschi J *et al.* (1984) Prospective study of the relationship between cervical neoplasia and herpes simplex type-2 virus. Herpes simplex type-2 antibody presence in sera taken at enrollment. *International Journal of Cancer* 33: 61–66.

Wald A, Zeh J, Selke S *et al.* (1995) Virologic characteristics of subclinical and symptomatic genital herpes infections. *New England Journal of Medicine* 333: 770–775.

Wald A, Zeh J, Barnum G *et al.* (1996) Suppression of subclinical shedding of herpes simplex virus type-2 with acyclovir. *Annals of Internal Medicine* 124: 8–15.

Wald A, Zeh J, Selke S *et al.* (2000) Reactivation of genital herpes simplex virus type-2 infection in asymptomatic seropositive persons. *New England Journal of Medicine* 342: 844–850.

Whitley D, Smith NA, Matthews S *et al.* (1999) Human herpes virus 8: seroepidemiology among women and detection in the genital tract of seropositive and negative women. *Journal of Infectious Diseases* 179: 234–236.

Whitley RJ, Nahmias AJ, Visinte AM *et al.* (1980) The natural history of herpes simplex virus infection of mother and newborn. *Pediatrics* 66: 489–494.

Williams W, Kimberlin D, Whitley R *et al.* (2006) Valacyclovir therapy to reduce recurrent genital herpes in pregnant women. *American Journal of Obstetrics and Gynecology* 194: 774–781.

Workowski KA, Levine WC, Wasserheit JN (2002) US Center for Disease Control and Prevention Guidelines for the treatment of sexually transmitted diseases: an opportunity to unify clinical and public health practice. *Annals of Internal Medicine* 137: 255–262.

Cervical neoplasia: natural history and pathology

CHAPTER 18

Epidemiology and the role of human papillomaviruses

Anita Koushik and Eduardo L.F. Franco

INTRODUCTION

Invasive cervical cancer (ICC) is one of the most common malignant neoplastic diseases affecting women. Most cases arise basically from two main histological lineages depending on whether they originate in squamous or in glandular cervical epithelium. Squamous cell carcinomas (SCC) account for almost 80% of all ICCs, while glandular malignancies, or adenocarcinomas (ADC), make up the bulk of the remainder (10–15%) (Schiffman and Brinton, 1995). The early phase of the natural history of ICC begins as a slow process of disruption of the normal maturation of the epithelium surrounding the transformation zone of the uterine cervix. This phase is invariably asymptomatic and can be discovered only through cytological examination using the Papanicolaou technique (the Pap test) and with confirmation via a colposcopic examination and biopsy of the suspected lesion.

The early stage of SCC is generally known as cervical intraepithelial neoplasia (CIN), according to the classification scheme of the World Health Organization (WHO), or as a squamous intraepithelial lesion (SIL), as per the recently revised Bethesda classification system (Solomon et al., 2002). Similarly, precursors to ADC exist; however, they are less well characterised (Ferenczy, 1997). In these earlier preinvasive stages, described in Chapter 21, the process is limited to degrees of differentiation within the epithelium. These lesions can therefore be treated. However, if left untreated, the lesions will develop into in situ cervical cancer or CIN3. This is represented by a full-thickness loss of cellular differentiation within the epithelium. Subsequently, it may traverse the lining formed by the basement membrane, which separates the epithelium from the underlying connective tissue, and become invasive.

DESCRIPTIVE EPIDEMIOLOGY OF INVASIVE CERVICAL CANCER

Global importance of ICC

An estimated 493 000 new cases of ICC are diagnosed each year worldwide, representing nearly 10% of all female cancers.

Its incidence is eighth overall among all cancer sites, regardless of gender, and is second among women, after breast cancer (Ferlay et al., 2004). The burden of cervical cancer is greatest in developing countries, where over 80% of cases occur. The highest risk areas for ICC are in southern and eastern Africa, Central America and the Caribbean, with average incidence rates exceeding 30 per 100 000 women per year (standardised per the age structure of the world population of 1960). Risk in western Europe and North America is relatively low at less than 10 new cases annually per 100 000 women.

Every year, an estimated 273 000 deaths from ICC occur worldwide, with over four-fifths of them in developing countries (Ferlay et al., 2004). In general, there is a correlation between incidence and mortality across all regions, but some areas seem to have a disproportionately higher mortality, such as Africa. Less than 50% of women affected by ICC in developing countries survive longer than 5 years, whereas the 5-year survival rate in developed countries is about 66%. Moreover, ICC generally affects multiparous women in the early postmenopausal years. In high-fertility developing countries, these women are the primary source of moral and educational values for their school-aged children. The premature loss of these mothers has important social consequences for the community.

Trends in the incidence of ICC

Overall, ICC incidence and mortality rates have declined during the last 50 years, particularly in western nations (Parkin et al., 2001), primarily as a consequence of the increased availability of Pap smear screening programmes and possibly due to the decline in fertility rates during the last four decades. In the US, the National Cancer Institute's Surveillance, Epidemiology, and End Results (SEER) programme has systematically collected information on all cancer cases diagnosed since 1973 in the states of Connecticut, Hawaii, Iowa, New Mexico and Utah and in the metropolitan areas of Detroit, Atlanta, San Francisco-Oakland and Seattle-Puget Sound (National Cancer Institute, 2002). In 1992, counties in the Los Angeles and San Jose-Monterey areas were added. The programme's

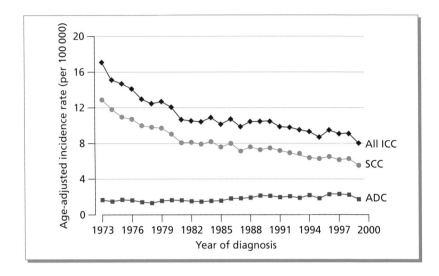

Fig. 18.1 Incidence rates of ICC (all subtypes), and SCC and ADC separately, in all SEER registration areas (1973–1999). Rates are standardised according to the age structure of the year 2000 US population and expressed per 100 000 women.

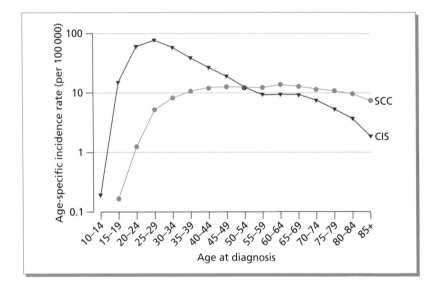

Fig. 18.2 Age-specific incidence rates of SCC and CIS in all SEER registration areas (1992–1999). Rates are standardised according to the age structure of the year 2000 US population and expressed per 100 000 women.

stringent quality control ensures very high rates of histopathological verification for registered cases.

Figure 18.1 depicts the decreasing incidence rates since 1973 in SEER registration areas for ICC, as well as separately for SCC and ADC. Of note is that this trend has occurred for all racial groups in the US; however, rates among black women are consistently higher than in other groups. There is an indication that the marked decline in rates of ICC seen until the mid-1980s has been slowing down in recent years. Potentially affecting the trend is the increase in rates of ADC and also of adenosquamous carcinomas of the cervix, which has been seen in many western populations (Vizcaino *et al.*, 1998). These two histological subtypes tend to be less detectable by cytological screening as their preinvasive lesions are usually less accessible in the endocervical canal and because of the lack of uniform criteria to recognise endocervical cytological abnormalities (Ferenczy, 1997).

Figure 18.2 shows age-specific incidence rates of SCC and carcinoma *in situ* (CIS)/CIN3, the immediate precursor to invasive SCC, in SEER areas averaged over the 1992–1999 period. The risk of ICC rises rapidly between the ages of 20 and 44 years, thereafter followed by a levelling off and then a slight decline in the incidence rates. This is in contrast to the peak incidence of CIS/CIN3, which exceeds the highest rate of ICC and occurs at ages 25 to 29 years, leaving a gap between peak incidence rates for CIS/CIN3 and SCC of approximately 15 years. Figure 18.3 shows that the gap in peak incidence between preinvasive adenocarcinoma *in situ* (AIS) and ADC is also approximately 15 years, with the age peak for ADC at around 45–49 years and at 30–34 years for AIS.

Survival

The importance of cervical cancer is further highlighted by the fact that the overall survival of patients with this neoplasm

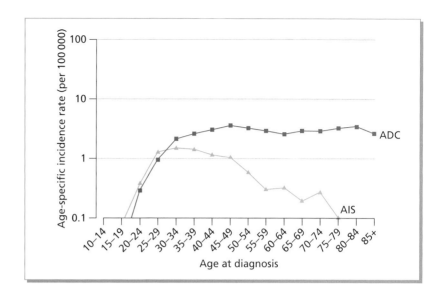

Fig. 18.3 Age-specific incidence rates of ADC and AIS in all SEER registration areas (1992–1999). Rates are standardised according to the age structure of the year 2000 US population and expressed per 100 000 women.

Table 18.1 Relative survival rates by time since diagnosis of ICC in SEER registration areas (1992–1999).

Population	Relative survival rate (%)		
	1-year	2-year	5-year
Total US population	89	80	70
White	89	81	71
Black	84	72	60

Source: National Cancer Institute's SEER Program.

is relatively short compared with, for instance, breast cancer patients. A relative survival rate is the ratio of the observed survival rate to the expected survival rate for the population from which the cervical cancer patients originated. The expected rate is based on mortality rates for the total female population of the same age composition. It is thus assumed that the presence of ICC is the only factor that distinguishes the cancer patient cohort from the general population, with the relative survival rate indicating the probability that patients will escape death due to causes associated with their diagnosed cancer.

Table 18.1 shows relative survival rates by time since cancer diagnosis in the SEER registration areas. Black women in the US appear to be at a disadvantage in terms of survival from ICC. Not only is the incidence of disease greater but the survival expectancy is also meaningfully lower than that of white women. Five-year survival rates are 71% for whites and 60% for blacks, after having improved dramatically until the mid-1970s. The gains in survival among black women did not continue in recent years, and there is an indication that survival rates have even declined, further widening the gap between races (Franco, 1997).

Aetiology

Sexually transmitted disease model for ICC

Prominent among the classical risk factors for ICC and its precursors is the role of certain measures of sexual activity, namely number of sexual partners and age at first intercourse (Herrero, 1996). The sexual behaviour of the woman's male partners has also long been recognised as a critical factor (Singer *et al.*, 1976). Case–control studies have shown that the number of sexual partners reported by the husbands or partners of the female subjects is a strong predictor of cervical cancer risk that contributes additional independent information relative to that of the number of male partners that a woman may have reported (Zunzunegui *et al.*, 1986; Brinton *et al.*, 1989a). In addition, some cohort studies have shown that wives of penile cancer patients are at increased risk of developing cervical cancer later in life (Graham *et al.*, 1979; Smith *et al.*, 1980). Such findings are further supported by results from correlation studies, in which strong associations have been found between cervical and penile cancer using mortality and morbidity data (Li *et al.*, 1982; Franco *et al.*, 1988). The correlation between the rates of these two cancers even exceeds in statistical strength that of smoking-related cancers (Franco *et al.*, 1988). Finally, it has been elegantly shown that the between-country differences in the distribution of numbers of sexual partners reported by the husbands of cervical cancer patients and control subjects further explains disease risk profiles between Spain and Colombia (Bosch *et al.*, 1996; Muñoz *et al.*, 1996).

The role of male circumcision has been raised by many authors over the last 40 years, especially in respect of the low risk of wives of circumcised men. The IARC multicentric study on cervical cancer (Muñoz *et al.*, 2002) examined penile HPV prevalence in circumcised and uncircumcised men. The woman's risk of cervical cancer was estimated according to the husband's circumcision status, and it was shown that circumcised men were about three times less likely to harbour HPV DNA in their penile specimens than uncircumcised men. It would seem that circumcision reduces the risk of genital HPV infection, retention and transmission and also the risk of cervical cancer in female partners. This seems to be particularly true for women whose male consort has a history of multiple sexual partners and of sexually transmitted disease (Castellsague *et al.*, 2002a). However, other studies have failed to report a lower prevalence of HPV DNA in the penis of circumcised males (Weaver *et al.*, 2004).

Although a consistent and coherent picture of the epidemiology and pathogenesis of HPV infection has developed over the past two decades, less is known about these infections in men (Partridge and Koutsky, 2006). A comprehensive review of HPV infections in men has recently been assembled by Partridge and Koutsky (2006).

The consistency of the sexually transmitted disease model for cervical neoplasia led much of the laboratory and epidemiological research in attempting to identify the putative microbial agent or agents acting as the relevant aetiological factor. Research conducted during the late 1960s and 1970s attempted to unveil an aetiological role for the herpes simplex viruses (HSV). Although HSV was proven to be carcinogenic *in vitro* and *in vivo*, clinical studies eventually demonstrated that only a fraction of cervical carcinomas contained traces of HSV DNA, and epidemiological studies initially failed to demonstrate an association between HSV and cervical cancer (reviewed by Franco, 1991a).

A role for human papillomaviruses (HPV) in the sexually transmitted disease model of ICC was proposed in the mid-1970s (zur Hausen, 1976), leading to an abundance of both epidemiological and laboratory research. However, strong evidence for an aetiological role of HPV was slow in coming, largely because of the inconsistency in epidemiological findings (reviewed by Franco 1991b). Contributing to the incoherence in the results of early research was the fact that the prevalence of HPV DNA in cervical tumour specimens, detected using DNA hybridisation techniques, was low and variable, ranging from 15% to 92% (Muñoz *et al.*, 1988). However, with the advent of polymerase chain reaction (PCR) techniques, which have much greater sensitivity than nonamplified DNA hybridisation methods, strong molecular epidemiological evidence for the central role played by HPV in cervical carcinogenesis emerged (Koutsky *et al.*, 1992; Muñoz *et al.*, 1992; Schiffman *et al.*, 1993).

It is now well established that infection with high oncogenic risk HPV types is the central causal factor in ICC (Walboomers *et al.*, 1999). Relative risks for the association between HPV and cervical cancer are in the 20–70 range, which are among the strongest statistical relations ever identified in cancer epidemiology. Both retrospective and prospective epidemiological

studies have demonstrated the unequivocally strong association between viral infection and risk of malignancy, both CIN and invasive disease (Bosch *et al.*, 2002). Furthermore, results from successive analyses using meticulous testing by PCR detection methods of a large collection of cervical tumour specimens assembled internationally showed that HPV DNA is present in 99.7% of cases (Bosch *et al.*, 1995; Walboomers *et al.*, 1999). Given sufficient sensitivity and adequate tumour sampling, it is likely that virtually all cervical tumours contain HPV DNA (Walboomers and Meijer, 1997).

Role of HPV

HPVs are small, double-stranded DNA viruses of approximately 55 nm with an icosahedral protein capsid containing 72 capsomers (Fig. 18.4). The genome is circular and contains 7500–8000 basepairs. Taxonomically, papillomaviruses used to be a subfamily in the Papovaviridae family but are now grouped independently as a family, the Papillomaviridae, affecting both cutaneous and mucosal epithelia (Fig. 18.5). As infectious agents, they are highly specific to their hosts. Different HPVs are classified as types on the basis of DNA sequence homology in particular genes, specifically L1, which codes for the viral capsid, and E6 and E7, both of which have

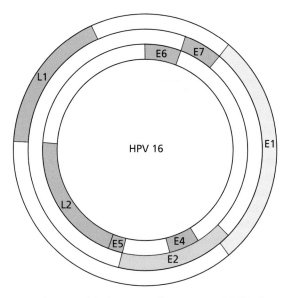

Fig. 18.4 Schematic of the human papillomavirus 16 (HPV 16) genome, showing the arrangement of the major non-structural and capsid genes. The three circles correspond to the three reading frames in which a sense strand can be translated. There are no known gene products produced by the antisense strand. Viral protein early 4 (E4) is encoded by a messenger RNA transcript that includes the initial amino acids of the E1 gene. The region between late 1 (L1) and E6 is an important transcription regulatory region — the mRNAs encoding most non-structural (E6, E7, E1, E2, E4 and E5) and capsid (L1 and L2) genes originate in this region. Most papillomavirus genomes resemble HPV 16 in general organisation. From Frazer (2004) with permission from Nature Publishing Group.

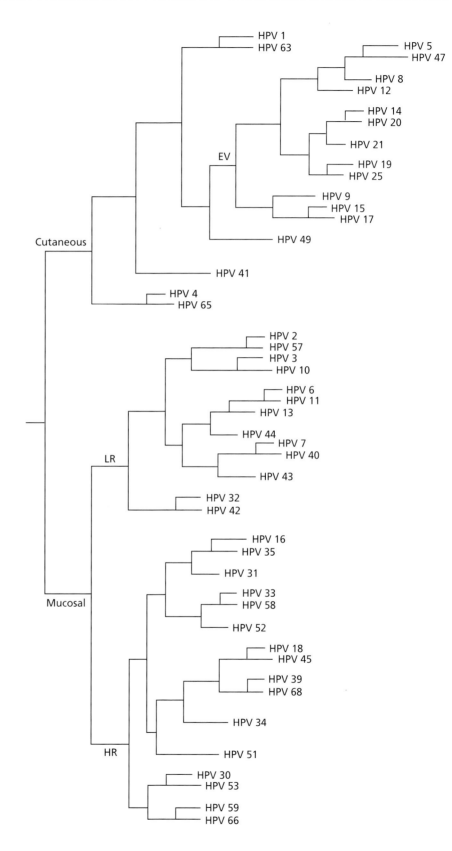

Fig. 18.5 Chart showing the classification of cutaneous and mucosal HPV types.

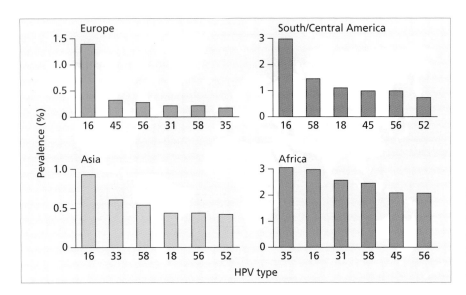

Fig 18.6 Prevalence of the six most common high-risk HPV types in female population-based samples (sexually active, cytologically normal women, aged 15–74 with a valid PCR result) by region. From the IARC multicentre HPV prevalence survey, 1995–2002 (IARC, 2003).

important carcinogenic functions (discussed below). More than 150 different HPV types have been catalogued so far (zur Hausen, 2000), of which over 40 infect the epithelial lining of the anogenital tract.

In 1995, the World Health Organization's International Agency for Research on Cancer (IARC), in its monograph series of carcinogenicity evaluation, classified HPV types 16 and 18 as carcinogenic to humans, HPV types 31 and 33 as probably carcinogenic, and other HPV types (except 6 and 11) as possibly carcinogenic (IARC Working Group, 1995). This classification was made conservatively on the basis of the available published evidence until 1994. Subsequent research has permitted the classification of more HPV types according to oncogenicity, or the risk they pose for cancer development, primarily based on their frequency of association with cervical tumours, as well as phylogenetic relatedness to known high- and low-risk types (i.e. 16 or 18, and 6 or 11 respectively). The best evidence for an epidemiological classification of HPV type-specific oncogenicity was provided by recent research from the IARC multicentre case–control studies, which utilised information pooled from 11 case–control studies (Muñoz *et al.*, 2003). On the basis of type-specific odds ratios and prevalence of types by case or control status, 15 HPV types have been deemed as oncogenic or high risk (16, 18, 31, 33, 35, 39, 45, 51, 52, 56, 58, 59, 68, 73 and 82), three types are considered as probable high-risk types (26, 53 and 66), and 12 types are classified as low risk (6, 11, 40, 42, 43, 44, 54, 61, 70, 72, 81 and CP6108). Low-risk HPV types may cause subclinical lesions known as flat condylomata or clinically visible benign lesions known as acuminate condylomata. The remaining HPV types are considered to have undetermined oncogenic risk. HPV types 16 and 18 are by far the most common HPV types and together account for 60% of the HPV-positive ICC specimens (Clifford *et al.*, 2003). The worldwide distribution of HPV types varies from country to country (Fig. 18.6).

Recently Clifford *et al.* (2005) examined the type-specific distribution across four world regions as well as the risk of being infected with low- and high-risk HPV types according to region (Figs 18.7–18.10).

The carcinogenic mechanism following HPV infection (see Chapter 19) involves the expression of two major viral oncogenes, E6 and E7, which produce proteins that interfere with tumour-suppressor genes controlling the cell cycle. Once viral DNA becomes integrated into the host's genome, E6 and E7 become upregulated. While E7 complexes with the cell growth regulator retinoblastoma (Rb) protein, causing an uncontrolled cell proliferation (Munger *et al.*, 2001), binding of E6 to the p53 protein promotes the degradation of the latter, exempting the deregulated cell from undergoing p53-mediated control (Mantovani and Banks, 2001). The degradation of p53 by E6 leads to loss of DNA repair function and prevents the cell from undergoing apoptosis. The infected cell can no longer stop further HPV-related damage and becomes susceptible to additional mutations and genomic instability. Interestingly, the effect of the E6 and E7 proteins on p53 and Rb has been shown to occur only with high-risk HPVs but not with low-risk HPVs (Dyson *et al.*, 1989).

Clinical, subclinical and latent HPV infections are the most common sexually transmitted viral diseases today (Cox, 1995). Asymptomatic HPV infection can be detected in 5–20% of sexually active women of reproductive age (Bosch *et al.*, 2002). In most cases, genital HPV infection is transient or intermittent (Hildesheim *et al.*, 1994; Moscicki *et al.*, 1998; Ho *et al.*, 1998a; Franco *et al.*, 1999; Liaw *et al.*, 2001); only a small proportion of those positive for a given HPV type tend to harbour the same type in subsequent specimens. In addition, prospective epidemiological studies have indicated that the risk of subsequent CIN increases substantially for women who develop persistent, long-term infections with high-risk HPV types (Koutsky *et al.*, 1992; Ho *et al.*, 1998a;

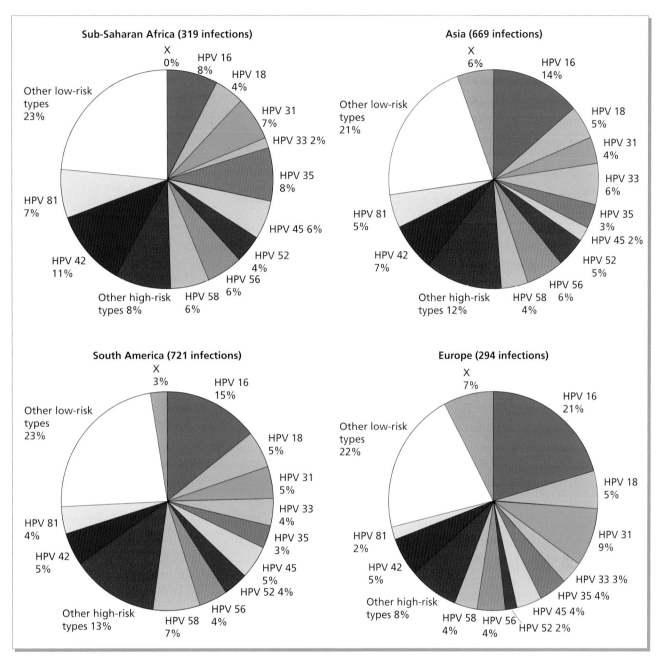

Fig. 18.7 Percentage distribution of various high- and low-risk HPV types in four continents. From Clifford (2005), with permission from Elsevier.

Nobbenhuis *et al.*, 1999; Ylitalo *et al.*, 2000; Moscicki *et al.*, 2001; Schlecht *et al.*, 2001), suggesting that only persistent infections trigger carcinogenic development. However, a recent publication (Strickler *et al.*, 2005) has shown that women in whom HPV may not be detected and in whom it is assumed it has been cleared may still be at some risk. It would seem as though HPV can be reactivated after lying quiet within the cervix for many years, making these women, especially those who are immunocompromised, vulnerable to cervical cancer. A study of 2500 women that were followed up every 6 months for an average of 3 years (the median number of semi-annual

follow-up visits was six) showed that those infected with the human immunodeficiency virus (HIV) virus were much more likely to be infected with HPV and at some point HPV became undetectable, most likely as a result of immune suppression and control. However, 29 women with HIV who also had HPV infection and in whom HPV was undetectable at a first follow-up visit were found, at a second follow-up visit, to show positivity for HPV. These women had been sexually inactive from the time that HPV had become undetectable to the time that it became detectable again. This suggests that women with HPV, and perhaps other women with suppressed immune

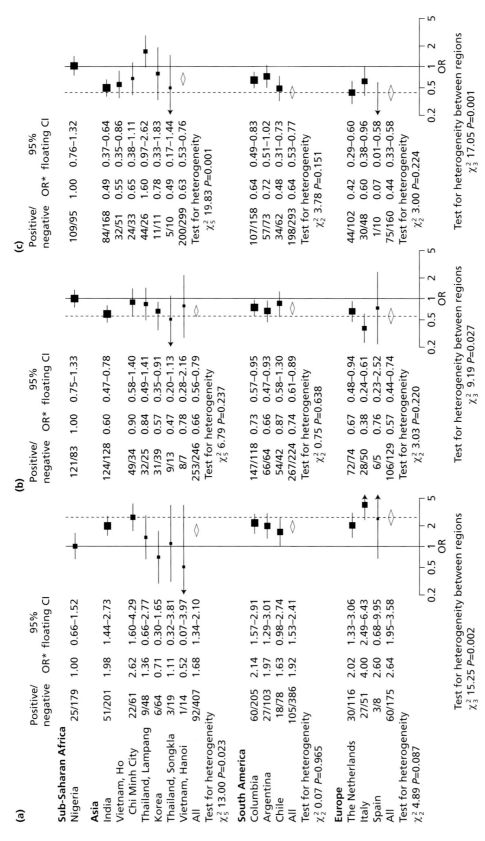

Fig. 18.8 Relative risk of infection with HPV 16 (a), high-risk HPV types other than HPV 16 (b) and low-risk HPV types (c) associated with geographic region. From Clifford (2005), with permission from Elsevier.

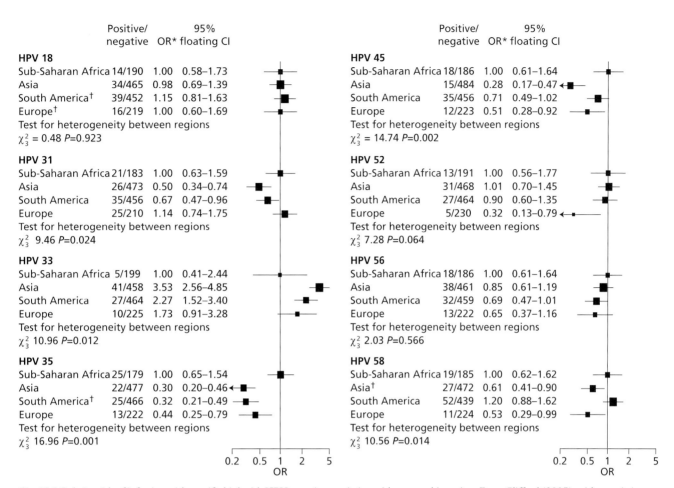

	Positive/ negative	OR*	95% floating CI
HPV 18			
Sub-Saharan Africa	14/190	1.00	0.58–1.73
Asia	34/465	0.98	0.69–1.39
South America[†]	39/452	1.15	0.81–1.63
Europe[†]	16/219	1.00	0.60–1.69
Test for heterogeneity between regions $\chi^2_3 = 0.48$ $P=0.923$			
HPV 31			
Sub-Saharan Africa	21/183	1.00	0.63–1.59
Asia	26/473	0.50	0.34–0.74
South America	35/456	0.67	0.47–0.96
Europe	25/210	1.14	0.74–1.75
Test for heterogeneity between regions χ^2_3 9.46 $P=0.024$			
HPV 33			
Sub-Saharan Africa	5/199	1.00	0.41–2.44
Asia	41/458	3.53	2.56–4.85
South America	27/464	2.27	1.52–3.40
Europe	10/225	1.73	0.91–3.28
Test for heterogeneity between regions χ^2_3 10.96 $P=0.012$			
HPV 35			
Sub-Saharan Africa	25/179	1.00	0.65–1.54
Asia	22/477	0.30	0.20–0.46
South America[†]	25/466	0.32	0.21–0.49
Europe	13/222	0.44	0.25–0.79
Test for heterogeneity between regions χ^2_3 16.96 $P=0.001$			

	Positive/ negative	OR*	95% floating CI
HPV 45			
Sub-Saharan Africa	18/186	1.00	0.61–1.64
Asia	15/484	0.28	0.17–0.47
South America	35/456	0.71	0.49–1.02
Europe	12/223	0.51	0.28–0.92
Test for heterogeneity between regions $\chi^2_3 = 14.74$ $P=0.002$			
HPV 52			
Sub-Saharan Africa	13/191	1.00	0.56–1.77
Asia	31/468	1.01	0.70–1.45
South America	27/464	0.90	0.60–1.35
Europe	5/230	0.32	0.13–0.79
Test for heterogeneity between regions χ^2_3 7.28 $P=0.064$			
HPV 56			
Sub-Saharan Africa	18/186	1.00	0.61–1.64
Asia	38/461	0.85	0.61–1.19
South America	32/459	0.69	0.47–1.01
Europe	13/222	0.65	0.37–1.16
Test for heterogeneity between regions χ^2_3 2.03 $P=0.566$			
HPV 58			
Sub-Saharan Africa	19/185	1.00	0.62–1.62
Asia[†]	27/472	0.61	0.41–0.90
South America	52/439	1.20	0.88–1.62
Europe	11/224	0.53	0.29–0.99
Test for heterogeneity between regions χ^2_3 10.56 $P=0.014$			

Fig. 18.9 Relative risk of infection with specific high-risk HPV types in association with geographic region. From Clifford (2005), with permission from Elsevier.

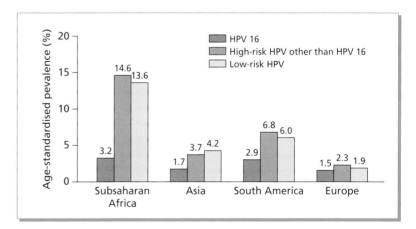

Fig. 18.10 Age-standardised prevalence (percentage) of low- and high-risk HPV types in four continents. From Clifford (2005), with permission from Elsevier.

systems, harbour undetectable HPV infections that become active once their immunity is compromised. In the Strickler *et al.* (2005) study, this was related to rising plasma HIV RNA levels and falling CD4+ T-cell counts.

Risk factors for HPV infection that have been identified in various cross-sectional and prospective cohort studies include number of sexual partners (lifetime and recent), age at first intercourse, smoking, oral contraceptive (OC) use and parity (Koutsky, 1997; Moscicki *et al.*, 2001; Sellors *et al.*, 2003; Winer *et al.*, 2003). Results have been inconsistent, partly owing to the fact that different populations have been studied. Furthermore, risk factor profiles have been found to differ depending on whether high-risk or low-risk infections were being examined (Franco *et al.*, 1995; Richardson *et al.*, 2000;

Giuliano *et al.*, 2002). Nonetheless, the most consistent determinant of incident HPV infection is age, with most studies indicating a sharp decrease in risk after the age of 30 years (Rousseau *et al.*, 2000; Giuliano *et al.*, 2002; Sellors *et al.*, 2003). The decrease in risk of HPV infection with increasing age seems to be independent of changes in sexual behaviour, suggesting the role of immune response.

Other risk factors

Prior to the identification of HPV as a causal agent, other lines of research, aside from that pertaining to sexual behaviours and sexually transmitted infections, identified environmental factors such as parity, the use of oral OCs and smoking as risk factors for ICC.

As HPV is present in virtually all cervical tumours, other determinants of risk cannot be considered as independent of HPV infection. However, given that infection by HPV alone is not sufficient to lead to the development of ICC or its precursors, other agents must be involved in the carcinogenic process. Thus, current epidemiological research centres on identifying factors that influence whether an HPV infection will clear spontaneously or progress further towards malignant disease. The environmental factors once thought to exert an independent role in cervical carcinogenesis are now being examined as potential cofactors mediating the central role played by HPV. The following section, along with Table 18.2, provides a brief summary of the findings regarding HPV cofactors in cervical carcinogenesis. Given that HPV is a necessary cause, case–control analyses restricted to HPV-positive women provide the best information on the role of cofactors in increasing the risk of ICC, given that HPV is present. The most important study in that respect is the IARC multicentre case–control studies where data from up to 10 studies have been pooled.

Parity

A high number of live births has consistently been found to be a risk factor for ICC, independently of factors related to sexual behaviours (e.g. age at first intercourse). An association with parity is plausible in the sense that multiple pregnancies may have a cumulative traumatic or immunosuppressive effect

Table 18.2 Evidence for the effect of various established and suspected risk factors for cervical cancer and associated methodological challenges.

| Risk factor | Association* | | Putative or proven nature of the aetiological relationship | Challenges |
	Strength	Consistency		
HPV infection	+++	+++	Central necessary cause for disease development	Identifying the relevant causal type at aetiologically relevant exposure window, defining latency
Parity	++	++	Influence of hormonal changes on HPV-infected cells; influence of immune system and response to HPV; traumatic event leading to changes in cervix	Control of confounding by sexual behavioural factors
OC use	+	+	Hormonal influences on HPV-infected cells or progression	Control of confounding by sexual behavioural factors
Smoking	++	+++	Tobacco-related carcinogens may directly influence carcinogenesis; influence on local immune response to HPV	Control of confounding by sexual behavioural factors
Diet	+	++	Effect of antioxidants quenching reactive radicals; modulation of cell growth and differentiation	Measurement of diet and micronutrient levels; definition of latency
HSV 2, *C. trachomatis*	+	+	Inflammatory response induced by sexually transmitted infections may facilitate HPV infection	Control of confounding by sexual behavioural factors
HIV	+	++	Impairment of immunity leads to establishment of persistent HPV infection	Disentangle effects of sexual behaviour and decreased immunity
HLA polymorphisms	+	+	Interindividual variability in immune response to HPV infection	Low power to detect associations with specific alleles and haplotypes
Codon 72 p53 polymorphism	++	+/−	Biological variability in binding of E6 to p53	Genotyping misclassification; confounding by race; selection biases

*The number of plus signs for the strength of the association indicates the relative magnitude of the underlying relative risk for the association, whereas, for consistency, it denotes the degree of the evidence based on the extent with which the association was found to be replicated in multiple studies.

on the cervix, thereby facilitating the acquisition of HPV infection (Schneider *et al.*, 1987), or that pregnancy-induced hormonal effects on the cervix could affect HPV genome elements that are responsive to progesterone (Pater *et al.*, 1994). In general, there is a linear trend in the parity–risk relationship as seen in large studies in North America and Latin America (Brinton *et al.*, 1987, 1989b). Investigation restricted to HPV-positive women in the IARC multicentre pooled analysis confirmed this relationship for both SCC and ADC, indicating that, among HPV-infected women, high parity further increases the risk of ICC (Muñoz *et al.*, 2002). However, the trend of increasing risk with increasing parity appears to be specific to SCC. A relative risk of 3.8 for SCC was observed for having had seven or more full-term pregnancies, relative to none. In a recent case–control study of HPV-seropositive participants, increasing parity was associated with an increased risk of SCC (Shields *et al*, 2004). Similar increased risks and trends have been observed for CIN among HPV-positive women, although with less consistency (Castellsague *et al.*, 2002b). In a prospective study, following women positive for high-risk HPV for the development of high-grade CIN or ICC, no association was observed, although the overall parity among the cohort was relatively low (Castle *et al.*, 2002).

Oral contraceptives

An increased risk of ICC among OC users has been observed, particularly among long-term users, after adjustment for most potential confounders (Delgado-Rodriguez *et al.*, 1992). The association seems to be somewhat stronger for ADC than for SCC (reviewed by Brinton, 1992; Schiffman *et al.*, 1996). The plausibility of the association rests on the potential for hormonal effects in HPV-containing cervical cells, as it has been shown that steroid stimulation may trigger viral oncogene-related events that may culminate in the integration of the virus into the host's genome (Pater *et al.*, 1994). Observed risks have appeared to be higher for CIN, particularly for recent OC use. However, such associations may be due to detection bias, as OC users tend to undergo more frequent gynaecological examinations than non-users, thereby enhancing detection of early disease (Irwin *et al.*, 1988). The effect of long-term OC use was evident among HPV-positive women in the IARC multicentre study, where an increased risk of ICC of approximately threefold was observed for those using OCs for 5 years or more, relative to never-users (Moreno *et al.*, 2002). However, more recent findings suggested that long-term OC use among HPV-positive women is inversely associated with SCC risk (Shields *et al*, 2004). In studies of CIN among HPV-positive cases and controls, an increased risk was observed in some studies but not in others (Castellsague *et al.*, 2002b). In one study, a particularly strong association was observed for adenocarcinoma *in situ* (relative risk = 17.1 for current OC use) (Lacey *et al.*, 1999). Results from a prospective follow-up of HPV-positive women showed no association

with current OC use at baseline (Castle *et al.*, 2002); however, duration of OC use was not assessed in that study.

Smoking

Tobacco smoking is a well-known risk factor for ICC and CIN (reviewed by Winkelstein, 1990). A role for smoking, independent of sexual behaviours, has been observed for CIN, with some studies demonstrating a positive trend with number of cigarettes smoked and duration of smoking and lower risks for former smokers (Brisson *et al.*, 1994; de Vet *et al.*, 1994; Kjellberg *et al.*, 2000), while others have failed to find an association with cigarette smoking (Koutsky *et al.*, 1992; Olsen *et al.*, 1995; Sasagawa *et al.*, 1997; Schiff *et al.*, 2000). Smoking seems to be a more important risk factor for higher grades of CIN (Cuzick *et al.*, 1990a; Parazzini *et al.*, 1992; Schiffman *et al.*, 1993; Brisson *et al.*, 1994; Ho *et al.*, 1998b), suggesting that this variable acts at a later stage in the natural history of cervical neoplasia. In fact, results from a recent study comparing women with SCC and CIS/CIN3 revealed that the odds of being an ever-smoker were higher among women with SCC and with CIS/CIN3, suggesting that smoking may be involved in disease progression (Thomas *et al.*, 2002). Among analyses restricted to HPV-positive women, an approximately twofold increased risk for ICC as well as CIN comparing ever- vs. never-smokers and also current vs. never-smokers has consistently been observed (Castellsague *et al.*, 2002b; Shields *et al.*, 2004). In another study, the prospective risk of development of high-grade CIN or ICC among HPV-positive women was increased by at least threefold for being a current or former smoker at baseline (Castle *et al.*, 2002).

A direct carcinogenic action of cigarette smoking on the cervix is conceivable as nicotine metabolites can be found in the cervical mucus of smokers (Schiffman *et al.*, 1987). Another plausible mechanism for smoking in cervical carcinogenesis is via the suppression of local immune response to HPV infection (Cox, 1995; Palefsky and Holly, 1995). Curiously, smoking seems to exert a protective effect against the development of persistent HPV infection (Hildesheim *et al.*, 1994; Ho *et al.*, 1998a), a critical intermediate endpoint in the genesis of cervical lesions. The biological rationale for this finding is not clear.

Diet

Much attention has been given to the role of dietary factors and serum micronutrients in the aetiology of ICC (García-Closas *et al.*, 2005). Epidemiological studies of CIN and ICC risk have been relatively consistent, indicating protective effects for consumption of fruits and vegetables, beta-carotene and vitamins A, C and E (Brock *et al.*, 1988; VanEenwyk *et al.*, 1991; 1992; Liu *et al.*, 1993; Potischman and Brinton, 1996; Kwasniewska *et al.*, 1998), although no associations were identified in some studies (Ziegler *et al.*, 1991; Kjellberg *et al.*, 2000). In addition, in two others studies a positive, rather than an inverse, association was observed with dietary beta-carotene (de Vet *et al.*, 1991; Shannon *et al.*, 2002). Other nutrients that have been shown to be inversely associated with risk include lycopene (VanEenwyk *et al.*, 1991; Palan *et al.*, 1996), tocopherols (Cuzick *et al.*, 1990b; Palan *et al.*, 1991; Kwasniewska *et al.*, 1997) and folates (VanEenwyk *et al.*, 1992; Kwasniewska *et al.*, 1997, 1998; Goodman *et al.*, 2001). Associations with retinol are less consistent (de Vet *et al.*, 1991; Liu *et al.*, 1995; Palan *et al.*, 1996), although results from a recent study suggest that foods rich in vitamin A and retinol may not only reduce the risk of *in situ* and invasive lesions, but perhaps also reduce the rate of progression from *in situ* to invasive cancer (Shannon *et al.*, 2002).

There is ample biological plausibility for a protective effect of diet in the genesis of cervical neoplasia. Carotenoids, tocopherols and ascorbic acid are potent antioxidants that can quench intracellular reactive radicals, thus potentially preventing DNA damage (Giuliano, 2000). Beta-carotene, in particular, may have an additional favourable property as a metabolic precursor to retinoic acid, which acts by modulating epithelial cell growth and differentiation. Dietary factors may also have a role in cervical immunity (Cox, 1995; Potischman and Brinton, 1996). However, assessing the effect of nutritional factors is complicated by methodological difficulties in the measurement of circulating micronutrients, in obtaining reasonably accurate diet intake information from interviews, as well as possible confounding by some risk factors, such as smoking and OC use (Giuliano, 2000).

Other sexually transmitted infections

Although attention to sexually transmitted infections (STIs) as a risk factor for ICC diminished following the discovery of HPV, there has recently been an interest in re-evaluating the role of STIs, particularly HSV type 2 (HSV 2) and *Chlamydia trachomatis*, as possible HPV cofactors. A possible mechanism whereby STIs could act as an HPV cofactor is by inducing local inflammation, thus facilitating the establishment of HPV infection via breaches in the cervical epithelium.

In general, an association between *C. trachomatis* and ICC and its precursors has been relatively consistent (de Sanjose *et al.*, 1994; Koskela *et al.*, 2000; Anttila *et al.*, 2001), although residual confounding by HPV cannot be ruled out. In a recent study involving countries from the IARC multicentre study (Brazil and Philippines), a relative risk of 2.1 for *C. trachomatis* seropositivity was observed among HPV-positive women (Smith *et al.*, 2002). Furthermore, the effect appeared to be more relevant for SCC than for ADC.

An increased risk for HSV 2 seropositivity, adjusted for HPV status, has also been shown (de Sanjose *et al.*, 1994; Thomas *et al.*, 2001), although this has not been consistent (Peng *et al.*, 1991; Ferrera *et al.*, 1997; Lehtinen *et al.*, 2002). A meta-analysis of longitudinal nested case–control studies also showed no overall association between HSV 2 and development of ICC or high-grade CIN (Lehtinen *et al.*, 2002). However, in the IARC case–control studies of HPV-positive women, an increased risk of twofold and threefold for SCC and ADC, respectively, was observed due to HSV 2 seropositivity.

Among HIV-infected women, HPV-associated diseases, including genital warts and malignancies of the lower anogenital tract, and latent HPV infection per se are particularly common (Wright, 1997; Jay and Moscicki, 2000; Conley *et al.*, 2002). HIV infection impairs cell-mediated immunity, thus increasing the risk of infections such as HPV. HPV prevalence estimates among HIV-positive women in various studies are in the range of 40–95%, whereas the equivalent range in HIV-negative women is 23–55%. The equivalent figures for CIN prevalence estimates are 10–36% and 1–12% respectively (Langley *et al.*, 1996; Rezza *et al.*, 1997; Maiman *et al.*, 1998; Massad *et al.*, 1999; Ellerbrock *et al.*, 2000; Moscicki *et al.*, 2000). In late 1992, because of the frequency of such coincidental findings, the Centers for Disease Control expanded the list of AIDS-defining conditions to include ICC. It also included high-grade CIN among the clinical categories for surveillance of HIV-positive women (Centers for Disease Control, 1993). A meta-analysis of several studies published between 1986 and 1998 indicated that HPV and HIV infection seems to interact synergistically to increase the risk of CIN, with some further mediation by the degree of immunosuppression (Mandelblatt *et al.*, 1999). With the successful adoption of antiretroviral therapy in the last few years, women are surviving longer with their HIV disease. Little is known, however, about the potential impact of HIV therapy on the natural history of SIL among HIV-infected women.

Non-environmental cofactors

Characteristics related to the host and the virus itself have been investigated in terms of influencing cervical carcinogenesis. The human leucocyte antigen (HLA) genes, whose protein products are involved in antigen presentation to T cells, play a role in the regulation of the cell-mediated Th-1 immune response. Certain HLA alleles or haplotypes seem to be involved in susceptibility to HPV infection and cervical neoplasia, probably by regulating the immune response against HPV infection and ultimately interfering in the establishment of productive persistent infections and cervical lesions (Hildesheim and Wang, 2002). The most consistent finding is an increased risk of HPV infection and cervical disease in individuals with the DQB1*03 allele (Odunsi *et al.*, 1995, 1996; Breitburd *et al.*, 1996; Odunsi and Ganesan, 1997; Hildesheim *et al.*, 1998; Maciag *et al.*, 2000). This association has been observed in European and American populations. An increased risk of CIN and ICC has also been associated with the DRB1*15 allele and the related DRB1*1501–DQB1*0602 haplotype among Hispanic and Swedish patients (Apple *et al.*, 1994, 1995; Sanjeevi *et al.*, 1996). Separate studies have also found an increased CIN risk among carriers of the haplotype DQA1*0102–DQB1*0602 in Norwegian

(Helland *et al.*, 1998) and Swedish (Sanjeevi *et al.*, 1996) populations. Conversely, protective effects have been observed for the DRB1*13 alleles among German, American and French populations (Breitburd *et al.*, 1996; Hildesheim *et al.*, 1998; Madeleine *et al.*, 2002). Although numerous studies in geographically diverse populations have found associations with these alleles, several inconsistencies nonetheless exist.

Another host marker of interest is a polymorphism in codon 72 of the p53 gene, which codes for two structurally distinct forms of the p53 protein depending on the DNA sequence (Matlashewski *et al.*, 1987). Specifically, the amino acid arginine is replaced by proline at codon 72, thereby altering the structure of the wild-type protein (Harris *et al.*, 1986; Matlashewski *et al.*, 1987). The association between this polymorphism and cervical disease has received considerable attention following experimental research demonstrating that the arginine form of the p53 protein was more susceptible than the proline form to binding and degradation by the HPV-E6 oncoprotein (Storey *et al.*, 1998). In addition, it was shown that women with cancer were more likely to be homozygous for arginine compared with control subjects. Although some subsequent investigations have detected similar increased risks resulting from arginine homozygosity in different populations, the majority of studies have been unable to corroborate the original results (reviewed by Jee *et al.*, 2004; Koushik *et al.*, 2004).

Viral characteristics, apart from HPV type, have been found to influence carcinogenesis. For instance, levels of HPV, or viral load, have been associated with the risk of cervical neoplasia. In some studies, a high level of HPV DNA has been associated with higher grade lesions (Morrison *et al.*, 1991; Bosch *et al.*, 1993), although more recent work indicates that high viral loads were more predictive of lower grade CIN (Schlecht *et al.*, 2003) but not of high-grade CIN (Lorincz *et al.*, 2002). Other studies indicate that a high viral load is associated with persistent HPV infections (Brisson *et al.*, 1996; Swan *et al.*, 1999).

Additionally, there is evidence that particular HPV intratype variants may differ in terms of oncogenic potential. Isolates of a given HPV type that have up to 2% nucleotide variation in specific regions of the genome are designated as molecular variants (Bernard *et al.*, 1994). HPV 16 has been studied extensively, and more than 40 molecular variants have been described (Chan *et al.*, 1992; Ho *et al.*, 1993; Bernard *et al.*, 1994; Yamada *et al.*, 1995). Sequence analysis of HPV 16, focusing on the non-coding long control region of the viral genome, has led to the identification of five major classes of HPV 16 variants based on geographical relatedness: European, two African variants, Asian and Asian-American (Ho *et al.*, 1993). In most studies, a higher risk of CIN was observed as a result of the presence of non-European variants of HPV 16 compared with European variants (Xi *et al.*, 1997, 2002; Villa *et al.*, 2000). However, in a study of Mexican women, risk of ICC seemed to be more associated with Asian-American

variants than with European variants (Berumen *et al.*, 2001). Variants involving the coding regions of the HPV genome have also been found to result in varying oncogenic potential (Villa, 1997). A well-known nucleotide variation is that of position 350 in the E6 gene of HPV-16. In a few studies, the variant with the nucleotide G at 350 was associated with high-grade lesions or progression of CIN (Londesborough *et al.*, 1996; Zehbe *et al.*, 1998); however, this was not observed in other studies (Bontkes *et al.*, 1998; Brady *et al.*, 1999; Hu *et al.*, 1999; Nindl *et al.*, 1999).

Current and future research

During the last 20 years, the concerted effort among virologists, epidemiologists and clinical researchers has helped to elucidate the role of infection by certain types of HPV as the necessary cause of ICC. This has opened new frontiers for preventing a disease that is responsible for substantial morbidity and mortality, particularly among women living in resource-poor countries. Research on two prevention fronts has already begun in several populations in the form of preliminary trials assessing the efficacy of HPV vaccines (Harper *et al.*, 2004; Villa *et al.*, 2005) and of studies of the value of HPV testing in ICC screening. Progress on both counts is very promising. While the benefits of vaccination against HPV infection as a cervical cancer prevention tool are at least a decade into the future, the potential benefits of HPV testing in screening for this disease can be realised now in most populations.

Primary prevention of cervical neoplasia can also be achieved through prevention and control of genital HPV infection. Health promotion strategies geared at a change in sexual behaviour targeting all STIs of public health significance can be effective in preventing genital HPV infection (Franco *et al.*, 2001). Although there is consensus that symptomatic HPV infection (genital warts) should be managed via treatment, counselling and partner notification, active case finding of asymptomatic HPV infection is currently not recommended as a control measure. Further research is needed to determine the effectiveness of such a strategy and the significance of such infections concerning a woman's subsequent cancer risk.

Research on HPVs has progressed at a fast pace. The HPV–cervical cancer model has become a paradigm of progress in cancer research and among neoplastic diseases with infectious origins (Franco *et al.*, 2004). We have reached the point where preventing ICC via vaccination against HPV infection is in the foreseeable future. However, screening programmes are still of great importance and will continue to be so in the future (Franco and Harper, 2005). Existing cytology-based screening programmes that seem to work need to be constantly assessed for quality and coverage. Ongoing research on the efficacy and cost-effectiveness of HPV testing as a mass screening tool will help countries to decide on the best approach for secondary prevention of ICC and will probably lead to reduced morbidity and mortality from this disease.

REFERENCES

Anttila T, Saikku P, Koskela P *et al.* (2001) Serotypes of *Chlamydia trachomatis* and risk for development of cervical squamous cell carcinoma. *Journal of the American Medical Association* 285: 47–51.

Apple RJ, Erlich HA, Klitz W *et al.* (1994) HLA DR-DQ associations with cervical carcinoma show papillomavirus-type specificity. *Nature Genetics* 6: 157–162.

Apple RJ, Becker TM, Wheeler CM *et al.* (1995) Comparison of human leukocyte antigen DR-DQ disease associations found with cervical dysplasia and invasive cervical carcinoma. *Journal of the National Cancer Institute* 87: 427–436.

Bernard HU, Chan SY, Delius H (1994) Evolution of papillomaviruses. *Current Topics in Microbial Immunology* 186: 33–54.

Berumen J, Ordonez RM, Lazcano E *et al.* (2001) Asian-American variants of human papillomavirus 16 and risk for cervical cancer: a case–control study. *Journal of the National Cancer Institute* 93: 1325–1330.

Bontkes HJ, van Duin M, de Gruijl TD *et al.* (1998) HPV 16 infection and progression of cervical intra-epithelial neoplasia: analysis of HLA polymorphism and HPV 16 E6 sequence variants. *International Journal of Cancer* 78: 166–171.

Bosch FX, Muñoz N, de Sanjose S *et al.* (1993) Human papillomavirus and cervical intraepithelial neoplasia grade III/carcinoma in situ: a case–control study in Spain and Colombia. *Cancer Epidemiology Biomarkers and Prevention* 2: 415–422.

Bosch FX, Manos MM, Muñoz N *et al.* (1995) Prevalence of human papillomavirus in cervical cancer — a worldwide perspective. *Journal of the National Cancer Institute* 87 (11): 796–802.

Bosch FX, Castellsague X, Muñoz N *et al.* (1996) Male sexual behavior and human papillomavirus DNA: key risk factors for cervical cancer in Spain. *Journal of the National Cancer Institute* 88: 1060–1067.

Bosch FX, Lorincz A, Muñoz N *et al.* (2002) The causal relation between human papillomavirus and cervical cancer. *Journal of Clinical Pathology* 55: 244–265.

Brady CS, Duggan-Keen MF, Davidson JA *et al.* (1999) Human papillomavirus type 16 E6 variants in cervical carcinoma: relationship to host genetic factors and clinical parameters. *Journal of General Virology* 80 (Pt 12): 3233–3240.

Breitburd F, Ramoz N, Salmon J *et al.* (1996) HLA control in the progression of human papillomavirus infections. *Seminars in Cancer Biology* 7: 359–371.

Brinton LA (1992) *Epidemiology of Cervical Cancer — Overview*. Lyon: IARC Scientific Publications, pp. 3–23.

Brinton LA, Hamman RF, Huggins GR *et al.* (1987) Sexual and reproductive risk factors for invasive squamous cell cervical cancer. *Journal of the National Cancer Institute* 79: 23–30.

Brinton, LA, Reeves WC, Brenes MM *et al.* (1989a) The male factor in the etiology of cervical cancer among sexually monogamous women. *International Journal of Cancer* 44: 199–203.

Brinton LA, Reeves WC, Brenes MM *et al.* (1989b) Parity as a risk factor for cervical cancer. *American Journal of Epidemiology* 130: 486–496.

Brisson J, Morin C, Fortier M *et al.* (1994) Risk factors for cervical intraepithelial neoplasia: differences between low- and high-grade lesions. *American Journal of Epidemiology* 140: 700–710.

Brisson J, Bairati I, Morin C *et al.* (1996) Determinants of persistent detection of human papillomavirus DNA in the uterine cervix. *Journal of Infectious Diseases* 173: 794–799.

Brock KE, Berry G, Mock PA *et al.* (1988) Nutrients in diet and plasma and risk of in situ cervical cancer. *Journal of the National Cancer Institute* 80: 580–585.

Castellsague X, Bosch FX, Muñoz N *et al.* (2002a) Male circumcision, penile human papillomavirus infection and cervical cancer in female partners. *New England Journal of Medicine* 346: 1105–1112.

Castellsague X, Bosch FX, Muñoz N (2002b) Environmental co-factors in HPV carcinogenesis. *Virus Research* 89: 191–199.

Castle PE, Wacholder S, Lorincz AT *et al.* (2002) A prospective study of high-grade cervical neoplasia risk among human papillomavirus-infected women. *Journal of the National Cancer Institute* 94: 1406–1414.

Centers for Disease Control (1993) 1993 revised classification system for HIV infection and expanded surveillance case definition for AIDS among adolescents and adults. *Journal of the American Medical Association* 269: 729–730.

Chan SY, Ho L, Ong CK *et al.* (1992) Molecular variants of human papillomavirus type 16 from four continents suggest ancient pandemic spread of the virus and its coevolution with humankind. *Journal of Virology* 66: 2057–2066.

Clifford GM, Gallus S, Herrero R, *et al.* (2005) Worldwide distribution of human papillomavirus types in cytologically normal women in the International Agency for Research on Cancer HPV prevalence surveys: a pooled analysis. *Lancet* 366: 991–998.

Clifford GM, Smith JS, Plummer M *et al.* (2003) Human papillomavirus types in invasive cervical cancer worldwide: a meta-analysis. *British Journal of Cancer* 88: 63–73.

Conley LJ, Ellerbrock TV, Bush TJ *et al.* (2002) HIV-1 infection and risk of vulvovaginal and perianal condylomata acuminata and intraepithelial neoplasia: a prospective cohort study. *Lancet* 359: 108–113.

Cox JT (1995) Epidemiology of cervical intraepithelial neoplasia: the role of human papillomavirus. *Bailliere's Clinical and Obstetric Gynaecology* 9: 1–37.

Cuzick J, Singer A, De Stavola BL *et al.* (1990a) Case–control study of risk factors for cervical intraepithelial neoplasia in young women. *European Journal of Cancer* 26: 684–690.

Cuzick J, De Stavola BL, Russell MJ *et al.* (1990b) Vitamin A, vitamin E and the risk of cervical intraepithelial neoplasia. *British Journal of Cancer* 62: 651–652.

de Sanjose S, Muñoz N, Bosch FX *et al.* (1994) Sexually transmitted agents and cervical neoplasia in Colombia and Spain. *International Journal of Cancer* 56: 358–363.

de Vet HC, Knipschild PG, Grol ME *et al.* (1991) The role of beta-carotene and other dietary factors in the aetiology of cervical dysplasia: results of a case–control study. *International Journal of Epidemiology* 20: 603–10.

de Vet HC, Sturmans F, Knipschild PG (1994) The role of cigarette smoking in the etiology of cervical dysplasia. *Epidemiology* 5: 631–633.

Delgado-Rodriguez M, Sillero-Arenas M, Martin-Moreno JM *et al.* (1992) Oral contraceptives and cancer of the cervix uteri. A meta-analysis. *Acta Obstetrica et Gynecologica Scandinavica* 71: 368–376.

Dyson N, Howley PM, Munger K *et al.* (1989) The human papilloma virus-16 E7 oncoprotein is able to bind to the retinoblastoma gene product. *Science* 243: 934–937.

Ellerbrock TV, Chiasson MA, Bush TJ *et al.* (2000) Incidence of cervical squamous intraepithelial lesions in HIV-infected women. *Journal of the American Medical Association* 283: 1031–1037.

Ferlay J, Bray F, Pisani P *et al.* (2004) *GLOBOCAN 2002: Cancer Incidence, Mortality and Prevalence Worldwide.* IARC CancerBase No. 5, version 2.0. Lyon: IARC Press.

Ferenczy A (1997) Glandular lesions: an increasing problem. In: Franco EL, Monsonego J (eds) *New Developments in Cervical Cancer Screening and Prevention.* Oxford: Blackwell, pp. 122–130.

Ferrera A, Baay MF, Herbrink P *et al.* (1997) A sero-epidemiological study of the relationship between sexually transmitted agents and cervical cancer in Honduras. *International Journal of Cancer* 73: 781–785.

Franco EL (1991a) Viral etiology of cervical cancer: a critique of the evidence. *Review of Infectious Disease* 13: 1195–1206.

Franco EL (1991b) The sexually transmitted disease model for cervical cancer: incoherent epidemiologic findings and the role of misclassification of human papillomavirus infection. *Epidemiology* 2: 98–106.

Franco EL (1997) Epidemiology of uterine cancers. In: Meisels A, Morin C (eds) *Cytopathology of the Uterus,* 2nd edn. Chicago: American Society of Clinical Pathologists, pp. 301–324.

Franco EL, Harper DM (2005) Vaccination against human papillomavirus infection: a new paradigm in cervical cancer control. *Vaccine* 23: 2388–2394.

Franco EL, Campos-Filho N, Villa LL *et al.* (1988) Correlation patterns of cancer relative frequencies with some socioeconomic and demographic indicators in Brazil: an ecologic study. *International Journal of Cancer* 41: 24–29.

Franco EL, Villa LL, Ruiz A *et al.* (1995) Transmission of cervical human papillomavirus infection by sexual activity: differences between low and high oncogenic risk types. *Journal of Infectious Diseases* 172: 756–763.

Franco EL, Villa LL, Sobrinho JP *et al.* (1999) Epidemiology of acquisition and clearance of cervical human papillomavirus infection in women from a high-risk area for cervical cancer. *Journal of Infectious Diseases* 180: 1415–1423.

Franco EL, Duarte-Franco E, Ferenczy A (2001) Cervical cancer: epidemiology, prevention and the role of human papillomavirus infection. *Canadian Medical Association Journal* 164: 1017–1025.

Franco EL, Correa P, Santella RM *et al.* (2004) Role and limitations of epidemiology in establishing a causal association. *Seminars in Cancer Biology* 14: 413–426.

Frazer IH (2004) Prevention of cervical cancer through papillomavirus vaccination. *Nature Reviews Immunology* 4: 46–54.

García-Closas R, Castellsague X, Bosch X *et al.* (2005) The role of diet and nutrition in cervical carcinogenesis: a review of recent evidence. *International Journal of Cancer* 117: 629–637.

Giuliano AR (2000) The role of nutrients in the prevention of cervical dysplasia and cancer. *Nutrition* 16: 570–573.

Giuliano AR, Papenfuss M, Abrahamsen M *et al.* (2002) Differences in factors associated with oncogenic and nononcogenic human papillomavirus infection at the United States–Mexico border. *Cancer Epidemiology Biomarkers and Prevention* 11: 930–934.

Goodman MT, McDuffie K, Hernandez B *et al.* (2001) Association of methylenetetrahydrofolate reductase polymorphism C677T and dietary folate with the risk of cervical dysplasia. *Cancer Epidemiology Biomarkers and Prevention* 10: 1275–1280.

Graham S, Priore R, Graham M *et al.* (1979) Genital cancer in wives of penile cancer patients. *Cancer* 44: 1870–1874.

Harper DM, Franco EL, Wheeler C *et al.* GlaxoSmithKline HPV Vaccine Study Group (2004) Efficacy of a bivalent L1 virus-like particle vaccine in prevention of infection with human papillomavirus types 16 and 18 in young women: a randomised controlled trial. *Lancet* 364: 1757–1765.

Harris N, Brill E, Shohat O *et al.* (1986) Molecular basis for heterogeneity of the human p53 protein. *Molecular and Cellular Biology* 6: 4650–4656.

zur Hausen H (1976) Condylomata acuminata and human genital cancer. *Cancer Research* 36: 794.

zur Hausen H (2000) Papillomaviruses causing cancer: evasion from host-cell control in early events in carcinogenesis. *Journal of the National Cancer Institute* 92: 690–698.

Helland A, Olsen AO, Gjoen K *et al.* (1998) An increased risk of cervical intra-epithelial neoplasia grade II–III among human papillomavirus positive patients with the HLA-DQA1*0102–DQB1*0602 haplotype: a population-based case–control study of Norwegian women. *International Journal of Cancer* 76: 19–24.

Herrero R (1996) Epidemiology of cervical cancer. *Journal of the National Cancer Institute Monograph* 1–6.

Hildesheim A, Wang SS (2002) Host and viral genetics and risk of cervical cancer: a review. *Virus Research* 89: 229–240.

Hildesheim A, Schiffman M, Scott DR *et al.* (1998) Human leukocyte antigen class I/II alleles and development of human papillomavirus-related cervical neoplasia: results from a case–control study conducted in the United States. *Cancer Epidemiology Biomarkers and Prevention* 7: 1035–1041.

Hildesheim A, Schiffman MH, Gravitt PE *et al.* (1994) Persistence of type-specific human papillomavirus infection among cytologically normal women. *Journal of Infectious Diseases* 169: 235–240.

Ho GY, Bierman R, Beardsley L *et al.* (1998a) Natural history of cervicovaginal papillomavirus infection in young women. *New England Journal of Medicine* 338: 423–428.

Ho GY, Kadish AS, Burk RD *et al.* (1998b) HPV 16 and cigarette smoking as risk factors for high-grade cervical intra-epithelial neoplasia. *International Journal of Cancer* 78: 281–285.

Ho L, Chan SY, Burk RD *et al.* (1993) The genetic drift of human papillomavirus type 16 is a means of reconstructing prehistoric viral spread and the movement of ancient human populations. *Journal of Virology* 67: 6413–6423.

Hu X, Guo Z, Tianyun P *et al.* (1999) HPV typing and HPV16 E6-sequence variations in synchronous lesions of cervical squamous-cell carcinoma from Swedish patients. *International Journal of Cancer* 83: 34–37.

IARC Working Group (1995) *Human Papillomaviruses.* IARC Monographs on the evaluation of carcinogenic risks to humans, Vol. 64. Lyon: World Health Organization, International Agency for Research on Cancer.

Irwin KL, Rosero-Bixby L, Oberle MW *et al.* (1988) Oral contraceptives and cervical cancer risk in Costa Rica. Detection bias or causal association? *Journal of the American Medical Association* 259: 59–64.

Jay N, Moscicki AB (2000) Human papillomavirus infections in women with HIV disease: prevalence, risk, and management. *AIDS Readings* 10: 659–668.

Jee SH, Won SY, Yun JE *et al.* (2004) Polymorphism p53 codon-72 and invasive cervical cancer: a meta-analysis. *International Journal of Gynaecology and Obstetrics* 85: 301–308.

Kjellberg L, Hallmans G, Ahren AM *et al.* (2000) Smoking, diet, pregnancy and oral contraceptive use as risk factors for cervical intraepithelial neoplasia in relation to human papillomavirus infection. *British Journal of Cancer* 82: 1332–1328.

Koskela P, Anttila T, Bjorge T *et al.* (2000) *Chlamydia trachomatis* infection as a risk factor for invasive cervical cancer. *International Journal of Cancer* 85: 35–39.

Koushik A, Platt RW, Franco EL (2004) p53 codon 72 polymorphism and cervical neoplasia: a meta-analysis review. *Cancer Epidemiology Biomarkers and Prevention* 13: 11–22.

Koutsky L (1997) Epidemiology of genital human papillomavirus infection. *American Journal of Medicine* 102: 3–8.

Koutsky LA, Holmes KK, Critchlow CW *et al.* (1992) A cohort study of the risk of cervical intraepithelial neoplasia grade 2 or 3 in relation to papillomavirus infection. *New England Journal of Medicine* 327: 1272–1278.

Kwasniewska A, Tukendorf A, Semczuk M (1997) Content of alpha-tocopherol in blood serum of human papillomavirus-infected women with cervical dysplasias. *Nutrition and Cancer* 28: 248–251.

Kwasniewska A, Charzewska J, Tukendorf A *et al.* (1998) Dietary factors in women with dysplasia colli uteri associated with human papillomavirus infection. *Nutrition and Cancer* 30: 39–45.

Lacey JV, Jr, Brinton LA, Abbas FM *et al.* (1999) Oral contraceptives as risk factors for cervical adenocarcinomas and squamous cell carcinomas. *Cancer Epidemiology Biomarkers and Prevention* 8: 1079–1085.

Langley CL, Benga-De E, Critchlow CW *et al.* (1996) HIV-1, HIV-2, human papillomavirus infection and cervical neoplasia in high-risk African women. *AIDS* 10: 413–417.

Lehtinen M, Koskela P, Jellum E *et al.* (2002) Herpes simplex virus and risk of cervical cancer: a longitudinal, nested case–control study in the nordic countries. *American Journal of Epidemiology* 156: 687–692.

Li JY, Li FP, Blot WJ *et al.* (1982) Correlation between cancers of the uterine cervix and penis in China. *Journal of the National Cancer Institute* 69: 1063–1065.

Liaw KL, Hildesheim A, Burk RD *et al.* (2001) A prospective study of human papillomavirus (HPV) type 16 DNA detection by polymerase chain reaction and its association with acquisition and persistence of other HPV types. *Journal of Infectious Diseases* 183: 8–15.

Liu T, Soong SJ, Wilson NP *et al.* (1993) A case–control study of nutritional factors and cervical dysplasia. *Cancer Epidemiology Biomarkers and Prevention* 2: 525–530.

Liu T, Soong SJ, Alvarez RD *et al.* (1995) A longitudinal analysis of human papillomavirus 16 infection, nutritional status, and cervical dysplasia progression. *Cancer Epidemiology Biomarkers and Prevention* 4: 373–380.

Londesborough P, Ho L, Terry G *et al.* (1996) Human papillomavirus genotype as a predictor of persistence and development of high-grade lesions in women with minor cervical abnormalities. *International Journal of Cancer* 69: 364–368.

Lorincz AT, Castle PE, Sherman ME *et al.* (2002) Viral load of human papillomavirus and risk of CIN3 or cervical cancer. *Lancet* 360: 228–229.

Maciag PC, Schlecht NF, Souza PS *et al.* (2000) Major histocompatibility complex class II polymorphisms and risk of cervical cancer and human papillomavirus infection in Brazilian women. *Cancer Epidemiology Biomarkers and Prevention* 9: 1183–1191.

Madeleine MM, Brumback B, Cushing-Haugen KL *et al.* (2002) Human leukocyte antigen class II and cervical cancer risk: a population-based study. *Journal of Infectious Diseases* 186: 1565–1574.

Maiman M, Fruchter RG, Sedlis A *et al.* (1998) Prevalence, risk factors, and accuracy of cytologic screening for cervical intraepithelial neoplasia in women with the human immunodeficiency virus. *Gynecological Oncology* 68: 233–239.

Mandelblatt JS, Kanetsky P, Eggert L *et al.* (1999) Is HIV infection a cofactor for cervical squamous cell neoplasia? *Cancer Epidemiology Biomarkers and Prevention* 8: 97–106.

Mantovani F, Banks L (2001) The human papillomavirus E6 protein and its contribution to malignant progression. *Oncogene* 20: 7874–7887.

Massad LS, Riester KA, Anastos KM *et al.* (1999) Prevalence and predictors of squamous cell abnormalities in Papanicolaou smears from women infected with HIV-1. Women's Interagency HIV Study Group. *Journal of Acquired Immune Deficiency Syndrome* 21: 33–41.

Matlashewski GJ, Tuck S, Pim D *et al.* (1987) Primary structure polymorphism at amino acid residue 72 of human p53. *Molecular and Cellular Biology* 7: 961–963.

Moreno V, Bosch FX, Muñoz N *et al.* (2002) Effect of oral contraceptives on risk of cervical cancer in women with human papillomavirus infection: the IARC multicentric case–control study. *Lancet* 359: 1085–1092.

Morrison EA, Ho GY, Vermund SH *et al.* (1991) Human papillomavirus infection and other risk factors for cervical neoplasia: a case–control study. *International Journal of Cancer* 49: 6–13.

Moscicki AB, Shiboski S, Broering J *et al.* (1998) The natural history of human papillomavirus infection as measured by repeated DNA testing in adolescent and young women. *Journal of Pediatrics* 132: 277–284.

Moscicki AB, Ellenberg JH, Vermund SH *et al.* (2000) Prevalence of and risks for cervical human papillomavirus infection and squamous intraepithelial lesions in adolescent girls: impact of infection with human immunodeficiency virus. *Archives of Pediatric and Adolescent Medicine* 154: 127–134.

Moscicki AB, Hills N, Shiboski S *et al.* (2001) Risks for incident human papillomavirus infection and low-grade squamous intraepithelial lesion development in young females. *Journal of the American Medical Association* 285: 2995–3002.

Munger K, Basile JR, Duensing S *et al.* (2001) Biological activities and molecular targets of the human papillomavirus E7 oncoprotein. *Oncogene* 20: 7888–7898.

Muñoz N, Bosch X, Kaldor JM (1988) Does human papillomavirus cause cervical cancer? The state of the epidemiological evidence. *British Journal of Cancer* 57: 1–5.

Muñoz N, Bosch FX, de Sanjose S *et al.* (1992) The causal link between human papillomavirus and invasive cervical cancer: a population-based case–control study in Colombia and Spain. *International Journal of Cancer* 52: 743–749.

Muñoz N, Castellsague X, Bosch FX *et al.* (1996) Difficulty in elucidating the male role in cervical cancer in Colombia, a high-risk area for the disease. *Journal of the National Cancer Institute* 88: 1068–1075.

Muñoz N, Franceschi S, Bosetti C *et al.* (2002) Role of parity and human papillomavirus in cervical cancer: the IARC multicentric case–control study. *Lancet* 359: 1093–1101.

Muñoz N, Bosch FX, de Sanjose S *et al.* (2003) Epidemiologic classification of human papillomavirus types associated with cervical cancer. *New England Journal of Medicine* 348: 518–527.

National Cancer Institute (2002) *Surveillance, Epidemiology, and End Results (SEER) Program.* Bethesda, MD: National Cancer Institute.

Nindl I, Rindfleisch K, Lotz B *et al.* (1999) Uniform distribution of HPV 16 E6 and E7 variants in patients with normal histology, cervical intra-epithelial neoplasia and cervical cancer. *International Journal of Cancer* 82: 203–207.

Nobbenhuis MA, Walboomers JM, Helmerhorst TJ *et al.* (1999) Relation of human papillomavirus status to cervical lesions and consequences for cervical-cancer screening: a prospective study. *Lancet* 354: 20–25.

Odunsi KO, Ganesan TS (1997) The roles of the human major histocompatibility complex and human papillomavirus infection in cervical intraepithelial neoplasia and cervical cancer. *Clinical Oncology (Royal College of Radiologists)* 9: 4–13.

Odunsi K, Terry G, Ho L *et al.* (1995) Association between HLA DQB1*03 and cervical intra-epithelial neoplasia. *Molecular Medicine* 1: 161–171.

Odunsi K, Terry G, Ho L *et al.* (1996) Susceptibility to human papillomavirus-associated cervical intra-epithelial neoplasia is determined by specific HLA DR-DQ alleles. *International Journal of Cancer* 67: 595–602.

Olsen AO, Gjoen K, Sauer T *et al.* (1995) Human papillomavirus and cervical intraepithelial neoplasia grade II–III: a population-based case–control study. *International Journal of Cancer* 61: 312–315.

Palan PR, Mikhail MS, Basu J *et al.* (1991) Plasma levels of antioxidant beta-carotene and alpha-tocopherol in uterine cervix dysplasias and cancer. *Nutrition and Cancer* 15: 13–20.

Palan PR, Mikhail MS, Goldberg GL *et al.* (1996) Plasma levels of beta-carotene, lycopene, canthaxanthin, retinol, and alpha- and tau-tocopherol in cervical intraepithelial neoplasia and cancer. *Clinics in Cancer Research* 2: 181–185.

Partridge JM, Koutsky LA (2006) Genital human papillomavirus infection in men. *Lancet Infectious Diseases* 6: 21–31.

Palefsky JM, Holly EA (1995) Molecular virology and epidemiology of human papillomavirus and cervical cancer. *Cancer Epidemiology Biomarkers and Prevention* 4: 415–428.

Parazzini F, La Vecchia C, Negri E *et al.* (1992) Risk factors for cervical intraepithelial neoplasia. *Cancer* 69: 2276–2282.

Parkin DM, Bray FI, Devesa SS (2001) Cancer burden in the year 2000. The global picture. *European Journal of Cancer* 37 (Suppl. 8): S4–66.

Pater MM, Mittal R, Pater A (1994) Role of steroid hormones in potentiating transformation of cervical cells by human papillomaviruses. *Trends in Microbiology* 2: 229–234.

Peng HQ, Liu SL, Mann V *et al.* (1991) Human papillomavirus types 16 and 33, herpes simplex virus type 2 and other risk factors for cervical cancer in Sichuan Province, China. *International Journal of Cancer* 47: 711–716.

Potischman N, Brinton LA (1996) Nutrition and cervical neoplasia. *Cancer Causes and Control* 7: 113–126.

Rezza G, Giuliani M, Branca M *et al.* (1997) Determinants of squamous intraepithelial lesions (SIL) on Pap smear: the role of HPV infection and of HIV-1-induced immunosuppression. DIANAIDS Collaborative Study Group. *European Journal of Epidemiology* 13: 937–943.

Richardson H, Franco E, Pintos J *et al.* (2000) Determinants of low-risk and high-risk cervical human papillomavirus infections in Montreal University students. *Sexually Transmitted Diseases* 27: 79–86.

Rousseau MC, Franco EL, Villa LL *et al.* (2000) A cumulative case–control study of risk factor profiles for oncogenic and nononcogenic cervical human papillomavirus infections. *Cancer Epidemiology Biomarkers and Prevention* 9: 469–476.

Sanjeevi CB, Hjelmstrom P, Hallmans G *et al.* (1996) Different HLA-DR-DQ haplotypes are associated with cervical intraepithelial neoplasia among human papillomavirus type-16 seropositive and seronegative Swedish women. *International Journal of Cancer* 68: 409–414.

Sasagawa T, Dong Y, Saijoh K *et al.* (1997) Human papillomavirus infection and risk determinants for squamous intraepithelial lesion and cervical cancer in Japan. *Japanese Journal of Cancer Research* 88: 376–384.

Schiff M, Becker TM, Masuk M *et al.* (2000) Risk factors for cervical intraepithelial neoplasia in southwestern American Indian women. *American Journal of Epidemiology* 152: 716–726.

Schiffman MH, Brinton LA (1995) The epidemiology of cervical carcinogenesis. *Cancer* 76: 1888–1901.

Schiffman MH, Haley NJ, Felton JS *et al.* (1987) Biochemical epidemiology of cervical neoplasia: measuring cigarette smoke constituents in the cervix. *Cancer Research* 47: 3886–3888.

Schiffman MH, Bauer HM, Hoover RN *et al.* (1993) Epidemiologic evidence showing that human papillomavirus infection causes most cervical intraepithelial neoplasia. *Journal of the National Cancer Institute* 85: 958–964.

Schiffman MH, Brinton LA, Devesa SS *et al.* (1996) Cervical cancer. In: Schottenfeld D, Fraumeni JF (eds) *Cancer Epidemiology and Prevention.* New York: Oxford University Press, pp. 1090–1116.

Schlecht NF, Kulaga S, Robitaille J *et al.* (2001) Persistent human papillomavirus infection as a predictor of cervical intraepithelial neoplasia. *Journal of the American Medical Association* 286: 3106–3114.

Schlecht NF, Trevisan A, Duarte-Franco E *et al.* (2003) Viral load as a predictor of the risk of cervical intraepithelial neoplasia. *International Journal of Cancer* 103: 519–524.

Schneider A, Hotz M, Gissmann L (1987) Increased prevalence of human papillomaviruses in the lower genital tract of pregnant women. *International Journal of Cancer* 40: 198–201.

Sellors JW, Karwalajtys TL, Kaczorowski J *et al.* (2003) Incidence, clearance and predictors of human papillomavirus infection in women. *Canadian Medical Association Journal* 168: 421–425.

Shannon J, Thomas DB, Ray RM *et al.* (2002) Dietary risk factors for invasive and in-situ cervical carcinomas in Bangkok, Thailand. *Cancer Causes and Control* 13: 691–699.

Shields TS, Brinton LA, Burk RD *et al.* (2004) A case–control study of risk factors for invasive cervical cancer among US women exposed to oncogenic types of human papillomavirus. *Cancer Epidemiology Biomarkers and Prevention* 13: 1574–1582.

Singer A, Reid BL, Coppleson M (1976) A hypothesis: the role of a high-risk male in the etiology of cervical carcinoma: a correlation of epidemiology and molecular biology. *American Journal of Obstetrics and Gynecology* 126: 110–115.

Smith JS, Muñoz N, Herrero R *et al.* (2002) Evidence for *Chlamydia trachomatis* as a human papillomavirus cofactor in the etiology of invasive cervical cancer in Brazil and the Philippines. *Journal of Infectious Diseases* 185: 324–331.

Smith PG, Kinlen LJ, White GC *et al.* (1980) Mortality of wives of men dying with cancer of the penis. *British Journal of Cancer* 41: 422–428.

Solomon D, Davey D, Kurman R *et al.* (2002) The 2001 Bethesda System: terminology for reporting results of cervical cytology. *Journal of the American Medical Association* 287: 2114–2119.

Stewart BW, Kleihues P (eds) (2003) *World Health Organization: World Cancer Report.* Lyon: International Agency for Research on Cancer.

Storey A, Thomas M, Kalita A *et al.* (1998) Role of a p53 polymorphism in the development of human papillomavirus-associated cancer. *Nature* 393: 229–234.

Strickler HD, Burk RD, Fazzari M *et al.* (2005) Natural history and possible reactivation of human papillomavirus in human immuno-deficiency virus-positive women. *Journal of the National Cancer Institute* 97: 577–586.

Swan DC, Tucker RA, Tortolero-Luna G *et al.* (1999) Human papillomavirus (HPV) DNA copy number is dependent on grade of cervical disease and HPV type. *Journal of Clinical Microbiology* 37: 1030–1034.

Thomas DB, Qin Q, Kuypers J *et al.* (2001) Human papillomaviruses and cervical cancer in Bangkok. II. Risk factors for in situ and invasive squamous cell cervical carcinomas. *American Journal of Epidemiology* 153: 732–739.

Thomas DB, Ray RM, Qin Q (2002) Risk factors for progression of squamous cell cervical carcinoma in-situ to invasive cervical cancer: results of a multinational study. *Cancer Causes and Control* 13: 683–690.

VanEenwyk J, Davis FG, Bowen PE (1991) Dietary and serum carotenoids and cervical intraepithelial neoplasia. *International Journal of Cancer* 48: 34–38.

VanEenwyk J, Davis FG, Colman N (1992) Folate, vitamin C, and cervical intraepithelial neoplasia. *Cancer Epidemiology Biomarkers and Prevention* 1: 119–124.

Villa LL (1997) Human papillomaviruses and cervical cancer. *Advances in Cancer Research* 71: 321–341.

Villa LL, Sichero L, Rahal P *et al.* (2000) Molecular variants of human papillomavirus types 16 and 18 preferentially associated with cervical neoplasia. *Journal of General Virology* 81: 2959–2968.

Villa LL, Costa RL, Petta CA *et al.* (2005) Prophylactic quadrivalent human papillomavirus (types 6, 11, 16, and 18) L1 virus-like particle vaccine in young women: a randomised double-blind placebo-controlled multicentre phase II efficacy trial. *Lancet Oncology* 6: 271–278.

Vizcaino AP, Moreno V, Bosch FX *et al.* (1998) International trends in the incidence of cervical cancer. I. Adenocarcinoma and adenosquamous cell carcinomas. *International Journal of Cancer* 75: 536–545.

Walboomers JM, Meijer CJ (1997) Do HPV-negative cervical carcinomas exist? *Journal of Pathology* 181: 253–254.

Walboomers JM, Jacobs MV, Manos MM *et al.* (1999) Human papillomavirus is a necessary cause of invasive cervical cancer worldwide. *Journal of Pathology* 189: 12–19.

Weaver BA, Thing Q, Homers KK *et al.* (2004) Evaluation of genital sites and sampling techniques for detection of human papillomavirus DNA in men. *Journal of Infectious Diseases* 189: 677–685.

Winer RL, Lee SK, Hughes JP *et al.* (2003) Genital human papillomavirus infection: incidence and risk factors in a cohort of female university students. *American Journal of Epidemiology* 157: 218–226.

Winkelstein W (1990) Smoking and cervical cancer—current status: a review. *American Journal of Epidemiology* 131: 945–957; discussion 958–960.

Wright TC, Jr (1997) Papillomavirus infection and neoplasia in women infected with human immunodeficiency virus. In: Franco, EL,

Monsonego J (eds) *New Developments in Cervical Cancer Screening and Prevention.* Oxford: Blackwell, pp. 131–143.

Xi LF, Koutsky LA, Galloway DA *et al.* (1997) Genomic variation of human papillomavirus type 16 and risk for high grade cervical intraepithelial neoplasia. *Journal of the National Cancer Institute* 89: 796–802.

Xi LF, Carter JJ, Galloway DA *et al.* (2002) Acquisition and natural history of human papillomavirus type 16 variant infection among a cohort of female university students. *Cancer Epidemiology Biomarkers and Prevention* 11: 343–351.

Yamada T, Wheeler CM, Halpern AL *et al.* (1995) Human papillomavirus type 16 variant lineages in United States populations characterized by nucleotide sequence analysis of the E6, L2, and L1 coding segments. *Journal of Virology* 69: 7743–7753.

Ylitalo N, Josefsson A, Melbye M *et al.* (2000) A prospective study showing long-term infection with human papillomavirus 16 before the development of cervical carcinoma in situ. *Cancer Research* 60: 6027–6032.

Zehbe I, Wilander E, Delius H *et al.* (1998) Human papillomavirus 16 E6 variants are more prevalent in invasive cervical carcinoma than the prototype. *Cancer Research* 58: 829–833.

Ziegler RG, Jones CJ, Brinton LA *et al.* (1991) Diet and the risk of in situ cervical cancer among white women in the United States. *Cancer Causes and Control* 2: 17–29.

Zunzunegui MV, King MC, Coria CF *et al.* (1986) Male influences on cervical cancer risk. *American Journal of Epidemiology* 123: 302–307.

FURTHER READING

Elfgren K, Rylander E, Radberg T *et al.* (2006) Colposcopic and histopathologic evaluation of women participating in population-based screening for human papillomavirus deoxyribonucleic acid persistance. *American Journal of Obstetrics and Gynecology* 193: 650–657.

Goldie SJ, Kohli M, Grima D *et al.* (2004) Protected clinical benefits and cost-effectiveness of a human papillomavirus 16/18 vaccine. *Journal of the National Cancer Institute* 96: 604–615.

Khan MJ, Castle P, Lorincz AT (2005) The elevated 10-year risk of cervical precancer and cancer in women with human papillomavirus (type 16 or 18) and the possible utility of type-specific HPV testing in clinical practice. *Journal of the National Cancer Institute* 97: 1072–1079.

Rousseau MC, Abrahamowicz M, Villa LL *et al.* (2003) Predictors of cervical coinfection with multiple human papillomavirus types. *Cancer Epidemiology Biomarkers and Prevention* 12 (10): 1029–1037.

Schlecht NF, Platt RW, Negassa A *et al.* (2003) Modeling the time dependence of the association between human papillomavirus infection and cervical cancer precursor lesions. *American Journal of Epidemiology* 158 (9): 878–886.

Schlecht NF, Platt RW, Duarte-Franco E *et al.* (2003) Human papillomavirus infection and time to progression and regression of cervical intraepithelial neoplasia. *Journal of the National Cancer Institute* 95: 1336–1343.

CHAPTER 19

Molecular basis of cervical neoplasia

Frank Stubenrauch and Thomas Iftner

INTRODUCTION

Papillomaviruses are widespread among higher vertebrates, but reveal a strict species specificity, and transmission from non-primates to humans has not been reported. In general, they cause local epithelial infections, with the exception of animal fibropapilloma viruses [e.g. bovine papillomavirus (BPV)], where the infection can also be found in the dermis. Viral spread to distant body sites does not occur.

Papillomaviruses are small icosahedral particles with a diameter of 55 nm, belonging to the family of Papillomaviridae, have no envelope and consist of a capsid composed of 72 capsomeres which accommodates the viral genome. The capsomeres are made of two structural proteins: the 57-kDa late protein L1, which accounts for 80% of the viral particle and is considered to be a group-specific antigen, and the 43- to 53-kDa minor capsid protein L2. Virus-like particles (VLPs) can be produced by expressing L1 alone or in combination with L2 with the help of mammalian or non-mammalian expression systems. They represent empty capsids that closely resemble authentic virions morphologically and immunologically. Systemic immunisation with L1 VLPs has been found to induce high titres of neutralising antibodies that are conformation dependent and type specific. 'Proof of principle' clinical trials using VLPs as a vaccine have been performed successfully (Koutsky *et al.*, 2002; Billich, 2003; Harper *et al.*, 2004; Villa *et al.*, 2005) and are currently extended. Because of the absence of an envelope, papillomaviruses are relatively stable and remain infectious in the environment for weeks to months. They are also resistant to organic solvents, and heat treatment to 56°C causes only a minor loss of infectivity.

CLASSIFICATION OF PAPILLOMAVIRUSES

Earlier attempts to classify human papillomaviruses (HPV) were based on the rather strict tropism of certain HPV types for cornifying squamous epithelium (cutaneous types, e.g. HPV 1, 5, 8) or mucosal epithelium (mucosal types, e.g. HPV 6, 16, 31), with some types strongly linked to distinctive clinical presentations. However, this classification is overly simple and is incorrect in some cases as demonstrated by the presence of the so-called 'mucosal' type HPV 6 in cornifying genital warts. Another attempt to group papillomaviruses is the classification into skin types causing vulgar warts (e.g. HPV 1) and genital types affecting primarily the anogenital area (e.g. HPV 6, 16, 18). Again, this classification is rather artificial, because HPV 16 can also be found in nail-bed carcinomas on the hands. The modern classification into different papillomavirus types according to the International Committee on the Taxonomy of Viruses is based on DNA nucleotide sequence differences within the L1 major capsid gene (de Villiers *et al.*, 2004). Using this definition, more than 100 types of papillomaviruses have been described. Papillomaviruses that share more than 60% homology in L1 are grouped together in genera (α to π). For example, the genus α-papillomavirus includes all accepted high-risk viruses, low-risk viruses and several unclassified types, whereas the genus beta-papillomaviruses includes all known papillomaviruses associated with the disease epidermodysplasia verruciformis. Genera are further subdivided into species (e.g., $\alpha9$ includes HPV 16, 31, 33, 35, 52 and 58), whose members share 71–89% homology in L1 (de Villiers *et al.*, 2004).

Recent studies have shown that HPV DNA can be found in 99.7% of all cervical carcinomas, with HPV types 16, 18, 45 and 31 being the most frequent ones (Bosch *et al.*, 1995; Walboomers *et al.*, 1999). Based on these observations, the genital HPVs have been divided into a group associated with a high risk of cervical cancer development – the 'high-risk' HPVs (HPV 16, 18, 26, 31, 33, 35, 39, 45, 51, 52, 53, 56, 58, 59, 66, 68, 73 and 82) – and a second group having a low carcinogenic potential – the 'low-risk' HPVs (HPV 6, 11, 40, 42, 43, 44, 54, 61, 72 and 81) (Muñoz *et al.*, 2003). It has now been proven beyond reasonable doubt that infection with a high-risk HPV is a necessary prerequisite for the development of cervical cancer (Bosch *et al.*, 2002), and the World Health Organization (WHO) has declared HPV 16, 18, 31, 33, 35, 39, 45, 51, 52, 56, 58, 59, and 66 as class I carcinogens (Cogliano *et al.*, 2005) for humans.

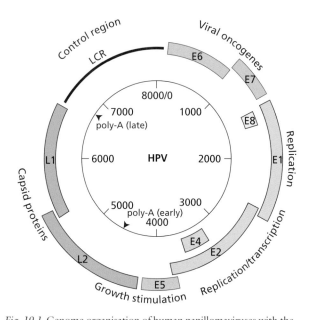

Fig. 19.1 Genome organisation of human papillomaviruses with the open reading frames (E1–E8, L1, L2) and the long control region (LCR).

STRUCTURE OF THE HPV GENOME

The HPV genome consists of a double-stranded 8-kbp DNA molecule, which is associated with cell-derived histone proteins that produce a nucleosome-like superhelical twisted structure. The relative arrangement of the 8–10 open reading frames (ORFs) within the genome is conserved within all papillomavirus types. One speciality of papillomaviruses is that the partly overlapping ORFs are arranged on only one DNA strand. To increase their coding capacities, HPVs make use of alternative splicing of primary transcripts to generate multiple proteins from one ORF or to generate fusion proteins consisting of parts from different reading frames. The genome can be divided into three regions: the long control region (LCR), the region of early proteins (E1–E8) and the region of late proteins (L1 and L2). In accordance with this, two RNA poly-A addition sites, one for the early protein transcripts and one for the late protein transcripts, are always present. An example of the genome organisation of human papillomaviruses is given in Figure 19.1.

The long control region (LCR)

The size of the LCR varies from 500 to 1000 bp between different HPVs. There are no conserved ORFs in this area of the genome, but it does contain several control elements, which regulate HPV DNA replication and gene expression. Some of these are promoter elements, such as a TATA box and a CAAT box, while others are binding sites for general transcription factors of cellular origin, such as NF1, AP1 and SP1, or cyto-

keratin and corticosteroid-responsive elements. Binding sites for the viral E2 regulatory protein can be found in the LCR with the number and the arrangement differing between human papillomaviruses causing anogenital lesions and those that do not. The viral origin of replication is located at the 3′ end of the LCR and consists of binding sites for the viral E1 and E2 proteins.

The proteins of papillomaviruses

The E1 protein

The nucleotide sequence of the E1 gene is highly conserved among the different HPV types. The E1 ORF codes for several proteins with molecular weights ranging from 68 to 85 kDa. These are responsible for the replication of the viral genome and possess adenosine triphosphatase (ATPase) and helicase activities. However, they have only a weak ability to bind to the origin of replication. In the majority of HPVs, the E1 binding site (E1BS) is located between two A+T-rich sequences, which are variable in length and show little sequence conservation between HPV types. These are then flanked by three binding sites for E2 proteins (E2BSs), which act to stabilise the binding of E1 and promote viral DNA replication (Wilson *et al.*, 2002).

The E2 protein

The E2 ORF codes for several forms of DNA-binding proteins that are required for DNA replication and the regulation of transcription. They recognise the DNA sequence motif 5′-ACCG NNNN CGGT-3′, which constitutes the E2 binding site (E2BS). Most HPVs have three high-affinity E2BSs located close to the origin of replication, two of which are required for efficient DNA replication. Binding to this site is achieved by the carboxy-terminus of the E2 protein (DNA-binding domain), whereas the transactivation domain is located in the amino-terminus. E2 proteins always bind DNA as dimers, with dimerisation domains identified in both the carboxy-terminus and the amino-terminus. The transactivation and DNA-binding domains are connected through a third 'linker' domain, which, in contrast to the well-conserved carboxy- and amino-termini, varies in composition and size between different HPV types.

The positive effect of the E2 protein on HPV DNA replication results from an interaction with the E1 protein at the origin of replication, by which E1 binding is enhanced. Another function of the E2 proteins in high-risk anogenital HPVs is to repress transcription of the E6 and E7 genes by preventing the formation of the preinitiation complex of transcription at the p97 promoter through sterical hindrance.

Recently, a new E2 protein consisting of a fusion of the product of the small E8 ORF with part of the E2 protein has been described for HPVs. This E8^E2C fusion protein is able to repress transcription as well as viral DNA replication from a range of extrachromosomal origins (Stubenrauch *et al.*, 2000, 2001; Zobel *et al.*, 2003), and it is therefore believed to play a major role in the maintenance of the latent state observed in the basal cells of the infected epithelium.

Other early proteins: E3, E4, E5 and E8

The E3 ORF is present in only a few HPV types, and the function of the E3 protein is not known.

The E4 ORF lies in the early region of the genome, although it appears to be expressed in a late stage of the infectious cycle. E4 proteins are expressed from suprabasal cell layers to terminally differentiated keratinocytes, but E4 is not a structural protein. Recent results point to an interaction of E4 with keratins, which induce a collapse of the cytokeratin network and may play a role in the release of virus during a lytic infection. Other studies describe a role for E4 in G2 arrest and HPV DNA replication.

The E5 ORF is not present in all HPVs. The E5 proteins of HPV 6, HPV 16 and BPV have been shown to cause morphological transformation of rodent fibroblasts and to increase the proliferative capacity of human keratinocytes by interaction with the epidermal growth factor receptor (EGFR), leading to the subsequent stimulation of cellular DNA synthesis.

The E8 ORF does not lead to the generation of a single E8 protein, but rather it is part of a fusion protein with part of the E2 protein (see comments for the E2 protein above).

The viral oncogenes E6 and E7

Transcription of the E6 and E7 genes is a consistent feature in cervical carcinomas and was the first indication of an important role for these genes in HPV-associated tumorigenesis. The E6 and E7 genes of HPV 16 and HPV 18 have been confirmed as potent viral oncogenes, and their transforming and immortalising abilities have been demonstrated in tissue culture experiments and experimental animal models (Münger *et al.*, 1992; zur Hausen 1996; Münger and Howley, 2002).

The E6 protein

The E6 ORF encodes a small protein of approximately 150 amino acids resulting in a molecular weight of 16–18 kDa. Alternative splicing of E6 transcripts generates truncated E6 proteins (E6*I and E6*II), which is a unique feature of high-risk HPVs, and these proteins may modulate the E6 promoter, giving rise to an autoregulatory feedback loop. The full-length E6 protein includes a potential zinc-binding motif (cys-x-x-cys) which, complexed with Zn^{2+} ions, is capable of binding to DNA. The E6 protein of high-risk anogenital types shows only weak oncogenic potential by itself in most established cell lines, with the exception of mammary epithelial cells and rodent fibroblasts, and cooperation with the E7 protein is required for the full transforming/immortalising capacity. The key mechanism of high-risk E6 is its ability to inhibit the function of p53, a tumour-suppressor protein, by binding and

enhancing its degradation through the ubiquitin pathway. This results in a dramatic shortening of the half-life of p53 from 3 hours to 20 minutes with a corresponding decrease in its biological function. For the ubiquitination of p53, E6 recruits a cellular protein called E6-associated protein (E6-AP), which acts as an E3–ubiquitin–protein ligase (Huibregtse *et al.*, 1991). In contrast, in non-infected eukaryotic cells, the ubiquitin-mediated proteolysis of p53 is triggered by the hdm-2 protein. In high-risk HPV-infected cells, the formation of the E6–p53–E6AP complex therefore replaces the control of p53 by hdm-2. This is reflected in the low level of p53 protein in cervical carcinoma cells, which is reduced two- to threefold compared with normal epithelial cells.

Independently of the E6AP-dependent degradation of the p53 protein, high-risk E6 proteins downregulate p53-dependent transcriptional control, which appears to result from the targeting of CBP/p300, a p53 co-activator, by E6. Furthermore, E6 appears to be able to activate the cellular enzyme telomerase in differentiated cells. Telomerase is an enzyme that counteracts the continuous shortening of the chromosome's telomeres which occurs naturally during replication of the cellular genome. This shortening correlates with cell ageing, and the prevention of chromosome shortening results in an increased lifespan for the affected cell (Mantovani and Banks, 2001).

While E6 proteins from low-risk genital HPV, cutaneous HPV and animal papillomavirus types do not bind to p53 or do not induce its degradation, the corresponding E7 proteins do bind to Rb, albeit at a reduced affinity (Münger *et al.*, 1989; Gage *et al.*, 1990; Schmitt *et al.*, 1994; Elbel *et al.*, 1997).

The E7 protein

The E7 ORF encodes for a small protein of about 100 amino acids (10 kDa). E7 is the major transforming oncogene of human papillomaviruses, and its activity is mediated through its ability to bind cellular proteins of the pRB family which, in concert with the E2F family of transcription factors, control cell replication (Davies *et al.*, 1993; Boyer *et al.*, 1996). Binding of E7 to the active form of pRB leads to the release of E2F transcription factors and a progression into the S-phase of the cell cycle with subsequent cell replication (Dyson *et al.*, 1989, 1992; Chellappan *et al.* 1992). E7 also forms complexes with cyclins A and E as well as with p21 and p27 (Dyson *et al.* 1992; Tommasino *et al.*, 1993; McIntyre *et al.*, 1996; Zerfass-Thome *et al.*, 1996; Funk *et al.*, 1997; Jones *et al.*, 1997). Both low- and high-risk HPV types prevent cell cycle exit of infected cells during differentiation, suggesting common mechanisms of action by these viral proteins (Halbert *et al.*, 1992; Cheng *et al.*, 1995; Ruesch and Laimins, 1998). Rb has been implicated in the regulation of differentiation of several types of tissues, making it plausible that this is one of the important targets of a viral infection (Yee *et al.*, 1998).

Taken together, the E7 protein causes the infected cell to enter S-phase to generate a cellular environment that allows the amplification of the viral DNA. This induces a number of cellular responses, such as stabilisation of the p53 protein, which would lead to programmed cell death via apoptosis. To counteract the cellular response to E7, high-risk papillomaviruses encode the E6 protein, which causes the degradation of p53. It is unclear at present how low-risk or cutaneous viruses, whose E6 proteins are unable to interfere with p53, but whose E7 proteins bind to pRB, overcome the p53-mediated apoptosis.

REPLICATION CYCLE IN THE INFECTED EPITHELIUM

The initial infection by HPV probably occurs in the basal layer of stratified epithelium (Fig. 19.2).

Following entry into the cell, HPV genomes are established as extrachromosomal elements in the nucleus. Upon cell division, one of the daughter cells migrates away from the basal layer and initiates a programme of differentiation. This leads to amplification of the viral DNA, expression of capsid proteins and, finally, to the production of progeny virus. The other daughter cell stays in the basal layer and provides a reservoir of

viral DNA, which may contribute to viral persistence. In normal epithelia, cells exit the cell cycle as they begin to differentiate. In many epithelia, the nuclei are no longer active and are degraded in suprabasal layers. As HPVs rely on cellular enzymes to replicate their genomes, one major consequence of an HPV infection is a blockage of cell cycle exit. HPV-infected cells undergo an incomplete S-phase in differentiated suprabasal cells to replicate HPV genomes to high levels (Laimins, 1996). In the high-risk HPV types, the blockage of cell cycle exit and induction of S-phase in differentiated suprabasal cells is mediated by the E6 and E7 proteins (Halbert *et al.*, 1992; Cheng *et al.*, 1995; Ruesch and Laimins, 1998).

HPVs maintain their genomes at 10–100 virus copies per infected cell over long periods of time *in vitro*, and this is thought to reflect viral DNA replication in basal cells *in vivo*. In these cells, viral DNA replication is not restricted by the mechanisms controlling cellular DNA replication, but is limited by copy number control mechanisms. The HPV 31 E8^E2C protein represents the major inhibitor of viral DNA replication in basal cells. Because of its functions as a transcriptional and replication repressor, E8^E2C might contribute to the establishment of latent infections.

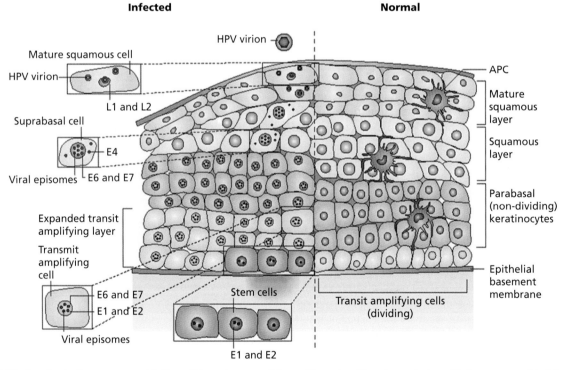

Fig. 19.2 The location in the squamous epithelium of the main stages of the papillomavirus life cycle: cervical stratified squamous epithelial cell architecture and the expression of human papillomavirus (HPV) proteins after infections. Daughter cells of the epithelial stem cells divide along the basement membrane and then mature vertically through the epithelium without further division (right side). After the introduction of HPV into stem cells in the basal layer of the epithelium, expression of viral non-structural proteins occurs. Under the regulation of these proteins, the dividing cell population expands vertically, and epithelial cell differentiation is delayed and is less complete. Viral proteins are expressed sequentially with differentiation as shown; the mature virions are produced only in the most superficial layers of the epithelium. Intraepithelial antigen-presenting cells (APCs) are depleted in the HPV-infected epithelium. From Frazer (2004), with kind permission from Nature Publishing Group.

Disturbances of the replication control of high-risk HPV may have implications for the progression of high-risk HPV-induced lesions *in vivo*, as the viral DNA is extrachromosomal in precursor lesions but is found integrated into the host chromosomes in the majority of invasive cancers. As no common integration site(s) have been identified, integration does not generally target proto-oncogenes or tumour-suppressor genes of the host cell. On the other hand, it has been observed that deletions and rearrangements of the integrated viral DNA occur. A model was proposed which suggests that the inactivation of the E2 gene releases E6/E7 oncogene expression from negative control. However, no evidence has been presented so far that, indeed, increased E6/E7 expression is necessary for the progression of HPV-induced lesions. Viral DNA integration could simply be a consequence of an environment that does not support HPV DNA replication. This is supported by observations that long-term extrachromosomal replication of high-risk HPV DNA has not been achieved in established HPV-positive or -negative tumour cell lines but occurs almost exclusively in normal human keratinocytes.

CERVICAL NEOPLASIA: TRANSIENT VERSUS PERSISTENT INFECTIONS

Nearly 30 HPV types infect the genital tract, and a subset of these are the aetiological agents of cervical cancers. Some 99.7% of cervical malignancies contain HPV sequences, and at least 13 types (HPV 16, 18, 31, 33, 35, 39, 45, 51, 52, 56, 58, 59, 66) are defined as class I carcinogenic to humans.

In contrast, HPV 6 and 11 are classified as possibly carcinogenic because of their association with laryngeal cancer, while HPV 40, 42, 43, 44, 54, 61, 70, 72 and 81 are termed low-risk types as infections of the genital tract by these viruses are not associated with the development of anogenital malignancies (Cogliano *et al.*, 2005). HPV 16 is the most prevalent type, found in 56–64% of the cases and also in 25–29% of the control subjects. HPV 18 is found in 3.7–20% of the cases in Europe but is more common in Asia and Africa (Muñoz *et al.*, 2003).

Transient genital HPV infections are quite common in young sexually active women (prevalence 11–20%). Many infections are subclinical and resolve, and most lesions that develop are self-limiting proliferations (low-grade squamous intraepithelial lesions, LSILs) and resolve spontaneously. Nevertheless, a minority of women develop persistent infections with focally high levels of high-risk HPV DNA. Some of these progress to high-grade squamous intraepithelial lesions (HSILs), and some HSILs progress to invasive carcinomas. LSIL is usually the reflection of a clinically apparent transient productive infection with HPV. Although the epithelium shows minor histological abnormalities, terminal differentiation of keratinocytes, which is a necessity for progeny production, takes place. The key question therefore is what events prohibit the completion of the natural viral life cycle. It has been known for quite a time that HPV can cause latent infections. Evidence from immunosuppressed patients and children with laryngeal papillomatosis suggests that true latent HPV infections, at least for some viral types, do exist (Berg and Lampe, 1981; Steinberg *et al.*, 1983; Sillman *et al.*, 1984; Blohme and Brynge, 1985; Ferenczy *et al.*, 1985; Penn, 1986; de Villiers *et al.*, 1997). Several early studies demonstrated the presence of HPV DNA in the absence of morphological changes characteristic of HPV infections, but this did not provide compelling evidence of a latent state (Syrjanen, 1989; Nuovo *et al.*, 1992). If HPV latency is defined only as the presence of viral DNA in the absence of differentiation-dependent virion production, it would be equivalent to persistency. However, not all latent infections are persistent, but some persistent infections are not truly latent in the sense that clinical symptoms such as SILs may develop (see Table 19.1).

An example of a true latent state comes from treatments for laryngeal papillomatosis. Despite the removal of infected tissues by laser treatments, and the confirmation that HPV 11 is not present in adjoining tissues, papillomas consistently and rapidly recur (Ferenczy *et al.*, 1985). How could a latent state for HPV occur *in vivo*? Such a latent state may require the presence of infected cells that fail to differentiate. For instance, an infected stem cell could remain dormant and so achieve a state of an abortive latent infection. The failure of the infected cell to enter the cell cycle could depend on the activities or levels of viral proteins such as E6 and E7 or could be due to the lack of an external signal that allows stem cells to enter the cell cycle. If such a cell starts to divide because of wound healing processes or during metaplastic events, the

Table 19.1 Classification of infections.

Type of infection	Infection state	Symptoms	Progression risk
Transient	Latent	No lesion	?
	Productive	LSIL	Low
	Abortive	Fast-developing HSIL in young women	Medium
Persistent	Latent	No lesion	?
	Productive	Persisting LSIL for > 2 years	Low
	Abortive	HSIL	High

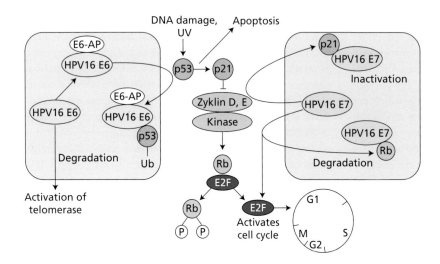

Fig. 19.3 Schematic illustration of the action of E6 and E7 oncoproteins of the anogenital high-risk HPV 16.

viral genome is distributed to the daughter cells, and the viral oncogenes may impede the terminal differentiation of the later ones, resulting in lesions with multiple layers of dividing cells called HSILs.

Cell transformation by E6 and E7 proteins

The important role of a continuous expression of the E6/E7 oncogenes for the immortalised phenotype was demonstrated by experiments with HPV containing cell lines in which E6/E7 expression was inhibited by inducible antisense constructs and which showed an inhibition of growth (von Knebel Doeberitz *et al.*, 1988, 1992) and a loss of the ability to induce tumours in animals. More recent studies using overexpression of E2- or siRNA-mediated gene silencing of E6 and/or E7 supported these findings. Although the E7 proteins of HPV 16 by themselves are able to immortalise primary foreskin keratinocytes (Halbert *et al.*, 1991, 1992; Sedman *et al.*, 1991, 1992), the efficiency of immortalisation can be dramatically increased by co-expression of the HPV 16 E6 protein. The cell-transforming ability of the E6 and E7 proteins strongly correlates with their capacity to bind cell cycle control proteins, such as members of the retinoblastoma family (pRb, p107, p130) and p53, which exhibit tumour-suppressor functions (Münger *et al.*, 1989; Barbosa *et al.*, 1991).

The main function of the pRb proteins in non-HPV-infected cells is to control entry into the S-phase of the cell cycle by sequestering transcription factors of the E2F protein family, which activate S-phase-specific genes with E2F binding sites in their promoters or enhancers (Fig. 19.3). After mitogenic stimulation of cells, the pRb protein is phosphorylated by cyclin-dependent kinases, leading to a release of E2F transcription factors from the pRb proteins, which then promote transcription of genes with E2F binding sites, resulting in cell replication. In HPV-infected cells, the HPV E7 protein binds to pRb and also leads to a release of E2F, favouring uncontrolled

cell growth. As a defence mechanism, the HPV-infected cell activates the p53 protein by post-translational stabilisation in order to lengthen its half-life from 20 minutes to 3 hours with a corresponding increase in its biological effects. One of the functions of p53 is the triggering of programmed cell death (apoptosis) and the activation of p21, which inhibits the cyclin-dependent kinases responsible for phosphorylation of pRb. However, in order to overcome this, the E6 proteins of high-risk HPVs have evolved to bind the p53 protein and cause its ubiquitin-dependent degradation (Scheffner *et al.*, 1990; Werness *et al.*, 1990; Beer-Romero *et al.*, 1997; Talis *et al.*, 1998; Mantovani and Banks, 2001). Inactivation of Rb by high-risk HPV E7 proteins induces an E2F-dependent entry into S-phase of the cell cycle. However, it also induces an E2F-dependent p53-driven apoptosis, as shown in experiments in which E7 was expressed in the absence of E6. Free E2F proteins upregulate the p19 ARF protein, which inactivates mdm-2, which is the natural counteractor of p53. For HPV to overcome the E7-induced G1 arrest and apoptosis, the E6 protein both replaces the function of mdm-2 and blocks p53-mediated pathways. In HPV-infected cells, there is a complete switch from hdm-2-mediated degradation of p53 to E6-AP-mediated degradation. While hdm-2 seems to be responsible for maintaining low p53 levels in uninfected cells, this function of hdm-2 is completely abrogated in HPV-infected cells expressing E6. Interestingly, E6-AP, a cellular protein that has no known p53 regulatory function in uninfected cells, becomes the main degradation factor for p53 in infected cells (Mantovani and Banks, 2001). In addition, it has been shown that the E6 proteins of some HPV types bind to a component of the single-strand break DNA repair complex and thereby inhibit its efficiency (Iftner *et al.*, 2002). A persistently infected cell therefore undergoes continuous cell division and is not only no longer able to react in response to DNA damage with G1 arrest or apoptosis, but is also impeded in DNA repair, which clearly supports its pathway to malignancy.

VIRAL AND HOST RISK FACTORS

Human leucocyte antigen haplotypes

The factors that determine whether an HPV infection is cleared or persists and that increase the risk of cervical cancer are not very well defined, but cellular immunity plays a major role. Altered HLA class I allele findings in cervical cancer have long been recognised, and the presence of specific HLA class II alleles may be decisive for the risk for cervical cancer. In the case of HLA class I A2 (Montoya *et al.*, 1998), B44 (Bontkes *et al.*, 1998) and HLA-B7, negative associations (Duggan-Keen *et al.*, 1996) have been described. The most likely underlying mechanism is the allele-specific downregulation of these antigens during cervical carcinogenesis. Downregulation of HLA-B7 on cervical cancer cells is associated with worse survival compared with normal expression of this antigen (Duggan-Keen *et al.*, 1996). In addition, the existence of HPV 16 variants with E6 mutations affecting HLA-A2 and -B7 binding motifs suggests that lack of CD8-restricted epitopes may enable the virus to escape the immune response (Ellis *et al.*, 1995; Yamada *et al.*, 1995).

A large number of human studies have focused on the association of HLA class II and SILs or cervical cancer, and several HLA class II haplotypes were found to be associated with disease, for example DQw3 increases and DR13 (DRB1*1301; Hildesheim and Wang, 2002) decreases the risk for cervical cancer in general. Some associations were found to be type specific, for example DR15 increases the risk for HPV 16-carrying cancer and DR7 may be either protective or increase the risk.

Cellular gene polymorphism

In addition to the functional assessment of differences in the immune response to HPV infections, natural polymorphisms or genetic variations between individuals in important cellular genes seem to constitute separate risk factors. For example, the wild-type p53 protein exhibits a common polymorphism at amino acid 72, resulting in either a proline residue (p53Pro) or an arginine residue (p53Arg) at this position.

This codon 72 polymorphism of the p53 gene has recently been proposed to increase the risk of cervical cancer by Storey *et al.* (1998), who reported that individuals with an Arg/Arg genotype at codon 72 of the p53 gene had a sevenfold increased risk of cervical cancer. However, in a large number of ongoing studies, substantial concern has been raised about a significant role for this polymorphism in the susceptibility to HPV-associated carcinogenesis. Whereas few studies were confirmative (Zehbe *et al.*, 2001), a large body of other studies contradicted this finding (Hayes *et al.*, 1998; Helland *et al.*, 1998; Hildesheim *et al.*, 1998; Josefsson *et al.*, 1998; Lanham *et al.*, 1998; Minaguchi *et al.*, 1998; Rosenthal *et al.*,

1998; Giannoudis *et al.*, 1999; Klaes *et al.*, 1999). A possible reason for the conflicting data could be large differences in the frequency of Arg72 homozygosity in the different populations studied, which made it difficult to define suitable control groups. Another pitfall is the source of DNA used to assess the p53 polymorphism, which differs greatly between the individual reports using peripheral blood lymphocytes, cervical epithelial cells or tumour biopsies. The use of the last source is a cause of erroneous results, because loss of one allele at the p53 locus is a frequent phenomenon of tumour cells, but not of the normal cells within the same patient. Interestingly, a very recent study in patients with the hereditary disease Fanconia anaemia, which is an autosomal recessive disorder characterised by congenital malformations, bone marrow failure and the development of squamous cell carcinomas (SCCs), adds further support to a role for the p53 codon 72 polymorphism as a risk factor for HPV-associated SCC development (Kutler *et al.*, 2003). It was shown that Fanconi anaemia patients with homozygosity for codon 72 p53Arg had a 5.6-fold increased risk of developing HPV-associated cancers compared with Fanconi anaemia patients who did not have Arg72 homozygosity. Unfortunately, however, although vulvar cancer cases were included, no cases of cervical cancer could have been studied in this analysis.

A possible solution to the still unclear role of p52 polymorphisms could be results of more recent analyses showing a trend for an increased frequency of p53 arginine homozygotes among cervical carcinoma patients carrying HPV 16 types with a specific mutation in the E6 gene (a T to G transition at basepair 350, resulting in an amino acid change at position 83 from a leucine to a valine; Brady *et al.*, 1999). A significant over-representation of HPV 16 350G/T variants was also evident in p53 Arg/Arg Dutch women with cervical cancer, which points to an increased carcinogenic effect of HPV 16 350T variants in the context of specific p53 genotypes.

Several other groups have attempted to identify further specific genetic polymorphisms associated with cervical cancer [e.g. MTHFR (Goodman *et al.*, 2001), WAFI (Harima *et al.*, 2001) and IL-10 (Stanczuk *et al.*, 2001)]. Given the large effort and sample size required, however, more data will have to be collected in the future to come to conclusive results.

Loss of heterozygosity

There is a substantial body of literature regarding chromosomal abnormalities in cervical cancer. Although chromosomal aberrations have been identified consistently (Southern and Herrington, 1998; Lazo, 1999; Kaufmann *et al.*, 2002), such as loss of heterozygosity (LOH) at chromosome 3p, 6, 11, 13, 16, 17 and 19, and chromosomal gains at 3q, identifying the target genes (oncogenes/tumour-suppressor genes) affected in these areas will be the next major goal.

Viral variants

Although there are more than 100 HPV types identified, studies on variants in viral genes mainly relate to the E6 gene of HPV type 16 (HPV 16) (Hecht *et al.*, 1995; Lizano *et al.*, 1997; Villa *et al.*, 2000; Chan *et al.*, 2002). It has been reported that HPV 16 variants with nucleotide alterations within the E6 gene, referred to as non-prototype-like variants, are more frequently associated with high-grade CIN and cervical cancer than wild-type genomes (Xi *et al.*, 1997; Zehbe *et al.*, 1998a), although this phenomenon could be population dependent (Zehbe *et al.*, 1998b; Nindl *et al.*, 1999). Based on regional differences, HPV 16 variants have been termed European (E), Asian-American (AA), African (Af1 and Aft) and North American (NA) (Yamada *et al.*, 1997).

Interestingly, a significant over-representation of HPV 16 350G/T variants was detected in cervical cancers of women with a p53 Arg/Arg polymorphism, and a possible differentially oncogenic effect of HPV 16 350G/T variants, which is influenced by the p53 genotype, was therefore suggested (van Duin *et al.*, 2000). Another E6 variant was described, the 131G variant, which was found to be present in 9.6% of cervical carcinoma patients ($n = 94$), of whom 78% had the HLA-B7 allele, already identified as a possible risk factor. Most of the studies performed did not consider other variations that may occur in the E6/E7 region or in other regions of the HPV genome. Therefore, the current risk observed, which is associated with viral variants in general, might be an underestimation. Furthermore, this risk might be influenced by other genomic alterations, and future studies have to be performed to decipher the underlying mechanisms.

Viral load

A number of cross-sectional epidemiological studies using the semi-quantitative HC2 technique (Iftner and Villa, 2003) have demonstrated an association between increasing viral load with HR-HPV types and the risk of cervical cancer. However, estimates of viral copy numbers depend directly on the total input of cells, and adjustment for cellular load is an absolute requirement that is frequently not fulfilled, as in the case of HC2. Using type-specific real-time quantitative polymerase chain reaction (PCR), others (Swan *et al.*, 1999; Ylitalo *et al.*, 2000) have reported a specific association of high viral load with HPV 16 infections that was consistently associated with an increased risk of progression. High copy numbers of 10^7 copies/pg of cellular DNA in patients with normal cytology were found to be increased with the severity of the lesions by a factor of 100 in CIN2/3 patients (Swan *et al.*, 1999). Interestingly, these associations have not been found for other HPV genotypes (Swan *et al.*, 1997; Abba *et al.*, 2003). Only few longitudinal data are available (Ylitalo *et al.*, 2000; Lorincz *et al.*, 2002), and these need to be extended.

Recently, van Duin *et al.* (2002) reported that viral load for HPV 16 in women with normal and abnormal smears is an indicator of incident CIN2/3. Unfortunately, little is known about the relationship of viral load to types other than HPV 16 and cervical neoplasia.

Viral DNA integration

HPV DNA is maintained as an episome in benign infections, whereas integrated HPV genomes are frequently detected in CIN3, cervical cancer and derived cell lines, and it was proposed that this integration event confers a certain growth advantage on the infected cells by activating the expression of the viral oncogenes (zur Hausen, 2000). The current model suggests that the inactivation of the E2 gene as a consequence of integration releases E6/E7 oncogene expression from E2-mediated negative control. However, no evidence has been presented so far that increased E6/E7 expression is indeed necessary for the progression of HPV-induced lesions. Viral DNA integration could simply be a consequence of an environment that does not support HPV DNA replication. This is reinforced by observations that long-term extrachromosomal replication of HR-HPV DNA has not been achieved in established HPV-positive or -negative tumour cell lines, but occurs almost exclusively in normal human keratinocytes (Meyers *et al.*, 1992). Furthermore, a number of studies reported exclusively episomal HPV 16 DNA in 20–70% of cervical cancers (Fuchs *et al.*, 1989; Matsukura *et al.*, 1989; Cullen *et al.*, 1991; Pirami *et al.*, 1997) and in high percentages (75–97%) of CIN3. Therefore, it remains unclear whether HPV integration is simply a consequence of loss of normal epithelial cell differentiation capacity and biologically conveys no further risk downstream or whether the integration event indeed contributes to progression. A full review of this mechanism and others in human HPV-induced oncogenesis has been published by Münger *et al.* (2004).

Epigenetic events

Epigenetic events are those that alter gene expression (e.g. phenotype) without a change in the DNA sequence and include hypermethylation or hypomethylation of genes (e.g. the addition or removal of a methyl group). For example, recent studies (Dong *et al.*, 2001; Virmani *et al.*, 2001) have identified the silencing of tumour-suppressor genes via promoter hypermethylation in HPV-infected host cells as a frequent human epigenetic event. Because of the potential implications for the activity of viral oncogenes or cellular tumour-suppressor genes such as TSLC1 (tumour suppressor in lung cancer), which reveals reduced expression in cervical cancer because of promoter methylation (Steenbergen *et al.*, 2004), continued investigation of epigenetic events in HPV-infected lesions is warranted.

SUMMARY

The persistent infection with one of the HPV types classified as class I carcinogenic for humans, HPV 16, 18, 31, 33, 35, 39, 45, 51, 52, 53, 56, 58, 59 and 66 is a necessary risk factor for the development of cervical cancer. Usually, infections with human papillomaviruses (HPV) are of a transient nature, lead to the production of progeny viruses and take place only in differentiated epithelium. Following entry into basal epithelial cells, HPV genomes are established as autonomously replicating extrachromosomal elements, and a low level of HPV gene expression occurs. Upon differentiation of infected cells, productive replication and expression of capsid genes is induced, resulting in the synthesis of progeny virions. Any event inhibiting the normal differentiation of the epithelium or the prevention of the normal sequence of viral replication may lead to the development of persistent initially latent infections, which can become persistently active as the result of a compromised immune status or other hitherto unknown factors. In persistently active infected cells, HPV DNA and even viral proteins are present, but no differentiation-dependent synthesis of virions occurs. The development of a long-term persistent infection is the decisive factor for the progressive course of the disease, and the identification of factors supporting this development is of major importance. A full review has recently been published by IARC (2005) with the conclusion that 'there is sufficient evidence that testing for human papillomavirus infection as a primary screening modality can reduce cervical cancer incidence and mortality rates'.

ACKNOWLEDGEMENT

The authors wish to thank Professor I. Frazer for permission to reproduce Figure 19.2 from his original article in *Nature Reviews Immunology* (2004).

REFERENCES

Abba MC, Mouron SA, Gomez MA *et al.* (2003) Association of human papillomavirus viral load with HPV16 and high-grade intraepithelial lesion. *International Journal of Gynecological Cancer* 13: 154–158.

Barbosa MS, Vass WC, Lowy DR *et al.* (1991) In vitro biological activities of the E6 and E7 genes vary among human papillomaviruses of different oncogenic potential. *Journal of Virology* 65: 292–298.

Beer-Romero P, Glass S, Rolfe M (1997) Antisense targeting of E6AP elevates p53 in HPV-infected cells but not in normal cells. *Oncogene* 14: 595–602.

Berg JW, Lampe JG (1981) High-risk factors in gynaecologic cancer. *Cancer* 48: 429–441.

Billich A (2003) HPV vaccine MedImmune/GlaxoSmithKline. *Current Opinion in the Investigation of Drugs* 4: 210–213.

Blohme I, Brynger H (1985) Malignant disease in renal transplant patients. *Transplantation* 39: 23–25.

Bontkes HJ, Walboomers JM, Meijer CJ *et al.* (1998) Specific HLA class I down-regulation is an early event in cervical dysplasia associated with clinical progression. *Lancet* 351: 187–188.

Bosch XF, Manos MM, Muñoz N *et al.*(1995) Prevalence of human papillomavirus in cervical cancer: a worldwide perspective. *Journal of the National Cancer Institute* 87: 796–802.

Bosch XF, Lorincz A, Muñoz N *et al.* (2002) The causal relation between human papillomavirus and cervical cancer. *Journal of Clinical Pathology* 55: 244–265.

Boyer SN, Wazer DE, Band V (1996) E7 protein of human papilloma virus-16 induces degradation of retinoblastoma protein through the ubiquitin–proteasome pathway. *Cancer Research* 56: 4620–4624.

Brady CS, Duggan-Keen MF, Davidson JA *et al.* (1999) Human papillomavirus type 16 E6 variants in cervical carcinoma: relationships to host genetic factors and clinical parameters. *Journal of General Virology* 80: 3233–3240.

Chan PK, Lam CW, Cheung TH *et al.* (2002) Association of human papillomavirus type 58 variant with the risk of cervical cancer. *Journal of the National Cancer Institute* 94: 1249–1253.

Chellappan S, Kraus VB, Kroger B *et al.* (1992) Adenovirus E1A, simians virus 40 tumor antigen, and human papillomavirus E7 protein share the capacity to disrupt the interaction between transcription factor E2F and the retinoblastoma gene product. *Proceedings of the National Academy of Sciences of the USA* 89: 4549–4553.

Cheng S, Schmidt-Grimminger DC, Murant T *et al.* (1995) Differentiation-dependent up-regulation of the human papillomavirus E7 gene reactivates cellular DNA replication in suprabasal differentiated keratinocytes. *Genes and Development* 9: 2335–2349.

Cogliano V, Baan R, Straif K *et al.* and the IARC Monograph Working Group (2005) Carcinogenicity of human papillomaviruses. *Lancet Oncology* 6: 204.

Cullen AP, Reid R, Campion M *et al.* (1991) Analysis of the physical state of different human papillomavirus DNAs in intraepithelial and invasive cervical neoplasm. *Journal of Virology* 65: 606–612.

Davies R, Hicks R, Crook T *et al.* (1993) Human papillomavirus type 16 E7 associates with a histone H1 kinase and with p107 through sequences necessary for transformation. *Journal of Virology* 67: 2521–2528.

de Villiers EM, Lavergne D, McLaren K *et al.*(1997) Prevailing papillomavirus types in non-melanoma carcinomas of the skin in renal allograft recipients. *International Journal of Cancer* 73: 356–361.

de Villiers EM, Fauquet C, Broker TR *et al.* (2004) Classification of papillomaviruses. *Virology* 324: 17–27.

Dong SM, Kim HS, Rha SH *et al.* (2001) Promoter hypermethylation of multiple genes in carcinoma of the uterine cervix. *Clinics in Cancer Research* 7: 1982–1986.

Duggan-Keen MF, Keating PJ, Stevens FR *et al.* (1996) Immunogenetic factors in HPV-associated cervical cancer: influence on disease progression. *European Journal of Immunogenetics* 23: 275–284.

Dyson N, Howley PM, Münger K *et al.* (1989) The human papilloma virus-16 E7 oncoprotein is able to bind to the retinoblastoma gene product. *Science* 243: 934–937.

Dyson N, Guida P, Munger K *et al.* (1992) Homologous sequences in adenovirus E1A and human papillomavirus E7 proteins mediate interaction with the same set of cellular proteins. *Journal of Virology* 66: 6893–6902.

Elbel M, Carl S, Spaderna S *et al.* (1997) A comparative analysis of the interactions of the E6 proteins from cutaneous and genital papillomaviruses with p53 and E6AP in correlation of their transforming potential. *Virology* 239: 132–149.

Ellis JR, Keating PJ, Baird J et al.(1995) The association of an HPV16 oncogene variant with HLA-B7 has implications for vaccine design in cervical cancer. *Nature Medicine* 1:464–470.

Ferenczy A, Mitao M, Nagai N et al. (1985) Latent papillomavirus and recurring genital warts. *New England Journal of Medicine* 313: 784–788.

Fraser IH (2004) Prevention of cervical cancer through papillomavirus vaccination. *Nature Immunology* 4: 46–54.

Fuchs PG. Girardi F, Pfister H (1989) Human papillomavirus 16 DNA in cervical cancers and in lymph nodes of cervical cancer patients: a diagnostic marker for early metastases? *International Journal of Cancer* 43: 41–44.

Funk JO, Waga S, Harry JB et al. (1997) Inhibition of CDK activity and PCNA-dependent DNA replication by p21 is blocked by interaction with the HPV-16 E7 oncoprotein. *Genes and Development* 11: 2090–2100.

Gage JR, Meyers C, Wettstein FO (1990) The E7 proteins of the nononcogenic human papillomavirus type 6b (HPV-6b) and of the oncogenic HPV-16 differ in retinoblastoma protein binding and other properties. *Journal of Virology* 64: 723–730.

Giannoudis A, Graham DA, Southern SA et al. (1999) p53 codon 72 ARG/PRO polymorphism is not related to HPV type or lesion grade in low- and high-grade squamous intraepithelial lesions and invasive squamous carcinoma of the cervix. *International Journal of Cancer* 83: 66–69.

Goodman MT, McDuffie K, Hernandez B et al.(2001) Association of methylenetetrahydrofolate reductase polymorphism C677T and dietary folate with the risk of cervical dysplasia. *Cancer Epidemiology Biomarkers and Prevention* 10: 1275–1280.

Halbert CL, Demers GW, Galloway DA (1991) The E7 gene of human papillomavirus type 16 is sufficient for immortalization of human epithelial cells. *Journal of Virology* 65: 473–478.

Halbert CL, Demers GW, Galloway DA (1992) The E6 and E7 genes of human papillomavirus type 6 have weak immortalising activity in human epithelial cells. *Journal of Virology* 66: 2125–2134.

Harima Y, Sawada S, Nagata K et al. (2001) Polymorphism of the WAF1 gene is related to susceptibility to cervical cancer in Japanese women. *International Journal of Molecular Medicine* 7: 261–264.

Harper DM, Franco EL, Wheeler CM et al. (2004) Efficacy of a bivalent L1 virus-like particle vaccine in prevention of infection of human papillomavirus type 16 and 18 in young women; a randomised controlled trial. *Lancet* 364: 1757–1765.

Hayes VM, Hofstra RAM, Buys CH et al. (1998) Homozygous arginine-72 in wild type p53 and risk of cervical cancer. *Lancet* 351: 1756.

Hecht JL, Kadish AS, Jiang G et al. (1995) Generic characterization of the human papillomavirus (HPV) 18 E2 gene in clinical specimens suggests the presence of a subtype with decreased oncogenic potential. *International Journal of Cancer* 60: 369–376.

Helland A, Olsen AO, Gjoen K et al. (1998) An increased risk of cervical intra-epithelial neoplasia grade II–III among human papillomavirus positive patients with the HLA-DQA1*0102–DQB1*0602 haplotype: a population-based case–control study of Norwegian women. *International Journal of Cancer* 76: 19–24.

Hildesheim A, Wang SS (2002) Host and viral genetics and risk of cervical cancer: a review. *Virus Research* 89: 229–240.

Hildesheim A, Schiffman M, Brinton LA et al. (1998) p53 polymorphism and risk of cervical cancer. *Nature* 396: 531–532.

Huibregtse JM, Scheffner M, Howley PM (1991) A cellular protein mediates association of p53 with the E6 oncoprotein of human papillomavirus types 16 or 18. *EMBO Journal* 10: 4129–4135.

IARC World Health Organization (2005) *IARC Handbooks of Cancer Prevention, Vol. 10: Cervical Cancer Screening.* Lyon: IARC Press.

Iftner T, Elbel M, Schopp B et al. (2002) Interference of papillomavirus E6 protein with single-strand break repair by interaction with XRCC1. *EMBO Journal* 21 (17): 4741–4748.

Iftner T, Villa LL (2003) Human papillomavirus technologies. *Journal of the National Cancer Institute Monographs* 31: 80–88.

Jones DL, Alani RM, Munger K (1997) The human papillomavirus E7 oncoprotein can uncouple cellular differentiation and proliferation in human keratinocytes by abrogating p21Cip1-mediated inhibition of cdk2. *Genes and Development* 11: 2101–2111.

Josefsson AM, Magnusson PK, Ylitalo N et al. (1998) p53 polymorphism and risk of cervical cancer. *Nature* 396: 531.

Kaufmann AM, Backsch C, Schneider A et al. (2002) HPV induced cervical carcinogenesis: molecular basis and vaccine development. *Zentralblatt für Gynäkologie* 124: 511–524.

Klaes R, Ridder R, Schaefer U et al. (1999) No evidence of p53 allele-specific predisposition in human papillomavirus-associated cervical cancer. *Journal of Molecular Medicine* 77: 299–302.

Koutsky LA, Ault KA, Wheeler CM et al. (2002) A controlled trial of a human papillomavirus type 16 vaccine. *New England Journal of Medicine* 347:1645–1651.

Kutler DI, Wreesmann VB, Goberdhan A et al. (2003) Human papillomavirus DNA and p53 polymorphisms in squamous cell carcinomas from Fanconi anemia patients. *Journal of the National Cancer Institute* 95: 1718–1721.

Laimins LA (1996) Human papillomaviruses target differentiating epithelium for virion production and malignant conversion. *Seminars in Virology* 7: 305–313.

Lanham S, Campbell I, Watt P et al. (1998) p53 polymorphism and risk of cervical cancer. *Lancet* 352: 1631.

Lazo PA (1999) The molecular genetics of cervical carcinoma. *British Journal of Cancer* 80: 2008–2018.

Lizano M, Berumen J, Guido MC et al. (1997) Association between human papillomavirus type 18 variants and histopathology of cervical cancer. *Journal of the National Cancer Institute* 89: 1227–1231.

Lorincz AT, Castle PE, Sherman ME et al. (2002) Viral load of human papillomavirus and risk of CIN3 or cervical cancer. *Lancet* 360: 228–229.

McIntyre MC, Ruesch MN, Laimins LA (1996) Human papillomavirus E7 oncoproteins bind a single form of cyclin E in a complex with cdk2 and p107. *Virology* 215: 73–82.

Mantovani F, Banks L (2001) The human papillomavirus E6 protein and its contribution to malignant progression. *Oncogene* 20: 7874–7887.

Matsukura T, Koi S, Sugase M (1989) Both episomal and integrated forms of human papillomavirus type 16 are involved in invasive cervical cancers. *Virology* 172: 63–72.

Meyers C, Frattini MG, Hudson JB et al. (1992) Biosynthesis of human papillomavirus from a continuous cell line upon epithelial differentiation. *Science* 257: 971–973.

Minaguchi T, Kanamori Y, Matsushima M et al. (1998) No evidence of correlation between polymorphism at codon 72 of p53 and risk of cervical cancer in Japanese patients with human papillomavirus 16/18 infection. *Cancer Research* 58: 4585–4586.

Montoya L, Saiz I, Rey G *et al.* (1998) Cervical carcinoma: human papillomavirus infection and HLA-associated risk factors in the Spanish population. *European Journal of Immunogenetics* 25: 329–337.

Münger K, Howley PM (2002) Human papillomavirus immortalization and transformation functions. *Virus Research* 89: 213–228.

Münger K, Phelps WC, Bubb V *et al.* (1989) The E6 and E7 genes of the human papillomavirus type 16 together are necessary and sufficient for transformation of primary human keratinocytes. *Journal of Virology* 63: 4417–4421.

Münger K, Scheffner M, Huibregtse JM *et al.* (1992) Interactions of HPV E6 and E7 with tumor suppressor gene products. *Cancer Surveys* 12: 197–217.

Münger K, Baldwin A, Edwards KM *et al.* (2004) Mechanisms of human papillomavirus-induced oncogenesis (review). *Journal of Virology* 78 (21): 11451–11460.

Muñoz N, Bosch FX, de Sanjose S *et al.* (2003) Epidemiologic classification of human papillomavirus types associated with cervical cancer. *New England Journal of Medicine* 348: 518–527.

Nindl I, Rindfleisch K, Lotz B *et al.* (1999) Uniform distribution of HPV 16 E6 and E7 variants in patients with normal histology, cervical intra-epithelial neoplasia and cervical cancer. *International Journal of Cancer* 82: 203–207.

Nuovo GJ, Becker J, Margotta M *et al.* (1992) Histological distribution of polymerase chain reaction-amplified human papillomavirus 6 and 11 DNA in penile lesions. *American Journal of Surgical Pathology* 16: 269–275.

Penn I (1986) Cancers of the anogenital region in renal transplant recipients. Analysis of 65 cases. *Cancer* 58: 611–616.

Pirami L, Giache V, Becciolini A (1997) Analysis of HPV 16, 18, 31 and 35 DNA in pre-invasive and invasive lesions of the uterine cervix. *Journal of Clinical Pathology* 50: 600–604.

Rosenthal AN, Ryan A, Al-Jehani RM *et al.* (1998) p53 codon 72 polymorphism and risk of cervical cancer in UK. *Lancet* 352: 871–975.

Ruesch MN, Laimins LA (1998) Human papillomavirus oncoproteins alter differentiation-dependent cell cycle exit on suspension in semi-solid medium. *Virology* 250: 19–29.

Scheffner M, Werness BA, Huibregtse JM *et al.* (1990) The E6 oncoprotein encoded by human papillomavirus types 16 and 18 promotes degradation of p53. *Cell* 63: 1129–1136.

Schmitt A, Harry JB, Rapp B *et al.* (1994) Comparison of the properties of the E6 and E7 genes of low- and high-risk cutaneous papillomaviruses reveals strongly transforming and high Rb-binding activity for the E7 protein of the low-risk human papillomavirus type 1. *Journal of Virology* 68: 7051–7059.

Sedman SA, Barbosa M, Vass WC *et al.* (1991) The full length E6 protein of human papillomavirus type 16 has transforming and trans-activating activities and cooperates with E7 to immortalise keratinocytes in culture. *Journal of Virology* 65: 4860–4866.

Sedman SA, Hubbert NL, Vass WC *et al.* (1992) Mutant p53 can substitute for human papillomavirus type 16 E6 in immortalization of human keratinocytes but does not have E6-associated trans-activation or transforming activity. *Journal of Virology* 66: 4201–4208.

Sillman F, Stanek A, Sedlis A *et al.* (1984) The relationship between human papillomavirus and lower genital intraepithelial neoplasia in immunosuppressed women. *American Journal of Obstetrics and Gynecology* 150: 300–308.

Southern SA, Herrington CS (1998) Molecular events in uterine cervical cancer. *Sexually Transmitted Infection* 74: 101–109.

Stanczuk GA, Sibanda EN, Perrey C *et al.* (2001) Cancer of the uterine cervix may be significantly associated with a gene polymorphism coding for increased IL-10 production. *International Journal of Cancer* 94: 792–794.

Steenbergen RD, Kramer D, Braakhuis BJ *et al.* (2004) TSLC1 gene silencing in cervical cancer cell lines and cervical neoplasia. *Journal of the National Cancer Institute* 96: 296–305.

Steinberg BM, Topp WC, Schneider PS *et al.* (1983) Laryngeal papillomavirus infection during clinical remission. *New England Journal of Medicine* 308: 1261–1264.

Storey A, Thomas M, Kalita A *et al.* (1998) Role of a p53 polymorphism in the development of human papillomavirus-associated cancer. *Nature* 393 (6682): 229–234.

Stubenrauch F, Hummel M, Iftner T *et al.* (2000) The E8E2C protein, a negative regulator of viral transcription and replication, is required for extrachromosomal maintenance of human papillomavirus type 31 in keratinocytes. *Journal of Virology* 74: 1178–1186.

Stubenrauch F, Zobel T, Iftner T (2001) The E8 domain confers a novel long-distance transcriptional repression activity on the E8^E2C protein of high-risk human papillomavirus type 31. *Journal of Virology* 75: 4139–4149.

Swan DC, Tucker RA, Holloway BP *et al.* (1997) A sensitive, type-specific, fluorogenic probe assay for detection of human papillomavirus DNA. *Journal of Clinical Microbiology* 35: 886–891.

Swan DC, Tucker RA, Tortolero-Luna G *et al.* (1999) Human papillomavirus (HPV) DNA copy number is dependent on grade of cervical disease and HPV type. *Journal of Clinical Microbiology* 37: 1030–1034.

Syrjanen KJ (1989) Epidemiology of human papillomavirus (HPV) infections and their associations with genital squamous cell cancer. *APMIS* 97: 957–970.

Talis AL, Huibregtse JM, Howley PM (1998) The role of E6AP in the regulation of p53 protein levels in human papillomavirus (HPV)-positive and HPV-negative cells. *Journal of Biological Chemistry* 273: 6439–6445.

Tommasino M, Adamczewski JP, Carlotti F *et al.* (1993) HPV16E7 protein associates with the protein kinase p33CDK2 and cyclin A. *Oncogene* 8: 195–202.

van Duin M, Snijders PJ, Vossen MT *et al.* (2000) Analysis of human papillomavirus type 16 E6 variants in relation to p53 codon 72 polymorphism genotypes in cervical carcinogenesis. *Journal of General Virology* 81: 317–325.

van Duin M, Snijders PJ, Schrijnemakers HF *et al.* (2002) Human papillomavirus 16 load in normal and abnormal cervical scrapes: an indicator of CIN II/III and viral clearance. *International Journal of Cancer* 98: 590–595.

Villa LL, Sichero L, Rahal P *et al.* (2000) Molecular variants of human papillomavirus types 16 and 18 preferentially associated with cervical neoplasia. *Journal of General Virology* 81: 2959–2968.

Villa LL, Costa RL, Petta CA *et al.* (2005) Prophylactic quadrivalent human papillomavirus (Type 6, 11, 16 and 18) L1 virus-like particle vaccine in young women: a randomised double blind placebo-controlled multi-centre phase 2 efficacy trial. *Lancet Oncology* 615: 256–257.

Virmani AK, Muller C, Rathi A *et al.* (2001) Aberrant methylation during cervical carcinogenesis. *Clinics in Cancer Research* 7: 584–589.

von Knebel-Döberitz M, Oltersdorf T, Schwarz E *et al.* (1988) Correlation of modified human papillomavirus early gene expression with altered growth properties in C4-1 cervical carcinoma cells. *Cancer Research* 48: 3780–3786.

von Knebel-Döberitz M, Rittmüller C, zur Hausen H *et al.* (1992) Inhibition of tumourigenicity of cervical cancer cells in nude mice by HPV E6–E7 anti-sense RNA. *International Journal of Cancer* 51: 831–834.

Walboomers JMM, Jacobs MV, Manos MM *et al.*(1999) Human papillomavirus is a necessary cause of invasive cervical cancer worldwide. *Journal of Pathology* 189: 12–19.

Werness BA, Levine AJ, Howley PM (1990) Association of human papillomavirus types 16 and 18 E6 proteins with p53. *Science* 248: 76–79.

Wilson VG, West M, Woytek K *et al.* (2002) Papillomavirus E1 proteins: form, function, and features. *Virus Genes* 24: 275–290.

Xi LF, Koutsky LA, Galloway DA *et al.* (1997) Genomic variation of human papillomavirus type 16 and risk for high grade cervical intraepithelial neoplasia. *Journal of the National Cancer Institute* 89: 796–802.

Yamada T, Manos MM, Peto J *et al.* (1995) Human papillomavirus type 16 sequence variation in cervical cancers: a worldwide perspective. *Journal of Virology* 71: 2463–2472.

Yee AS, Shih HH, Tevosian SG (1998) New perspectives on retinoblastoma family functions in differentiation. *Frontiers in Bioscience* 3: D532–D547.

Ylitalo N, Sorensen P, Josefsson AM *et al.* (2000) Consistent high viral load of human papillomavirus 16 and risk of cervical carcinoma in situ: a nested case–control study. *Lancet* 355: 2194–2198.

Zehbe I, Voglino G, Delius H *et al.* (1988a) Risk of cervical cancer and geographical variations of human papillomavirus 16 E6 polymorphisms. *Lancet* 352: 1441–1442.

Zehbe I, Wilander E, Delius H *et al.* (1998b) Human papillomavirus 16 E6 variants are more prevalent in invasive cervical carcinoma than the prototype. *Cancer Research* 58: 829–833.

Zehbe I, Voglino G, Wilander E *et al.* (2001) p53 codon 72 polymorphism and various human papillomavirus 16 E6 genotypes are risk factors for cervical cancer development. *Cancer Research* 61: 608–611.

Zerfass-Thome K, Zwerschke W, Mannhardt B *et al.* (1996) Inactivation of the cdk inhibitor p27KIP1 by the human papillomavirus type 16 E7 oncoprotein. *Oncogene* 13: 2323–2330.

Zobel T, Iftner T, Stubenrauch F (2003) The papillomavirus E8-E2C protein represses DNA replication from extrachromosomal origins. *Molecular and Cellular Biology* 23: 8352–8362.

zur Hausen H (1996) Roots and perspectives of contemporary papillomavirus research. *Journal of Cancer Research and Clinical Oncology* 122 (1): 3–13.

zur Hausen H (2000) Papillomaviruses causing cancer: evasion from host-cell control in early event in carcinogenesis. *Journal of the National Cancer Institute* 92: 690–698.

CHAPTER 20

Angiogenesis in cervical neoplasia

Peter W. Hewett and Asif Ahmed

INTRODUCTION

Squamous cervical cancer arises from the metaplastic epithelium of the transformation zone and develops slowly through progressive dysplastic changes to carcinoma *in situ* and invasive cancer. Cervical intraepithelial neoplasia is (CIN) divided into three stages according to the degree of epithelial dysplasia and differentiation, and the lesions are accessible to colposcopic biopsy, making it relatively easy to monitor disease progression. Low-grade CIN may spontaneously regress, or not progress further, and the malignant potential of CIN3 is 36% over 20 years (McIndoe *et al.*, 1984). There is considerable controversy surrounding the possible overtreatment of patients with mild cervical abnormalities, which are often excised or ablated, and markers of those lesions that will progress would be of great prognostic value (Shafi and Luesley, 1995); see Chapters 28A and B. Adenocarcinomas account for approximately 20% of invasive cervical cancers, and their incidence is increasing, notably among women under 35 years old, with no evidence of a reduction since the introduction of mass screening programmes (Chilvers, 1994; Zheng *et al.*, 1996; Waggoner, 2003).

Over the past few decades, significant advances have been made in understanding the molecular genetics underlying the development of human cancers. However, we are still far from constructing complete sequelae of events leading to the development of invasive cervical cancer. There are many associated risk factors, including number of sexual partners, parity, oral contraceptive use and smoking (Green *et al.*, 2003), but persistent human papillomavirus (HPV) 16 and 18 infection is the most significant factor in the aetiology of this disease (Haverkos *et al.*, 2000; zur Hausen, 2002). HPV E6 and E7 early proteins activate oncogenes such as c-*fos* and inactivate the tumour-suppressor genes, p53 and retinoblastoma protein (Rb) (see Chapter 19). However, additional genetic alterations may be required to maintain a malignant phenotype. For example, the presence of H-*ras* mutations in CIN2 and 3 is implicated in very rapid malignant progression within 2 years (Alonio *et al.*, 2003).

This chapter will consider the regulation and significance of angiogenesis and lymphangiogenesis in the development, diagnosis and treatment of cervical neoplasia. It will focus on the gross vascular changes that occur in late CIN, which have been recognised for many years, and the significant increases in microvessel density (MVD) associated with these changes. Factors that initiate angiogenesis in CIN will be considered, and the role of the vascular endothelial growth factor (VEGF) family will be discussed. Consideration of angiogenesis and lymphangiogenesis may provide some further evidence as to the fundamental aetiological mechanisms inherent in the cause of cervical neoplasia.

MECHANISMS OF NEW VESSEL GROWTH

Vasculogenesis

Blood vessels develop initially by the process of vasculogenesis, which involves the *in situ* differentiation of endothelial cells from mesenchymal precursors (Risau and Flamme, 1995). In early development, haemangioblasts differentiate to give rise to the blood and endothelial cells, which coalesce to form a primary capillary plexus and are then remodelled acquiring perivascular cells [smooth muscle cells (SMCs) and pericytes] to form the major vessels (aorta and great veins) (Risau and Flamme, 1995). The vascular network is extended by angiogenesis, a process that continues in the cycling endometrium, wound healing and various pathologies (Risau, 1997). Although originally thought to be limited to embryological development, it is now apparent that vasculogenesis also occurs in the adult through the release of endothelial progenitor cells (EPCs) from the bone marrow under the control of circulating factors such as VEGF and the angiopoietins. Circulating EPCs are incorporated at sites of both physiological and pathological angiogenesis and contribute to developing vessels (Asahara *et al.*, 1999).

Angiogenesis

This is a highly regulated process involving coordinated endothelial cell proliferation, migration, tube formation and remodelling to form new blood vessels (Risau, 1997; Carmeliet, 2000). It is typically viewed as the sprouting of new vessels from postcapillary venules, with local vasodilation, vascular leakage and basement membrane degradation preceding the proliferation and migration of endothelial cells into the surrounding extracellular matrix (ECM) and the formation of tubes (canalisation). These subsequently anastomose and are remodelled acquiring mesenchymal perivascular cells to form differentiated vascular networks (Risau, 1997; Carmeliet, 2000). However, blood vessels are also generated through vessel elongation (endothelial cell rolling) and 'intussusception', in which pre-existing vessels are divided by longitudinal folding or invading tissue columns (Burri and Tarek, 1990; Patan, 1998; Carmeliet, 2000). In addition, existing collateral arteries are remodelled and extended in ischaemia by the distinct process of *arteriogenesis*, which requires different cues and is dependent on blood flow and leucocyte invasion (Carmeliet, 2000).

Lymphangiogenesis

The discovery of the lymphangiogenic factors VEGF-C and VEGF-D (see below) and the transcription factor Prox-1 (Wigle and Oliver, 1999) has shed new light on the formation of lymphatic vessels. In the fetus, lymphatic vessels sprout from the lymphatic sacs, derived from the jugular and perimesonephric large central veins. Further lymphatic vessels may develop through a process analogous to vasculogenesis with the *in situ* differentiation of mesenchymal lymphangioblasts into lymphatic endothelial cells (Karkkainen *et al.*, 2001). This process may continue in the adult through the release of circulating lymphatic endothelial progenitors (Schoppmann *et al.*, 2002).

Tumour angiogenesis

Since the pioneering work of Dr Judah Folkman and colleagues in the early 1970s, tumour angiogenesis has been recognised as a critical factor in the malignant progression of tumours (Folkman, 1971; Folkman and Hanahan, 1991). The supporting vasculature of tumours not only delivers oxygen and essential nutrients to the growing tumour cells but also provides a route for metastatic spread (Liotta *et al.*, 1991). The development of tumours has conventionally been considered to follow a prevascular phase in which the growth of the primary tumour is restricted to a few millimetres in diameter as a result of the diffusion limit of oxygen (Folkman and Hanahan, 1991). The tumour may remain dormant for many years before acquiring the ability to stimulate neovascularisation through the production of angiogenic factors (Holmgren *et al.*, 1995; Holmgren, 1996). This model appears to be consistent with the development of tumours that arise in epithelial tissues such as breast, colon and cervix where the malignant cells are separated from the supporting vasculature by a basement membrane (Hanahan *et al.*, 1996). However, recent evidence

suggests that primary tumours or metastases developing in highly vascular tissues such as the lung can grow initially by parasitising the pre-existing host vasculature (Holmgren, 1996). This may subsequently regress, leaving an avascular tumour that cannot grow further without acquiring an angiogenic phenotype and inducing new vessel growth (Holash *et al.*, 1999).

In the majority of healthy adult tissues, the rate of endothelial cell division is extremely low, and vascular quiescence is maintained by a predominance of angiogenic inhibitors such as thrombospondin-1 and the close association of endothelial and perivascular cells (Hanahan, 1997; Holash *et al.*, 1999; Carmeliet, 2000). However, in the presence of elevated concentrations of pro-angiogenic factors and/or reduced levels of angiogenesis inhibitors, endothelial cell cycle time can be reduced from years to just a few days. Angiogenesis is therefore controlled dynamically by the local tissue concentrations of pro- and anti-angiogenic factors. Stimuli that alter the local balance of pro- and anti-angiogenic factors in favour of blood vessel formation are thought to constitute 'angiogenic switches' (Folkman and Hanahan, 1991; Hanahan *et al.*, 1996). Physiological factors such as tissue hypoxia or the activation of oncogenes (e.g. H-*ras*, *src*, *HER-2/neu*) or loss of tumour-suppressor gene expression (e.g. p53, Rb, p16) in malignancy may trigger the development of new vessels (Carmeliet and Jain, 2000; Rak and Klement, 2000; Rak *et al.*, 2000).

ASSESSING ANGIOGENESIS IN TUMOURS

It was Weidner and colleagues who first demonstrated a correlation between MVD, as an indicator of tumour angiogenesis, and survival in breast cancer (Weidner *et al.*, 1991; Weidner, 1993), and it has since been found to have prognostic significance in many human cancers. MVD is conventionally determined in regions of high vascularity ('vascular hotspots') in histological sections stained with an endothelial marker such as von Willebrand factor (VWF) or CD31 (Weidner *et al.*, 1991). Tumours are often highly heterogeneous with regard to microvessel content, and vascular hotspots are found by scanning the histological section under low magnification; vessels are then counted at higher magnification by independent observers or automated digital analysis. While this technique has proved to be a useful indicator of tumour angiogenesis, it is important to recognise its limitations: (i) it is invasive requiring a biopsy; (ii) only a small part of a larger tumour may be sampled; and (iii) histological sections are essentially two-dimensional, and vessel counts may be exaggerated by the presence of tortuous vessels. Alternative non-invasive continuous methods are being developed to give a more accurate measurement of angiogenesis throughout the tumour. For example, in the cervix, transvaginal power Doppler ultrasound blood flow measurements have been used to assess angiogenesis (Hawighorst *et al.*, 1998). In the future, it may be possible to monitor levels of angiogenic factors in the circulation or wet cell-based screens to identify early cervical lesions requiring treatment.

ANGIOGENESIS AND CERVICAL CANCER

Premalignant cervical lesions

The association of gross vascular changes, visible as epithelial punctation and mosaicism, in CIN3 has been recognised for many years and utilised as colposcopic diagnostic indicators (Stafl and Mattingly, 1975) (Fig. 20.1). We (Dobbs *et al.*, 1997) and others (Smith-McCune and Weidner, 1994; Guidi *et al.*, 1995; Dellas *et al.*, 1997; Obermair *et al.*, 1997; Smith-McCune *et al.*, 1997; Ozalp *et al.*, 2003) identified increases in MVD in the stroma subtending the dysplastic epithelium with grade of CIN, indicating that angiogenesis occurs early in disease progression. We observed progressive increases in MVD with malignancy, which were significant even in low- to moderate-grade CIN (1 and 2) compared with normal cervical tissue from patients undergoing hysterectomy (Dobbs *et al.*, 1997). However, Guidi and colleagues (1995) and Smith-McClune and Weidner (1994) found that increases in MVD reached significance only in high-grade CIN3 and invasive squamous cell carcinomas, but used adjacent benign/normal tissue as controls. Similarly, Obermair *et al.* (1997) reported a significant increase in MVD between CIN1/CIN2 and CIN3 but did not examine MVD in normal cervix. The subepithelial stroma of non-dysplastic epithelium adjacent to CIN lesions has since been shown to have significantly higher MVD than cervical tissue with no evidence of CIN from hysterectomy

patients (Smith-McCune *et al.*, 1998). Conversely, other studies have not observed elevated MVD in carcinoma *in situ* compared with normal control tissues (Leung *et al.*, 1994; Abulafia *et al.*, 1996).

In addition to human cervical neoplasia, Smith McCune and colleagues (1997) also examined MVD in an elegant multistage murine model of squamous carcinogenesis where HPV

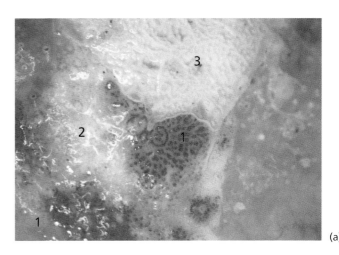

(a)

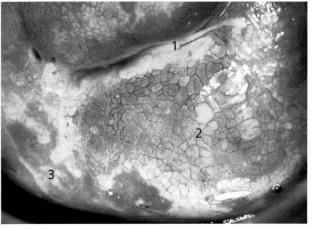

(b)

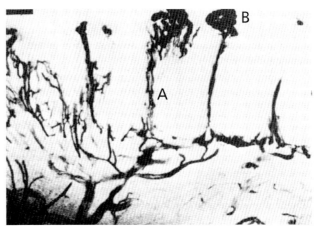

(c)

Fig. 20.1 (*right*) (a) Capillaries within premalignant epithelium (CIN) are seen through the colposcope as end-on red points (1). The term punctation is used to describe this appearance, which represents the dilated and often twisted and irregular terminating vessels of a particular hairpin-type appearance. They can be elongated and arranged in a prominent punctated pattern. They are associated with all the changes of CIN. In this colpophotograph, the white epithelium seen at (2) and (3) represents the presence of human papillomavirus (HPV) within this tissue. (b) This colpophotograph shows the appearance of capillaries within the epithelium in a wall-like structure that subdivides blocks of tissue in a honeycomb fashion and is called a mosaic pattern. Capillaries are arranged parallel to the surface, thereby forming this quasi-pavement-like appearance, and they enclose a vascular field that ranges from small to large and may be regular or irregular. (1) in this photograph shows the abnormal premalignant tissue (CIN) extending into the endocervix and at (2) the classical mosaic pattern is seen, with the boundary of the abnormal tissue in the region of (3). (c) This photomicrograph (angiography using alkaline phosphatase, 125-μm section) demonstrates that the mosaic vessel forms basket-like structures that surround blocks of neoplastic cells. The figure shows these coiled intraepithelial capillaries at (A) with numerous subepithelial vessels ending in a capillary network beneath the epithelium at (B).

16 early genes are expressed in the basal squamous epithelium under the control of the keratin 14 promoter. Angiogenesis occurred in the local supporting endothelium adjacent to the neoplastic epithelium in a similar manner to that observed in the early premalignant stages of human squamous carcinogenesis, and further increases in MVD were noted in high-grade premalignant lesions.

Invasive cancers of the cervix

The prognostic significance of MVD in invasive cervical cancers may depend on tumour type, stage and treatment regimen. However, in the majority of studies, high MVD is associated with reduced patient survival (Schlenger *et al.*, 1995; Wiggins *et al.*, 1995; Abulafia *et al.*, 1996; Bremer *et al.*, 1996; Dinh *et al.*, 1996; Dellas *et al.*, 1997; Kaku *et al.*, 1998; Obermair *et al.*, 1998). For example, a high MVD has been reported to predict an increased rate of recurrence (Dinh *et al.*, 1996) and represents a strong independent prognostic indicator of disease-free/ overall survival (Dellas *et al.*, 1997; Obermair *et al.*, 1998) in FIGO stage IB squamous cell carcinoma (SCC). In more advanced (FIGO IB–IVA) cervical cancers, MVD was found to be the strongest independent prognostic indicator (Schlenger *et al.*, 1995; Wiggins *et al.*, 1995). Conversely, a high MVD has been shown to predict improved patient survival following chemotherapy (Kohno *et al.*, 1993), and both improved (Siracka *et al.*, 1988) and reduced (Schlenger *et al.*, 1995; Cooper *et al.*, 1999) survival following radiotherapy. Other studies report no correlation between MVD and prognosis in SCC (Rutgers *et al.*, 1995), or poorer recurrence-free interval in tumours with a low MVD (Kainz *et al.*, 1995).

Fewer studies have examined the impact of MVD on adenocarcinomas of the cervix. In one study of 56 early invasive cervical adenocarcinomas (FIGO I and II), Kaku and colleagues (1998) reported significant increases in MVD associated with ascites cytology, and high MVD was an independent negative prognostic indicator for progression-free survival and overall survival. In addition, patients with the more aggressive adenoma malignum had higher MVD than those with typical cervical adenocarcinomas. Lee and colleagues (2002) examined 37 adenocarcinomas and found MVD to be associated with shorter survival, although it did not reach prognostic significance.

Angiogenic factors in cervical cancer

The malignant progression of cervical carcinoma is associated with increased levels of circulating angiogenic factors. Chopra *et al.* (1998) reported that the serum concentrations of angiogenin, interleukin (IL) 2, IL-6, IL-7, IL-8, IL-10, basic fibroblast growth factor, tumour necrosis factor-α (TNF-α), transforming growth factor-β and granulocyte–monocyte colony-stimulating factor are elevated during the malignant

progression of cervical cancer. In addition to growth factors and cytokines, steroid hormones also modulate the expression of genes involved in angiogenesis and metastasis, and the phase of the menstrual cycle at the time of surgery may significantly affect patient survival (Formenti *et al.*, 2000). In cervical cancer tissue, inhibitor of metalloproteinase (MMP)-2 and COX-2 expression are significantly higher during the proliferative phase of the cycle. Estrogen is also reported to promote vasculogenesis, enhancing the mobilisation and incorporation of bone marrow-derived EPCs into injured carotid vessels (Iwakura *et al.*, 2003).

The vascular endothelial growth factor (VEGF) family is critically required for the development and maintenance of blood and lymphatic vessels (Neufeld *et al.*, 1999; Carmeliet and Collen, 2000). Six VEGF family members (VEGF-A, -B, -C, -D and -E and placenta growth factor/PlGF) have been identified and bind with high affinity to one or more of three tyrosine kinase receptors: Flt-1 (VEGFR-1), KDR/Flk-1 (VEGFR-2) and Flt-4 (VEGFR-3) and with lower affinity to neuropilins (NP-1 and NP-2) (Neufeld *et al.*, 2002) and heparan sulphate-containing proteoglycans (Fig. 20.2). They are pleiotropic, eliciting a wide range of activities in endothelial cells, including proliferation, migration and survival. VEGF-A was the first family member to be identified as the potent vascular permeability-inducing activity produced by tumour cells (Senger *et al.*, 1983). There are at least six human VEGF isoforms ($VEGF_{121}$, $VEGF_{145}$, $VEGF_{162}$, $VEGF_{165}$, $VEGF_{189}$ and $VEGF_{206}$) produced by alternative mRNA splicing that show differing affinities for heparan sulphate, which determines their bioavailability (Houck *et al.*, 1991; Tischer *et al.*, 1991; Charnock-Jones *et al.*, 1993).

In endothelial cells, the major activities of VEGF are mediated by KDR/Flk-1 (Waltenberger *et al.*, 1994; Neufeld *et al.*, 1999). Flt-1 (VEGFR-1) activation upregulates urokinase plasminogen activator and plasminogen activator inhibitor-1 expression (Lymboussaki *et al.*, 1998) and, in part, regulates vascular permeability (Stacker *et al.*, 1999a; Luttun *et al.*, 2002a). Flt-1 is also produced as a soluble truncated receptor (sFlt-1) that sequesters VEGF and acts as a dominant-negative inhibitor of VEGF receptor signalling (Kendall *et al.*, 1996) (Fig. 20.3). Evidence from transgenic mice carrying null or lack of function VEGF receptor mutations indicates that KDR is essential for vasculogenesis (Shalaby *et al.*, 1995), whereas Flt-1 limits the differentiation of haemangioblasts into endothelial cells (Fong *et al.*, 1995, 1999; Hiratsuka *et al.*, 1998). During development, Flt-1 acts primarily as a decoy receptor regulating VEGF availability as: (i) mice lacking both the Flt-1-specific ligands, VEGF-B and PlGF, develop normally; (ii) PlGF expression is virtually absent in the embryo; and (iii) Flt-1 is produced mainly as the soluble receptor during development (Carmeliet *et al.*, 2001). However, activated Flt-1 associates with the p85 subunit of phosphatidylinositol 3-kinase (PI3-kinase), phospholipase C

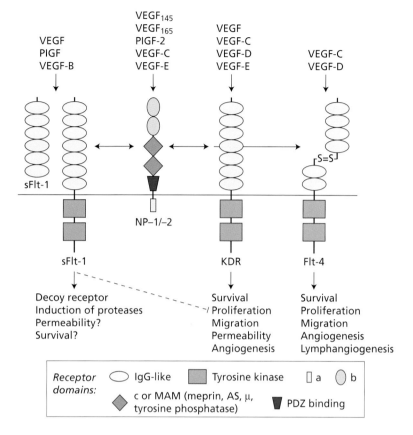

Fig. 20.2 The interactions of the VEGFs with their high-affinity tyrosine kinase receptors, Flt-1, KDR and Flt-4, and accessory receptors, neuropilin-1 and -2 (NP-1/-2). Flt-1, KDR and Flt-4 possess seven immunoglobulin-like loops in the extracellular domain and an intracellular split tyrosine kinase domain and bind VEGFs selectively. NP-1 and NP-2 bind VEGF and PlGF in an isoform-specific manner and interact with Flt-1, KDR and Flt-4 to modulate their activity. Signalling diversity is increased further by the expression of VEGF homo- and heterodimers and the formation of heterodimeric receptor complexes.

(Cunningham *et al.*, 1997; de Vries *et al.*, 1992) and Src (Waltenberger *et al.*, 1994), and we and others have shown that Flt-1 negatively regulates KDR/Flk-1-induced proliferation, via the PI3-kinase pathway (Ahmed *et al.*, 1997; Rahimi *et al.*, 2000; Zeng *et al.*, 2001), promoting the organisation of endothelial cells into capillary-like tube networks (Bussolati *et al.*, 2001). In addition, we have shown that PlGF promotes the long-term survival and stability of capillary-like tube formation in retinal microvessel endothelial cells (Cai *et al.*, 2003).

Flt-1 is an important mediator of pathological angiogenesis

Recent evidence has highlighted the importance of Flt-1 signalling in adult pathologies. The growth of Lewis lung tumours overexpressing PlGF-2 is inhibited in transgenic mice expressing truncated Flt-1 lacking the tyrosine kinase domains (Hiratsuka *et al.*, 2001), and embryonic stem cell-derived tumours growing in PlGF$^{(-/-)}$ mice are small and poorly vascularised (Carmeliet *et al.*, 2001). Flt-1 is also present on monocytes, which migrate and express tissue factor in response to VEGF and PlGF (Clauss *et al.*, 1996). A significant component of Flt-1 activity in pathological conditions may therefore be due to its ability to promote an inflammatory response rather than its direct effect on the endothelium (Carmeliet *et al.*, 2001; Luttun *et al.*, 2002b).

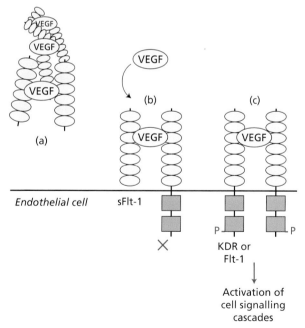

Fig. 20.3 sFlt-1 regulates VEGF availability and activity. (a) It acts as a sink, sequestering its ligands, VEGF, PlGF and VEGF-B, and preventing binding to Flt and KDR. (b) sFlt-1 also acts in a dominant-negative manner to block the formation of Flt-1 and KDR homo- and heterodimers and so prevent (c) their transphorylation/activation.

The recent clinical failure of several KDR tyrosine kinase inhibitors and the success of general VEGF blockade with humanised anti-VEGF antibody (Avastin/Bevacizumab) (Ferrara, 2004) underline the importance and therapeutic potential of the Flt-1 receptor in pathological angiogenesis. Blocking antibodies against Flt-1 suppress tumour angiogenesis (Luttun *et al.*, 2002b), and angiozyme, a ribozyme targeted to Flt-1, has demonstrated good efficacy *in vivo*, producing more pronounced tumour inhibition than a ribozyme against KDR (Weng and Usman, 2001).

VEGF EXPRESSION IN CIN AND INVASIVE CERVICAL CANCER

In common with most tumours, VEGF is a key angiogenic factor in cervical cancer. We observed increased VEGF protein in dysplastic cervical epithelium accompanied by increased MVD in the stroma subtending the epithelial lesion (Dobbs *et al.*, 1997). This concurs with the study by Guidi and colleagues (1995) showing increases in VEGF mRNA in dysplastic epithelium by *in situ* hybridisation. Smith-McCune *et al.* (1997) examined VEGF expression in a multistage model of cervical carcinogenesis (see above), in which expression of HPV 16 early genes in the basal squamous epithelium resulted in a progressive increase in VEGF expression with severity of the epithelial dysplasia/neoplasia.

High levels of VEGF mRNA expression are reported to correlate with MVD in early invasive cervical cancers (Kodama *et al.*, 1999). Although cytosolic VEGF protein is a marker of pelvic lymph node involvement and an independent prognostic indicator in early-stage cervical carcinoma (Cheng *et al.*, 2000), Kodama and colleagues (1999) found no significant difference in VEGF mRNA levels with respect to lymph node metastasis, depth of stromal invasion, tumour size and parametrial or vaginal involvement in patients with invasive cervical cancer. In contrast, Tjalma *et al.* (1998) found an inverse relationship between MVD and VEGF expression in invasive SCC. In adenocarcinomas of the cervix, MVD has also been correlated with VEGF expression (Tokumo *et al.*, 1998; Loncaster *et al.*, 2000).

VEGF expression appears to be a common characteristic of cervical tumour cells. In one study, VEGF-A mRNA was detected in all cervical cancer cell lines investigated (Ueda *et al.*, 2001). Levels of VEGF secretion may in part account for differences in the behaviour of adenocarcinomas and SCC, such as the propensity of adenocarcinomas to metastasise earlier by both lymphatic and haematogenous routes (Santin *et al.*, 1999). While levels of VEGF mRNA are reported to be similar in different histological types (Kodama *et al.*, 1999), the amount of VEGF protein secreted by adenocarcinoma biopsies or established cell lines is reported to be significantly greater than SCC biopsies or cell lines (Santin *et al.*, 1999). In tissue sections, Tokumo and colleagues (1998) found VEGF

expression to be higher in adenocarcinomas (19 cases) than in SCC (51), and correlated with MVD. Conversely, in another study, greater VEGF expression was reported in SCC (94) compared with albeit a small number (5) of adenocarcinomas (Loncaster *et al.*, 2000).

Host cells in the tumour stroma also provide an important source of VEGF. Factors released by the tumour cells, such as epidermal growth factor (EGF) and platelet-derived growth factor, may act indirectly to stimulate cells in the stroma to produce VEGF. In particular, tumour-infiltrating macrophages produce large amounts of VEGF (McLaren *et al.*, 1996) and are associated with increased MVD in endometrial cancer (Hashimoto *et al.*, 2000). A recent study has highlighted the role of tumour-derived fibroblasts, which secrete significantly more VEGF under both normoxic and hypoxic conditions than cervical tumour cell lines (Pilch *et al.*, 2001).

REGULATION OF VEGF EXPRESSION IN CERVICAL CANCER

VEGF expression is regulated by tissue hypoxia, growth factors, cytokines and hormones. The most notable of these is hypoxia, which induces VEGF transcription via hypoxia-inducible factor-1α, and also increases VEGF mRNA stability (Shweiki *et al.*, 1992; Goldberg and Schneider, 1994; Stein *et al.*, 1995; Carmeliet *et al.*, 1998). However, while hypoxia may be an important regulator of VEGF expression in CIN, no correlation was found between VEGF expression and hypoxia in invasive cervical carcinomas (Raleigh *et al.*, 1998; West *et al.*, 2001).

Oncogenes

The activation of oncogenes, including mutant *ras*, EGF receptor family, c-*myc* and v-*src*, or loss of tumour-suppressor genes such as *P53* is often associated with increased VEGF expression (Carmeliet and Jain, 2000; Lopez-Ocejo *et al.*, 2000; Rak and Klement, 2000; Rak *et al.*, 2000). For example, the loss of wild-type p53 increased VEGF expression in fibroblasts from a Li–Fraumeni patient (Dameron *et al.*, 1994), and transfection of wild-type p53 in endometrial cancer cells reduced VEGF secretion (Fujisawa *et al.*, 2003). In cervical adenocarcinomas, p53 mutations correlate with high VEGF expression (Lee *et al.*, 2002). Mutant *ras* induces VEGF production in tumour cells (Rak *et al.*, 2000), and the presence of H-*ras* in CIN2 and 3 is implicated in very rapid malignant progression within 2 years (Alonio *et al.*, 2003). The expression of the EGF receptor-2 (*HER-2/neu/*c-*erbB*-2) is associated with angiogenesis and VEGF upregulation in several tumour types (Petit *et al.*, 1997; Yen *et al.*, 2000; Lee *et al.*, 2002), and this appears to be related to functional changes in Sp-1 transcription factor activity (Finkenzeller *et al.*, 2004). Although overexpression of *HER-2* is not common in invasive SCC (Rosty *et al.*, 2004), VEGF levels were significantly greater in HER-2-positive tumours (Tokumo *et al.*, 1998). In adenocarcinomas of the cervix, HER-2 expression is frequently associated with poor prognosis (Kihana *et al.*, 1994), and significant increases in VEGF expression are detected in HER-2-positive adenocarcinomas (Lee *et al.*, 2002).

HPV infection

HPV infection may promote VEGF expression both directly and indirectly. The HPV 16 and 18 E6 and E7 early viral proteins transform target cells (Woodworth *et al.*, 1988; Barbosa and Schlegel, 1989; Munger *et al.*, 1989) (see Chapter 19). E7 inactivates p53 and Rb (Dyson *et al.*, 1989; Werness *et al.*, 1990), and E6 induces c-*fos* and c-*myc* (Morosov *et al.*, 1994; Kinoshita *et al.*, 1997). The loss of wild-type p53 and Rb and increased expression of c-*myc* and c-*fos* have all been shown to induce VEGF expression in epithelial cells (Carmeliet and Jain, 2000; Rak and Klement, 2000; Rak *et al.*, 2000). Indeed, exogenous E7 increases VEGF production in cervical cancer lines and the angiogenic/inflammatory cytokines TNF-α, IL-1β and IL-6 in macrophages (Le Buanec *et al.*, 1999). It is interesting to note that IL-6 promotes the growth of human cervical (C33A) tumours through the induction of VEGF, which enhanced their angiogenic activity with little direct effect on C33A proliferation *in vitro* (Wei *et al.*, 2003). More recently, HPV 16 E6-positive cells were found to express high levels of VEGF mRNA, and E6 protein induced VEGF promoter activity in both human keratinocytes and mouse fibroblasts in a p53- and EGF-independent manner (Lopez-Ocejo *et al.*, 2000). It appears that E6 may activate VEGF transcription directly via a regulatory region containing four Sp-1 transcription factor binding sites required for constitutive VEGF expression.

Ovarian steroids

The distribution of VEGF correlates with estrogen expression in the mouse uterus (Shweiki *et al.*, 1993), and both estradiol and progestins induce VEGF expression in the rat (Cullinan-Bove and Koos, 1993). The VEGF gene promoter contains estrogen response elements (Tischer *et al.*, 1991), and treatment of breast cancer cells with 17β-estradiol induces a four-fold increase in VEGF mRNA levels mediated through estrogen receptor-α/Sp1 and estrogen receptor-β/Sp3 interactions with GC-rich motifs in the VEGF promoter (Stoner *et al.*, 2004). Estrogen also promotes the recruitment of macrophages and increases their VEGF production and indirectly stimulates VEGF expression in stromal cells (Lebovic *et al.*, 2000; Losordo and Isner, 2001).

The transformation zone is highly sensitive to estrogens, and HPV 16 infection is reported to result in an eightfold increase in the conversion of estradiol to 16α-hydroxyestrone, which in turn enhances HPV gene expression and so may pro-

mote transformation (de Villiers, 2003). Estrogen receptor expression decreases markedly in the later stages of CIN, whereas progesterone receptor levels increase with the progression of CIN (Kanai *et al.*, 1998). However, only 27–28% of cervical carcinomas are progesterone receptor positive and 20–25% estrogen receptor positive (Ghandour *et al.*, 1994; Kanai *et al.*, 1998). Moreover, estrogen responsiveness correlates with disease-free survival in adenocarcinomas (Ghandour *et al.*, 1994), and VEGF levels are unaffected by the phase of the cycle in cervical cancer (Formenti *et al.*, 2000). It is therefore likely that sex steroids have a significant effect on VEGF expression only in early cervical lesions.

LYMPHANGIOGENESIS AND CERVICAL CANCER

VEGF-C and VEGF-D

In contrast to the rest of the VEGF family, VEGF-C and VEGF-D undergo proteolytic processing to increase their affinity for Flt-4 and enable them to bind KDR/Flk-1 (Joukov *et al.*, 1997; Stacker *et al.*, 1999b) (Fig. 20.2). Flt-4$^{(-/-)}$ null mice die at embryonic day 9.5 as a result of vascular insufficiency, demonstrating that Flt-4 is required for vascular development (Kaipainen *et al.*, 1995; Dumont *et al.*, 1998). However, by embryonic day 13.5, Flt-4 becomes restricted to the developing lymphatic vessels. In the adult, Flt-4 is abundant in lymphatic endothelium and is also present in the fenestrated capillaries and venules of endocrine tissues (Pajusola *et al.*, 1992; Partanen *et al.*, 2000). When overexpressed in the skin of transgenic mice, both human VEGF-C and VEGF-D induce the development of lymphatic and blood vessels (Veikkola *et al.*, 2001), but they show only partially overlapping patterns of expression, indicating that they may perform distinct biological functions.

Lymphatic vessels provide an important route for tumour spread and, owing to high intratumoral interstitial pressures, most tumour cell invasion occurs via lymphatics at the tumour periphery. The lymphangiogenic activity of VEGF-C and VEGF-D in experimental tumour models indicates that newly formed lymphatics may play an important role in this process (Karpanen *et al.*, 2001; Mandriota *et al.*, 2001; Jain *et al.*, 2002; Stacker *et al.*, 2002). In several types of human tumour, such as breast, colorectal and cervix, high VEGF-C and/or VEGF-D expression has been linked to poor prognosis. For example, we recently reported that VEGF-D is an independent indicator in colorectal cancer (White *et al.*, 2002).

While the induction of angiogenesis is clearly a critical step in malignant progression, the first detectable disseminated disease in most tumours, including those of the cervix, occurs in the local lymph nodes (Van Trappen *et al.*, 2001). Lymph node involvement significantly affects the prognosis of cervical cancer patients and forms an integral part of tumour staging. The identification of novel lymphatic markers such as Flt-4

(Pajusola *et al.*, 1992), the CD44-related hyaluronan receptor LYVE-1 (Banerji *et al.*, 1999) and the mucoprotein podoplanin (Breiteneder-Geleff *et al.*, 1999), have facilitated the measurement of lymphatic vessel density (LVD) and its impact on the prognosis of cancer patients.

In early-stage invasive SCC, increased LVD is associated with the presence of inflammatory cells and lymphatic invasion but not with lymph node involvement (Birner *et al.*, 2001; Schoppmann *et al.*, 2001). The observed association of high LVD and improved patient survival in these studies may be due to an enhanced immune response as the presence of dendritic cells is associated with improved patient survival in cervical cancer (Bethwaite *et al.*, 1996). However, in a subsequent study, Schoppmann and colleagues (2002) demonstrated that a subset of activated tumour-associated macrophages in cervical cancers produced large amounts of VEGF-C and VEGF-D, and co-expressed Flt-4. The local density of macrophage-expressing VEGF-C and VEGF-D was associated with significant lymphangiogenesis in the stroma surrounding the tumour and lymphatic spread. It also appears that a small fraction of circulating CD34/CD133-positive monocytes co-express Flt-4 and may contribute to developing lymphatic vessels in an analogous manner to vasculogenesis in the adult (Schoppmann *et al.*, 2002).

Van Trappen and colleagues (2003) observed significant increases in VEGF-C and/or VEGF-D and Flt-4 expression in CIN3 and SCC compared with CIN1/2, indicating a switch to a lymphangiogenic phenotype prior to invasion. In addition to the endothelium of lymphatic vessels, a subset of blood vessels, Flt-4, was also detected in the cytoplasm of neoplastic cells, suggesting that VEGF-C/-D may modify tumour cell activity in an autocrine manner. VEGF-C transcripts in cervical cancer are reported to be upregulated by 130-fold (Van Trappen *et al.*, 2002) and, in cervical cancer cell lines, VEGF-C secretion correlates with MMP-2 expression and their ability to invade basement membrane proteins *in vitro* (Ueda *et al.*, 2001). Ueda and colleagues subsequently found VEGF-C expression to be significantly higher in tumours exhibiting deep stromal invasion and lymphatic involvement, and an independent factor in pelvic lymph node metastasis in cervical cancer (Ueda *et al.*, 2001, 2002). Hashimoto *et al.* (2001) observed markedly increased VEGF-C mRNA levels in the invasive cervical cancers of patients with pelvic lymph node metastases and lymphovascular space involvement, and high VEGF-C expression was an indicator of poor prognosis.

The acquisition of angiogenic phenotype and lymphatic invasion is a critical step in cervical tumour progression, and the VEGFs are central to these processes. The measurement of angiogenic/lymphangiogenic factors or associated vascularity may provide a basis for more accurate diagnostic tests for CIN and invasive cancers to tailor individual patient treatment. The clinical development of agents that inhibit VEGF and/or cognate receptors may provide new cancer treatments to prevent tumour growth and metastasis.

SUMMARY

Tumours require an adequate blood supply for growth and haematological spread. The gross vascular changes that occur in late cervical intraepithelial neoplasia (CIN2/3) have been recognised for many years, and significant increases in microvessel density (MVD) are associated with these later stages of CIN. In invasive cervical cancers, high MVD is reported to represent an independent prognostic indicator of disease-free/overall survival. The identification of factors that initiate angiogenesis in CIN may provide valuable prognostic markers to identify those lesions that will progress and require further treatment. The vascular endothelial growth factor (VEGF) family plays a central role in coordinating both new blood and lymphatic vessel growth and maintenance. Increased VEGF expression is associated with MVD in CIN and correlates with prognosis in invasive cancers. Lymphatic invasion and the subsequent development of lymph node metastases are important prognostic factors in cervical cancer. The identification of novel lymphatic vessel markers and growth factors, VEGF-C and VEGF-D, has facilitated the study of lymphangiogenesis in cervical tumours and may provide novel diagnostic markers. It is hoped that the development of agents that selectively target the VEGF ligands and receptors will generate new therapies to limit tumour growth and metastases.

ACKNOWLEDGEMENTS

Figures 20.1a–c are taken from Singer A., Monaghan J.M. (eds) *Lower Genital Tract Precancer*, 2nd edn, Oxford: Blackwell Science, 2000, with thanks.

REFERENCES

Abulafia O, Triest WE, Sherer DM (1996) Angiogenesis in squamous cell carcinoma in situ and microinvasive carcinoma of the uterine cervix. *Obstetrics and Gynecology* 88: 927–932.

Ahmed A, Dunk C, Kniss *et al.* (1997) Role of VEGF receptor-1 (Flt-1) in mediating calcium-dependent nitric oxide release and limiting DNA synthesis in human trophoblast cells. *Laboratory Investigation* 76: 779–791.

Alonio LV, Picconi MA, Dalbert D *et al.* (2003) Ha-ras oncogene mutation associated to progression of papillomavirus induced lesions of uterine cervix. *Journal of Clinical Virology* 27: 263–269.

Asahara T, Masuda H, Takahashi T *et al.* (1999) Bone marrow origin of endothelial progenitor cells responsible for postnatal vasculogenesis in physiological and pathological neovascularization. *Circulation Research* 85: 221–228.

Banerji S, Ni J, Wang SX *et al.* (1999) LYVE-1, a new homologue of the CD44 glycoprotein, is a lymph-specific receptor for hyaluronan. *Journal of Cell Biology* 144: 789–801.

Barbosa MS, Schlegel R (1989) The E6 and E7 genes of HPV-18 are sufficient for inducing two-stage in vitro transformation of human keratinocytes. *Oncogene* 4: 1529–1532.

Bethwaite PB, Holloway LJ, Thornton A *et al.* (1996) Infiltration by immunocompetent cells in early stage invasive carcinoma of the uterine cervix: a prognostic study. *Pathology* 28: 321–327.

Birner P, Schindl M, Obermair A *et al.* (2001) Lymphatic microvessel density as a novel prognostic factor in early-stage invasive cervical cancer. *International Journal of Cancer* 95: 29–33.

Breiteneder-Geleff S, Soleiman A, Kowalski H *et al.* (1999) Angiosarcomas express mixed endothelial phenotypes of blood and lymphatic capillaries: podoplanin as a specific marker for lymphatic endothelium. *American Journal of Pathology* 154: 385–394.

Bremer GL, Tiebosch AT, van der Putten HW *et al.* (1996) Tumor angiogenesis: an independent prognostic parameter in cervical cancer. *American Journal of Obstetrics and Gynecology* 174: 126–131.

Burri PH, Tarek MR (1990) A novel mechanism of capillary growth in the rat pulmonary microcirculation. *Anatomical Record* 228: 35–45.

Bussolati B, Dunk C, Grohman M *et al.* (2001) Vascular endothelial growth factor receptor-1 modulates vascular endothelial growth factor-mediated angiogenesis via nitric oxide. *American Journal of Pathology* 159: 993–1008.

Cai J, Ahmad S, Jiang WG *et al.* (2003) Activation of vascular endothelial growth factor receptor-1 sustains angiogenesis and Bcl-2 expression via the phosphatidylinositol 3-kinase pathway in endothelial cells. *Diabetes* 52: 2959–2968.

Carmeliet P (2000) Mechanisms of angiogenesis and arteriogenesis. *Nature Medicine* 6: 389–395.

Carmeliet P, Collen D (2000) Molecular basis of angiogenesis. Role of VEGF and VE-cadherin. *Annals of the New York Academy of Sciences* 902: 249–262; discussion 262–24.

Carmeliet P, Jain RK (2000) Angiogenesis in cancer and other diseases. *Nature* 407: 249–257.

Carmeliet P, Dor Y, Herbert JM *et al.* (1998) Role of HIF-1alpha in hypoxia-mediated apoptosis, cell proliferation and tumour angiogenesis. *Nature* 394: 485–490.

Carmeliet P, Moons L, Luttun A *et al.* (2001) Synergism between vascular endothelial growth factor and placental growth factor contributes to angiogenesis and plasma extravasation in pathological conditions. *Nature Medicine* 7: 575–583.

Charnock-Jones DS, Sharkey AM, Rajput-Williams J *et al.* (1993) Identification and localization of alternately spliced mRNAs for vascular endothelial growth factor in human uterus and estrogen regulation in endometrial carcinoma cell lines. *Biology of Reproduction* 48: 1120–1128.

Cheng WF, Chen CA, Lee CN *et al.* (2000) Vascular endothelial growth factor and prognosis of cervical carcinoma. *Obstetrics and Gynecology* 96: 721–726.

Chilvers C (1994) Oral contraceptives and cancer. *Lancet* 344: 1378–1379.

Chopra V, Dinh TV, Hannigan EV (1998) Circulating serum levels of cytokines and angiogenic factors in patients with cervical cancer. *Cancer Investigations* 16: 152–159.

Clauss M, Weich H, Breier G *et al.* (1996) The vascular endothelial growth factor receptor Flt-1 mediates biological activities. Implications for a functional role of placenta growth factor in monocyte activation and chemotaxis. *Journal of Biological Chemistry* 271: 17629–17634.

Cooper RA, West CM, Wilks DP *et al.* (1999) Tumour vascularity is a significant prognostic factor for cervix carcinoma treated with radiotherapy: independence from tumour radiosensitivity. *British Journal of Cancer* 81: 354–358.

Cullinan-Bove K, Koos RD (1993) Vascular endothelial growth factor/vascular permeability factor expression in the rat uterus: rapid stimula-

tion by estrogen correlates with estrogen-induced increases in uterine capillary permeability and growth. *Endocrinology* 133: 829–837.

Cunningham SA, Arrate MP, Brock TA *et al.* (1997) Interactions of FLT-1 and KDR with phospholipase C gamma: identification of the phosphotyrosine binding sites. *Biochemical and Biophysical Research Communications* 240: 635–639.

Dameron KM, Volpert OV, Tainsky MA *et al.* (1994) Control of angiogenesis in fibroblasts by p53 regulation of thrombospondin-1. *Science* 265: 1582–1584.

Dellas A, Moch H, Schultheiss E *et al.* (1997) Angiogenesis in cervical neoplasia: microvessel quantitation in precancerous lesions and invasive carcinomas with clinicopathological correlations. *Gynecological Oncology* 67: 27–33.

de Villiers EM (2003) Relationship between steroid hormone contraceptives and HPV, cervical intraepithelial neoplasia and cervical carcinoma. *International Journal of Cancer* 103: 705–708.

de Vries C, Escobedo JA, Ueno H *et al.* (1992) The fms-like tyrosine kinase, a receptor for vascular endothelial growth factor. *Science* 255: 989–991.

Dinh TV, Hannigan EV, Smith ER *et al.* (1996) Tumor angiogenesis as a predictor of recurrence in stage Ib squamous cell carcinoma of the cervix. *Obstetrics and Gynecology* 87: 751–754.

Dobbs SP, Hewett PW, Johnson IR *et al.* (1997) Angiogenesis is associated with vascular endothelial growth factor expression in cervical intraepithelial neoplasia. *British Journal of Cancer* 76: 1410–1415.

Dumont DJ, Jussila L, Taipale J *et al.* (1998) Cardiovascular failure in mouse embryos deficient in VEGF receptor-3. *Science* 282: 946–949.

Dyson N, Howley PM, Munger K *et al.* (1989) The human papilloma virus-16 E7 oncoprotein is able to bind to the retinoblastoma gene product. *Science* 243: 934–937.

Ferrara N (2004) Vascular endothelial growth factor as a target for anticancer therapy. *Oncologist* 9 (Suppl. 1): 2–10.

Finkenzeller G, Weindel K, Zimmermann W *et al.* (2004) Activated Neu/ErbB-2 induces expression of the vascular endothelial growth factor gene by functional activation of the transcription factor Sp 1. *Angiogenesis* 7: 59–68.

Folkman J (1971) Tumor angiogenesis: therapeutic implications. *New England Journal of Medicine* 285: 1182–1186.

Folkman J, Hanahan D (1991) Switch to the angiogenic phenotype during tumorigenesis. *Princess Takamatsu Symposium* 22: 339–347.

Fong GH, Rossant J, Gertsenstein M *et al.* (1995) Role of the Flt-1 receptor tyrosine kinase in regulating the assembly of vascular endothelium. *Nature* 376: 66–70.

Fong GH, Zhang L, Bryce DM *et al.* (1999) Increased hemangioblast commitment, not vascular disorganization, is the primary defect in flt-1 knock-out mice. *Development* 126: 3015–3025.

Formenti S, Felix J, Salonga D *et al.* (2000) Expression of metastases-associated genes in cervical cancers resected in the proliferative and secretory phases of the menstrual cycle. *Clinical Cancer Research* 6: 4653–4657.

Fujisawa T, Watanabe J, Kamata Y *et al.* (2003) Effect of p53 gene transfection on vascular endothelial growth factor expression in endometrial cancer cells. *Experimental Molecular Pathology* 74: 276–281.

Ghandour FA, Attanoos R, Nahar K *et al.* (1994) Immunocytochemical localization of oestrogen and progesterone receptors in primary adenocarcinoma of the cervix. *Histopathology* 24: 49–55.

Goldberg MA, Schneider TJ (1994) Similarities between the oxygen-sensing mechanisms regulating the expression of vascular endothelial growth factor and erythropoietin. *Journal of Biological Chemistry* 269: 4355–4359.

Green J, Berrington de Gonzalez A, Sweetland S *et al.* (2003) Risk factors for adenocarcinoma and squamous cell carcinoma of the cervix in women aged 20–44 years: the UK National Case–Control Study of Cervical Cancer. *British Journal of Cancer* 89: 2078–2086.

Guidi AJ, Abu-Jawdeh G, Berse B *et al.* (1995) Vascular permeability factor (vascular endothelial growth factor) expression and angiogenesis in cervical neoplasia. *Journal of the National Cancer Institute* 87: 1237–1245.

Hanahan D (1997) Signaling vascular morphogenesis and maintenance. *Science* 277: 48–50.

Hanahan D, Christofori G, Naik P *et al.* (1996) Transgenic mouse models of tumour angiogenesis: the angiogenic switch, its molecular controls, and prospects for preclinical therapeutic models. *European Journal of Cancer* 32A: 2386–2393.

Hashimoto I, Kodama J, Seki N *et al.* (2000) Macrophage infiltration and angiogenesis in endometrial cancer. *Anticancer Research* 20: 4853–4856.

Hashimoto I, Kodama J, Seki N *et al.* (2001) Vascular endothelial growth factor-C expression and its relationship to pelvic lymph node status in invasive cervical cancer. *British Journal of Cancer* 85: 93–97.

Haverkos H, Rohrer M, Pickworth W (2000) The cause of invasive cervical cancer could be multifactorial. *Biomedical Pharmacotherapy* 54: 54–59.

Hawighorst H, Knapstein PG, Knopp MV *et al.* (1998) Uterine cervical carcinoma: comparison of standard and pharmacokinetic analysis of time–intensity curves for assessment of tumor angiogenesis and patient survival. *Cancer Research* 58: 3598–3602.

Hiratsuka S, Minowa O, Kuno J *et al.* (1998) Flt-1 lacking the tyrosine kinase domain is sufficient for normal development and angiogenesis in mice. *Proceedings of the National Academy of Sciences of the USA* 95: 9349–9354.

Hiratsuka S, Maru Y, Okada A *et al.* (2001) Involvement of Flt-1 tyrosine kinase (vascular endothelial growth factor receptor-1) in pathological angiogenesis. *Cancer Research* 61: 1207–1213.

Holash J, Maisonpierre PC, Compton D *et al.* (1999) Vessel cooption, regression, and growth in tumors mediated by angiopoietins and VEGF. *Science* 284: 1994–1998.

Holmgren L (1996) Antiangiogenesis restricted tumor dormancy. *Cancer Metastasis Review* 15: 241–245.

Holmgren L, O'Reilly MS, Folkman J (1995) Dormancy of micrometastases: balanced proliferation and apoptosis in the presence of angiogenesis suppression. *Nature Medicine* 1: 149–153.

Houck KA, Ferrara N, Winer J *et al.* (1991) The vascular endothelial growth factor family: identification of a fourth molecular species and characterization of alternative splicing of RNA. *Molecular Endocrinology* 5: 1806–1814.

Iwakura A, Luedemann C, Shastry S *et al.* (2003) Estrogen-mediated, endothelial nitric oxide synthase-dependent mobilization of bone marrow-derived endothelial progenitor cells contributes to reendothelialization after arterial injury. *Circulation* 108: 3115–3121.

Jain RK, Munn LL, Fukumura D (2002) Dissecting tumour pathophysiology using intravital microscopy. *Nature Reviews Cancer* 2: 266–276.

Joukov V, Sorsa T, Kumar V *et al.* (1997) Proteolytic processing regulates receptor specificity and activity of VEGF-C. *EMBO Journal* 16: 3898–3911.

Kainz C, Speiser P, Wanner C *et al.* (1995) Prognostic value of tumour microvessel density in cancer of the uterine cervix stage IB to IIB. *Anticancer Research* 15: 1549–1551.

Kaipainen A, Korhonen J, Mustonen T *et al.* (1995) Expression of the fms-like tyrosine kinase 4 gene becomes restricted to lymphatic endothelium during development. *Proceedings of the National Academy of Sciences of the USA* 92: 3566–3570.

Kaku T, Hirakawa T, Kamura T *et al.* (1998) Angiogenesis in adenocarcinoma of the uterine cervix. *Cancer* 83: 1384–1390.

Kanai M, Shiozawa T, Xin L *et al.* (1998) Immunohistochemical detection of sex steroid receptors, cyclins, and cyclin-dependent kinases in the normal and neoplastic squamous epithelia of the uterine cervix. *Cancer* 82: 1709–1719.

Karkkainen MJ, Jussila L, Ferrell RE *et al.* (2001) Molecular regulation of lymphangiogenesis and targets for tissue oedema. *Trends in Molecular Medicine* 7: 18–22.

Karpanen T, Egeblad M, Karkkainen MJ *et al.* (2001) Vascular endothelial growth factor C promotes tumor lymphangiogenesis and intralymphatic tumor growth. *Cancer Research* 61: 1786–1790.

Kendall RL, Wang G, Thomas KA (1996) Identification of a natural soluble form of the vascular endothelial growth factor receptor, FLT-1, and its heterodimerization with KDR. *Biochemical and Biophysical Research Communications* 226: 324–328.

Kihana T, Tsuda H, Teshima S *et al.* (1994) Prognostic significance of the overexpression of c-erbB-2 protein in adenocarcinoma of the uterine cervix. *Cancer* 73: 148–153.

Kinoshita T, Shirasawa H, Shino Y *et al.* (1997) Transactivation of prothymosin alpha and c-myc promoters by human papillomavirus type 16 E6 protein. *Virology* 232: 53–61.

Kodama J, Seki N, Tokumo K *et al.* (1999) Vascular endothelial growth factor is implicated in early invasion in cervical cancer. *European Journal of Cancer* 35: 485–489.

Kohno Y, Iwanari O, Kitao M (1993) Prognostic importance of histologic vascular density in cervical cancer treated with hypertensive intraarterial chemotherapy. *Cancer* 72: 2394–2400.

Le Buanec H, D'Anna R, Lachgar A *et al.* (1999) HPV-16 E7 but not E6 oncogenic protein triggers both cellular immunosuppression and angiogenic processes. *Biomedical Pharmacotherapy* 53: 424–431.

Lebovic DI, Shifren JL, Ryan IP *et al.* (2000) Ovarian steroid and cytokine modulation of human endometrial angiogenesis. *Human Reproduction* 15 (Suppl. 3): 67–77.

Lee JS, Kim HS, Jung JJ *et al.* (2002) Expression of vascular endothelial growth factor in adenocarcinomas of the uterine cervix and its relation to angiogenesis and p53 and c-erbB-2 protein expression. *Gynecological Oncology* 85: 469–475.

Leung KM, Chan WY, Hui PK (1994) Invasive squamous cell carcinoma and cervical intraepithelial neoplasia III of uterine cervix. Morphologic differences other than stromal invasion. *American Journal of Clinical Pathology* 101: 508–513.

Liotta LA, Steeg PS, Stetler-Stevenson WG (1991) Cancer metastasis and angiogenesis: an imbalance of positive and negative regulation. *Cell* 64: 327–336.

Loncaster JA, Cooper RA, Logue JP *et al.* (2000) Vascular endothelial growth factor (VEGF) expression is a prognostic factor for radiotherapy outcome in advanced carcinoma of the cervix. *British Journal of Cancer* 83: 620–625.

Lopez-Ocejo O, Viloria-Petit A, Bequet-Romero M *et al.* (2000) Oncogenes and tumor angiogenesis: the HPV-16 E6 oncoprotein activates the vascular endothelial growth factor (VEGF) gene promoter in a p53 independent manner. *Oncogene* 19: 4611–4620.

Losordo DW, Isner JM (2001) Estrogen and angiogenesis: a review. *Arteriosclerosis Thrombosis and Vascular Biology* 21: 6–12.

Luttun A, Brusselmans K, Fukao H *et al.* (2002a) Loss of placental growth factor protects mice against vascular permeability in pathological conditions. *Biochemical and Biophysical Research Communications* 295: 428–434.

Luttun A, Tjwa M, Moons L *et al.* (2002b) Revascularization of ischemic tissues by PlGF treatment, and inhibition of tumor angiogenesis, arthritis and atherosclerosis by anti-Flt1. *Nature Medicine* 8: 831–840.

Lymboussaki A, Partanen TA, Olofsson B *et al.* (1998) Expression of the vascular endothelial growth factor C receptor VEGFR-3 in lymphatic endothelium of the skin and in vascular tumors. *American Journal of Pathology* 153: 395–403.

McIndoe WA, McLean MR, Jones RW *et al.* (1984) The invasive potential of carcinoma in situ of the cervix. *Obstetrics and Gynecology* 64: 451–458.

McLaren J, Prentice A, Charnock-Jones DS *et al.* (1996) Vascular endothelial growth factor is produced by peritoneal fluid macrophages in endometriosis and is regulated by ovarian steroids. *Journal of Clinical Investigation* 98: 482–489.

Mandriota SJ, Jussila L, Jeltsch M *et al.* (2001) Vascular endothelial growth factor-C-mediated lymphangiogenesis promotes tumour metastasis. *EMBO Journal* 20: 672–682.

Morosov A, Phelps WC, Raychaudhuri P (1994) Activation of the c-fos gene by the HPV16 oncoproteins depends upon the cAMP-response element at −60. *Journal of Biological Chemistry* 269: 18434–18440.

Munger K, Werness BA, Dyson N *et al.* (1989) Complex formation of human papillomavirus E7 proteins with the retinoblastoma tumor suppressor gene product. *EMBO Journal* 8: 4099–4105.

Neufeld G, Cohen T, Gengrinovitch S *et al.* (1999) Vascular endothelial growth factor (VEGF) and its receptors. *FASEB Journal* 13: 9–22.

Neufeld G, Cohen T, Shraga N *et al.* (2002) The neuropilins: multifunctional semaphorin and VEGF receptors that modulate axon guidance and angiogenesis. *Trends in Cardiovascular Medicine* 12: 13–19.

Obermair A, Bancher-Todesca D, Bilgi S *et al.* (1997) Correlation of vascular endothelial growth factor expression and microvessel density in cervical intraepithelial neoplasia. *Journal of the National Cancer Institute* 89: 1212–1217.

Obermair A, Wanner C, Bilgi S *et al.* (1998) Tumor angiogenesis in stage IB cervical cancer: correlation of microvessel density with survival. *American Journal of Obstetrics and Gynecology* 178: 314–319.

Ozalp S, Yalcin OT, Oner U *et al.* (2003) Microvessel density as a prognostic factor in preinvasive and invasive cervical lesions. *European Journal of Gynaecological Oncology* 24: 425–428.

Pajusola K, Aprelikova O, Korhonen J *et al.* (1992) FLT4 receptor tyrosine kinase contains seven immunoglobulin-like loops and is expressed in multiple human tissues and cell lines. *Cancer Research* 52: 5738–5743.

Partanen TA, Arola J, Saaristo A *et al.* (2000) VEGF-C and VEGF-D expression in neuroendocrine cells and their receptor, VEGFR-3, in fenestrated blood vessels in human tissues. *FASEB Journal* 14: 2087–2096.

Patan S (1998) TIE1 and TIE2 receptor tyrosine kinases inversely regulate embryonic angiogenesis by the mechanism of intussusceptive microvascular growth. *Microvascular Research* 56: 1–21.

Petit AM, Rak J, Hung MC *et al.* (1997) Neutralizing antibodies against epidermal growth factor and ErbB-2/neu receptor tyrosine kinases down-regulate vascular endothelial growth factor production by tumor cells in vitro and in vivo: angiogenic implications for signal transduction therapy of solid tumors. *American Journal of Pathology* 151: 1523–1530.

Pilch H, Schlenger K, Steiner E *et al.* (2001) Hypoxia-stimulated expression of angiogenic growth factors in cervical cancer cells and

cervical cancer-derived fibroblasts. *International Journal of Gynecological Cancer* 11: 137–142.

Rahimi N, Dayanir V, Lashkari K (2000) Receptor chimeras indicate that the vascular endothelial growth factor receptor-1 (VEGFR-1) modulates mitogenic activity of VEGFR-2 in endothelial cells. *Journal of Biological Chemistry* 275: 16986–16992.

Rak J, Klement G (2000) Impact of oncogenes and tumor suppressor genes on deregulation of hemostasis and angiogenesis in cancer. *Cancer Metastasis Review* 19: 93–96.

Rak J, Mitsuhashi Y, Sheehan C *et al.* (2000) Oncogenes and tumor angiogenesis: differential modes of vascular endothelial growth factor up-regulation in ras-transformed epithelial cells and fibroblasts. *Cancer Research* 60: 490–498.

Raleigh JA, Calkins-Adams DP, Rinker LH *et al.* (1998) Hypoxia and vascular endothelial growth factor expression in human squamous cell carcinomas using pimonidazole as a hypoxia marker. *Cancer Research* 58: 3765–3768.

Risau W (1997) Mechanisms of angiogenesis. *Nature* 386: 671–674.

Risau W, Flamme I (1995) Vasculogenesis. *Annual Review of Cell and Developmental Biology* 11: 73–91.

Rosty C, Couturier J, Vincent-Salomon A *et al.* (2004) Overexpression/amplification of HER-2/neu is uncommon in invasive carcinoma of the uterine cervix. *International Journal of Gynecological Pathology* 23: 13–17.

Rutgers JL, Mattox TF, Vargas MP (1995) Angiogenesis in uterine cervical squamous cell carcinoma. *International Journal of Gynecological Pathology* 14: 114–118.

Santin AD, Hermonat PL, Ravaggi A *et al.* (1999) Secretion of vascular endothelial growth factor in adenocarcinoma and squamous cell carcinoma of the uterine cervix. *Obstetrics and Gynecology* 94: 78–82.

Schlenger K, Hockel M, Mitze M *et al.* (1995) Tumor vascularity — a novel prognostic factor in advanced cervical carcinoma. *Gynecological Oncology* 59: 57–66.

Schoppmann SF, Schindl M, Breiteneder-Geleff S *et al.* (2001) Inflammatory stromal reaction correlates with lymphatic microvessel density in early-stage cervical cancer. *Anticancer Research* 21: 3419–3423.

Schoppmann SF, Birner P, Stockl J *et al.* (2002) Tumor-associated macrophages express lymphatic endothelial growth factors and are related to peritumoral lymphangiogenesis. *American Journal of Pathology* 161: 947–956.

Senger DR, Galli SJ, Dvorak AM *et al.* (1983) Tumor cells secrete a vascular permeability factor that promotes accumulation of ascites fluid. *Science* 219: 983–985.

Shafi MI, Luesley DM (1995) Management of low grade lesions: follow-up or treat? *Bailliere's Clinical Obstetrics and Gynaecology* 9: 121–131.

Shalaby F, Rossant J, Yamaguchi TP *et al.* (1995) Failure of blood-island formation and vasculogenesis in Flk-1-deficient mice. *Nature* 376: 62–66.

Shweiki D, Itin A, Soffer D *et al.* (1992) Vascular endothelial growth factor induced by hypoxia may mediate hypoxia-initiated angiogenesis. *Nature* 359: 843–845.

Shweiki D, Itin A, Neufeld G *et al.* (1993) Patterns of expression of vascular endothelial growth factor (VEGF) and VEGF receptors in mice suggest a role in hormonally regulated angiogenesis. *Journal of Clinical Investigation* 91: 2235–2243.

Siracka E, Revesz L, Kovac R *et al.* (1988) Vascular density in carcinoma of the uterine cervix and its predictive value for radiotherapy. *International Journal of Cancer* 41: 819–822.

Smith-McCune KK, Weidner N (1994) Demonstration and characterization of the angiogenic properties of cervical dysplasia. *Cancer Research* 54: 800–804.

Smith-McCune K, Zhu YH, Hanahan D *et al.* (1997) Cross-species comparison of angiogenesis during the premalignant stages of squamous carcinogenesis in the human cervix and K14-HPV16 transgenic mice. *Cancer Research* 57: 1294–1300.

Smith-McCune KK, Zhu Y, Darragh T (1998) Angiogenesis in histologically benign squamous mucosa is a sensitive marker for nearby cervical intraepithelial neoplasia. *Angiogenesis* 2: 135–142.

Stacker SA, Vitali A, Caesar C *et al.* (1999a) A mutant form of vascular endothelial growth factor (VEGF) that lacks VEGF receptor-2 activation retains the ability to induce vascular permeability. *Journal of Biological Chemistry* 274: 34884–34892.

Stacker SA, Stenvers K, Caesar C *et al.* (1999b) Biosynthesis of vascular endothelial growth factor-D involves proteolytic processing which generates non-covalent homodimers. *Journal of Biological Chemistry* 274: 32127–32136.

Stacker SA, Achen MG, Jussila L *et al.* (2002) Lymphangiogenesis and cancer metastasis. *Nature Review of Cancer* 2: 573–583.

Stafl A, Mattingly RF (1975) Angiogenesis of cervical neoplasia. *American Journal of Obstetrics and Gynecology* 121: 845–852.

Stein I, Neeman M, Shweiki D *et al.* (1995) Stabilization of vascular endothelial growth factor mRNA by hypoxia and hypoglycemia and coregulation with other ischemia-induced genes. *Molecular and Cellular Biology* 15: 5363–5368.

Stoner M, Wormke M, Saville B *et al.* (2004) Estrogen regulation of vascular endothelial growth factor gene expression in ZR-75 breast cancer cells through interaction of estrogen receptor alpha and SP proteins. *Oncogene* 23: 1052–1063.

Tischer E, Mitchell R, Hartman T *et al.* (1991) The human gene for vascular endothelial growth factor. Multiple protein forms are encoded through alternative exon splicing. *Journal of Biological Chemistry* 266: 11947–11954.

Tjalma W, Van Marck E, Weyler J *et al.* (1998) Quantification and prognostic relevance of angiogenic parameters in invasive cervical cancer. *British Journal of Cancer* 78: 170–174.

Tokumo K, Kodama J, Seki N *et al.* (1998) Different angiogenic pathways in human cervical cancers. *Gynecological Oncology* 68: 38–44.

Ueda M, Terai Y, Kumagai K *et al.* (2001) Vascular endothelial growth factor C gene expression is closely related to invasion phenotype in gynecological tumor cells. *Gynecological Oncology* 82: 162–166.

Ueda M, Terai Y, Yamashita Y *et al.* (2002) Correlation between vascular endothelial growth factor-C expression and invasion phenotype in cervical carcinomas. *International Journal of Cancer* 98: 335–343.

Van Trappen PO, Gyselman VG, Lowe DG *et al.* (2001) Molecular quantification and mapping of lymph-node micrometastases in cervical cancer. *Lancet* 357: 15–20.

Van Trappen PO, Ryan A, Carroll M *et al.* (2002) A model for co-expression pattern analysis of genes implicated in angiogenesis and tumour cell invasion in cervical cancer. *British Journal of Cancer* 87: 537–544.

Van Trappen PO, Steele D, Lowe DG *et al.* (2003) Expression of vascular endothelial growth factor (VEGF)-C and VEGF-D, and their receptor VEGFR-3, during different stages of cervical carcinogenesis. *Journal of Pathology* 201: 544–554.

Veikkola T, Jussila L, Makinen T *et al.* (2001) Signalling via vascular endothelial growth factor receptor-3 is sufficient for lymphangiogenesis in transgenic mice. *EMBO Journal* 20: 1223–1231.

Waggoner SE (2003) Cervical cancer. *Lancet* 361: 2217–2225.

Waltenberger J, Claesson-Welsh L, Siegbahn A *et al.* (1994) Different signal transduction properties of KDR and Flt1, two receptors for vascular endothelial growth factor. *Journal of Biological Chemistry* 269: 26988–26995.

Wei LH, Kuo ML, Chen CA *et al.* (2003) Interleukin-6 promotes cervical tumor growth by VEGF-dependent angiogenesis via a STAT3 pathway. *Oncogene* 22: 1517–1527.

Weidner N (1993) Tumor angiogenesis: review of current applications in tumor prognostication. *Seminars in Diagnostic Pathology* 10: 302–313.

Weidner N, Semple JP, Welch WR *et al.* (1991) Tumor angiogenesis and metastasis — correlation in invasive breast carcinoma. *New England Journal of Medicine* 324: 1–8.

Weng DE, Usman N (2001) Angiozyme: a novel angiogenesis inhibitor. *Current Oncology Reports* 3: 141–146.

Werness BA, Levine AJ, Howley PM (1990) Association of human papillomavirus types 16 and 18 E6 proteins with p53. *Science* 248: 76–79.

West CM, Cooper RA, Loncaster JA *et al.* (2001) Tumor vascularity: a histological measure of angiogenesis and hypoxia. *Cancer Research* 61: 2907–2910.

White JD, Hewett PW, Kosuge D *et al.* (2002) Vascular endothelial growth factor-D expression is an independent prognostic marker for survival in colorectal carcinoma. *Cancer Research* 62: 1669–1675.

Wiggins DL, Granai CO, Steinhoff MM *et al.* (1995) Tumor angiogenesis as a prognostic factor in cervical carcinoma. *Gynecological Oncology* 56: 353–356.

Wigle JT, Oliver G (1999) Prox1 function is required for the development of the murine lymphatic system. *Cell* 98: 769–778.

Woodworth CD, Bowden PE, Doniger J *et al.* (1988) Characterization of normal human exocervical epithelial cells immortalised in vitro by papillomavirus types 16 and 18 DNA. *Cancer Research* 48: 4620–4628.

Yen L, You XL, Al Moustafa AE *et al.* (2000) Heregulin selectively upregulates vascular endothelial growth factor secretion in cancer cells and stimulates angiogenesis. *Oncogene* 19: 3460–3469.

Zeng H, Dvorak HF, Mukhopadhyay D (2001) Vascular permeability factor (VPF)/vascular endothelial growth factor (VEGF) receptor-1 down-modulates VPF/VEGF receptor-2-mediated endothelial cell proliferation, but not migration, through phosphatidylinositol 3-kinase-dependent pathways. *Journal of Biological Chemistry* 276: 26969–26979.

Zheng T, Holford TR, Ma Z *et al.* (1996) The continuing increase in adenocarcinoma of the uterine cervix: a birth cohort phenomenon. *International Journal of Epidemiology* 25: 252–258.

zur Hausen H (2002) Papillomaviruses and cancer: from basic studies to clinical application. *Nature Reviews Cancer* 2: 342–350.

CHAPTER 21

Pathology of neoplastic squamous lesions

Raji Ganesan and Terence P. Rollason

INTRODUCTION

Squamous carcinoma is the second commonest female malignancy worldwide, with an estimated incidence of perhaps 400 000 cases per year and 200 000 deaths (Parkin *et al.*, 1999; Pisani *et al.*, 1999; Lonky, 2002). In many countries in the developing world, it is the commonest malignancy in women. Cervical intraepithelial neoplasia (CIN) is far commoner than invasive carcinoma and, as perhaps 60% of low-grade CIN regresses and the overall, long-term risk of development of carcinoma from low-grade CIN is in the region of 1% (McIndoe *et al.*, 1984; Holowaty *et al.*, 1999), it can be appreciated that intraepithelial neoplastic lesions of the cervix and invasive carcinoma constitute a massive clinical and social challenge. In the UK, the incidence of invasive squamous carcinoma of the cervix is now less than 9 per 100 000 women per year, and this overall incidence has been falling for more than 30 years. An increase apparent in younger women (less than 35 years of age), seen in earlier decades, now appears to have been reversed. The aetiology and epidemiology of CIN and invasive carcinoma is dealt with elsewhere, but it should be stressed at this point that, while human papillomavirus (HPV) infection is now usually accepted as a necessary event preceding the development of cervical carcinoma, the reasons why, of the approximately 80% of women who will develop evidence of HPV infection during their lives, well in excess of 90% will develop no sequelae in terms of intraepithelial or invasive carcinoma are not understood.

The majority of deaths from cervical cancer occur in the fourth to sixth decades with a peak age incidence in women of 60–64 years. Historically, squamous carcinoma has been said to make up almost 90% of all primary neoplasms of the cervix, but adenocarcinoma is increasing proportionately in incidence and has risen from approximately 5% of cervical carcinomas in the 1950s to perhaps as many as 23% of all invasive tumours by the mid-1990s (Plaxe and Saltzstein, 1999). Obtaining accurate comparative numbers is dogged by difficulties in diagnostic practice, however, with some including all adenosquamous carcinomas in the glandular group and others undoubtedly putting a proportion of such tumours in the squamous category. One recent study suggests that there has been a greater than 40% decrease in the age-specific incidence of squamous carcinoma but an almost 30% increase in adenocarcinoma over a 20-year period (Smith *et al.*, 2000), and these tumours appear to be occurring in women younger than those typically developing squamous carcinoma. Some of this alteration is undoubtedly related to the effect of cervical screening, with the highest relative increase in adenocarcinoma seen in those countries with effective screening programmes.

CERVICAL INTRAEPITHELIAL SQUAMOUS NEOPLASIA (SQUAMOUS INTRAEPITHELIAL LESION)

Terminology in preinvasive cervical squamous neoplasia

There are now two terminologies in common use for intraepithelial neoplasia of the cervix. The earlier terminology, which has the advantage of longevity and previously widespread common usage, is the CIN terminology. This is still generally used in Great Britain. Under this classification, preinvasive cervical neoplasia of squamous type is divided into three grades. This classification superseded the older dysplasia/carcinoma *in situ* terminology (Cocker *et al.*, 1968) and was introduced, in part, because ploidy and clonality studies suggested that the dysplasia/carcinoma *in situ* spectrum was a single, continuous disease process (Richart, 1973; Fu *et al.*, 1983). Unfortunately, its introduction did not dispose of the inconsistencies in histological reporting inherent in the old system, and we now know that there is significant interobserver variability in the diagnosis and grading of CIN (Ismail *et al.*, 1989; Robertson, 1989; de Vet *et al.*, 1992). In general, the diagnosis of CIN3 is consistent and reproducible, but distinction between low-grade CIN and HPV infection alone is highly subjective, and separation of CIN1 and CIN2 is also unreliable. Similarly, problems occur in the separation of low-grade CIN from reactive and reparative conditions in the cervix. In Great Britain, the term recommended by the NHS Cervical Screening Programme for abnormalities of the cervix, where one cannot differentiate between true CIN and reactive conditions, is 'basal (epithelial) abnormalities of uncertain significance' (NHSCSP, 1999). It should be stressed that there is no clear evidence that CIN3 develops from CIN1, and it has been argued that CIN3 arises alongside CIN1 rather than from it (see below).

These problems in diagnostic consistency, together with inconsistencies and difficulties in histological subclassification of CIN into three grades (or cytological subclassification of dyskaryosis into mild, moderate and severe) and its separation from HPV-associated changes alone, has led to considerable recent national debate in the UK, which seems likely to lead to a simplification of the CIN and squamous dyskaryosis classification systems to bring them closer to the so-called Bethesda system, in common use in the USA.

The Bethesda classification system for reporting cervical and vaginal intraepithelial neoplasia was originally introduced as a cytological grading system (Solomon, 1989; Luff, 1992; Solomon *et al.*, 2002). Essentially, under this system, those changes related to HPV and CIN are classified into two grades. High-grade lesions (high-grade squamous intraepithelial lesion, HGSIL) are cytologically essentially comparable to moderate and severe dyskaryosis, and low-grade lesions (low-grade squamous intraepithelial lesion, LGSIL) to mild dyskaryosis or HPV effect alone. The low-grade squamous intraepithelial lesion in the Bethesda system would therefore be equivalent to either HPV effect alone and HPV effect with CIN1 or just CIN1 with or without warts, depending on the author, in the histological classification presently used, whereas high-grade squamous intraepithelial lesion would be equivalent to CIN2 and 3, with or without warts. It was hoped that this classification would reflect the now widely held view that, biologically, HPV with or without CIN1 represents a biologically distinct group with a high likelihood of regression and essentially a productive HPV infection, whereas CIN2 and 3 represent a true neoplastic process. The HPV alone and with CIN1 subgroups also have the same dominant HPV subtypes and ploidy levels.

The major problem with the adoption of the Bethesda SIL system relates to those cases that show HPV effect alone. While the histological differentiation of HPV effect alone from HPV effect and CIN1 may be very difficult, it is possible in many cases, and there is a theoretical and practical difficulty in considering HPV effect alone, without other features of intraepithelial neoplasia, as a continuum in the neoplastic process. Further work is really needed on the outcome of the two-tier system compared with what is essentially a four-tier system: HPV, CIN1, CIN2, CIN3. The Bethesda system also does not remove the difficulty in separating CIN1 from CIN2 and, as the cut-off point for surgical therapy is often at this point, it therefore leaves unaddressed one of the most difficult areas in histological interpretation.

Outcome for cases of CIN

It should be appreciated that, whether one uses the Bethesda or CIN classification for the histological features of squamous intraepithelial neoplasia, the disease is essentially a histological continuum from normal to high-grade CIN, and any subdivisions must inevitably be arbitrary. HPV-associated changes may be present in all grades of CIN and in non-neoplastic epithelium but are often most florid in association with CIN1. While it is inevitable that, conceptually, the impression is given that disease progresses from low to high grade, in fact, when there is high-grade CIN present histologically in the cervix, there is usually lower grade disease in other areas, and a complex interweaving pattern of low- and high-grade disease is commonly seen. While most have accepted that progression from low- to high-grade CIN precedes invasion, other work suggests that high-grade CIN may develop *de novo* at the margins of low grade (Burghardt, 1991; Koss, 1992). Cytological correlation with histological findings depends closely on the extent of high-grade disease, as well as the actual grade of CIN.

Historical studies on outcome for CIN are very difficult to interpret as methodology varies greatly. They suggest that around 45–60% of CIN1 regresses, 22–45% persists without progression and 10–16% progresses to CIN3. A literature review by Östör (1993) suggested that around 1% progresses to invasive carcinoma. Around 28–40% of CIN2 lesions regress, 20–40% persist, perhaps 17–50% progress to CIN3 and 5% to invasion and perhaps a third of CIN3 regresses and between 10% and 15% probably progresses to invasion (Östör, 1993). Others put the risk for CIN3 progressing at 20–30% (Chang, 1990). The unfortunate outcome of studies at the National Women's Hospital in New Zealand showed that persisting abnormal smears after a histological diagnosis of CIN3 led to a 25-fold increased risk of developing invasive carcinoma compared with women with no history of CIN, whereas a woman in whom destruction of carcinoma *in situ* was successful had a relative risk of approximately three times. Studies from the same unit showed that, after 20 years, 36% of women with an original diagnosis of CIN3, mostly on cone biopsies, would, if they continued to have abnormal smears, develop invasive carcinoma. The rate at 10 years was 18% (McIndoe *et al.*, 1984). Other data have suggested that CIN may take 10 or more years to become invasive. In truth, the interval between CIN3 and invasive carcinoma is probably highly variable and has been put at 3–10 years (Barron *et al.*, 1978), but there appears to be a group of women who develop invasive carcinoma much more quickly and even a small group who may not ever have an interval between normal and invasive disease of a duration that allows its detection cytologically, histologically or colposcopically.

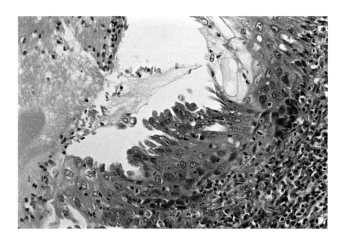

Fig. 21.1 Immature squamous metaplasia with superadded inflammatory and reactive changes. The squamous epithelium here shows marked nuclear reactive changes related to inflammation superimposed on pre-existing immature metaplasia. This pattern can be very difficult to separate from true CIN.

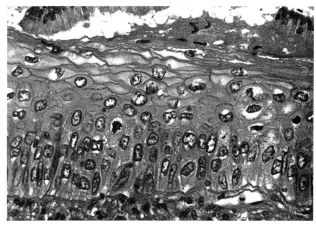

Fig. 21.2 CIN1. The epithelium shows a degree of nuclear abnormality throughout the full thickness of the epithelium, but undifferentiated epithelial cells are confined to the lower third. These cells show increased nuclear pleomorphism, an increased nuclear–cytoplasmic ratio and nuclear enlargement. Warty changes are also seen in the form of koilocytes with enlarged nuclei and perinuclear halos.

Histological features and grading of CIN

The physiological changes seen in the cervix have been alluded to elsewhere in this volume and will not be repeated here. It should be noted, however, that several of these changes may cause considerable difficulties in the separation of CIN from benign conditions. In particular, immature squamous metaplasia (Fig. 21.1), severe atrophic changes, marked reactive changes and thinning of the epithelium and post-traumatic artefacts may all cause major difficulties and are discussed later in this chapter.

CIN is characterised by abnormal cellular proliferation, abnormal epithelial maturation and cytological atypia. To diagnose CIN histologically, it is necessary that there is, throughout the full thickness of the epithelium, some degree of nuclear abnormality. Grading depends, to a considerable extent, on the level in the epithelium where cytoplasmic maturation begins and the level to which undifferentiated ('basaloid') cells extend. In CIN1, the abnormalities are most severe and obvious in the basal third of the epithelium, which is usually replaced, in part or all of its height, by undifferentiated epithelial cells (Fig. 21.2).

The nuclear abnormalities that are seen include nuclear pleomorphism, an increase in nuclear–cytoplasmic ratio, nuclear enlargement and nuclear hyperchromasia. In CIN1, the degree of nuclear pleomorphism in the upper part of the epithelium is mild, as is the increase in nuclear size and the degree of hyperchromasia. Some would argue that an abnormally high level of mitotic figures beyond the lower third of the epithelium is useful in differentiating low-grade CIN from HPV effect alone, but warty changes of themselves may lead to high mitotic figures. Abnormal mitotic figures are generally accepted to be

evidence of CIN. In CIN1, cytoplasmic maturation is limited to the upper two-thirds of the epithelium. The actual variation in the patterns of the epithelium, which most pathologists would regard as CIN1, are wide, and this, together with the difficulty in differentiating CIN1 at one end of the continuum from warty changes alone and at the other end from CIN2, means that the diagnosis is a very subjective one. This has been shown by numerous studies. CIN1 can be found, as can higher degrees of CIN, in mature squamous epithelium, immature epithelium and atrophic epithelium and is usually accompanied by HPV-associated changes, in particular koilocytes.

There is at least as much subjectivity in differentiating true koilocytes from cellular glycogen vacuolation and superadded reactive changes as in separating HPV effect from CIN1, making the Bethesda system just as subjective, at the lower end of the scale, as the CIN system.

In those cases where the epithelium is very thinned or partially lost, one cannot grade the CIN, and the recommendation usually made is that this should be reported as 'ungradable CIN due to epithelial thinning'. The histological diagnosis of CIN2 and 3 (high-grade SIL) is considerably more robust than that of CIN1. In CIN2, nuclear atypia and pleomorphism are generally greater than in CIN1 and, although some nuclear atypia extends through the full thickness of the epithelium, it is usual for cytoplasmic maturation to commence in the middle third. In cases of CIN3, again the nuclear atypia increases with either no cytoplasmic maturation and complete replacement of the epithelium by dedifferentiated cells or maturation only in the upper third (Fig. 21.3). Mitotic activity usually increases as the grade of CIN increases, but this is not always the case.

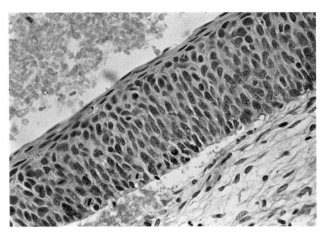

Fig. 21.3 CIN3. The whole thickness of the epithelium is replaced by essentially undifferentiated cells with pleomorphic nuclei showing hyperchromasia, nuclear enlargement and loss of nuclear polarity. Mitoses are common in the basal layers, but are often seen throughout the thickness of the epithelium in CIN3.

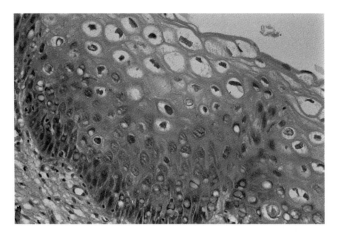

Fig. 21.4 HPV effect. Koilocytes are seen in the epithelium. These show nuclear enlargement, irregular nuclear outlines and perinuclear clearing of the cytoplasm. These are the classical features of HPV infection.

Ploidy in high-grade CIN appears to be correlated with outcome, with aneuploid lesions having higher risk of progression (Hering *et al.*, 2000). Some workers have suggested that abnormal mitoses mean high-grade CIN (Richart, 1990).

HPV-ASSOCIATED CHANGES

The key histological feature of HPV infection is koilocytosis. A koilocyte is a cell with a wrinkled nuclear outline, nuclear enlargement, a usually mild degree of nuclear hyperchromasia and sharply etched perinuclear cytoplasmic clearing. Koilocytes are usually most strikingly seen in the upper layers of the epithelium and in lower grades of CIN. While a very consistent feature of HPV infection, it is now known that koilocytosis is not pathognomonic of HPV and may be seen for a number of other reasons. To avoid overdiagnosis, koilocytes must show nuclear enlargement and atypia. Other features of HPV infection include cellular multinucleation in squamous cells, individual cell keratinisation, parakeratosis, acanthosis and papillomatosis (Fig. 21.4). Those examples of HPV effect that show a papillary outline and an exophytic pattern are usually referred to as condylomata acuminata. Koilocytosis and its associated warty features may make differentiation from CIN extremely difficult and sometimes impossible. While this usually relates to the differential diagnosis of CIN1, there are also cases where the warty changes may produce a very monomorphic nuclear pattern in the epithelium where differentiation of HPV effect, even from CIN3, may prove very difficult. It is likely in the future that ancillary staining, for example with p16, may be helpful in such cases. p16 staining may also be useful in differentiating atrophy from CIN, and proliferation markers may also help in this regard.

OTHER HISTOLOGICAL MIMICS OF CIN

There are a number of normal and abnormal, non-neoplastic variations in the squamous epithelium of the cervix that cause difficulties in the differential diagnosis of CIN. The commonest of these is squamous metaplasia, where the reserve cell hyperplasia evident early in the process may be mistaken for cellular dedifferentiation and CIN in thinned epithelium or, when early squamous differentiation is already evident, the variability in the cellular orientation and the mild nuclear enlargement that is seen may cause problems in differentiation from low-grade CIN. Nuclear pleomorphism and hyperchromasia should be absent, as should loss of cellular polarity but, as the squamous metaplasia is often in the area of the cervix most affected by inflammatory and traumatic changes, this may cause superadded difficulties (Fig. 21.1). The term atypical immature metaplasia is confusing and best avoided.

Atrophy in the squamous epithelium due to low estrogen levels may be a potent mimic of even high-grade CIN. The age of the patient and knowledge of the relative estrogenic state may be useful, as may careful assessment of the epithelium, where the cells can be seen to be generally of parabasal type with epithelial thinning present. While a mild degree of hyperchromasia is usually seen, pleomorphism should be absent or limited in extent, and cellular polarity is usually retained. The site of the atrophic epithelium, i.e. usually towards the vaginal portion of the cervix rather than the squamocolumnar junction, may be very helpful and, in problematic cases, the use of p16 may, in the future, prove useful. Many pathologists would also use Ki67 staining to determine the rate of proliferation. A simpler method of differentiation is to look carefully for mitoses, particularly above the basal layer. In atrophic epithelia, mitoses are usually absent or very sparse and those present are basal.

Basal cell hyperplasia is the presence of an increase in the thickness of the basal layers of the epithelium, often associated with some nuclear enlargement and mild hyperchromasia. This is a very common finding which is related to any form of trauma, infection or irritation of the cervix and may be over-diagnosed as CIN1. There is, however, no significant nuclear pleomorphism, no abnormal mitoses are seen and often the cause of the basal hyperplasia will be evident in the underlying or adjacent tissue.

Particularly in elderly patients, the squamous epithelium of the ectocervix and transformation zone may take on a very monomorphic pattern with little differentiation in the upper layers. It may then closely resemble the transitional epithelium of the urogenital tract. Such 'transitional cell metaplasia' may be widespread and may involve epidermidised crypts. The similarity to transitional epithelium may extend to the nuclei taking on a regular, ovoid pattern with nuclear grooving, but the cells lack excessive mitotic activity, hyperchromasia and true nuclear pleomorphism.

SQUAMOMUCOSAL INTRAEPITHELIAL LESION OF THE ENDOCERVIX (SMILE)

This condition, which has also been called adenosquamous carcinoma *in situ* and multilayered cervical glandular intra-epithelial neoplasia (CGIN), shows replacement of the surface epithelium or crypt epithelium of the cervix by neoplastic cells, usually throughout the epithelial thickness, which do not form glands, but have intracellular mucin vacuoles present. There is still debate about the nature of this condition, some regarding it as an uncommon precursor of adenosquamous carcinoma, others as an intermediate pattern between CIN and CGIN, and others as a variant of CGIN with multilayering of the epithelium. It is usually seen in association with CIN and CGIN and shows the nuclear pleomorphism, increased mitotic rate and loss of polarity typical of an intraepithelial neoplastic lesion. It should be noted that examples of CIN3, particularly involving crypts, may have smaller amounts of mucin within the cellular cyto-plasm, presumably due to its uptake from the lumen, and also residual endocervical cells may be caught up in foci of CIN, or remain on their surface, in zones of immature metaplasia, which may cause problems with differentiation from SMILE.

BASAL (EPITHELIAL) ABNORMALITIES OF UNCERTAIN SIGNIFICANCE

This label has been recommended for those cases in which there is slight nuclear pleomorphism near to the basal layers of the epithelium, where this cannot be explained by inflamma-tion or other pathology adjacent, or cases where the presence of severe inflammation and reparative change makes it imposs-ible to exclude CIN1. While this concept is a useful one, it is not a diagnostic term that is frequently employed by patho-

logists. Some recent data suggest that outcome from the point of view of prognosis is similar to that of CIN1 (Heatley, 2001).

HISTOLOGICAL VARIANTS OF CIN3

Several different patterns of high-grade CIN exist and, in the past, a distinction has been made by some authors between small cell non-keratinising (anaplastic), large cell non-keratinising and keratinising types, similar to the typing of invasive squam-ous carcinoma (Poulsen *et al.*, 1975; Buckley *et al.*, 1982). There is some association of type with site in the cervix, in that the small cell variant tends to be found more commonly towards the endocervical margin of the squamocolumnar junction and within the canal, whereas the keratinising type is often seen on the ectocervix (Fig. 21.5). Some have also employed the term 'differentiated CIN' for those cases where, despite the presence of apparently high-grade CIN, differenti-ation begins in the middle or even lower third of the epithe-lium and there is abundant eosinophilic cytoplasm above this point. There is no evidence at present that any of these sub-divisions is of clinical relevance.

THE SITES OF CIN WITHIN THE CERVIX

It is well recognised that CIN tends to occur at and adjacent to the squamocolumnar junction and commonly extends into the underlying crypts (Anderson and Hartley, 1980) (Fig. 21.6). CIN is also twice as frequent on the anterior lip of the cervix and often more extensive here. It rarely involves the lateral cervical margins early in the disease. This topography is similar to the distribution and extent of cervical eversion and

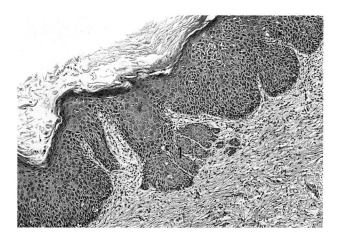

Fig. 21.5 Keratinising-type, high-grade CIN in the congenital transformation zone. The pleomorphism and loss of polarity of high-grade CIN is seen in the epithelium, but the epithelium is differentiating nonetheless towards the surface and shows overlying keratinisation. The residual papillary pattern of the congenital transformation zone is also seen centrally (1).

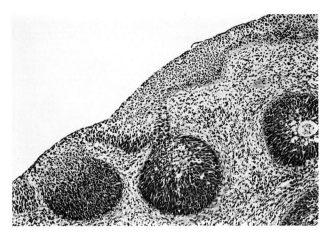

Fig. 21.6 CIN3 with crypt involvement. The surface epithelium of the transformation zone and the underlying crypts are replaced by CIN showing full-thickness undifferentiated cells. This appearance can, to the unwary, be mistaken for invasive squamous carcinoma.

transformation zone formation (Richart, 1965). It tends to stop abruptly at the native squamous epithelium of the portio. Extension along the endocervical canal tends to vary with grade and, rarely, even the endometrium and fallopian tubes may show replacement of the epithelium by high-grade CIN. More than 80% of cases of CIN3 show some crypt involvement, and this may be to the full crypt depth, i.e. up to 7 mm (or presumably even more in those cervices with deep, cystic, dilated crypts). In Anderson and Hartley's study (1980), mean depth of involvement was 1.24 mm and maximum 5.2 mm, with the mean plus three standard deviations being a depth of 3.8 mm. Clearly, this crypt involvement is of considerable importance in deciding treatment modality, as any undestroyed CIN deep in crypts may be cut off from the overlying surface epithelium and therefore be cytologically silent. It may then develop into an occult invasive carcinoma. Degree and depth of involvement of crypts by CIN tends to increase with increasing grade of CIN (Abdul-Karim *et al.*, 1982). It is also well known that the larger the area of CIN on the cervix, the more likely there is to be high-grade CIN present and, in fact, lesion size correlates closely with the cytology of the lesion.

Two main theories on the mode of development and extension of CIN exist. The first suggests that the disease arises multifocally and the foci then coalesce. The alternative theory is that the disease arises at one site and spreads laterally by lifting the adjacent epithelium (Richart, 1965). Clonality studies have supported the latter concept (Larson *et al.*, 1997). More recent work on HPV infection suggests that low- and high-grade CIN, when associated with high-risk HPV infection, may be monoclonal, whereas low-grade CIN associated with low-risk HPV types may be polyclonal (Park *et al.*, 1996). It is generally now felt that the disease arises in basal cells of the transformation zone rather than in endocervical reserve cells.

EARLY INVASIVE SQUAMOUS CARCINOMA

Terminology in early invasive squamous carcinoma is problematic, and the commonly used term microinvasive carcinoma tends to mean different things to different people. In Britain, microinvasive carcinoma is usually taken to be synonymous with FIGO stages IA1 and 2, i.e. up to 5 mm depth of invasion and 7 mm diameter, but, elsewhere, particularly in the United States, the cut-off point for the diagnosis of microinvasive carcinoma is often the limit of FIGO stage IA1 disease, i.e. 3 mm in depth, and cases with vessel involvement have been excluded. Some also have not used lateral dimension cut-off points, and others have used volume criteria alone to make the diagnosis. Methods of measurement of depth of invasion (see later) have also varied. It is therefore wise to avoid the use of the term microinvasive carcinoma and utilise the latest FIGO staging system (Table 21.1), with an indication in the histological report of the exact dimensions of the early invasive tumour.

The concept of microinvasive carcinoma was introduced by Mestwerdt in 1947 to indicate small tumours, less than 5 mm depth of extension into the stroma, which carried a much better prognosis than larger stage I lesions (Mestwerdt, 1951). It should be noted that the presence of lymphatic or blood vessel permeation adjacent to the early invasive tumour, while it is important that it is identified and commented on in the histological report, does not alter the FIGO staging of the tumour. Neither is the stage affected by extension of multifocal tumours to the isthmus or lower body of the uterus, while still meeting the size criteria for stage IA carcinoma, although this is a very uncommon finding except for the extension of CIN3 adjacent to early invasive carcinoma.

The earliest stage of stromal invasion is represented by tiny buds of squamous cells, which often have an altered morphology compared with the overlying zone of, usually high-grade, CIN from which they arise. It should be noted, however, that there is not always CIN3 in the overlying epithelium, and invasion may arise from CIN1. These small invasive tongues show what is often referred to as paradoxical differentiation, i.e. an increase in cytoplasmic eosinophilia and amount of cytoplasm relative to the nucleus with some apparent reduction in the pleomorphism of the nuclei compared with the overlying CIN (Fig. 21.7). Adjacent to the invasive epithelium, there may be a loose and oedematous pattern to the stroma with a chronic inflammatory cell infiltrate, but this is by no means always seen. The pattern described above was often referred to in the past as 'early stromal invasion' (ESI) and constituted the major proportion of examples of stage IA1 disease in the previous FIGO classification (prior to 1995).

There is, of course, a point at which one cannot be certain whether a tumour bud has broken through into the stroma, and a useful term for those examples of CIN with an agitated irregular base and some cytoplasmic eosinophilia is

Table 21.1 Carcinoma of the cervix uteri — staging.

FIGO stages	Description	TNM categories
	Primary tumour cannot be assessed	TX
	No evidence of primary tumour	T0
0	Carcinoma *in situ* (preinvasive carcinoma)	Tis
I	Cervical carcinoma confined to uterus (extension to corpus should be disregarded)	T1
IA	Invasive carcinoma diagnosed only by microscopy. All macroscopically visible lesions (even with superficial invasion) are stage IB/T1b	T1a
IA1	Stromal invasion no greater than 3.0 mm in depth and 7.0 mm or less in horizontal spread	T1a1
IA2	Stromal invasion more than 3.0 mm and not more than 5.0 mm with a horizontal spread 7.0 mm or less[a]	T1a2
IB	Clinically visible lesion confined to the cervix or microscopic lesion greater than IA2/T1a2	T1b
IB1	Clinically visible lesion 4.0 cm or less in greatest dimension	T1b1
IB2	Clinically visible lesion more than 4 cm in greatest dimension	T1b2
II	Tumour invades beyond the uterus but not to pelvic wall or to lower third of the vagina	T2
IIA	Without parametrial invasion	T2a
IIB	With parametrial invasion	T2b
III	Tumour extends to pelvic wall/or involves lower third of vagina and/or causes hydronephrosis or non-functioning kidney	T3
IIIA	Tumour involves lower third of vagina with no extension to pelvic wall	T3a
IIIB	Tumour extends to pelvic wall and/or causes hydronephrosis or non-functioning kidney	T3b
IVA	Tumour invades mucosa of bladder or rectum and/or extends beyond true pelvis[b]	T4
IVB	Distant metastasis	M1

Taken from FIGO Committee on Gynecologic Oncology (2000) *International Journal of Gynecology and Obstetrics* 70: 209–262, 223.
[a]The depth of invasion should not be more than 5 mm taken from the base of the epithelium, either surface or glandular, from which it originates. The depth of invasion is defined as the measurement of the tumour from the epithelial stromal junction of the adjacent most superficial epithelial papilla to the deepest point of invasion. Vascular space involvement, venous or lymphatic, does not affect classification.
[b]The presence of bullous oedema is not sufficient to classify a tumour as T4.

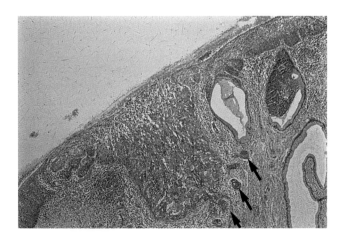

Fig. 21.7 Early invasive squamous carcinoma. Arising from squamous epithelium, showing high-grade CIN, are tiny buds of early invasive squamous epithelium (early stromal invasion, arrowed).

'questionable early stromal invasion'. Al-Nafussi and Hughes (1994) showed that there was a high likelihood of identifying early invasion when CIN3 was extensive and there was widespread, deep extension into endocervical crypts and also when

there was necrotic material in the lumina of the crypts with intraepithelial squamous maturation and expansion of the crypt width.

From these minor buds of squamous epithelium, there is essentially a continuum of changes seen up to large invasive squamous carcinomas, and the FIGO classification applies arbitrary points of separation of tumour into two subgroups within stage Ia. The major determinant of point of separation of the subgroups should be outcome (see below).

Differential diagnosis of early invasive carcinoma

Apart from differentiation from inflammatory changes producing irregularities of the epithelial base and CIN3-like carcinoma, there are two pregnancy-related changes that may cause diagnostic problems. The first of these is focal decidualisation of the cervix (deciduosis). This occurs commonly in pregnancy and may be colposcopically mistaken for carcinoma. Histologically too, the large, pale stromal cells may be confused with early invasive foci. Appreciation of the lack of nuclear pleomorphism and poorly demarcated nature of the change is key to the diagnosis. Focal pseudodecidualisation, due to exogenous hormones, may lead to similar problems.

It is not commonly appreciated that the endocervix is a very common site for the occurrence of placental site plaques or nodules. The fact that these may persist for several years after pregnancy may also mislead. Histologically, the nuclear pleomorphism and cellular morphology may superficially resemble early invasive squamous carcinoma, but the lack of mitotic activity, eosinophilic stroma, circumscription and presence of multinucleate or clear cells may all help in differentiation, as may immunohistochemistry.

Prognostic factors in early invasive squamous carcinoma

Tumour dimensions and volume

It is accepted that tumour depth of invasion for squamous carcinoma of the cervix is closely allied to prognosis. This, of course, is the underlying basis of the FIGO staging system within stage 1. As indicated previously, however, it must be accepted that the points of cut-off for various stages should reflect prognostic groups as closely as possible. In essence, those tumours with invasion into the stroma less than 1.0 mm in depth have no risk of metastasis, whereas those between 3 and 5 mm perhaps have a 6–8% risk of nodal metastases and, between 1 and 3 mm, probably in the region of 1–2%. What is probably even more important is the actual extent of the interface of the invasive tumour with the adjacent stoma, and this is better measured by a three-dimensional assessment of the tumour volume. Extensive work on this problem by Burghardt and Holzer (1977) suggested that, without vessel invasion, there is no significant risk of metastasis below a tumour volume of 500 mm^3, although in the case of those tumours with lymphatic involvement, the position is less clear (Burghardt, 1978). Measuring the volume accurately is a lengthy and time-consuming process, however, and requires the knowledge of the maximum depth and lateral extent of tumour in all the blocks taken, together with the width of the individual block. A rough assessment of volume can be made without step sections, provided the block width is roughly known and the tumour dimensions in each block. This method has an acceptable accuracy for clinical purposes and would, if widely applied, allow a larger proportion of patients to be treated conservatively. It should be stressed that those methods that depend upon mathematical formulae, for example that of a truncated cone, are really much less acceptable, in that they tend to considerably overestimate the volume of tumour present.

To apply the FIGO staging criteria accurately, it is imperative that the measurements employed are determined exactly in accordance with the definitions in the staging system (see below).

Lateral (horizontal) extent of tumour appears to correlate with the presence of residual tumour in post-cone hysterectomy specimens (Sedlis *et al.*, 1979). Takeshima *et al.* (1999) found that, overall, 18% of stage IA tumours were upgraded to IB on the basis of lateral spread of more than 7 mm, but this varied from 6% for stage IA1 to 61% for IA2.

Excision margins

The presence of neoplasia at the resection plane of a cone biopsy is a very important prognostic factor, but data are very difficult to interpret as often invasive disease at the margins of a cone is used as well as CIN to predict the risk of recurrent/residual disease in the hysterectomy specimen. If both categories are included, then perhaps 4% with clear margins will have residual disease in the hysterectomy compared with 35–80% with involved margins (Wright *et al.*, 2002a). The situation after large loop excision of the transformation zone (LLETZ) is less clear, but the margins are still likely to be of importance.

Vessel involvement

The data available in the literature on outcome related to lymphatic or small blood vessel involvement in the cervix are very conflicting with variations in incidence between 10% and 30% for stage IA and between 12% and 57% for IB (Wright *et al.*, 2002b). The incidence of capillary space involvement varies greatly depending on the number of sections examined. Roche and Norris (1975) suggested that, in tumours with invasion of between 2 and 5 mm, almost 60% may have capillary space involvement and, in their study, none of these showed lymph node involvement on radical hysterectomy and lymphadenectomy. Other workers (e.g. Burghardt, 1982) did, however, show that the presence of lymphatic vessel involvement increased the risk of metastasis and that this was related to tumour size (Roman *et al.*, 1998). It has been suggested that vessel invasion may account for those very rare cases of lymph node metastasis in tumours invading to a depth of 1 mm or less (van Nagell *et al.*, 1983; Collins *et al.*, 1989). Artefactual spaces in the tissue due to processing may mimic the appearance of vessel invasion. Some have suggested that the use of immunohistochemistry, for example CD31 antigen, may help here, and newer markers are becoming available (Birner *et al.*, 2001). While it is difficult to summarise the overall literature on vessel invasion, it might be argued that it is really only in stage IA2 and IB1 tumours that vessel invasion affects outcome, and there is still no clear, generally accepted guidance on altering therapy dependent upon vessel invasion, although it is common for clinicians to treat examples of stage IA2 disease with vessel invasion by radical therapy.

Growth pattern

The growth pattern of invasive tumours, beyond the limits of early stromal invasion, varies greatly, and attempts have been made to separate the invasive patterns into a so-called spray growth pattern and a pushing or broad growth pattern but, unfortunately, it is very common to see both these growth patterns within an individual tumour. There have been reports that growth pattern may be important in predicting recurrence (Schumaker and Schwarz, 1989; Kristensen *et al.*, 1999), and Boyes *et al.* (1970) suggested that confluence of invasive groups of tumour cells carried an increased risk of metastatic spread, when compared with the finger-like growth pattern seen more commonly in very small tumours. It has been common, however, to use the term 'confluent' in different ways and also, at least in early-stage tumours, confluence of the tumour appears to be a surrogate marker of tumour size. Other workers, e.g. Roche and Norris (1975), found no association between growth pattern and vessel invasion and, overall, there is still considerable doubt over its significance in the stage IA subgroup. To our knowledge, no studies on mathematical measurement of variation in marginal characteristics of tumours of the cervix exist with outcome data.

Histological reporting of early invasive squamous carcinoma

In the histological report on such cases, it is strongly advised (NHSCSP, 1999) that the following information is included in all reports:

1 The nature and pattern of the invasive tumour, i.e. a small confluent tumour or non-confluent tiny tongues of invasion resembling 'early stromal invasion'.

2 Tumour depth of invasion, as measured from the base of the overlying parent epithelium or, if there is no intact overlying epithelium, from the base of the nearest intact epithelium and, where the tumour involves and arises from a crypt, from its point of origin from the crypt epithelial base. It is defined as 'the measurement of the tumour from the epithelial–stromal junction of the adjacent most superficial epithelial papilla to the deepest point of invasion' (Table 21.1). Where small invasive foci are seen in the stroma with no site of origin apparent, then the tumour depth should again be measured from the nearest overlying surface epithelial base. If the surface of a small carcinoma is ulcerated, it is impossible to measure how much tissue has been lost, and one should not simply include such tumours in the stage IA group without qualification and clarification.

4 The width of the tumour measured in the section in which the width is the greatest. This width should be measured from the edge at which invasion is first seen to the most distant edge at which invasion can be detected and should include tiny foci of early stromal invasion at the margins. In the opinion of the author, it should not include entirely separate foci in multifocal disease, but others argue for the summation of the width of all foci.

5 The presence or absence of vascular permeation (lymphatic or capillary) should be recorded.

6 In tumours that are large enough to allow differentiation to be assessed, the grade of the tumour should be noted.

7 Clear comment should be made as to whether both the invasive tumour and any adjacent CIN or CGIN are fully excised on all the relevant margins.

The term microinvasive carcinoma and substaging within stage I should not be applied to small cell neuroendocrine tumours or peripheral neuroectodermal tumours of the cervix,

no matter how small the lesion is. These tumours require aggressive therapy. It must also be stressed that one cannot make a diagnosis of stage IA1 or 2 carcinoma on a punch biopsy, and the diagnosis cannot be made if the margins of the loop or cold knife conisation specimen are involved by invasive tumour. The histology report in such cases should simply state the extent of the tumour in the available tissue and indicate clearly that the margins are involved and therefore full measurement cannot be made and more advance disease excluded.

As the lateral extent of the tumour most likely derives its value prognostically as a surrogate measure of volume, it is important to recognise that, if a tumour involves more than two tissue blocks, it potentially may be greater than 7 mm in extent in the third dimension and, in the authors' opinion, such tumours should not be placed in the stage IA category. It is necessary to have a knowledge of the width, on average, of the blocks (from a knowledge of the width of the specimen and the number of blocks obtained from it) to allow this assessment; for example, if 2-mm-wide blocks were taken, the tumour would still be within the limits of stage IA disease until four blocks were involved, whereas three blocks could exceed the limit if the block width was 3 mm, which is, in practice, commoner.

INVASIVE SQUAMOUS CARCINOMA AND ITS VARIANTS

Squamous cell carcinoma not otherwise specified (NOS)

Gross pathology

Squamous carcinoma may present as an ulcerated or elevated granular area with contact bleeding, leading to intermenstrual or postmenopausal bleeding or discharge (Fig. 21.8), or may be a polypoid, exophytic tumour mass, but a proportion of

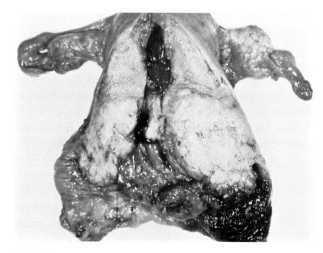

Fig. 21.8 Squamous carcinoma of the cervix. The cervix shows a very large squamous carcinoma extending through its full thickness and involving the portio vaginalis.

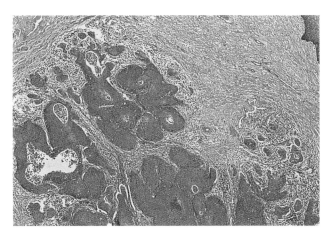

Fig. 21.9 Invasive squamous cell carcinoma. Classical features of invasive squamous carcinoma are seen with tongues of malignant squamous epithelium infiltrating the cervical stroma as irregular angulated foci at the margins of larger tumour masses.

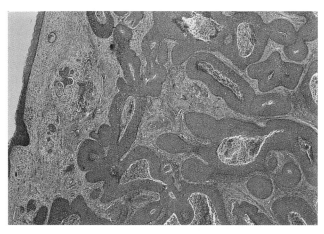

Fig. 21.10 Squamous carcinoma of the cervix with CIN3-like growth pattern. This squamous carcinoma is extensively infiltrating the cervical stroma, but retains a generally rounded outline with keratinous debris in the centre of the cell nests, mimicking the appearance of CIN3. Clearly invasive foci with angular margins can be seen focally, however, particularly in the superficial part of the tumour.

tumours also present as deeply infiltrating carcinomas extending along the cervical canal (so-called barrel carcinomas of the cervix). The majority of carcinomas involve the external os. Separating tumours into nodular infiltrative and ulcerative infiltrative seems to have no prognostic value. Clinical staging of squamous carcinoma is a subjective and inaccurate process, and it is now usual prior to surgery to stage carcinomas in the UK by combined clinical, pathological and radiological means and to finally allocate tumour stage on the basis of the main resection specimen wherever possible.

Histological features

Considerable variation in growth pattern, differentiation and cellular morphology is seen within the squamous carcinoma category and even within individual tumours. Most infiltrate as irregular islands or tongues of squamous cells, showing increasing differentiation towards the centre of the islands and irregular ragged margins to the tumour cell groups (Fig. 21.9). Keratin pearls may be seen within the cell groups – the keratinising variant. Non-keratinising tumours usually appear more pleomorphic and may be more mitotically active. A second variant of non-keratinising carcinoma is composed of smaller, basaloid cells with more nuclear hyperchromasia. Between the groups, there is usually a prominent stromal reaction with inflammatory cells often numerous, but other tumours may grow as more rounded, confluent, solid tumour masses or as partly cystic tumour masses with central cavities and necrosis. Occasionally, tumour infiltration may be predominantly by single cells. The inflammatory and stromal response may be very variable. In some cases, even without a so-called glassy cell morphology, there may be a very prominent eosinophilic infiltrate in the stroma.

Some tumours very closely mimic the appearances of crypt involvement by CIN (Al-Nafussi and Monaghan, 2000). Such

tumours may often be recognised by the necrotic debris within the rounded tumour cell aggregates and by the focal areas of marginal irregularity and tongue-like infiltration usually present on extensive examination (Fig. 21.10). When viewed at low power, they also show a very marked alteration in the apparent crypt architecture. It should be stressed that no clear prognostic difference is evident between these individual cell types within the pure squamous carcinoma group (Zaino *et al.*, 1992).

Recently, WHO has recommended classifying squamous carcinomas into only keratinising and non-keratinising groups, avoiding the use of the term 'small cell squamous carcinoma', which was previously the third type recognised, and reserving the term small cell carcinoma for neuroendocrine tumours, which have a much poorer prognosis. There has, however, been debate as to whether even small cell squamous carcinoma may be an aggressive variant. It must be stressed that individually keratinising cells will be seen even in non-keratinising carcinomas, although even one squamous pearl makes a carcinoma keratinising in some eyes, and it is important not to include entirely undifferentiated carcinomas in the squamous group simply because they are composed of large cells.

There has been considerable debate in the literature around the use of the term 'adenosquamous carcinoma' and relative outcome for this tumour. This entity is dealt with under glandular lesions of the cervix, and it will suffice to comment here that there is no overall agreement on when to use the term. Most would agree that, when a tumour shows clear-cut squamous differentiation, together with undoubted focal gland formation and mucin production, then this has to be regarded as an adenosquamous carcinoma. The question arises as to what diagnosis should be used in those cases that just show a very occasional rudimentary acinus, or droplets of intracellular mucin in an otherwise obviously squamous tumour. It is likely that these problems underlie the difficulty in determining whether adenosquamous carcinomas have a poorer prognosis than pure squamous. At present, probably the best assessment of the overall literature is that adenosquamous carcinomas tend to occur in a somewhat younger age group than squamous carcinomas NOS and may have an increased risk of nodal metastasis, but there is no clear-cut evidence that they have poorer overall outcome. There is some suggestion that, within the adenosquamous group, there may be a subgroup of more aggressive tumours, occurring in young women, which may possibly be definable by the use of adjunctive studies, such as EGFR (Hale *et al.*, 1993).

Histological grading of squamous carcinoma is generally and widely applied, and it is surprising, therefore, that no generally accepted method of grading exists, and outcome related to grade and type is still unclear (Zaino *et al.*, 1992). In general, grade is unlikely to affect the treatment modality offered, but grading is useful to allow retrospective review of outcome, and future modification of the grading method may allow more prognostic information to be derived. The most widely used grading system is a modification of Broder's original system that divides tumours into three grades based upon the extent of keratinisation, cellular pleomorphism and mitotic activity among other characteristics (Wright *et al.*, 2002b). In essence, however, when one uses the three-grade system of well, moderately and poorly differentiated, the specific criteria used are very loose and relate more to degree of differentiation of the predominant cell present (Stock *et al.*, 1994). More than half of tumours fall into the moderately differentiated group with the other 40% or so evenly divided between poorly and well differentiated. Interpreting historical data on outcome by grade is fraught with problems because, often, tumours within individual groups were of different stage or size, but it is likely that a two-group classification would be more useful prognostically, i.e. low and high grade.

The stromal inflammatory reaction to invasive carcinoma usually comprises predominantly lymphocytes and plasma cells, although where there is necrosis, polymorphs are often very prominent. Some workers have suggested a better outcome for tumours with a very prominent stromal response (Abell, 1973; Hasumi *et al.*, 1977; van Nagell *et al.*, 1978), but this is not a generally accepted prognostic marker. A florid eosinophil or giant cell stromal response may also be seen, and it has been suggested that those tumours with a florid giant cell reaction may have a better prognosis, although again this remains to be confirmed by more definitive studies.

The effect of patient age on survival is not entirely clear. Early studies suggested that older patients had an improved survival, but the study by Meanwell *et al.* (1988) showed younger women to have a better prognosis. What data exist perhaps suggest that younger women with high-stage tumours have a poorer outcome (Wright *et al.*, 2002b).

Histological reporting of squamous carcinomas

As for stage IA carcinomas, all histological reports should grade and determine the lateral extent and depth of invasion of the tumour and also comment on the presence or absence of vessel invasion. Adequacy of excision should always be assessed with regard to the vaginal, deep cervical and parametrial margins, and comment on the presence or absence of involvement of the parametria, vagina, isthmus or uterine corpus should be included. It has been suggested that it is also useful to determine the distance of clearance not only from the deep cervical margin but also from the deep cervical–stromal interface. The presence or absence of nodal metastases should be clearly stated together with the total number of nodes identified in each anatomical group.

Local and metastatic spread

Squamous carcinoma of the cervix spreads by direct extension into adjacent structures, followed by lymphatic invasion then, less commonly, blood vessel invasion and implantation. It spreads into the body of the uterus and, more commonly, directly into the vagina, outwards to the parametrial tissues (and by metastasis into parametrial nodes) and sidewalls of the pelvis, involving the ureters, and also through the deep cervical planes to involve the bladder and rectum. Lymph node metastases occur most frequently in the external iliac, hypogastric and obturator nodes, followed less commonly by the common iliac, parametrial and paracervical nodes. Involvement of para-aortic and inguinal nodes is infrequent (Plentl and Friedman, 1971; Piver and Chung, 1976) and in isolation is rare (Morice *et al.*, 2000). Between 25% and 50% of patients with stage 1B and 2 carcinomas will be found to have lymph node metastases. Deaths resulting from cervical carcinoma are usually due to local effects and, in particular, destruction of adjacent structures and occlusion of the ureters. The proportion of patients dying of ureteric obstruction and renal failure has decreased considerably since the 1970s due to improvements in irradiation.

Variants of squamous carcinoma

Verrucous carcinoma

Verrucous carcinomas of the cervix appear to be very rare (Faaborg *et al.*, 1979; Tiltman and Atad, 1982; Kashimura *et al.*, 1984), and many of the comments made in the literature are derived by extrapolation from the behaviour, etc. of this tumour at other sites. Some have questioned their true nature in the female genital tract (Robertson *et al.*, 1993). Essentially, verrucous carcinomas are exophytic, large, papillary tumours with minimal nuclear atypia, usually confined to the basal layers of the epithelium, and often with a rather pale overall epithelial cellular appearance. Tumours previously termed giant condylomata acuminata and Buschke–Lowenstein tumours appear to be the same lesion. Verrucous carcinomas have evidence of co-existent HPV infection (Gissman *et al.*, 1982). It is not clear whether they develop from pre-existing condylomata. They are bulky fungating tumours, sometimes show ulceration and often produce a foul smell and discharge. They appear to grow slowly and very rarely produce nodal or distant metastases (Lucas *et al.*, 1974), but compress and destroy adjacent structures. They are commonly locally advanced at the time of treatment. The tumour margin is rounded and well defined without infiltrative tongues. The stroma usually shows a mixed inflammatory cell infiltrate, which may be prominent but, as there are no infiltrating tumour foci within the stroma, there is not a prominent desmoplastic response.

They may cause diagnostic difficulties with simple exophytic squamous carcinomas, so-called warty carcinomas and with the very rare squamous papilloma of the cervix. Very large, simple condylomata acuminata may also be very difficult to differentiate from verrucous carcinoma, and a large, deep biopsy is necessary to allow an accurate diagnosis (Jennings and Barclay, 1972; Isaac, 1976). Treatment of this condition is by wide surgical excision, but lymphadenectomy is generally considered unnecessary. Local infiltration may be extensive, reaching into the endometrium and pelvic tissues. It has been argued that inadequate irradiation may cause anaplastic transformation of such tumours (Krauz and Perez-Meza, 1966; Faaborg *et al.*, 1979; Tiltman and Atad, 1982; Kashimura *et al.*, 1984) but, for vulval tumours, debate surrounds the use of radiotherapy to reduce tumour size and allow easier surgery.

Warty squamous carcinoma

This recently described variant of squamous cell carcinoma is similar to the identically named vulval tumour (Rastkar *et al.*, 1982). It shows marked cytoplasmic vacuolation and nuclear changes resembling koilocytosis, but the infiltrative margin is similar to that of squamous cell carcinoma 'NOS' rather than verrucous carcinoma. The importance of the diagnosis appears to be that this tumour variant may have a relatively good outcome, although data are at present very limited.

Lymphoepithelioma-like carcinoma

This tumour occurs in women over a wide age range (20 to more than 60 years), and presentation and the overall macroscopic appearances are similar to those of squamous carcinoma NOS, although macroscopically the tumour margins tend to be well circumscribed. It is an uncommon tumour (Hafiz *et al.*, 1985; Mills *et al.*, 1985; Halpin *et al.*, 1989; Weinburg *et al.*, 1993; Tseng *et al.*, 1997; Lopez-Rios *et al.*, 2000) and is composed of very poorly defined groups of irregular undifferentiated cells lying in, and divided up by, sheets of lymphocytes. The pattern is very similar to that of so-called lymphoepithelioma of the nasopharynx. The malignant epithelial cells have a moderate to large amount of poorly delimited, eosinophilic cytoplasm, which gives the tumour cell aggregates the appearance of syncytia. Nuclei are similar in size with prominent nucleoli and granular chromatin. Most of the lymphocytes on immunohistochemistry are T cells, and the undifferentiated carcinoma cells show immunohistochemical marker positivity as squamous cells.

The major reason for differentiating this tumour type, apart from the need to separate it from lymphoma and from non-malignant conditions, is that it would appear to have a much better prognosis than squamous carcinoma NOS. There is no clear evidence at present that it has the same degree of radiosensitivity shown by nasopharyngeal carcinomas. Hasumi *et al.* (1977) showed that only around 5% of patients with lymphoepithelioma had positive regional nodes, but further studies are necessary to determine the overall prognosis of this tumour variant. Unlike lymphoepitheliomas in the nasopharyngeal region, determination of Epstein–Barr virus (EBV) status in cervical tumours has yielded conflicting results (Martorell *et al.*, 2002). Weinburg *et al.* (1993) failed to find EBV genomic material in lymphoepithelioma-like carcinoma of the cervix, but Tseng *et al.* (1997) found that 11 of 15 carcinomas had EBV genomic material but only 3 of 15 had HPV DNA. Lopez-Rios *et al.* (2000) did not find EBV in the single case they analysed. As the study by Tseng *et al.* (1997) was on an Asian population, there may be geographical variation in the nature of this tumour and in its causation.

The differential diagnosis of lymphoepithelioma-like carcinoma includes conditions with a major inflammatory cell component such as postoperative spindle cell nodule, inflammatory pseudotumour, lymphomas and pseudolymphomatous lesions (Wright *et al.*, 2002b).

Papillary squamotransitional (squamous) cell carcinoma

This is a relatively rare variant of cervical carcinoma. Originally, these tumours were felt to represent transitional cell carcinomas (Randall *et al.*, 1986; Albores-Saavedra and Young, 1995). More recently, they have been divided into predominantly squamous, mixed squamous–transitional and predominantly transitional (Koenig *et al.*, 1997), but no definite difference in prognosis is seen between the three types. The immunohistochemical pattern of the tumours is, in fact, more in keeping with squamous carcinoma than with transitional cell carcinoma of the urinary tract.

Histologically, these tumours have multilayered, papillary epithelium resembling either transitional cell carcinoma of the bladder or high-grade CIN. Foci of usual squamous carcinoma are often found adjacent. The tumour columns arising from the base of the papillae often extend deep into the cervix, and the cores of the papillae may also be invaded. Behaviour appears to be similar to that of squamous carcinoma NOS, although it has been suggested that the tumour may show a particular tendency for unusually late recurrence (Randall *et al.*, 1988). The major importance of accurate diagnosis is that it may be mistaken histologically for papillary CIN or a condyloma.

Prognostic histological factors in cervical squamous carcinoma

Clinical stage of tumour is the most significant prognostic factor in cervical cancer. When stage is allowed for, grade of tumour has little value. In stages IB and IIA, for surgically treated tumours, the tumour size is important in determining the risk of nodal metastasis and survival. Within a single stage tumour volume, depth of invasion and lateral extent, cervical stromal tumour-free rim, nodal metastases and parametrial extension are all important (Inoue, 1984; Hale *et al.*, 1991; Smiley *et al.*, 1991; Zaino *et al.*, 1992; Sevin *et al.*, 1996; Stockler *et al.*, 1996; Zreik *et al.*, 1996). In a US Gynaecologic Oncology Group (GOG) study, patients whose tumours invaded only the inner third of the cervical stroma had a 98% 5-year progression-free rate, whereas those with outer third involvement had a 63% rate (Zaino *et al.*, 1992). Lymphatic or vessel blood vessel permeation would appear to be an important risk factor for lymph node metastasis, in particular for patients with stage IB disease (Barber *et al.*, 1978; van Nagell *et al.*, 1978; Crissman *et al.*, 1985; Buckley *et al.*, 1988; Hale *et al.*, 1991; Smiley *et al.*, 1991; Kainz *et al.*, 1994). In patients without nodal metastases, it also appears to predict a group with a higher risk of relapse [a relative risk of 2.5:1 in the study by Stockler *et al.* (1996)]. In the same GOG study quoted above, 5-year progression-free survival was 70% with and 83% without lymphovascular space invasion (Zaino *et al.*, 1992). Van Nagell *et al.* (1978) found that lymph node metastases increased from 6% to 34% of patients without and with vessel involvement, and Barber *et al.* (1978) found that 5-year survival varied from almost 60% in patients with radical hysterectomy with vascular involvement to 90% without vascular involvement, in the stage IB group. Others have found a 2.5-fold increased risk of relapse in those with vessel invasion (Stockler *et al.*, 1996).

Oncogene studies have generally produced conflicting results. Oncogene overexpression is common in cervical cancer (Zhang *et al.*, 2002). A relationship between prognosis and C-erb-B2 overexpression (Hale *et al.*, 1992; Soh *et al.*, 2002) and EGF-r overexpression (Hale *et al.*, 1993) has been reported. Other workers suggest C-erb-B2 measurement may be of value in adenocarcinomas but not squamous cancers (Mandai *et al.*, 1995). Other suggested prognostic factors include CD44 (Speiser *et al.*, 1977), vessel density (Lenczewski *et al.*, 2002) and levels of angiogenesis (Tjalma *et al.*, 1998).

HPV 18-positive tumours would appear to have a poorer prognosis than others (Burger *et al.*, 1993, 1996; Rose *et al.*, 1995), with some reporting a 2.5-fold increase in risk of

recurrence when detected by Southern blot analysis (Walker *et al.*, 1989). There has been some debate whether the presence of concurrent pregnancy alters outcome for squamous carcinomas. Hacker *et al.* (1982) found that delaying definitive surgery for up to 2 months did not affect outcome and that overall prognosis by stage for cervical cancer in pregnancy was similar to that of non-pregnant women, but a group with more advanced disease was suggested to have a poorer prognosis. They suggest that the apparently favourable prognosis noted by some workers was actually due to a greater proportion of early-stage tumours in pregnancy.

REFERENCES

Abdul-Karim FW, Fu YS, Reagan JW *et al.* (1982) Morphometric study of intraepithelial neoplasia of uterine cervix. *Obstetrics and Gynecology* 60: 210–214.

Abell MR (1973) Invasive carcinoma of the uterine cervix. In: Norris HJ, Hertig AI, Abell MR (eds) *The Uterus.* Baltimore: Williams & Wilkins, pp. 413–456.

Albores-Saavedra J, Young RH (1995) Transitional cell neoplasms (carcinomas and inverted papillomas) of the uterine cervix. A report of five cases. *American Journal of Surgical Pathology* 19: 1138–1145.

Al-Nafussi AI, Hughes DE (1994) Histological features of CIN3 and their value in predicting invasive microinvasive squamous carcinoma. *Journal of Clinical Pathology* 47: 799–804.

Al-Nafussi AI, Monaghan H (2000) Squamous cell carcinoma of the cervix with CIN3-like growth pattern: an under-diagnosed lesion. *International Journal of Gynaecological Cancer* 10: 95–99.

Anderson MC, Hartley RB (1980) Cervical crypt involvement by intraepithelial neoplasia. *Obstetrics and Gynecology* 55: 546–550.

Barber HRK, Sommers SC, Rotterdam H *et al.* (1978) Vascular invasion as a prognostic factor in stage 1b cancer of the cervix. *Obstetrics and Gynecology* 52: 343–348.

Barron BA, Cahill MC, Richart RM (1978) A statistical model of the natural history of cervical neoplastic disease: the duration of carcinoma in situ. *Gynecologic Oncology* 6: 196–205.

Birner P, Obermair A, Schindl M *et al.* (2001) Selective immunohistochemical staining of blood and lymphatic vessels reveals independent prognostic influence of blood and lymphatic vessel invasion in early-stage cervical cancer. *Clinical Cancer Research* 7: 93–97.

Boyes DA, Worth JA, Fidler HK (1970) The results of treatment of 4389 cases of preclinical cervical squamous carcinoma. *Journal of Obstetrics and Gynaecology of the British Commonwealth* 77: 769–780.

Buckley CH, Butler EB, Fox H (1982) Cervical intraepithelial neoplasia. *Journal of Clinical Pathology* 35: 1–13.

Buckley CH, Beards CS, Fox H (1988) Pathological prognostic factors in cervical cancer with particular reference to patients under the age of 40 years. *British Journal of Obstetrics and Gynaecology* 95: 47–56.

Burger JPM, Hollema H, Gouw AS *et al.* (1993) Cigarette smoking and human papillomavirus in patients with reported cervical cytological abnormality. *British Medical Journal* 306: 749–752.

Burger RA, Monk BJ, Kurosaki T *et al.* (1996) Human papillomavirus type 18: association with poor prognosis in early stage cervical cancer. *Journal of the National Cancer Institute* 88: 1361–1368.

Burghardt E (1978) Microcarcinoma of the cervix uteri. *Wiener Klinische Wochenschrift* 90: 477–485.

Burghardt E (1982) Diagnostic and prognostic criteria in cervical microcarcinoma. *Clinics in Oncology* 1: 323–333.

Burghardt E (1991) *Colposcopy—Cervical Pathology*. New York: Thieme Medical Publishers.

Burghardt E, Holzer E (1977) Diagnosis and treatment of microinvasive carcinoma of the cervix uteri. *Obstetrics and Gynecology* 49: 641–653.

Chang AR (1990) Carcinoma-in-situ of the cervix and its malignant potential. A lesson from New Zealand. *Cytopathology* 1: 321–328.

Cocker J, Fox H, Langley FA (1968) Consistency in the histological diagnosis of epithelial abnormalities of the cervix uteri. *Journal of Clinical Pathology* 21: 67–70.

Collins HS, Burke TW, Woodward JE *et al.* (1989) Widespread lymph node metastases in a patient with microinvasive cervical carcinoma. *Gynecologic Oncology* 34: 219–221.

Crissman JD, Makuch R, Budhraja M (1985) Histopathologic grading of squamous cell carcinoma of the uterine cervix. *Cancer* 55: 1590–1596.

De Vet HCW, Knipschild PG, Schouten HJA *et al.* (1992) Sources of interobserver variation in histopathological grading of cervical dysplasia. *Journal of Clinical Epidemiology* 45: 785–790.

Faaborg LL, Smith ML, Newland JR (1979) Case report: uterine cervical and vaginal verrucous squamous cell carcinoma. *Gynecologic Oncology* 8: 104–109.

Fu YS, Reagan JW, Richart RM (1983) Precursors of cervical cancer. *Cancer Surveys* 2: 359–382.

Gissman L, de Villiers EM, Zur Hausen H (1982) Analysis of human genital warts (condyloma acuminata) and other genital tumours for human papillomavirus type 6 DNA. *International Journal of Cancer* 29: 143–146.

Hacker NF, Berek JS, Lagasse LD *et al.* (1982) Carcinoma of the cervix associated with pregnancy. *Obstetrics and Gynecology* 59: 735–746.

Hafiz MA, Kragel PJ, Toker C (1985) Carcinoma of the uterine cervix resembling lymphoepithelioma. *Obstetrics and Gynecology* 66: 829–831.

Hale RJ, Wilcox FL, Buckley CH *et al.* (1991) Prognostic factors in uterine cervical carcinoma: a clinicopathological analysis. *International Journal of Gynecological Cancer* 1: 19–23.

Hale RJ, Buckley CH, Fox H *et al.* (1992) Prognostic value of c-erbB-2 expression in uterine cervical carcinoma. *Journal of Clinical Pathology* 45: 594–596.

Hale RJ, Buckley CH, Gullick WJ *et al.* (1993) Prognostic value of epidermal growth factor receptor expression in cervical carcinoma. *Journal of Clinical Pathology* 46: 149–153.

Halpin TF, Hunter RE, Cohen MB (1989) Lymphoepithelioma of the uterine cervix. *Gynecologic Oncology* 34: 101–105.

Hasumi K, Sugano H, Sakamoto G *et al.* (1977) Circumscribed carcinoma of the uterine cervix, with marked lymphocytic infiltration. *Cancer* 39: 2503–2507.

Heatley MK (2001) The prognosis in cervical epithelial changes of uncertain significance is similar to that of cervical intraepithelial neoplasia grade I. *Journal of Clinical Pathology* 54: 474–475.

Hering B, Horn LC, Nenning H *et al.* (2000) Predictive value of DNA cytometry in CIN1 and 2. Image analysis of 193 cases. *Annals of Quantitative Cytology and Histology* 22: 333–337.

Holowaty P, Miller AB, Rohan T *et al.* (1999) Natural history of dysplasia of the uterine cervix. *Journal of the National Cancer Institute* 91: 252–258.

Inoue T (1984) Prognostic significance of the depth of invasion relating to nodal metastases, parametrial extension, and cell types. A study of 628 cases with stage IB, IIA, and IIB cervical carcinoma. *Cancer* 54: 3035–3042.

Isaac JH (1976) Verrucous carcinoma of the female genital tract. *Gynecologic Oncology* 4: 259–269.

Ismail SM, Colclough AB, Dinnen JS *et al.* (1989) Observer variation in histopathological diagnosis and grading of cervical intraepithelial neoplasia. *British Medical Journal* 298: 707–710.

Jennings RH, Barclay DL (1972) Verrucous carcinoma of the cervix. *Cancer* 30: 430–434.

Kainz C, Gitsch G, Tempfer C *et al.* (1994) Vascular space invasion and inflammatory stromal reaction as prognostic factors in patients with surgically treated cervical cancer stage IB to IIB. *Anticancer Research* 14: 2245–2248.

Kashimura M, Tsukamoto N, Matsukuma K *et al.* (1984) Verrucous carcinoma of the uterine cervix: report of a case with follow-up of 6 1/2 years. *Gynecologic Oncology* 19: 204–215.

Koenig C, Turnicky RP, Kankam CF *et al.* (1997) Papillary squamo-transitional cell carcinomas of the cervix: a report of 32 cases. *American Journal of Surgical Pathology* 21: 915–921.

Koss LG (1992) *Diagnostic Cytology and its Histopathologic Basis*, Vol. 1, 4th edn. Philadelphia: Lippincott, pp. 383–387.

Krauz FT, Perez-Meza C (1966) Verrucous carcinoma: clinical and pathologic studies of 105 cases involving oral cavity, larynx and genitalia. *Cancer* 19: 26–38.

Kristensen GB, Abeler VM, Risberg B *et al.* (1999) Tumor size, depth of invasion and grading of the invasive tumor front are the main prognostic factors in early squamous cell cervical carcinoma. *Gynecologic Oncology* 74: 245–251.

Larson AA, Liao SY, Stanbridge EJ *et al.* (1997) Genetic alterations accumulate during cervical tumorigenesis and indicate a common origin for multifocal lesions. *Cancer Research* 57: 4171–4176.

Lenczewski A, Terlikowski SJ, Sulkowski M (2002) Prognostic significance of CD34 expression in early cervical squamous cell carcinoma. *Folia Histochemica Cytobiologica* 40: 205–206.

Lonky NM (2002) Reducing death from cervical cancer. Examining the prevention paradigms. *Obstetric and Gynecological Clinics of North America* 29: 599–611.

Lopez-Rios F, Migeul PS, Bellas C *et al.* (2000) Lymphoepithelioma-like carcinoma of the uterine cervix: a case report studied by in situ hybridization and polymerase chain reaction for Epstein–Barr virus. *Archives of Pathology and Laboratory Medicine* 124: 746–747.

Lucas WE, Benirschke K, Lebherz RB (1974) Verrucous carcinoma of the female genital tract. *American Journal of Obstetrics and Gynecology* 119: 435–440.

Luff RD (1992) The Bethesda system for reporting cervical/vaginal cytologic diagnoses—report of the 1991 Bethesda workshop. *American Journal of Clinical Pathology* 98: 152–154.

McIndoe WA, McLean MA, Jones RW *et al.* (1984) The invasive potential of carcinoma in situ of the cervix. *Obstetrics and Gynecology* 64: 451–454.

Mandai M, Konishi I, Koshiyama M *et al.* (1995) Altered expression of nm23-H1 and c-erbB-2 proteins have prognostic significance in adenocarcinoma but not in squamous cell carcinoma of the uterine cervix. *Cancer* 75: 2523–2529.

Martorell MA, Julian JM, Calabrig C *et al.* (2002) Lymphoepithelioma-like carcinoma of the uterine cervix. *Archives of Pathology and Laboratory Medicine* 126: 1501–1505.

Meanwell CA, Kelly KA, Wilson S *et al.* (1988) Young age as a prognostic factor in cervical cancer: analysis of population based data from 10 022 cases. *British Medical Journal* 296: 386–391.

Mestwerdt G (1951) Elective Therapie des Mikrokarzinoms am collum uteri? *Zentralblatt für Gynaekologie* 73: 558–567.

Mills SE, Austin MB, Randall ME (1985) Lymphoepithelioma-like carcinoma of the uterine cervix: a distinctive, undifferentiated carcinoma with inflammatory stroma. *American Journal of Surgery and Pathology* 9: 883–889.

Morice P, Sabourin JC, Pautier P *et al.* (2000) Isolated paraaortic node involvement in stage IB/II cervical carcinoma. *European Journal of Gynaecology and Oncology* 21: 123–125.

National Health Service Cervical Screening Programme (1999) *Histopathology Reporting in Cervical Screening* (publication no. 10).

Östör AG (1993) Natural history of cervical intraepithelial neoplasia: a critical review. *International Journal of Gynecological Pathology* 12: 186–192.

Park TJ, Richart RM, Sun X-W *et al.* (1996) Association between HPV type and clonal status of cervical squamous intraepithelial lesions (SIL). *Journal of the National Cancer Institute* 88: 355–358.

Parkin DM, Pisani P, Ferlay J (1999) Estimates of the worldwide incidence of 25 major cancers in 1990. *International Journal of Cancer* 80: 827–841.

Pisani P, Parkin DM, Bray F *et al.* (1999) Estimates of the worldwide mortality from 25 cancers in 1990. *International Journal of Cancer* 83: 18–29.

Piver MS, Chung WS (1976) Prognostic significance of cervical lesion size and pelvic node metastases in cervical carcinoma. *Obstetrics and Gynecology* 46: 507–510.

Plaxe SC, Saltzstein SL (1999) Estimates of the duration of the preclinical phase of cervical adenocarcinoma suggests that there is ample opportunity for screening. *Gynecologic Oncology* 75: 55–61.

Plentl AE, Friedman EA (1971) *Lymphatic System of the Female Genitalia*. Philadelphia: Saunders.

Poulsen HE, Taylor CW, Sobin LH (1975) *Histological Typing of Female Genital Tract Tumours. International Histological Classification of Tumours, no. 13.* Geneva: World Health Organization.

Randall ME, Anderson WA, Mills SE *et al.* (1986) Papillary squamous cell carcinoma of the uterine cervix: a clinicopathologic study of nine cases. *International Journal of Gynecological Pathology* 5: 1–10.

Randall ME, Constable WC, Hahn SS *et al.* (1988) Results of the radiotherapeutic management of carcinoma of the cervix with emphasis on the influence of histologic classification. *Cancer* 62: 48–53.

Rastkar G, Okagaki T, Twiggs LB *et al.* (1982) Early invasive and in-situ warty carcinoma of the vulva: clinical, histologic and electron microscopic study with particular reference to viral association. *American Journal of Obstetrics and Gynecology* 143: 814–820.

Richart RM (1965) Colpomicroscopic studies of the distribution of dysplasia and carcinoma in-situ on the exposed portion of the human uterine cervix. *Cancer* 18: 950.

Richart RM (1973) Cervical intraepithelial neoplasia: a review. In: Sommers SC (ed.) *Pathology Annual*. East Norwalk: Appleton-Century-Crofts, pp. 301–328.

Richart RM (1990) A modified terminology for cervical intraepithelial neoplasia. *Obstetrics and Gynecology* 75: 131–133.

Robertson AJ (1989) Histopathological grading of cervical intraepithelial neoplasia (CIN) — is there need for a change? *Journal of Pathology* 159: 273–275.

Robertson DI, Maung R, Duggan MA (1993) Verrucous carcinoma of the genital tract: is it a distinct entity? *Canadian Journal of Surgery* 36: 147–151.

Roche WD, Norris HJ (1975) Microinvasive carcinoma of the cervix: the significance of lymphatic invasion and confluent patterns of stromal growth. *Cancer* 36: 180–186.

Roman LD, Felix JC, Muderspach LI *et al.* (1998) Influence of quantity of lymph-vascular space invasion on the risk of nodal metastases in women with early stage squamous cancer of the cervix. *Gynecologic Oncology* 68: 220–225.

Rose BR, Thompson CH, Simpson JM *et al.* (1995) Human papillomavirus deoxyribonucleic acid as a prognostic indicator in early-stage cervical cancer: a possible role for type 18. *American Journal of Obstetrics and Gynecology* 173: 1461–1468.

Schumaker A, Schwarz R (1989) Histopathologic and tumor-metric studies of stage Ia cervix cancer. *Zentralblatt für Gynäkologie* 111: 516–523.

Sedlis A, Sall S, Tsukuda Y *et al.* (1979) Microinvasive carcinoma of the uterine cervix: a clinicopathological study. *American Journal of Obstetrics and Gynecology* 133: 64–74.

Sevin BU, Lu Y, Bloch DA *et al.* (1996) Surgically defined prognostic parameters in patients with early cervical carcinoma: a multivariate tree analysis. *Cancer* 78: 1438–1446.

Smiley LM, Burke TM, Silva EG *et al.* (1991) Prognostic factors in stage IB squamous cervical cancer patients with low risk for recurrence. *Obstetrics and Gynecology* 77: 271–275.

Smith HO, Tiffany MF, Qualls CR *et al.* (2000) The rising incidence of adenocarcinoma relative to squamous cell carcinoma of the uterine cervix in the United States — a 24 year population based study. *Gynecologic Oncology* 78: 97–105.

Soh LT, Heng D, Lee JW *et al.* (2002) The relevance of oncogenes as prognostic markers in cervical cancer. *International Journal of Gynecological Cancer* 12: 465–474.

Solomon D (1989) The 1988 Bethesda system for reporting cervical/vaginal cytological diagnoses. *Acta Cytologica* 33: 567–574.

Solomon D, Davey D, Kurman R *et al.* (2002) The 2001 Bethesda system: terminology for reporting results of cervical cytology. *Journal of the American Medical Association* 287: 2114–2119.

Speiser P, Wanner C, Tempfer C *et al.* (1997) CD44 is an independent prognostic factor in early-stage cervical cancer. *International Journal of Cancer* 74: 185–188.

Stock RJ, Zaino R, Bundy BN *et al.* (1994) Evaluation and comparison of histopathologic grading systems of epithelial carcinoma of the uterine cervix: Gynecologic Oncology Group studies. *International Journal of Gynecological Pathology* 13: 99–108.

Stockler M, Russell P, McGahan S *et al.* (1996) Prognosis and prognostic factors in node-negative cervix cancer. *International Journal of Gynecological Cancer* 6: 477–482.

Takeshima N, Yanoh K, Tabata T *et al.* (1999) Assessment of the revised International Federation of Gynecology and Obstetrics staging for early invasive squamous cervical cancer. *Gynecologic Oncology* 74: 165–169.

Tiltman AJ, Atad J (1982) Verrucous carcinoma of the cervix with endometrial involvement. *International Journal of Gynecological Pathology* 1: 221–226.

Tjalma W, van Marck E, Weyler J *et al.* (1998) Quantification and prognostic relevance of angiogenic parameters in invasive cervical cancer. *British Journal of Cancer* 78: 170–174.

Tseng CJ, Pao CC, Tseng LH *et al.* (1997) Lymphoepithelioma-like carcinoma of the uterine cervix: association with Epstein–Barr virus and human papillomavirus. *Cancer* 80: 91–97.

van Nagell JR, Donaldson ES, Wood EG *et al.* (1978) The significance of vascular invasion and lymphocytic infiltration of invasive cervical cancer. *Cancer* 41: 228–234.

van Nagell JR, Greenwell N, Powell DF *et al.* (1983) Microinvasive carcinoma of the cervix. *American Journal of Obstetrics and Gynecology* 145: 981–991.

Walker J, Bloss JD, Liao SY *et al.* (1989) Human papillomavirus genotype as a prognostic indicator in carcinoma of the uterine cervix. *Obstetrics and Gynecology* 74: 781–785.

Weinburg E, Hoisington S, Eastman AY *et al.* (1993) Uterine cervical lymphoepithelioma-like carcinoma—absence of Epstein–Barr virus genomes. *American Journal of Clinical Pathology* 99: 195–199.

Wright CW, Kurman RJ, Ferenczy A (2002a) Precancerous lesions of the cervix. In: Kurman RJ (ed.) *Blaustein's Pathology of the Female Genital Tract*, 5th edn. New York: Springer.

Wright CW, Ferenczy A, Kurman RJ (2002b) Carcinoma and other tumours of the cervix. In: Kurman RJ (ed.) *Blaustein's Pathology of the Female Genital Tract*, 5th edn. New York: Springer.

Zaino RJ, Ward S, Delgado G *et al.* (1992) Histopathologic predictors of the behaviour of surgically treated stage IB squamous cell carcinoma of the cervix. *Cancer* 69: 1750–1758.

Zhang A, Maner S, Betz R *et al.* (2002) Genetic alterations in cervical carcinoma: frequent low level amplifications of oncogenes are associated with human papillomavirus infection. *International Journal of Cancer* 101: 427–433.

Zreik TG, Chambers JT, Chambers SK (1996) Parametrial involvement, regardless of nodal status: a poor prognostic factor for cervical cancer. *Obstetrics and Gynecology* 87: 741–746.

CHAPTER 22

The pathology of glandular cervical lesions

Raji Ganesan, the late Andrew G. Östör and Terence P. Rollason

ADENOCARCINOMA OF THE CERVIX

Introduction

Adenocarcinomas are the commonest primary carcinomas of the endocervix. Adenocarcinoma of the endocervix and its variants account for an increasing proportion of cervical carcinomas. A recent study has shown that, over the past 24 years, the incidence of all cervical cancer and squamous cell carcinoma has continued to decline. An almost 30% increase in the age-adjusted incidence rate of adenocarcinoma has been noted since 1973 with a 95% proportional increase relative to squamous cell carcinomas. Thus, the proportion of adenocarcinoma relative to squamous cell carcinoma and all cervical cancers has doubled (Smith *et al.*, 2000). Part of the rise has been in younger women with an 8–10% increase in women below 35 years of age. Recognising these tumours, awareness of their morphological variants and knowledge of their differential diagnosis are imperative.

Adenocarcinomas of the cervix are a heterogeneous group of neoplasms with a variety of histological patterns; sometimes cell types and patterns are admixed in the same tumour. Most primary endocervical adenocarcinomas are of the endocervical cell type. Smaller numbers are mucinous, endometrioid, clear cell, serous or mesonephric in type. Other carcinomas occurring in the endocervix with a notable glandular component are adenosquamous carcinomas and their variants – glassy cell carcinomas, adenoid basal carcinoma and adenoid cystic carcinoma. Endocervical, mucinous and endometrioid carcinomas taken together account for 45–90% of all invasive adenocarcinomas of the cervix.

The cell of origin of primary adenocarcinomas of the cervix is thought to be the pluripotent reserve cell of the columnar epithelium, which normally lines the endocervical surface and crypts. Epidemiological risk factors for adenocarcinoma of the cervix are similar to those for squamous cell carcinomas (Parazinni *et al.*, 1988). Associations include multiple sexual partners, young age at first intercourse and an interval of more than 5 years since the last screening cervical smear. They are all associated with the presence of CIN, although cervical glandular intraepithelial neoplasia (CGIN; adenocarcinoma *in situ*) is regarded as the immediate forerunner of invasive adenocarcinoma. Human papillomavirus (HPV), particularly HPV 16 and 18, has been found in association with cervical adenocarcinomas (Leminen *et al.*, 1991; Arends *et al.*, 1993) with a disproportionate representation of HPV 18 compared with squamous carcinoma. Some studies have shown an association of adenocarcinomas with oral contraceptive use, particularly for periods greater than 10 years but, when adjustments are made to include sexual history, screening history and HPV status, there is no clear increase in risk due to contraceptive use alone (Parazzini *et al.*, 1988).

Clinical aspects of the management of CGIN are discussed in Chapter 32.

Classification of adenocarcinomas

Classifications of cervical adenocarcinomas vary; our own preferred classification is given in Table 22.1 (Clement and Scully, 1982; Fu *et al.*, 1987; Young and Clement, 2002). Although a single pattern predominates in most lesions, a tumour may exhibit more than a single morphological type.

Early invasive adenocarcinoma

In contrast to the extensive work on 'microinvasive' (stage 1A) squamous cell carcinoma, the glandular counterpart, microinvasive adenocarcinoma (MIA), has been little discussed in the literature. Ever since the concept of microinvasion was introduced by Mestwerdt in 1947, there has been a tacit assumption that only squamous lesions be included. Mestwerdt, however, did not specify a cell type in tumours. He defined the depth of stromal invasion as up to 5 mm. Two of the most commonly used definitions, that of the Society of Gynecological Oncologists (SGO, USA) and that of the International Federation of Gynaecology and Obstetrics (FIGO), do not specifically refer to cell type. The Japanese Joint Study Committee for staging gynaecological cancer includes only squamous lesions.

A number of individual authors have also attempted to define MIA. Some have used 1 mm, others 2 and 3 mm, but

Table 22.1 Classification of primary neoplasms of the cervix —
glandular and those including a glandular component.

1. *In situ* carcinoma — CGIN
    a. Low grade
    b. High grade
        i. Endocervical
        ii. Endometrioid
        iii. Intestinal
        iv. Stratified mucinous intraepithelial lesion (SMILE)
        v. Serous
        vi. Clear cell
2. Invasive carcinoma
    a. Pure adenocarcinomas
        i. Endocervical or usual-type NOS including villoglandular carcinoma
        ii. Mucinous carcinoma including signet ring and intestinal type
        iii. Endometrioid carcinoma
        iv. Minimum deviation carcinoma (including endometrioid and clear cell variants)
        v. Clear cell carcinoma
        vi. Serous carcinoma
        vii. Mesonephric carcinoma
    b. Carcinomas with a glandular component
        i. Adenosquamous carcinoma including glassy cell variant
        ii. Adenoid basal carcinoma
        iii. Adenoid cystic carcinoma

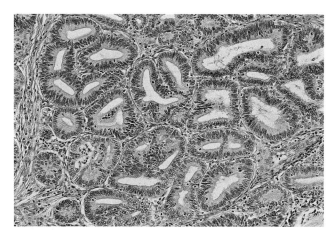

Fig. 22.1 High-grade CGIN/MIA characterised by loss of apical
mucin, nuclear stratification and vigorous mitotic activity. The degree
of glandular crowding makes separation of invasive from *in situ* disease
extremely difficult here.

most use 5 mm. Further measurements (length, width, area)
have been ignored except by Burghardt and Holzer (1977)
and, more recently, by Kaspar and associates (1993), who
proposed a volume of 500 mm³ or less for glandular lesions,
similar to microinvasive squamous carcinoma.

Clinical features

MIA is far less common than its squamous counterpart,
accounting for 12% of microinvasive carcinoma. The average
age of patients is 39 years, approximately 7 years younger
than the peak incidence of frankly invasive adenocarcinoma.
Although there are no reliable cytologic criteria for MIA, most
present with abnormal smears, atypical glandular cells being
present in up to 66% of cases (Mulvany and Östör, 1997). A
few complain of vaginal bleeding or discharge. Occasionally,
MIA is an incidental finding in a large loop excision of the
transformation zone (LLETZ), conisation or hysterectomy
specimen. MIA is usually not evident colposcopically; it may
arise from deep crypts or in the canal out of range of the colposcope, thus escaping early detection.

Pathology

MIA often shows marked glandular irregularity with effacement
of the normal glandular architecture and tumour extension
beyond the deepest normal crypt. Cribriform, papillary or solid
patterns may be present. There may be a stromal response in
the form of oedema, a chronic inflammatory infiltrate or a
desmoplastic reaction; lymphovascular space involvement may
be seen.

Distinguishing MIA from CGIN may be very difficult
(Fig. 22.1). Apart from stromal/vascular invasion, none of
the features noted in MIA is pathognomonic. A dense chronic
inflammatory infiltrate around CGIN is not uncommon and,
conversely, a stromal reaction may not be seen in all cases of
MIA. Both cribriform and papillary patterns are common in
CGIN. Superficial foci of MIA limited within the normal crypt
field do occur. For these reasons, in 15–20% of cases, it is
impossible to distinguish between CGIN and MIA.

However, several characteristic growth patterns are encountered. Tiny finger-like processes may extend into the stroma
from the base of the epithelium, or detached cellular clusters

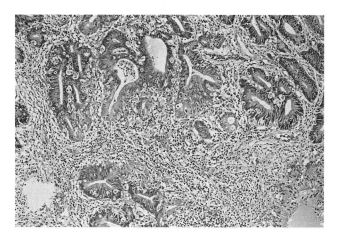

Fig. 22.2 Microinvasive cervical adenocarcinoma. There are closely
packed glands lined by pseudostratifed epithelium with cells showing
anisonucleosis, coarse chromatin and mitotic activity. There are foci of
microinvasion showing cells with increased eosinophilic cytoplasm and
a stromal reaction arising from the CGIN.

may be found lying free in the stroma. The individual cells in this pattern of invasion are large with more voluminous pink cytoplasm, as in early stromal invasion by squamous cell carcinoma (Fig. 22.2). 'Crab-like' invasion also occurs with irregular claws of neoplastic glands invading an altered stroma. A cribriform pattern of numerous rounded aggregates of neoplastic glands perforated by small spaces may be seen. Intraglandular papillae may be prominent. 'Bulky outgrowth' resembles the similar pattern seen in early invasive squamous cell carcinoma. The tumour invades on a broad front with a relatively discrete demarcation from the adjacent stroma. Solid growth is seen with only a minor glandular component, the presence of which may need to be enhanced by mucin stains. The most difficult pattern to evaluate is what may be called 'naked invasion', which closely resembles diffusely infiltrating adenocarcinoma of the endometrium. In this pattern, well-differentiated glands are found, singly or in groups, in a completely unaltered fibromuscular stroma. Evidence supporting the invasive nature of such lesions, aside from the depth of the glands, is their frequent association with frank invasion elsewhere in the same specimen. This problem is well illustrated by Fu *et al.* (1987).

All histological types seen in adenocarcinomas are generally encountered in MIA. The most common is the endocervical type followed by endometrioid carcinoma. Other subtypes include the intestinal, clear cell and serous adenocarcinomas.

Having established the presence of invasion, the depth of invasion and the width of the tumour may also be very difficult to assess. In most cases, the depth has to be measured from the surface rather than from the point of origin. Thus, tumour thickness, rather than 'depth of invasion', is often all that can be measured.

Much has been written about the topography and multicentricity of CGIN. Some authorities believe that CGIN and MIA are situated high up in the endocervical canal and are often multicentric. Therefore, they conclude that CGIN and MIA need long cylindrical cone biopsies if that modality is selected as the treatment of choice (Brand *et al.*, 1987; Östör *et al.*, 1997; Anderson and Arffmann, 1989). The little information available on MIA, however, suggests that most cases arise in the transformation zone, as does CGIN, and 'skip lesions' are rare and unlikely to be missed by conisation. According to Fluhmann (1961), the part of the cervix corresponding to a duct of an exocrine gland is called 'the cleft', and the part corresponding to the acinus is called the 'tunnel'. Using this terminology, Noda and associates (1983) found that MIA of the endocervical type originates from the primary cleft, and the less common endometrioid type from the deepest tunnels.

Diagnosis and treatment
A definitive diagnosis of MIA can never be made on punch biopsy alone, but requires a large LLETZ, cold-knife cone biopsy or hysterectomy specimen. Some workers feel that loop excision procedures are contraindicated in the diagnosis and

treatment of glandular abnormalities of the cervix (Benedet *et al.*, 2000). Such biopsies are often fragmented, making orientation impossible. In addition, thermal damage frequently interferes with microscopic interpretation. Both these factors may preclude adequate assessment of margins and even the diagnosis of invasion. Diathermy of the base after loop excision may destroy any disease that is left behind, making accurate staging impossible. Others feel that a well-performed LLETZ procedure can produce specimens equally as good as small cold-knife conisation (Tseng *et al.*, 1997).

In a recent literature review by one of the authors (Östör, 2000), where MIA was referred to as a tumour with less than 5 mm depth of invasion, there were only 436 patient reports found from which meaningful clinicopathological data could be extracted. Nevertheless, at least 126 patients had a radical hysterectomy and, although not always specifically stated, none appeared to have parametrial involvement. At least 155 patients had one or both ovaries removed and none had ovarian neoplasia, either primary or secondary. Of the 219 patients with pelvic lymph node dissection, five (2%) had metastases. However, the figure of 2% is almost certainly lower, as some authors did not specify the number of lymphadenectomies (Sivanesaratnam *et al.*, 1993). There were 15 recurrences (it was not possible to determine what numbers were central or lateral) and six patients died of their tumour. The mean survival in the largest series was 4 years. The relationship of capillary-like space involvement, lymph node metastasis and recurrence could not be determined because most reports did not state their presence or absence. Only 21 patients were treated by conisation alone, including five who also had pelvic lymph node dissection; seven of these were followed for 4 years with no recurrence.

The author concluded that, when the tumour does not invade beyond 5 mm in depth, there is no capillary-like space involvement, the margins are free and the cone biopsy has been totally embedded, conservative therapy is acceptable (Yaegeshi *et al.*, 1994).

However, the data suggest that MIA behaves in the same manner as its squamous counterpart. Only one-third of patients with MIA are eligible for cold-knife conisation as conservative treatment because of compromised margins. To be treated successfully, the cone biopsy must be adequately sampled. The role for loop excision procedures in the management of glandular neoplasms requires further study, the main problem being assessment of the state of the margins due to fragmentation and/or diathermy artefact.

ADENOCARCINOMA OF USUAL ENDOCERVICAL TYPE

Clinical features

The presenting symptom of invasive adenocarcinoma is bleeding in about two-thirds of cases. Some are asymptomatic and detected on routine cervical smears.

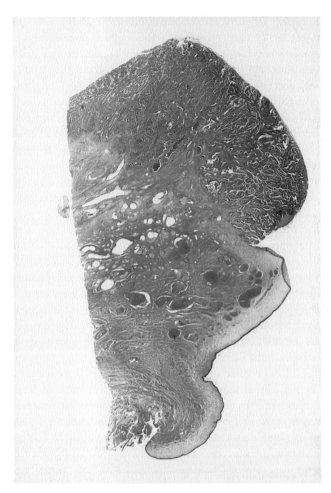

Fig. 22.3 A very low-power view showing an adenocarcinoma of the cervix arising at the transformation zone.

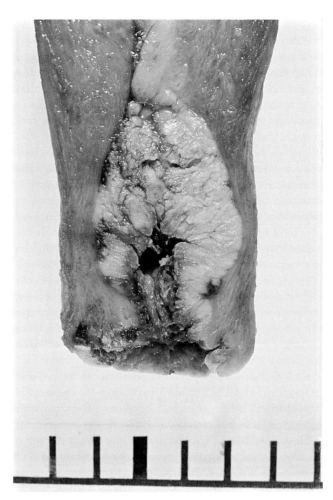

Fig. 22.4 A macroscopic specimen showing the cervix and lower uterus with an endocervical carcinoma presenting as a deeply infiltrative tumour in the upper part of the canal. Lesions such as this one may be clinically inapparent.

Pathology

On gross examination about half the patients have a fungating, polypoid or papillary mass (Fig. 22.3). The cervix may be diffusely enlarged or nodular. In about 15% of patients, the lesion is clinically inapparent and, although such lesions are usually early cancers, occasionally deeply invasive lesions arising high in the canal are not obvious on gross examination (Fig. 22.4). As in squamous carcinomas, circumferential involvement may result in a barrel-shaped cervix.

Adenocarcinomas, of the usual endocervical type, account for about 80% of all adenocarcinomas of the cervix. This type of adenocarcinoma may contain little or no demonstrable intracellular mucin, although the cytoplasm is often pale. Many experts therefore categorise these tumours separately from those that show overt mucinous morphology (Young and Clement, 2002) (Fig. 22.5). The arrangement of glands varies and can assume a tightly packed pattern of small acinar structures or produce cystically dilated glands. Malignant glands may be arranged in a complex racemose fashion, bearing resemblance to the normal endocervical crypts, or have an infiltrative pattern of randomly arranged elements. Sometimes, they retain a lobular pattern. A papillary pattern can be seen on the surface and should not lead to a diagnosis of villoglandular papillary adenocarcinoma in the absence of the other classical features of that tumour.

These tumours may elicit very little stromal reaction, but careful examination will reveal a desmoplastic stromal reaction at least focally. Solid areas can be seen in this type of adenocarcinoma but usually only form a minor component. Nuclear atypia is usually significant. Although not overtly mucinous, the cells have a characteristic pale eosinophilic cytoplasm with brisk mitotic and apoptotic activity.

Grading of adenocarcinomas

Grading of adenocarcinomas of the cervix has been done either by nuclear grade, architectural grade or a combination

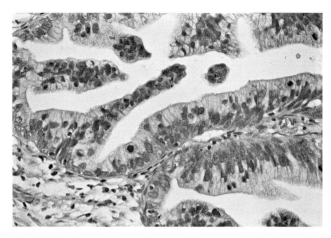

Fig. 22.5 Usual type adenocarcinoma of the cervix with the lining cells with clear mucinous cytoplasm, nuclear stratification and brisk mitotic activity. Intracellular mucin is more prominent here than in many examples.

of the two. Architectural grade is based on the degree of gland formation. If less than 50% of the area of the tumour shows a pattern of acini and/or tubules, the tumour is regarded as poorly differentiated. If 10–50% of the tumour forms glands and tubules, it is designated as moderately differentiated. If more than 90% of the area of the neoplasm shows tubule or gland formation, it is designated as a well-differentiated adenocarcinoma.

By nuclear grading, oval nuclei with evenly dispersed chromatin are regarded as grade 1 adenocarcinomas, those with markedly enlarged nuclei with coarse chromatin and prominent nucleoli are considered grade 3, and those with features in between grade 1 and grade 3 are designated grade 2.

Architectural grading is more widely used than nuclear grade but, as a large proportion of adenocarcinomas at this site show well-formed and widespread glands, it offers rather poor prognostic separation. Many upgrade the architectural grade by one if nuclear atypia is disproportionate.

Histological reporting of adenocarcinomas

All histological reports should grade and determine the lateral extent and depth of invasion of the tumour and also comment on the presence or absence of vessel invasion. Adequacy of excision should always be assessed with regard to the vaginal, deep cervical and parametrial margins, and comment on the presence or absence of involvement of the parametria, vagina, isthmus or uterine corpus should be included. It has been suggested that it is also useful to determine the distance of clearance not only from the deep cervical margin but also from the deep cervical–stromal interface. The presence or absence of nodal metastases should be clearly stated together with the total number of nodes identified in each anatomical group.

Local and metastatic spread

Adenocarcinoma of the cervix spreads in a manner similar to that of squamous cell carcinoma. Direct spread to contiguous structures, i.e. the uterine corpus, vagina and parametrium, and through deep cervical planes to the bladder and rectum is seen. At the time of discovery of the tumour, about 85% of the patients have disease confined to the cervix (stage I) or extending to the parametrium or upper vagina (stage II). Lymphovascular spread first occurs to pelvic obturator and external iliac nodes followed by involvement of common iliac and, least frequently, inguinal and para-aortic nodes. Autopsy study of fatal cases suggests a higher rate of metastasis to the adrenal gland and para-aortic lymph nodes than in fatal cases of squamous cell carcinoma (Drescher *et al.*, 1989). The commonest secondary sites of extrapelvic disease are in the peritoneum, para-aortic lymph nodes, lung and pleura (Horowitz *et al.*, 1988).

VARIANTS OF ADENOCARCINOMA

Villoglandular adenocarcinoma

This variant of adenocarcinoma occurs predominantly in younger women. It has been associated with an excellent prognosis, with most patients, including those treated conservatively, being alive and well without recurrence at 7–77 months of follow-up (Young and Scully, 1989). Recent studies, however, question this uniformly good prognosis and show an association of vascular involvement with lymph node metastasis and death. Superficial biopsy may not reveal an underlying second tumour type of aggressive biological behaviour.

Histologically, this tumour is characterised by a surface papillary component of variable thickness (Jones *et al.*, 1993). The papillae are usually tall and thin, but the stroma may be prominent (Fig. 22.6). They are lined by cells that are stratified

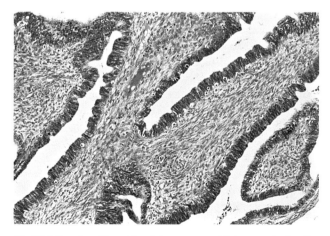

Fig. 22.6 Broad papillae with cellular stroma and lining neoplastic cells with very little pleomorphism are seen in this villoglandular carcinoma. The stroma maybe less prominent and papillae thinner than in this case.

and non-mucinous in type. The cells have no more than mild to moderate cytological atypia, and occasional mitotic figures may be seen. A greater degree of nuclear atypia militates against this good prognostic variant of endocervical carcinoma. The appearances of this tumour may be strikingly similar to those of villous adenomas of the colon. When an invasive component of tumour is present, the glands are typically elongated and branching in character. Sometimes, the invasive component can appear very low grade. Unfavourable features are deep invasion, the presence of vascular invasion, large tumour volume and an associated additional tumour type.

Mucinous adenocarcinoma

This group of endocervical carcinomas is characterised by the presence of abundant mucin in the malignant cells. Goblet cells, neuroendocrine cells and even Paneth cells are seen. The mucin-containing cells can either form acinar and glandular structures or may invade insidiously as single cells. In the latter, the intracytoplasmic mucin distends the cells and produces a peripherally located, flattened nucleus – a signet ring cell. Mucinous carcinomas are usually easily diagnosable because their component glandular structures are both architecturally and cytologically malignant. The main differential diagnosis is with mucinous metastatic carcinoma. Unlike primary carcinomas, metastatic carcinomas tend to have extensive vascular invasion, and the tumour tends to grow from outside within rather than from within outwards.

Adenoma malignum (minimum deviation adenocarcinoma)

This variant of adenocarcinoma has a deceptively benign appearance (Young and Scully, 1993). It usually has a mucinous phenotype, although endometrioid and other variants have been described. They are uncommon tumours and account for only 1–3% of all endocervical carcinomas (Gilks *et al.*, 1989). These tumours are more likely than other types of endocervical carcinomas to be associated with synchronous or metachronous ovarian carcinomas – the most likely associated tumours are mucinous adenocarcinomas and sex cord tumours with annular tubules (SCTAT). Both minimum deviation adenocarcinoma (MDA) and SCTAT have been strongly associated with Peutz–Jeghers syndrome (McGowan *et al.*, 1980).

In MDA, the malignant glands are lined by a mucinous epithelium that has basal nuclei and apical mucin, closely mimicking the appearance of the normal endocervical glands. The glands, however, are deeply infiltrative, have lost their lobularity and bear an abnormal relationship to deep vessels. Thorough sampling, as is possible on a hysterectomy specimen, usually reveals at least some foci of more conventional appearing adenocarcinoma, especially deeper in the tumour, or foci of perineural or vascular invasion (Gilks *et al.*, 1989).

Other important clues to accurate diagnosis, even if focal, are periglandular stromal oedema, vascular and perineural invasion. Recent studies suggest that women with MDA have survival rates similar to those of women with well-differentiated adenocarcinomas of the cervix.

Gastric mucins – with periodic acid–Schiff (PAS)-positive sialomucin predominant – have been shown to be present in MDA. Interestingly, a benign lesion sometimes presenting with similar symptoms, including a watery vaginal discharge, is lobular endocervical glandular hyperplasia. This lesion has been shown to react with antibodies to pyloric gland-type mucins. This association raises the possibility that lobular endocervical glandular hyperplasia may precede adenoma malignum.

A newly described morphological variant – microcystic endocervical adenocarcinoma – can be considered as a variant of minimal deviation carcinoma. These endocervical adenocarcinomas have a prominent cystic component that may, on superficial examination, bear a resemblance to benign endocervical lesions, notably to tunnel clusters or deep Nabothian cysts (Tambouret *et al.*, 2000). The lining epithelium is similar to the usual endocervical-type adenocarcinoma. Although the architecture is deceptively benign, the lining cells show nuclear hyperchromasia, atypia and chromatin abnormalities along with significant mitotic activity. There is an association with antecedent abnormal cervical smears and CGIN. Focally, at least, conventional invasive adenocarcinoma can usually be seen, offering diagnostic help.

Endometrioid carcinoma

These tumours of the cervix are morphologically identical to the endometrioid type of endometrial carcinomas. Absence of intracellular mucin in this phenotype is a feature that results in resemblance to the usual type of endocervical adenocarcinomas. Frequency of reporting of endometrioid carcinomas of the cervix varies from series to series with figures as high as 50% or as low as 7%. This is due to the great subjectivity in differentiating endometrioid from usual-type endocervical adenocarcinoma of the cervix (McCluggage, 2002; Young and Clement, 2002). Endometrioid adenocarcinomas of the cervix have tubular glands and may have a surface papillary component. They often have foci of squamous (morular) metaplasia. Sometimes, they have a very benign appearance and merit the designation of a minimum deviation carcinoma of endometrioid type.

While the clinical outcome of these tumours may not differ significantly from usual-type endocervical adenocarcinomas, it is important to rule out a primary endometrial carcinoma with cervical involvement. An unusual pattern of spread of endometrial carcinomas has been reported recently (Tambouret *et al.*, 2003). Deeply invasive cervical glandular proliferation of widely spaced glands devoid of stromal reaction was seen. In all cases, an obvious carcinoma of the uterine corpus was present. Recognition of this pattern in a cervical biopsy specimen may be difficult.

Clear cell adenocarcinoma

These tumours account for approximately 4% of all adenocarcinomas of the cervix. This type of carcinoma has an established association with diethylstilbestrol (DES) exposure – in this setting, it occurs in young women (Young and Scully, 1998). However, this morphology was well documented before the DES era and continues to be recognised now in the post-DES period. Sporadic cases occur generally in postmenopausal women. There are three morphological patterns of clear cell carcinoma, tubulocystic, solid and papillary. The acini are lined by hobnail, eosinophilic or clear cells. The stroma is often hyalinised, sometimes extensively. The lining cells are pleomorphic.

Outcome for early sporadic clear cell carcinomas is probably similar to that for adenocarcinoma of the usual type, but higher stage tumours appear to have a more aggressive course.

Serous papillary carcinoma

This is an uncommon form of cervical adenocarcinoma that bears a strong resemblance to the commoner serous carcinoma of the ovary. The diagnosis can usually be made firmly only on a hysterectomy specimen when it is apparent that the endometrium and ovaries are uninvolved. The tumour is characterised by papillary tufts lined by cells with pronounced cytonuclear atypia, cellular budding and sometimes psammoma body formation (Fig. 22.7). Differentiation from villoglandular carcinoma is especially important as the poor prognosis associated with serous carcinomas contrasts with the good outcome in villoglandular carcinoma despite the shared papillary morphology. Serous carcinoma has a high rate of recurrence (Costa *et al.*, 1995); prognosis in the later stages is grim.

Mesonephric adenocarcinoma

These are extremely rare neoplasms that arise from mesonephric – Wolffian duct – remnants present in the lateral aspects of the cervix (Clement *et al.*, 1995). They form tubular structures characteristically with a PAS-positive, diastase-resistant, eosinophilic luminal secretion. They may resemble clear cell carcinomas and are distinguished from them by presenting as tumours arising deep in the wall of the cervix at the site where benign mesonephric remnants can be seen. Discrimination from benign proliferations of the mesonephric duct is achieved by recognising solid epithelial sheets, loss of stroma between glands, a focal cribriform pattern and an infiltrative rather than lobular glandular arrangement (Ferry and Scully, 1990). Mesonephric carcinomas can be pure adenocarcinomas or may have an admixed spindle cell component, which resembles endometrial stroma. Mesonephric carcinomas appear to have a propensity for late recurrence (Clement *et al.*, 1995).

Adenosquamous carcinoma

These are tumours that contain a mixture of malignant squamous and glandular cells (Fig. 22.8). These account for between 5% and 45% of cervical carcinomas depending on the vigour with which mucin is sought in apparently squamous carcinomas and the diagnostic criteria used. Some make the diagnosis simply on the presence of intracellular mucin; others require clear squamous and glandular differentiation. The significance of identifying this tumour lies in the fact that they appear to metastasise to pelvic lymph nodes more often

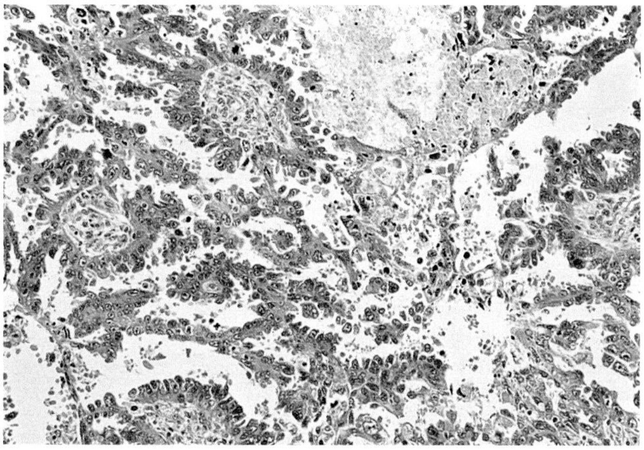

Fig. 22.7 Serous papillary adenocarcinoma — papillary structures of varying sizes are lined by pleomorphic cells. Many of the cells have a hobnail appearance.

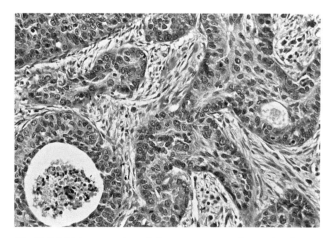

Fig. 22.8 A high-power view of adenosquamous carcinoma showing glandular and squamous differentiation within the invasive islands of tumour.

than squamous or adenocarcinomas. However, despite this increased frequency of metastasis, the prognosis of adenosquamous carcinoma has not been clearly worse than that of patients with squamous carcinomas of the same stage (Yazigi *et al.*, 1990).

Glassy cell carcinoma

This is a poorly differentiated form of adenosquamous carcinoma with distinctive morphological characteristics. The growth pattern histologically appears syncytial. The component cells have a granular ground glass cytoplasm (hence the term glassy cell), distinct cell membranes, prominent nucleoli and vesicular nuclei. Mitotic figures are abundant. The stroma is infiltrated by large numbers of inflammatory cells with a heavy component of eosinophils. Rarely, keratin formation, abortive lumen formation and intracytoplasmic mucin are noted. Prognosis of these tumours is poor with survival rates as low as 50% at 5 years in patients with stage I disease.

Adenoid basal carcinoma

These rare tumours are composed of small uniform cells arranged in lobules (Brainard and Hart, 1998). At the periphery of these nests, the cells show nuclear palisading. Lumina are seen in some of the larger nests, and these can show a mucinous, clear cell or squamotransitional pattern to the lining cells. Nuclear atypia is usually minimal, mitotic activity low, and there is no stromal reaction to the tumour. The lesion is often associated with CIN of the overlying epithelium, and these cases may be detected as a result of cervical screening. They are also associated with the presence of co-existent adenoid cystic carcinomas, adenosquamous carcinomas and squamous cell carcinomas of the cervix. Overall, the prognosis of adenoid basal carcinomas is excellent – no deaths have been reported (Ferry and Scully, 1988). Many prefer not to regard these as malignant and suggest an alternative designation of basal cell epithelioma.

Adenoid cystic carcinoma

These patients usually present with an obvious cervical mass. On histology, the tumour is composed of cells that are arranged in nests with at least a focal cribriform pattern. The resemblance to the salivary gland cancers with the same name is enhanced by the presence of hyaline basement membrane-like material in the 'gland' lumina. A solid, trabecular and cord-like pattern may also be seen. Nuclear atypia is significant, mitotic activity usually brisk and necrosis often present in the malignancy. A stromal response in the form of myxoid areas or fibroblastic proliferation is also seen. The main differential diagnosis – clinically significant as adenoid cystic carcinomas have a worse prognosis – is adenoid basal carcinoma.

IMMUNOHISTOCHEMISTRY RELEVANT TO DIAGNOSIS AND PROGNOSIS OF ENDOCERVICAL ADENOCARCINOMAS

In differentiation of CGIN from its benign mimics, proliferation markers, CEA, CD44 and other immunohistochemical stains, have been used. In distinction between high-grade CGIN and benign conditions such as microglandular hyperplasia and tubo-endometrioid metaplasia (TEM), MIB-1 is of value. Generally, in benign lesions, only scattered nuclei are positive, whereas in high-grade CGIN, positivity is seen in more than 50% of nuclei. P16 is also of use because it is diffusely and strongly positive in CGIN but negative or only weakly positive in most benign lesions except TEM. There, it is occasionally positive (McCluggage, 2002).

Immunohistochemistry with monoclonal carcinoembryonic antigen (CEA) may be useful in distinguishing reactive from neoplastic cervical lesions – the latter are believed to show diffuse cytoplasmic staining. Pitfalls are that benign glands may show focal luminal staining, adenoma malignum may show no staining or very focal staining, and microglandular hyperplasia may show cytoplasmic positivity, especially in areas of immature squamous metaplasia.

Recent studies have shown that gastric mucins are present in adenoma malignum, and these may be detected by HIK1083, a monoclonal antibody against gastric mucin. Normal endocervical glands are consistently negative, although usual-type endocervical adenocarcinomas may show focal positivity.

Immunohistochemistry may be useful to separate endocervical from endometrial primary carcinomas (Castrillon *et al.*, 2002; McCluggage *et al.*, 2002). This is relevant because the treatment of the two lesions is different, and a diagnosis of endometrial carcinoma may result in undertreatment of an endocervical primary. The panel of antibodies used are vimentin, estrogen and progesterone receptors, and CEA. Endometrial carcinomas show lateral border membrane positivity for vimentin and nuclear positivity for ER and PR. Endocervical carcinomas are generally negative for these markers but show cytoplasmic positivity with CEA.

More recently, CD10 and calretinin have been studied in endocervical glandular lesions (McCluggage *et al.*, 2003). Most endocervical glandular lesions were found to be negative with calretinin except mesonephric carcinomas. CD10 stained mesonephric remnants and mesonephric carcinomas, but positive staining of usual-type endocervical carcinomas and endometrioid endometrial carcinomas limited its specificity.

BENIGN AND TUMOUR-LIKE CONDITIONS

Since the renaissance of CGIN in the 1980s, (first described in 1953), there has been enormous interest in its protean mimics. While most of these have been well known to most practising pathologists, they have been better delineated

Table 22.2 Benign and tumour-like lesions.

Normal variants
Metaplasias
Hormonal
Hyperplastic
Iatrogenic
Infective
Mucin extravasation
Regeneration
Polyps

Table 22.3 Normal variants.

Tunnel clusters
Mesonephric remnants
Papillary endocervicitis
Deep glands and cysts
Ectopias

and refined. The classification of these entities appears in Table 22.2.

Normal variants

Adenocarcinomas of the cervix can be confused morphologic-ally with a wide variety of benign lesions. Most benign lesions are located superficially, lack lobulation, have a well-demarc-ated margin and do not show any stromal response. Malignant lesions generally show deep invasion, have an infiltrative out-line, have a stromal response at the irregularly infiltrative edge and show cytonuclear atypia (Young and Clement, 2002). While these guidelines ring true in most situations, there are notable exceptions such as the deceptively bland appearance of adenoma malignum or the marked cytological atypia seen in Arias–Stella reaction. Noteworthy benign proliferations, particularly those that mimic malignancy, are discussed below.

A number of structures that are normally present in the cervix may pose diagnostic problems (Table 22.3).

Tunnel clusters

This incidental finding, commonly encountered in hysterec-tomy specimens, was first and extensively described by Fluhmann in 1961. He recognised two varieties, cystic (type A) and non-cystic (type B) (Fig. 22.9). Cystic clusters are grossly visible in just under half the cases. The majority are multiple. A tunnel cluster is a discrete rounded aggregate of 20–50 oval, round or irregular, closely packed tubules of vary-ing sizes. The lining cells are columnar mucin-secreting when cystic and flattened or cuboidal when non-cystic. Although the nuclei are bland and mitoses are typically absent (as in normal endocervical mucosa), nuclear atypia and mitoses have rarely been observed. Tunnel clusters are believed to be

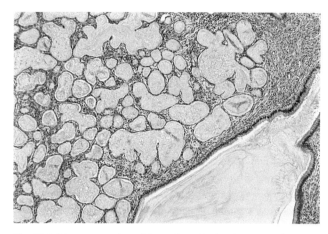

Fig. 22.9 A low-power view of the endocervix showing a tunnel cluster (type B). It is composed of a lobular group of dilated benign endocervical crypts in the superficial endocervical stroma.

involutional in nature and are of no clinical significance. Although mistaking these for adenoma malignum (minimal deviation adenocarcinoma) is highly unlikely, the lack of a mass, tubular pattern and lack of stromal response favour a benign process (Daya and Young 1995; Jones and Young, 1996).

Mesonephric remnants

Mesonephric remnants are found in about 10% of conisa-tion or hysterectomy specimens. They are usually incidental findings, although abnormal cytology may be the initial pre-sentation in some cases. The incidence rises if many lateral blocks are taken or if cone biopsies are serially sectioned, as the distal portion of the mesonephric duct runs laterally on either side of the cervix. The remnants are small, round, tubular structures lined by bland mucin-free cuboidal cells, which clas-sically contain PAS-positive, diastase-resistant intraluminal secretions. They may be mistaken for adenoma malignum and mesonephric carcinoma.

Papillary endocervicitis

This is an incidental microscopic finding of no clinical signi-ficance. The elongated finger-like endocervical fronds, which appear as grape-like villi in three dimensions, are supported by an inflamed stroma. It usually does not pose any problem in differential diagnosis.

Deep glands and cysts

Otherwise typical endocervical glands or their cystic counter-parts (Nabothian cysts) occasionally extend deeply into or through the cervical wall. Such cysts may have a striking gross honeycomb-like appearance. In contrast to adenocarcinoma, especially adenoma malignum, the glands and cysts are usually widely spaced, have bland nuclear features and lack stromal response.

Table 22.4 Metaplasias.

Tubal (ciliated)
Tubo-endometrioid
Serous papillary
Intestinal
Endometriosis
Endocervicosis

Table 22.5 Hyperplasias.

Simple
Atypical
Reserve cell
Lobular endocervical glandular
Diffuse laminar
Mesonephric remnant
Microglandular

Ectopias

Rare examples of ectopic prostate, sebaceous glands or breast tissue have been reported (Larraza-Hernandez *et al.*, 1997; Nucci *et al.*, 2000; McCluggage *et al.*, 2006).

Metaplasias

Cervical metaplasias that may mimic pre- or neoplastic lesions are listed in Table 22.4.

Metaplasia is defined as the change or metamorphosis of one differentiated type of epithelium into another. Columnar epithelium undergoing squamous metaplasia is a universal event in the cervix. Tubal metaplasia and its variants are also common, to the extent that some observers regard them as normal. The glands are disposed especially in the upper reaches of the cervix. The glands are usually multiple and may resemble tubal epithelium (ciliated metaplasia), a mixture of tubal and endometrial epithelium (tubo-endometrioid metaplasia) or endometrial glands (endometrioid metaplasia). Tubo-endometrioid metaplasia is particularly common following cold-knife conisation or destructive surgery on the cervix (Ismail, 1991). In contrast to CGIN, with which they may be confused, epithelial stratification, nuclear atypia, mitoses, cytoplasmic vacuolation and apoptosis are all absent (Oliva *et al.*, 1995). They are almost always incidental findings, although at times their presence may be suspected by abnormal cytology smears. Adenocarcinoma is distinguished by a lack of invasion. In endometriosis, the affected glands are invested by endometrial stroma. Ciliated CGIN, a recently described entity, may also cause confusion.

Endometriosis and endocervicosis

Cervical endometriosis may be superficial (mucosal) or deep. Superficial endometriosis is unrelated to generalised (deep) endometriosis and is believed to occur on a metaplastic basis. However, as it is often found following procedures on the cervix, implantation of menstrual endometrium is an alternative mechanism (Baker *et al.*, 1999). Although usually an incidental finding of no clinical significance, the patients may sometimes present with abnormal smears.

Endocervicosis refers to the presence of ectopic, benign-appearing, endocervical-like glands. The outer wall of the cervix may rarely be affected as part of the more common bladder involvement, in which case adenoma malignum may be simulated. The latter, however, always involves the cervical mucosa as well (Clement and Young, 1992).

Hormonal changes

Arias–Stella reaction

The Arias–Stella reaction is typically an incidental finding in up to 10% of pregnant women (Cove, 1979). It may also be observed in polyps and can be seen in endocervical glands as well as in foci of cervical endometriosis. The nuclei show pleomorphism and occasional mitotic activity. Abundant clear and eosinophilic cytoplasm is seen. The differential diagnosis is with clear cell carcinoma. However, the atypia in Arias–Stella reaction is random and focal. The reaction may be confused with CGIN, especially in punch biopsies or clear cell adenocarcinoma.

Hyperplasias

The various forms of endocervical hyperplasias (Table 22.5) are differentiated from adenocarcinoma by their orderly arrangement and bland nuclei.

Simple hyperplasia

There is generalised overgrowth of normal endocervical mucosa to be distinguished from adenoma malignum by the features listed above.

Lobular endocervical glandular hyperplasia

This is usually an incidental finding in women in the reproductive period. There is a lobular proliferation of small to moderate-sized glands centred on a larger central gland. Cystic glands may be prominent (Nucci *et al.*, 1999). The intervening stroma varies from normal to mildly cellular. This condition may be distinguished from adenoma malignum by its superficial location, lobular arrangement, absence of atypia, mitoses and stromal reaction.

Diffuse laminar endocervical glandular hyperplasia

This is a rare incidental finding in women of reproductive age characterised by a circumscribed band-like proliferation of closely packed endocervical glands sharply demarcated from the underlying stroma. An intense stromal chronic inflammatory infiltrate is usually present (Jones *et al.*, 1991). It is distinguished from adenoma malignum by its well-circumscribed border and absence of invasion.

Microglandular hyperplasia

First described in 1967, this condition is characterised by proliferation of endocervical glandular epithelium lacking significant nuclear atypia, with the formation of closely packed, small or occasionally cystically dilated glands, containing mucin and acute inflammatory cells. The lesion occurs most commonly in women who are pregnant or are receiving the oral contraceptive pill or progestins. However, it may occur in the absence of all the above factors. It is usually an incidental finding, but may rarely present as a polyp. The glands are lined by low columnar, cuboidal or flattened cells, frequently showing subnuclear vacuolation. The nuclei are small and regular, with inconspicuous nucleoli. Mitoses are absent or rare. Focal squamous metaplasia may be present. Unusual microscopic features include: (i) solid, reticular and trabecular patterns; (ii) a pseudoinfiltrative pattern due to strands of epithelium entrapped in an oedematous, myxoid or hyalinised stroma; (iii) spindle-shaped cells, polygonal cells with abundant eosinophilic cytoplasm and signet ring-like cells; and (iv) nuclei showing mild pleomorphism. The differential diagnosis is clear cell adenocarcinoma or rare endocervical-type adenocarcinoma with a microcystic pattern (Young and Scully, 1992). Features favouring a neoplasm include a mass, cells with glycogen-rich cytoplasm, marked nuclear atypia, mitoses, invasion and strong immunoreactivity to CEA.

Mesonephric hyperplasia

Like mesonephric remnants (see above), mesonephric hyperplasia is almost always an incidental finding in women of reproductive age. The tubules are most commonly arranged in a lobular pattern (80% of cases), or they may be diffusely disposed, or there may be hyperplasia of the main duct, parts of which are usually seen in all types (Ferry and Scully, 1990). The histology is very similar to that of mesonephric remnants, except for crowding. Mitoses are absent. In mesonephric duct hyperplasia, the duct is lined by epithelium showing intraluminal papillary tufts (Seidman and Tavassoli, 1995). Occasionally, mesonephric carcinomas may arise in an area of florid mesonephric hyperplasia. The differential diagnosis is adenoma malignum or clear cell carcinoma. Features favouring mesonephric hyperplasia include its deep location, mucin-free cytoplasm, absence of stromal response and negative staining with CEA (Ferry and Scully, 1990). Features favouring a clear cell carcinoma include a mass, solid and/or papillary patterns, presence of intracytoplasmic mucin, hobnail cells, marked nuclear atypia and numerous mitoses. Differentiation from a true mesonephric carcinoma may be extremely difficult.

Iatrogenic changes

Diathermy/cautery effect

Thermal artefacts are commonly seen with the widespread use of the LLETZ procedure. Similar changes may be produced by laser surgery. The heat-affected nuclei in the columnar epithelium may be misinterpreted as dysplasia. Thus, the cells are stratified, often heaped up into as many as 10 layers, and are compressed with hyperchromatic and elongated nuclei with smudged chromatin. The history in such cases facilitates the diagnosis.

Post-cone changes

Tubo-endometrioid metaplasia is virtually always present in hysterectomy specimens removed after conisation and has been discussed above.

Radiation-induced atypia

Such changes are common, especially after brachytherapy (intracavity irradiation). The co-existence of epithelial and stromal changes helps in the diagnosis.

Infective changes

A number of viral infections of the columnar epithelium may mimic dysplasia because of their cytopathic effect. Nevertheless, patients with these afflictions are rarely biopsied so they do not often pose diagnostic challenges. Virus-affected cells are more likely to be seen in Pap smears as incidental findings. They are more commonly seen in immune-suppressed women.

Adenovirus rarely affects the cervix but may result in abnormal cytology and histology due to small eosinophilic, lobulated, intranuclear inclusions, clearing of nuclear chromatin with prominent nuclear membranes and a perinuclear halo. In contrast to the above viruses, multinucleate giant cells and nuclear 'ground glass' appearance are not seen. Adenoviruses can be distinguished from chlamydia and lymphogranuloma venereum as these have intracytoplasmic inclusions. The presence of the virus can be confirmed by immunoperoxidase staining.

PROGNOSTIC HISTOLOGICAL FACTORS IN CERVICAL ADENOCARCINOMAS

Survival rates for cervical adenocarcinoma are significantly influenced by stage, histological subtype, tumour grade, the presence of positive lymph nodes and tumour size. The prognosis of adenocarcinoma relative to squamous cell carcinoma has been the subject of debate. Many studies have shown that, independent of stage and grade, the outcome of adenocarcinomas is poorer than that of squamous cell carcinomas (Kilgore *et al.*, 1988). Even node-negative, early-stage adenocarcinomas have been suggested to recur more commonly than squamous cell carcinoma. Adenocarcinoma has bee shown to metastasise relatively more frequently. These observations are not uniform, and others have shown that histological type has no prognostic effect on stage IB disease.

Age at diagnosis has been suggested to influence prognosis only below the age of 30 years (Kilgore *et al.*, 1988) or above the age of 80 years in stage I disease. The 5-year survival in patients under 30 years of age in one study was about 40%, in contrast to > 80% 5-year survival in older patients, but most studies have shown that age is not an independent prognostic factor (Hopkins *et al.*, 1988).

In almost all studies, stage of disease at diagnosis is the most important prognostic variable (Kilgore *et al.*, 1988). The 5-year survival rates noted in these studies varied from 60–90% in stage I disease to 44–66% in stage II, 25–29.5% in stage III and 0–5.3% in stage IV disease.

Involvement of lymph nodes also emerges as a significant prognostic factor in multivariate analyses. The 5-year survival rate in stage I disease drops from around 82% in node-negative cases to about 28% when metastatic nodal disease is found. This impact of lymph node disease on survival is not significant at higher stages (Hopkins *et al.*, 1988; Leminen *et al.*, 1990; Bertrand *et al.*, 1987). The presence of lymphovascular space invasion is a poor prognostic factor in disease greater than stage I.

The size of the lesion measured as the maximum tumour dimension has been found to have direct correlation with prognosis (Kilgore *et al.*, 1988). The cut-off point used in studies varies from 2 to 5 cm. This differs slightly from tumour volume measurements made in estimating prognosis in early invasive adenocarcinomas. Tumour size over 3 cm has been shown as a poor prognostic factor irrespective of stage.

Some have shown no significant difference in survival rate between usual-type adenocarcinoma, adenosquamous carcinoma and clear cell adenocarcinoma. In another review of 203 patients with adenocarcinoma of the cervix, the following types were identified: endocervical, 94 (46%); adenosquamous, 67 (33%); papillary, 21 (11%); clear cell, 16 (8%); and mucoid, 5 (4%). The histological subtype did not significantly influence survival (Hopkins *et al.*, 1988). There has been some evidence from other studies that high-stage clear cell carcinomas have a poorer prognosis than adenocarcinoma not otherwise specified (NOS).

Histological grade has been shown in several studies to have a direct correlation with the survival rate; for grade 1 tumours, it is reported at about 60%, whereas among patients with high-grade tumours only about 10% survive. Leminen *et al.* (1990), however, failed to show a correlation of grade with prognosis.

REFERENCES

Anderson ES, Arffmann E (1989) Adenocarcinoma in situ of the uterine cervix: a clinico-pathologic study of 36 cases. *Gynecologic Oncology* 35: 1–7.

Arends MJ, Donaldson YK, Duvall E *et al.* (1993) Human papillomavirus type 18 associates with more advanced cervical neoplasia than human papillomavirus type 16. *Human Pathology* 24: 432–437.

Baker PM, Clement PB, Bell DA *et al.* (1999) Superficial endometriosis of the uterine cervix: a report of 20 cases of a process that may be confused with endocervical glandular dysplasia or adenocarcinoma in situ. *International Journal of Gynecological Pathology* 18: 198–205.

Benedet JL, Bender H, Jones H III (2000) FIGO staging classifications and clinical practice guidelines in the management of gynaecological cancers. *International Journal of Gynecology and Obstetrics* 70: 209–262.

Bertrand M, Lickrish GM, Colgan TJ (1987) The anatomic distribution of cervical adenocarcinoma in situ: implications for treatment. *American Journal of Obstetrics and Gynecology* 157: 21–25.

Brainard JA, Hart WR (1998) Adenoid basal epitheliomas of the uterine cervix: a reevaluation of distinctive cervical basaloid lesions currently classified as adenoid basal carcinoma and adenoid basal hyperplasia. *American Journal of Surgical Pathology* 22: 965–975.

Burghardt E, Holzer E (1977) Diagnosis and treatment of microinvasive carcinoma of the cervix uteri. *Obstetrics and Gynecology* 49: 641–653.

Castrillon DH, Lee KR, Nucci MR (2002) Distinction between endometrial and endocervical adenocarcinoma: an immunohistochemical study. *International Journal of Gynecologic Pathology* 21: 4–10.

Clement PB, Scully RE (1982) Carcinoma of the cervix: histologic types. *Seminars in Oncology* 9: 251–264.

Clement PB, Young RH (1992) Endocervicosis of the urinary bladder: a report of six cases of a benign müllerian lesion that may mimic adenocarcinoma. *American Journal of Surgical Pathology* 16: 533–542.

Clement PB, Young RH, Keh P *et al.* (1995) Malignant mesonephric neoplasms of the uterine cervix. A report of eight cases, including four with a malignant spindle cell component. *American Journal of Surgical Pathology* 19: 1158–1177.

Costa MJ, McIlnay KR, Trelford J (1995) Cervical carcinoma with glandular differentiation: histological evaluation predicts disease recurrence in clinical stage I or II patients. *Human Pathology* 26: 829–837.

Cove H (1979) The Arias–Stella reaction occurring in the endocervix in pregnancy: recognition and comparison with an adenocarcinoma of the endocervix. *American Journal of Surgical Pathology* 3: 567–568.

Daya D, Young RH (1995) Florid deep glands of the uterine cervix: another mimic of adenoma malignum. *American Journal of Clinical Pathology* 103: 614–617.

Drescher CW, Hopkins MP, Roberts JA (1989) Comparison of the pattern of metastatic spread of squamous cell cancer and adenocarcinoma of the uterine cervix. *Gynecologic Oncology* 33: 340–343.

Ferry JA, Scully RE (1988) 'Adenoid cystic' carcinoma and adenoid basal carcinoma of the uterine cervix. A study of 28 cases. *American Journal of Surgical Pathology* 12: 134–144.

Ferry JA, Scully RE (1990) Mesonephric remnants, hyperplasia and neoplasia in the uterine cervix. A study of 49 cases. *American Journal of Surgical Pathology* 14 (12): 1100–1111.

Fluhmann CF (1961) Focal hyperplasia (tunnel clusters) of the cervix uteri. *Obstetrics and Gynecology* 17: 206–214.

Fu YS, Berek JS, Hilborne LD (1987) Diagnostic problems of in situ and invasive adenocarcinomas of the uterine cervix. *Applied Pathology* 5: 47–56.

Gilks CB, Young RH, Aguirre P *et al.* (1989) Adenoma malignum (minimal deviation adenocarcinoma) of the uterine cervix. A clinico-pathological and immunohistochemical analysis of 26 cases. *American Journal of Surgical Pathology* 13: 717–729.

Hopkins MP, Schmidt RW, Roberts JA *et al.* (1988) The prognosis and treatment of stage I adenocarcinoma of the cervix. *Obstetrics and Gynecology* 72: 915–921.

Horowitz IR, Jacobson LP, Zucker PK *et al.* (1988) Epidemiology of adenocarcinoma of the cervix. *Gynecologic Oncology* 31: 25–31.

Ismail SM (1991) Cone biopsy causes cervical endometriosis and tubo-endometrioid metaplasia. *Histopathology* 18: 107–114.

Jones MA, Young RH (1996) Endocervical type A (noncystic) tunnel clusters with cytologic atypia: a report of 14 cases. *American Journal of Surgical Pathology* 20: 1312–1318.

Jones MA, Young RH, Scully RE (1991) Diffuse laminar endocervical glandular hyperplasia: a report of seven cases. *American Journal of Surgical Pathology* 15: 1123–1129.

Jones MW, Silverberg SG, Kurman RJ (1993) Well-differentiated villo-glandular adenocarcinoma of the uterine cervix: a clinicopathological study of 24 cases. *International Journal of Gynecologic Pathology* 12 (1): 1–7.

Kaspar HG, Dinh TV, Doherty MG *et al.* (1993) Clinical implications of tumour volume measurement in Stage I adenocarcinoma of the cervix. *Obstetrics and Gynecology* 81: 296–300.

Kilgore LC, Soong SJ, Gore H *et al.* (1988) Analysis of prognostic features in adenocarcinoma of the cervix. *Gynecologic Oncology* 31: 137–153.

Larraza-Hernandez O, Molberg KH, Lindberg G *et al.* (1997) Ectopic prostatic tissue in the uterine cervix. *International Journal of Gynecologic Pathology* 16: 291–293.

Leninen A, Paavonen J, Forss M *et al.* (1990) Adenocarcinoma of the uterine cervix. *Cancer* 65: 53–59.

Leninen A, Paavonen J, Vesterinen E *et al.* (1991) Human papillomaviruses 16 and 18 in adenocarcinoma of the uterine cervix. *American Journal of Clinical Pathology* 95: 647–652.

McCluggage WG (2002) Recent advances in immunohistochemistry in gynaecological pathology. *Histopathology* 40: 309–326.

McCluggage WG, Sumathi VP, McBride HA *et al.* (2002) A panel of immunohistochemical stains, including carcinoembryonic antigen, vimentin, and estrogen receptor, aids the distinction between primary endometrial and endocervical adenocarcinomas. *International Journal of Gynecologic Pathology* 21: 11–15.

McCluggage WG, Oliva E, Herrington CS *et al.* (2003) CD10 and calretinin staining of endocervical glandular lesions, endocervical stroma and endometrioid adenocarcinomas of the uterine corpus: CD10 positivity is characteristic of, but not specific for, mesonephric lesions and is not specific for endometrial stroma. *Histopathology* 43: 144–149.

McCluggage WG, Ganesan R, Herschowitz L *et al.* (2006) Ectopic prostatic tissue in the uterine cervix and vagina: report of a series with detailed immunohistochemical analysis. *American Journal of Surgical Pathology* 30: 209–215.

McGowan L, Young RH, Scully RE (1980) Peutz–Jeghers syndrome with 'adenoma malignum' of the cervix. A report of two cases. *Gynecologic Oncology* 10: 125–133.

Mestwerdt G (1947) Fruhdiagnose des Kollumkarzinoms. *Zentralb Gynaekologie* 69: 326.

Mulvany N, Östör A (1997) Microinvasive adenocarcinoma of the cervix: a cytohistopathologic study of 40 cases. *Diagnostic Cytopathology* 16: 430–436.

Noda K, Kimura K, Ikeda M *et al.* (1983) Studies on the histogenesis of cervical adenocarcinoma. *International Journal of Gynecologic Pathology* 1: 336–346.

Nucci MR, Clement PB, Young RH (1999) Lobular endocervical glandular hyperplasia, not otherwise specified: a clinicopathologic analysis of thirteen cases of a distinctive pseudoneoplastic lesion and comparison with fourteen cases of adenoma malignum. *American Journal of Surgical Pathology* 23: 886–891.

Nucci MR, Ferry JA, Young RH (2000) Ectopic prostate in uterine cervix: a report of 2 cases and review of ectopic prostate tissue. *American Journal of Surgical Pathology* 24: 1224–1230.

Oliva E, Clement PB, Young RH (1995) Tubal and tubo-endometrioid metaplasia of the uterine cervix: unemphasized features that may cause problems in differential diagnosis. A report of 25 cases. *American Journal of Clinical Pathology* 103: 618–623.

Östör AG (2000) Early invasive adenocarcinoma of the uterine cervix. *International Journal of Gynecological Pathology* 19: 29–38.

Östör AG, Rome R, Quinn M (1997) Microinvasive adenocarcinoma of the cervix: a clinicopathologic study of 77 women. *Obstetrics and Gynecology* 89: 88–93.

Parazzini F, La Vecchia C, Negri E *et al.* (1988) Risk factors for adenocarcinoma of the cervix: a case–control study. *British Journal of Cancer* 57: 201–204.

Seidman JD, Tavassoli FA (1995) Mesonephric hyperplasia of the uterine cervix: a clinicopathologic study of 51 cases. *International Journal of Gynecological Pathology* 14: 293–299.

Smith HO, Tiffany MF, Qualls CR *et al.* (2000) The rising incidence of adenocarcinoma relative to squamous cell carcinoma of the uterine cervix in the United States—a 24 year population based study. *Gynecologic Oncology* 78: 97–105.

Sivanesaratnam V, Sen DK, Jayalakshmi P *et al.* (1993) Radical hysterectomy and pelvic lymphadenectomy for early invasive cancer of the cervix—14-year experience. *International Journal of Gynaecological Cancer* 3: 231–238.

Tambouret R, Bell DA, Young RH (2000) Microcystic endocervical adenocarcinomas: a report of eight cases. *American Journal of Surgical Pathology* 24: 369–375.

Tambouret R, Clement PB, Young RH (2003) Endometrial endometrioid adenocarcinoma with a deceptive pattern of spread to the uterine cervix: a manifestation of stage IIb endometrial carcinoma liable to be misinterpreted as an independent carcinoma or a benign lesion. *American Journal of Surgical Pathology* 27: 1080–1088.

Tseng C-J, Horng S-G, Soong Y-K (1997) Conservative conization for microinvasive carcinoma of the cervix. *American Journal of Obstetrics and Gynaecology* 176: 1009–1010.

Yaegashi N, Sato S, Inoue Y (1994) Conservative surgical treatment in cervical cancer with 3 to 5 mm stromal invasion in the absence of confluent invasion and lymph-vascular space involvement. *Gynecologic Oncology* 54: 333–337.

Yazigi R, Sandstad J, Muñoz AK *et al.* (1990) Adenosquamous carcinoma of the cervix: prognosis in stage IB. *Obstetrics and Gynecology* 75: 1012–1015.

Young RH, Scully RE (1989) Villoglandular papillary adenocarcinoma of the uterine cervix. *Cancer* 63: 1773–1779.

Young RH, Scully RE (1992) Uterine carcinomas simulating

microglandular hyperplasia. A report of six cases. *American Journal of Surgical Pathology* 16: 1092–1097.

Young RH, Scully RE (1993) Minimal-deviation endometrioid adeno-carcinoma of the uterine cervix. A report of five cases of a distinctive neoplasm that may be misinterpreted as benign. *American Journal of Surgical Pathology* 17: 660–665.

Young RH, Scully RE (1998) Cancer risk in women exposed to diethyl-stilbestrol in utero. *Journal of the American Medical Association* 280: 630–634.

Young RH, Clement PB (2002) Endocervical adenocarcinoma and its variants: their morphology and differential diagnosis. *Histopathology* 41: 185–207.

Cervical neoplasia: screening

CHAPTER 23

Emotional aspects of cervical neoplasia screening and management

Theresa Freeman-Wang and Amali Lokugamage

INTRODUCTION

The feeling of anxiety is an intrinsic part of the human condition. It is a natural response to certain environmental and psychological factors. An awareness of the effect is found in one of the first literary narratives, the *Epic of Gilgamesh*, which dates to the Babylonian and Sumerian civilisations in the second and third millennia BC. The feeling of anxiety, in the sense of an inner experience of intense anguish, is associated with self-awareness and the appreciation of one's own individuality and responsibility.

In philosophy, Plato emphasised the separation between reason and the passions. He divided the soul into three parts: the rational functions located in the head; courage and anger located in the area of the heart; and desires assigned to the lower part of the body. The last two formed the basis of the conception of the passions, which laid the basis for the later detailed development of the theory of the passions and encompassed the concept of fear.

Western philosophical thought has been strongly influenced by early Christian teachings such as those of St Paul, in which he emphasised a person's individuality. Thus, as soon as man became responsible for himself, he was subject to guilt from failing to meet his responsibilities. Responsibility gave both solace and dignity, but also anxiety. This idea of guilt remains central to the contemporary conceptions of anxiety in the nineteenth to twenty-first centuries.

Prior to 1950, there was relatively little research on human anxiety, mainly because of the complexity of the phenomena, the lack of appropriate measuring tools and the ethical problems of inducing anxiety in laboratory settings.

Since then, conceptual advances have clarified anxiety as a theoretical construct, and a number of scales for measuring anxiety have been developed.

The term anxiety is most commonly used to describe an unpleasant emotional state or condition. It is also used to describe relatively stable differences in anxiety proneness as a personality trait. These concepts of state and trait anxiety were first introduced by Cattell and Rickells (1968) and elaborated by Spielberger (1983). Originally developed in 1966, modified in 1972 (Spielberger, 1972) and later in 1979 (Spielberger, 1980), the Spielberger Trait Anxiety Inventory (STAI) remains the most commonly used psychological tool for assessing anxiety.

To the clinician, hospitals and clinics are familiar friendly places, and a colposcopic examination is a minor investigative procedure used to detect an abnormality which, if found, can be effectively treated. What health care providers frequently overlook is that this is not a view shared by patients, who find attending hospital and undergoing investigative and therapeutic procedures very stressful.

Much of the psychosocial and psychosexual impact associated with investigation for an abnormal smear stems from fear and unfounded guilt. Being told of an abnormal smear result compounds a woman's fears, as it poses a triple threat — to her mortality, her sexuality and her fertility — and may have a lasting negative effect on her body image and self-esteem. For some, the distress begins with the first invitation to attend for cervical screening.

THE PSYCHOSOCIAL IMPACT OF CERVICAL SCREENING

Screening in general involves actively seeking to identify a disease or predisease condition in people who are presumed, and presume themselves, to be healthy. Screening healthy people without informing them about the magnitude of the inherent risks of screening is ethically unjustifiable (Skrabanek, 1988). One of the inherent disadvantages of screening is the generation of anxiety in those being screened.

Since the introduction of the National Health Service Cervical Screening Programme (NHSCSP) in 1988 in the UK, both the incidence of and deaths from cervical cancer have reduced by 7% per year, as described in Chapter 25. Countries that lack an effective screening programme continue to have high rates of cervical cancer. Indeed, worldwide, this largely preventable disease affects almost 500 000 women per year. Of these, around 350 000 will die. In this context and despite criticism of the accuracy of the current screening test, it is understandable that, as health professionals, we view cervical screening as a positive medical intervention. However, many of the women invited to participate in the programme have a poor understanding of their anatomy, of how and why a smear is taken and of what the results of the test mean. They often think the purpose of the test is to detect cancer rather than prevent it.

An early study following the introduction of the NHSCSP in 1988 showed that some women thought the invitation for a smear meant their general practitioner already knew they had cancer (Nathoo, 1988). In a survey of 600 women in London, 71% thought cervical screening was to detect cancer, while only 11% understood that it was to prevent cervical cancer.

Recent studies assessing women's knowledge of cervical screening have been more encouraging, with 62–97% of women understanding the purpose of screening. However, only 52% of them realised that a 'normal result' meant low risk rather than no risk (Marteau *et al.*, 2001).

Women are often unaware that the likelihood of being recalled for a repeat test following routine screening is relatively high at 1 in 12. Thirty per cent of women estimated the chance of recall as between 1 in 100 and 1 in 1000 women (Marteau *et al.*, 2001). In addition, the widely published risk factors for cervical cancer and premalignancy associated with sexual activity including early age at first intercourse, multiple sexual partners and a history of sexually transmitted infection lead to the belief, often erroneous, of female 'promiscuity' as a major cause of an abnormal cervical smear result. Against this background, an abnormal result becomes a stigmatising event. It is therefore not surprising that the receipt of any abnormal smear result can have a seriously negative effect on women (Stoate, 1989; Wolfe *et al.*, 1992; Bell *et al.*, 1995).

On being told of an abnormal smear result, women are confronted by a threat to their mortality because the word 'cancer' has been used. For many, this word induces a greater dread than that of other diseases which may carry a worse prognosis and, once heard, pervades all thinking (Austoker, 1994). Added to this is the implication that treatment may affect future child-bearing potential. Beresford and Gervaize (1986) were one of the first groups of researchers to show that all women given an abnormal smear result feared they had cancer. On a scale of mild, moderate or severe intensity, for 70% of women, this fear was graded as severe. Almost 70% expressed a high level of concern about the potential loss of their reproductive potential, about the procedure itself and a fear of loss of bodily integrity. In addition to these fears, women reported other behavioural symptoms of distress, including sleep disturbances, irritability, crying, outbursts of anger and difficulty with sexual relationships.

As well as the fear of discovering pathology, the pelvic examination itself is generally considered to be one of the most anxiety-provoking common medical procedures. All women experience a range of negative feelings towards gynaecological examination. For some, the process is both physically and emotionally traumatising. Women rarely overcome the feeling of personal intrusion, regardless of the number of previous examinations experienced. Added to their embarrassment and feelings of vulnerability and helplessness is the fear of physical discomfort and pain from the investigation and treatment they may undergo. Adverse psychosexual effects of an abnormal smear have been reported in several studies (Schmale and Iker, 1971; Goodkin *et al.*, 1986; Campion *et al.*, 1988; Posner and Vessey, 1988; McDonald *et al.*, 1989; Marteau *et al.*, 1990; Lerman *et al.*, 1991; Nugent *et al.*, 1993; Roberts and Blunt, 1994; Gath *et al.*, 1995; Mould *et al.*, 1995; Jones *et al.*, 1996). Women perceive a challenge to their sexuality because cervical cancer may be considered a sexually transmitted disease, with inherent judgemental and negative associations. Campion *et al.* (1988) showed a significant increase in the frequency of negative feelings towards sexual intercourse and a reduction in spontaneous interest in sex following diagnosis and treatment of an abnormal smear. Posner and Vessey (1988) found that 65 (43%) of the 150 women they interviewed experienced 'disturbed' sexual relationships, including abstaining from or pain during intercourse due to tension. For some, there was concern that the changes discovered by the cervical smear could be transmitted to or were gained from their sexual partner. Consequently, an abnormal smear result may lead to feelings of low self-esteem and negative body image.

These fears, particularly of embarrassment and pain, remain important reasons that women give for not participating in a cervical screening programme. Ultimately, women have the right to choose whether or not they wish to be part of the programme, but they should have access to accurate information to enable them to arrive at an informed decision. In countries where screening exists, health care providers need to be able to explain in an understanding and empathetic manner:

1 the purpose of screening;
2 the likelihood of a positive or negative result;
3 the uncertainties and risks of screening;
4 the follow-up plans and availability of support services.

In this balance of providing accurate information, it is also important for women to be made aware that cervical cancer presents most commonly in those who have not been screened.

THE PSYCHOSOCIAL IMPACT OF HUMAN PAPILLOMAVIRUS (HPV) TESTING

Human papillomaviruses are ubiquitous in sexually active populations and infect more than 80% of women of reproductive age at some point (Syrjanen *et al.*, 1988; Oster, 1993). As discussed elsewhere, they are also a necessary component in the pathogenesis of cervical neoplasia (Bosch *et al.*, 2002). There has been a plethora of studies not only evaluating the association between HPV and cervical premalignancy, but assessing the application of HPV testing to clinical and laboratory management.

Although HPV testing has not as yet been incorporated into the NHSCSP, it is common practice as a method of triage of atypical squamous cells of uncertain significance (ASCUS) smears within the screening programme in the United States, and the literature shows that it has a potentially valuable role both as a test of cure post treatment and in primary screening, especially in areas currently without screening and where financial and manpower resources are limited. However, the potential distress of HPV testing in relation to cervical screening is only now being considered (Cuzick *et al.*, 2001). Indeed, the psychological sequelae of being given the diagnosis of an HPV infection have previously concentrated on visible genital warts rather than high-risk oncogenic types or have failed to distinguish between the two (Filiberti *et al.*, 1993; Reitano, 1997; Conaglen *et al.*, 2001).

Filiberti *et al.*'s (1993) small study of 51 women with a primary HPV infection showed that 57% of the study group experienced deterioration in their relationships following the first diagnosis of a wart virus infection. This was because of the diagnosis itself, the fear of transmitting it to a partner, the forced use of condoms or the development of dyspareunia. Nine women stopped having intercourse, and four felt the diagnosis alone contributed to the ending of their current relationship. In contrast, although Conaglen *et al.* (2001) showed that the diagnosis of HPV infection was associated with psychological difficulties, this was no different from those associated with other sexually transmitted infections or even those with no active diagnosis.

As has been shown to be the case for cervical screening in general, relatively few women have an understanding of the significance of an HPV infection (Syrjanen *et al.*, 1988; Oster, 1993; Waller *et al.*, 2004). Most of the studies to date assessing knowledge of HPV have been from the United States. All have shown consistently low awareness of HPV and a poor knowledge of its mode of transmission (Vail-Smith and White, 1992; Yacobi *et al.*, 1999; Lambert, 2001). One of the few studies from the UK is a recent survey by Pitts and Clarke among employees of a university in the north of England; only 30% ($n = 120$) of those responding to the questionnaires ($n = 400$) had heard of HPV infection prior to the study. Of these, only 16.7% ($n = 67$) had a good working knowledge of HPV testing and the meaning of HPV positivity (Pitts and Clarke, 2002).

A series of recent UK papers from McCaffery *et al.* (2003) have examined both awareness and attitudes to HPV testing among purposively selected samples of women from different ethnic backgrounds (Waller *et al.*, 2003, 2004; McCaffery *et al.*, 2003). Using focus group discussions, the authors elicited women's attitudes towards HPV testing in the context of cervical cancer prevention. Their findings indicate that, although some women welcomed the possible introduction of HPV testing, they were not fully aware of the sexually transmitted nature of cervical cancer and expressed anxiety, confusion and stigma about HPV as a sexually transmitted infection. The term 'wart virus', often used by medical professionals to describe high-risk HPV to women, appeared to exacerbate stigma and confusion. Testing positive for HPV raised concerns about women's sexual relationships in terms of trust, fidelity, blame and protection, particularly for women in long-term monogamous relationships. Participation in HPV testing also had the potential to communicate messages of distrust, infidelity and promiscuity to women's partners, family and community. Concern about the current lack of available information about HPV was clearly expressed, and public education about HPV was seen as necessary for the whole community, not only women.

Although there is understandable anxiety associated with HPV positivity, one might expect that being told a negative result in the context of a borderline/ASCUS or mildly dyskaryotic smear and the associated very low risk of developing cervical cancer would be reassuring. However, Maissi *et al.* (2004) addressed this in a cross-sectional questionnaire study. Variables that predicted anxiety in HPV-positive women were younger age, higher perceived risk of cervical cancer and reporting a lack of understanding of the meaning of the test result. While women with normal test results had significantly less anxiety ($P = 0.028$), among women with an abnormal smear result, those testing HPV negative were no less anxious than those women with an abnormal smear result who were not tested for HPV ($P = 0.949$).

The evidence shows a strong link between persistent high-risk oncogenic HPV infection and the development of cervical premalignancy and malignancy. That this viral infection is sexually transmissible is also clear. What remains difficult is how best to convey this information and so appropriately inform the public without creating stigma or adding to the anguish of many women. Two recent studies have examined this problem and, in the study from McCaffery *et al.* (2004), the findings suggested that testing positive for HPV may have an adverse psychosocial impact with increased anxiety, distress and concern about sexual relationships. McCaffery and her group suggested that the outcomes of HPV testing need much further investigation and must be considered alongside clinical and economic decisions to include HPV testing in routine screening. In a further study, Waller *et al.* (2005) showed that women's understanding of HPV varied considerably, even after participation in testing, and they suggested that the way this information is presented to women is crucial in minimising the negative psychological impact of testing positive and also ensuring that participation in future screening remains high. Therefore, it would seem obvious that more research is needed to examine this area and to assess how to avoid the anxiety, distress and concern of a positive result and to provide reassurance for those with a negative result.

ANXIETY IN RELATION TO COLPOSCOPY AND TREATMENT

As already mentioned, the STAI is one of the most commonly used psychological tools to assess anxiety (Spielberger *et al.*, 1970). The range for scoring is 20–80. The average score for an adult woman is 35. Scores above 49 are found in patients with a diagnosis of an anxiety disorder. In 1992, Marteau *et al.* conducted a series of studies at The Royal Free Hospital in London, assessing anxiety levels in different situations. Very high levels of anxiety in women attending for colposcopy were confirmed, with a mean score of 51.2 (Marteau *et al.*, 1990). This score was higher than anxiety levels experienced by pregnant women attending the hospital for antenatal care who had been told of an abnormal alpha-fetoprotein level screening for fetal abnormality (STAI = 47) and higher than that in women the night before undergoing major surgery (STAI = 41). The level of distress highlighted by this study was more strongly related to anticipation of the procedure than the outcome. Women's main concerns were that the procedure would be uncomfortable and painful and that they were uncertain as to what it would involve. There was no relationship between the anxiety scores and the severity of the referred problem or the perceived seriousness of the problem.

The advent of large loop excision of the transformation zone (LLETZ or LEEP) in the late 1980s brought about a marked change in colposcopic practice. Traditionally, women were referred, had a colposcopic assessment and possible punch biopsy. They were then reviewed with the results and arrangements made for attendance for treatment at a subsequent visit. LLETZ facilitated the introduction of a 'see and treat' policy whereby a woman referred with an abnormal smear could undergo colposcopic assessment and treatment, if required, at the same initial visit. Gunasekera *et al.* (1990) suggested this might be associated with fewer adverse psychological sequelae because there were fewer return visits.

Some studies have suggested that high levels of distress at colposcopy are transient. Gath *et al.* (1995) assessed anxiety levels prior to and at 4 and 32 weeks following the first colposcopic appointment. Ninety per cent of women reported shock, panic and horror in the first week after receiving an abnormal smear result. Asked about their experience of colposcopy, 51% described pain, embarrassment, shock or distress. One-third of women with a sexual partner reported deterioration in their relationships. However, by 32 weeks, only 4% said this state had persisted. Transient or not, the distress suffered by women attending for colposcopy remains significant. This problem needs to be addressed not only to improve women's experience of the whole process, but also because of the potential psychophysiological role that the feelings of stress and hopelessness may play in the promotion of cervical intraepithelial neoplasia (CIN) to invasive cancer (Goodkin *et al.*, 1986).

PSYCHONEUROIMMUNOLOGY AND THE CERVIX

It is known that the acquisition of the most oncogenic types of HPV is necessary for the development of CIN. However, the relationship is complex and still not fully understood. As mentioned previously, up to 80% of sexually active women get HPV infection, but only a few will develop CIN. In these women, persistence of HPV, i.e. failure or the immune system to clear the infection, is probably a significant risk factor. This observable fact is clearly seen in women infected with human immunodeficiency virus (HIV), but may occur in situations where there are more subtle forms of depressed immunity.

It is known that emotional state, and in particular the response to stress, can modify capacity to cope with infection, autoimmunity and cancer. Ill-defined effects of several forms of stressful life events on the immune system have been reported, but accurate correlations and measurements have thus far been elusive (Bartrop *et al.*, 1977; Ader *et al.*, 1995; Kiecolt-Glaser and Glaser, 1995). The term psychoneuroimmunology has been coined for this area of multidisciplinary work.

Progression from infection with HPV to cervical cancer may involve a 'permissive' host environment, in which the immune response is mobilised in an inappropriate manner. In this scenario, the immune system would mount a suboptimal response to infection by HPV. This would then result in 'viral tolerance', which would allow the virus to persist in the tissues. Alternatively, the virus may tamper with the intracellular mechanism inside an infected cell and thus sabotage the immune response completely. Later reactivation may occur, under conditions in which oncogenic viral potential will manifest more readily. Because of the increasing awareness that an immunological interpretation may contribute to the pathogenesis of CIN, vaccine-based strategies are already at an exciting stage of development (Kibur *et al.*, 2000). However, greater understanding of immunopermissive conditions may broaden the scope of other possible interventions.

There is now widespread acknowledgement that the immune system does not act in an autonomous fashion. Homeostatic immune function is part of a dynamic interaction with other systems, including in particular neurological and endocrine systems.

Existing research measuring T-cell activation has demonstrated an abnormal response to adverse psychological events (Byrnes *et al.*, 1998). There have also been attempts to document changes in cytokine profile, looking at several interleukins (e.g. IL-2, IL-4, IL-10, IL-12) (Clerici *et al.*, 1997; Jacobs *et al.*, 1998; Bontkes *et al.*, 1999). Emotional stress can result in the release of glucocorticoids, which can depress immunity; hence, the endocrine system can also have an impact on the immune system (Cacioppo *et al.*, 1995; Webster *et al.*, 2002). More recently, it has become clear that the cytokine (and chemokine) pathways do impinge upon the neurological pathways directly, with intracerebral 'macrophages' – the microglia – playing a key role in the complex feedback required (Denicoff *et al.*, 1987). It has been postulated that cytokines play a direct role locally in the cervix; however, it may be that the systemic quantitative levels of these mediators are not only easier to measure but also a more accurate reflection of the biological activity within the important psychoneuroimmune circuit (Mota *et al.*, 1999). There remains much to discern about how end-organ immunological factors vary with systemic immunological factors.

Several reviews have been conducted in this area. However, the studies have been of variable methodological quality. Restricted ranges of psychosocial and immunological variables have been measured, small numbers of participants have been included, and samples have been taken not always from the general population, but rather from highly selective clinical groups. For instance, a study (Byrnes *et al.*, 1998) that looked at 36 women who were HIV positive, and thereby at risk of recurrent HPV infection as a result of their special clinical status, used only two psychosocial variables: stressful life events and pessimism. The former of these variables was measured by way of a truncated 10-item questionnaire that was insufficiently comprehensive, whereas previous life event checklists contain 40 or more items (Holmes and Rahe, 1967). Therefore, it was not surprising that frequencies of life events were found to be unrelated to immunological parameters, given the reduced adequacy of the measure used. The standardised measure of pessimism, however, did reveal a borderline significant relationship (independent of the effects of other variables) with cytotoxic T-cell counts. The latter may be difficult to interpret in these patients in view of well-known effects of HIV infection. The same research group followed on with another publication of similar sample size. This did show an association between life stress, particularly bereavement, and progression and/or persistence of CIN disease (Pereira *et al.*, 2003). A larger study of 342 subjects conducted in the Netherlands (Tiersma *et al.*, 2004), found no association between tests of psychosocial variables and the grade of CIN. However, this study also found no correlation with traditional risk factors, e.g. smoking, number of sexual partners before the age of 20 years and oral contraceptive use. The methodology of comparing psychosocial traits and all grades of CIN did not take into account lag time for development of disease, which may have had a considerable residual confounder effect.

MEDICAL ANTHROPOLOGY AND BIOMEDICAL RESEARCH

There is a bewildering array of immunological and psychological risk factors that could potentially be tested in psychoneuroimmunological studies. Anthropological literature suggests that medical anthropologists have a valuable role in the act of hypothesis generation for research projects (Yoder, 1997).

Western biomedicine assumes that the biomedical model is the norm. However, anthropological project input allows the model to stretch to include categories from pre-existing historical base health care models that incorporate a mind–body link.

Other health care models that follow a mind–body paradigm could offer psychosocial risk factors for research workers to investigate. Such systems include traditional Chinese medicine, Aruyveda and homeopathy, which lack scientific plausibility as yet, but are nevertheless based on hundreds or thousands of years of observational data (Sharma, 2004). The paucity of scientific evidence in these fields needs to be addressed with rigorously conducted studies. All the aforementioned medical systems place disease within a holistic picture of the patient, which includes emotional as well as physical profiles. Present emotional state, past emotional insults and the emotional traits of their parents are considered as part of the aetiology of any disease state and vice versa. The emotions indicate a foundation of vulnerability on which other physical factors can cause illness. For instance, in homeopathy, personalities or life situations that lead to a psychological state that predisposes to cancer include subjugation, self-martyrdom and 'people pleasing' with inability to stand up and demand respect from others. Furthermore, with respect to cervical cancer, homeopaths postulate that the former psychological attributes tend to occur within the framework of a patient feeling intuitively that she may be a victim of possible infidelity. Practitioners from these other traditions of medicine claim that the psychosocial mechanisms of their health care models lie outside the dualistic mind and body schism of western philosophical thought founded by René Descartes. Psychoneuroimmunology allows potential bridge-building between the dualistic and holistic health care ideologies, as it assesses the whole person to a greater extent than previous scientific frameworks.

INTERVENTIONS TO REDUCE ANXIETY

The anxieties and distress experienced by women receiving an abnormal smear result and attending for colposcopy are well documented (Beresford and Gervaize, 1986; Posner and Vessey, 1988; McDonald *et al.*, 1989; Marteau *et al.*, 1990; Nugent *et al.*, 1993; Palmer *et al.*, 1993; Gath *et al.*, 1995; Jones *et al.*, 1996; Tomaino-Brunner *et al.*, 1996, 1998; Fylan, 1998; Freeman-Wang *et al.*, 2001; Paraskevaidis *et al.*, 2001; Idestrom *et al.*, 2003). Despite this and the many studies looking at potential helpful interventions, there has been little change in the levels of stress created or in compliance with cervical screening or follow-up once part of the programme. Most strategies have concentrated on the provision of accurate information both because this has been shown to reduce anxiety and because it empowers patients to make informed choices and so be involved in the management of their own condition. However, other factors can also be important. In a survey in an inner London area with a large ethnic population,

25% of women stated that, if there was the guaranteed availability of a female practitioner, they would attend for a cervical smear (Schwartz *et al.*, 1989).

Marteau *et al.* (2001) showed that, in relation to the provision of information, women in receipt of a clear simple account of the meaning of an abnormal smear result and the colposcopy procedure were less anxious and more reassured by the subsequent consultation than those receiving either no information or those receiving a complex explanatory booklet. Adequate pre-visit information is particularly important (Byrom *et al.*, 2002). Colposcopy clinics offering a 'see and treat' policy or a LLETZ procedure at the first appointment for women referred with high-grade smears have become common practice in the UK. Within the NHSCSP, this management has the benefit of reducing waiting times but, contrary to Gunasekera's assumption, can be associated with even higher levels of anxiety. In a pilot study in a colposcopy unit introducing a 'see and treat' policy in place of the traditional 'select and treat' policy, anxiety levels as measured with the STAI were 51.2 in the 'select and treat' group but 58.6 in the 'see and treat' group. Again, written or visual pre-visit information in the form of a short explanatory video can lead to significant reductions in the levels of anxiety experienced (Gardeil and Turner, 1995; Freeman-Wang *et al.*, 2001). There is also evidence that a one-stop service for the management of women with low-grade abnormalities, although associated with similar levels of anxiety at the actual visit, is associated with less anxiety and negative emotions 1 week after the consultation (Naik *et al.*, 2001).

Behavioural implications of interventions

Ultimately, reducing the incidence of cervical cancer cannot rely exclusively on traditional secondary screening. Primary prevention and changes in health-related behaviour are equally important. Sexual health in the UK has deteriorated in recent years with further increases in HIV and other sexually transmitted infections (STIs) reported in 2002 (Brown *et al.*, 2004). Diagnoses of new HIV infections have doubled from 1997 to 2002, mainly driven by heterosexuals who acquired their infection abroad. So, if the UK is not doing well in this regard, then developing countries have an almost insurmountable challenge. As HPV is a sexually transmitted agent, campaigns to reduce other STIs could be potentially beneficial. Condoms may not provide full protection as the virus is transmitted through skin-to-skin contact, although consistent use of condoms is likely to reduce the risk of infection (Waller *et al.*, 2004).

Some studies have found that a woman's number of sexual partners and the sexual behaviour of women's male partners are risk factors for HPV infection. Despite epidemiological evidence for the role of men's sexual behaviour in women's cancer risk, this factor has been relatively neglected in psy-

chosocial literature (Waller *et al.*, 2004). Further studies are required in this area, although accurate data may be hard to gather due to partner reluctance to participate.

The link between the numbers of women's sexual partners and viral transmission may be quite immunologically complex, as illustrated in studies relating to HIV infection. It has been well documented that some female sex workers in Kenya and Thailand are resistant to HIV infection. This may involve HIV-specific cervicovaginal antibody responses in a minority of highly exposed HIV-seronegative women in association with other protecting factors, such as local production of HIV-suppressive chemokines (Belec *et al.*, 2001; Kaul *et al.*, 2001). In addition, a key epidemiological correlate of late seroconversion was a reduction in sex work over the preceding year. Paradoxically, in persistently uninfected control subjects, a break from sex work was associated with a loss of HIV-specific CD8+ responses. Psychoneuroimmunological circuits may be implicated in these phenomena, but there has been little work in this area to date.

Vaccination is one of the cornerstones of public health interventions and, in the long term, prevention of HPV is likely to rely on vaccination. However, vaccine uptake and herd immunity levels in any given community are vulnerable to cultural beliefs. The recent measles, mumps and rubella (MMR) vaccine controversy demonstrates that, despite scientific evidence, there has been individual refusal and some public resistance to the vaccine based on fears, rumour and concern about vaccine safety. Indeed, there are other examples of public resistance in vaccination history with particular respect to a perceived 'threat to feminine fertility'. Fertility is a status symbol in poorer societies, in developing countries where a woman's social status is low. An example of this is a failed vaccination programme in Cameroon. In 1990, a rumour that public health workers were administering a vaccine to sterilise girls and women spread throughout Cameroon. Schoolgirls leapt from windows to escape the vaccination teams, and the colonial vaccination campaign (part of the Year of Universal Child Immunisation) was aborted (Feldman-Savelsberg *et al.*, 2000). Future vaccination programmes need to be sensitive to cultural views on female reproduction and the historical perspective of other public health interventions in the geographical region.

CONCLUSION

Holland and Stewart (1990) defined screening as 'actively seeking to identify a disease or pre-disease condition in people who are presumed and presume themselves to be healthy'. This is justifiable only if the condition is an important health problem and the intervention is both acceptable to the public and effective. The evidence shows the benefit of cervical screening and the potential benefits of HPV testing, but this is not without cost. Screening may cause significant anxiety, even for those who are disease free. The advent of HPV testing now brings a sexually transmissible agent into the forum of cervical screening and thus adds a new layer of complexity to the delivery of this service. Explaining that HPV infection is common, often transient and may be purely a reflection of sexual activity needs to be seen as an important public health issue. People need to be aware that exposure to the virus does not necessarily reflect promiscuity or infidelity. Studies in psychoneuroimmunology may further our understanding of biobehavioural and psychosocial factors associated with cervical neoplasia. More research is needed to provide a clear picture to the public of our understanding of cervical cancer as a rare complication of HPV infection, which is a common occurrence.

Further UK data from the HPV pilot study organised by the NHSCSP, the Trial of Management of Borderline and other Low-grade Abnormal smears (TOMBOLA) and A Randomised Trial of HPV Testing in Primary Cervical Screening (ARTISTIC) trials should provide further valuable information to help in assessing the place of HPV testing within an already well-organised cervical screening programme.

Overall, the evidence lends support to the introduction of HPV testing for primary screening in countries currently without an organised programme but, again, for the long-term success of cervical screening, the potential psychosocial sequelae should not be overlooked.

REFERENCES

Ader R, Cohen N, Felten D (1995) Psychoneuroimmunology: interactions between the nervous system and the immune system (review; 55 refs). *Lancet* 345 (8942): 99–103.

Austoker J. (1994) Cancer prevention in primary care. Screening for cervical cancer. *British Medical Journal* 309 (6949): 241–248.

Bartrop RW, Luckhurst E, Lazarus L *et al.* (1997) Depressed lymphocyte function after bereavement. *Lancet* 1 (8016): 834–836.

Belec L, Ghys PD, Hocini H *et al.* (2001) Cervicovaginal secretory antibodies to human immunodeficiency virus type 1 (HIV-1) that block viral transcytosis through tight epithelial barriers in highly exposed HIV-1-seronegative African women. *Journal of Infectious Diseases* 184 (11): 1412–1422.

Bell S, Porter M, Kitchener H *et al.* (1995) Psychological response to cervical screening. *Preventive Medicine* 24 (6): 610–616.

Beresford J, Gervaize P (1986) The emotional impact of abnormal Pap smears on patients referred for colposcopy. *Colposcopy and Gynecologic Laser Surgery* 2 (2): 83–87.

Bontkes HJ, de Gruijl TD, Walboomers JM *et al.* (1999) Immune responses against human papillomavirus (HPV) type 16 virus-like particles in a cohort study of women with cervical intraepithelial neoplasia. II. Systemic but not local IgA responses correlate with clearance of HPV-16. *Journal of General Virology* 80 (Pt 2): 409–417.

Bosch FX, Lorincz A, Muñoz N *et al.* (2002) The causal relation between human papillomavirus and cervical cancer. *Journal of Clinical Pathology* 55 (4): 244–265.

Brown AE, Sadler KE, Tomkins SE *et al.* (2004) Recent trends in HIV and other STIs in the United Kingdom: data to the end of 2002 (review; 95 refs). *Sexually Transmitted Infections* 80 (3): 159–166.

Byrnes DM, Antoni MH, Goodkin K *et al.* (1998) Stressful events, pessimism, natural killer cell cytotoxicity, and cytotoxic/suppressor T cells in HIV+ black women at risk for cervical cancer. *Psychosomatic Medicine* 60 (6): 714–722.

Byrom J, Clarke T, Neale J *et al.* (2002) Can pre-colposcopy sessions reduce anxiety at the time of colposcopy? A prospective randomised study. *Journal of Obstetrics and Gynaecology* 22 (4): 415–420.

Cacioppo JT, Malarkey WB, Kiecolt GJK *et al.* (1995) Heterogeneity in neuroendocrine and immune responses to brief psychological stressors as a function of autonomic cardiac activation. *Psychosomatic Medicine* 57 (2): 154–164.

Campion M, Brown J, McCance D *et al.* (1988) Psychosexual trauma of an abnormal cervical smear. *British Journal of Obstetrics and Gynaecology* 195: 175–181.

Cattell RB, Rickels K (1968) The relationship of clinical symptoms and IPAT-factored tests of anxiety, regression and asthenia: a factor analytic study. *Journal of Nervous and Mental Diseases* 146 (2): 147–160.

Clerici M, Merola M, Ferrario E *et al.* (1997) Cytokine production patterns in cervical intraepithelial neoplasia: association with human papillomavirus infection (see comments). *Journal of the National Cancer Institute* 89 (3): 245–250.

Conaglen HM, Hughes R, Conaglen JV *et al.* (2001) A prospective study of the psychological impact on patients of first diagnosis of human papillomavirus. *International Journal of STD and AIDS* 12 (10): 651–658.

Cuzick J, Sasieni P, Davies P *et al.* (2001) A systematic review of the role of human papillomavirus testing within a cervical screening programme (review; 280 refs). *Health Technology Assessment* 3 (14): i–iv.

Denicoff KD, Rubinow DR, Papa MZ *et al.* (1987) The neuropsychiatric effects of treatment with interleukin-2 and lymphokine-activated killer cells. *Annals of Internal Medicine* 107 (3): 293–300.

Feldman-Savelsberg P, Ndonko FT, Schmidt-Ehry B (2000) Sterilizing vaccines or the politics of the womb: retrospective study of a rumor in Cameroon. *Medical Anthropology Quarterly* 14 (2): 159–179.

Filiberti A, Tamburini M, Stefanon B *et al.* (1993) Psychological aspects of genital human papillomavirus infection: a preliminary report. *Journal of Psychosomatic Obstetrics and Gynaecology* 14 (2): 145–152.

Freeman-Wang T, Walker P, Linehan J *et al.* (2001) Anxiety levels in women attending colposcopy clinics for treatment for cervical intraepithelial neoplasia: a randomised trial of written and video information. *British Journal of Obstetrics and Gynaecology* 108 (5): 482–484.

Fylan F (1998) Screening for cervical cancer: a review of women's attitudes, knowledge, and behaviour (see comments) (review; 83 refs). *British Journal of General Practice* 48 (433): 1509–1514.

Gardeil F, Turner MJ (1995) The case for selective 'see and treat' in patients referred for colposcopy (see comments). *International Journal of STD and AIDS* 6 (6): 418–421.

Gath D, Hallam N, Mynors-Wallis L *et al.* (1995) Emotional reactions in women attending a UK colposcopy clinic. *Journal of Epidemiology and Community Health* 49: 79–83.

Goodkin K, Antoni M, Blaney P (1986) Stress and hopelessness in the promotion of cervical intraepithelial neoplasia to invasive squamous cell carcinoma of the cervix. *Journal of Psychosomatic Research* 30: 67–76.

Gunsasekera P, Phipps J, Lewis B (1990) Large loop excision of the transformation zone (LLETZ) compared to carbon dioxide laser in the treatment of CIN: a superior mode of treatment. *British Journal of Obstetrics and Gynaecology* 97: 995–998.

Holland WW, Stewart S (1990) *Screening in Health Care: Benefit or Bane?* London: Nuffield Provincial Hospitals Trust.

Holmes TH, Rahe RH (1967) The social readjustment rating scale. *Journal of Psychosomatic Research* 11 (2): 213–218.

Idestrom M, Milsom I, Andersson-Ellstrom A (2003) Women's experience of coping with a positive Pap smear: a register-based study of women with two consecutive Pap smears reported as CIN1. *Acta Obstetrica et Gynecologica Scandinavica* 82 (8): 756–761.

Jacobs N, Giannini SL, Doyen J *et al.* (1998) Inverse modulation of IL-10 and IL-12 in the blood of women with preneoplastic lesions of the uterine cervix. *Clinical and Experimental Immunology* 111 (1): 219–224.

Jones MH, Singer A, Jenkins D (1996) The mildly abnormal cervical smear: patient anxiety and choice of management. *Journal of the Royal Society of Medicine* 89 (5): 257–260.

Kaul R, Rowland-Jones SL, Kimani J *et al.* (2001) Late seroconversion in HIV-resistant Nairobi prostitutes despite pre-existing HIV-specific CD8+ responses (comment). *Journal of Clinical Investigation* 107 (3): 341–349.

Kibur M, Af GV, Pukkala E *et al.* (2000) Attack rates of human papillomavirus type 16 and cervical neoplasia in primiparous women and field trial designs for HPV16 vaccination. *Sexually Transmitted Infections* 76 (1): 13–17.

Kiecolt-Glaser JK, Glaser R (1995) Psychoneuroimmunology and health consequences: data and shared mechanisms (review; 50 refs). *Psychosomatic Medicine* 57 (3): 269–274.

Lambert EC (2001) College students' knowledge of human papillomavirus and effectiveness of a brief educational intervention. *Journal of the American Board of Family Practice* 14 (3): 178–183.

Lerman C, Miller S, Scarborough R *et al.* (1991) Adverse psychologic consequences of positive cytologic cervical screening. *American Journal of Obstetrics and Gynecology* 163 (3): 658–662.

McCaffery K, Forrest S, Waller J *et al.* (2003) Attitudes towards HPV testing: a qualitative study of beliefs among Indian, Pakistani, African-Caribbean and white British women in the UK. *British Journal of Cancer* 88 (1): 42–46.

McCaffery K, Waller J, Forrest S *et al.* (2004) Testing positive for human papillomavirus in routine cervical screening examination of psychosocial impact *British Journal of Obstetrics and Gynaecology* 111 (2): 1437–1443.

McDonald TW, Neutens JJ, Fischer LM *et al.* (1989) Impact of cervical intraepithelial neoplasia diagnosis and treatment on self-esteem and body image. *Gynecologic Oncology* 34 (3): 345–349.

Maissi E, Marteau TM, Hankins M *et al.* (2004) Psychological impact of human papillomavirus testing in women with borderline or mildly dyskaryotic cervical smear test results: cross sectional questionnaire study. *British Medical Journal* 328 (7451): 1293.

Marteau TM, Walker P, Giles J *et al.* (1990) Anxieties in women undergoing colposcopy. *British Journal of Obstetrics and Gynaecology* 97 (9): 859–861.

Marteau TM, Senior V, Sasieni P (2001) Women's understanding of a 'normal smear test result': experimental questionnaire based study. *British Medical Journal* 322 (7285): 526–528.

Mota F, Rayment N, Chong S *et al.* (1999) The antigen-presenting environment in normal and human papillomavirus (HPV)-related premalignant cervical epithelium. *Clinical and Experimental Immunology* 116 (1): 33–40.

Mould TA, Rodgers ME, Singer A (1995) The psychological reaction of women to a colposcopy clinic (letter; comment). *British Journal of Obstetrics and Gynaecology* 102 (5): 428–429.

Naik R, Bang-Mohammed K, Tjalma WA *et al.* (2001) The feasibility of a one-stop colposcopy clinic in the management of women with low grade smear abnormalities: a prospective study. *European Journal of Obstetrics, Gynecology and Reproductive Biology* 98 (2): 205–208.

Nathoo V (1988) Investigation of non-responders at a cervical screening clinic in Manchester. *British Medical Journal (Clinical Research Edition)* 296 (6628): 1041–1042.

Nugent LS, Tamlyn-Leaman K, Isa N *et al.* (1993) Anxiety and the colposcopy experience. *Clinical Nursing Research* 2 (3): 267–277.

Oster AG (1993) Natural history of cervical intraepithelial neoplasia: a critical review. *International Journal of Gynecological Pathology* 12: 186–192.

Palmer AG, Tucker S, Warren R *et al.* (1993) Understanding women's responses to treatment for cervical intra-epithelial neoplasia. *British Journal of Clinical Psychology* 32 (Pt 1): 101–112.

Paraskevaidis E, Malamou-Mitsi V, Koliopoulos G *et al.* (2001) Expanded cytological referral criteria for colposcopy in cervical screening: comparison with human papillomavirus testing. *Gynecologic Oncology* 82 (2): 355–359.

Pereira DB, Antoni MH, Danielson A *et al.* (2003) Life stress and cervical squamous intraepithelial lesions in women with human papillomavirus and human immunodeficiency virus. *Psychosomatic Medicine* 65 (3): 427–434.

Pitts M, Clarke T (2002) Human papillomavirus infections and risks of cervical cancer: what do women know? *Health Education Research* 17 (6): 706–714.

Posner T, Vessey M (1988) *Prevention of Cervical Cancer: The Patient's View*. London: King's Fund Publishing Office.

Reitano M (1997) Counselling patients with genital warts. *American Journal of Medicine* 102 (5A): 38–43.

Roberts RA, Blunt SM (1994) The psychological reaction of women to a colposcopy clinic (see comments). *British Journal of Obstetrics and Gynaecology* 101 (9): 751–752.

Schmale A, Iker H (1971) Hopelessness as a predictor of cervical cancer. *Social Science and Medicine* 5: 95–100.

Schwartz M, Savage W, George J *et al.* (1989) Women's knowledge and experience of cervical screening: a failure of health education and medical organisation. *Community Medicine* 46: 499–507.

Sharma Y (2004) *Spiritual Bioenergetics of Homeopathic Materia Medica*, 1st edn. Middlesex: Academy of Light Ltd.

Skrabanek P (1988) Cervical cancer screening: the time for reappraisal. *Canadian Journal of Public Health* 79 (2): 86–89.

Spielberger CD (1972) *Anxiety: Current Trends in Theory and Research*. New York, NY: Academic Press.

Spielberger CD (1980) *Test Anxiety Inventory: Preliminary Professional Manual*. Palo Alto, CA: Consulting Psychologists Press.

Spielberger CD (1983) *Manual for the State–Trait Anxiety Inventory*. Palo Alto, CA: Consulting Psychologists Press.

Stoate H (1989) Can health screening damage your health? *Journal of the Royal College of General Practitioners* 39 (322): 193–195.

Syrjanen K, Mantyjarvi R, Saarikoski S *et al.* (1988) Factors associated with progression of cervical human papillomavirus (HPV) infections into carcinoma in situ during a long-term prospective follow-up. *British Journal of Obstetrics and Gynaecology* 95 (11): 1096–1102.

Tiersma ES, van der Lee ML, Peters AA *et al.* (2004) Psychosocial factors and the grade of cervical intra-epithelial neoplasia: a semi-prospective study. *Gynecologic Oncology* 92 (2): 603–610.

Tomaino-Brunner C, Freda MC, Runowicz CD (1996) 'I hope I don't have cancer': colposcopy and minority women. *Oncology Nursing Forum* 23 (1): 39–44.

Tomaino-Brunner C, Freda MC, Damus K *et al.* (1998) Can precolposcopy education increase knowledge and decrease anxiety? *Journal of Obstetric, Gynecologic and Neonatal Nursing* 27 (6): 636–645.

Vail-Smith K, White DM (1992) Risk level, knowledge, and preventive behavior for human papillomaviruses among sexually active college women. *Journal of the American College of Health* 40 (5): 227–230.

Waller J, McCaffery K, Forrest S *et al.* (2003) Awareness of human papillomavirus among women attending a well woman clinic. *Sexually Transmitted Infection* 79 (4): 320–322.

Waller J, McCaffery KJ, Forrest S *et al.* (2004) Human papillomavirus and cervical cancer: issues for biobehavioral and psychosocial research. *Annals of Behavioural Medicine* 27 (1): 68–79.

Waller J, McCaffery K, Nazroo J *et al.* (2005) Making sense of information about HPV in cervical screening: a qualitative study. *British Journal of Cancer* 92 (2): 265–270.

Webster JI, Tonelli L, Sternberg EM (2002) Neuroendocrine regulation of immunity. *Annual Review of Immunology* 20: 125–163.

Wolfe C, Doherty I, Raju KS *et al.* (1992) First steps in the development of an information and counselling service for women with an abnormal smear result. *European Journal of Obstetrics, Gynecology and Reproductive Biology* 45 (3): 201–206.

Yacobi E, Tennant C, Ferrante J *et al.* (1999) University students' knowledge and awareness of HPV. *Preventive Medicine* 28 (6): 535–541.

Yoder PS (1997) Negotiating relevance: belief, knowledge and practice in international health projects. *Medical Anthropology Quarterly* 11 (2): 131–146.

CHAPTER 24

Cytology of normal and neoplastic cervical epithelium

Alastair R.S. Deery

INTRODUCTION

Morphology of cells and histological sections is a visual art. The guidance for its interpretation is founded upon repeated observation and association. There is no single source of such guidance but it is generally possible to discern a consensus of expert views about the more rudimentary appearances. Given that the images of cells and tissues are dependent on microscopic resolution and stain colour and that their description relies on accurate and sometimes inspired verbal depiction, it is evident that there may be more than one truth.

Long and hard-gained experience of histopathological outcomes is the only sure support for regarded cytopathological opinion. This appears to suggest a 'gold standard'. The quality of gold is always graded however and a 'pure' histopathological opinion is as hard to obtain. The cellular pathologist must look carefully at tissues resulting from smear predictions directly, or as part of review, throughout their period of practice. Failure to do this leads to much of the variance in expert opinions on cytological materials. The colposcopist has the task of weighing cytological prediction against histological findings derived from clinically directed biopsies and must establish future colposcopic opinions upon their correlation. Often enough, there is not a match between a single smear and a single biopsy. In less usual cases, there may be no match between many smears and multiple biopsies. Only persistent and fastidious audit, of experience of many cases, will forge or improve that colposcopic opinion. The colposcopist's acknowledgement of the variability, in number, quality and appropriateness, of smears and biopsies will grow together with an awareness of the underlying variability in reporting from colleagues.

The cytological descriptions and opinions expressed in this chapter will not be agreed by all, but are based on a continuous experience of the author, of predicting histological outcomes from smear appearances and subsequent histopathological review of biopsy materials from the same cases, over 20 years. The intention is to give reliable visual and verbal description to cell occurrences and appearances and broad guidance to their clinical interpretation.

CONVENTIONAL DIRECT SMEAR: EXFOLIATIVE AND SCRAPE CERVICAL CYTOLOGY

Normal contents and appearances of smears

Metaplastic squamous cells

A cervical smear is taken from the cervical transformation zone, with a vaginal speculum in place and with the jaws of the speculum widened to allow a satisfactory view of the cervical os. What is less obvious and rarely remarked is that the os is unfolded by the vaginal pull of the blades of the speculum, so that the smear-taking implement (Fig. 24.1) is placed within or over the transformation zone [i.e. the area of the cervical epithelium visually boundaried: laterally by the indistinct line of the original squamous epithelium (OSE) of the ectocervix and centrally by the irregular and interrupted line of transition to endocervical epithelium, the 'new squamocolumnar junction' (SCJ) (Fig. 24.2)]. This ensures that most of the squamous cell component of any properly taken cervical smear is composed of mature but metaplastic squamous cells. Once this has been understood, the historically interminable cytological

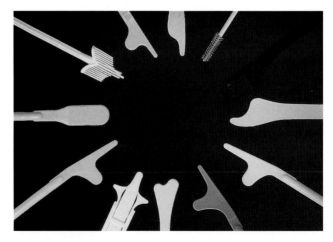

Fig. 24.1 Clock-face display of a full range of cervical smear implements variably designed to produce an exfoliative and scrape cell sample.

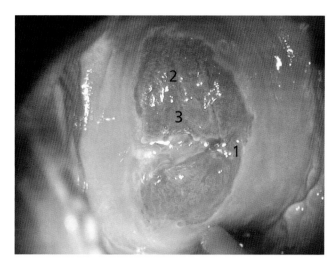

Fig. 24.2 The cervical transformation zone (TZ). The lateral boundary of the OSE (original squamous epithelium) is at (1) with the TZ composed of a mixture of metaplastic squamous (2) and original endocervical columnar epithelium (3).

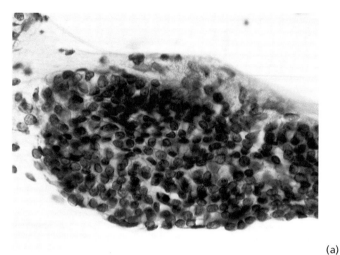

(a)

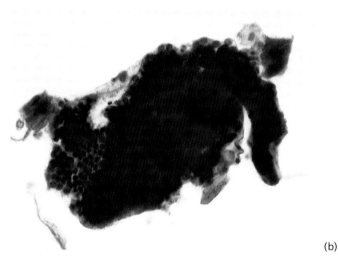

(b)

Fig. 24.4 Endocervical cells in a conventional (a) and ThinPrep smear (b). The cells may appear as a raft of oriented cells much like a picket fence, as an obliquely seen sheet or, here, as a honeycomb with the intercellular borders creating an ordered array. In liquid-based preparations (b) the thickness of the fragments is often paradoxically more striking due to the compaction of partial alcohol fixation in the vial fluid.

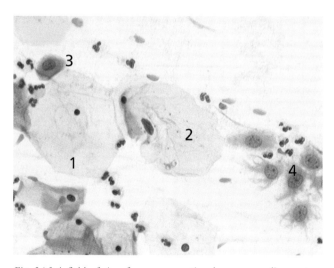

Fig. 24.3 A field of view from a conventional smear revealing mature squamous cells (1); intermediate squamous cells (2); and an immature parabasal squamous cell (3). Note the cytoplasmic processes of a group of immature metaplastic squamous cells from an actively migrating area of squamous metaplasia (4). The latter are the cells that many cytologists seek as an indicator of adequacy, which is a fundamental misunderstanding of the cell appearances in a typical cervical cytology sample.

debate, concerning the imperfect recognition of immature metaplastic squamous cells, is revealed as redundant. The presence or absence of cytologically recognisable, immature metaplastic cells does not meaningfully qualify the adequacy of the smear (Fig. 24.3).

Endocervical cells

Endocervical cells (Fig. 24.4a and b) are present in a smear taken from the transformation zone. Exfoliation brings these

cells into the cervical mucus and the scrape action of a spatula or implement may additionally pull sheets or strips of these cells into the smear. These cells are poorly recorded in many systems of reporting, i.e. Bethesda, Pap, BSCC. Some reporting systems include the presence or absence of endocervical cells as a measure of adequacy and this has led to the combined use of a 'scrape smear' and an endocervical brush. These concerns have usually focused on older women with 'new' squamocolumnar junctions, lying within the invisible part of the cervical canal (Fig. 24.5), or in previously treated cervices, or with the wider concern to detect endocervical adeno-carcinoma *in situ* (AIS) or cervical glandular intraepithelial neoplasia (CGIN) in mind. It is remarkable, then, that there

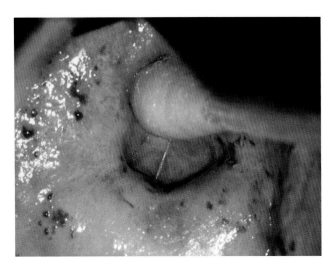

Fig. 24.5 Cervix at colposcopy of a post menopausal woman, showing only squamous mucosa because the SCJ (squamocolumnar junction) is in the endocervical canal and not visible.

edly introduce several new problems of interpretation for cytologists, e.g. distorted endocervical sheets, endometrioid and tubal metaplastic cells, endometrial fragments. All of these can considerably reduce the specificity of cytological reporting and consequently increase the yield of negative cone biopsies. An extended tip spatula or ectocervical brush/broom (extended tips at 2, 3, 4, 5, 7, 8, 11 and 12 o'clock/brush at 10 o'clock, Fig. 24.1) is equally able to afford detection of all neoplastic lesions as a rigid scrape spatula in combination with an endocervical brush (at 1 o'clock, Fig. 24.1) (Buntinx and Brouwers, 1997), despite the added assurance that cytologists feel by seeing what they deem to be a more prolific normal endocervical cell component within the resultant smear. Likewise any benefit of endocervical curettage is unproven. AIS is found most often right at the squamocolumnar junction, as is CIN (Östör *et al.*, 1984). With good cytological screening and interpretation the apparent sensitivities for either lesion are in fact similar (Schoolland *et al.*, 2002). Statistically, however, AIS is much more frequently of small volume and may often be confined to part of the thickness of a single 3-mm-thick block of the excised cervix. High-grade CIN lesions usually cover a larger area of the cervix. The exfoliative and scrape samples of abnormal cells are thereby proportionately reduced in endocervical glandular neoplasia. Early studies of liquid-based cytology (LBC), revealing reduced detection of AIS, emphasise the reduction in numbers of cells offered by a process-dependent sample of a sample (Roberts *et al.*, 1999) (Fig. 24.6a and b). As history shows in many programmes around the world, only expert knowledge and persistent education about endocervical glandular cell appearances will improve cytological detection of AIS to the same levels as CIN3 uniformly (Roberts *et al.*, 2005). Audit of the last 5 years in the author's own laboratory compared

are no studies that evidence an improved ability to cytologically detect either cervical intraepithelial neoplasia (CIN) or AIS (by histological outcome) with the additional use of an endocervical brush, specifically.

Most studies, and meta-analyses of studies, of smear implements have been of poor design and have oddly used, as a proxy for the ability to detect dyskaryosis, the presence of endocervical cells (Martin-Hirsch *et al.*, 2000). Yet a well-controlled study of histological outcomes at colposcopy has shown no significant relationship between different samplers' abilities to procure endocervical cells and the effective smear prediction of CIN (Metcalf *et al.*, 1994). On the other hand, specific attempts to sample the endocervical canal undoubt-

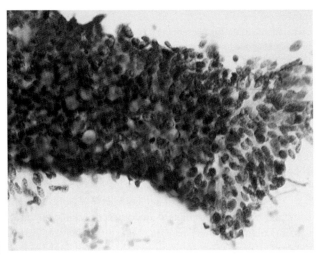

(a)

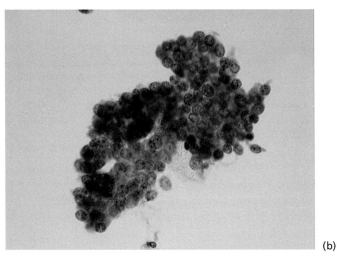

(b)

Fig. 24.6 Adenocarcinoma *in situ* (AIS) in a conventional (a) and a ThinPrep smear (b). With fewer and more compacted cellular aggregates the detection and interpretation is typically more difficult in liquid-based samples.

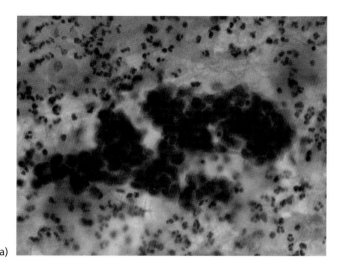
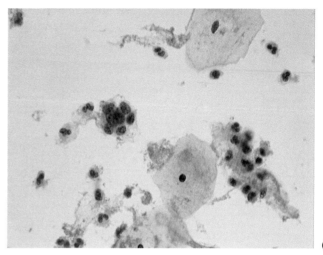

(a)

(b)

Fig. 24.7 Endometrial cells in a conventional (a) and ThinPrep smear (b). In the latter, endometrial cells can look much like severe squamous dyskaryosis.

'apparent sensitivities' of a single high-grade referral smear, of 77% for CIN3 versus 79% for AIS, measured against all histological diagnoses of CIN3 and AIS over the period. However, in 48% of AIS there was combined high-grade squamous/glandular disease, and in 85% of that fraction of cases the smear predicted a high-grade squamous lesion only. The lesson is clear that in the presence of very abnormal cells there remains a difficulty in accurately interpreting some of them as showing also glandular differentiation. During the audit period, the ratio of AIS to CIN3 was 1:34, on probabilities favouring a squamous interpretation. A single extended-tip wooden spatula had been in use for all samples during the period. This bias has great importance for the colposcopist, who likewise would see predominantly squamous lesions when performing diagnostic or therapeutic procedures.

Endometrial cells

Endometrial cells (Fig. 24.7a and b) are poorly reported or are unreliably noted within cervical smears generally and, indeed, can be very difficult to recognise in small numbers or even when in large microbiopsies (because of exfoliating fragment thickness and consequent obscuration of cell detail and relationships). The range of 'normal' appearances of endometrial cells, with their usual exfoliative degenerative changes, IUCD associated changes, functional hormonal changes, metaplastic appearances, 'inflammatory' associated changes and regenerative and iatrogenic hyperplastic changes, make the business of excluding neoplasia highly inaccurate. Compromise clinical guidance has been almost universally adopted: to advise the referral and investigation of the presence of 'normal' endometrial cells in a smear occurring after day 12 calculated from day 1 of the last menstrual period in any woman over 40 years of age (Bethesda System, 2001; see Solomon *et al.*, 2002). Given

the range of possible cytological confusions in interpreting the presence and appearances of endometrial cells, smears should be taken after this time has elapsed, as close to mid-cycle as possible, though this seems difficult to organise in gynaecology and colposcopy clinics. The frequent absence of clinical information regarding the last menstrual period, within the smear request, clearly does not assist the smear report.

Atrophic smears

Atrophic smears (Fig. 24.8a and b) or immature incompletely estrogenised smears come from a variety of situations. A common misconception is that these smears frequently lack endocervical cells. This is in fact not usually the case, but the differences between sheets of endocervical cells and parabasal or immature squamous cells may become reduced and therefore difficult for some to interpret. Stripped (of cytoplasm) trails of endocervical cell nuclei may defeat correct recognition. The parabasal squamous cells may be in thick microbiopsies, because of the increased fragility of attachment of the epithelium, and because of their high nuclear–cytoplasm ratio these may closely mimic high-grade CIN, but do not show mitoses.

Sometimes the problem is reversed and high-grade CIN in an atrophic smear may be assumed to be just the expected normal parabasal squamous biopsies. If there is genuine difficulty, then the custom of 'estrogenising' the epithelium for a few days with local pessaries, followed by a gap of several days to clear the debris from these effects and a repeat smear, has great value in promoting differentiation of normal squamous cells and revealing any still immature or atypical mature high-grade CIN by contrast (Fig. 24.9a and b).

Similar atrophic appearances, with some important differences, may be seen rarely in anorexia, in transsexuals treated with estrogens and in women on anti-estrogen treatment

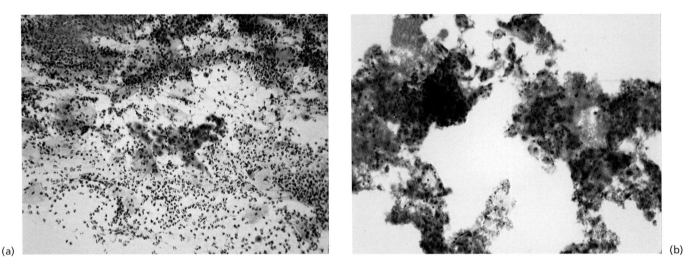

(a)

(b)

Fig. 24.8 Atrophic conventional smear (a) and ThinPrep smear (b). The arrangements of cells in a liquid-based preparation are often more clumped, ragged and obscured by accompanying red cell clots.

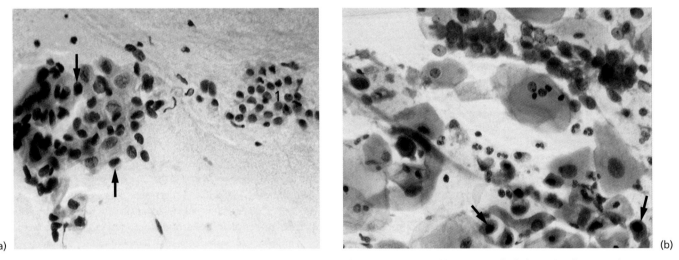

(a)

(b)

Fig. 24.9 A conventional atrophic smear (a) with sheets of normal endocervical cells (1) and atypical but uncertainly dyskaryotic cells present in close association (arrows). After estrogen pessaries a further smear (b) reveals a partly mature smear pattern and by contrast the dyskaryotic cells are now more clearly seen and interpreted as high-grade dyskaryosis predicting at least cervical intraepithelial neoplasia (CIN) 2 (arrows). This is an underused strategy.

for breast cancer, but most probably and commonly in the post-partum period. Certainly for most women a smear should be avoided for 3 months after delivery, but in some, the period of relatively immature smears can be for up to 9 months. The recommencement of periods is, not unexpectedly, the best guide. Clearly the presence of previous abnormality overrides this issue. Clinical information concerning any hormonal treatments, particularly anti-estrogens (e.g. tamoxifen), is very important, to defray adverse assessment of some of these cellular changes. The small blue 'reserve' or parabasal cells seen with the latter are particularly prone to be confused with one pattern of high grade small cell, CIN (Fig. 24.10). Nuclear enlargement is a frequent feature of intermediate cells within atrophic or partly mature smears, but without increased

nuclear chromasia or abnormality of nuclear detail and the lack of nuclear envelope irregularity. Such cells often give rise to ASC-US or borderline or minor squamous atypia smear reports. They are commonly associated with hormone therapy, which is nearly universal and very rarely with folate deficiency. The morbidity in the screened population, as a consequence of subsequent LLETZ or LEEP procedures, at a time when the new squamocolumnar junction is often within the canal, is very considerable and must be avoided. The only way to avoid these unwelcome interventions is for cytologists to know about and recognise the frequency of such appearances in atrophic smears (Fig. 24.11). Too often, they do not. Having a defined threshold set of parameters for the recognition of dyskaryosis is critical (see TPNS criteria below).

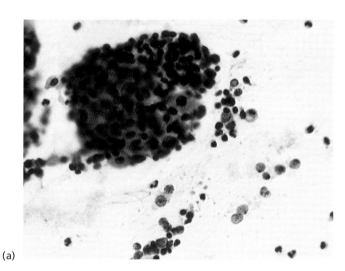

(a)

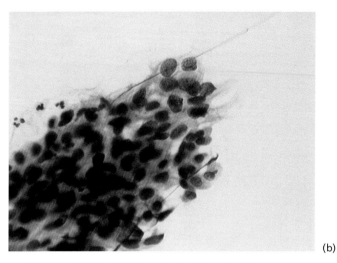

(b)

Fig. 24.10 Small blue 'reserve cells' within the cervical smear of a tamoxifen-treated woman (a) that might be confused with small-cell severe dyskaryosis (b) within conventional smears.

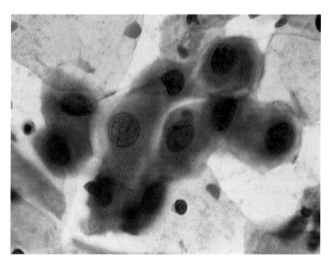

Fig. 24.11 A perimenopausal smear with a small sheet of intermediate squamous cells showing merely nuclear enlargement but no other features of dyskaryosis. The chromatin is unremarkable and the nuclear envelopes smooth. Too often cytologists include these cells as borderline nuclear changes (BNC) or atypical squamous cells — undertermined significance (ASC-US).

Fig. 24.12 Ciliated cell metaplasia in the endocervical component of a cervical smear. There is multinucleation (1) due to cell fusion, terminal cilial insertions forming terminal bars (2), apical supranuclear cytoplasmic separation (3) leading to apical cell separation (ciliacytophthoria), nuclear enlargement and chromatin smudging (4), which may lead to mistaken interpretation of cells as dyskaryotic or atypical. The frequency of this metaplasia in normal smears is hugely underestimated.

Cytolytic smears

Cytolytic smears, where the squamous cell cytoplasm has been stripped and dispersed from around the remaining bare squamous nuclei, are a feature of late cycle smears with increasing progestogenic effects. Younger women on depot progestogens, women on combined pills and older peri-menopausal women, or those on hormone replacement therapy including progestogens, may all have exaggeratedly cytolytic smears. Such smears offer relative difficulties in separating smear cell components, thereby complicating some cytological notions of

adequacy. Separated nuclei may also prove difficult to accept as normal. The remedy is to take the smear as close to mid-cycle as possible and to simply avoid smears on other occasions. This is a critical clinical issue for smear takers, which is commonly ignored.

Metaplastic endocervical cells

Metaplastic endocervical cells of ciliated appearance (tubal metaplasia) are frequent (> 25% of smears) in cervical smears

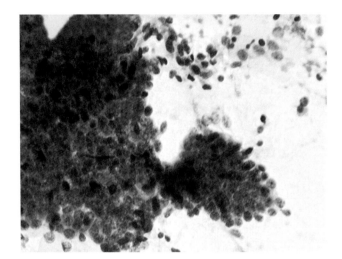

Fig. 24.13 Endometrial metaplasia in a cervical smear with small crowded compact angulated cells and mitoses. These unusual appearances are a mimic of adenocarcinoma *in situ* (AIS).

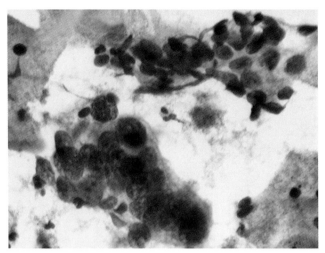

Fig. 24.14 Atypical ciliated cell metaplasia associated closely in a microbiopsy with features of adenocarcinoma *in situ* (AIS) within a conventional smear. However described or categorised, atypical tubal metaplasia requires referral for LLETZ or LEEP.

(Fig. 24.12). Both Papanicolaou and Koss thought them normal constituents of the upper endocervical canal. No histological studies confirm this assertion. These cells may be seen either in orientated rafts or dissociated – in the latter case they require careful observation and skilled interpretation. Endometrioid metaplasias are much less frequent (< 1%) (Fig. 24.13). Atypical ciliated cell metaplasia may be closely associated with AIS (Fig. 24.14) in the same smear. There is not yet enough accurate cytological or histological description of the normal cervix, or pathological correlation of these metaplastic occurrences and appearances.

'Goblet cell' or partial intestinal type metaplasia is normally seen, very rarely, among sheets of endocervical cells in smears. Histologically, goblet cell metaplasia may be seen in a small percentage of AIS/CGIN or endocervical adenocarcinoma either focally or more extensively. In such instances goblet cell metaplasia may even be seen in adjacent areas of normal endocervical epithelium, without other changes of AIS/CGIN. The occurrence of this type of metaplasia in otherwise morphologically normal endocervical biopsies or smears has been denied in the literature (McCluggage, 2003), but does occur (Fig. 24.15a and b).

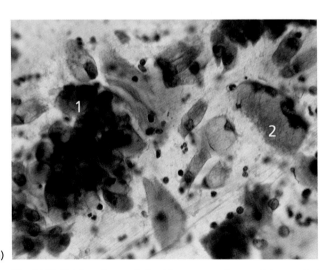

(a)

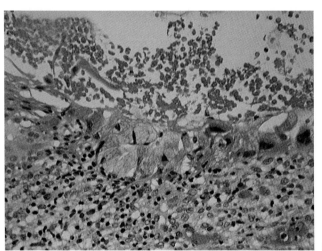

(b)

Fig. 24.15 Goblet cell metaplasia without any nuclear atypia in a cervical smear (a). Note the 'port-hole' like goblet cells in the endocervical sheet (1) and individual flask-shaped mucus-containing cells arranged longitudinally (2). In (b) is the squamocolumnar junction of a histological section of the LLETZ biopsy in the same case. The goblet cells are arrowed. There is no cervical glandular intraepithelial neoplasia (CGIN) or adenocarcinoma *in situ* (AIS). This is a normal but infrequent metaplasia that is more usually associated with AIS or adenocarcinoma.

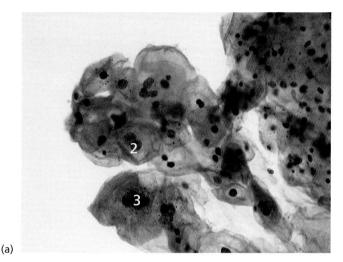 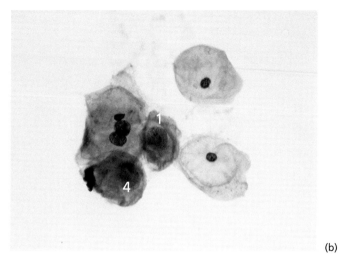

Fig. 24.16 Koilocytotic atypia or dyskaryotic koilocytes in a conventional (a) and ThinPrep smear (b). There is perinuclear vacuolation (1), multinucleation smear (2), nuclear enlargement (3), nuclear increased chromatin and abnormal texture (4).

Abnormal contents and appearances

Specific infections

A range of organisms might be reported from time to time in smears, e.g. the bacteria responsible for bacterial vaginosis, *Candida, Trichomonas*, Actinomycetes, herpes simplex, cytomegalovirus, *Chlamydia*, mycobacteria, *Enterobius vermicularis, Schistosoma haematobium* or *japonicum, Aspergillus flavus*, even *Pediculus pubis*, and are valid, usually specific, if sometimes exotic rarities, with often unexpected clinical value. Characteristic accompanying cellular changes are described in the figure legends.

Human papillomavirus

The cytopathic effect of human papillomavirus is the 'koilocyte' (named by Koss, 1961 and Koss and Durfee, 1956), described originally as 'perinuclear cavitation' (Papanicolaou, 1954). This degenerative cytoplasmic hole is *always* accompanied by nuclear enlargement, increased nuclear chromatin (at even the same chromatin density the larger nucleus contains more condensed stainable nucleoprotein), multinucleation and dyskeratosis (abnormal or inappropriate individual cell keratinisation) (Fig. 24.16a and b). The koilocytotic vacuolar degeneration seen only in relatively mature squamous cell cytoplasm should have a discrete or sharp margin irregularly surrounding the nucleus and at some variable distance from it (Fig. 24.17a and b). This was characterised as a viral cytopathic effect in association with condyloma acuminatum, in two studies simultaneously (Purola and Savia, 1977; Zur Hausen, 1977), and has paradoxically caused some consternation and confusion since.

The majority of pathologists would not accept that a portion of cervical intraepithelial change that they had laboured to judge 'neoplastic' could now simply prove to be 'infective hyperplasia', even when a previous generation of pathologists familiar only with degrees of 'dysplasia' had thought much of so-called CIN1 in the new CIN spectrum just 'basal cell hyperplasia'. After the recognition of HPV, then, some 10 years after apparent consensus concerning the compromise continuum known as CIN, the histopathological dogma became to interpret the grade of CIN and separately note the presence of 'koilocytotic changes'. It also became possible to report lesions that contained koilocytotic changes only. For the cytopathologist, a small problem was immediately apparent. All koilocytes have observable nuclear atypia or 'dyskaryosis', consisting of nuclear enlargement, hyperchromasia (increased condensed stainable chromatin) and some degree of nuclear envelope irregularity (though probably only subsequent degenerative shrinkage). Their nuclear changes are identical to the lower band of the spectrum of increasingly severe nuclear chromatin and envelope changes termed 'dyskaryosis' or 'atypia'.

It is obvious from longitudinal studies of low-grade histological lesions, whether koilocytosis only, or CIN1 and koilocytosis, or CIN1 without koilocytosis (or even the big proportion of CIN2), that similar large fractions of each category appear to regress or fail to progress, suggesting infection alone (Syjainen, 1996). Their HPV profiles are similar. Some cytologists insist that koilocytosis be divided into those with 'dyskaryotic' nuclear changes and those without. This insistence has misdirected much koilocytotic change into 'borderline nuclear changes' (BNC) in the UK (Buckleigh *et al.*, 1994; Deery, 2003), while within 'Bethesda' guidance it is uniformly directed into LSIL (low-grade squamous intraepithelial lesion) along with predicted CIN1 (Kurman and Solomon, 1994). Clearly these arguments are clinically and morphologically insoluble. Simultaneous identification of HPV type, integration

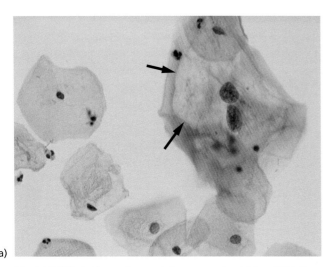
(a)

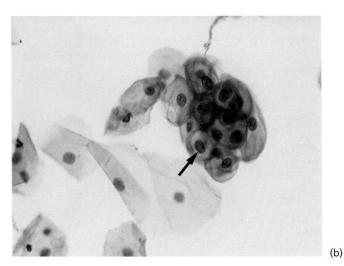
(b)

Fig. 24.17 The koilocytotic vacuole in a conventional (a) and ThinPrep smear (b) with a sharp irregular margin around the clear degenerated area of the cell cytoskeleton (arrows) (see also Fig. 28A.2a and b).

and copy number of the viral genome and associated oncogene and oncoprotein expression, by immuno-cytochemistry and by DNA and RNA analysis, are all necessary (Castle *et al.*, 2003; Sherman *et al.*, 2003). Recent studies (Kahn *et al.*, 2005) indicate that there is an elevated risk over 10 years for development of CIN/cancer in those infected with HPV types 16 and/or 18. There would seem to be a clinical utility in the identification of HPV subtypes in management. This subject is discussed in detail in Chapters 28A and B, which deal specifically with tumour markers.

CERVICAL INTRAEPITHELIAL SQUAMOUS NEOPLASIA

Problems with cytology?

The essence of cervical cytology has always been to identify 'dyskaryosis' or 'atypia' in the nuclei of cervical epithelial cells, with the intention of allowing effective but conservative intervention and treatment of cervical pre-cancer at a significant point in its progression. When the smear is taken appropriately and when the cytology is performed by specialist cytologists of all grades, then the results, in terms of sensitivity and specificity, are as good as in any alternative field of exfoliative cytology. Within organised screening programmes the results are singular and irrefutable (Austin and McLendon, 1997; Quinn *et al.*, 1999). No other screening method for any cancer has demonstrated comparable success.

Though there is, perhaps surprisingly, little evidence that relates screener smear numbers directly with levels of sensitivity or specificity, it is certain that there must be a 'boundary' relationship: beyond a certain number of smears, screening misses increase. It is no accident that the pressures to technologically 'improve' cervical cytology have come from the

processing of high smear numbers per screener, driven mainly by commercial factors. Little evidence to bolster US perceptions of poor sensitivity for conventional cytology, versus LBC, has been transferable to other screening settings outside the USA (MSAC, 2002; NICE, 2003). Some improvements in productivity are afforded by the reduced screenable areas of the preparations. Uniquely in the UK, because of an initially arbitrarily higher cell threshold for adequacy and critically the loss of relationship between the number of cells in the final preparation and the number in the initial vial sample, the concept of actual or global sample adequacy is removed and inadequacy rates are reduced dramatically by LBC, i.e. eight- to tenfold (NICE, 2003). Any actual increases in detection rates are evidenced scantily, if at all, by meta-analyses of historical cohort studies with adequate histological outcomes (Arbyn *et al.*, 2004). Two large studies have commented on the low sensitivity of exfoliative cytology (Fahey *et al.*, 1995; Agency for Health Care Policy and Research, 1999). No randomised prospective comparative studies have been published to date. However, the subjects of sensitivity and specificity in relation to cytology are fully discussed in Chapters 25 and 28A respectively.

Dyskaryotic ('atypical' or 'abnormal' or 'dysplastic') squamous cells

Dyskaryosis is often considered a descriptive cytological term applied to a squamous nuclear appearance predicting CIN. This term when qualified by an adjective, i.e. mild, moderate or severe, intends to be discrete in its predictive value. By biopsy outcome in routine practice, it falls some way short. It is no different, therefore, from other descriptors. When applied to an abnormal or atypical squamous cell nucleus, it is in fact a global interpretation of a nuclear appearance, which has at least three major separate characteristic observable and measurable descriptive features or points:

- Relative nuclear enlargement (by comparison with nuclear–cytoplasmic ratios observed in normal squamous cells of similar maturity) is best assessed 'in smear' by relative nuclear diameter (*not* nuclear area).
- Hyperchromasia (increased haematoxylin staining) is recognised by an increase in nuclear chromatin staining *alongside simultaneous discernible changes in chromatin texture*, or stainable nucleoprotein configuration. Degenerate dyskaryotic nuclei in some staining conditions can have little or no increased staining but nonetheless often retain visible alteration in texture, i.e. 'pale cell dyskaryosis'.
- Fine nuclear envelope irregularities are not a feature of the threshold, mild grade of dyskaryotic change, but are a feature of higher grades. Distinguishable coarser, degenerative nuclear envelope collapse, with folding, is a common feature of lower grades.

What strikes the screeners' eyes first, as they screen a smear, is any increase in relative nuclear size. This, by the way, is never enough for dyskaryosis.

Much of BNC (UK), ASC-US (atypical squamous cells–undetermined significance) (Bethesda System, 2001), minor non-specific changes (NHMRC, 1994) and Pap IIIa (Soost, 1989) might be correctly expunged if this isolated change were appropriately interpreted as negative. The desire to be inclusive of all possible lesions is at the great expense of the specificity of cytology prediction. The morbidity attached to earlier unjustified and not necessarily reassuring gynaecological intervention is universal.

To return to nuclear size: area measurements of enlarged squamous nuclei have been made by various authors in respect of otherwise dyskaryotic nuclei and compared with normal squamous cell nuclei, from normal cells of similar maturation. This is too elaborate for normal use. Relative nuclear diameters can be more specifically and quickly assessed during active microscopy.

1 The diameter of any mildly dykaryotic nucleus is approximately 1.5 times (150%) the size of a normal squamous cell nucleus of similar maturity, usually mature or nearly mature (1 point). The diameter of a moderately or severely dyskaryotic nucleus is usually twice or more than twice (200%) the size of a normal cell nucleus of similar maturity, usually immature or parabasal (2 points).

2 Simultaneously a screener will assess hyperchromasia and texture of chromatin within the enlarged nuclei. A mildly dyskaryotic nucleus will have some hyperchromasia by comparison with other adjacent cells but the texture of chromatin may be little altered (1 point). A moderately or severely dyskaryotic nucleus will have a much more striking degree of hyperchromasia along with coarser textural alteration (1 or 2 points). In mature cell patterns from the surface of CIN lesions, apoptotic nuclei predominate and there may seem little

difference in the intensity of staining of similar, dense, collapsed chromatin, whether actually mild or severe dyskaryosis. The degree of actual nuclear diameter enlargement is then the key. Degenerate, pale immature dyskaryotic cells may not actually appear hyperchromatic. Again nuclear size, chromatin texture and envelope irregularity will add points and grade these as at least moderate dyskaryosis.

3 Nuclear envelope irregularity requires higher power microscopy and is a feature of some cells that are usually severely, but occasionally only moderately, dyskaryotic. Mildly dyskaryotic nuclei will always gain 0 points in this parameter. Mild irregularity will score 1 point, and severe irregularities requiring continual adjustment in the fine focus in order to follow the contour of the whole nuclear envelope will score 2 points. Quick movements of the fine focus of the microscope, bringing different points of the envelope into sharp focus, will make the nucleus appear to move or 'dance' from one plane of focus to a subjacent or suprajacent one. This is a vital aspect of the assessment of this nuclear parameter and is a fundamental limitation of single plane digital imaging and, therefore, existing scanning technologies.

This simple three-point nuclear scoring system (TPNS), using these three parameters, can be a guide until, in some practitioners, aptitude and experience take over. The system correctly separates all smear patterns of dyskaryosis (Figs 24.18–24.21), at least into low and high grade, if not always mild/moderate/severe. Borderline/ASC-US never scores more than 1 point (Fig. 24.22a and b) and can be adopted or discarded according to circumstances (e.g. atrophic smears) and experience. Mild dyskaryosis will always score 2 and predict CIN1 (Fig. 24.23a and b). Moderate dyskaryosis will always score 3 or 4 and predict at least CIN2 (Fig. 24.24a and b). Severe dyskaryosis will score 4, 5 or 6, usually 5 or 6, and predict CIN3 (Fig. 24.25a and b). HPV changes alone will nearly always score 2 (Fig. 24.26). Table 24.1 summarises this TPNS for assessing squamous dyskaryosis or atypia and is easily memorised.

Invasive features of squamous cancers in smears

Among the earliest published reports of the use of microscopy in the diagnosis of tumours during the 1840s and 1850s, and before biopsies and sections of hardened tissue had been developed, is an account of the diagnosis of two cases of squamous carcinoma of the neck of the uterus, intriguingly by looking at the cytology of the ulcer surfaces in smears (Donaldson, 1853). Before that, an account of the diagnostic cytology of ulcerated lesions in general was published by Bennett in Edinburgh in 1845. This was 73 years before Papanicolaou's first publication of the results of his cytological studies on cervical cancer in 1928. The cytological features of ulcerated squamous carcinoma are ulcer slough (red cells, neutrophils, necrotic cell debris, fibrin), with vital tumour

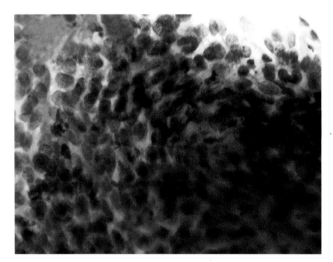

Fig. 24.18 A thick microbiopsy composed of dyskaryotic squamous cells in a conventional smear revealing increased nuclear size (score 2), hyperchromasia and textural chromatin coarsening (score 2), fine nuclear envelope irregularity (score 1) and mitoses. Total score 5 out of 6 = severe dyskaryosis and predicts cervical intraepithelial neoplasia (CIN)3.

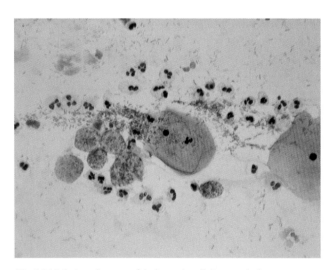

Fig. 24.19 Stripped group of dyskaryotic cells in a cervical smear without visible cytoplasm but with large nuclei (score 2), pale degenerate but altered chromatin pattern (score 1) and irregular nuclear envelopes (score 2). Total score 5 out of 6 = severe dyskaryosis.

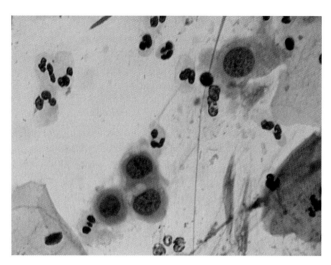

Fig. 24.20 Scattered individual or 'sprinkle pattern' dyskaryotic cells with large nuclei (score 2), hyperchromasia (score 2) and nuclear irregularity (score 1). Total score 5 out of 6 = severe dyskaryosis.

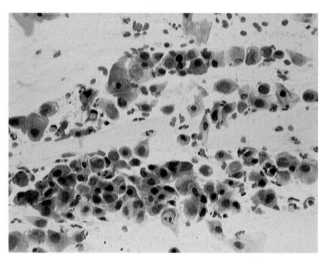

Fig. 24.21 An air-dried area of a conventional smear revealing nonetheless dyskaryotic cells with nuclear enlargement (score 2), hypochromasia but chromatin pattern irregularity (score 1) but no nuclear envelope irregularity (score 0). Total score 3 out of 6 = moderate dyskaryosis and predicts cervical intraepithelial neoplasia (CIN)2.

Terminology

There has been much parochial defence of trivial differences in descriptive terms for abnormal cells and interpretations. Classifications of precancerous lesions have diverged even more in recent decades, with unilateral evolution of different nomenclatures within different national screening programmes. An international terminology conference needs to resolve these issues and force an agreed nomenclature, which will allow comparison of published studies. Since the Bethesda System 2001 is the most recent and exhaustive of these terminologies

cells and dying (apoptotic) tumour cells fallen in: 'tumour diathesis'. The reliability of these findings in the presence of ulcer caused by cancer of the cervix is as close to 100% (i.e. about 90%, from Uyar *et al.*, 2003) as any expert opinion, on anything, ever got (Fig. 24.27a and b). The value of such cytology upon the event of colposcopy is very considerable, in the early stages of cancer. It advises the colposcopist *not* to undertake small biopsies, which may mislead because of their superficiality and lack of subepithelial stroma.

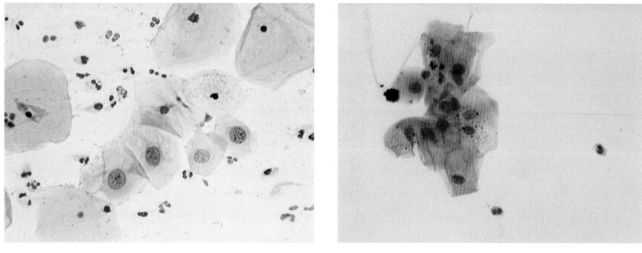

(a)   (b)

Fig. 24.22 Borderline cells or atypical squamous cells — undertermined significance (ASC-US) in a conventional (a) and ThinPrep smear (b).
Nuclear enlargement (score 1).

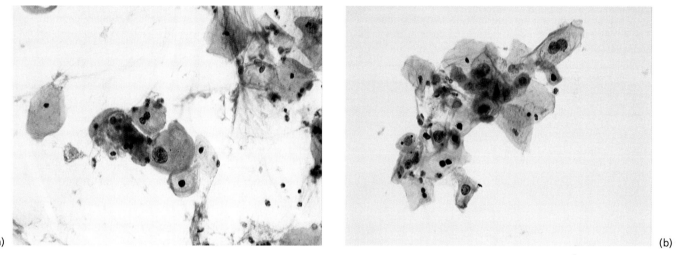

(a)   (b)

Fig. 24.23 Mildly dyskaryotic cells in a conventional (a) and ThinPrep smear (b). Nuclear enlargement (score 1), nuclear chromatin increase and
altered distribution (score 1). Total score 2 out of 6 = mild dyskaryosis. Accompanying koilocytotic changes and other HPV (human papillomavirus)
effects are almost invariably present.

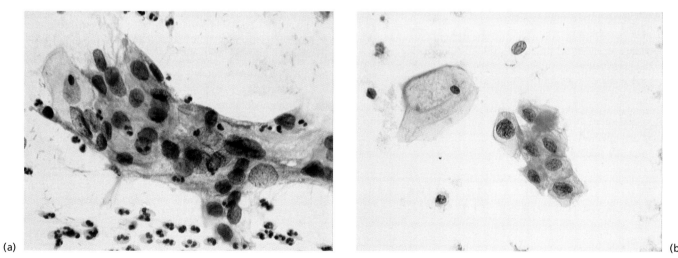

(a)   (b)

Fig. 24.24 Moderate dyskaryosis in a conventional (a) and ThinPrep smear (b). There is nuclear enlargement (score 2), nuclear hyperchromasia
and altered distribution (score 2) but no nuclear irregularity (score 0). Total score 4 out of 6 = moderate dyskaryosis and predicts at best cervical
intraepithelial neoplasia (CIN)2.

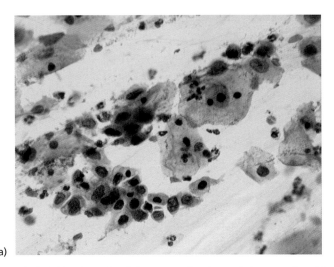

(a)

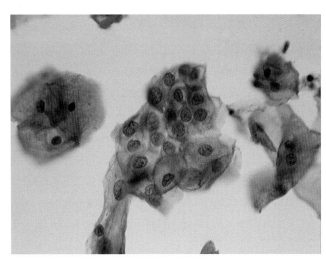

(b)

Fig. 24.25 Dyskaryotic cells in a conventional smear in large numbers (a) and typically separated into small groups within a ThinPrep smear (b). Despite differences in fixation; enlargement, hyperchromasia and nuclear irregularity all score 6 and are interpreted equally as cervical intraepithelial neoplasia (CIN)3.

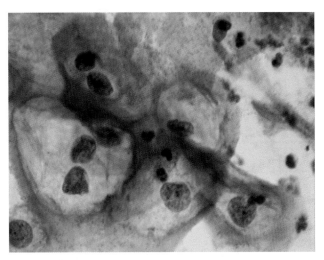

Fig. 24.26 Koilocytotic cells are invariably dyskaryotic (score 1 each for nuclear enlargement and altered chromatin). Nuclear folding due to post-hydropic shrinkage is coarse and has no relation to fine irregularity related to cellular anaplasia.

it would seem to be the best basis for discussion, adaptation and universal adoption. The accepted classifications are presented in Table 24.2.

CERVICAL GLANDULAR INTRAEPITHELIAL NEOPLASIA (CGIN/AIS)

History

Adenocarcinoma *in situ* (AIS) of the cervix was described histologically in 1953 by Friedell and McKay, in two case findings of atypical endocervical glandular lesions, one in a

patient with co-existent CIN3 and another with adjacent adenocarcinoma. In 1952, Helper *et al.* had described *in situ* atypical glandular cells adjoining invasive adenocarcinoma of the cervix, but did not offer the observation a name. Earlier pathologists had alluded to, or partly described, the occurrence of such lesions in endocervical glands, at least as far back as Gustav Hauser in 1890, but had not associated their significance with subsequent adenocarcinoma. Description of some of the cytological features of AIS followed in 1970, with Barter and Waters. Further publications (Krumins *et al.*, 1977; Bousfield *et al.*, 1980; Ayer *et al.*, 1987) identified the main cytological criteria that are standard in current use. As the range of recognisable possible precursor lesions has grown, so new terminological preferences, to allow for lesser cytological and histological appearances, have appeared, e.g. 'endocervical dysplasia' (Bousfield *et al.*, 1980), 'cervical intraepithelial glandular neoplasia' (CIGN) (Gloor and Hurlimann, 1986), 'atypical hyperplasia' (Hopkins *et al.*, 1988). Suffice to state that there is a broad current consensus concerning a usually focal, endocervical glandular atypia that occurs usually right at the squamocolumnar junction, which can be called AIS or high-grade CGIN, and that this is the precursor lesion for most endocervical adenocarcinomas. The lesser lesions are often shorter length, with perhaps less cytological atypia in some instances — certainly less histological architectural volume and disturbance — and can be variably termed histologically as 'atypical hyperplasia' (glandular dysplasia) or even 'low-grade CGIN'.

Probably only a broad single category of atypical endocervical cells, with various arrangements, is seen in smears, and these eventually partially reflect and attract a variety of histological appearances and opinions in the subsequent histology. As with squamous CIN, the numbers of cells and the

Table 24.1 Three-point nuclear score (TPNS) for squamous dyskaryosis/atypia.

	Nuclear diameter of similar maturity cells	Nuclear chromasia/texture	Nuclear envelope irregularity	Diathesis: pleomorphism, apoptosis, dyscohesion, nucleolation	Three-point nuclear score (TPNS)
Normal	100% 0 point	Fine even 0 point	Regular folded 0 point	Nil	0 point
Borderline ASC-US	~ 150% 1 point	Fine even 0 point	Regular folded 0 point	Nil	1 points
Mild dyskaryosis LSIL	~ 150% 1 point	Fine even increased 1 point	Regular folded 0 point	Nil	2 points
Moderate dyskaryosis HSIL	> 200% 2 points	Fine, coarse increased 1 or 2 points	Regular, irregular, folds, indent 0 or 1 points	Nil	3 or 4 points
Severe dyskaryosis HSIL	> 200% 2 points	Fine, coarse increased 1 or 2 points	Regular, irregular, indented 1 or 2 points	Nil or nucleoli	5 or 6 points
Severe dyskaryosis ? Invasive	> 200% 2 points	Coarse, irregular increased 1 or 2 points	Irregular, indented 2 points	Dyscohesive necrotic nucleolated pleomorphic 1 or 2 points	7 or 8 points

ASC, atypical squamous cells; HSIL, high-grade squamous intraepithelial lesion; LSIL, low-grade squamous intraepithelial lesion; US, undetermined significance.

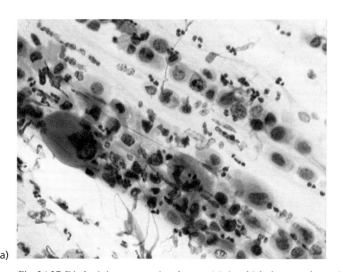 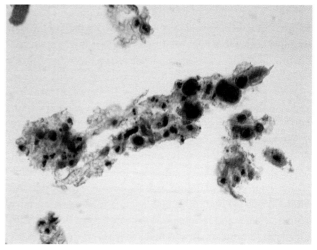

(a) (b)

Fig. 24.27 Diathesis in a conventional smear (a), in which the severely atypical and dying tumour cells are easily seen within exfoliative trails. Diathesis that is difficult to interpret in a ThinPrep smear (b) owing to aggregation and compaction during vial partial fixation.

interpreted severity of their cytological appearance may not reflect the histological lesion extent or severity.

Different experiences in the ability to detect AIS are evidenced within separate cytological programmes. The experience within the United States, which has lately evolved the multistranded Bethesda System 2001 (Solomon *et al.*, 2002), boasts four categories of possible 'atypical glandular cells' (AGC not specified or AGC favour reactive; AGC favour AIS;

AIS; adenocarcinoma), and these separations shine dimly by outcome. Most, even very recent, studies in US publications reveal no discernible specificity in outcome, for all but the most severe category (Lee *et al.*, 1997; Deery, 2003; Renshaw *et al.*, 2004), the majority of outcomes revealing squamous disease or entirely benign pathology. By contrast Australian publications, also with four categories (atypical endocervical cells (AEC), ?AIS, AIS, adenocarcinoma) (Australian Government

Table 24.2 Comparative terminologies 2005 index.

Papanicolaou Northern Europe	Bethesda 2001 (USA)	BSCC 2005 (UK)
Inadequate 0	Inadequate	Inadequate
Negative I	Negative	Negative
Atypical II	ASC-US, ASC-HG AGC-NOS, AGC-?AIS	BNC-LG squamous, BNC-HG squamous BNC-glandular
Suspicious of neoplasia III	LSIL	Mild dyskaryosis
Suggestive of neoplasia IV	HSIL AGC favour AIS	Moderate dyskaryosis, severe dyskaryosis, ?glandular neoplasia
Invasive V	Invasive squamous adenocarcinoma	Severe dyskaryosis, ?invasive, ?glandular neoplasia

AEC, atypical endocervical cells; AGC, atypical glandular cells; AIS, adenocarcinoma *in situ*; ASC, atypical squamous cells; BNC, borderline nuclear changes; HG, high-grade; HSEA, high-grade squamous epithelial abnormality; HSIL, high-grade squamous intraepithelial lesion; LG, low-grade; LSEA, low-grade squamous epithelial abnormality; LSIL, low-grade squamous intraepithelial lesion; NOS, n ot otherwise specified; US, undetermined significance.

Department of Health and Ageing, 2003), manage to show good apparent sensitivity relative to CIN3 (Schoolland *et al.*, 2002), but very good specificity and postive predictive value (PPV) (Roberts *et al.*, 2000, 2005) for all but the AEC category. Indeed, with PPVs averaging just below or well above 50% for AIS or adenocarcinoma arising out of the ?AIS and AIS categories respectively there will be an argument for reducing to three categories, by merging the top two, in that programme soon. In both these two categories clinicians might soon confidently resort to laser/knife/needle cone biopsy of 25 mm length.

Most of the rest of the world lies in between these two ends of the published performance range (Mathers *et al.*, 2002; Kirwan *et al.*, 2004; Wilson and Jones, 2004). In the UK, in the near future, common sense should allow a revision to three categories: BNC-G (glandular cells), CGIN (AIS) and ?adenocarcinoma. Clearly, adequate guidance for early colposcopy, while acknowledging that colposcopy cannot 'see' AIS often (Wright *et al.*, 2002) and systematic category audit (of both morbidity and histological outcomes) must be established for all categories that are adopted in any screening setting.

AIS or HGCGIN

When endocervical cells are atypical, or dyskaryotic, because of exfoliation or dislodgement from underlying AIS, then the microarchitecture of the normal cohesive arrangements is disturbed (Figs 24.28–24.30). The cells within sheets lose their ordered non-overlapped 'honeycomb' appearance and appear more crowded, with nuclear superimposition or overriding, forming densely nucleated microbiopsies, clusters or crowded strips, if seen on edge. These microbiopsies of the AIS lesion often contain enough conserved architectural detail within conventional smears (but less available in liquid-based preparations) to allow identification of microtubules or cribriform associations of adjacent glandular spaces, or papilliform structures. There is uniform nuclear enlargement (1.5 nuclear diameters) by comparison with normal endocervical cells, hyperchromasia usually without macronucleolation, soft sometimes barely visible nuclear envelopes and increased numbers of mitoses. At the margins of these crowded clusters and tubular arrangements there is commonly retained polarity, the apical cytoplasmic margins of adjacent cells pointing in one direction. The pseudostratification seen in histological examples of AIS, where cells seem to pile up upon a seemingly unchanged length of basement membrane, often results in smear microbiopsies, with successive palisades or arcades of polarised crowded cells stepping down towards the cluster margins again. 'Feathering' is a term utilised by Ayer *et al.* (1987), to describe the characteristic orientation of drawn-out, or stretched, polarised, parallel, fragile endocervical cells and sometimes stripped, bare atypical nuclei, whose cytoplasm is completely detached, at the periphery of these crowded clusters or strips.

Atypical hyperplasia (glandular dysplasia) or LGCGIN

Some have proposed a range of lesser, histological lesions, in endocervical cells (Krumins *et al.*, 1977; Bousefield *et al.*, 1980; Gloor and Hurlimann, 1986; Fox and Buckley, 1999) and others have suggested a number of uncertainly recognisable cytological appearances which might predict these in smears (Goff *et al.*, 1992; Siziopikou *et al.*, 1997; Cenci *et al.*, 2000; Lee, 2002). There is undoubtedly a range of 'borderline' histological appearances that, because of extreme focality and minimal architectural disturbance, pathologists find

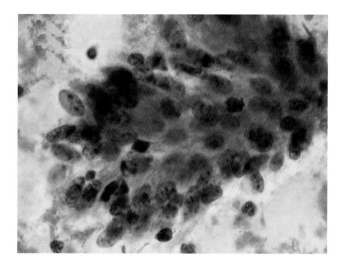

Fig. 24.28 Papilliform arrangement of crowded overlapping hyperchromatic endocervical cells with enlarged nuclei and mitoses typical of adenocarcinoma *in situ* (cervical glandular intraepithelial neoplasia) [AIS (CGIN)]. Conventional smear.

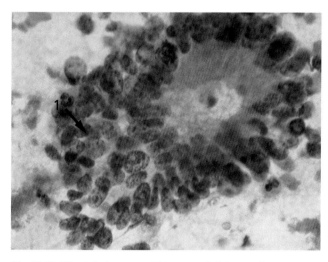

Fig. 24.29 Microtubular space within a crowded cluster of hyperchromatic enlarged endocervical cells typical of adenocarcinoma *in situ* (cervical glandular intraepithelial neoplasia) [AIS (CGIN)]. A mitosis is arrowed at (1). Conventional smear.

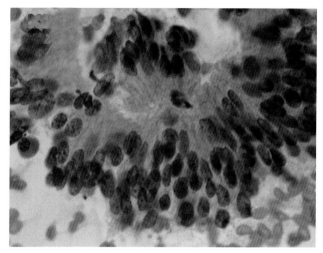

Fig. 24.30 Feathered fragile marginal atypical endocervical cells so often characteristic of adenocarcinoma *in situ* (cervical glandular intraepithelial neoplasia) [AIS (CGIN)]. Feathering is also seen in endometrioid and tubal metaplasia and must be accompanied by cellular atypia as here. Conventional smear.

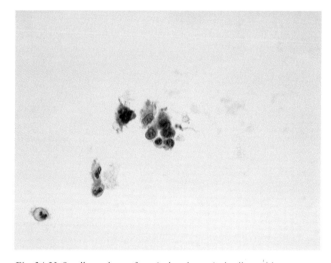

Fig. 24.31 Small numbers of atypical endocervical cells unable to evidence a disturbed microarchitecture but with cytological characteristics of adenocarcinoma *in situ* (cervical glandular intraepithelial neoplasia) [AIS (CGIN)]. Even careful and experienced observation may overlook such cells. ThinPrep smear.

difficult to describe as small foci of AIS. When such lesions exfoliate or are dislodged into smear samples, it is unusual that, when recognised, they look any different from AIS. The degree of individual cellular atypia or dyskaryosis is no different, but there are often only a few small strips or dispersed cells (Fig. 24.31).

Features of adenocarcinoma

All of the above, plus three of the following features:
- dyscohesion and associated 'diathesis' (ulcer slough with separated cells);
- anisocytosis (cell to cell variability and irregularity);
- anisonucleosis (nucleus to nucleus variability and nuclear irregularity);
- anisonucleolinosis (macronucleoli and nucleolar outline irregularity);
- abnormal mitotic figures;
- apoptotic nuclear bodies and cytoplasmic debris.

Infrequent cervical tumour cytology

Other types of infrequent primary cervical tumour give rise to abnormal smears and the cytologist must be alert to these

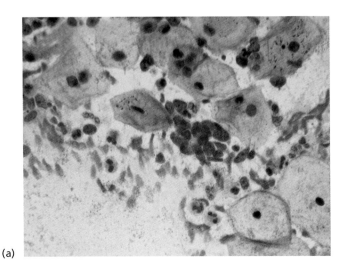

(a)

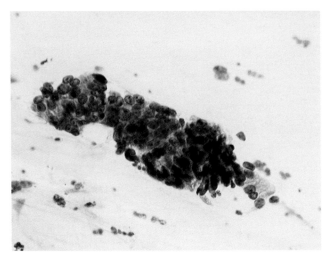

(b)

Fig. 24.32 Conventional smear containing moulded atypical small cell carcinoma (a) and separately seen crowded microbiopsies of nucleolated atypical endocervical cells from a synchronous endocervical adenocarcinoma (b).

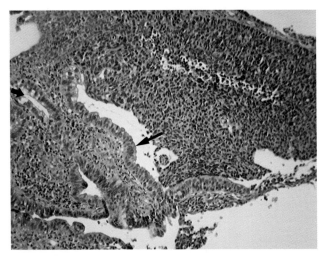

Fig. 24.33 Histological section of a cervical wedge biopsy from the same case as Figure 24.32 showing grade 1 adenocarcinoma (thick arrow) and intimately associated anaplastic small-cell carcinoma effacing one side of a malignancy glandular space and invading stroma (thin arrow).

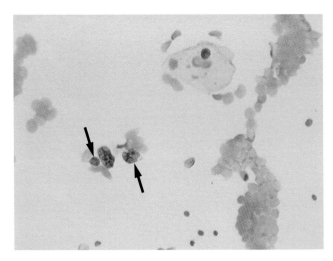

Fig. 24.34 Cytospin preparation from a 26-year-old woman: smear spatula broken off into culture medium and resuspended and cytocentrifuged. A scattered population of centrocytoid lymphoid blast cells is present and cleaved small lymphocytes (arrows).

appearances of course. Many of these appearances dictate a very different clinical approach and the abnormal cells can be overlooked entirely if not recognised specifically. Examples of anaplastic small cell carcinoma, a MALToma and a lymphoblastic (Burkitt's) lymphoma, presenting in screening smears in young women (under 30 years), are described in the accompanying legends to the figures (Figs 24.32–24.37).

Liquid-based cytology

General

Suspending cells in a fluid medium is an imitation of one of the earliest naturally discovered ways of looking at cells. Body cavity fluids, urine samples and cerebrospinal and joint fluids were all sedimented or crudely centrifuged or filtered by pathologists from the very beginnings of cytology in the nineteenth century and before it was possible to look at solid tissues. With the invention of methods of looking at sections of solid tissue, diagnostic cytology continued at its own pace to accommodate slight changes in methods of preparation of cells for microscopy. Always the goal has been easier visualisation of cell detail, but generally also with the least disturbance to their natural relationships to other accompanying cells. Where the sample is an exfoliative one, i.e. naturally lost from an epithelial or mesothelial surface, then the intercellular relationships are tenuous but perhaps important to preserve. A trail of dissociated cells in natural exudates, such as in mucous or mucopurulent or serofibrinous exudates, e.g. as in a diathe-

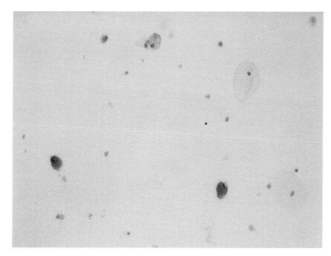

Fig. 24.35 CD20 B-cell immunocytochemical marker stains these cells in a separate parallel cytospin preparation, proving they are B lymphoid cells.

sis from an ulcerated cancer surface, nonetheless has interpretable, 'geological' features – perhaps of placement, juxtaposition and loose association of cell types – that allow a probable conclusion to be reached. If these cells are collected and subsequently dispersed in a liquid phase then the underlying associations are destroyed, in proportion to the completeness of the dispersal (Fig. 24.38a and b).

Liquid-based cytology paradox

* To make the best interpretation, one wishes to transfer a cell sample that is as complete as possible (e.g. use of a low-absorption plastic implement plus fluid collecting medium).
* But ensuring the sample of the sample remains complete

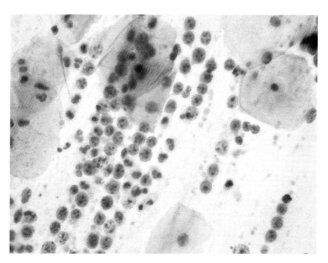

Fig. 24.37 Figure of a field from a routine cervical smear, which contained numerous trails of monotonous intermediate sized, multiply nucleolated lymphoid blasts with nuclear hofs and a tendency to mould where aggregated. The patient was in her mid-20s. The features are of Burkitt or Burkitt-like lymphoblastic lymphoma. The patient was HIV negative (with acknowledgment and thanks to the cytopathology staff of Laverty's laboratory, Sydney, Australia).

or as representative as possible requires even dispersal of the sample (mass-dependent, vortex suspension or density-dependent preparation of cellular component of the dispersed phase) and then mathematically proportional sampling [vortexing fluid followed by filter transfer (Cytyc, Fig. 24.39); or sedimentation, until extinction, of the suspended phase (SurePath, Fig. 24.40); or direct cytocentrifugation of suspension with absorption (drying) of fluid phase (Cytospin, Fig. 24.41)].

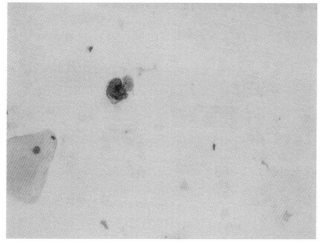

(a)

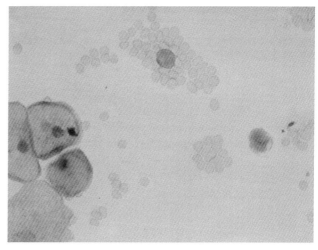

(b)

Fig. 24.36 (a) An immunostained cytospin for κ-immunoglobulin light chain, which is positive on the same population of lymphoid cells. Compare with (b), which is stained for λ light chain, which is absent on tumour cells. These two stains confirm the lymphoid population is clonally restricted and further immunostains confirmed a phenotype of marginal zone primary B-cell lymphoma of cervix (CD20-, 79a-, 21-, BCL2-positive; CD3-, 5-, 10-, cyclin D1-negative).

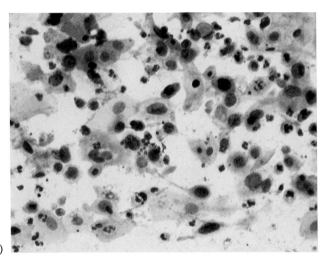

(a)

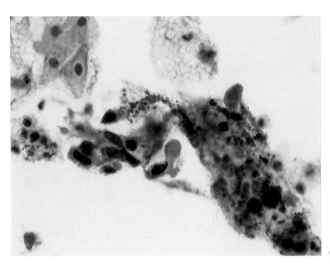

(b)

Fig. 24.38 Diathesis in a conventional smear (a) identified easily by close association among dyscohesive groups of pleomorphic and necrotic dyskaryotic cells. In a ThinPrep smear (b), by comparison, the cells are found in partly fixed exudates and the significance of their placement is lost.

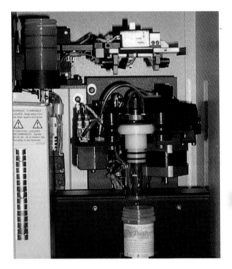

Fig. 24.39 T2000 ThinPrep filter processor.

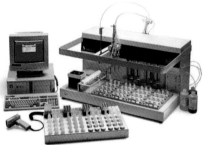

Fig. 24.40 SurePath Prepstain cell sedimentation processor.

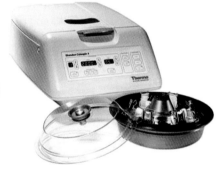

Fig. 24.41 Cytospin cytocentrifuge processor.

• The resultant aliquot selected for examination, while striving to be representative of a more complete initial sample, is necessarily more dissociated, contains fewer total and abnormal cells and inevitably reduces best interpretation.

Cellular appearances with liquid-based cytology
Partial fixation of cells

The appearances of cells and cell nuclei are always very dependent on whether you initially fix (i.e. coagulate and condense their proteins) before or after placing them on a glass slide for staining and light microscopic inspection. LBC mediums all contain dilute, closely related, methanol or ethanol-based alcoholic fixatives, the selection of which has been arbitrary, in order to preserve cells for a period of time (not necessary in

intrahospital-based diagnostic practice, where time delays are minimal), to allow the sample to be transported (pre-fixation). The cells are incompletely fixed.

Conventional cervical smears are best treated by immediate plunge fixation in a container of 95% alcohol for a period of perhaps 20 minutes (post-fixation). Subsequently they can be transported in alcohol-containing plastic receptacles. A common compromise, which is in widespread use throughout the world, but is not of comparable result, is alcohol spray fixation, with an included wax preservative to protect the cellular material during transport. The protective material is then removed, or not, in the laboratory by alcohol immersion. A critical difference is that LBC slides are partially pre-fixed before allowing cells on to slide surfaces, and the cells and their nuclei do

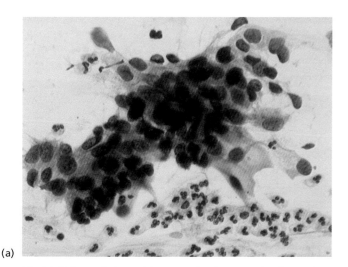
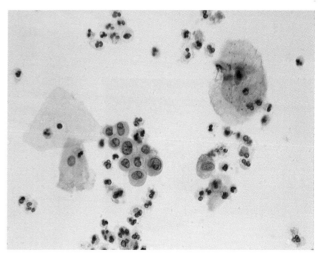

(a)

(b)

Fig. 24.42 Severe dyskaryosis in conventional smear with cell spreading and good post-spread fixation of chromatin (a) compared with appearances of similar cells in a ThinPrep smear with pre-fixation contraction (b). These cells are incompletely fixed and show pallor of chromatin staining.

not spread as much as in a conventional smear. Commercially the differences have been packaged for LBC as 'better fixation', which misrepresents a disadvantage as an advantage. Slightly flatter cells with flatter nuclei, with the above advantages of retained associations and larger actual numbers, are better to 'read' accurately (Fig. 24.42a and b).

A liquid-based cytology preparation is not a 'thin layer'

Current commercial methods produce a varying cell thickness not dissimilar to conventional smears. Many chunky blocks of cells remain, tethered within mucoid or bloody smears. These remain as impenetrable to the eye as the thickest sheets of cells within conventional smears. Atrophic smears with copious contracted (pre-fixed) exudates, are arguably less accessible than ever. Squamous diatheses (which would indicate invasive

cancer) are gathered in from their characteristic sprawl to occupy small clumps, from which there is greater difficulty in teasing out atypical cellular detail. Microbiopsies of endocervical cells are often tightly compacted, cells more crowded and overlapped with thick margins, making it very taxing to pick out atypical microarchitecture, which has been the mainstay of such accurate predictions of AIS or CGIN as there are (Fig. 24.43a and b). Individual cells and small strips of cells then become more important, but can be very scarce.

Why change to liquid-based cytology?

So why are pathologists and gynaecologists are attracted to alternatives to manual, skilled, labour-intensive screening of cervical smears? If one can reduce the area of slide to be screened but maintain the sensitivity and thereby increase

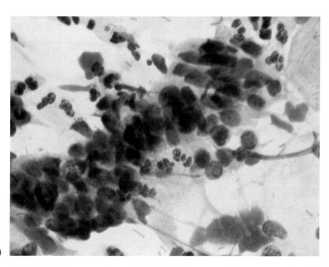
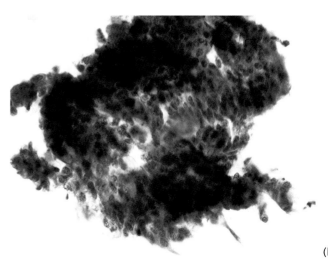

(a)

(b)

Fig. 24.43 Adenocarcinoma *in situ* (AIS) compared in a conventional (a) and ThinPrep smear (b) from the same patient. The conventional smear appearance is much easier to interpret.

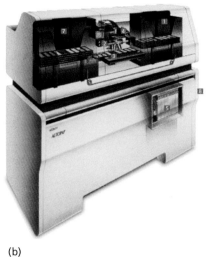

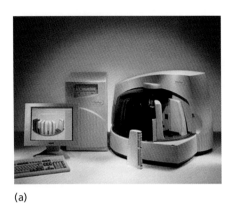

(a)   (b)

Fig. 24.44 A ThinPrep scanner and review station (a) and a SurePath scanner (b).

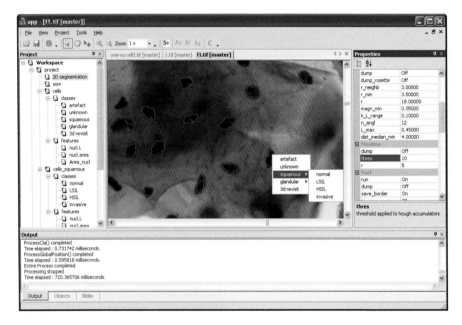

Fig. 24.45 Screenshot of a real-time multi-parameter software program for analysing automated digitised smears (conventional and liquid-based cervical cytology slides) and intended to replace manual screening.

the numbers of slides screened, then productivity is increased (maybe). Importantly, most 'quality' measures indirectly measure productivity. In the UK, for example, turnaround times for smear results have often failed to meet nationally set targets. If the slides can be machine pre-scanned (Fig. 24.44) more easily (or quickly), and if this automation puts fewer slides or similar numbers faster through available subsequent human screeners, then productivity may be increased. Even if you must retrain screeners and pathologists and allow them a phase of re-experiencing the new slide preparations, but eventually they achieve a similar predictive rate and better productivity, then this may outweigh the costs. In the UK's early experience of trial of LBC, one can reduce inadequate rates and, in these special circumstances, one can diminish intrusive examinations and smears and increase consumer satisfaction with the screening programme. Health economists argue that the costs/ benefits are in favour of LBC (Sherlaw-Johnson *et al.*).

For the first time it is possible to examine simultaneously the same cervical cell sample, by multiple other analytical technologies. It is noted that multiple smears from the same cervical sample do not always show the same cytological features, however these technologies add diagnostic and prognostic value to morphological features (Fig. 24.45). Alternative non-cytological developments for automated cell and nucleic acid and protein analysis, inadvertently made possible by conjuring a liquid analysate, are now an overriding goal.

REFERENCES

Agency for Health Care Policy and Research (1999) *Evaluation of Cervical Cytology*, AHCPR Publication No. 99-E010 (Evidence report — Technology Assessment No. 5), US Department of Health and Human Services.

Arbyn M, Abarca M, Delvenne P *et al.* (2004) Meta-analysis of the test accuracy of liquid-based versus conventional cytology. Presented at the 15th International Congress of Cytology, Santiago de Chile. www.iph.fgov.be.

Austin RM, McLendon WW (1997) The Papanicolaou smear. Medicine's most successful cancer screening procedure is threatened. *Journal of the American Medical Association* 277: 754–755.

Australian Government Department of Health and Ageing (2003) *Performance Measures for Australian Laboratories Reporting Cervical Cytology*. Canberra: Australian Government Department of Health and Ageing.

Australian Health Technology Advisory Committee (AHTAC) (1998) *Review of Automated and Semi-automated Cervical Screening Devices*. Canberra: AHTAC. Available at: www.csp.nsw.gov.au/downloads/review_automated_sem.pdf (accessed July 2005).

Ayer B, Pacey F, Greenberg M, Bousfield L (1987) The cytologic diagnosis of adenocarcinoma in situ of the cervix uteri and related lesions. 1. Adenocarcinoma in situ. *Acta Cytologica* 31: 397–411.

Barter RA, Waters ED (1970) Cyto and histo-morphology of cervical adenocarcinoma in situ. *Pathology* 2: 33–40.

Bennett JH (1845) Introductory address to a course of lectures on histology and the use of the microscope. *Lancet* 1: 517–22.

Bousfield L, Pacey F, Young Q, Krumins I, Osborn R (1980) Expanded cytologic criteria for the diagnosis of AIS of the cervix and related lesions. *Acta Cytologica* 24: 283–296.

Buckleigh CH, Herbert A, Johnson J *et al.* (1994) Borderline nuclear changes in cervical smears: guidelines on their recognition and management. *Journal of Clinical Pathology* 47: 481–492.

Buntinx F, Brouwers M. (1997) Relation between sampling device and detection of abnormality in cervical smears: a meta-analysis of randomised and quasi-randomised studies. *British Medical Journal* 314: 1277.

Castle PE, Solomon D, Schiffman M *et al.* (2005) Human papillomavirus type 16 infections and 2-year absolute risk of cervical precancer in women with equivocal or mild cytologic abnormalities. *Journal of the National Cancer Institute* 97: 1066–1071.

Cenci M, Mancini R, Nofroni I *et al.* (2000) Endocervical atypical cells of undetermined significance. I. Morphometric and cytological charcterisation of cases that 'cannot rule out carcinoma in situ'. *Acta Cytologica* 44: 319–326.

Cervical Screening Wales (2003) *Liquid-based Cytology Pilot Project. Project Report*. Cervical Screening Wales, November 2003, www.cancerscreening.org.uk

Deery A. (2003) Atypical squamous cells (USA); atypical glandular cells (USA); borderline nuclear changes (UK); low-grade epithelial abnormality: subcategory: minor non-specific changes (AUS modified Bethesda); inconclusive: possible high-grade epithelial abnormality (AUS modified Bethesda); Pap Class III (Germany). *Cytopathology* 14: 1–4.

Donaldson F (1853). The practical application of the microscope to the diagnosis of cancer. *American Journal of Medical Science* 25: 43–70.

Fahey MT, Irwig L, Macaskill P (1995) Meta-analysis of pap test accuracy. *American Journal of Epidemiology* 141: 680–689.

Fox H, Buckley CH (1999) Working party of the Royal College of Pathologists and the NHS Cervical Screening Programme. *Histopathology Reporting in Cervical Screening*. Sheffield: NHSCSP No. 10, 16–36.

Friedell GH, McKay DG (1953) Adenocarcinoma in situ of the endocervix. *Cancer* 6: 887–97.

Gloor E, Hurlimann J (1986) Cervical intraepithelial glandular neoplasia (adenocarcinoma and glandular dysplasia). *Cancer* 58: 1272–1280.

Goff BA, Atanosoff P, Brown E *et al.* (1992) Endocervical glandular atypia in Papanicolaou smears. *Obstetrics and Gynaecology* 79: 101–104.

Hauser G (1890) *Das Zylinderepithelkarzinom des Magens und des Dickdarms*. Jena.

Helper TK, Dockerty MB, Randall L (1952). Primary adenocarcinoma of the cervix. *American Journal of Obstetrics and Gynecology* 63: 800–808.

Hopkins MP, Robert JA, Schmidt RW (1988). Cervical adenocarcinoma in situ. *Obstetrics and Gynaecology* 842–844.

Kahn MJ, Castle PE, Lorincz A *et al.* (2005) The elevated 10-year risk of cervical precancer and cancer in women with human papillomavirus (HPV) type 16 or 18 and the possible utility of type-specific HPV testing in clinical practice. *Journal of the National Cancer Institute* 97: 1072–1079.

Kirwan JM, Herrington CS, Smith PA *et al.* (2004) A retrospective clinical audit of cervical smears reported as glandular neoplasia. *Cytopathology* 15: 188–194.

Koss LG (1961) *Diagnostic Cytology and its Histopathologic Bases*, 1st edn, Philadelphia: J.B. Lippincott.

Koss LG and Durfee GR (1956) Unusual patterns of squamous epithelium of the uterine cervix: cytologic and pathologic study of koilocytotic atypia. *Annals of the New York Academy of Sciences* 63: 1245–1253.

Krane JF, Granter SR, Trask CE *et al.* (2001) Papanicolaou smear sensitivity for the detection of adenocarcinoma of the cervix. A study of 49 cases. *Cancer (Cancer Cytopathology)* 93: 8–15.

Krumins I, Young Q, Pacey F, Bousfield L, Mulhearn L (1977) The cytologic diagnosis of adenocarcinoma of the cervix uteri. *Acta Cytologica* 21: 320–329.

Kurman RJ, Solomon D (1994) *The Bethesda System for Reporting Cervical/Vaginal Cytologic Diagnoses: Definitions, Criteria and Explanatory Notes for Terminology and Specimen Adequacy*. New York: Springer-Verlag.

Lee KR, Minter LJ, Granter SR (1997) Papanicolaou smear sensitivity for adenocarcinoma in situ of the cervix. A study of 34 cases. *American Journal of Clinical Pathology* 107: 30–35.

Lee KR, Darragh TM, Joste NE *et al.* (2002) Atypical glandular cells of undertermined significance (AGUS). Interobserver reproducibility in cervical smears and corresponding thin-layer preparations. *American Journal of Clinical Pathology* 117: 96–102.

McCluggage WG (2003). Endocervical glandular lesions: controversial aspects and ancillary techniques. *Journal of Clinical Pathology* 56: 164–73.

Martin-Hirsch P, Jarvis G, Kitchener H *et al.* (2000) Collection devices for obtaining cervical cytology samples. *Cochrane Database of Systematic Reviews* 2: CD001036.

Mathers ME, Johnson SJ, Wadehra V (2002) How predictive is a cervical smear suggesting glandular neoplasia? *Cytopathology* 13: 83–91.

Medical Services Advisory Committee (MSAC) (2002) *Liquid-Based Cytology for Cervical Screening.* Canberra: MSAC.

Metcalf KS, Sutton J, Moloney MD *et al.* (1994) Which cervical sampler? A comparison of four methods. *Cytopathology* 5: 219–25.

Mitchell HS (2003) How much cervical cancer is being prevented? (letter). *Medical Journal of Australia* 178: 298.

National Health and Medical Research Council for the Organised Approach to Preventing Cancer of the Cervix (1994) *Guidelines for the Management of Women with Screen-detected Abnormalities.* Canberra: Australian Government Publishing Service.

National Institute of Clinical Excellence (NICE) (2003). *Guidance on the Use of Liquid-based Cytology for Cervical Screening. Technology Appraisal Guidance No. 69.* London: NICE.

Östör AG, Pagano R, Davoren RAM *et al.* (1984) Adenocarcinoma in situ of the cervix. *International Journal of Gynaecology* 3:179–190.

Papanicolaou GN (1928) New cancer diagnosis. In: *Proceedings of the Third Race Betterment Conference,* Battle Creek, MI: Race Betterment Foundation, pp. 528–534.

Papanicolaou G (1954) *Atlas of Exfoliative Cytology.* Cambridge, MA: Published for the Commonwealth Fund by Harvard University Press.

Purola E, Savia F (1977) Cytology of gynaecologic condyloma acuminatum. *Acta Cytologica* 21: 26–31.

Quinn M, Babb P, Jones J, Allen E (1999) Effect of screening on incidence and mortality from cancer of the cervix in England. *British Medical Journal* 318: 904–8.

Renshaw AA, Mody DR, Lozano RL *et al.* (2004) Detection of adenocarcinoma in situ of the cervix in Papanicolaou tests. Comparison of diagnostic accuracy with other high-grade lesions. *Archives of Pathology and Laboratory Medicine* 128: 153–157.

Roberts JM, Thurloe JK, Bowditch RC *et al.* (1999) Comparison of ThinPrep and Pap smear in relation to prediction of adenocarcinoma in situ. *Acta Cytologica* 43: 74–80.

Roberts JM, Thurloe JK, Bowditch RC *et al.* (2000). Subdividing atypical glandular cells of undetermined significance according to the Australian modified Bethesda system: Analysis of outcomes. *Cancer (Cancer Cytopathology)* 90: 87–95.

Roberts JM, Thurloe JK, Biro C *et al.* (2004) Follow up of cytologic predictions of endocervical glandular abnormalities: Histologic outcomes in 123 cases. *Journal of Lower Genital Tract Disease* 9: 71–77.

Schoolland M, Segal A, Allpress S *et al.* (2002) Adenocarcinoma in situ of the cervix. Sensitivity of detection by cervical smear. *Cancer (Cancer Cytopathology)* 96: 330–337.

Sherlaw-Johnson C, Phillips Z (2004) An evaluation of liquid-based cytology and human papillomavirus testing in the UK. *British Journal of Cancer* 91: 84–91.

Sherman ME, Lorincz AT, Scott DR *et al.* (2003) Baseline cytology, human papilloma testing, and risk for cervical neoplasia: a 10-year cohort analysis. *Journal of the National Cancer Institute* 95: 46–52.

Siziopikou KP, Wang HH, Abu-Jawdeh G (1997) Cytological features of neoplastic lesions in endocervical glands. *Diagnostic Cytopathology* 17: 1–7.

Solomon D, Davey D, Kurman R *et al.* (2002) The 2001 Bethesda System: terminology for reporting results of cervical cytology. *Journal of the American Medical Association* 287: 2114–2119.

Soost HJ (1989) Nomenklatur und Befundwiedrgabe in der gynaekologischen Zytologie. In: Schenk U and Soost H-J (eds) *Referatbund der 10. Fortbildungstagung fur klinische Zytologie.* Munich: Springer-Verlag, pp. 306–314.

Syjainen KJ (1996) Spontaneous evolution of intraepithelial lesions according to the grade and type of the implicated HPV. *European Journal of Obstetrics, Gynecology and Reproductive Biology* 65: 45–51.

Uyar DS, Eltabbakh GH, Mount SL (2003) Positive predictive value of liquid based and conventional cervical Papanicolaou smears reported as malignant. *Gynecology and Oncology* 89: 227–232.

Wilson C, Jones H (2004) An audit of cervical smears reported to contain atypical glandular cells. *Cytopathology* 15: 181–187.

Wright TC Jr, Cox JT, Massad LS *et al.* (2002) for the 2001 ASCCP-sponsored consensus conference 2001. Consensus guidelines for the management of women with cervical cytological abnormalities. *Journal of the American Medical Association* 287: 2120–2129.

Zur Hausen H (1977) Human papilloma viruses and their possible role in squamous cell carcinomas. *Current Topics in Microbiology and Immunology* 78: 1–30.

CHAPTER 25

Cytological screening for cervical neoplasia

Julietta Patnick

INTRODUCTION

Death rates from cervical cancer have fallen worldwide as a result of systematic cytological screening (Robles *et al.*, 1996; Levi *et al.*, 2000) over the last 30–40 years. However, one of the most dramatic falls has been in England and Wales, where the death rates from cervical cancer in young women have halved since 1988 when a national call–recall system was introduced (Quinn *et al.*, 1999; Sasieni *et al.*, 2003). This system, in the form of a computerised recall system, has targeted women between 20 and 64 years, who receive an invitation every 3–5 years according to local policies. If they produce abnormal smears, they are triaged to immediate colposcopy and/or retesting (Sasieni and Adams, 1999). This programme has achieved remarkable success in respect of coverage, with 80.6% of eligible women screened in 2003/2004. Indeed, another success of this particular programme has been the prevention of nearly 5000 deaths per year from cervical cancer in the UK over the subsequent 20 years. These figures have been estimated by Peto *et al.* (2004) using age cohort modelling. Indeed, Peto *et al.* (2004) argue that a cervical cancer epidemic has been prevented by cytological screening.

In order to explain the continued success of this and many other such cervical cancer screening programmes, a number of factors, as listed below, will be discussed. These are:

1 the requirements of an adequate screening programme;
2 the development of successful screening programmes; and
3 the future directions of screening programmes.

REQUIREMENTS OF AN ADEQUATE SCREENING PROGRAMME

There are internationally well-recognised criteria for the introduction of a screening programme. These were developed for WHO in 1968 by Wilson and Jungner and, while they postdate the development of cervical screening, they provide a framework in which the suitability of cervical cancer as a disease to be screened for can be considered. The overall requirement is that the benefits outweigh the harms, but Wilson and Jungner identified a number of more detailed requirements which, ideally, should all be addressed in order to produce an efficient screening programme. These are:

- that the disease studied is an important health problem;
- that the proposed screening test is appropriate and suitable for screening for the particular disease;
- that the proposed test is acceptable to the target population;
- that the sensitivity and specificity of the screening test are known;
- that the psychological, physical and financial costs of the screening programme are considered;
- that the natural history of the disease to be screened for is well understood, with an identifiable preclinical phase.

That the disease studied is an important health problem

The first criterion is that the disease in question should be an important health problem. This is certainly the case worldwide where cervical cancer accounts for 12% of all cancers in women. It is estimated that there are 470 600 new cases and 233 400 deaths from cervical cancer each year. It is the second most common cancer in women worldwide. However, these bald figures mask the fact that, in developed countries, the disease is largely controlled by screening, and 80% of cases are now found in developing countries where it is the most common female cancer (Ferlay *et al.*, 2001).

That the proposed screening test is suitable

That there should be a suitable test is the next requirement. Papanicolaou and Traut first described the cytology smear, or 'Pap' test, in 1943 (Papanicolaou and Traut, 1943). If this technology were discovered today, undoubtedly it would be tested with a randomised controlled trial (RCT). Given the vintage of the test, this was never done. However, its suitability for the early detection of cervical abnormalities has now been demonstrated clearly, and it would be unethical to undertake such a trial today. In 1986, the International Agency for Research on Cancer (IARC) published *Screening for Cancer of the Uterine Cervix* (IARC Scientific Publications

No. 76). This collated evidence from around the world that demonstrated the effectiveness of exfoliative cytology for cervical cancer screening and considered what might be optimum ages and frequencies for screening. Laara *et al.* (1987) contrasted the experience across those countries in Scandinavia where screening was taking place and those where it was not practised widely. Recently, the IARC updated its consideration of the evidence on cervical cancer screening and reported that there was sufficient evidence that screening by conventional cytology had reduced cervical cancer incidence and mortality rates. It estimated that, among well-screened women aged 35–64 years, screening prevented 80% of cervical cancers (IARC, 2005).

That the proposed test be acceptable to the target population

Jungner and Wilson (1968) also stated that the test offered should be an acceptable test to its target population. So far as the 'Pap' smear is concerned, its effectiveness in controlling cervical cancer in a population is largely determined by the proportion of women who are tested. The acceptability of the 'Pap' test can be seen in the large numbers of women who accept the test when it is offered. In England, over 80% of women aged 25–64 years have had a test in the last 5 years (DOH Statistical Bulletin, 2003); see Figure 25.1. Germany and Sweden similarly report 3-year coverage rates of 80% or more (van Ballegooijen *et al.*, 2000). In the United States, rates of 79.9% are reported for women over 25 years of age (Breen *et al.*, 2001).

That the sensitivity and specificity of the screening test be known

Jungner and Wilson (1968) suggest that the sensitivity and the specificity of the smear test should be known. It cannot be calculated with the accuracy that would be available had the technique been subjected to the rigours of the RCT. In addition, as the smear is used to screen for a preclinical condition, which might resolve naturally, the finding of a cytological abnormality is not definite proof of a cancer averted. While the specificity is generally agreed to be over 90%, the sensitivity has been variously estimated to be in the range 50–80% (Fahey *et al.*, 1995; Nanda *et al.*, 2000). In recent times, the limited sensitivity of the test has been acknowledged openly. However, the cumulative sensitivity of three successive smears is over 90%, thus emphasising the importance of regular screening. Previously, however, it was often said that every cervical cancer was preventable. Women were not generally told that an abnormality could be missed in case this deterred them from accepting screening. These strategies led to overexpectation and to frequent legal action when a woman who had attended for screening later developed cervical cancer.

That costs of the screening programme are considered

Financial

The costs of the programme have to be considered in financial, psychological and physical terms. In financial terms, it has generally proved difficult to obtain the full and accurate costs of cervical screening because so many different elements of a health system are involved. However, in England, in 1998, the National Audit Office estimated that the NHS Cervical Screening Programme, which was screening almost 4 million women a year out of a total population of 50 million people, was costing £137 million (Comptroller and Auditor General, 1998). This cost included everything from calling the women for screening to colposcopically directed treatment for those who needed it. While this cost might seem high, it is suggested that a cervical cancer epidemic may well have been averted, and that the programme in the UK as a whole (population

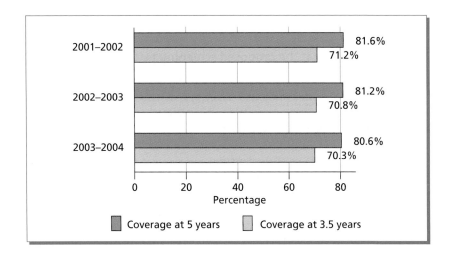

Fig. 25.1 Coverage of screening programmes — women aged 25–64 years. From the *Annual Review of the NHS Cervical Screening Programme*, 2004.

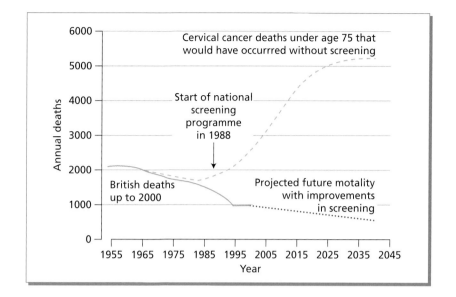

Fig. 25.2 Projected cervical cancer deaths in women younger than 75 years without any screening (England and Wales). The dashed line represents cervical cancer deaths that would have happened after 1987 without screening. The solid line shows annual deaths from 1953 to 2002. The dotted line denotes model fitted to data up to 1987. The arrow indicates the start of national screening in 1988. From Peto *et al.* (2004), with permission from Elsevier.

60 million) is preventing around 11 000 cancers a year and around 5000 deaths a year each year for the next 30 years among women born since 1950 (Peto *et al.*, 2004) (Fig. 25.2).

Physical and psychological

The physical and psychological effects of cervical cytology should not be underestimated. The test itself may be embarrassing and sometimes uncomfortable, but it is not harmful. The colposcopic assessment of women with abnormal cytology has similar characteristics, with possibly greater psychological effects as referral to a clinic is required. Colposcopically directed treatment carried out by trained colposcopists is both effective and safe with minimal complications or recurrence rates.

A number of reports have documented the psychological effects of cervical screening, and that there is anxiety associated with the test and with colposcopy (Marteau *et al.*, 1990, 2001; Marteau, 1993; Crombie *et al.*, 1995); see Chapter 23. However, for most women, the greater the understanding of the procedure and the rationale behind it, the less the associated fear. Nevertheless, two-thirds of women report being alarmed on receipt of an abnormal smear result, and a quarter of women to being 'shocked or devastated'. To this end, great care must be taken when explaining the implications of cervical screening in order to minimise psychological harm and increase the woman's understanding of the benefits and limitations of screening.

That natural history of the disease is well understood

Further requirements of Wilson and Jungner are that the natural history of the disease should be well understood and that there should be a well-recognised preclinical period for screening tests to target. It was clearly understood by Papanicolaou that abnormal changes in the cervix could be seen well before a cancer became established, and that treatment of these changes could prevent the cancer from developing. As time has passed, understanding of the progression from very low-grade, borderline change through to cervical intraepithelial neoplasia (CIN)3 and invasive cervical cancer has grown. Over the years, a number of theories have been put forward to account for these changes. Although the natural history is still not fully understood, it is clear that human papillomavirus (HPV) is necessary for the initiation of neoplastic change in association with other risk factors (see Chapters 18 and 19). Links with sexual activity and smoking were recognised as leading to a higher risk of cervical abnormalities and cervical cancer. In the past decade, however, HPV has been recognised as necessary to the development of a cervical cancer, and a number of high-risk types of HPV have been identified (Walboomers *et al.*, 1999).

DEVELOPMENT OF A SUCCESSFUL SCREENING PROGRAMME

Demonstrating the value of the cytology smear

Following the publication of Papanicolaou's paper, some individual doctors began to pick up on the technique. In 1949, in British Columbia, an organised screening programme was started with the aim initially of demonstrating the value of the cytology smear in a defined population. Over the next decade, it became a mass screening programme. This was followed by the development of screening programmes around the world. By the early 1960s, for example, there were screening programmes in much of Scandinavia, and there was increasing advocacy of the 'Pap' smear in other countries such as the United States. In the UK, screening started in Aberdeen in Scotland, and the first guidance on cervical screening was issued by the Department of Health in 1966.

By the mid-1980s, considerable evidence had been accumulated confirming that the 'Pap' smear was effective in reducing the incidence of and mortality from cervical cancer. However, this has only been brought about in recent years by the high coverage of the populations screened, often achieved through the introduction of a call and recall system. When the IARC brought the evidence together, in 1986, it was estimated that, if all women were screened, 5-yearly cervical screening could reduce the incidence of cervical cancer by around 84%, and 3-yearly screening by around 91% (Day, 1986).

Standardising age range and frequency of screening

The age group at which cytology screening should be directed and the frequency of screening have not yet been standardised. In the US, annual 'Pap' smears have often been recommended from the onset of sexual activity or around the age of 18 years. In contrast, in the Netherlands, screening is 5-yearly and commences at the age of 30 years. For countries with more limited resources, a single cervical smear, if timed correctly and sufficient population coverage is achieved, has been estimated to lead to a reduction of 50% in cervical cancer incidence (Miller, 1992). For any given population, the target age and frequency of screening must be determined taking into account the resources available. However, the IARC now states that, for women aged over 50 years, a 5-year screening interval is considered appropriate, whereas, for women aged 25–49 years, a 3-year rather than a 5-year interval might be considered in countries with the necessary resources. It does

not recommend annual screening at any age (IARC, 2005). Sasieni *et al.* (2003), in examining evidence from the UK audit of screening histories, have shown that the relative risk (RR) of cancer as a function of time clearly shows the advantage of 3-yearly over 5-yearly screening for the younger age group. They calculated the time since the last negative smear at 6-monthly intervals and noted the substantial jump (approximately two-fold) that existed on either side of the 3- to 5-year time scale. They also estimated that, in each age group, the estimated RR 3–3.5 years after a negative smear was greater than that after 3.5–4 years (Fig. 25.3).

Controversy surrounding date of commencement

The age of commencement of screening has been controversial because of the high rate of low-grade abnormalities seen in younger women, which can lead to frequent treatment. While the treatment has a low complication rate, clearly the consequences of a complication are greater for a young woman who has not yet completed her family than for an older woman for whom preservation of fertility is no longer an issue.

The UK study by Sasieni *et al.* (2003) (Table 25.1) demonstrated that the NHS programme was achieving little, if any, benefit by starting screening at 20 years and, considering that more harm might be being done than good, in 2003 England changed its starting age for screening from 20 to 25 years. At the other end of the age scale, many countries take women over 60 or 65 years out of their programmes. This is due to a number of factors. In the past, these women have been poor attenders for screening, good-quality smears are difficult to obtain in women so far past the menopause and, if they have had regular smears with a normal outcome in the past, particularly if they have had two negative smears in the last 10 years, women aged 65 years or over are considered to be at low risk of developing cervical cancer (IARC, 2005).

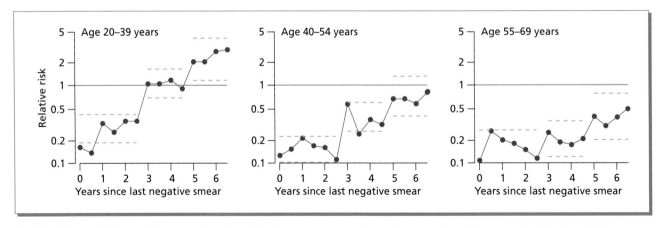

Fig. 25.3 Relative risk of cervical cancer as a function of time since last operationally negative smear. The risks are calculated in 6-monthly intervals. The horizontal dotted lines mark the 95% confidence bands on the relative risks for 0–3, 3–5 and 5+ years. All estimates are relative to the risk in women who have never had a negative smear. From Sasieni *et al.* (2003), with permission of Cancer Research UK.

Table 25.1 Age distribution of invasive, microinvasive and unknown stage cases from the audit conducted by Sasieni *et al.* (2003) compared with all UK cervical cancer registrations. From Sasieni *et al.* (2003), with permission of Cancer Research UK.

Age group (years)	Stage			Total	Registrations of UK 1993–97 (%)
	1A	*1B+*	*Unknown*	*Total*	
< 20	0 (0.0%)	1 (0.1%)	0 (0.0%)	1 (0.0%)	0.1
20–24	18 (3.3%)	13 (0.8%)	3 (0.6%)	34 (1.3%)	1.3
25–39	291 (54.2%)	425 (24.6%)	157 (32.1%)	873 (31.7%)	28.7
40–54	156 (29.1%)	481 (27.9%)	147 (30.0%)	784 (28.5%)	26.9
55–69	61 (11.4%)	386 (22.4%)	93 (18.9%)	540 (19.6%)	19.8
70+	11 (2.0%)	420 (24.3%)	90 (18.4%)	521 (18.9%)	23.2
Total	537 (100%)	1726 (100%)	490 (100%)	2753 (100%)	100

Opportunistic versus organised screening

Opportunistic versus organised screening has been another argument. High rates of coverage can be achieved even with opportunistic screening. As we have seen, the US reports 79.9% (Breen *et al.*, 2001). However, in all countries where opportunistic screening is the main form of delivery, costs are generally higher than in organised programmes for the same amount of benefit (Schaffer *et al.*, 1995). A major problem with opportunistic rather than systematically organised programmes is that the women who are not reached in this way tend to be the higher risk women. Yet, it must be acknowledged that, even in a situation such as that of the UK, where the service is both organised and free, there are still high-risk women who prove hard to reach. Finally, the IARC considers that opportunistic programmes may do more harm than organised programmes because of the greater likelihood of overscreening and overtreatment (IARC, 2005).

When do we consider that a screening programme has failed?

The reasons for a cervical screening programme failing were defined in 1986 by Jocelyn Chamberlain (1986) for IARC. These were failure to reach the women at risk, failure to screen the population sufficiently frequently, failure to follow up identified abnormalities and, finally, failure to pick up abnormalities on the smear. The last factor has been the subject of further exercises to examine why abnormalities that were present either did not appear on the slide (sampling/smear-taker error) or were not reported if they were on the slide (laboratory error). The importance of quality assurance cannot be overemphasised and, without it, standards of screening will not be maintained. Nevertheless, the cytology smear has proved an effective means of cervical cancer control over most of the developed world.

FUTURE DIRECTIONS OF SCREENING PROGRAMMES

New technologies

Cervical screening, having changed little for half a century, is now moving very quickly in a number of directions with new technologies being employed. These include liquid-based cytology (LBC), testing of cytology specimens for HPV status and employment of real-time screening techniques such as those described in Chapter 27.

Liquid-based cytology (see also Chapter 24)

Here, the cells from the cervix, instead of being smeared onto a glass slide and fixed by the smear-taker, are placed in a vial of liquid in which they are preserved until they reach the laboratory. In the laboratory, the specimen is processed to produce a thin layer of cells that is a random sample of those in the specimen. This, it is argued, improves the sensitivity of the test and produces lower rates of inadequate tests (Sherman *et al.*, 1998; Hutchinson *et al.*, 1999). Large pilot studies in the UK, for example, have examined the cost-effectiveness of LBC and the practicalities of using it routinely instead of the conventional cytology smear. The UK historically had particularly high inadequate smear rates of almost 10%. This was perhaps because of the long screening interval of 5 years for much of the country. These studies led to the decision to convert the entire programme to LBC because of the advantages to the UK programmes where the introduction of LBC should see a dramatic fall in unsatisfactory cytology specimens (Moss *et al.*, 2002). The introduction of LBC also offers the opportunity to retrain smear-takers, and deficiencies here, which would obviously also contribute to inadequate smears, can then be addressed.

In the US, the majority of cytology screening is now undertaken using LBC rather than conventional cytology. With the thin, even layer of cells presented by LBC slides, the use of automation to assist in reporting of cervical cytology, something which has been researched since the 1950s, is becoming a reality.

HPV status evaluation (see Chapters 18 and 26)

Testing cervical cytology specimens for HPV status has become a great deal easier with the move to LBC, which facilitates adjunctive tests. Following the development of the first reliable commercial test for the presence of high-risk HPV, a number of research projects examined the method of using knowledge of HPV status in a cervical screening context. The first of these to report considered the use of testing for high-risk HPV types to triage women with atypical squamous cells of uncertain significance (ASCUS) or low-grade squamous intraepithelial lesion (LSIL) cytology into two groups, those who needed referral and those who could safely be left to routine cytology (Manos *et al.*, 1999; Solomon *et al.*, 2001). Because a high proportion of women with LSIL tests were HPV positive, such triaging proved unhelpful but, for women whose smears were reported as showing ASCUS, this was potentially useful, and this strategy is now being introduced in several areas of the world. The presence of a very high negative predictive value (98–99%) in respect of an ASCUS smear means that the vast majority of women with this cytological finding can be screened at longer intervals, and also the emotional overlay inherent in the diagnosis of an abnormal cytology can be allayed by the reassurance given by a negative HPV DNA test. Likewise, its use in assessing 'test of cure' after treatment of a cervical abnormality can lead to longer follow-up screening intervals and reduction in anxiety in the follow-up period after treatment.

The place of testing for high-risk HPV as part of the initial testing in the screening programme is as yet unclear. The IARC has now stated that 'there is sufficient evidence that testing for human papillomavirus infection as the primary screening modality can reduce cervical cancer incidence and mortality rates' and that the efficacy can be expected to be at least as good as that of conventional cytology (IARC, 2005). This, however, remains to be demonstrated. It is often suggested that HPV testing should be used in conjunction with cytology, with action taken if either test is positive. An alternative strategy is to use HPV testing as the first-line test, and cytology might be used for triage on those women who have tested HPV positive.

Implications of HPV testing (see Chapter 26)

The clinical utility of HPV testing and its cost-effectiveness clearly need defining. The psychological consequences of cervical screening also need re-evaluating if HPV testing is to be used. Generally, HPV is sexually transmitted and, while there has always been a link between cervical cancer and sexual activity, there have not been the social implications that might be brought into play when the infection itself is screened for or found.

Real-time screening techniques (see Chapter 27)

The employment of real-time devices has enormous potential in that the identification of cervical lesions is instantaneous, with the benefit of potentially immediate treatment. The application of these real-time (feedback) techniques to the screening programme would also allow for immediate counselling, management and referral and, in situations where loss to recall is a concern, this technology could potentially allow the screening diagnosis and treatment of cervical disease to be performed immediately. Whether the accuracy of these real-time devices is device dependent is discussed in detail in Chapter 27.

Developing world (see Chapter 29)

For the developing world, it may be that another tactic altogether has to be adopted. Whether HPV testing or cytology is used, a sample must be obtained, reported in a laboratory and then, if necessary, the woman found again and treated. The difficulties of doing this in a developing world situation, together with the difficulty in finding the technical and other resources needed for laboratory-based testing, have led to the investigation of the use of visual inspection with the application of either acetic acid (VIA) or Lugol's iodine (VILI) as a potential screening technique (see Chapter 29). At the moment, there is only limited evidence of efficacy, but use of these techniques for the early detection of preclinical, high-grade cervical abnormalities and their immediate treatment could play a major role in the control of cervical cancer in the developing country setting (Sankaranarayanan *et al.*, 1999; Mandelblatt *et al.*, 2002).

Vaccines (see Chapter 44)

HPV vaccines (see Chapter 44) are not yet available commercially, but promising results have been published, and it is predicted that they will be available by 2006/7 (Koutsky *et al.*, 2002; Harper *et al.*, 2004). Indeed, in a recent publication from Harper *et al.* (2004), it was shown that a bivalent HPV vaccine was efficacious in preventing the incident and persistent cervical infections associated with HPV 16 and HPV 18 and their associated cytological abnormalities and lesions. Recently, Villa *et al.* (2005) have reported a randomised, double-blind, placebo-controlled phase II trial that was done to assess the efficacy of a prophylactic quadrivalent vaccine targeted at HPV types, 6, 11, 16 and 18 with an L1 virus-like particle vaccine that was given to young women. This specific vaccine targeted HPV types that were associated with 70% of cervical cancers (types 16 and 18) and with 90% of genital warts (types 6 and 11). The results showed that the combined incidence of persistent infections or disease that were associated with the specific types fell by 90% (95% CI 71–97, $P < 0.0010$) in those given the vaccine compared with the young women who were given placebo.

Harper *et al.* (2006) recently presented data showing sustained efficacy of up to 4.5 years of a bivalent L1 virus-like particle vaccine, although the numbers in the trial were small and conclusions concerning cross-protection have been questioned.

These vaccines hold great promise and may offer the most appropriate strategy for the developing world, where the question of reaching adolescents in significant numbers to be effective is causing much concern and debate (Biddlecom *et al.*, 2006).

In the developed world, it is not anticipated that any vaccine currently under development will entirely replace a screening programme, but much depends on the duration of protection after vaccination. Vaccine type will also be key factor. The vaccines under consideration include at least the most common types, 16 and 18. However, these by no means account for all cervical cancers. Certain HPV types are prevalent in some parts of the world and almost unknown in others. The behaviour of the other risk types once the two or more most common high-risk types are controlled is also unknown.

SUMMARY

Cervical screening is an extremely effective technique that can prevent the majority of cervical cancers. The basic cytological technique has changed little until recently, but there is now a plethora of developments which could even see the end of screening in due course as a better method of controlling cervical cancer is found. Until such time, however, improved screening techniques will be brought into use as research demonstrates their effectiveness. Nothing, however, will be effective unless high coverage of the population is achieved and maintained.

REFERENCES

Biddlecom A, Bankole A, Patterson K (2006) Vaccines for cervical cancer: reaching adolescents in sub-Saharan Africa. *Lancet* 367: 1299–1300.

Breen N, Wagener DK, Brown ML *et al.* (2001) Progress in cancer screening over a decade: results of cancer screening from the 1987, 1992, and 1998 National Health Interview Surveys. *Journal of the National Cancer Institute* 93: 1704–1713.

Chamberlain J (1986) for the IARC Working Group on Cervical Cancer Screening. Reasons that some screening programmes fail to control cervical cancer. In: Hakama M, Miller AB, Day NE (eds) *Screening for Cancer of the Uterine Cervix.* IARC Scientific Publications No. 76. Lyon: International Agency for Research on Cancer, pp. 161–168.

Comptroller and Auditor General (1998) *The Performance of the NHS Cervical Screening Programme in England.* London: The Stationery Office.

Crombie IK, Orbell S, Johnston G *et al.* (1995) Women's experiences at cervical screening. *Scottish Medical Journal* 40 (3): 81–82.

Day NE (1986) for IARC Working Group on Cervical Cancer Screening. The epidemiological basis for evaluating different screening policies. In: Hakama M, Miller AB, Day NE (eds) *Screening for Cancer of the Uterine Cervix.* IARC Scientific Publications No. 76. Lyon: International Agency for Research on Cancer, pp. 199–212.

DoH Statistical Bulletin (2003) *Cervical Screening Programme, England: 2002–3.* London: Department of Health.

Fahey MT, Irwig L, Macaskill P (1995) Meta-analysis of Pap-test accuracy. *American Journal of Epidemiology* 141: 680–689.

Ferlay J, Bray F, Pisani P *et al.* (2001) *Cancer Incidence, Mortality and Prevalence Worldwide.* GLOBOCAN 2000, Version 1.0. IARC Cancer Base no. 5. Lyon: IARC Press.

Harper DM, Franco EL, Wheeler C *et al.* (2004) Efficacy of a bivalent L1 virus-like particle vaccine in prevention of infection with human papillomavirus types 16 and 18 in young women; a randomised controlled trial. *Lancet* 364: 1757–1765.

Harper DM, Franco EI, Wheeler C *et al.* (2006) Sustained efficacy of up to 4.5 years of a bivalent L1 virus-like particle vaccine. *Lancet* 367: 1247–1255.

Hutchinson ML, Zahniser DJ, Sherman ME *et al.* (1999) Utility of liquid-based cytology for cervical carcinoma screening: results of a population-based study conducted in a region of Costa Rica with a high incidence of cervical carcinoma. *Cancer* 87 (2): 48–55.

IARC (2005) *Cervical Cancer Screening. IARC Handbook of Cancer Prevention 10.* Lyon: International Agency for Research on Cancer.

Jungner Y, Wilson JMG (1968) *Principles and Practice of Screening for Disease.* WHO Working Paper 34. Geneva: WHO.

Koutsky LA, Ault KA, Wheeler CM *et al.* (2002) A controlled trial of a human papillomavirus type 16 vaccine. *New England Journal of Medicine* 347 (21): 1645–1651.

Laara E, Day NE, Hakama M (1987) Trends in mortality from cervical cancer in the Nordic countries: association with organised screening programmes. *Lancet* 1 (8544): 1247–1249.

Levi F, Lucchini F, Negri E *et al.* (2000) Cervical cancer mortality in young women in Europe: patterns and trends. *European Journal of Cancer* 36 (17): 2266–2271.

Mandelblatt JS, Lawrence WF, Gaffikin L *et al.* (2002) Costs and benefits of different strategies to screen for cervical cancer in less-developed countries. *Journal of the National Cancer Institute* 94 (19): 1469–1483.

Manos MM, Kinney WK, Hurley LB *et al.* (1999) Identifying women with cervical neoplasia: using human papillomavirus DNA testing for equivocal Papanicolaou results. *Journal of the American Medical Association* 281: 1605–1610.

Marteau TM (1993) Management of mildly dyskaryotic smears. *Lancet* 342 (8874): 814.

Marteau TM, Walker P, Giles J *et al.* (1990) Anxieties in women undergoing colposcopy. *British Journal of Obstetrics and Gynaecology* 97 (9): 859–861.

Marteau TM, Senior V, Sasieni P (2001) Women's understanding of a 'normal smear test result': experimental questionnaire based study. *British Medical Journal* 322 (7285): 526–528.

Miller AB (1992) *Cervical Cancer Screening Programmes: Managerial Guidelines.* Geneva: WHO.

Moss SM, Gray A, Legood R *et al.* (2002) *Evaluation of HPV/LBC Cervical Screening Pilot Studies.* First report to the Department of

Health on evaluation of LBC (http://www.cancerscreening.nhs.uk/cervical/lbc-pilot-evaluation.pdf).

Nanda K, McCrory DC, Myers ER *et al.* (2000) Accuracy of the Papanicolaou test in screening for and follow-up of cervical cytologic abnormalities: a systematic review. *Annals of Internal Medicine* 132: 810–819.

Papanicolaou G, Traut HF (1943) *The Diagnosis of Uterine Cancer by the Vaginal Smear.* New York: Commonwealth Fund.

Peto J, Gilham C, Fletcher O *et al.* (2004) The cervical cancer epidemic that screening has prevented in the UK. *Lancet* 364 (9430): 249–256.

Quinn M, Babb P, Jones J *et al.* (1999) Effect of screening on incidence of and mortality from cancer of cervix in England: evaluation based on routinely collected statistics. *British Medical Journal* 318: 904–908.

Robles SC, White F, Peruga A (1996) Trends in cervical cancer mortality in the Americas. *Bulletin of the Pan American Health Organization* 30 (4): 290–301.

Sankaranarayanan R, Shyamalakumary B, Wesley R *et al.* (1999) Visual inspection with acetic acid in the early detection of cervical cancer and precursors. *International Journal of Cancer* 80: 161–163.

Sasieni P, Adams J (1999) Effect of screening on cervical cancer mortality in England and Wales: analysis of trends with an age period cohort model. *British Medical Journal* 318: 1244–1245.

Sasieni P, Adams J, Cuzick J (2003) Benefit of cervical screening at different ages: evidence from the UK audit of screening histories. *British Journal of Cancer* 89 (1): 88–93.

Schaffer P, Anthony S, Allemand H (1995) Would a higher frequency of tests lead to the prevention of cervical cancer? In: Monsonego J (ed.) *Papillomavirus in Human Pathology.* Rome: Ares Serona Symposia, pp. 193–204.

Sherman ME, Mendoza M, Lee KR *et al.* (1998) Performance of liquid-based, thin-layer cervical cytology: correlation with reference diagnoses and human papillomavirus testing. *Modern Pathology* 11 (9): 837–843.

Solomon D, Schiffman M, Tarone R (2001) Comparison of three management strategies for patients with atypical squamous cells of undetermined significance: baseline results from a randomized trial. *Journal of the National Cancer Institute* 93: 293–299.

van Ballegooijen M, van den Akker-van Marle E, Patnick J *et al.* (2000) Overview of important cervical cancer screening process values in European Union (EU) countries, and tentative predictions of the corresponding effectiveness and cost-effectiveness. *European Journal of Cancer* 36 (17): 2177–2188.

Villa LL, Costa RLR, Petta CA *et al.* (2005) Prophylactic quadrivalent human papillomavirus (types 6, 11, 16 and 18) L1 virus-like particle vaccine in young women: a randomised double-blind placebo-controlled multicentre phase II efficacy trial. *Lancet Oncology* 6: 271–278.

Walboomers JM, Jacobs MV, Manos MM *et al.* (1999) Human papillomavirus is a necessary cause of invasive cervical cancer worldwide. *Journal of Pathology* 189 (1): 12–19.

CHAPTER 26

Screening for cervical cancer using HPV tests

Andrea R. Spence and Eduardo L.F. Franco

INTRODUCTION

Screening for cervical cancer using the Papanicolaou (Pap) smear with the concomitant worldwide decline in incidence and mortality from this neoplasm is truly one of the successes of contemporary, preventive medicine. These improvements are especially pronounced in more developed countries (Peto, 2004). Despite the success of the Pap smear, it has several limitations; the most predominant drawback is its relatively low sensitivity. This has led to a deluge of research into improvements to the conventional Pap smear and into the development of novel screening methods.

Research into the use of human papillomavirous (HPV) DNA testing as a potential cervical cancer screening tool emerged in the late 1980s (Deligeorgi-Politi et al., 1986) following the gradual realisation of the putative causal role of HPV in the genesis of cervical neoplasia. The initial objective of most of this research was simply to detect the virus as an end in itself (reviewed by Schiffman, 1992); however, it was eventually realised that the standardised molecular testing of exfoliated cervical cells for the presence of HPV DNA could have clinical utility as a screening test for identifying cervical cancer precursors (Lorincz et al., 1990; Wilbur and Stoler, 1991; Lorincz, 1992). Further, it was believed that HPV testing could have several advantages over conventional Pap cytological screening including greater reproducibility and greater amenability to automation, which would naturally lend itself to high-volume testing in clinical laboratories. Lastly, the use of HPV testing addresses the concerns about the quality of Pap smears in terms of both cervical specimen smear preparation in the clinical setting and the ultimate processing and reading of smears within cytopathology laboratories. These postulates all bolstered the rationale for using HPV testing as an adjunct to Pap cytology (Reid and Lorincz, 1991; Reid et al., 1991). However, opposing views in defence of Pap cytology as a solo and sufficient screening test also appeared at the time (Nuovo and Nuovo, 1991; Beral and Day, 1992). More recently, Pap cytology has been characterised not only as a sufficient screening test, but also as a likely necessary component of future screening programmes based on HPV or visual testing, on account of the low relative specificity of non-cytological methods (Suba and Raab, 2004).

HISTORICAL BACKGROUND

The last 25 years have brought a dramatic evolution in the sophistication of techniques to detect the presence of HPV in cervical cell specimens. These techniques progressed temporally as follows: (i) simple scoring of koilocytes (a type of cytopathic effect taken to indicate the presence of HPV in the host epithelial cells) present in cervical smears (Komorowski and Clowry, 1976) to (ii) immunocytochemical staining (Syrjanen and Pyrhonen, 1982); non-amplified nucleic acid hybridisation methods, such as (iii) dot blot (Parkkinen et al., 1986), (iv) Southern blot (Okagaki et al., 1983) and (v) filter in situ hybridisation (Schneider et al., 1985); signal-amplified, immunoassay-based nucleic acid hybridisation techniques such as the (vi) Hybrid Capture™ (HC) assay (Farthing et al., 1994); and (vii) a variety of type-specific (Dallas et al., 1989) and general or consensus primer (Gregoire et al., 1989; Manos et al., 1989; Snijders et al., 1990; Roda Husman et al., 1995; Kleter et al., 1998; Gravitt et al., 2000) polymerase chain reaction (PCR) techniques. Further, adaptations of the solution-based, non-amplified hybridisation and PCR protocols have been used to detect HPV DNA in histological sections or smears, to allow for correlation of the presence of the virus with particular target cells. Molecular pathology studies have employed these in situ techniques to a certain extent (Gupta et al., 1985; Nuovo et al., 1991), but their use as cervical cancer screening tools never gained popularity.

Serological assays to detect antibodies to HPV capsid or functional protein antigens have also received attention as investigational tools in epidemiological and clinical studies (Jochmus-Kudielka et al., 1989; Galloway, 1992). However, as with in situ assays, they have not been considered as potential candidates for cervical cancer screening. Serology detects humoral immune response to HPV antigens, which may reflect cumulative exposure to HPV infection acquired through genital and non-genital mucosal sites, thereby negating its suitability as a screening tool. Early clinical studies used non-amplified DNA hybridisation methods (without signal amplification) to gauge the screening utility of HPV testing to identify and manage cervical lesions. Such methods are no longer used, however, because of their insufficient sensitivity and specificity for epidemiological and clinical studies (Franco, 1992; Schiffman and Schatzkin, 1994).

Despite the fact that several biotechnology companies are presently developing HPV DNA diagnostic systems for clinical use, only a limited number of them are available commercially or have yet been subjected to rigorous scrutiny by major clinical studies. The exceptions are the commercially available HC assays and some of the PCR protocols. These HPV testing techniques are the most established methods as they have been the primary focus of numerous screening studies over the last decade.

HPV testing has a history of use in empirical studies investigating cancer aetiology and in natural history studies of cervical cancer development. The more clinically relevant role of HPV testing is related to cervical cancer screening and management and can be further defined as per the specific clinical and public health niche. First, primary screening refers to an attempt to detect the presence of cervical cancer precursors or cervical cancer among asymptomatic women without a prior referral diagnosis (Franco, 2003a). Secondly, HPV testing also has a role as a screening triage tool. In this case, HPV testing is used for the detection of cancer precursors or invasive cancer among women who have had an abnormal Pap smear that requires further evaluation. Thirdly, HPV testing can also be used as a surveillance tool for recurrent cervical lesions. The following overview will focus on the more entrenched HPV testing methods, namely HC and some of the PCR protocols, in their role as primary screening tools.

POLYMERASE CHAIN REACTION

PCR involves the repetitive replication of a target sequence of DNA flanked on each end by a pair of specific oligonucleotide primers, which initiate the polymerase-catalysed chain reaction. Primers can be type specific or consensus (also known as general). The latter primers target conserved DNA regions in the HPV genome and, hence, are able to amplify sequences from several different HPV types. The amplified DNA products are then stained with ethidium bromide and separated by agarose or acrylamide gel electrophoresis. This allows for the presumptive verification of the expected molecular weight of the amplified target, thus confirming positivity. Verification can also be done by methods that further probe the post-amplification products for their sequence homology with the target. Dot blot, Southern blot or line strip hybridisation are used to do this and generally result in improved molecular sensitivity and specificity compared with electrophoresis and staining (Gravitt and Manos, 1992; Gravitt *et al.*, 1998). Finally, use of restriction enzymes to analyse the fragment length

signatures in combination with probe hybridisation (Bernard *et al.*, 1994) and direct DNA sequencing provides the highest possible resolution to distinguish among HPV types present in a biological specimen.

The continuous cycle of denaturation, annealing and replication involved in PCR results in an exponential amplification in the number of copies of target DNA sequence. Consequently, the molecular sensitivity of PCR is extremely high, allowing for the detection of fewer than 10 copies of HPV in a mixture. Hence, PCR has a lower threshold of molecular detection for HPV DNA than the HC assay discussed below. This very high sensitivity of PCR is actually the very factor limiting its clinical relevance. Molecular threshold does not correlate directly with clinical sensitivity and specificity (Snijders *et al.*, 2003). Further, the prolific nature of PCR can produce millions of copies of a DNA target from a single molecule, hence rendering the testing environment extremely vulnerable to contamination with HPV sequences from airborne droplets and aerosolised reaction mixtures. This could lead to contamination of other specimens and control samples. In fact, cross-contamination was a major problem in some of the early applications of PCR in HPV testing. Accordingly, extreme vigilance must be taken in PCR testing laboratories in order to minimise the potential for contamination. One of the most important procedures to achieve this goal is the separation of preamplification and postamplification areas.

Judicious analysis of sequence homology among different genes of distinct HPV types using software that aligns DNA sequences will reveal countless segments that could serve as candidates for PCR primer design. In fact, many type-specific and consensus HPV testing PCR protocols have been published in the last 15 years. However, because of the requirements for validation, reproducibility and general acceptability, relatively few have become well established to the point of being widely used in clinical and epidemiological studies. Primer systems targeting sequences in the L1, El, E6 and E7 genes have been the most common in the literature. Because of their well-conserved sequences, L1 and El have been targeted by the consensus primer protocols. E6 and E7, on the other hand, have more sequence variation among HPV genotypes, which makes them less desirable as targets for amplification of a broad spectrum of HPV types (Gravitt and Manos, 1992). The most widely used PCR protocols are of the consensus or general primer (degenerate or non-degenerate) type. These primers can potentially amplify sequences of multiple HPV types with one primer set in one reaction pass. The size of the amplified product is the same regardless of the HPV type present in the starting mixture, and thus electrophoresis cannot serve to reveal the actual type present in the sample. The post-amplification hybridisation or sequencing techniques described above must be used to provide positive identification of the HPV type or types originally present in the specimen. Three consensus primer systems (and their technical variations) based on L1 sequence detection have become popular in the clinical and epidemiological literature. They can detect essentially all types of HPV that infect the mucosal areas of the lower genital and upper aerodigestive tracts. Two of them, the MY09/11 (Manos *et al.*, 1989) and the GP5/6 (Snijders *et al.*, 1990; Van den Brule *et al.*, 1990) systems, have evolved into technical variants with better primer composition and internal oligonucleotide probing, such as the PGMY09/11 (Gravitt *et al.*, 1998, 2000) and the GP5+/6+ (Roda Husman *et al.*, 1995; Jacobs *et al.*, 1995, 1997; Van den Brule *et al.*, 2002) protocols. Over the years, the original radioactively labelled hybridisation probes were also gradually phased out in favour of biotinylated probes and enzyme immunoassay formats. The third protocol is known as SPF10 LiPA, for line probe assay based on the SPF10 primer set (Kleter *et al.*, 1998; Quint *et al.*, 2001). Although these three consensus protocols amplify targets within the L1 gene of HPV, they do so for segments of considerably different sizes: 450 basepairs (bp) for MY09/11, 140 bp for GP5/6 and 65 bp for SPF10 LiPA. The size of the amplified product is not a trivial matter. Although discrimination of sequence homology is better for longer gene segments and thus would in theory permit improved HPV typing resolution, shorter fragments tend to yield better sensitivity in severely degraded specimens, such as paraffin-embedded, archival tumour tissue. Damage is often pronounced in DNA extracted from such archival specimens, resulting in DNA fragments of less than 200 bp. In these circumstances, a protocol targeting a short fragment, such as GP5/6+ and SPF10 LiPA, tends to yield fewer false-negative results (Gravitt and Manos, 1992).

The newly developed Roche prototype microwell plate assay (Roche MWP) is also based on a consensus primer design. It amplifies a short fragment of the L1 gene of high-risk type HPV (170 bp, compared with 450 bp obtained with PGMY09/11). The amplicon is bound to the wells of a microtitre well plate (MWP) and visualised by colorimetric detection with Roche AMPLICOR chemistry. Because it amplifies a shorter fragment, it is considered to be more sensitive than PGMY09/11 PCR and also amenable for poorly preserved specimens. In fact, it has also been reported that these primers detect about 13% more HPV in cervical smears than the PGMY primers (Iftner and Villa, 2003). Similar to the HC2 test discussed below, the Roche MWP system was designed for 13 high-risk types only (HPV 16, 18, 31, 33, 35, 39, 45, 51, 52, 56, 58, 59 and 68).

There is a vast amount of literature discussing the reproducibility and agreement of HPV testing results among the above three popular PCR protocols, as well as between them and HC2 (discussed below) for overall HPV detection. While agreement at the overall positivity level may be considered adequate in clinical settings, concordance at the level of type detection leaves much to be desired (Qu *et al.*, 1997; Kleter *et al.*, 1998, 1999; Peyton *et al.*, 1998; Swan *et al.*, 1999;

Gravitt *et al.*, 2000; Castle *et al.*, 2002, 2003; Van Doom *et al.*, 2002).

HYBRID CAPTURE™ ASSAY

The Hybrid Capture (HC) system (Digene, Inc., Gaithersburg, MD, USA) is the only HPV test currently approved by the US Food and Drug Administration (FDA). The HC assay, which has gone through two major iterations, has been the one most often employed in clinical investigations of HPV testing. The HC system is a nucleic acid hybridisation assay with signal amplification for the qualitative detection of the DNA of high-risk, cancer-associated HPV types in cervical specimens. HPV detection is performed with a combined RNA probe mix and, hence, determination of specific HPV type(s) is not possible. The first-generation HC assay (HC1) was a tube-based detection system and probed for only nine of the high-risk HPV types: 16, 18, 31, 33, 35, 45, 51, 52 and 56. The improved second-generation HC system (HC2), which is based on a microplate assay layout, targets 13 high-risk HPV types: 16, 18, 31, 33, 35, 39, 45, 51, 52, 56, 58, 59 and 68. Probes for high-risk HPV types are typically referred to as probe B, and the probe set for a few non-oncogenic HPV types (6, 11, 42, 43, 44) is designated probe A. The utility of probe A has not been sufficiently investigated in clinical or epidemiological studies.

HC2 includes a sampler kit with a special cervical brush shaped like a cone and a vial with specimen transport medium (STM). This conical brush allows for optimal sampling of cells from both ecto- and endocervix, if used as directed (Fig. 26.1). The brush should be gently inserted into the cervical canal, fully rotated three times, carefully removed without touching the vaginal wall and then inserted into the collection tube containing STM. The tip is then broken, the tube is closed and then sent to the laboratory for analysis (Fig. 26.2). Specimens in STM can be held at room temperature for up to 2 weeks and

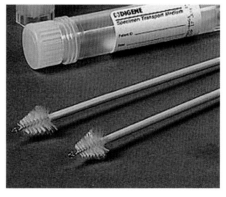

Fig. 26.1 The Hybrid Capture 2 HPV DNA test cervical sampler (Digene), showing the conical brush that is inserted into both endo- and ectocervix.

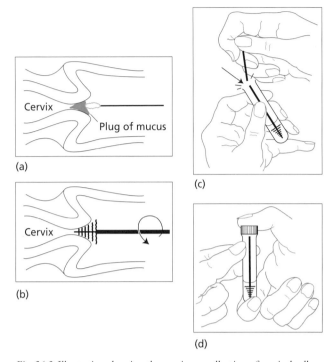

(a)

(b)

(c)

(d)

Fig. 26.2 Illustration showing the specimen collection of cervical cells from ecto- and endocervix, showing the use of a cervical swab to clean the cervix (a) and the insertion of the conical brush into the endo- and ectocervix (b). The specimen is then placed into the STM collection bottle, the tip is broken (c) and the tube then closed and sent to the laboratory for analysis (d). A brush specifically developed for the ThinPrep® test system can also be used with the cell sample being analysed cytologically and the resultant fluid tested for HPV DNA.

can be stored for another week at 4°C. If not analysed in the first 3 weeks after collection, they can be stored at –20°C for up to 3 months.

The initial step of immersing the collected sample into the STM ruptures the exfoliated cervical cells which are present, resulting in a release of host and HPV DNA molecules (Fig. 26.3). The HPV DNA then hybridises with the corresponding RNA probe, resulting in the formation of DNA–RNA hybrids which reflect the composition of HPV types present in the mixture. This hybridisation step occurs in solution inside the wells of a 96-well plastic microtitration plate that were previously coated with universal polyclonal immunoglobulin (Ig) G antibodies that are specific for RNA–DNA hybrids, regardless of sequence homology. Any such hybrids will then be captured by the solid phase-bound antibodies, hence the name 'hybrid capture'. Any unbound molecules are washed away, and the bound RNA–DNA hybrids are labelled with anti-RNA–DNA hybrid antibodies which are covalently linked with the enzyme alkaline phosphatase. After further washing to remove the unbound molecules, a solution containing a chemiluminescent dioxetane compound is added to the wells. Dephosphorylation of the substrate by the alkaline phosphatase produces a luminescent reaction in solution (Fig. 26.3). The intensity of the light emitted, which is proportional to the amount of HPV DNA originally present in the specimen, is measured by a special luminometer provided with the system, and readings are transferred directly into a software program where the results are analysed.

The reaction signal of any given specimen is then expressed in a relative scale known as relative light units (RLU for short) (Fig. 26.4). RLU is the ratio of light emitted from the sample compared with the mean reactivity measured in triplicate wells

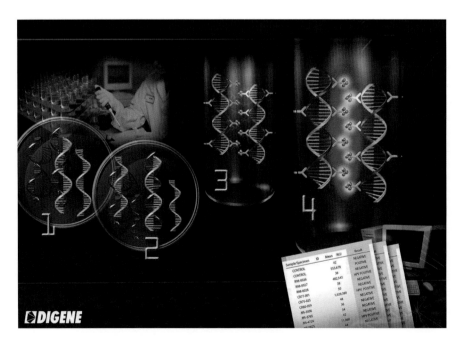

Fig. 26.3 The Hybrid Capture process (Digene). The stages of the detection of HPV DNA are illustrated and described in the text. Briefly they are (1) denature specimen, (2) hybridise with RNA probe, (3) capture and detect hybrids, and (4) luminescence.

Loc.	Sample/Specimen ID	RLU	Mean RLU	%CV	RLU/CO	Manipulated?	Result
A1	NC	62					
B1	NC	50					
C1	NC	54	55.33	11.04	0.18		NC
D1	CB	302					
E1	CB	282					
F1	CB	320	301.33	6.30	1.00		PC
G1	173	352	352.00	not used	1.16		High Risk +
H1	128	388	388.00	not used	1.28		High Risk +
A2	157	74	74.00	not used	0.24		–
B2	163	90	90.00	not used	0.29		–
C2	141	132	132.00	not used	0.43		–
D2	190	136	136.00	not used	0.45		–
E2	137	196	196.00	not used	0.65		–
F2	49	116	116.00	not used	0.38		–
G2	144	92	92.00	not used	0.30		–
H2	121	8954	8954.00	not used	29.71		High Risk +
A3	126	70	70.00	not used	0.23		–
B3	188	76	76.00	not used	0.25		–
C3	147	84	84.00	not used	0.27		–
D3	123	150	150.00	not used	0.49		–
E3	155	108	108.00	not used	0.35		–
F3	41	116	116.00	not used	0.38		–
G3	38	9868	9868.00	not used	32.74		High Risk +
H3	?xx	40	40.00	not used	0.13		–
A4	192	110	110.00	not used	0.36		–
B4	152	92	92.00	not used	0.30		–
C4	60	98	98.00	not used	0.32		–
D4	17	214	214.00	not used	0.71		–
E4	78	956	956.00	not used	3.17		High Risk +
F4	64	124	124.00	not used	0.41		–
G4	145	786	786.00	not used	2.60		High Risk +

Fig. 26.4 A specimen print-out showing the reaction signalled within the specimen expressed in a relative scale known as relative light units (RLU). It can be seen that specimens yielding RLUs ≥ 1 are considered as positive.

with a positive control containing 0.3 pg of HPV DNA per mL. Specimens yielding RLUs greater than or equal to 1.0 are considered positive. Some studies have questioned the validity of this cut-off point using receiver operating characteristic (ROC) curve analysis (Schiffman *et al.*, 2000). In most clinical settings, the manufacturer (Digene) certifies the laboratory that intends to perform HC2 testing, thus ensuring quality control.

HC2 has many attractive features. First, HC2 is easy to perform in clinical practice and is amenable to automation, which makes it attractive for high-volume screening use. In fact, Digene has developed a robotic assay workstation named Rapid Capture System™. This robot station performs specimen transfer, all pipetting operations, incubations, shakings and washings. However, the denaturation of specimens in the sample device tubes still has to be performed by hand. This automatic station increases the accuracy of the test and allows a single user to test 352 specimens within 4 hours. Further, because the RLU signal is proportional to the amount of HPV DNA present in the specimen, the HC2 assay has occasionally been used to infer viral load, on a semi-quantitative scale (Clavel

et al., 1998; Sun *et al.*, 2001; Cuzick *et al.*, 2003). Importantly, HC2, which is based on signal amplification, is less prone to cross-specimen contamination than the PCR protocols which involve target amplification. This precludes the need for special laboratory facilities to avoid cross-contamination (Coutlee *et al.*, 1997). In addition, although Digene supplies both the oncogenic probe mix (probe B) and the non-oncogenic mix (probe A), only the former is used in clinical practice to screen for cervical lesions as the latter has no clinical utility for cervical cancer screening, thus reducing the cost and time needed to test for the presence of HPV.

Moreover, it is noteworthy that, at the standard FDA-approved cut-off of 1 pg/mL (RLU ≥ 1.0) and even at higher discriminant levels, there is cross-reactivity between certain HPV types not present as targets in the probe B set (e.g. 53, 66, 67, 73) and the RNA probes used as reagents in that probe (Peyton *et al.*, 1998; Vernon *et al.*, 2000; Howard *et al.*, 2002, 2004). Cross-reactivity with non-cancer-causing types would have an adverse impact on test specificity in settings with high prevalence of the aforementioned low-risk types.

On the other hand, cross-reactivity with other high-risk types not represented in the probe B set may be beneficial for test sensitivity (Castle *et al.*, 2003). A successor to HC2, named hybrid capture 3 (HC3), is now under development. The primary distinction between these two techniques is that a first implementation of HC3 used biotinylated DNA oligonucleotides specific to certain DNA sequences to capture the HPV DNA–RNA hybrids and immobilise them on the wells of the plate that had been coated with streptavidin rather than with bound antibodies used in HC2. This manoeuvre should decrease the possibility of cross-reactivity discussed above (Castle *et al.*, 2003).

SENSITIVITY AND SPECIFICITY OF HPV ASSAYS

A multitude of studies have been published that assessed the diagnostic performance of the various hybrid capture techniques and PCR protocols. Only a subset of them provided direct comparisons with Pap cytology in detecting high-grade precancerous lesions and clearly specified the type of population, i.e. whether it was a primary screening or secondary triage study. Instead, the vast majority of studies either did not provide data on cytology or presented data on mixed patient series that could not be unequivocally designated as screening or triage settings. Table 26.1 describes the main features of selected published studies that provided data on the comparison of HPV testing with Pap cytology in primary screening for cervical cancer and its precursor. Table 26.2 shows estimates of sensitivity and specificity for HPV testing and for Pap cytology in the same studies.

There is tremendous potential for variability in study results which, not unexpectedly, arises in part from the enormous variation across studies in relation to investigational design, chosen study population and methodology. Most studies assessed HPV test performance on the basis of prevalent lesions using simple cross-sectional designs or retrospective case series, and some assessed both prevalent and seemingly short-term incident lesions based on cross-sectional investigations with extended follow-up (ALTS, 2003a,b). Lesion definitions varied across studies and included either cervical intraepithelial neoplasia (CIN)1 (low-grade squamous intra-epithelial lesion, LSIL) or CIN2/3 (high-grade squamous intraepithelial lesion, HSIL) or worse lesions. In most studies, diagnoses were histologically confirmed on specimens obtained by colposcopy-guided biopsy although, in some studies, the colposcopic result was used if no biopsy was taken. The majority of these studies were clinic based, but some involved recruitment from the community. None of the studies was based on long-term follow-up for more relevant endpoints, such as incidence of CIN2/3 or cancer or mortality from invasive cervical cancer. There were no randomised controlled trials (RCTs); instead, all investigations were split sample studies based on the simultaneous testing for HPV and cytology or for additional tests. Split sample studies get their name from the fact that the cervical specimen collected in single or multiple exfoliative procedures using a swab, a cytobrush or other collection devices is split into several subsamples for testing. Studies varied in terms of timing of collection, collection method or whether or not visual methods for cervical inspection were used as adjunct screening techniques. All the studies estimated specificity on women free of histologically demonstrable squamous lesions.

Although for many of the studies presented in Tables 26.1 and 26.2 the purpose was the comparison of HPV testing with other screening technologies for cervical cancer (primarily the Pap test), the following discussion refers only to the results for HPV testing. On average, HC2 has greater sensitivity but lower specificity for CIN2/3 than does PCR. HPV testing tends to be more sensitive when specimen sampling is done by the clinician than when performed by the woman herself. In general, sensitivity is greater for CIN2/3 than for CIN1 (these results are not noted in Table 26.2). In some studies, the combination of cytology and HPV testing attained very high sensitivity and negative predictive values (approaching 100%) (reviewed by Franco, 2003). A testing combination with such a high negative predictive value could potentially allow increasing screening intervals safely, e.g. from 1–3 years to 3–5 years, depending on the population and risk profile. The drawback of this approach is the loss in specificity with respect to either test in isolation due to the excessive number of patients who would need to be referred for colposcopy. Resource-rich countries can absorb the extra costs related to the secondary triage of cases that will be referred via a dual testing screening approach because this strategy may be cost saving upon long-term assessment, via the reduced patient flow for primary screening clinics. Economic models based on valid estimates of screening efficacy across different settings are urgently needed to assess the potential benefit of combined screening in relation to its costs.

A few large RCTs of HPV testing in primary cervical cancer screening are currently ongoing. Of note are the UK HPV in Addition to Routine Testing (HART) investigation (Cuzick *et al.*, 2003), the Dutch POBASCAM trial (Bulkmans *et al.*, 2004), the UK 'A Randomised Trial In Screening To Improve Cytology' (ARTISTIC) (H. Kitchener, personal communication), the Osmanabad trial in India (R. Sankaranarayanan, personal communication), the Italian trial (G. Ronco, personal communication) and the Canadian Cervical Cancer Screening Trial (CCCaST) (Mayrand *et al.*, 2006).

VALIDITY ISSUES IN COMPUTING SENSITIVITY AND SPECIFICITY

Selection biases and other issues affect the computation of sensitivity and specificity. This is the case with most of the

Table 26.1 Characteristics of selected studies that provided data on the comparison of HPV testing with Pap cytology in primary screening for cervical cancer and its precursor lesions.

Study (first author, year)	Country, study site	Study size	Age (years)	HPV test	Study features
Cuzick, 1995	UK, London	2009	20–45	Type-specific PCR (16, 18, 31, 33)	Women free of cytological abnormalities at enrolment
Cuzick, 1999	UK, London	2981	35+	HC1, HC2, MY09/11 PCR	Women free of cytological abnormalities at enrolment
Kuhn, 2000	South Africa, Cape Town	2944	35–65	HC1, HC2	Unscreened population, community recruitment
Ratnam, 2000	Canada, Newfoundland	2098	18–69	HC1, HC2	Multiple screening practices, 10% random sample of Pap−/HPV− women referred for colposcopy
Schiffman, 2000	Costa Rica, Guanacaste	8554	18–90+	HC1, HC2	Population-based, HPV positivity not a criterion for colposcopy referral
Wright, 2000	South Africa, Cape Town	1365	35–65	HC2	Subset of sample in Kuhn (2000)
Schneider, 2000	Germany, East Thuringia	4761	18–70	GP5+/6+ PCR	Multiple screening practices, cross-sectional plus 8 months' follow-up testing
Belinson, 2001	China, Shanxi	1997	35–45	HC2	Unscreened population, community recruitment, all women underwent colposcopy
Blumenthal, 2001	Zimbabwe, Harare	2073	25–55	HC2	Completed recruitment (irrespective of HIV serostatus) of study in Womack (2000); all women underwent colposcopy
Clavel, 2001	France, Reims	7932	15–76	HC2	Women free of cytological abnormalities at enrolment, cross-sectional plus 15 months' follow-up testing; HPV positivity alone not a criterion for immediate colposcopy referral
Kulasingam, 2002	US, Washington State	4075	18–50	HC2, MY09/11 PCR	Family planning clinic recruitment, ThinPrep cytology, 41% random samples of Pap−/HPV− women referred for colposcopy
Petry, 2003	Germany, Hannover and Tuebingen	8466	30+	HC2 AND PCR with three different primer sets (PPF1/PPF2, PPF1/CP5, CP4/CP5)	Primary screening network of clinics and gynaecological practices: patients attending routine cervical screening stratified to be representative of all Germany. Bias controlled
Salmeron, 2003	Mexico, Morelos	7868	15–85	HC2	Women attending opportunistic screening. Self-collected vaginal compared with clinician-collected cervical samples. Those positive for HPV or by cytology were referred for colposcopy and biopsy
Cuzick, 2003	UK, five centres	10 385	30–60	HC2	Randomised controlled trial in women free of cytological abnormalities at enrolment
Sankaranarayanan, 2004	India, Kolkata, Mumbai, Trivandrum	18 035	25–65	HC2	Women attending primary screening in four different sites in India. All subjects investigated by colposcopy and, when necessary, underwent a biopsy. Averted verification bias in the design

Table 26.2 Estimates of screening performance indices from studies that provided data on the comparison of HPV testing with Pap cytology* in primary screening for cervical cancer and its precursor lesions.

Study (first author, year)	Sensitivity		Specificity		Comments
	HPV	Pap	HPV	Pap	
Cuzick, 1995	75	46	96	96	
Cuzick, 1999	95	79	94	99	HPV indices based on HC2 ($n = 1703$)
Kuhn, 2000	88	78	82	97	LSIL in histology excluded, HPV indices based on HC2 ($n = 424$)
	73		88		LSIL in histology excluded, HPV indices based on HC1 ($n = 2861$)
Ratnam, 2000	68	27	91	96	All ages, bias adjusted**, specificity includes CIN1
	82	40	94	97	30+ years, bias adjusted**, specificity includes CIN1
Schiffman, 2000	88	78	89	94	Conventional cytology and HC2, all ages
	93		80		HC2, ages 18–30
	81		90		HC2, ages 31–40
	93		94		HC2, age > 40
Wright, 2000	84	61	83	96	Clinician-collected cervical samples
	66		81		Self-collected cervical samples
Schneider, 2000	89	20	94	99	Bias adjusted**
Belinson, 2001	95	87	85	94	ThinPrep cytology
Blumenthal, 2001	80	44	61	91	Bias controlled**
Clavel, 2001	100	68	87	95	All ages, paired set with conventional cytology ($n = 2281$)
	100	88	86	93	All ages, paired set with ThinPrep cytology ($n = 5651$)
	100	58	90	96	Age > 30, paired set with conventional cytology ($n = 1550$)
	100	84	88	95	Age > 30, paired set with ThinPrep cytology ($n = 4121$)
Kulasingam, 2002	91/88	57	73/79	90	All ages, detection of ≥ CIN3, HPV tests: HC2/PCR, bias adjusted**
	74/70	46	71178	89	Age < 30, detection of ≥ CIN2, HPV tests: HC2/PCR, bias adjusted**
	63/57	36	83/87	96	Age ≥ 30, detection of ≥ CIN2, HPV tests: HC2/PCR, bias adjusted**
Petry, 2003	98	44	95	98	CIN2/3+, bias adjusted**
	97	46	95	98	CIN3+, bias adjusted**
Salmeron, 2003	93	59	92	98	CIN2/3+, clinician-collected cervical samples
	71		89		CIN2/3+, self-collected vaginal samples
Cuzick, 2003	98	72	93	99	For entire cohort entered into randomisation
Sankaranarayanan, 2004	46	37	92	87	Kolkata
	69	70	94	99	Mumbai
	81	72	95	98	Trivandrum

*LSIL threshold (majority of studies) or LSIL or persistent ASCUS (Kulasingam, 2002). Unless otherwise indicated, results are based on conventional cytology. Unless otherwise stated, estimates shown are for CIN2/3 lesions or worse as disease outcome.
**Verification bias: bias controlled denotes verification of disease status among all participants, and bias adjusted denotes correction of estimates based on the verification of disease status in a random sample of test-negative women.

studies in Table 26.2; thus, results must be interpreted with caution. Specifically, the sensitivity and specificity estimates derived from the majority of these studies are affected by and were not corrected for verification bias, which renders the values relative, not absolute, estimates. Verification bias occurs whenever the probability of disease verification via the gold standard is dependent on the screening test result (Franco, 2000). In general, such studies used a design in which only women with one or more positive screening tests were referred for colposcopy and biopsy, which prevented the unbiased estimation of absolute sensitivity and specificity. These studies relied on the fact that, with two or more tests, there were always combinations of either Pap-negative or HPV-negative women with verified disease status available for analysis. However, the biasing effects of the unequal verification of disease status can be strong and may lead to estimates of screening efficacy that cannot be generalised for cost considerations and other public health uses (Franco, 2000). Some studies either prevent verification bias through the application of the gold standard of disease verification to all women or correct for it through the extrapolation of the screening results from a random fraction of women with negative screening tests to those without colposcopic verification. A few of the studies in Table 26.2, as indicated, corrected for this bias.

An inherent assumption of dealing with the issue of verification bias is that colposcopy-directed biopsies, the gold standard, are perfectly accurate in revealing the presence of cervical dysplasia. Studies that either avoided or adjusted for this putative bias made this assumption and then ascertained the distribution of diseased and non-diseased women to allow the computation of adjusted estimates of screening efficacy. While the approach is correct for its intended purpose, researchers should be cognisant of the fact that a simple colposcopy or even a colposcopy-guided biopsy cannot provide a guarantee that an existing lesion will be detected. In some test-negative women, the colposcopist cannot visualise lesional tissue and may decide that the colposcopic impression of no disease alone serves as a definitive diagnosis. However, this may not be a wise decision because a lesion could be hidden in the endocervical canal and not be visible. It is possible to reduce this potential impediment by adopting a policy that blind biopsies should be collected every time colposcopies are performed. However, even then, it is still possible that a fraction of the existing lesions will remain undetected due to their size or location. Therefore, in any cross-sectional survey of screening efficacy, the ethically acceptable gold standard for cervical lesions (colposcopy-guided biopsies) is an imperfect one because of inadequate sampling of the entire cervical tissue that is at risk for squamous cell malignancy. One could speculate that only a more aggressive diagnostic approach, such as an extensive histological examination of serial sections from cone biopsies or from specimens collected via the loop electrosurgical excision procedure (LEEP) or via the large loop excision of the transformation zone (LLETZ), would approach the definition of an acceptable gold standard of disease. However, adopting such an approach even in a sample of test-negative women would be both unethical and impractical.

Even if tissue sampling could be done optimally with respect to lesion site and time of development, there is also the possibility of misclassification of lesion outcome status that exists even with histopathological ascertainment. Studies that involve multiple expert pathologists indicate that the reproducibility in grading histopathology specimens is not high, even with large specimens, such as LEEP or LLETZ tissue samples. Therefore, in order to minimise the possibility of lesion misclassification, it is optimal for studies to have a panel of several pathologists, rather than a lone pathologist, to review each case and come to a consensus diagnosis.

In addition, at present, the design of screening efficacy studies is evolving from the traditional cross-sectional design with single-opportunity sampling to long-term, repeated sampling extending over several years. As a result, disease case definition will become a more dynamic process, requiring the juxtapositioning of screening and diagnostic test results obtained from multiple samples collected over time. This process involves combining the results from different diagnostic approaches, which may be differentially triggered by the severity of the lesion grade presumed by the test (HPV or cytology), e.g. colposcopy with simple biopsy for equivocal or low-grade lesions, LEEP or LLETZ for high-grade lesions, etc. These are the challenges faced by long-term natural history investigations of HPV and cervical neoplasia. These studies have the added complexity of having to differentiate between lesion progression and regression, prevalent and incident lesions, and relating them to screening test performance. The estimation of sensitivity and specificity in these studies involves the combination of diagnostic information over multiple samples, which greatly lessens the probability that any lesions are missed by the pitfalls described above for a cross-sectional study relying on colposcopy-guided biopsies alone. On the other hand, the repeated sampling layout of these investigations precludes the need for invasive diagnostic procedures among women testing consistently negative for both HPV and Pap over many visits. The longitudinal nature of the investigation ends up providing the test and diagnostic data that approach the true distribution of disease dynamics conditional on study duration. Therefore, correction for verification bias is not a critical issue in these longitudinal studies with intensive follow-up of test-negative women and repeated histological sampling of test-positive cases. However, these studies do have to contend with the issue of distinguishing between prevalent and incident lesions to properly assign the distribution of disease for the purposes of gauging screening test efficacy.

Another issue that affects the screening performance of HPV tests is the method used to collect the cervical specimen, i.e. clinician or self-collected. In theory, clinician-collected cervical specimens are ideal in terms of sampling exfoliated cells from the cervix. Therefore, clinical correlations between lesion severity and the presence of HPV should be optimal in such specimens. Those studies in Table 26.2 that included both clinician collection and self-sampling found that the former had slightly greater sensitivity than the latter. However, self-sampling is a viable alternative to clinician-collected samples as the former has several potential benefits over the latter, such as greater convenience for women and it may be more acceptable to some women who have reservations about gynaecological examinations based on social or religious grounds. Ultimately, self-sampling may result in greater adherence to screening recommendations. There may also be monetary savings to self-sampling. Thus, as long as the loss of screening accuracy is not substantial, it will be outweighed by the benefits of self-sampling (Sellors *et al.*, 2000). Further, self-sampling of genital specimens remains an attractive option in developing countries or in remote regions where health care providers cannot be available at point of care settings. However, issues of validity, acceptability and training represent key obstacles for a wider application of self-sampling.

IMPACT OF HPV TESTING

Cost-effectiveness analyses based on US economic figures estimate that the costs for conventional cytology, liquid-based cytology and HPV testing via HC2 range as follows: US$12–75, US$20–80 and US$30–200 respectively (Goldie *et al.*, 2004). Therefore, at present, HPV testing is one of the most expensive methods of cervical cancer screening. This, along with the fact that it is not a public domain technology, as is cervical cytology, is a major obstacle to the widespread use of HPV testing. The cost-effectiveness of HPV testing is heavily dependent on assumptions related to the intrinsic cost of the test, infrastructure available in the target setting where the screening will be implemented, length of interval between screening visits and the existing expenditures incurred by quality assurance imposed by local legislation. More studies are needed in low-, middle- and high-income countries to assess effectiveness as a function of these variables.

The cervical cytological specimen used for HPV testing is the same as that collected for the conventional Pap test. The physical act of collecting exfoliated cervical cells is only mildly discomforting to the patient and carries only very minimal risk. On the other hand, little is known about the psychological and emotional impact of receiving a positive HPV test result. With the advent of HPV testing and its increasing clinical use, there has been a gradual shift in how the medical and public health community considers cervical cancer prevention. Specifically, cervical cancer prevention has shifted from an oncological perspective to a paradigm in which a sexually transmitted infection is now the focus (Franco, 2003). If it were eventually implemented in primary screening for cervical cancer, testing for HPV would result in a large proportion of women who would have to be told that they harbour a sexually transmitted viral infection that can ultimately cause cancer. It should be noted that HPV infections, especially in women younger than 30 years, are extremely common; the age-dependent prevalence among sexually active young women ranges from 5% to 40% (Ley *et al.*, 1991; Bauer *et al.*, 1993; Melkert *et al.*, 1993). Fortunately, most HPV infections are very transient, and it is estimated that a newly diagnosed HPV infection will usually clear within 12–18 months in 80% of women (Ho *et al.*, 1998; Franco *et al.*, 1999; Thomas *et al.*, 2000; Liaw *et al.*, 2001). Therefore, it is debatable whether conveying a

woman's HPV status would bring any benefit other than the certainty of full disclosure about the incidental finding of a health status item for a screening participant. The vast majority of such women will not be required to change their lifestyle or be referred for a more aggressive diagnostic work-up on the basis of this information (as their infection will be found to be transient). There is a dearth of research on the merits and consequences of conveying this information to women, so it is imperative that future studies investigate the potential negative impact of imparting this information to the screening public. Much research is also needed to enable a better understanding of the dynamics of sexual transmission of HPV infection so that health providers can convey meaningful information on risk to couples.

An important theoretical and practical concern with the use of HPV testing in cancer screening is the potential for a breakdown in quality control safeguards if too many commercial test suppliers end up entering the market without a minimal level of regulatory control of performance standards by health care or government agencies. Currently, there are only a few commercial suppliers of HPV diagnostic systems. The two major players in the field (Digene, Roche) can absorb the costs of strict quality control standards in reagent batch production and performance characteristics by passing on the costs to the consumers or their health insurers, private or public. However, it is conceivable that a diminishing market share and subsequent reduction in the cost of testing may force test manufacturers to relax their standards of quality. Such a scenario could prove disastrous in many respects as there are theoretically many more variables that can affect the performance of HPV testing than there are sources of variation that need to be controlled in Pap cytology screening. It is imperative, therefore, that early performance and proficiency standards be agreed upon by public health agencies involved with quality assurance of cervical cancer screening.

A recent study by Cuzick *et al.* (2006) supported the concept that HPV testing as the sole primary test for cervical cancer screening, with cytology reserved for women who test positive for HPV, was feasible and scientifically valid. Cuzick's study of 60 000 women in Europe and North America clearly showed the increased sensitivity of HPV testing over cytology (96.1% vs 53%) for detecting high-grade epithelial disease.

FUTURE DEVELOPMENTS

Future developments will revolve around improvements in screening technologies, especially in advance rapid testing. In 2003, PATH (Programme for Appropriate Technologies in Health) and its parent organisations began a new project to develop two biochemical screening tests for the prevention of cervical cancer. This was part of the START project (Screening Technologies to Advance Rapid Testing). They realised that visual tests such as visual inspection with acetic acid (VIA) or

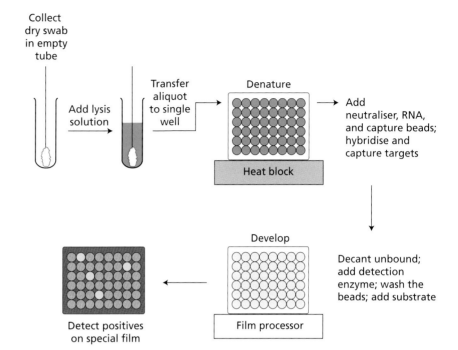

Fig. 26.5 Diagrammatic representation of the process involved in the recently developed hybrid capture technique which will reduce analysis time to 2.5 hours.

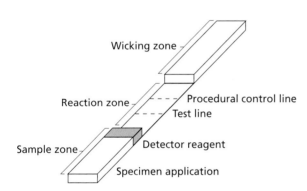

Fig. 26.6 Lateral flow strip designed to detect E6 protein from oncogenic types of HPV in less than 20 minutes (Arbor Vita Corporation, Sunnydale, CA, USA).

with Lugol's iodine (VILI) are promising alternatives to cervical cytology for primary screening in scarce resource settings. They realised that new rapid biochemical assays were needed in these environments. Two such assays are currently under research and development in an effort led by PATH, which is a non-profit organisation based in Seattle.

One test is being developed as a rapid batch assay for the DNA of oncogenic types of HPV in partnership with Digene Corporation (Gaithersburg, MD, USA), building on the HC2 assay technology to produce a test that can be performed with minimal training and equipment in less than 2.5 hours (Fig. 26.5).

The other assay, a lateral flow strip (Fig. 26.6), is under development by PATH in collaboration with Arbor Vita

Corporation (Sunnydale, CA, USA) to detect E6 protein from oncogenic types of HPV in less than 20 minutes.

The aims of these new tests are to be accurate, reproducible, acceptable to women and providers, affordable and available to the public health sector in low- and middle-income countries at a preferential price compared with the private sector. It is hoped that rapidly available results will allow reduction in the number of visits that women need to make to health care providers, as further management can be accomplished at the same visit as screening.

CONCLUSION

HPV testing has opened up a new frontier in cervical cancer screening. HPV testing has provided health care professionals with additional information upon which to base their medical decisions in order to be better able to provide their patients with the best preventive and diagnostic care. However, HPV testing is a frontier that still holds many unanswered questions, both practical and theoretical. For example, what is the appropriate age at which HPV testing should be initiated? What are the optimal management algorithms for the various combinations of Pap and HPV results that can potentially occur? What is the feasibility of HPV testing in less economically developed nations? What are the psychosocial ramifications on women and their partners of receiving a positive HPV test result? These and many other questions need to be answered by the research community. Undoubtedly, in the years to come, we will witness further advancements and refinements in the methodology of HPV testing techniques and, with the probable availability of HPV vaccines in the future, the whole realm of cervical cancer prevention will be revolutionised.

ACKNOWLEDGEMENTS

The authors wish to thank Dr John Sellors, the Project Director of the SMART Programme, for his contribution in respect of the two new rapid biochemical assays at present being coordinated by the PATH organisation in Seattle, WA, USA.

REFERENCES

ASCUS-LSIL Triage Study (ALTS) Group (2003a) A randomized trial on the management of low-grade squamous intraepithelial lesion cytology interpretations. *American Journal of Obstetrics and Gynecology* 188: 1393–1400.

ASCUS-LSIL Triage Study (ALTS) Group (2003b) Results of a randomized trial on the management of cytology interpretations of atypical squamous cells of undetermined significance. *American Journal of Obstetrics and Gynecology* 188: 1383–1392.

Bauer HM, Hildesheim A, Schiffman MH *et al.* (1993) Determinants of genital human papillomavirus infection in low-risk women in Portland, Oregon. *Sexually Transmitted Diseases* 20: 274–278.

Belinson J, Qiao YL, Pretorius R *et al.* (2001) Shanxi Province Cervical Cancer Screening Study: a cross-sectional comparative trial of multiple techniques to detect cervical neoplasia. *Gynecologic Oncology* 83: 439–444.

Beral V, Day NE (1992) Screening for cervical cancer: is there a place for incorporating tests for the human papillomavirus? In: Muñoz N, Bosch FX, Shah KV *et al.* (eds) *The Epidemiology of Human Papillomavirus and Cervical Cancer.* Lyon: IARC Scientific Publications, pp. 263–269.

Bernard HU, Chan SY, Manos MM *et al.* (1994a) Identification and assessment of known and novel human papillomaviruses by polymerase chain reaction amplification, restriction fragment length polymorphisms, nucleotide sequence, and phylogenetic algorithms. *Journal of Infectious Diseases* 170: 1077–1085.

Blumenthal PD, Gaffikin L, Chirenje ZM *et al.* (2001) Adjunctive testing for cervical cancer in low resource settings with visual inspection, HPV, and the Pap smear. *International Journal of Gynecology and Obstetrics* 72: 47–53.

Bulkmans NW, Rozendaal L, Snijders PJ *et al.* (2004) POBASCAM, a population-based randomized controlled trial for implementation of high-risk HPV testing in cervical screening: design, methods and baseline data of 44,102 women. *International Journal of Cancer* 110: 94–101.

Castle PE, Schiffman M, Gravitt PE *et al.* (2002) Comparisons of HPV DNA detection by MY09/11 PCR methods. *Journal of Medical Virology* 68: 417–423.

Castle PE, Lorincz AT, Scott DR *et al.* (2003) Comparison between prototype hybrid capture 3 and hybrid capture 2 human papillomavirus DNA assays for detection of high-grade cervical intraepithelial neoplasia and cancer. *Journal of Clinical Microbiology* 41: 4022–4030.

Clavel C, Bory JP, Rihet S *et al.* (1998) Comparative analysis of human papillomavirus detection by hybrid capture assay and routine cytologic screening to detect high-grade cervical lesions. *International Journal of Cancer* 75: 525–528.

Clavel C, Masure M, Bory JP *et al.* (2001) Human papillomavirus testing in primary screening for the detection of high-grade cervical lesions: a study of 7932 women. *British Journal of Cancer* 84: 1616–1623.

Coutlee F, Mayrand MH, Provencher D *et al.* (1997) The future of HPV testing in clinical laboratories and applied virology research. *Clinics in Diagnostic Virology* 8: 123–141.

Cuzick J, Szarewski A, Terry G *et al.* (1995) Human papillomavirus testing in primary cervical screening. *Lancet* 345: 1533–1536.

Cuzick J, Beverley E, Ho L *et al.* (1999) HPV testing in primary screening of older women. *British Journal of Cancer* 81: 554–558.

Cuzick J, Szarewski A, Cubie H *et al.* (2003) Management of women who test positive for high-risk types of human papillomavirus: the HART study. *Lancet* 362: 1871–1876.

Cuzick J, Clavel C, Petry KU (2006) Overview of the European and North American studies on HPV testing in primary cervical cancer screening. *International Journal of Cancer* 119: 1095–1101.

Dallas PB, Flanagan JL, Nightingale BN *et al.* (1989) Polymerase chain reaction for fast, nonradioactive detection of high- and low-risk papillomavirus types in routine cervical specimens and in biopsies. *Journal of Medical Virology* 27: 105–111.

de Cremoux P, Coste J, Sastre-Garau X *et al.* (2003) Efficiency of the hybrid capture 2 HPV DNA test in cervical cancer screening. A study by the French Society of Clinical Cytology. *American Journal of Clinical Pathology* 120: 492–499.

Deligeorgi-Politi H, Mui KK, Trotta K *et al.* (1986) Immunocytochemical localization of human papilloma virus and cytomorphologic correlation in smears and biopsies of cervical flat condylomata. *Diagnostic Cytopathology* 2: 320–325.

Farthing A, Masterson P, Mason WP *et al.* (1994) Human papillomavirus detection by hybrid capture and its possible clinical use. *Journal of Clinical Pathology* 47: 649–652.

Franco EL (1992) Measurement errors in epidemiologic studies of human papillomavirus and cervical cancer. In: Muñoz N *et al.* (eds) *The Epidemiology of Human Papillomavirus and Cervical Cancer.* IARC scientific publication no. 119. Oxford: Oxford University Press, pp. 181–197.

Franco EL (2000) Statistical issues in human papillomavirus testing and screening In: Carr J (ed.) *Human Papillomavirus.* Philadelphia: W.B. Saunders, pp. 345–367.

Franco EL (2003a) Chapter 13: Primary screening of cervical cancer with human papillomavirus tests. *Journal of the National Cancer Institute Monograph* 31: 89–96.

Franco EL (2003b) Are we ready for a paradigm change in cervical cancer screening? *Lancet* 362: 1866–1867.

Franco EL, Villa LL, Sobrinho JP *et al.* (1999) Epidemiology of acquisition and clearance of cervical human papillomavirus infection in women from a high-risk area for cervical cancer. *Journal of Infectious Diseases* 180: 1415–1423.

Galloway DA (1992) Serological assays for the detection of HPV antibodies. In: Muñoz N, Bosch FX, Shah KV *et al.* (eds) *The Epidemiology of Human Papillomavirus and Cervical Cancer.* Lyon: IARC Scientific Publications, pp. 147–161.

Goldie SJ, Kohli M, Grima D *et al.* (2004) Projected clinical benefits and cost-effectiveness of an HPV 16/18 vaccine. *Journal of the National Cancer Institute* 96: 604–615.

Gravitt PE, Manos MM (1992) Polymerase chain reaction-based methods for the detection of human papillomavirus DNA. In: Muñoz N, Bosch FX, Shah KV *et al.* (eds) *The Epidemiology of Human Papillomavirus and Cervical Cancer.* Lyon: IARC Scientific Publications, pp. 121–133.

Gravitt PE, Peyton CL, Apple RJ *et al.* (1998) Genotyping of 27 human papillomavirus types by using L1 consensus PCR products by a single-hybridization, reverse line blot detection method. *Journal of Clinical Microbiology* 36: 3020–3027.

Gravitt PE, Peyton CL, Alessi TQ *et al.* (2000) Improved amplification of genital human papillomaviruses. *Journal of Clinical Microbiology* 38: 357–361.

Gregoire L, Arella M, Campione-Piccardo J *et al.* (1989) Amplification of human papillomavirus DNA sequences by using conserved primers. *Journal of Clinical Microbiology* 27: 2660–2665.

Gupta J, Gendelman HE, Naghashfar Z *et al.* (1985) Specific identification of human papillomavirus type in cervical smears and paraffin sections by in situ hybridization with radioactive probes: a preliminary communication. *International Journal of Gynecological Pathology* 4: 211–218.

Ho GY, Bierman R, Beardsley L *et al.* (1998) Natural history of cervicovaginal papillomavirus infection in young women. *New England Journal of Medicine* 338: 423–428.

Howard M, Sellors J, Kaczorowski J (2002) Optimizing the hybrid capture II human papillomavirus test to detect cervical intraepithelial neoplasia. *Obstetrics and Gynecology* 100 (5 Pt 1): 972–980.

Howard M, Sellors J, Kaczorowski J *et al.* (2004) Optimal cutoff of the hybrid capture II human papillomavirus test for self-collected vaginal, vulvar, and urine specimens in a colposcopy referral population. *Journal of Lower Genital Tract Diseases* 8: 33–37.

Iftner T, Villa LL (2003) Chapter 12: Human papillomavirus technologies. *Journal of the National Cancer Institute Monograph* 31: 80–88.

Jacobs MV, Roda Husman AM, Van den Brule AJ *et al.* (1995) Group-specific differentiation between high- and low-risk human papillomavirus genotypes by general primer-mediated PCR and two cocktails of oligonucleotide probes. *Journal of Clinical Microbiology* 33: 901–905.

Jacobs MV, Snijders PJ, Van den Brule AJ *et al.* (1997) A general primer GP5+IGP6(+)-mediated PCR-enzyme immunoassay method for rapid detection of 14 high-risk and 6 low-risk human papillomavirus genotypes in cervical scrapings. *Journal of Clinical Microbiology* 35: 791–795.

Jochmus-Kudielka I, Schneider A, Braun R *et al.* (1989) Antibodies against the human papillomavirus type 16 early proteins in human sera: correlation of anti-E7 reactivity with cervical cancer. *Journal of the National Cancer Institute* 81: 1698–1704.

Kleter B, van Doom LJ, ter Schegget J *et al.* (1998) Novel short-fragment PCR assay for highly sensitive broad-spectrum detection of anogenital human papillomaviruses. *American Journal of Pathology* 153: 1731–1739.

Kleter B, van Doom LJ, Schrauwen L *et al.* (1999) Development and clinical evaluation of a highly sensitive PCR-reverse hybridization line probe assay for detection and identification of anogenital human papillomavirus. *Journal of Clinical Microbiology* 37: 2508–2517.

Komorowski R, Clowry L, Jr (1976) Koilocytotic atypia of the cervix. *Obstetrics and Gynecology* 47: 540–544.

Kuhn L, Denny L, Pollack A *et al.* (2000) Human papillomavirus DNA testing for cervical cancer screening in low-resource settings. *Journal of the National Cancer Institute* 92: 818–825.

Kulasingam SL, Hughes JP, Klviat NB *et al.* (2002) Evaluation of human papillomavirus testing in primary screening for cervical abnormalities: comparison of sensitivity, specificity, and frequency of referral. *Journal of the American Medical Association* 288: 1749–1757.

Ley C, Bauer HM, Reingold A *et al.* (1991) Determinants of genital human papillomavirus infection in young women. *Journal of the National Cancer Institute* 83: 997–1003.

Liaw KL, Hildesheim A, Burk RD *et al.* (2001) A prospective study of human papillomavirus (HPV) type 16 DNA detection by polymerase chain reaction and its association with acquisition and persistence of other HPV types. *Journal of Infectious Diseases* 183: 8–15.

Lorincz A (1992) Detection of human papillomavirus DNA without amplification: prospects for clinical utility. In: Muñoz N, Bosch FX, Shah KV *et al.* (eds) *The Epidemiology of Human Papillomavirus and Cervical Cancer.* Lyon: IARC Scientific Publications, pp. 135–145.

Lorincz AT, Schiffman MH, Jaffurs WJ *et al.* (1990) Temporal associations of human papillomavirus infection with cervical cytologic abnormalities. *American Journal of Obstetrics and Gynecology* 162: 645–651.

Manos MM, Ting Y, Wright DK *et al.* (1989) Use of polymerase chain reaction amplification for detection of genital papillomavirus. *Cancer Cell* 29: 20–27.

Mayrand MH, Duarte-Franco E, Coutlée F *et al.* for the CCCaST Study Group (2006) Randomized study of human papillomavirus testing versus Pap cytology in the primary screening for cervical cancer precursors: design, methods and preliminary accrual results of the Canadian Cervical Cancer Screening Trial (CCCaST). *International Journal of Cancer* (in press).

Melkert PW, Hopman E, van den Brule AJ *et al.* (1993) Prevalence of HPV in cytomorphologically normal cervical smears, as determined by the polymerase chain reaction, is age-dependent. *International Journal of Cancer* 53: 919–23.

Nuovo GJ, Nuovo J (1991) Should family physicians test for human papillomavirus infection? An opposing view. *Journal of Family Practice* 32: 188–192.

Nuovo GJ, MacConnell P, Forde A *et al.* (1991) Detection of human papillomavirus DNA in formalin-fixed tissues by in situ hybridization after amplification by polymerase chain reaction. *American Journal of Pathology* 139: 847–854.

Okagaki T, Twiggs LB, Zachow KR *et al.* (1983) Identification of human papillomavirus DNA in cervical and vaginal intraepithelial neoplasia with molecularly cloned virus-specific DNA probes. *International Journal of Gynecological Pathology* 2: 153–159.

Parkkinen S, Mantyjarvi R, Syrjanen K *et al.* (1986) Detection of human papillomavirus DNA by the nucleic acid sandwich hybridization method from cervical scraping. *Journal of Medical Virology* 20: 279–288.

Peto K (2004) The cervical cancer epidemic that screening has prevented in the UK. *Lancet* 364 (9430): 249–256.

Petry KU, Menton S, Menton M *et al.* (2003) Inclusion of HPV testing in routine cervical cancer screening for women above 29 years in Germany: results for 8466 patients. *British Journal of Cancer* 88: 1570–1577.

Peyton CL, Schiffman M, Lorincz AT *et al.* (1998) Comparison of PCR- and hybrid capture-based human papillomavirus detection systems using multiple cervical specimen collection strategies. *Journal of Clinical Microbiology* 36: 3248–3254.

Qu W, Jiang G, Cruz Y *et al.* (1997) PCR detection of human papillomavirus: comparison between MY09/MY11 and GP5+/GP6+ primer systems. *Journal of Clinical Microbiology* 35: 1304–1310.

Quint WG, Scholte G, van Doorn LJ *et al.* (2001) Comparative analysis of human papillomavirus infections in cervical scrapes and biopsy specimens by general SPF(10) PCR and HPV genotyping. *Journal of Pathology* 194: 51–58.

Ratnam S, Franco EL, Ferenczy A (2000) Human papillomavirus testing for primary screening of cervical cancer precursors. *Cancer Epidemiology Biomarkers and Prevention* 9: 945–951.

Reid R, Lorincz AT (1991) Should family physicians test for human papillomavirus infection? An affirmative view. *Journal of Family Practice* 32: 183–188.

Reid R, Greenberg MD, Lorincz A *et al.* (1991) Should cervical cytologic testing be augmented by cervicography or human papillomavirus deoxyribonucleic acid detection? *American Journal of Obstetrics and Gynecology* 164: 1461–1469.

Roda Husman AM, Walboomers JM, Van den Brule AJ *et al.* (1995) The use of general primers GP5 and GP6 elongated at their T ends with adjacent highly conserved sequences improves human papillomavirus detection by PCR. *Journal of General Virology* 76 (Pt 4): 1057–1062.

Salmeron J, Lazcano-Ponce E, Lorincz A *et al.* (2003) Comparison of HPV-based assays with Papanicolaou smears for cervical cancer screening in Morelos State, Mexico. *Cancer Causes and Control* 14: 505–512.

Sankaranarayanan R, Chatterji R, Shastri SS *et al.* IARC Multicenter Study Group on Cervical Cancer Prevention in India (2004) Accuracy of human papillomavirus testing in primary screening of cervical neoplasia: results from a multicenter study in India. *International Journal of Cancer* 112: 341–347.

Schiffman MH (1992) Validation of hybridization assays: correlation of filter in situ, dot blot and PCR with Southern blot. In: Muñoz N, Bosch FX, Shah KV *et al.* (eds) *The Epidemiology of Human Papillomavirus and Cervical Cancer.* Lyon: IARC Scientific Publications, pp. 169–179.

Schiffman MH, Schatzkin A (1994) Test reliability is critically important to molecular epidemiology: an example from studies of human papillomavirus infection and cervical neoplasia. *Cancer Research* 54: 1944s–1947s.

Schiffman M, Herrero R, Hildesheim A *et al.* (2000) HPV DNA testing in cervical cancer screening: results from women in a high-risk province of Costa Rica. *Journal of the American Medical Association* 283: 87–93.

Schneider A, Kraus H, Schuhmann R *et al.* (1985) Papillomavirus infection of the lower genital tract: detection of viral DNA in gynecological swabs. *International Journal of Cancer* 35: 443–448.

Schneider A, Hoyer H, Lotz B *et al.* (2000) Screening for high-grade cervical intra-epithelial neoplasia and cancer by testing for high-risk HPV, routine cytology or colposcopy. *International Journal of Cancer* 89: 529–534.

Sellors JW, Lorincz AT, Mahony JB *et al.* (2000) Comparison of self-collected vaginal, vulvar and urine samples with physician-collected cervical samples for human papillomavirus testing to detect high-grade squamous intraepithelial lesions. *Canadian Medical Association Journal* 163: 513–518.

Snijders PJ, Van den Brule AJ, Schrijnemakers HF *et al.* (1990) The use of general primers in the polymerase chain reaction permits the detection of a broad spectrum of human papillomavirus genotypes. *Journal of General Virology* 71 (Pt 1): 173–181.

Snijders PJ, van den Brule AJ, Meijer CJ (2003) The clinical relevance of human papillomavirus testing: relationship between analytical and clinical sensitivity. *Journal of Pathology* 201: 1–6.

Suba EJ, Raab SS (2004) Papanicolaou screening in developing countries: an idea whose time has come. *American Journal of Clinical Pathology* 121: 315–320.

Sun CA, Lai HC, Chang CC *et al.* (2001) The significance of human papillomavirus viral load in prediction of histologic severity and size of squamous intraepithelial lesions of uterine cervix. *Gynecologic Oncology* 83: 95–99.

Swan DC, Tucker RA, Tortolero-Luna G *et al.* (1999) Human papillomavirus (HPV) DNA copy number is dependent on grade of cervical disease and HPV type. *Journal of Clinical Microbiology* 37: 1030–1034.

Syrjanen KJ, Pyrhonen S (1982) Immunoperoxidase demonstration of human papilloma virus (HPV) in dysplastic lesions of the uterine cervix. *Archives of Gynecology* 233: 53–61.

Thomas KK, Hughes JP, Kuypers JM *et al.* (2000) Concurrent and sequential acquisition of different genital human papillomavirus types. *Journal of Infectious Diseases* 182: 1097–1102.

Van den Brule AJ, Snijders PJ, Gordijn RL *et al.* (1990) General primer-mediated polymerase chain reaction permits the detection of sequenced and still unsequenced human papillomavirus genotypes in cervical scrapes and carcinomas. *International Journal of Cancer* 45: 644–649.

Van den Brule AJ, Pol R, Fransen-Daalmeijer N *et al.* (2002) GP5+/6+ PCR followed by reverse line blot analysis enables rapid and high-throughput identification of human papillomavirus genotypes. *Journal of Clinical Microbiology* 40: 779–787.

van Doorn LJ, Quint W, Kleter B *et al.* (2002) Genotyping of human papillomavirus in liquid cytology cervical specimens by the PGMY line blot assay and the SPF(10) line probe assay. *Journal of Clinical Microbiology* 40: 979–983.

Vernon SD, Unger ER, Williams D (2000) Comparison of human papillomavirus detection and typing by cycle sequencing, line blotting, and hybrid capture. *Journal of Clinical Microbiology* 38: 651–655.

Wilbur DC, Stoler MH (1991) Testing for human papillomavirus: basic pathobiology of infection, methodologies, and implications for clinical use. *Yale Journal of Biological Medicine* 64: 113–125.

Womack SD, Chirenje ZM, Gaffikin L *et al.* (2000) HPV-based cervical cancer screening in a population at high risk for HIV infection. *International Journal of Cancer* 85: 206–210.

Wright TC, Jr, Denny L, Kuhn L *et al.* (2000) HPV DNA testing of self-collected vaginal samples compared with cytologic screening to detect cervical cancer. *Journal of the American Medical Association* 283: 81–86.

CHAPTER 27

Real-time devices for the screening and diagnosis of cervical neoplasia

Karen Canfell and Carl Chow

INTRODUCTION

Traditional methods of cervical cancer detection involve cytological screening, followed by referral to colposcopy for the evaluation of smear-detected abnormalities. The colposcopist inspects the cervix using low-powered magnification, with contrast enhancement between normal and abnormal epithelium achieved via the topical application of agents such as aqueous acetic acid and Lugol's iodine solution. A biopsy may be indicated, and further follow-up and treatment is based on the colposcopic examination and the pathology result. Although the traditional screening, referral and treatment process has proved very effective in reducing overall cervical cancer incidence if implemented within a coordinated programme (Quinn *et al.*, 1999), the process is not a fail-safe method of detecting and treating all cervical abnormalities. At the screening stage, the cytological smear is known to suffer from sensitivity limitations (Nanda *et al.*, 2000). Diagnostic assessment inevitably relies on the subjective interpretation of the magnified and illuminated colposcopic image, despite the implementation of standardised training, accreditation and quality assurance systems in some jurisdictions (Department of Health UK, 2001; see Chapter 30). This leads to variability in the colposcopic diagnosis and in management decisions (Etherington *et al.*, 1997). A consequent level of inaccuracy in the localisation of biopsy site contributes to a significant false-negative rate for cervical biopsy (Skehan *et al.*, 1990).

Several approaches to improving the accuracy of cervical disease detection have been considered. For cervical screening, technological improvements to cytology include liquid-based cytology and automated cytological evaluation systems. A number of new approaches to cervical screening and diagnosis have also emerged and include HPV DNA testing, the use of molecular markers and real-time devices. Real-time devices utilise *in vivo* measurement techniques and computerised analysis to provide immediate feedback to the clinician. They incorporate optical and/or electrical biosensors, which are linked to software processing systems designed to classify tissue types. The technology relies on changes in primary tissue characteristics, such as cellular composition, cellular morpho-

logy and vascular structure, which can be used to distinguish between various types of normal and abnormal cervical epithelium. Secondary (or derived) effects of these primary characteristics, which can be measured directly, include tissue reflectance and absorbance, tissue autofluorescence, the intensity and direction of backscattered light and the electrical properties of the tissue.

Two major applications have been proposed for real-time devices. The first is in cervical cancer screening, where the device is used by the health practitioner for routine screening. In this situation, real-time technology is likely to be introduced initially as an adjunct to cervical cytology although, in the longer term, the technology has the potential to operate as an autonomous screening test. The second major application is as a tool for the colposcopist, with the device used as an aid to identifying and classifying abnormal tissue locations on the cervix. Depending on the clinical setting, this information can potentially be used either to guide the choice of biopsy site or to facilitate see-and-treat protocols. One of the major benefits associated with real-time devices is the automation, and consequent standardisation, of the test process. In effect, these devices have the potential to bring the expertise of the specialist gynaecologist to a wider group of practitioners. The second major advantage is in the provision of instantaneous feedback to the clinician or screener. For screening applications, real-time feedback allows immediate counselling, management and referral. In situations where loss-to-recall is a concern, the technology could potentially allow the screening, diagnosis and treatment of cervical disease to take place within a single clinical session.

The accuracy of real-time devices for classifying cervical disease is device dependent, and is intrinsically dependent on two major factors. The first is the specific choice of biosensor, or combination of biosensors, used for assessing cervical tissue. In general terms, the chosen biosensor must have several key characteristics. It must be capable of reliable and reproducible measurement, and it must discriminate between the various types of normal and abnormal cervical tissue. The second major factor in real-time device accuracy is the processing software used to convert the information obtained from the biosensor(s) into a clinically relevant tissue classification. The software must be capable of integrating the information obtained from the biosensors, and it must be able to deal with measurement artefacts induced, for example, by background ambient illumination or device movement during data acquisition. The software must detect such artefacts, filter them out and, if appropriate, signal to the clinician that corrective action is required.

The first part of this chapter will review the various types of optical and electrical biosensors used in real-time devices and discuss the software used to process information obtained from biosensors. The second part of the chapter will discuss some considerations for the clinical assessment of real-time devices. The final section of the chapter will review seven specific real-time technologies that have been reported in the literature, discussing the biosensors, system configuration and clinical application in each case.

BIOSENSORS AND PROCESSING SOFTWARE FOR REAL-TIME DEVICES

Primary tissue characteristics in cervical disease

The pathophysiological changes of cervical pre-cancer and cancer involve alterations in cellular structure and vascularisation that result in differences in the optical and electrical properties of the cervical tissue. Histologically, precancerous cervical

intraepithelial neoplasia (CIN) lesions are associated with nuclear changes, cellular differentiation abnormalities and abnormal mitotic figures, with the grading of CIN1–3 based on the extent of epithelial involvement (Anderson, 1985). CIN may also be associated with neovascularisation and increasing abnormalities of the intracellular junctions. At a cellular level, these alterations progressively affect structure, nuclear size, capillary perfusion and haemoglobin concentration. Invasive squamous cell carcinoma is classified on the basis of the degree of differentiation and the specific cell type predominating within the tumour, and is associated with giant bizarre cells, necrotic tissue and neovascularisation (Leung *et al.*, 1994).

A biological sensor (or biosensor) is a measurement system applied to tissue that has the property of varying as the tissue type changes. The measurement system generally incorporates a form of tissue excitation, and the response of the tissue to stimulation is measured (Fig. 27.1). The two major classes of sensor technologies used for cervical tissue classification are optical and electrical sensors. One of the main challenges of real-time device development is in the particular choice of sensor and an assessment of its discrimination capability for normal and abnormal tissue types.

Optical biosensors

Optical biosensors are, conceptually, an automated extension of visual colposcopic methods. Diagnostic colposcopy uses

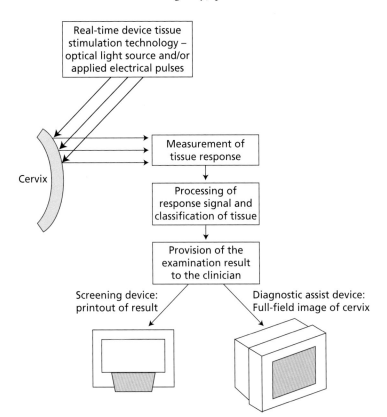

Fig. 27.1 Real-time device (RTD) operation.

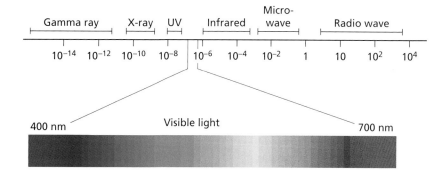

Fig.27.2 The electromagnetic spectrum. Real-time devices generally operate within the ultraviolet (UV), visible and infrared regions of the spectrum.

contrast agents, magnification and visual filters to assess the vascularisation, margins and colour of cervical lesions. In an analogous fashion, optical biosensors use the spectral characteristics of tissue to assess lesion morphology or tissue structure. The main characteristics of an optical biosensor are the form of spectral excitation used and the frequencies at which the spectral response is measured, as the properties of light waves vary with frequency. The frequencies of most interest for real-time device design are the ultraviolet, visible light and infrared regions of the electromagnetic spectrum (Fig. 27.2).

Developments in optical technology include the refinement of laser and optical fibre-based excitation systems, which enable precise targeting of the tissue for excitation. The tissue response can be elucidated either by a fibre-optic probe detector, which encompasses a particular spectral band, or by an imaging system. The form of optical excitation and the choice of spectral parameters must be chosen carefully in order to maximise the tissue discrimination potential. For cervical tissue classification, the three major classes of optical techniques reported in the current literature are fluorescence spectroscopy, direct reflectance and optical backscattering.

Tissue fluorescence

The term *fluorescence* refers to the emission of light when tissue is illuminated with incident radiation in the ultraviolet or visible spectral regions. Fluorescence depends on the absorption of a relatively high-energy light photon, resulting in the excitation of molecular constituents of the tissue. Eventually, relaxation occurs and, if this is due to a radiative process, a photon is released from the tissue, with emission generally occurring within 10 ns of absorption (Roa, 1995). At higher intensities, two or more photons may be absorbed sequentially or simultaneously, resulting in fluorescence that has a shorter wavelength (higher frequency) than the incident light.

The fluorescent response of tissue varies in spectral content for various tissue types and, therefore, fluorescent biosensors have the potential to differentiate between normal and malignant tissue (Alfano *et al.*, 1984). Tissue fluorescence, which yields metabolic and structural information, may be enhanced with the use of a photosensitive dye such as haematoporphyrin derivative, which is preferentially taken up by abnormal tissue.

Fluorescence using photosensitive dyes has been explored for the cervix (Bogaards *et al.*, 2002). However, the focus for cervical applications has been in the area of *autofluorescence*, in which the administration of photosensitive agents is not required. The degree of abnormality is reflected by a decreased autofluorescence from the collagen fibres of the underlying stroma as the epithelial thickness increases in progressive CIN, coupled with an increase in the oxyhaemoglobin attenuation of fluorescence as vascularity increases, and an increase in the relative contribution of reduced nicotinamide dinucleotide phosphate [NAD(P)H] fluorescence (Ramanujam *et al.*, 1994a; Drezek *et al.*, 2001). Therefore, the autofluorescence response tends to decrease in magnitude as the degree of cervical abnormality increases (Ramanujam *et al.*, 1994a,b, 1996). Autofluorescence levels may also depend upon other factors, for example levels appear to be increased in postmenopausal women, indicating changes in collagen cross-linking patterns in this group (Brookner *et al.*, 2003; Gill *et al.*, 2003). However, measurements appear to be robust with respect to fibre-optic probe pressure (Rivoire *et al.*, 2004). A major technical problem with the measurement of tissue autofluorescence is the low level of the response signal, which may be three to four orders of magnitude weaker than the excitation signal.

Direct reflectance and optical backscattering

Light reflected by tissue consists of *direct* or *Fresnel* reflection from the surface and *backscattered* light from within the tissue (Fig. 27.3). Direct reflectance is a result of a step change in refractive index between tissue and air, and contains information related to surface topology and structure. A proportion of the incident light enters the tissue, where absorption and scattering processes together determine the penetration depth. Most incident light will be scattered and redirected multiple times before being absorbed or backscattered from the tissue (Frank *et al.*, 1989). The scattering process provides information about bulk tissue structures, intracellular organelles, vascularity and changes in biochemistry (Anderson, 1991; Richards-Kortum and Servick-Muraca, 1996; Drezek *et al.*, 2003a). For example, the volume fraction of mitochondria and melanin granules within cells affects both the total intensity and the angular distribution of the scattered light (Dunn

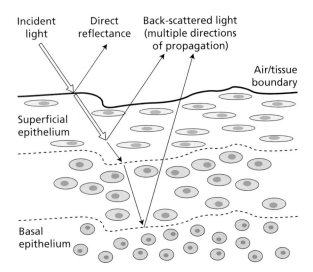

Fig. 27.3 Direct reflectance and back-scattering of light in cervical epithelium.

and Richards-Kortum, 1996). In addition, a dependency on epithelial depth has been identified, with scattering decreasing from the superficial to intermediate layers and increasing in the basal and parabasal layers (Arifler *et al.*, 2003). Therefore, characteristics such as the intensity and spatial distribution of remitted light vary between normal tissue and CIN, as a consequence of the changes associated with the progressive development of cervical abnormalities.

The geometry of tissue excitation and detection of backscattered light can be controlled using either a tissue-contacting optical fibre probe or a non-tissue-contacting optical array. As the distance between the light emitter and the detector is reduced, the light arriving at the detector is more likely to result from direct, rather than multiple, backscattering events. Therefore, the device optics must be carefully designed such that the separation distance between the light emitter and the detector allows the optimal detection of backscattered light.

Electrical measurements

A current flows between two electrodes in contact with tissue when an electrical voltage is applied. The current undergoes an exponential decay in magnitude during the time of voltage application, and the shape of the current curve and the rate of decay are dependent on features of the electrode–tissue interface, the capacitance (or charge-storing capability) of the tissue, the tissue resistance (or the opposition offered to the flow of current) and the frequency of the applied voltage signal. The electrical impedance is dependent upon both resistance and capacitance. The dielectric properties of a tissue segment are related to the additive effects of local resistances and capacitances at the cellular and structural level. As the degree of abnormality increases, the intracellular structure becomes

divided into zones with varying dielectric properties, and the dielectric properties of extracellular structures also change (Thornton *et al.*, 1991). Therefore, measurements of electrical decay curves, or direct measurements of impedance, can be used to distinguish between normal and abnormal cervical tissue. The important parameters for disease detection using electrical impedance measurements have been found to be cell size and shape distribution, the nuclear-to-cytoplasmic ratio and the extracellular space (Walker *et al.*, 2003). Of necessity, devices using electrical measurements must incorporate tissue-contacting elements.

Tissue classification technology

Real-time device processing software

Real-time devices are generally designed to collect a large volume of digitised data, which is unlikely to be interpretable by the clinician in its raw form. Therefore, the data must be processed to arrive at the final device output or display at the end of the cervical examination. The processing software to convert and condense the biosensor signals into a clinical output is termed a *tissue classification algorithm*. If the tissue classification algorithm has been previously 'trained' to classify the biosensor signals according to a suitable diagnostic reference standard, the algorithmic software is referred to as an *expert system*.

Expert systems have increasingly been used in medical applications to mimic the operation of a qualified human expert in recognition tasks. The potential benefits of expert systems include faster, simpler, standardised, objective and more cost-effective diagnoses, and they are well suited to screening and diagnostic applications. The use of expert systems has been explored in many areas of medicine, including the classification of magnetic resonance spectra (Howells *et al.*, 1992), the analysis of computerised tomography (CT) scan images (Dhawan and Juvvadi, 1990), the classification of liver disease (Bayazitoglu *et al.*, 1992), melanoma detection (Dhawan, 1998) and connective tissue disease diagnosis (Porter *et al.*, 1988).

Expert system training

Expert system training is the process of algorithmically connecting the values of input biosensor parameters to a diagnostic standard for cervical disease. The system must learn to 'recognise' particular combinations of biosensor parameters as associated with particular tissue types. In order to perform expert system training effectively, a large number of training tissue exemplars are required in order to characterise intersubject and intrasubject variability properly. It is desirable that these are obtained from a large group of women, preferably from geographically diverse regions, and ensuring that women with a range of ages are represented in the training set. These considerations ensure that expert system training is a labour-intensive process. For example, the TruScreen screening system (Polartechnics Limited, Sydney, Australia) was trained on a data set of more than 1500 women and, in each case, multiple digital images of the cervix were extensively analysed. Site-specific colposcopic and histological diagnoses were painstakingly matched to the biosensor data obtained at each site. The analysis of multiple tissue areas from each woman in the training data set was then used in the construction of the expert system tissue classification algorithm.

CLINICAL ASSESSMENT OF REAL-TIME DEVICES

Device application and clinical trial implications

Clinical data for real-time devices must be collected and evaluated in the context of the ultimate application of the device. The appropriate measures of performance vary with the application and, therefore, it is not possible to compare directly the performance of a device designed as a colposcopy tool with a device designed for general screening. For colposcopy applications, one of the appropriate measures of accuracy is the sensitivity and specificity of tissue discrimination at specific local regions (or 'spots') on the cervix, as the task of the device is to identify abnormal tissue locations for biopsy or treatment. However, integrative software algorithms are required in order to interpret the data from multiple tissue spots measured on the same cervix in a fashion that will lead to an accurate result for overall diagnosis or for screening purposes. Studies reporting only on tissue spot accuracy cannot assess the efficacy of such critical patient-level roll-up software.

For screening applications, device performance must be assessed from the perspective of accurately identifying the relatively small number of women with cervical lesion(s) from within the general population. A 'patient-level' perspective is appropriate for screening applications, as the task of the device is to identify women with abnormal cervical lesions, rather than identifying the location of the lesions themselves. This distinction is important, as spot-level assessments will tend to inflate specificity compared with a patient-level assessment. As an example of this effect, consider a device with a demonstrated specificity of 90% on a tissue spot-level basis, where the device measures 20-mm^2 tissue spots on the ectocervix. A specificity of 90% corresponds to an approximate false-positive rate of 10% and, therefore, for 10% of the measurements conducted on normal tissue, the device will inappropriately signal a tissue abnormality. If a minimum of 10 tissue spots are required in order to cover the ectocervical area then, on average, at least one tissue spot per woman will have a false-positive result. This effect possibly contributed to the dramatic loss of specificity reported by Belinson *et al.* (2002) in a trial of a fluorescence-based device in a screening population in rural China. In this study, the device examination involved measurements from eight areas on the cervix. The overall patient-level sensitivity reported was 94% for the identification of women with CIN2/3, but the device achieved an overall specificity of only 9%. Other possible explanations for the poor specificity include the fact that the device was used without prior application of acetic acid solution, and that the population included a large number of women with chronic cervicitis (Belinson *et al.*, 2002).

Transition from proof-of-principle to full-scale evaluation

A critical transition must be made between proof-of-principle clinical experimentation and full-scale clinical evaluation of new real-time technologies. Generally, real-time devices are initially developed by examining tissue biosensor measurements at local regions on the cervix. Therefore, proof-of-principle studies have focused on assessing the accuracy of the *in vivo* technology in correctly identifying spot regions of abnormal tissue (Coppleson *et al.*, 1994; Wunderman *et al.*, 1995). However, full-scale clinical evaluation of automated screening technology must directly assess overall screening accuracy, and ideally provide some comparative information against cervical cytology (Singer *et al.*, 2003). For devices designed as tools for the colposcopist, proof-of-principle studies have tended to involve many spot measurements performed on different areas of the cervix in a small number of women. However, full-scale evaluation of the diagnostic technology requires that independent measurements are performed across a population of women large enough to assess patient-level sensitivity and specificity with a narrow 95% confidence interval.

Study design considerations

Another important factor in assessing the potential benefits of real-time methods is the amount and quality of the available clinical data. Study characteristics that should be taken into consideration include the population in which the study was conducted, the number of subjects included in the study and the choice of reference diagnosis against which the performance of the device is to be assessed. Generally, colposcopically directed biopsy or fully sectioned large loop excision histology is considered the optimal reference standard. Of particular concern for real-time device studies is the issue of masking the clinician to the results of the device assessment. In normal clinical practice, the results of the real-time device are available immediately. Therefore, within the clinical study, the result could influence the choice of biopsy site, thus leading to verification bias in the assessment of sensitivity. One approach to dealing with this issue is to encrypt the device results and decode them after the clinical session has been completed. Another measure that should be considered for the elimination of bias is the masking of the study histologist to the real-time device result (Singer *et al.*, 2003).

Because the presence of CIN in the general population is relatively low, studies of screening devices may be designed to incorporate a proportion of women recruited from the colposcopy clinic environment. The inclusion of a group 'enriched' for disease abnormalities allows the more precise assessment of real-time device sensitivity, whereas specificity can be assessed on the group of women ultimately found to be normal from both recruitment streams. In such a trial, masking the study histologist to the referral information should be considered, as it is critical that the reference diagnosis for all women in the study is derived independently of the recruitment stream.

REAL-TIME DEVICE TECHNOLOGIES

This section will review the available literature on seven real-time devices for cervical pre-cancer and cancer detection. The review will not cover technologies designed to provide structural images of tissue, such as reflectance confocal microscopy (RCM) and optical coherence tomography (OCT) systems but, rather, will focus on systems that immediately provide the primary practitioner or colposcopist with clinical feedback. Each of the devices uses a particular combination of biosensors, as shown in Table 27.1. The seven technologies are: (i) the *TruScreen*™ (Polartechnics Limited, Sydney, NSW, Australia), which uses a combination of direct reflectance, optical backscattering and electrical measurements in a system designed for cervical screening; (ii) the University of Sheffield device (Brown *et al.*, 2000), which uses electrical impedance measurements and has potential application to screening; (iii) the *Cerviscan*™ (LifeSpex, Bothell, WA, Australia), which uses tissue autofluorescence; (iv) the *Colpoprobe*™ (MediSpectra, Lexington, MA, USA), which uses autofluorescence and optical backscattering; (v) the *Multimodal Hyperspectral Imaging (MHI) System*™ (SpectRx, Norcross, GA, USA), which uses autofluorescence and direct reflectance; (vi) the *Trimodal Spectroscopy (TMS) System* (Georgakoudi *et al.*, 2002), which uses autofluorescence, direct reflectance and backscattering; and (vii) the FORTH (Crete, Greece) device (Balas *et al.*, 1999; Balas, 2001), which uses optical backscattering.

The four systems that use tissue autofluorescence (Cerviscan, Colpoprobe, the MHI system and the TMS system) appear to be primarily targeted towards use during colposcopy. They provide a spectral map of the cervix, enabling precise visualisation of lesion morphology, so that the colposcopist can pinpoint the optimal location for biopsy and improve the colposcopic grading of lesions. Because differences in fluorescence emission spectra from normal and abnormal cervical tissues appear to increase in the presence of acetic acid (Agrawal *et al.*, 1999), the potential performance of fluorescence-based devices in a screening situation (without acetic acid applica-

tion) is unclear. To date, the clinical assessment of fluorescence devices has focused on women with previous abnormal Pap smear results referred for colposcopic evaluation.

TruScreen

The TruScreen device uses a combination of directly reflected light, backscattered light and electrical decay curves as biosensors for a general screening instrument (Quek *et al.*, 1998; Coppleson *et al.*, 2000). The device incorporates optical fibre technology and electrical connections in a probe-shaped handpiece (Fig. 27.4) and is designed to be used without the application of aqueous acetic acid. The 5-mm-diameter distal tip of the handpiece is covered with a disposable tissue-contacting element designed to protect against cross-infection and applied to the cervix. Tissue is illuminated at four discrete wavelengths in the visible and infrared regions of the spectrum. In addition, the system incorporates electrical measurements of decay curves. In general, the rate of electrical decay is inversely proportional to the degree of abnormality on the cervix. Pulses of 0.8 V are applied for 100 μs, and the electrical decay curve is assessed by sampling the magnitude at various points and by integrating the area underneath the curve. Figure 27.5 shows sample electrical decay curves for normal and abnormal cervical tissue types. These electrical measurements are complementary to the optical signals also measured by the TruScreen system.

The biosensor measurements are repeated at the rate of 14 times per second, and various parameters are extracted from each of the biosensor signals. The information is filtered, sampled and processed by a microcomputer within a portable console to extract the parameters of greatest value for tissue discrimination. Several hundred parameters are processed per second, and a tissue discrimination algorithm classifies the tissue on the basis of the values of the multiple parameters. Real-time feedback in the form of indicator lights on the back of the handpiece guides the operator through the examination process, which involves moving the tip of the handpiece

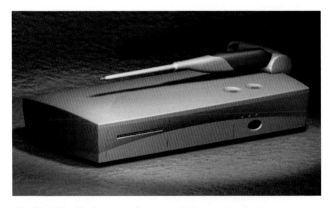

Fig. 27.4 The TruScreen real-time cervical screening device.

Table 27.1 Comparison of real-time device technologies.

	Device configuration			Biosensors			
Real-time device (RTD) technology	Requires application of acetic acid solution?	Includes vaginal probe in contact with cervix?	Other system components	Tissue fluorescence	Direct reflectance	Optical backscattering	Electrical measurements
(1) TruScreen	No	Yes — 5-mm-diameter probe, covered by a disposable cervical contact sensor element. Probe is moved across cervix	Probe is connected to a portable console which prints out a screening result	–	+	+	+
(2) University of Sheffield device	No	Yes — 5-mm-diameter cervical contact probe. Probe is moved across cervix	Probe is connected to a computer	–	–		+
(3) Cerviscan	Yes	Yes — 25-mm-diameter probe, covered by a disposable cervical contact element. Probe fits over cervical area	Probe is connected to a xenon arc lamp light source and a computer	+	–	–	–
(4) Colpoprobe	Yes	No — non-cervical contact optical head accessory mounted on a colposcope	Optical head is connected to a laser fluorescent light source and a computer	+	–	+	–
(5) MHI system	Yes	Yes — cervical contact probe mounted on a customised vaginal speculum. Probe fits over cervical area	Probe is connected to a xenon arc lamp light source and a computer	+	+	–	–
(6) TMS system	Yes	Yes — flexible optical cervical contact probe	Fast excitation–emission matrix (EEM) instrument used to record optical spectra. Data currently processed 'offline'	+	+	+	–
(7) FORTH device	Yes	No — non-cervical contact colposcope-mounted imaging system	Imaging system consists of a halogen light source, a ring fibre-optic bundle, a camera and a computer	–	–	+	–

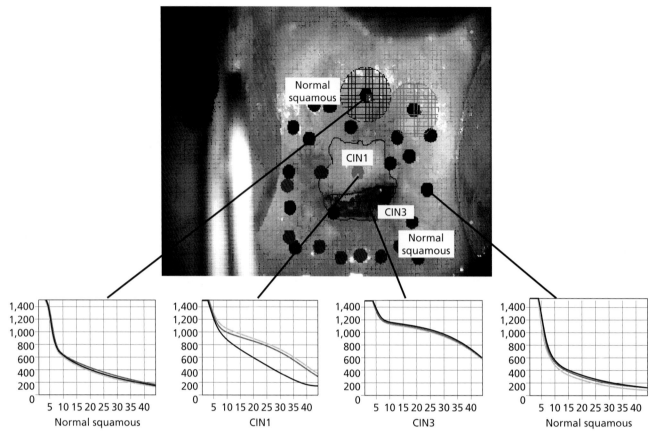

Fig. 27.5 Electrical decay curves. Electrical decay curves vary between normal and abnormal cervical tissue.

across the cervix and is performed in approximately 1 minute. When the examination is complete, the operator presses a button on the handpiece and the device prints out the final screening result. Difficulties in interpretation are resolved because the device provides a simple print-out at the end of the examination which records the screening result. This level of automation should allow the utilisation of the technology on a widespread basis, without the need for expert physicians. Therefore, this system is particularly suited to screening applications.

The first major clinical evaluation of TruScreen assessed the ability of a prototypic version of the device accurately to detect invasive cervical cancer (Singer, 1997). The trial, conducted in Recife, Brazil, involved two groups of women. Group 1 comprised 41 women presenting with symptomatic invasive cervical carcinoma of various stages. Group 2 comprised 45 women with a negative colposcopy and negative Papanicolaou smear. Histological analysis for the study was performed by a local pathologist and subsequently reviewed by an independent expert pathologist in the UK. The patient-level sensitivity and specificity of the prototypic TruScreen

device for histologically confirmed invasive cancer was found to be 98% and 91% respectively.

A subsequent clinical study examined the performance of TruScreen as a screening adjunct to the Pap smear for the detection of CIN (Singer *et al.*, 2003). Analysis on a patient-level basis was performed on a group of 651 subjects, the majority of whom were recruited from the general population. However, in order to enrich the study with a higher proportion of subjects with disease, 25% of subjects were recruited from the colposcopy clinic population. The sensitivities for histologically confirmed CIN2/3 lesions by TruScreen, Pap and TruScreen/Pap combined were 70%, 69% and 93% respectively. For histologically reported CIN1, the sensitivities of the TruScreen, Pap and combined test were 67%, 45% and 87%. The corresponding specificities were 81%, 95% and 80%, demonstrating that a loss of specificity was associated with the improvement in sensitivity in a screening setting. The improvement in sensitivity for the combined test compared with the Pap smear alone was statistically significant, and therefore this device is potentially a viable real-time adjunct to the Pap smear for cervical screening.

The University of Sheffield device

Electrical measurements have been used in a prototypical probing device for cervical screening, which utilises electrical impedance changes at eight frequencies of measurements (Brown *et al.*, 2000). The 5-mm-diameter probe incorporates four gold electrodes and is applied directly to the cervix, without the application of aqueous acetic acid. The electrical impedance depends on both tissue resistance and capacitance, and its variation with frequency depends on the underlying tissue composition. The tissue resistance depends primarily upon extracellular and intracellular current flow, whereas the capacitance is predominantly determined by cell membrane structure. In a group of 124 women referred to the colposcopy clinic for the evaluation of high-grade abnormal smears, high sensitivities and specificities for abnormal tissue were demonstrated on a tissue spot-level basis. When results for all tissue spot measurements taken on each woman were combined to determine a final patient-level result, the device was found to have sensitivity of 75% and specificity of 71%, although these results were obtained after excluding spot measurements with colposcopically identified columnar epithelium or immature metaplasia. Further clinical results on a general screening population are necessary to fully assess the potential of this electrical biosensor device for cervical screening.

Cerviscan

The Cerviscan cervical imaging system involves a large 25-mm-diameter probe which fits over the cervical area and is covered by a disposable tissue-contacting element. The system is used after the application of aqueous acetic acid and utilises a xenon lamp with bypass filters to excite the cervical tissue at multiple frequencies in the ultraviolet and visible light regions of the spectrum. The spectral data are processed and used to construct an 'abnormality index', which can be used to classify the region as either normal or abnormal. From the spectrally derived classification at each point on the cervix, a full-field image is constructed. A six-centre trial was performed to assess the performance of prototypes of the Cerviscan in women with a previously abnormal Pap smear test (Drezek *et al.*, 2003b). In 97 subjects, the device achieved sensitivity of 88% and specificity of 80% for distinguishing high-grade lesions from low-grade or normal lesions. A recent publication (Nath *et al.*, 2004) summarised a multicentre phase II screening trial that was primarily conducted to test data collection and patient examination procedures. A fibre-optic device measured fluorescence, excitation–emission matrices at one to three cervical sites in 58 women. A multivariate analysis algorithm correctly identified squamous normal tissue in 99% but columnar normal tissue in only 7%. It was felt that 'the study was successful as a pilot trial; the current algorithm for diagnosis identified squamous normal tissue very accurately but did less well for columnar tissue'. The authors believed that the 'screening trial of fluorescence and reflectance spectroscopy was successful', but obviously further clinical trials must be performed before the role of this device in a screening situation is determined.

Colpoprobe

Another real-time device technology using tissue fluorescence as a biosensor is the Colpoprobe, which incorporates a non-cervical contact laser fluorescence system attached to a colposcope and is used after the application of aqueous acetic acid (Burke *et al.*, 1999). The optical head attachment on the colposcope is connected via a set of optical fibres to a 337-nm ultraviolet laser light source, a spectral measurement device and a computer for analysis of the signals. The system also uses backscattered white light as a secondary biosensor. In a study involving women referred for evaluation of an abnormal smear, the system was found to perform at a sensitivity of 91% and specificity of 93% for discriminating between CIN2/3 lesions and normal squamous tissue. For distinguishing CIN1 from normal tissue, the sensitivity was 86% and specificity was 87% (Nordstrom *et al.*, 2001).

Recently, Huh *et al.* (2004) described the *in vivo* optical detection of high-grade epithelial disease on the whole cervix with the non-contact stereoscopic device. A total of 604 women were scanned with the device, which collected intrinsic fluorescence and broadband white light spectra and video images during routine colposcopic examination at six clinical centres. A statistically significant data set has been developed of intrinsic fluorescence and white light-induced cervical tissue spectra that was correlated to expert histopathological results. More than 10 000 measurements were taken, and the algorithm performance, according to the authors, demonstrated a sensitivity of approximately 90%. Using the multivariate classification algorithm, optical detection predicted 33% more high-grade epithelial lesions than did corresponding colposcopic examination. These encouraging results need to be confirmed in larger studies.

Multimodal hyperspectral imaging (MHI) system

A third device using tissue fluorescence is the multimodal hyperspectral imaging (MHI) system (Ferris *et al.*, 2001). A large-diameter cervical contact probe is applied over the cervix and mounted to a customised vaginal speculum. The probe is connected via optical fibres to a xenon arc lamp source for cervical illumination at multiple wavelengths, and also to a filter assembly, spectrograph and charge-coupled device (CCD) camera for detection of emitted and reflected signals. The device is designed to be used after the application of aqueous acetic acid. In addition to the fluorescent response, the device measures reflected light from the tissue, facilitating the detection of structural changes. The examination time is approximately 6 minutes, during which time multiple spectral measurements of the cervix are made.

Clinical studies of the MHI system focus on women with a previous abnormal Pap smear result or women referred for treatment or follow-up after treatment. In a study of 111 women performed on an initial model, the sensitivity of the system for the detection of high-grade CIN was compared with that of a Pap smear performed during colposcopy, with the threshold of detection for MHI adjusted so that the specificity matched that of the smear (Ferris *et al.*, 2001). The sensitivity and specificity of the MHI system were found to be 97% and 70%, respectively, on a patient-level basis. This result compares favourably with that of the Pap smear performed during colposcopy, which was found to have a sensitivity and specificity of 72% and 70%.

Trimodal spectroscopy (TMS) system

The trimodal spectroscopy (TMS) system uses an optical contact probe designed to measure fluorescence after excitation at 10 wavelengths, diffuse reflectance and scattered light (Georgakoudi *et al.*, 2002; Drezek *et al.*, 2003b). A feasibility study in 44 women referred for an abnormal Pap smear found that the information obtained from the three biosensors has the potential to improve disease detection (Georgakoudi *et al.*, 2002). Real-time operation of the processing software to combine information from the three biosensors has not yet been reported.

The FORTH/Crete device

The FORTH/Crete device uses the intensity of backscattered light to perform cervical imaging over a 10-minute period after the application of aqueous acetic acid (Balas *et al.*, 1999; Balas, 2001). The non-contact device does not incorporate a vaginal probe. The colposcope-mounted system is connected to a halogen light source, a ring fibre-optic bundle, a camera and a computer. The system uses digital processing to perform image contrast enhancement of acetowhite epithelium and to correct for glare produced by direct surface reflection off the epithelium. Ten images at different frequencies across the visual spectrum are captured and updated every 10 seconds as the examination progresses. The final result is a complete data set of the intensity of backscattered light captured for a range of incident light frequencies over time. Therefore, the time-dependent changes in aqueous acetic acid uptake are standardised and classified. These changes form the basis of a quantitative dynamic assessment of the interaction between the cervical epithelium and the applied acetic acid marker. The greatest contrast enhancement between normal and abnormal epithelium was found to be at a spectral band of approximately 525 nm. In this frequency band, absorption by the vascular plexus underlying the epithelium is almost complete, thus removing a source of noise for the epithelial backscattering measurements. In addition to assisting the colposcopist in mapping lesions and choosing the biopsy sites, this system should facilitate diagnostic colposcopy, whereby a lesion is classified and graded before performing a biopsy.

CONCLUSIONS

In vivo real-time technologies use biosensors that are sensitive to the underlying pathophysiological changes associated with cervical disease. Optical biosensors measure variations in tissue fluorescent emission, reflectance or backscattering, following illumination at multiple frequencies. Electrical biosensors rely on changes in electrical decay curves or tissue impedance, which are both related to the dielectric properties of tissue structures. Real-time instruments can be divided into two main categories — those designed for screening and those designed for cervical diagnostic applications. In general, real-time technologies that do not rely on the application of aqueous acetic acid solution and do not involve full-field imaging are more suited to screening applications. Two such technologies, the TruScreen and the prototypic University of Sheffield device, have been reviewed. Diagnostic devices provide an enhanced view of the cervix for the colposcopist, with the biosensor data used to supply information about lesion morphology and tissue structure. Five such devices, the Cerviscan, the Colpoprobe, the MHI system, the TMS system and the FORTH/Crete device, have been reviewed. The screening potential of these image-based real-time technologies is yet to be realised. However, several practical problems would need to be resolved before imaging-based real-time devices would be suitable for screening applications. These problems include the requirement for aqueous acetic acid application before the real-time device examination, the time required for acetowhite effects to be maximised, the time required for imaging (up to several minutes in some cases) and the interpretation of the result by a non-specialist screener. A practical screening test must involve an examination time of 1 minute or less. Furthermore, the eventual application of imaging-based real-time devices to screening must be assessed through clinical studies conducted in screening populations, which examine the performance of the device in terms of the overall accuracy of assessment of each woman, rather than concentrating only upon specific tissue locations.

New developments in sensor technology and expert system processing have made it possible to automate the process of identifying abnormal cervical tissue. This automation is expected to generate benefits in terms of increased standardisation and quality control of the screening and diagnostic process. In addition, *in vivo* real-time methods provide immediate feedback to the clinician, facilitating the discussion of management strategies with patients and potentially minimising the number of follow-up visits required. It is expected that these key benefits will drive the further technological development of real-time devices, and that a substantial body of clinical data will emerge on the performance of these systems. Providing that their potential can be realised, real-time devices are capable of significantly improving the accuracy and standardisation of cervical screening and diagnosis.

ACKNOWLEDGEMENT

The authors would like to thank Professor Malcolm Coppleson for critical review of an early draft of this chapter.

GLOSSARY

Autofluorescence Fluorescence resulting from endogenous elements within tissue and not dependent on the administration of contrast dyes.

Backscattering The process whereby tissue is illuminated and scattered light travels back towards the illumination source. Backscattering results from one or more interactions between the incident light and scattering centres within the tissue.

Biosensor A measurement system applied to tissue which has the property of varying as the tissue type changes.

Capacitance A measure of the ability of tissue to store an electric charge.

Cervical intraepithelial neoplasia (CIN) A histological classification of cervical premalignant lesions, graded in terms of severity from CIN1 to CIN3.

Dielectric properties The dielectric properties of a tissue segment are related to the additive effects of local resistances and capacitances associated with various intracellular and extracellular zones.

Direct (Fresnel) surface reflectance Reflected light resulting from a step change in refractive index between two media, which may be tissue and air or varying structures within the tissue.

Expert system A system designed to mimic the operation of human diagnostic expert(s), using a software-implemented classifier that 'learns' the correct classifications through a 'training' process.

Fluorescence The emission of light when tissue is illuminated.

Impedance The impedance of tissue is dependent on its electrical capacitance and resistance.

Infrared (IR) light Longer wavelength light with an approximate wavelength range of 700 nm to 1 mm.

Patient-level assessment An assessment of device performance on the basis of overall accuracy in identifying women harbouring abnormal lesions. This is contrasted with spot-level assessment.

Real-time devices Automated devices for cervical assessment that provide immediate feedback to the clinician. Real-time devices use biosensors to measure cervical tissue *in vivo* and process the results to classify cervical tissue using computerised analysis.

Resistance The opposition offered by tissue to the flow of electric current.

Spot-level assessment An assessment of device performance in the accurate classification of local tissue areas or 'spots'. This is contrasted with patient-level assessment.

Tissue classification algorithm Processing software designed to convert and condense biosensor signals into a clinically relevant output.

Ultraviolet (UV) light Shorter wavelength light with an approximate wavelength range of 100–400 nm.

Visible light Intermediate wavelength light with an approximate wavelength range of 400–700 nm.

REFERENCES

Agrawal A, Utzinger U, Brookner C *et al.* (1999) Fluorescence spectroscopy of the cervix: influence of acetic acid, cervical mucus, and vaginal medications. *Lasers in Surgery and Medicine* 25: 237–249.

Alfano RR, Tata DB, Cordero J *et al.* (1984) Laser induced fluorescence spectroscopy from native cancerous and normal tissue. *IEEE Journal of Quantum Electronics* QE-20: 1507–1511.

Anderson MC (1985) The pathology of cervical cancer. *Clinics in Obstetrics and Gynaecology* 12 (1): 87–119.

Anderson RR (1991) Polarized light examination and photography of the skin. *Archives of Dermatology* 127 (7): 1000–1005.

Arifler D, Guillaud M, Carraro A *et al.* (2003) Light scattering from normal and dysplastic cervical cells at different epithelial depths: finite-difference time-domain modeling with a perfectly matched layer boundary condition. *Journal of Biomedical Optics* 8: 484–494.

Balas C (2001) A novel optical imaging method for the early detection, quantitative grading, and mapping of cancerous and precancerous lesions of cervix. *IEEE Transactions on Biomedical Engineering* 48 (1): 96–104.

Balas CJ, Themelis GC, Prokopakis EP *et al.* (1999) In vivo detection and staging of epithelial dysplasias and malignancies based on the quantitative assessment of acetic acid–tissue interaction kinetics. *Journal of Photochemistry and Photobiology* 53: 153–157.

Bayazitoglu A, Smith JW, Johnson TR (1992) A diagnostic system that learns from experience. *Proceedings of the Annual Symposium of Computing in Applied Medical Care* 685–689.

Belinson J, Qiao Y, Pretorius R *et al.* (2001) Shanxi Province cervical cancer screening study: a cross-sectional comparative trial of multiple techniques to detect cervical neoplasia. *Gynecologic Oncology* 83 (2): 439–444.

Bogaards A, Aalders MC, Zeyl CC *et al.* (2002) Localization and staging of cervical intraepithelial neoplasia using double ratio fluorescence imaging. *Journal of Biomedical Optics* 7 (2): 215–220.

Brookner C, Utzinger U, Follen M *et al.* (2003) Effects of biographical variables on cervical fluorescence emission spectra. *Journal of Biomedical Optics* 8: 479–483.

Brown BH, Tidy JA, Boston K *et al.* (2000) Relation between tissue structure and imposed electrical current flow in cervical neoplasia. *Lancet* 355: 892–895.

Burke L, Modell M, Niloff J *et al.* (1999) Identification of squamous intraepithelial lesions: fluorescence of cervical tissue during colposcopy. *Journal of Lower Genital Tract Disease* 3 (3): 159–162.

Coppleson M, Reid B, Skladnev V *et al.* (1994) An electronic approach to the detection of pre-cancer and cancer of the uterine cervix: a preliminary evaluation of Polarprobe. *International Journal of Gynecological Cancer* 4: 79–83.

Coppleson M, Canfell K, Skladnev V (2000) The Polarprobe—an instantaneous optoelectronic approach to cervical screening. *Continuing Medical Education Journal of Gynecological Oncology* 5: 31–38.

Department of Health UK (2001) *Colposcopy Clinics, Referrals, Treatments and Outcomes (KC65)*. Department of Health IAR No. DH999–000329.

Dhawan AP (1988) An expert system for the early detection of melanoma using knowledge-based image analysis. *Analytic Quantitative Cytology and Histology* 10 (6): 405–416.

Dhawan AP, Juvvadi S (1990) Knowledge-based analysis and understanding of medical images. *Computing Methods and Programs in Biomedicine* 33: 221–239.

Drezek R, Sokolov K, Utzinger U *et al.* (2001) Understanding the contributions of NADH and collagen to cervical tissue fluorescence spectra: modeling, measurements, and implications. *Journal of Biomedical Optics* 6 (4): 385–396.

Drezek R, Guillaud M, Collier T *et al.* (2003a) Light scattering from cervical cells throughout neoplastic progression: influence of nuclear morphology, DNA content, and chromatin texture. *Journal of Biomedical Optics* 8: 7–16.

Drezek RA, Richards-Kortum R, Brewer MA *et al.* (2003b) Optical imaging of the cervix. *Cancer* 98: 2015–2027.

Dunn A, Richards-Kortum R (1996) Three-dimensional computation of light scattering from cells. *IEEE Journal of Selected Topics in Quantum Electronics* 2 (4): 898–905.

Etherington IJ, Luesley DM, Sahfi MI *et al.* (1997) Observer variability among colposcopists from the West Midlands region. *British Journal of Obstetrics and Gynaecology* 104 (12): 1380–1384.

Ferris DG, Lawhead RA, Dickman ED *et al.* (2001) Multimodal hyperspectral imaging for the non-invasive diagnosis of cervical neoplasia. *Journal of Lower Genital Tract Disease* 5 (2): 65–72.

Frank KH, Kessler M, Appelbaum K *et al.* (1989) Measurements of angular distributions of Rayleigh and Mie scattering events in biological models. *Physics in Medicine and Biology* 34 (12): 1901–1916.

Georgakoudi I, Sheets EE, Muller MG *et al.* (2002) Trimodal spectroscopy for the detection and characterization of cervical pre-cancers *in vivo*. *American Journal of Obstetrics and Gynecology* 186: 374–382.

Gill EM, Malpica A, Alford RE *et al.* (2003) Relationship between collagen autofluorescence of the human cervix and menopausal status. *Photochemistry and Photobiology* 77: 653–658.

Howells SL, Maxwell RJ, Peet AC *et al.* (1992) An investigation of tumor 1H nuclear magnetic resonance spectra by the application of chemometric techniques. *Magnetic Resonance Medicine* 28 (2): 214–236.

Huh WK, Cestero RM, Garcia FA *et al.* (2004) Optical detection of high-grade cervical intraepithelial neoplasia *in vivo*: results of a 604-patient study *American Journal of Obstetrics and Gynecology* 190: 1249–1257.

Leung KM, Chan WY, Hui PK (1994) Invasive squamous cell carcinoma and cervical intraepithelial neoplasia III of uterine cervix. Morphologic differences other than stromal invasion. *American Journal of Clinical Pathology* 101 (4): 508–513.

Nanda K, McCrory DC, Myers ER *et al.* (2000) Accuracy of the Papanicolaou test in screening for and follow-up of cervical cytologic abnormalities: a systematic review. *Annals of Internal Medicine* 132: 810–819.

Nath A, Rivoire K, Chang S *et al.* (2004) A pilot study for a screening trial of cervical fluorescent spectroscopy. *International Journal of Gynecological Cancer* 14: 1097–1107.

Nordstrom RJ, Burke L, Niloff JM *et al.* (2001) Identification of cervical intraepithelial neoplasia (CIN) using UV-excited fluorescence

and diffuse-reflectance tissue spectroscopy. *Lasers in Surgery and Medicine* 29: 118–127.

Porter JF, Kingsland LC, Lindberg DA *et al.* (1988) The AI/RHEUM knowledge-based computer consultant system in rheumatology. Performance in the diagnosis of 59 connective tissue disease patients from Japan. *Arthritis and Rheumatism* 31 (2): 219–226.

Quek SC, Mould T, Canfell K *et al.* (1998) The Polarprobe — emerging technology for cervical cancer screening. *Annals of the Academy of Medicine Singapore* 27: 717–721.

Quinn M, Babb P, Jones J *et al.* (1999) Effect of screening on incidence of and mortality from cancer of cervix in England: evaluation based on routinely collected statistics. *British Medical Journal* 318: 904–908.

Ramanujam N, Mitchell MF, Mahadevan A *et al.* (1994a) In vivo diagnosis of cervical intraepithelial neoplasia using 337-nm-excited laser-induced fluorescence. *Proceedings of the National Academy of Sciences of the USA* 91 (21): 10193–10197.

Ramanujam N, Mitchell MF, Mahadevan A *et al.* (1994b) Fluorescence spectroscopy: a diagnostic tool for cervical intraepithelial neoplasia (CIN). *Gynecologic Oncology* 52: 31–38.

Ramanujam N, Mitchell MF, Mahadevan A *et al.* (1996) Spectroscopic diagnosis of cervical intraepithelial neoplasia (CIN) *in vivo* using laser-induced fluorescence spectra at multiple excitation wavelengths. *Lasers in Surgery and Medicine* 19 (1): 63–74.

Richards-Kortum R, Sevick-Muraca E (1996) Quantitative optical spectroscopy for tissue diagnosis. *Annual Reviews of Physical Chemistry* 47: 555–606.

Rivoire K, Nath A, Cox D *et al.* (2004) The effects of repeated spectroscopic pressure measurements on fluorescence intensity in the cervix. *American Journal of Obstetrics and Gynecology* 191 (5): 1606–1617.

Roa RL (1995) Clinical laboratory: separation and spectral methods. In: Bronzino JD (ed.) *The Biomedical Engineering Handbook*. Boca Raton, FL: CRC/IEEE Press, pp. 1241–1248.

Singer A (1997) Clinical experience with the usage of the Polarprobe. Proceedings of the EUROGIN Third International Congress, 24–27 March 1997, Paris. Paris: European Research Organisation on Genital Infection and Neoplasia.

Singer A, Coppleson M, Canfell K *et al.* (2003) A real time optoelectronic device as an adjunct to the Pap smear for cervical screening: a multicenter evaluation. *International Journal of Gynecological Cancer* 13: 804–811.

Skehan M, Soutter WP, Lim K *et al.* (1990) Reliability of colposcopy and directed punch biopsy. *British Journal of Obstetrics and Gynaecology* 97 (9): 811–816.

Thornton BS, Hung WT, Irving J (1991) Relaxation distribution function of intracellular dielectric zones as an indicator of tumorous transition of living cells. *IMA Journal of Mathematical Applications in Medicine and Biology* 8 (2): 95–106.

Walker DC, Brown BH, Blackett AD *et al.* (2003) A study of the morphological parameters of cervical squamous epithelium. *Physiological Measurement* 24: 121–135.

Wunderman I, Coppleson M, Skladnev V *et al.* (1995) Polarprobe: a precancer detection instrument. *Journal of Gynecological Technology* 1 (2): 105–109.

Tumour markers in cervical cancer — I

John J. O'Leary, Katharine Astbury and Walter Prendiville

INTRODUCTION

Cervical cancer is the second most common malignancy in women worldwide. Each year, there are approximately 400 000 newly diagnosed cases and 250 000 deaths from the disease. Over the past 50 years, the introduction of cervical screening programmes, involving the use of the Papanicolaou (Pap) smear, has led to a dramatic reduction in cervical cancer incidence and death among women in the developed world. Human papillomavirus (HPV) is the major aetiological factor in the genesis of cervical neoplasia. Its role as a tumour biomarker in the management of these conditions will be discussed in this chapter as well as that of other products deemed to qualify as tumour markers.

HUMAN PAPILLOMAVIRUS (HPV)

The clinical utility of oncogenic high-risk (HR) HPV DNA testing

Before addressing the science of biomarkers for cervical precancer, it is worth considering the clinical significance of detecting 'high-risk' oncogenic HPV types. Figure 28A.1 details the powerful association existing between women testing positive for HPV and the lifetime risk of cervical cancer.

Three large studies, i.e. the ALTS Group (2003) trial in the USA, the HART study in the UK (Cuzick, 2002; Cuzick *et al.*, 2003) and the ALTS-like study in Germany (Petry *et al.*, 2003), have produced large comparative data sets on which to base guidelines for the appropriate clinical usage of HPV testing. There are circumstances where the evidence in favour of using the test is convincing [e.g. in the evaluation of the borderline nuclear activity smear (ASCUS equivalent) and after treatment for cervical intraepithelial neoplasia (CIN)], and there are circumstances where to use the test may be counterproductive (primary screening of young women). The question of whether the test should be used in older women for primary screening is more difficult because the decision rests not just on the particular qualities and characteristics of the test but also on its relative cost in a particular community (vs. colposcopy or cytology), as well as the prevalence of HPV and the acceptability of the test to the community in question. Also, an educational programme will be necessary wherever it is brought into use. Finally, there is the question of how the result is expressed.

Clinical usage of HPV testing

High-risk HPV (HR HPV) DNA testing as a primary screening tool in conjunction with or as an alternative to cytology

The effectiveness of systematic call and recall cervical screening

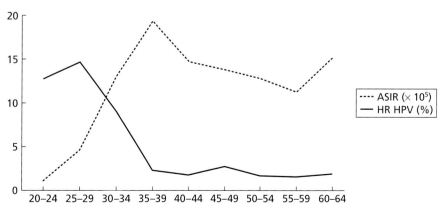

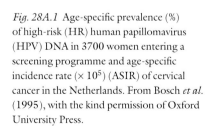

Fig. 28A.1 Age-specific prevalence (%) of high-risk (HR) human papillomavirus (HPV) DNA in 3700 women entering a screening programme and age-specific incidence rate ($\times 10^5$) (ASIR) of cervical cancer in the Netherlands. From Bosch *et al.* (1995), with the kind permission of Oxford University Press.

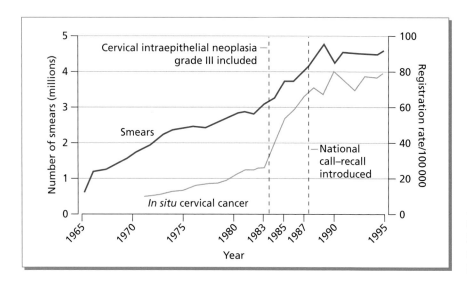

Fig. 28A.2 Age-standardised incidence of invasive cancer and coverage of screening, England 1971–1995. From Quinn *et al.* (1999) with the kind permission of the BMJ Publishing Group.

in order to detect (and then manage) precancerous lesions has been widely accepted as an effective intervention in many countries, such as England and Wales (see Chapter 25). The ability of screening programmes to reduce the incidence of, and mortality from, cervical cancer is now well established. Cervical cancer is still a leading cause of death worldwide but, in the developed world, where screening has been comprehensive, dramatic falls in death rates have been achieved. Although relatively late in starting a systematic screening programme, the UK has implemented a highly organised and deeply penetrative system. The results of such an organised and comprehensive approach have been dramatic and are described in Chapter 25. Since the introduction of the nationwide scheme in 1988, there has been a steady and continuing fall in both incidence and death rates from cervical cancer. Over the 15-year duration of the scheme, the number of women dying from cervical cancer has fallen by 60%, despite the increasing rates of CIN. Maximum protection has occurred relative to depth of penetration in the community (see Fig. 28A.2).

Limitations of cytology
It might seem foolish to tamper with such a successful programme, but cytology has relatively poor individual test sensitivity (Arbyn *et al.*, 2004). In a recent report, commissioned by the US Agency for Healthcare Research and Quality (1999) (Fig. 28A.3a and b), Myers *et al.* (2000) found an individual conventional smear's sensitivity to be 51%.

Even the recent development of liquid-based cytological testing has not helped to increase the sensitivity of cytological screening. Disappointing rates for sensitivity using this technology range from 61% to 95% (Hutchinson *et al.*, 1999; Clavel *et al.*, 2001; Kulasingam *et al.*, 2002). Also, glandular dysplasia is less amenable to cytological screening than squamous disease. Krane *et al.* (2001) have reported

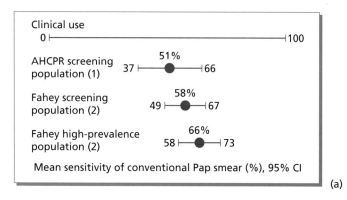

(a)

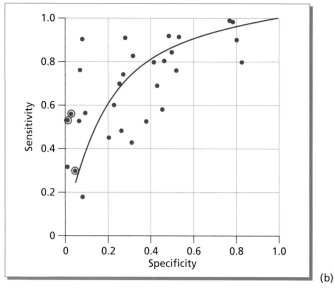

(b)

Fig. 28A.3 (a) Mean sensitivity of conventional Pap smear (%), 95% CI. (1) Agency for Healthcare Policy and Research (AHCPR) report: Evaluation of cervical cytology (1999), Durham, NC: Duke University. (2) Fahey *et al.* (1995). (b) ROC curve for cytology. Reproduced from the Duke University AHCPR Report (1999).

recently that the sensitivity of the Papanicolaou smear for the detection of adenocarcinoma ranges between 45% and 76%. This may be related to the difficulty in sufficiently sampling the entire endocervical canal, where the majority of glandular lesions occur.

Fortunately, the natural history of CIN is slow, and cytology's limitations are to some extent offset by a screening programme's repetitive nature. Also, even with compliant screening practice, some cancers will develop. Endocervical adenocarcinomas appear to be disproportionately common in women with cancer who have had adequate smear histories (Colgan *et al.*, 2001). Also, the expense of cytology-based screening, along with the difficulty of procuring adequate numbers of properly trained cytology screening technicians, may be partly responsible for the fact that many countries with rising cervical cancer rates have not yet established systematic programmes (including the UK's nearest neighbours France and Ireland).

With the limitations of exfoliative cytology obvious, the question has to be asked whether HR HPV DNA testing can be considered as an alternative or as an adjunctive technique to cytology in an endeavour to improve its sensitivity and overall performance. There are three main usages that have been proposed for HR HPV DNA testing, and these will be discussed below:

In an attempt to improve the sensitivity of cytological screening. In the most recent IARC monograph (2005), the consensus among experts was that:

> Primary screening of women older than 30 years of age utilising HPV testing yields, on average, about 10% to 20% greater sensitivity and 10% lower specificity than cytology (either conventional or liquid based). In some studies the combination of cytology and HPV testing (as independent or reflex testing) attained very high sensitivity and negative predictive value (approaching 100%), a testing combination with such a high predictive value could allow screening intervals to be increased, e.g. from the minimum of 3 years up to 5 years or longer, depending on the population and risk profile.

In talking about the combination of different modalities such as HR HPV DNA testing with cytology, it further states that:

> Adding a sensitive detection method for High Risk HPV DNA to cytology yields a substantial increase in test sensitivity and negative predictive value for CIN3 or cancer and probably allows an increase in screening intervals.

In the conclusions to their report, the experts state that:

> There is sufficient evidence that testing for human papillomavirus infection as a primary screening modality can reduce cervical cancer incidence and mortality rates.

Persistent oncogenic HPV infection is necessary for the development of cervical cancer (Wright and Schiffman, 2003). Fortunately, in those women who develop cancer, they do so many years after initial HPV recognition, and HPV negativity has been shown to allow for a far longer interscreening interval than that recommended with cytology programmes (Kulasingam *et al.*, 2002). If a combined HPV/cervical smear test were used, the evidence suggests a near 100% negative predictive value. The medicolegal protection afforded by this for any programme is apparent.

This debate is likely to continue. HR HPV DNA testing is also imperfect. A high proportion of young women, usually under 30–35 years of age will test positive for HPV (15–45%). The great majority of these women who are HPV positive are at very low risk of developing cervical cancer as their HPV will be innocuously cleared (Sherman *et al.*, 2003; Clavel *et al.*, 2004). Unless careful consideration is given to the potential psychological damage (see Chapter 23) associated with informing a large number of women that they have a 'cancer-causing virus', the introduction of HPV testing into primary screening of all women independent of age is unlikely to be broadly welcomed. Its selective use in women over 30 has real value.

The value of HR HPV DNA testing as a primary screening method is also described in detail in Chapter 26.

In the evaluation of the borderline nuclear abnormality (BNA) or ASCUS smear

While CIN3 occurs in less than 1% of all women tested in the UK, 6 or 7% will be reported with a BNA. This category roughly equates to the ASCUS term of the Bethesda system used in the USA, where over US$2.5 billion dollars are spent annually investigating this report. This equates to more than that spent on CIN2–3! Women expect dichotomy in their test result. The borderline abnormality or ASCUS smear report is the antithesis of this and represents a difficult clinical circumstance for both patient and clinician. Most BNA smears will revert to normal but a small number harbour covert CIN2–3.

Present management strategies: cytology dependent
A number of management strategies are available. Repeat cytology, usually at 6-monthly intervals until three successive smears are negative, has a poor sensitivity/specificity profile (Manos *et al.*, 1999; Shlay *et al.*, 2000; Lin *et al.*, 2000; Solomon *et al.*, 2001). Traditionally, women with persistent BNA cytologically have been referred for colposcopic evaluation. But colposcopy is relatively expensive and has poor interobserver variability at the lower end of the spectrum of CIN (Etherington *et al.*, 1997) even when utilising directed biopsies (Buxton *et al.*, 1991).

Place of HR HPV DNA testing
Against this background, HPV testing has some advantages.

The test will not distinguish between transient unimportant HPV presence and the persistent significant positivity. However, its real utility again rests with its negativity, with there being a very high negative predictive value of between 97% and 100%. In the large ALTS trial (2003), 3488 women with ASCUS were evaluated in a randomised controlled trial (RCT) of management strategies. HPV testing reduced the need for referral for colposcopy by 44% and had sensitivity for CIN2–3 of 96%. This compared with 44% for cytology alone. In a similar study of over 8000 women in Germany, Petry *et al.* (2003) found HPV negativity in 100% of women with high-grade CIN who had a cytological diagnosis of '*PAP I*' (roughly equates to BNA). But the trials of management in cytological abnormality are not entirely homogeneous. In attempting to better approach the truth, Arbyn *et al.* (2004) undertook a meta-analysis of RCTs investigating the comparative value of virology and cytology with ASCUS smear reports for their ability to detect high-grade CIN. After reviewing 15 studies, he attempted to collate differences in accuracy by assessing pooled ratio (HPV/cytology) sensitivities. He concluded that the Hybrid Capture 2 (HC2; Digene) method has improved accuracy (higher sensitivity and similar specificity) compared with repeat Pap smears using the threshold of ASCUS for an outcome of CIN2 or worse among women with equivocal cytology. The sensitivity of triage at higher cytology thresholds is poor.

In the follow-up of women treated for CIN (see Chapter 33)

Recommended routine

Current UK NHS clinical guidelines (NHSCSP, 2004) recommend cervical cytology at 6 and 12 months with annual cytology for a further 5 years. Colposcopy is widely used but not considered essential. In France, colposcopists are advised to perform cytology and colposcopy once at 3 months after treatment, after which cytology is advised 3-monthly for 1 year and annually thereafter. Variations on this theme are common in European and North American practice. The reason for this relatively intensive follow-up advice is that post-treatment residual or recurrent CIN is relatively common, ranging from 5% (Bigrigg *et al.*, 1990; Dobbs *et al.*, 2000) to 9% or 10% (Flannelly *et al.*, 1997; Chew *et al.*, 1999).

Risk of recurrence after treatment

Although cervical cancer is not common after treatment for CIN, Soutter *et al.* (1997) have shown that it is still five times more likely than in the population as a whole. For this reason, follow-up guidelines are indeed currently exhaustive. Fortunately, the great majority of lesions are discovered within the first 2 years of follow-up. Specific factors have been shown to be associated with an increased risk of recurrence. These include the presence of dysplasia at the endocervical margin (Mergui *et al.*, 1994; Gardeil *et al.*, 1997), age over 50 years at

treatment (Liu *et al.*, 2000; Flannelly *et al.*, 2001) and high parity (Liu *et al.*, 2000). These factors will highlight a population at relatively increased risk of having residual disease, but their absence does not confer absolute protection.

Place of HR HPV DNA testing

HPV testing has a place in the follow-up of CIN-treated women. In the Chua and Hjerpe (1997) study, there were no recurrences in women who tested HR HPV DNA negative, and 96% of those who had recurrent disease were HR HPV DNA positive. In 2001 and 2004, Paraskevaides and his group reported very similar data. In the latter publication, Paraskevaides *et al.* showed that, in 12 studies, 10 of which were prospective and two of which were case–control, HPV DNA testing after treatment predicted residual or recurrent CIN with higher sensitivity than cytology or histology of the section margins. They also showed that the specificity of the HPV DNA does not differ significantly from that of the other method, and they felt that, in future, there should be an evaluation of the role of HPV DNA typing and viral load in the follow-up of women treated for CIN. Again, it is the HR HPV DNA test's negative predictive value that is so powerful. It would seem sensible to incorporate this test in the post-treatment surveillance of women who have been treated for CIN (see Chapter 33).

HPV in the pathogenesis of cervical cancer: background to its role as a potential biomarker (see also Chapters 18 and 19)

The role of transforming genes (oncogenes) and tumour suppressor cellular mechanisms

High-risk HPV plays a pivotal role in the development of cervical cancer (Kirwan and Herrington, 2001). HPV contributes to neoplastic progression predominantly through the action of two viral oncoproteins, namely E6 and E7 (Giannoudis and Herrington, 2001). The combined expression of high-risk HPV E6 and E7 genes is necessary and sufficient for efficient immortalisation of primary squamous epithelial cells, and they are invariably expressed in HPV-positive cervical cancers (Munger and Howley, 2002). High-risk HPV E6 and E7 products interfere with critical cell cycle pathways including those governed by the tumour-suppressor proteins p53 and retinoblastoma protein (pRb). Dysregulation of these pathways results in the accumulation of DNA damage and the development of cervical cancer. The transforming functions of the viral E6 genes are mediated through their interactions with a variety of cellular suppressor proteins. These mechanisms have been covered fully in Chapters 18 and 19.

Potential biomarkers of cervical neoplasia

It can be seen that there are a number of clearly identified factors associated with the development of CIN and cervical cancer. The key to improving screening lies in the ability to develop a reliable test to identify one or more of these associated factors — either the detection of evidence of HPV infection itself or the changes effected at the RNA or protein level by infection with HPV. Thus, potential biomarkers can be divided into two categories:

1 markers that provide evidence of HPV infection;
2 host molecular markers of dyskaryosis.

Molecular markers that provide evidence of HPV infection
Positivity for high-risk HPV DNA is a marker for current or subsequent development of precursor lesions, with evidence of persistent HPV DNA being an even stronger predictive factor (Schiffman *et al.*, 2000; Bosch *et al.*, 2002; Muñoz *et al.*, 2003). The failure of conventional screening programmes to eradicate cervical cancer, a potentially preventable disease, has prompted the evaluation of the role of HPV testing in cervical cancer screening, as discussed in Chapter 26.

Methods of HPV testing A variety of methods exist for the detection, typing and quantification of HPV. To date, the most flexible and sensitive of all the HPV detection methods are the polymerase chain reaction (PCR)-based detection techniques. A variety of general or consensus HPV primers have been published, including GP5+/GP6+ (de Roda Husman *et al.*, 1995), SPF10, MYO9/11 (Perrons *et al.*, 2002) and PGMY (Coutlee *et al.*, 2002). These PCR assays allow the detection of a broad spectrum of HPV types in clinical samples using a single PCR. Once PCR amplification using consensus primers has been performed, specific HPV genotyping can be carried out using a variety of different methods. These methods include restriction fragment length polymorphisms (RFLP) analysis of consensus primer-amplified DNA and reverse hybridisation using line probe assays. Direct nucleic acid sequencing of PCR products and alignment of genomes by sequence comparisons can also be employed for HPV-specific genotyping. Real-time PCR, which is based on the detection and quantification of a fluorescent signal, can be employed for HPV viral load (VL) determination. Because PCR-based methods frequently entail the use of patented HPV sequences, the use of most PCR-based HPV detection and typing methods is limited to research.

Currently, the only HPV kit to have approval from the Food and Drug Administration (FDA) for *in vitro* diagnostic use is the Hybrid Capture 2 (HC2) test, manufactured by Digene Corporation Inc. (Gaithersburg, MD, USA; see Chapter 26). The HC2 test provides a positive or negative test result at a threshold of approximately 1 pg/mL. This assay employs HPV genotype-specific RNA probes, which bind to DNA targets. Hybrids, consisting of target HPV bound to RNA probes, are bound or 'captured' by antibodies recognising RNA–DNA hybrids. The addition of a second antibody tagged with alkaline phosphatase allows detection of the bound hybrid

using a chemiluminescence detection system. Within the HC2 system, genotype-specific HPV probes are mixed to form low-risk (6, 11, 42, 43, 44) and high/intermediate-risk (16, 18, 31, 33, 35, 39, 45, 51, 52, 56, 58, 59 and 68) HPV cocktails. The HC2 system provides an easy to use method, allowing triage of patients with HPV infection into low- and high-risk groups for the development of cervical dysplasia (Hubbard *et al.*, 2003). However, the HC2 test has some limitations including the inability to identify specific HPV types or mixed HPV infections. However, in clinical practice, the deficiencies do not significantly interfere with the management of the patient. In the United States, the Digene HC2 test is approved for use as an adjunct to the Papanicolaou test in cervical cancer screening rather than as a stand-alone screening test.

HPV mRNA testing as a marker of cervical dyskaryosis The incorporation of HPV DNA testing into primary screening remains controversial. While HPV testing shows high sensitivity in the detection of high-grade CIN, it has low specificity. This is because the vast majority of HPV infections are transient and, although they frequently produce temporal cytological changes, these are clinically non-significant. Worldwide, 50–60% of women contract an HPV infection during their lifetime. However, only 10–20% of such HPV infections become persistent and contribute to the development of high-grade precancerous lesions or cervical cancer (Ho *et al.*, 1995; Remmink *et al.*, 1995). This is particularly relevant to young women in their teens and 20s. It is possible that widespread use of HPV DNA testing will result in the classification of large numbers of women as being at risk even though their infections are likely to be transient. Such misclassification would result in overtreatment of lesions, unnecessary expenditure and considerable anxiety to patients. The persistent activity of HPV E6 and E7 oncogenes is a necessary prerequisite for the development and progression of high-grade cervical lesions and cervical cancer. Therefore, testing for HPV oncogenic activity rather than simply the presence of HPV DNA may be a more relevant clinical indicator for the development of cervical lesions and cervical cancer. The detection of HPV E6/E7 messenger RNA (mRNA) is an indicator of HPV oncogenic activity and may be used as a clinically predictive marker to identify women at risk of developing high-grade cervical dysplastic lesions and cervical carcinoma. HPV mRNA can be detected using the PreTect HPV-Proofer kit (NorChip, Norway). The HPV-Proofer kit is a molecular test kit based on real-time NASBA (nucleic acid sequence-based hybridisation) technology, which detects the presence of high-risk HPV types 16, 18, 31, 33 and 45. Although promising, there is to date only very limited information on its use in clinical practice, and its eventual role has yet to be defined. No large major clinical trials have been reported as yet using this technology.

Host molecular markers of cervical dyskaryosis

As mentioned previously, HPV infection is manifested by changes in the expression level of several host cell cycle regulatory proteins. Such differentially expressed host proteins and nucleic acids may have a role as 'biomarkers' of dysplastic cells. It is hoped that these biomarkers can be used in conjunction with conventional screening programmes to enhance diagnostic accuracy and reproducibility. Investigation of potential biomarkers may also help to unravel new pathways involved in the HPV-mediated pathogenesis of cervical dyskaryosis. The use of specific molecular biomarkers will also allow comparison of the efficacy of virus-like particle (VLP) vaccines and other HPV vaccine approaches in the future (Frazer, 2002; Fausch *et al.*, 2003).

To date, a wide array of molecular markers has been evaluated for their role in cervical screening including established proliferation markers such as proliferating nuclear cell antigen (PCNA) and Ki-67. However, both PCNA (see Chapter 28B) and Ki-67 have a number of recognised limitations. Staining for PCNA can be affected by a variety of factors including the method and duration of fixation time, the clone of antibody used, the half-life of the antigen and the effects of growth factors. Similarly, levels of expression of Ki-67 can be affected by a number of variables including nutrient deprivation. To date, studies concerning the clinical utility of Ki-67 as a marker of dysplasia remain inconsistent. The expression of the telomerase small subunit hTERT has also been extensively examined in cervical smear and biopsy samples. While an increasing level of hTERT transcripts is detected with increasing grade of dysplasia, false-negative and false-positive results have limited the clinical use of this marker in cervical cancer screening (Jarboe *et al.*, 2002). Three markers that have demonstrated the greatest potential are the DNA replication licensing proteins CDC6 and MCM5 (Williams *et al.*, 1998; Fujita *et al.*, 1999; Williams and Coleman, 1999; Bonds *et al.*, 2001) and the cyclin-dependent kinase inhibitor p16^{INK4} (Klaes *et al.*, 2001; Murphy *et al.*, 2003). There is a growing body of evidence to suggest that other members of the MCM family (minichromosome maintenance proteins), namely MCM2 and -3 (Ha *et al.*, 2004), also have potential as biomarkers. These MCM proteins will be discussed below. More recently, interest has also been firmly focused on CDT1, an MCM loading protein, and its inhibitor geminin (Wohlschlegel *et al.*, 2002; Tachibana *et al.*, 2005).

MINICHROMOSOME MAINTENANCE PROTEINS

In all eukaryotes, a conserved mechanism of DNA replication exists which ensures that DNA replication occurs only once in a single cell cycle (Diffley and Labib, 2002). This mechanism is often termed the 'licensing' of DNA replication (Takisawa *et al.*, 2000). DNA replication requires the regulated assembly of prereplicative complexes (pre-RC) onto DNA during the G1 phase of the cell cycle. These complexes are formed as a result of the loading of the minichromosome maintenance (MCM) proteins onto areas of cellular DNA known as origins of replication. These origins of replication are found scattered along the length of the chromosome. Pre-RCs render the chromatin competent or 'licensed' to replicate and, as part of the licensing process, bound MCM proteins mark all the chromatin that is to be replicated. Among the proteins known to assemble the MCM proteins onto the origins of replication is CDC6, a cell division cycle protein that has been shown to act as an MCM loading factor (Cook *et al.*, 2002; Shin *et al.*, 2003). More recently, it has been demonstrated that another cell cycle protein, CDT1, acts in conjunction with CDC6 to load the MCM complex onto the chromatin in the G1 phase of the cell cycle. In the S phase of the cell cycle, activation of the pre-RC leads to replication of all the DNA to which the MCM proteins are bound. During this process of DNA replication, the MCM proteins are phosphorylated and, as a result, the MCM complex becomes dissociated from the chromatin. The MCM proteins are then prevented from rebinding DNA until late mitosis, thus ensuring that DNA is replicated only once during each cell cycle. This inhibition of MCM–chromatin binding is achieved by the inactivation of the loading factors CDC6 and CDT1 (Lei and Tye, 2001).

The eukaryotic MCM family consists of six essential proteins (MCM2–7), all of which are necessary for replication fork progression (Shin *et al.*, 2003). The MCM proteins form a heterohexameric ring-shaped complex, which has helicase activity. It has been proposed that the MCM hexameric ring acts a rotary motor, which pumps DNA along its helicase axis, by simple rotation. Laskey and Madine (2003) have proposed a rotary pumping model for the helicase function of MCM proteins. This model is comparable to the movement of a threaded bolt through a nut (Laskey and Madine, 2003). Biological analysis of CDC6 suggests that it functions as a clamp loader in which ATP binding and hydrolysis induce conformational changes that result in the recruitment or loading of MCMs onto DNA (Shin *et al.*, 2003).

Dysregulation of DNA replication results in genomic instability and contributes to the malignant transformation of cells (Takisawa *et al.*, 2000; Ishimi *et al.*, 2003). It is therefore not surprising that changes in the expression pattern of these DNA 'licensing' proteins are frequently observed in dysplastic cells. It has been clearly demonstrated by a number of research groups that, in normal cells, CDC6 and the MCM proteins are present only during the cell cycle and that they are lost from the cell during quiescence and differentiation (Madine *et al.*, 2000; Stoeber *et al.*, 2001). However, a marked overexpression of MCM proteins and CDC6 is observed in dysplastic cells, where CDC6 and the MCM complex appear to remain bound to double-stranded DNA, thus allowing continued DNA replication. As a consequence, MCM5 and CDC6 have been proposed as specific biomarkers of proliferating cells. Dysplastic cells are characterised in functional terms as remaining in the cell cycle, and this would appear to explain the elevated levels of MCM and CDC6 expression seen in dysplastic cells. MCM protein expression has been examined extensively. Results have highlighted the potential use of MCM protein expression in the identification and/or diagnosis of several dysplastic and neoplastic conditions (Ohta *et al.*, 2001; Alison *et al.*, 2002; Davies *et al.*, 2002; Going *et al.*, 2002; Stoeber *et al.*, 2002; Davidson *et al.*, 2003).

MCM proteins as markers of cervical dysplasia

In normal cervical epithelium, MCM protein staining is limited to the basal proliferating layer and is absent in differentiated and quiescent cells (Williams *et al.*, 1998; Freeman *et al.*, 1999). In contrast, in cervical glandular and squamous dysplasia, MCM expression is dramatically increased, suggesting its potential as a biomarker of cervical dysplasia. Studies have revealed a strong correlation between the number of nuclei positive for MCM5 at the surface of dysplastic epithelium and the severity of dysplasia (Williams *et al.*, 1998; Freeman *et al.*, 1999). Figure 28A.4 illustrates MCM5 immunostaining in cervical squamous and glandular lesions and in invasive squamous cell carcinoma and adenocarcinoma of the cervix.

MCM5 has also been shown to stain exfoliated dysplastic cells within ThinPrep slides. This finding means that it has potential as a marker to be used in conjunction with the Pap smear. Although staining of morphologically normal metaplastic cells has been identified as a potential false positive in a number of isolated cases, these cells can easily be identified as normal by morphological criteria using the Pap stain. A striking increase in MCM5 protein expression is observed in cells showing histological HPV features. This may be due to the release of pRb inhibition of E2F as a result of the binding of HPV E7 oncoproteins. The transcription factor E2F then promotes transcription of MCM5 (Ohtani *et al.*, 1999) by its binding to MCM5 promoter sites. In accordance with this, our own group has demonstrated, using quantitative TaqMan reverse transcription (RT)-PCR, that MCM5 mRNA expression increases significantly with increasing severity of dysplasia. Minichromosome maintenance protein 7 (MCM7) has also been identified as a highly informative marker of cervical cancer. Diffuse and full epithelium thickness staining for MCM7 staining was observed in high-grade cervical epithelial lesions and in invasive cervical carcinoma (Williams *et al.*, 1998; Brake *et al.*, 2003).

In view of these findings, interest has turned to other members of the MCM family as potential markers of dyskaryosis. To date, there is evidence of increased staining for MCM2, -3 and -4

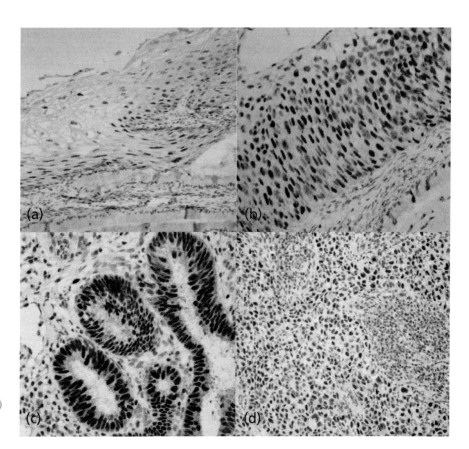

Fig. 28A.4 Four examples of immunohistochemical staining for MCM5. Immunostaining in (a) CIN1, (b) CIN3, (c) adenocarcinoma of the cervix, (d) invasive squamous carcinoma of the cervix.

in cervical cancer tissues (Freeman *et al.*, 1999; Ishimi *et al.*, 2003; Ha *et al.*, 2004). In a similar manner to our own assessment of levels of MCM5 mRNA, it has been demonstrated by RT-PCR that there is increased expression of MCM2 mRNA in cultured HeLa (HPV 18-positive cervical cancer) cells (Ishimi *et al.*, 2003). In addition, gene expression profiling experiments have shown upregulation of MCM proteins 2, 4 and 5 in cervical cancer cells when compared with normal cervical keratinocytes (Santin *et al.*, 2005). Gene expression profiling has also shown MCM6 to be upregulated in squamous and adenocarcinoma of the cervix when compared with normal cervical cells, and tissue microarrays have been used to confirm these results (Chen *et al.*, 2003).

It has also been suggested that the frequency of expression of the MCM proteins in cervical cancer specimens shows an inverse relationship to the degree of tumour differentiation (Freeman *et al.*, 1999). In addition, there is some evidence that the number of cells staining for MCM2 is significantly higher is cervical cancers that are resistant to radiotherapy than in those that are radiosensitive (Mukherjee *et al.*, 2001). These findings have led to the suggestion that the MCM proteins may have an additional role to play, both in assessing prognosis in women with cervical cancer and in determining their likely response to therapy.

CDC6 as a marker of cervical dyskaryosis

The MCM loading protein CDC6 shows a similar expression pattern to that which is seen in the MCM protein family itself, i.e. it is present in proliferating cells but absent in differentiated or quiescent cells. In normal cervical epithelium, CDC6 staining is absent or limited to the basal proliferative layer. However, CDC6 protein expression is dramatically upregulated in squamous and glandular cervical carcinomas and in the cervical carcinoma cell lines C33A, HeLa and CaSki. In 1998, using a polyclonal CDC6 antibody, Williams *et al.* (Williams and Coleman, 1999) identified CDC6 as a marker of dysplastic cervical cells in both cervical biopsies and smears. In subsequent studies employing CDC6 mouse monoclonal antibodies, carried out by Bonds *et al.* (2001) and by our own group, it was observed that CDC6 stains high-grade cervical lesions, although the proportion of positively stained lesional cells was lower than previously described. In lower grade lesions, CDC6 protein expression is weak or absent (Fig. 28A.5).

CDC6 is preferentially expressed in areas exhibiting histological HPV changes. This may suggest activation of genomic DNA replication processes by HPV-associated oncoproteins. Inactivation of pRb by HPV E7 releases inhibition of E2F and may result in transcriptional upregulation of CDC6. In agreement with this, our own group has demonstrated, using quantitative TaqMan RT-PCR, that CDC6 mRNA expression is increased significantly in dysplastic cells (Murphy *et al.*, 2005). It has been demonstrated in human cell lines that, in

order for re-replication to result from the overexpression of CDC6 and CDT1, inactivation of the tumour suppressor protein p53 is required (Vaziri *et al.*, 2003). Re-replication results in genomic instability and DNA damage. In cells with functional p53, this DNA damage results in activation of the p53 protein, which prevents re-replication by inducing G1 phase cell cycle arrest or, alternatively, by induction of apoptosis. High-risk HPV E6 oncoprotein targets p53 for proteolytic degradation. Thus, HPV-infected cells have developed a strategy that permits continued and prolonged re-replication despite the presence of DNA damage and overexpression of CDC6 protein. Interestingly, the expression pattern of CDC6 closely mirrors that of the high-risk HPV E6 oncoprotein, which is mainly expressed in higher grade lesions and invasive carcinomas. In this context, CDC6 overexpression appears to be a relatively late event in the 'dysplastic progression model'. CDC6 expression can be used as a marker of high-grade dysplasia in diagnostic cervical pathology and cervical cytology.

p16^INK4A

The CDKN2A gene located on chromosome 9p21 encodes the tumour suppressor protein p16^INK4A. This 16-kDa protein inhibits cyclin-dependent kinases 4 and 6, which phosphorylate the Rb (retinoblastoma) protein. Therefore, p16^INK4A functions to keep pRb bound to E2F, thus preventing transcriptional activation of the cell. A reciprocal relationship between p16^INK4A and pRb expression has been observed, suggesting the presence of a negative feedback loop allowing pRb to limit levels of p16^INK4A (Li *et al.*, 1994; Tam *et al.*, 1994; Yoshinouchi *et al.*, 2000). Thus, reduced or absent pRb function should result in enhanced p16^INK4A levels. Disruption of the p16^INK4A–pRb cell cycle regulatory pathway results in unrestricted proliferation, eventually contributing to the malignant transformation of cells (Akanuma *et al.*, 1999). Not surprisingly then, loss of p16^INK4A function represents a common pathway to tumorigenesis. p16^INK4A can be inactivated by a variety of different mechanisms including mutation, altered splicing, homozygous deletion (Kamb *et al.*, 1994) and promoter hypermethylation (Merlo *et al.*, 1995). The majority of these genetic alterations result in loss of p16^INK4A protein expression. However, overexpression of p16^INK4A protein in tumours has also been described.

p16^INK4A *as a marker of cervical dyskaryosis*

A marked overexpression of p16^INK4A is observed in precancerous and malignant cervical lesions. Upregulation of p16^INK4A in cervical lesions is believed to be a consequence of functional inactivation of pRb by HPV E7 protein (Sakaguuchi *et al.*, 1996). It has been suggested that p16^INK4A may be directly induced by the transcription factor E2F that is released from pRb after binding of HPV E7 (Khleif *et al.*, 2001). In concordance with this, a number of recent studies have

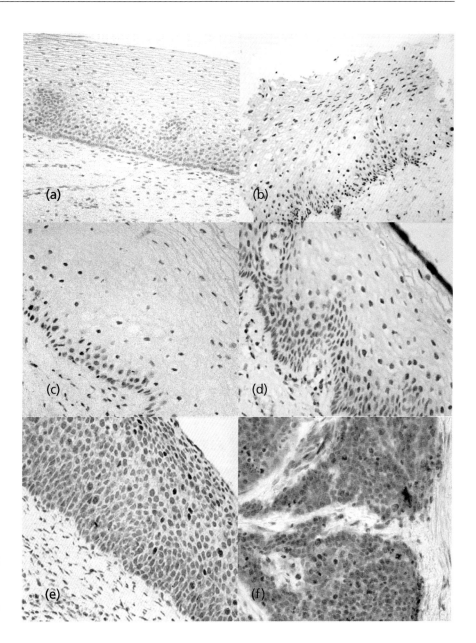

Fig. 28A.5 Immunohistochemical staining for CDC6. CDC6 immunostaining in (a) normal cervical epithelium, (b) CIN1, (c) basal CIN1, (d) CIN2 and (e) CIN2–3, (f) invasive squamous cell carcinoma.

reported a significant increase in p16^{INK4A} protein expression in a number of high-risk HPV-associated cancers including HPV-associated penile carcinomas (Ferreux *et al.*, 2003) and HPV-associated oral cancers (Fregonesi *et al.*, 2003). Although p16^{INK4A} upregulation in cervical lesions is believed to be a consequence of HPV infection, p16^{INK4A} upregulation in the C33A (HPV-negative) cell line (Murphy *et al.*, 2003) and in HPV-negative lesions (Milde-Langosch *et al.*, 2001) may indicate that an HPV-independent pathway also exists.

The expression pattern of p16^{INK4A} in dysplastic squamous and glandular cervical cells in tissue sections and in cervical smears has been extensively investigated (Sano *et al.*, 1998; Klaes *et al.*, 2001; Saqi *et al.*, 2002; Bibbo *et al.*, 2003; Negri *et al.*, 2003; Murphy *et al.*, 2003; Pientong *et al.*, 2003). In

normal cervical tissues, it has been demonstrated that all epithelial, metaplastic, endocervical, reactive and inflammatory regions do not exhibit any p16^{INK4A} staining. In addition, all normal regions adjacent to CIN lesions do not show any detectable p16^{INK4A} expression. In cervical biopsy sections, p16^{INK4A} identified dysplastic squamous and glandular lesions with a sensitivity rate of 99.9% and specificity rate of 100% (Murphy *et al.*, 2003). Figure 28A.6 demonstrates p16^{INK4A} immunostaining in squamous and glandular lesions and in invasive squamous cell carcinoma and adenocarcinoma of cervix. Figure 28A.7 illustrates p16^{INK4A} in exfoliated dysplastic cells.

It is now widely accepted that p16^{INK4A} is a sensitive and specific marker of squamous and glandular dysplastic cells of

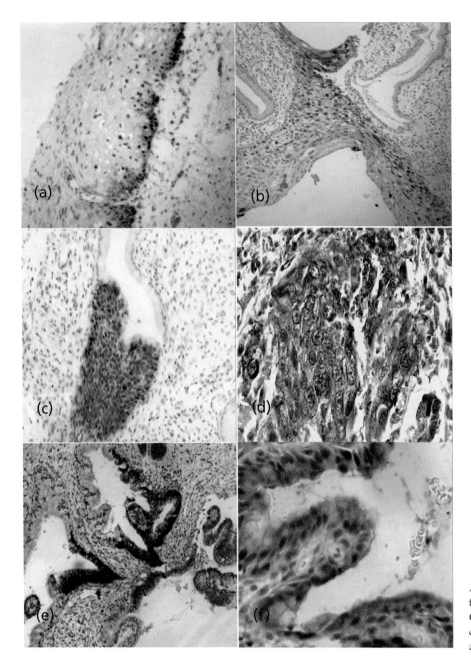

Fig. 28A.6 Immunohistochemical staining for p16^INK4A in (a) CIN1, (b) CIN2, (c) CIN3, (d) invasive squamous cell carcinoma, (e) cGIN, and (f) adenocarcinoma of the cervix.

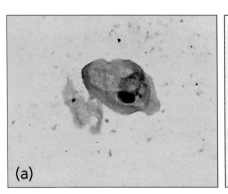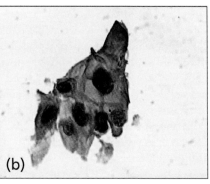

Fig. 28A.7 Immunocytochemical staining of exfoliated dysplastic cells in ThinPrep slides using p16^INK4A-specific antibody. p16^INK4A expression in a mild dyskaryotic cell (a) and in a mild to moderately dyskaryotic cell cluster (b).

the cervix and is a valuable adjunctive test in cervical cancer screening. One study published by Klaes *et al.* (2001) involving five experienced pathologists clearly demonstrated that the use of p16^{INK4A} immunostaining allows precise identification of CIN and cervical cancer lesions in cervical biopsy specimens and can significantly reduce false-negative and false-positive interpretation in cervical cancer screening.

While p16^{INK4A} has been determined to be a sensitive and specific marker of cervical adenocarcinoma and its precursor lesions, knowledge of p16^{INK4A} staining patterns in glandular mimic lesions such as tubo-endometrioid metaplasia (TEM), endosalpingiosis and prolapsed fallopian tube syndrome is vital. TEM is considered a benign histological lesion where endometrial or fallopian tube-type cells are present in the endocervical glands due to metaplasia. TEM can give rise to diagnostic difficulty when found at the transformation zone. It is vital that TEM is correctly recognised because histologically it may be misinterpreted as CGIN or adenocarcinoma *in situ* (AIS). Occasional p16^{INK4A} nuclear positivity and definite cytoplasmic staining is observed in TEM lesions (Murphy *et al.*, 2004). Intercalating tubal/peg cells are negative for p16^{INK4A} expression. While this type of staining in TEM lesions is easily distinguishable from the intense nuclear and cytoplasmic staining observed in CGIN, it is important to be aware of the difference in expression as this may pose a potential pitfall when using p16^{INK4A} staining to aid in CGIN and adenocarcinoma diagnosis. In addition, p16^{INK4A} stains

endosalpingiosis and fallopian tube epithelium, two other potential diagnostic pitfalls in cervical biopsy pathology and cytopathology. One possible suggestion put forward by Cameron *et al.* (2002) is to consider using a panel of antibodies composed of p16^{INK4A}, MIB1 and bcl2 in problematic endocervical glandular lesions to allow discrimination between benign mimics and CGIN. They describe how this panel can be used to discriminate TEM, endometriosis and microglandular hyperplasia from CGIN.

Santin *et al.* (2005) have recently demonstrated the upregulation of p16^{INK4A} at the mRNA level. cDNA microarray analysis of RNA extracted from cells derived from cervical cancer specimens showed a greater than ninefold upregulation of the *CDKN2A* gene, which encodes for p16^{INK4A}, when compared with the gene expression level found in normal cervical keratinocytes. This overexpression at the mRNA level was confirmed by quantitative RT-PCR. Further analysis confirmed that, in those cervical cancer cases where there was overexpression of *CDKN2A* at the mRNA level, this correlated with overexpression of the p16^{INK4A} protein on immunohistochemical analysis of the original tumour specimen.

Geminin and CDT1

Recently, interest has increasingly focused on geminin and CDT1 as potential markers of cervical cancer. CDT1 is known to act as an MCM loading protein in conjunction with CDC6

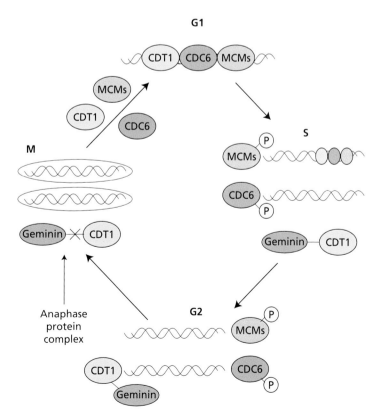

Fig. 28A.8 Role of geminin and CDT1 in regulating DNA replication.

(Saxena and Dutta, 2005). In the normal cell cycle, CDT1 is present in all proliferating cells during the G1 phase of the cell cycle. Together with CDC6, it is essential for the initiation of replication through the loading of the MCM proteins onto areas of DNA to be replicated. Once DNA replication is complete, the MCM proteins are prevented from rebinding DNA by a combination of high CDK2 levels and functional inactivation of their loading factors (Tachibana *et al.*, 2005). Inactivation of CDC6 is achieved by phosphorylation of the protein with subsequent export from the nucleus to the cytoplasm. In contrast, CDT1 is phosphorylated and degraded. Any CDT1 that escapes degradation is inhibited by geminin, which binds it tightly from the S phase to late mitosis. In late mitosis, geminin itself is degraded by the anaphase protein complex (APC), thus allowing the MCM protein complex to bind to the chromatin of each daughter cell in preparation for further DNA replication (Fig. 28A.8).

CDT1 has been shown to be upregulated at the mRNA level in cDNA microarray gene expression profiling experiments of cervical cancer specimens (Santin *et al.*, 2005). It remains to be seen whether this upregulation at the RNA level is translated into an increased production of CDT1 protein that could be detected immunohistochemically. Although geminin functions as an inhibitor of DNA replication, it has actually been shown to be paradoxically overexpressed in cervical cancer (Wohlschlegel *et al.*, 2002). While this result is unexpected, it has been replicated in a number of other malignancies (Gonzalez *et al.*, 2004). These findings would suggest that geminin warrants further investigation as a potential molecular marker in cervical dyskaryosis and malignancy.

THE FUTURE

Our increasing knowledge of the underlying pathogenesis of cervical cancer, combined with advances in molecular technologies including cDNA arrays and tissue microarrays, heralds the emergence of a 'molecular age' in cervical cancer prevention. The challenge that faces us is to extract, from the huge amounts of data that these technologies generate, information regarding novel biomarkers of cervical dysplasia. In conjunction with conventional screening and HPV testing, the use of biomarkers will ultimately result in a reduction in the number of false-positive and -negative smear results and, therefore, in a decrease in the overall cost of cervical cancer screening. In addition, it is hoped that this information will help to unravel further the pathogenesis of HPV infection and dysplastic progression, and ultimately improve the treatment of CIN and cervical cancer.

REFERENCES

Agency for Healthcare Policy and Research (1999) *Evaluation of Cervical Cytology.* AHCPR Publication No. 99-E010 (Evidence Report—Technology Assessment No. 5), US Department of Health and Human Services.

Akanuma D, Uzawa N, Yoshida MA *et al.* (1999) Inactivation patterns of the p16 (INK4a) gene in oral squamous cell carcinoma cell lines. *Oral Oncology* 35 (5): 476–483.

Alison MR, Hunt T, Forbes SJ (2002) Minichromosome maintenance (MCM) proteins may be pre-cancer markers. *Cancer* 50: 291–292.

ALTS Group (2003) Results of a randomized trial on the management of cytology interpretations of atypical squamous cells of undermined significance. *American Journal of Obstetrics and Gynecology* 188: 1383–1392.

Arbyn M, Dillner J, Van Ranst M *et al.* (2004) Virological versus cytology triage of women with equivocal Pap smears: a meta-analysis of the accuracy to detect high-grade intraepithelial neoplasia. *Journal of the National Cancer Institute* 96: 280–293.

Bibbo M, DeCecco J, Kovatich AJ (2003) P16INK4a as an adjunct test in liquid based cytology. *Analytical and Quantitative Cytology and Histology* 25 (1): 8–11.

Bigrigg MA, Codling BW, Pearson P *et al.* (1990) Colposcopic diagnosis and treatment of cervical dysplasia at a single clinic visit. *Lancet* 306: 229–231.

Bonds L, Baker P, Gup C *et al.* (2001) Immunohistochemical localization of CDC6 in squamous and glandular neoplasia of the uterine cervix. *Archives of Pathology and Laboratory Medicine* 126: 1162–1168.

Bosch FX, Manos MM, Muñoz N *et al.* (1995) Prevalence of human papillomavirus in cervical cancer: a worldwide perspective. International Biological Study on Cervical Cancer (IBSCC) Study Group. *Journal of the National Cancer Institute* 87: 796–802.

Bosch FX, Lorincz A, Muñoz N *et al.* (2002) The causal relation between human papillomavirus and cervical cancer. *Journal of Clinical Pathology* 55: 244–265.

Brake T, Connor JP, Petereit DG *et al.* (2003) Comparative analysis of cervical cancer in women and in a human papillomavirus-transgenic mouse model: identification of minichromosome maintenance protein 7 as an informative biomarker for human cervical cancer. *Cancer Research* 63 (23): 8173–8180.

Buxton EJ, Luesley DM, Shafi MI *et. al.* (1991) Colposcopically directed punch biopsy: a potentially misleading investigation. *British Journal of Obstetrics and Gynaecology* 98: 1273–1276.

Cameron RI, Maxwell P, Jenkins D *et al.* (2002) Immunohistochemical staining with MIB1, bcl2, and p16 assist in the distinction of cervical glandular intraepithelial neoplasia from tubo-endometrial metaplasia, endometriosis and microglandular hyperplasia. *Histopathology* 41: 313–321.

Chen Y, Miller C, Mosher R *et al.* (2003) Identification of cervical cancer markers by cDNA and tissue microarrays. *Cancer Research* 63: 1927–1935.

Chew GK, Jandial L, Paraskevaidis E *et al.* (1999) Pattern of CIN recurrence following laser ablation treatment on long term follow up. *International Journal of Gynecological Cancer* 9: 487–490.

Chua KL, Hjerpe A (1997) Human papillomavirus analysis as a prognostic marker following conization of the cervix uteri. *Gynecologic Oncology* 66: 108–113.

Clavel C *et al.* (2001) Human papillomavirus testing in primary screening for the detection of high-grade cervical lesions: a study of 7932 women. *British Journal of Cancer* 84: 1616–1623.

Colgan TJ, Austin RM, Davey DD (2001) The annual pap test: women's safety and public policy. *Cancer (Cancer Cytopathology)* 93: 81–85.

Cook JG, Park CH, Burke TW *et al.* (2002) Analysis of Cdc6 function in the assembly of mammalian prereplication complexes. *Proceedings of the National Academy of Sciences of the USA* 99 (3): 1347–1352.

Coutlee F, Gravitt P, Kornegay J *et al.* (2002) Use of PGMY primers in L1 consensus PCR improves detection of human papillomavirus DNA in genital samples. *Journal of Clinical Microbiology* 3: 902–907.

Cuzick J (2002) Role of HPV testing in clinical practice. *Virus Research* 89 (2): 263–269.

Cuzick JA, Szarewski A, Cubie H *et al.* (2003) Management of women who test positive for high-risk types of human papillomavirus: the HART study. *Lancet* 362: 1871–1876.

Davidson EJ, Morris LS, Scott IS *et al.* (2003) Minichromosome maintenance (Mcm) proteins, cyclin B1 and D1, phosphohistone H3 and in situ DNA replication for functional analysis of vulval intraepithelial neoplasia. *British Journal of Cancer* 88 (2): 257–262.

Davies RJ, Freeman A, Morris LS *et al.* (2002) Analysis of minichromosome maintenance proteins as a novel method for detection of colorectal cancer in stool. *Lancet* 359 (9321): 1917–1919.

de Roda Husman AM, Walboomers JM, van den Brule AJ *et al.* (1995) The use of general primers GP5 and GP6 elongated at their 3′ ends with adjacent highly conserved sequences improves human papillomavirus detection by PCR. *Journal of General Virology* 76 (4): 1057–1062.

Diffley JF, Labib K (2002) The chromosome replication cycle. *Journal of Cell Science* 115 (5): 869–872.

Dobbs SP, Asmussen T, Nunns D *et al.* (2000) Does histological incomplete excision of cervical intraepithelial neoplasia following large loop excision of transformation zone increase recurrence rates? A six-year cytological follow up. *British Journal of Obstetrics and Gynaecology* 107: 1298–1301.

Etherington IJ, Luesley DM, Shafi MI *et al.* (1997) Observer variability among colposcopists from the West Midlands region. *British Journal of Obstetrics and Gynaecology* 104 (12): 1380–1384.

Fahey MT, Irwig L, Macaskill P (1995) Meta-analysis of pap test accuracy. *American Journal of Epidemiology* 141: 680–689.

Fausch SC, Da Silva DM, Eiben GL *et al.* (2003) HPV protein/peptide vaccines: from animal models to clinical trials. *Frontiers in Bioscience* 8: 81–91.

Ferreux E, Lont AP, Horenblas S *et al.* (2003) Evidence for at least three alternative mechanisms targeting the p16INK4A/cyclin D/Rb pathway in penile carcinoma, one of which is mediated by high-risk human papillomavirus. *Journal of Pathology* 201: 109–118.

Flannelly G, Langhan H, Jandial L *et al.* (1997) A study of treatment failures following large loop excision of the transformation zone for the treatment of cervical intraepithelial neoplasia. *British Journal of Obstetrics and Gynaecology* 104 (6): 718–722.

Flannelly G, Bolger B, Fawzi H *et al.* (2001) Follow up after LLETZ: could schedule be modified according to risk of recurrence? *British Journal of Obstetrics and Gynaecology* 108: 1025–1030.

Frazer I (2002) Vaccines for papillomavirus infection. *Virus Research* 89 (2): 271–274.

Freeman A, Morris LS, Mills AD *et al.* (1999) Minichromosome maintenance proteins as biological markers of dysplasia and malignancy. *Clinics in Cancer Research* 5 (8): 2121–2132.

Fregonesi PA, Teresa DB, Duarte RA *et al.* (2003) p16(INK4A) immunohistochemical overexpression in premalignant and malignant oral lesions infected with human papillomavirus. *Journal of Histochemistry and Cytochemistry* 51 (10): 1291–1297.

Fujita M, Yamada C, Goto H *et al.* (1999) Cell cycle regulation of human Cdc 6 protein. *Journal of Biological Chemistry* 274: 25927–25932.

Gardeil F, Barry Walsh C, Prendiville W *et al.* (1997) Persistent intraepithelial neoplasia after excision for cervical intraepithelial neoplasia grade III. *Obstetrics and Gynaecology* 89 (3): 419–422.

Giannoudis A, Herrington SC (2001) Human papillomavirus variants and squamous neoplasia of the cervix. *Journal of Pathology* 193: 295–302.

Going JJ, Keith WN, Neilson L *et al.* (2002) Aberrant expression of minichromosome maintenance proteins 2 and 5, and Ki-67 in dysplastic squamous oesophageal epithelium and Barrett's mucosa. *Gut* 50 (3): 373–377.

Gonzalez MA, Tachibana KK, Chin S-F *et al.* (2004) Geminin predicts adverse clinical outcome in breast cancer by predicting cell-cycle progression. *Journal of Pathology* 204: 121–130.

Ha S-A, Shin SM, Namkoong H *et al.* (2004) Cancer-associated expression of minichromosome maintenance 3 gene in several human cancers and its involvement in tumourigenesis. *Clinics in Cancer Research* 10: 8386–8395.

Ho GY, Burk RD, Klein S *et al.* (1995) Persistent genital human papillomavirus infection as a risk factor for persistent cervical dysplasia. *Journal of the National Cancer Institute* 87 (18): 1365–1371.

Hutchinson ML, Zahniser DJ, Sherman ME *et al.* (1999) Utility of liquid-based cytology for cervical carcinoma screening: results of a population-based study conducted in a region of Costa Rica with a high incidence of cervical carcinoma. *Cancer (Cancer Cytopathology)* 87: 48–55.

International Agency for Research on Cancer (1995) Human papillomaviruses. In: *IARC Monographs on the Evolution of Carcinogenic Risks to Humans*, vol. 64. Lyon: IARC.

Ishimi Y, Okayasu I, Kato C *et al.* (2003) Enhanced expression of MCM proteins in cells derived from the uterine cervix. *European Journal of Biochemistry* 260 (6): 1089–1101.

Jarboe EA, Liaw KL, Thompson LC *et al.* (2002) Analysis of telomerase as a diagnostic biomarker of cervical dysplasia and carcinoma. *Oncogene* 21 (4): 664–673.

Kamb A, Gruis NA, Weaver-Feldhaus J *et al.* (1994) A cell cycle regulator potentially involved in genesis of many tumour types. *Science* 264: 436–440.

Khleif SN, DeGregori J, Yee CL *et al.* (2001) Inhibition of cyclin D-CDK4/CDK6 activity is associated with E2F-mediated induction of cyclin-kinase activity. *Proceedings of the National Academy of Sciences of the USA* 93: 4350–4354.

Kirwan JM, Herrington CS (2001) Human papillomavirus and cervical cancer: where are we now? *British Journal of Obstetrics and Gynaecology* 108: 1204–1213.

Klaes R, Friedrich T, Spitkovsky D *et al.* (2001) Overexpression of p16 as a specific marker for dysplastic and neoplastic epithelial cells of the cervix uteri. *International Journal of Cancer* 92: 276–284.

Krane JF, Granter SR, Trask CE *et al.* (2001) Papanicolaou smear sensitivity for the detection of adenocarcinoma of the cervix: a study of 49 cases. *Cancer* 93: 8–15.

Kulasingam SL *et al.* (2002) Evaluation of human papillomavirus testing in primary screening for cervical abnormalities: comparison of sensitivity, specificity, and frequency of referral. *Journal of the American Medical Association* 288: 1749–1757.

Laskey RA, Madine MA (2003) A rotary pumping model for helicase function of MCM proteins at a distance from replication forks. *EMBO Reports* 4 (1): 26–30.

Lei M, Tye B (2001) Initiating DNA synthesis: from recruiting to activating the MCM complex. *Journal of Cell Science* 114: 1447–1454.

Li Y, Nichols MA, Shay JW *et al.* (1994) Transcriptional repression of the D-type cyclin dependent kinase inhibitor p16 by retinoblastoma susceptibility gene product pRb. *Cancer Research* 54: 6078–6082.

Lin H-P, Huang YY, Wu HY *et al.* (2004) Method for testing for human papillomavirus infection in patients with cervical intraepithelial disease. *Journal of Clinical Microbiology* 42.

Liu WJ, Liu XS, Zhao KN *et al.* (2000) Papillomavirus virus-like particles for the delivery of multiple cytotoxic t-cell epitopes. *Virology* 273: 374–382.

Madine MA, Swietlik M, Pelizon C *et al.* (2000) The roles of the MCM, ORC, and Cdc6 proteins in determining the replication competence of chromatin in quiescent cells. *Journal of Structural Biology* 129 (2–3): 198–210.

Manos M, Kinney W, Hurley B *et al.* (1999) Identifying women with cervical neoplasia *Journal of the American Medical Association* 281 (917): 1605–1610.

Mergui JL, Tauscher P, Bergeron C *et al.* (1994) L'electronconisation a l'ansa diathermique (ECAD): indications et resultants. *Contraception, Fertility and Sex* 22: 53–59.

Merlo A, Herman JG, Mao L *et al.* (1995) 5′ CpG island methylation is associated with transcriptional silencing of the tumour suppressor p16/CDKN2/MTS1 in human cancers. *Nature Medicine* 1: 868–692.

Milde-Langosch K, Hagen M, Bamberger AM *et al.* (2001) Expression of cyclin-dependent kinase inhibitors p16MTS1, p21WAF1, and p27KIP1 in HPV-positive and HPV-negative cervical adenocarcinomas. *Virchow's Archive* 439 (1): 55–61.

Mukherjee G, Freeman A, Moore R *et al.* (2001) Biological factors and response to radiotherapy in carcinoma of the cervix. *International Journal of Gynaecological Cancer* 11 (3): 187–193.

Munger K, Howley PM (2002) Human papillomavirus immortalization and transformation functions. *Virus Research* 89: 213–228.

Muñoz N, Bosch FX, de Sanjose S *et al.* (2003) Epidemiologic classification of human papillomavirus types associated with cervical cancer. *New England Journal of Medicine* 348 (6): 518–527.

Murphy N, Ring M, Killalea AG *et al.* (2003) P16INK4A as a marker for cervical dyskaryosis: CIN and cGIN in cervical biopsies and ThinPrep™ smears. *Journal of Clinical Pathology* 56: 53–63.

Murphy N, Heffron CC, King B *et al.* (2004) p16^{INK4A} positivity in benign, premalignant and glandular lesions: a potential diagnostic problem. *Virchow's Archive* 445 (6): 610–615.

Murphy N, Ring M, Heffron CC *et al.* (2005) Quantitation of Cdc6 and MCM5 mRNA in cervical intraepithelial neoplasia and invasive squamous cell carcinoma of the cervix. *Modern Pathology* (Epub ahead of print).

Myers ER, McCrory DC, Subramanian S *et al.* (2000) Setting the target for a better cervical screening test: characteristics of a cost-effective test for cervical neoplasia screening. *Obstetrics and Gynecology* 96: 645–652.

Negri G, Egarter-Vigl E, Kasal A *et al.* (2003) p16INK4a is a useful marker for the diagnosis of the cervix uteri and its precursors: an immunohistological study with immunocytochemical correlations. *American Journal of Surgical Pathology* 27 (2): 187–193.

NHSCSP (2004) *Colposcopy and Programme Management: Guidelines for the NHS Cervical Screening Programme*. NHSCSP Publication No. 20.

Ohta S, Koide M, Tokuyama T *et al.* (2001) Cdc6 expression as a marker of proliferative activity in brain tumours. *Oncology Reports* 5: 1063–1066.

Ohtani K, Iwanaga R, Nakamura M *et al.* (1999) Cell growth-regulated expression of mammalian MCM5 and MCM6 genes mediated by transcription factor E2F. *Oncogene* 14: 2299–2309.

Paraskevaides E, Koliopoulos G, Malamou-Mitsi V *et al.* (2001) Large loop excision of the transformation zone for treating cervical intraepithelial neoplasia: a 12 year experience. *Anticancer Research* 21: 3097–3099.

Paraskevaidis E, Arbyn M, Sotiriadis A *et al.* (2004) The role of HPV DNA testing in the follow-up period after treatment for CIN. A systematic review of the literature/ *Cancer Treatment Review* 30 (2): 205–211.

Perrons C, Kleter B, Jelley R *et al.* (2002) Detection and genotyping of human papillomavirus DNA by SPF10 and MY09/11 primers in cervical cells taken from women attending a colposcopy clinic. *Journal of Medical Virology* 67 (2): 246–252.

Petry KU, Menton S, Menton M *et al.* (2003) Inclusion of HPV testing in routine cervical cancer screening for women above 29 years in Germany: results for 8466 patients. *British Journal of Cancer* 88: 1570–1577.

Pientong C, Ekalaksananan T, Swadpanich U *et al.* (2003) Immunocytochemical detection of p16INK4a protein in scraped cervical cells. *Acta Cytologica* 47 (4): 616–623.

Quinn M, Babb P, Jones J *et al.* (1999) Effect of screening on incidence of and mortality from cancer of cervix in England: evaluation based on routinely collected statistics. *British Medical Journal* 318: 904.

Remmink AJ, Walboomers JM, Helmerhorst TJ *et al.* (1995) The presence of persistent high-risk HPV genotypes in dysplastic cervical lesions is associated with progressive disease: natural history up to 36 months. *International Journal of Cancer* 61 (3): 306–311.

Sakaguchi M, Fujii Y, Hirabayashi H *et al.* (1996) Inversely correlated expression of p16 and Rb protein in non-small cell lung cancers: an immunohistochemical study. *International Journal of Cancer* 65: 442–445.

Sano T, Oyama T, Kashiwabara K *et al.* (1998) Overexpression of p16 protein associated with intact retinoblastoma protein expression in cervical cancer and cervical intraepithelial neoplasia. *Pathology International* 48: 580–588.

Santin AD, Fenghuang Z, Bignotti E *et al.* (2005) Gene expression profiles of primary HPV-16 and HPV-18 infected early stage cervical cancers and normal cervical epithelium: identification of novel candidate molecular markers for cervical cancer diagnosis and therapy. *Virology* 331: 269–291.

Saqi A, Pasha TL, McGrath CM *et al.* (2002) Overexpression of p16INK4A in liquid-based specimens (SurePath) as a marker of cervical dysplasia and neoplasia. *Diagnostic Cytopathology* 27 (6): 365–370.

Saxena S, Dutta A (2005) Geminin–Cdt1 balance is critical for genetic stability. *Mutation Research* 569: 111–121.

Schiffman M, Herrero R, Hildesheim A *et al.* (2000) HPV DNA testing in cervical cancer screening: results from women in a high-risk province of Costa Rica. *Journal of the American Medical Association* 283 (1): 87–93.

Sherman ME, Lorincz AT, Scott DR *et al.* (2003) Baseline cytology, human papillomavirus testing, and risk of cervical neoplasia: a 10 year cohort analysis. *Journal of the National Cancer Institute* 95: 46–52.

Shin JH, Grabowski B, Kasiviswanathan R *et al.* (2003) Regulation of minichromosome maintenance helicase activity by Cdc6. *Journal of Biological Chem*istry 278 (39): 38059–38067.

Shlay JC, Dunn T, Byers T *et al.* (2000) Prediction of cervical intra-epithelial neoplasia grade 2–3 using risk assessment and human papillomavirus testing in women with atypia on papanicolaou smears. *Obstetrics and Gynecology* 96 (3): 410–416.

Solomon D, Schiffman M, Tarone R (2001) Comparison of three management strategies for patients with atypical squamous cells of undetermined significance: baseline results from a randomized trial. *Journal of the National Cancer Institute* 93 (4): 293–299.

Soutter WP, de Barros Lopes A, Fletcher A *et al.* (1997) Invasive cervical cancer after conservative therapy for cervical intraepithelial neoplasia. *Lancet* 349 (9057): 978–980.

Stoeber K, Tlsty TD, Happerfield L *et al.* (2001) DNA replication licensing and human cell proliferation. *Journal of Cell Science* 114: 2027–2041.

Stoeber K, Swinn R, Prevost AT *et al.* (2002) Diagnosis of genitourinary tract cancer by detection of minichromosome maintenance 5 protein in urine sediments. *Journal of the National Cancer Institute* 94 (14): 1071–1079.

Tachibana KK, Gonzalez MA, Coleman N (2005) Cell-cycle-dependent regulation of DNA replication and its relevance to cancer pathology. *Journal of Pathology* 205: 123–129.

Takisawa H, Mimura S, Kubota Y (2000) Eukaryotic DNA replication: from pre-replication complex to initiation complex. *Current Opinion in Cell Biology* 12 (6): 690–696.

Tam SW, Shay JW, Pagano M (1994) Differential expression and cell cycle regulation of the cyclin dependant kinase inhibitor p16INK4A. *Cancer Research* 54: 5816–5820.

Vaziri C, Saxena S, Jeon Y *et al.* (2003) A p53-dependent checkpoint pathway prevents rereplication. *Molecules and Cells* 4: 997–1008.

Williams GH, Romanowski P, Morris L *et al.* (1998) Improved cervical smear assessment using antibodies against proteins that regulate DNA replication. *Proceedings of the National. Academy of Sciences of the USA* 99: 14932–14937.

Williams GH, Coleman N (1999) Minichromosome maintenance proteins as biological markers of dysplasia and malignancy. *Clinical Cancer Research* 5: 2121–2132.

Wohlschlegel JA, Kutok JL, Weng AP *et al.* (2002) Expression of geminin as a marker of cell proliferation in normal tissues and malignancy. *American Journal of Pathology* 161 (1): 267–273.

Wright EC, Schiffman M (2003) Adding a test for human papillomavirus DNA to cervical-cancer screening. *New England Journal of Medicine* 348: 489–490.

Yoshinouchi M, Hongo A, Takamoto N *et al.* (2000) Alteration of the CDKN2/P16 gene is not required for HPV-positive uterine cervical cell lines. *International Journal of Oncology* 16 (3): 537–541.

FURTHER READING

Bohmer G, Van den Brule AJ, Brummer O *et al.* (2003) No confirmed case of human papillomavirus DNA-negative cervical intraepithelial neoplasia grade 3 or invasive primary cancer if the uterine cervix among 511 patients. *American Journal of Obstetrics and Gynecology* 189 (1): 118–120.

Crook T, Wrede D, Tidy JA *et al.* (1992) Clonal p53 mutation in primary cervical cancer: association with human-papillomavirus-negative tumours. *Lancet* 339 (8801): 1070–1073.

Elfgren K, Jacobs M, Walboomers JM *et al.* (2002) Rate of human papillomavirus clearance after treatment of cervical intraepithelial neoplasia. *Obstetrics and Gynecology* 100 (5 Pt 1): 965–971.

Franco EL, Duarte-Franco E, Ferenczy A (2001) Cervical cancer: epidemiology, prevention and the role of human papillomavirus infection. *Canadian Medical Association Journal* 164 (7): 1017–1025.

Funk JO, Waga S, Harry JB *et al.* (1997) Inhibition of CDK activity and PCNA-dependent DNA replication by p21 is blocked by interaction with the HPV-16 E7 oncoprotein. *Genes and Development* 11 (16): 2090–2100.

Hopman EH, Rozendaal L, Voorhorst FJ *et al.* (2000) High risk human papillomavirus in women with normal cervical cytology prior to the development of abnormal cytology and colposcopy. *British Journal of Obstetrics and Gynaecology* 107 (5): 600–604.

Jacobs MV, Snijders PJ, Voorhorst FJ *et al.* (1999) Reliable high risk HPV DNA testing by polymerase chain reaction: an intermethod and intramethod comparison. *Journal of Clinical Pathology* 52: 498–503.

Lewin B (2000) *Genes VII.* Oxford: Oxford University Press.

Reshkin SJ, Bellizzi A, Caldeira S *et al.* (2000) Na$^+$/H$^+$ exchanger-dependent intracellular alkalinization is an early event in malignant transformation and plays an essential role in the development of subsequent transformation-associated phenotypes. *FASEB Journal* 14 (14): 2185–2197.

von Knebel Doberitz M (2002) New markers for cervical dysplasia to visualise the genomic chaos created by aberrant oncogenic papillomavirus infections. *European Journal of Cancer* 38: 2229–2242.

Walboomers JM, Jacobs MV, Manos MM *et al.* (1999) Human papillomavirus is a necessary cause of invasive cervical cancer worldwide. *Journal of Pathology* 189 (1): 12–19.

Tumour markers in cervical cancer — II

Michael Sindos and Narendra Pisal

INTRODUCTION

In countries that have implemented regular screening programmes to detect easily recognisable and treatable premalignant stages of cervical neoplasia, cervical cytology has been the successful screening tool employed. In many western countries that have adopted such programmes, the incidence and mortality of cervical cancer has dropped dramatically. Despite its success, exfoliative cytology is associated with certain drawbacks, mainly in respect of the significant false-negative and false-positive rate (Fahey *et al.*, 1995; Costa *et al.*, 2000; Cox *et al.*, 2003). It also detects a large number of minor abnormalities, where the likelihood of the presence of high-grade disease and subsequent progression to cervical cancer is low. In order to prevent one case of cervical cancer, 1000 women need to undergo regular cytological screening for 35 years (Raffle *et al.*, 2003). Therefore, it is essential to improve the accuracy and specificity of cervical screening by the introduction of other methods, which may be used in place of or in combination with cervical cytology. Human papillomavirus (HPV) and its role in the management of cervical neoplasia has been discussed in Chapter 28A.

Over the last few years, understanding of the molecular basis of cervical cancer and its associated natural history, particularly as it involves the central role played by HPV, has led to the availability of various molecular biomarkers. Before clinical cervical cancer develops, there is a long premalignant stage (cervical intraepithelial neoplasia, CIN), which allows for screening and intervention. The cellular, molecular and genetic changes associated with the development of cervical neoplasia are specific and offer great potential for improving the screening and diagnosis of cervical cancer. The techniques for detecting these changes are still being researched; however, in the future, it is hoped that they will improve the sensitivity and specificity of cervical cancer screening. The molecular markers of cervical neoplasia that will be discussed below are listed in Table 28B.1. However, some of them that are being used at present and are undergoing trials are shown diagrammatically in Figure 28B.1. The roles, again, of some of them, in causing intracellular dysfunction, especially in respect of

aberrant S-phase induction of cervical neoplasia, are seen diagrammatically in Figure 28B.2.

USE OF HPV AND ITS PRODUCTS AS TUMOUR MARKERS

This subject has been covered in detail in Chapter 28A and also in Chapter 26. However, certain key DNA, RNA or protein biomarkers arising as a result of the neoplastic process that involves HPV could predict the progressive character of the disease. Some of these markers could be used in screening, diagnosis and treatment. Examples of such progression markers are mRNA for viral oncoproteins E6 and E7, HPV DNA sequences integrated in the human genome, overexpression of cell cycle regulator proteins or proliferation protein markers or determinants of certain genetic or immunological profiles (Bibbo *et al.*, 2002; Hildesheim and Wang, 2002; Kadish *et al.*, 2002; Altiok, 2003; Wang *et al.*, 2003). Cyclin-dependent kinases (CDKs), cyclins and CDK inhibitors control the cell cycle and coordinate DNA synthesis, chromosome separation and cell division. These CDKs interact either directly or indirectly with the viral oncoproteins and play a major part in the neoplastic process.

PROLIFERATING CELL NUCLEAR ANTIGEN (PCNA)

PCNA is an S phase-associated nuclear protein that acts as a cofactor of DNA polymerase (Bravo *et al.*, 1987). Besides its use as an S-phase probe in flow cytometry, monoclonal antibodies to PCNA can be used on paraffin-embedded tissue, thus extending its application to cytology and histology (Garcia *et al.*, 1989; Landberg and Roos, 1991). The staining pattern is intranuclear. In normal cervical epithelium, rare basal epithelial cells stain but, in the setting of inflammation, the number of basal cells staining increases (Garcia *et al.*, 1989). Shurbaji *et al.* (1993) demonstrated that the highest level of the epithelium at which PCNA-positive nuclei were seen correlated with both the grade of dysplasia and the mitotic grade. Mittal *et al.* (1993) reported expression of

Table 28B.1 Potential molecular markers for cervical neoplasia.

Marker	Change	Family	Rationale
Protein markers			
p16^(INK4)	Increased	Cyclin-dependent kinase (CDK) inhibitor	E7-mediated degradation of the Rb gene yields enhanced transcription of the gene coding for p16
p53	Decreased	Anti-tumour regulating protein, involved in apoptosis	Viral E6 protein from oncogenic HPV types binds p53 facilitating its degradation
Ki-67	Increased	Cell proliferation marker	Abnormal cell proliferation beyond basal cell layers
PCNA	Increased	Cell proliferation marker	Abnormal cell proliferation beyond basal cell layers
Cyclin E	Increased	Protein associated with CDK2	Drives cells from G1 to S phase through phosphorylation of pRb and other targets
MCM5, CDC6, c-myc, TOP2A	Increased	Proliferation markers	Abnormal cell proliferation beyond basal cell layers
Telomerase	Increased	Nucleoprotein consisting of hTR (RNA) and hTERT (enzyme)	Controls length of telomeres and plays a role in cell immortalisation
RNA markers			
E7 or E6 mRNA	Presence	Viral mRNA transcripts of E6 or E7 gene from oncogenic HPV types	Presence indicates active expression of oncogenes
Brn-3a	Increased	POU family of mRNA	Increase indicates activation of E6/E7

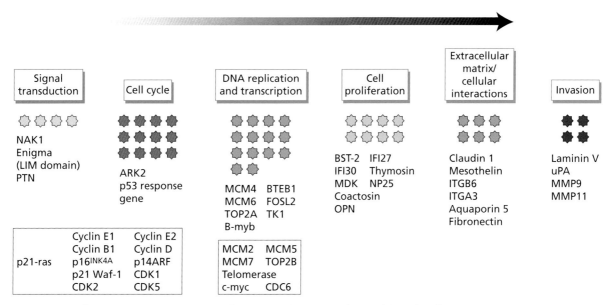

Fig. 28B.1 Diagram of some of the molecular markers of cervical neoplasia. From Chen *et al.* (2003), with permission.

PCNA in the basal and parabasal cells of normal ectocervix as well as 9/11 (82%) cases of squamous metaplasia. Expression in higher layers of the epithelium correlated with degree of CIN. Staining was markedly reduced in atrophy [outright negative staining in 5/6 (83.3%)] compared with normal epithelium. Eleven out of 12 (91.6%) high-grade lesions displayed staining in more than 35% of basal nuclei. Conversely, 35 out of 37 (94.6%) normal, metaplastic or atrophic epithelia displayed staining in less than 10% of this cell population. However, overlap in both the pattern of staining and the index of basal cell staining was seen between the low-grade lesions and squamous metaplasia (Mittal *et al.*, 1993). In another

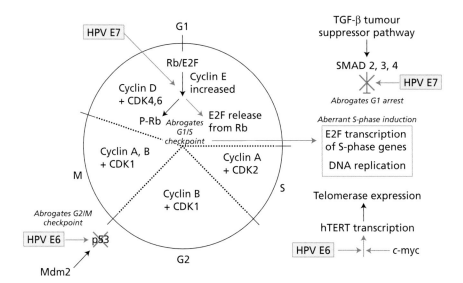

Fig. 28B.2 Aberrant S-phase induction in cervical neoplasia. From Malinowski (2005).

study, all cases of dysplasia had basal as well as suprabasal staining of dysplastic cells, which corresponded to and clearly delineated the grade of CIN (Raju, 1994). Nineteen cases of invasive squamous cell carcinoma were positive for more than 90% of nuclei, with localisation to the marginal (non-keratinised) tumour cells. The increased distribution of PCNA staining in basal cells of neoplasia suggests a departure from strict cell cycle regulation characteristic of normal epithelium. Concentration of staining to the marginal (immature) cell layers of carcinomas is characteristic of increased cell cycle in immature epithelium. Studies correlating PCNA staining with HPV DNA *in situ* hybridisation show that PCNA staining slightly precedes the accumulation of viral DNA, whereas PCNA-negative surface cells remain strongly HPV positive (Demeter *et al.*, 1994).

KI-67 (MIB-1)

The Ki-67 antigen is a non-histone protein that identifies proliferating cells. It is not phase specific, being expressed in all active parts of the cell cycle (Ki-67 is not expressed in G0) (Gerdes *et al.*, 1984). MIB-1 antibody, a monoclonal antibody produced using recombinant parts of the Ki-67 antigen as an immunogen, detects this antigen in paraffin sections (Cattoretti *et al.*, 1992; Key *et al.*, 1993). Ki-67 staining is intranuclear.

Like PCNA, Ki-67 staining spares all but rare basal cells in mature cervical squamous epithelium and concentrates in the second and third (suprabasal) cell layers (Konishi *et al.*, 1991). The basal and suprabasal cell populations conform, respectively, to the stem and transient amplifying cells, the latter signifying cells committed to differentiation (Watt, 1998). The index of Ki-67-positive cells is hormone dependent, roughly doubling (to approximately 50 per 100 parabasal cells) in the luteal phase of the menstrual cycle compared with the follicular phase. Basal cells and transformation zone reserve cells, which are otherwise negative for Ki-67, demonstrate focal positivity during the luteal phase and pregnancy (Konishi *et al.*, 1991).

HPV infection activates host cell cycle progression with increased cell cycle kinetics, and this phenomenon is reflected in an increased Ki-67 staining index. In a study of 59 cervical cone biopsy specimens taken from patients with CIN, the distribution and index of Ki-67 increased as a function of increasing grade, peaking in invasive carcinoma (Resnick *et al.*, 1996). Interestingly, squamous metaplasia specimens occasionally exhibited positive cells in all layers of the epithelium, but the index of staining was low relative to that of CIN specimens (never more than 25% of the total number of cells). Typically, parabasal and intermediate cell layers in low-grade lesions were Ki-67 positive, in contrast to all layers in high-grade lesions. In essence, the distinction of a CIN from non-neoplastic epithelium is based on the presence of Ki-67-positive cells in the upper epithelial layers of CIN.

Both CIN and atrophy are characterised by altered maturation, nuclear crowding and increased nuclear/cytoplasmic ratio. Postmenopausal epithelial alterations encompass both severe atrophy, which may be confused with CIN3, and milder disturbances in maturations that may mimic low-grade lesions (Jovanovic *et al.*, 1995). A third pattern characterised by sporadic, marked nuclear enlargement has been described in atrophic smears; these changes may occur in the absence of preinvasive disease and may resolve with topical estrogen therapy (Abati *et al.*, 1998). In a study comparing Ki-67 expression in elderly women, Mittal *et al.* (1999) showed that atrophic and neoplastic epithelia were easily distinguished by the much higher index of Ki-67 positivity in the latter (Fig. 28B.3). Atrophic changes were virtually devoid of Ki-67

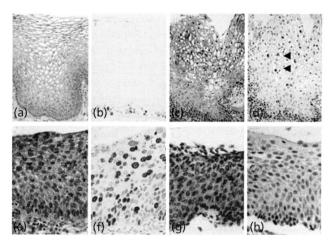

Fig. 28B.3 Distribution of MIB-1 positivity in normal mucosa. In mature squamous mucosa (a), staining is confined to nuclei in the second and third cell layers (transient amplifying cells), with occasional basal cell staining (b). In low-grade squamous lesions (c), staining is seen in areas of cytopathic effect in the upper epithelial layers (d, arrowheads), permitting distinction from normal epithelium. In CIN3 (e), staining is more diffuse and includes a higher index of cell nuclei (f). In atrophy (g), staining is markedly reduced or absent (h), permitting its distinction from CIN3. From Keating *et al.* (2001b).

positivity (Mittal *et al.*, 1999). Importantly, there was no significant difference in the expression of Ki-67 in biopsy specimens with and without inflammation. This study suggests a role for Ki-67 staining in resolving diagnostic problems associated with atrophy. Studies attempting to distinguish immature metaplasia from CIN using Ki-67 immunostaining found that it would be helpful only in a subset of HPV-positive cases that had a high degree of nuclear atypia and elevated Ki-67 index (Geng *et al.*, 1999).

TELOMERASE

Telomeres are repetitive DNA sequences at the ends of eukaryotic chromosomes that are shortened at each cell division. The shortening of telomeres is thought to be involved in cellular senescence, and severe loss in length may cause chromosome instability and cell death (Wright and Shay, 2000). Telomerase is a ribonucleoprotein enzyme composed of an RNA component (hTR) and a catalytic protein subunit (hTERT), which has a reverse transcriptase DNA polymerase activity that plays an important role in maintaining telomere length at chromosome ends (Meyerson *et al.*, 1997). In normal tissues, a small subset of cells has telomerase activity, including the proliferative basal zone of epithelia and some stromal cells (Kolquist *et al.*, 1998). Most premalignant and malignant tissues have increased telomerase activity, which is thought to contribute to their immortal phenotype.

The telomeric repeat amplification protocol (TRAP), a poly-

merase chain reaction (PCR) assay, is able to detect telomerase activity. Using this method, several authors detected telomerase activity in 100% of squamous cell carcinomas (SCC) (Shroyer *et al.*, 1998). In one study, more than 90% of CIN3 and approximately 50% of CIN1 specimens exhibited telomerase activity; however, 56% of reactive atypia and 18% of normal cervical mucosa samples were also positive, which may reflect normally increased proliferative activity (Anderson *et al.*, 1997).

The expression of telomerase at the single-cell level was assayed by *in situ* hybridisation for hTERT mRNA in tissue sections. hTERT is the rate-limiting subunit of the telomerase enzyme, and its expression correlates with enzyme activity, making it useful as a surrogate marker for telomerase activity (Takakura *et al.*, 1998). In normal cervical mucosa, hTERT expression was limited to basal and rare suprabasal cells with *in situ* hybridisation (Nakano *et al.*, 1998). Recently, this finding was confirmed by immunohistochemistry using an antibody against hTERT, which revealed that all levels of the lesional epithelium from CIN3 and SCC specimens exhibited high levels of telomerase. In contrast, the staining was confined to the basal layers in normal mucosa and was mixed in CIN1 (Frost *et al.*, 2000). In this study, a modified immunohistochemical staining protocol was used, which was problematic because of low expression levels coupled with high background staining of endocervical cells. The relationship between telomerase and HPV was demonstrated by Klingelhutz *et al.* (1996), who showed that HPV 16 E6 oncoprotein expression in human foreskin keratinocytes induced telomerase activity by a p53-independent mechanism (Klingelhutz *et al.*, 1996).

These findings suggest that telomerase plays a role in the development of cervical neoplasia. However, the clinical utility of this marker has been limited so far owing to its low expression levels, which make it difficult to detect with conventional immunohistochemical methods.

CYCLIN E

Cyclin E, through its interaction with CDK2, a cyclin-dependent kinase (CDK), and p27, a cyclin-dependent kinase inhibitor (CDKi), is involved with the passage through the critical G1–S checkpoint of the cell cycle (Dulic *et al.*, 1992; Knoblich *et al.*, 1994). The active cyclin E–CDK2 complex phosphorylates pRb, causing it to dissociate from E2F-1 (Lees *et al.*, 1992). It is E2F-1 which allows transcription of genes whose products are required for the S phase of the cell cycle (Cotran *et al.*, 1999). As cells progressing through this checkpoint are committed to completion of the cell cycle and replication, regulation of this transition is important to ensure the genetic fidelity of the cell, and it is at this point in the cell cycle that the tumour-suppressor p53, in the setting of DNA damage, is thought to induce G1 arrest via the cyclin-dependent kinase inhibitor p21, thereby allowing for DNA repair.

Interruption of the viral E1/E2 open reading frame (ORF) during HPV integration results in overexpression of the E6 and E7 viral genes of high-risk HPVs. The E6 protein binds and facilitates degradation of p53. An important consequence of binding of the E7 oncoprotein to pRb is displacement of the host E2F transcription factor, allowing progression through G1–S (Dyson *et al.*, 1989). This dysregulation of E2F activity appears to be reflected in increased transcription of the cyclin E gene (Fig. 28B.2) (Bolz *et al.*, 1996; Geng *et al.*, 1996). Studies have shown that cyclin E is upregulated by HPV 16 E7, and also interacts with the E1 gene product that is involved in viral replication (Martin *et al.*, 1998). Thus, cyclin E expression may be upregulated by E7 and, in turn, this upregulation may influence viral replication.

Several studies have shown an association between *in vivo* cyclin E staining and preinvasive and invasive cervical disease (Cho *et al.*, 1997; Dellas *et al.*, 1998; Quade *et al.*, 1998; Tae Kim *et al.*, 2000). In the 1997 study by Cho *et al.*, 15 of 23 (65%) histologically identified CINs, 17 of 39 (44%) invasive SCCs and two of six (33%) cervical adenocarcinomas were positive for cyclin E by immunohistochemistry with a mean staining index (% of positive nuclei) of 7.17%, 10.32% and 0.53% respectively. HPV types 16 and 18, detected by nested PCR, were identified in seven (30%) cases of CIN, eight (21%) SCCs and only one (17%) of the adenocarcinomas with a mean cyclin E index of 13.1%, 11.4% and 0.9% respectively. No cyclin E staining was observed in normal or metaplastic cervical tissue.

Quade *et al.* (1998) showed that 95% of normal or reactive epithelia were cyclin E negative, while over 95% of CIN1 exhibited nuclear staining, most typically in cells demonstrating a viral cytopathic effect. This association is of interest in as much as it conforms to the purported relationship between cyclin E expression and viral replication. Precisely what upregulates cyclin E in lesions associated with low-risk HPV types is not clear. Evidence that cyclin E staining is linked, directly or indirectly, to a viral cytopathic effect is seen in staining of 'immature' condylomata, which lack koilocytosis and also exhibit a much lower index of cyclin E staining. Expression in higher grade lesions is more variable, with approximately 50% staining positive for cyclin E in the study by Quade *et al.* (1998).

Tae Kim *et al.* (2000) demonstrated a statistically significant increase in the cyclin E index (CEI) (staining per 1000 cells) in 45 cases of invasive carcinoma (mean 12.3%) and CIN (7.1%) compared with a control group (1.2%) ($P < 0.05$ each). The invasive carcinomas included 39 SCCs, four adenocarcinomas and two adenosquamous carcinomas with cyclin E indexes of 15.5%, 4.6% and 9.2% respectively. High-risk HPV types, as detected by nested PCR, were positive in 31 cases of invasive carcinoma and negative in 14. The CEI for the HPV-negative cases was 19.9% on average, and was 40.7% in the HPV-positive cases ($P < 0.05$). For precursor lesions, staining

intensity by squamous intraepithelial lesion (SIL) group is not included nor is the pattern of cyclin E staining.

In a recent study of normal and abnormal cervical squamous epithelium, it was found that a histological diagnosis of SIL correlated strongly with cyclin E positivity ($P < 0.001$). Cyclin E was significantly more often full thickness in high-grade (H) SILs (78.1%) and in the lower half of the epithelium in low-grade (L) SILs (69.6%). Overall, 92.1% of lesions were cyclin E positive. Presence of HPV by PCR restriction fragment length polymorphism (RFLP) analysis correlated with cyclin E positivity, and the positive predictive value (PPV) of cyclin E for HPV was 88.7%. High-risk HPV type-specific infections were identified by cyclin E in 95% of cases. HPV risk categories (high vs. low) correlated with cyclin E positivity ($P = 0.03$) and pattern of staining ($P = 0.03$) Limitations in specificity included diffuse weak nuclear cyclin E staining in some normal or metaplastic epithelia (Keating *et al.*, 2001a).

Immunohistochemical staining of cyclin E is localised to the nucleus. Staining can also be seen in inflammatory cells as well as cervical stromal cells. Given this, interpretation of cervical epithelium with an inflammatory infiltrate can be difficult (Keating *et al.*, 2001b).

p16^INK4A (see also Chapter 28A)

p16^INK4, the *CDKN2A* gene product, is a cyclin-dependent kinase inhibitor that inhibits the CDK4/6 interaction with cyclin D1, thereby inhibiting progression through the G1–S transition checkpoint of the cell cycle. Also, in the normal cell, E2F-1 accumulation leads to induction (transcription) of p16^INK4 activity, thereby limiting G1 kinase activity by feedback inhibition.

The p16^CDKN2 gene is frequently altered in cell lines and some types of cancers (Nielsen *et al.*, 1999). However, inactivation of this gene does not appear to be important in the tumorigenesis of cervical cancer (Yoshinouchi *et al.*, 2000). On examination of 41 primary tumours and eight cell lines, Hirama *et al.* (1996) did not detect any deletions or mutations in this gene. Furthermore, in a study of 57 HPV-positive primary tumours and matched normal tissues and three HPV-positive cervical cancer-derived cell lines, there was no evidence for intragenic homozygous deletion or point mutation of the p16^INK4A gene as examined by PCR and direct sequencing (Kim *et al.*, 1998).

Previous studies have shown that p16INK4 is strongly expressed in almost all cervical cancers and that immunoreactivity for pRb is preserved, in contrast to the inverse relationship noted in other tumour types. In a study evaluating the expression of p16^INK4 and Rb proteins in 98 cervical neoplastic lesions, strong immunoreactivity for the p16^INK4 protein was observed in both the nuclei and the cytoplasm of all CIN and invasive cancer cases except several low-grade CIN lesions, and the expression of Rb protein was also demonstrated in scattered nuclei of neoplastic and normal cells in all cases investigated (Sano *et al.*, 1998a). This may relate to the fact that Rb function is altered by the E7 viral oncoprotein. Khleif *et al.* (1996) have shown that p16^{INK4} is expressed in cervical cancer cell lines in which the pRB is not functional as a consequence of HPV E7 oncoprotein activity, and that the resultant overexpression of E2F-1 induces the expression of a p16^{INK4}-related transcript. Precisely why p16^{INK4} overexpression occurs in HPV-associated lesions is not known, but a positive feedback linked to an increase in E2F transcription factor is a likely cause.

In a study of p16^{INK4} expression in two to eight samples from a normal cervix, Nielsen *et al.* (1999) demonstrated p16 staining in some areas of squamous metaplasia with only relatively few Ki-67-positive cells in these same areas. As described by Sano *et al.* (1998a), lesions scored as diffusely positive show strong homogeneous cytoplasmic staining, while those scored as focally positive show definite areas of cytoplasmic staining which tend to be in the basal one-third and lack the diffuse staining pattern. Non-neoplastic epithelia and some lesions associated with low-risk HPV types demonstrate variable and weak cytoplasmic immunoreactivity, which is quantitatively and qualitatively different from high-grade lesions, exhibiting a weak blush rather than strong granular staining.

Sano *et al.* (1998b) described uniform strong and diffuse staining for p16 in both nuclei and cytoplasm of all CIN3 and invasive cancer lesions, as well as those of many CIN1, in marked contrast to non-neoplastic lesions. They also demonstrated focal and scattered staining in most condylomas and approximately one-third of CIN1.

BRN-3A

Transcription of the viral genes encoding E6 and E7 oncoproteins is controlled by an upstream regulatory region (URR) of the virus genome, which is preferentially active in cells of cervical origin (Cripe *et al.*, 1987; Gloss *et al.*, 1987), but the majority of transcription factors that bind to this region are ubiquitously expressed (Fig. 28B.4).

The existence has been reported, however, of a cervical specific regulatory activity that is able to bind to a sequence (ATGCAATT) in the URR of HPV 16 and HPV 18 and to activate their expression specifically in cell lines of cervical origin (Dent *et al.*, 1991; Morris *et al.*, 1993). This sequence is absent in the URR of HPV 6 and HPV 11, which cause only benign warts. This activity is mediated by two distinct transcription factors, Brn-3a and Brn-3b, which were originally identified in neuronal cells (Lillycrop *et al.*, 1992; Gerrero *et al.*, 1993; Turner *et al.*, 1994) but were subsequently also demonstrated to be expressed in cervical cells (Lillycrop *et al.*, 1992). Brn-3a and Brn-3b are members of the POU family of transcription factors (Verrijzer and Van der Vliet, 1993; Wegner *et al.*, 1993) and are closely related to one another, although

they are encoded by distinct genes (Theil *et al.*, 1993). Interestingly, Brn-3a and Brn-3b have an antagonistic action on the activity of the URR, with Brn-3a stimulating transcription via the ATGCAATT motif, whereas Brn-3b suppresses transcription and interferes with activation by Brn-3a (Morris *et al.*, 1994).

Most importantly, Brn-3a plays a key role in maintaining the activity of the HPV URR in HPV-transformed cells and thereby also determines the growth characteristics of cervical cancer cells. Thus, inhibition of Brn-3a expression in an HPV-transformed cell line reduces both HPV E6 gene expression and growth rates, saturation density and anchorage-independent growth (Ndisang *et al.*, 1999). Moreover, these cervical cells with reduced Brn-3a expression are unable to form tumours when grown in nude mice, whereas the control cells with normal Brn-3a levels readily do so (Ndisang *et al.*, 2001). These effects are only observed in cervical cells expressing HPV, whereas reduction of Brn-3a levels in cervical cells transformed by other means has no effect. Thus, Brn-3a exerts its effect via modulating HPV gene expression, which in turn modulates tumour cell growth.

Ndisang *et al.* (1998) reported that Brn-3a is overexpressed approximately 300-fold in cervical biopsies taken from women with CIN3 lesions compared with women without detectable cervical abnormality. In contrast, Brn-3b levels were similar within the two groups (Ndisang *et al.*, 1998). This therefore suggests that elevated expression of Brn-3a may play a key role in inducing transcription of the genes encoding E6 and E7 in women with HPV 16 or HPV 18 infection, resulting in cervical cancer. The elevation of Brn-3a levels in women with CIN3 is not confined to the area of abnormality, but is also observed in adjacent apparently normal areas (Ndisang *et al.*, 1998) and, indeed, throughout the cervix of such women (Ndisang *et al.*, 2000). This suggests that the elevation in Brn-3a levels is not a consequence of cellular transformation because, in this case, it would be confined to the abnormal region of the cervix. Rather, it suggests that a proportion of women may have elevated Brn-3a levels as a result of genetic or environmental (for example, cigarette smoking) reasons and would therefore be particularly prone to cervical transformation following infection with HPV, with the tumour appearing at the junction of the ectocervix and endocervix where HPV and cervical tumours are particularly localised. Ndisang *et al.* (2006a) showed that Brn-3a differentially regulates HPV 16 variants, which are associated with different risks of progression to cervical carcinoma.

Sindos *et al.* (2003a) demonstrated recently that Brn-3a levels can also be measured in Pap smears and that its presence is frequently associated with the presence of HPV mRNA positivity. They also demonstrated that the mean Brn-3a levels show statistically significant correlation with the histological diagnosis and the colposcopic impression (Sindos *et al.*, 2003a). Brn-3a levels in Pap smears may be of considerable diagnostic

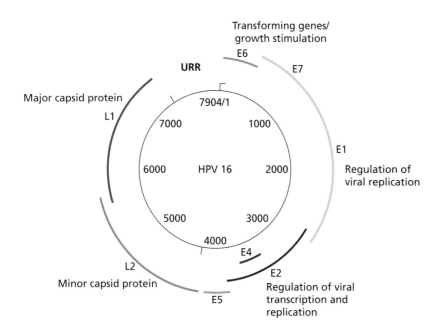

Fig. 28B.4 The upstream regulatory region (URR) controls the transcription of the viral genes encoding E6 and E7 oncoproteins.

value in identifying women requiring further follow-up or treatment (Sindos *et al.*, 2003b), as it detects activation of oncogenic HPV viruses rather than simply detect their presence, as is currently being done (Clavel *et al.*, 2001). The ability of Brn-3a to predict for cervical disease seems to be independent of the geographical characteristics of the population (Ndisang *et al.*, 2006b).

CDC6 AND MCM

Cell division cycle (CDC6) protein and minichromosome maintenance (MCM) protein play essential roles in eukaryotic DNA replication. Several studies have highlighted the potential of these proteins as molecular markers of dysplastic and malignant cells in histopathological diagnosis. The mode of expression of CDC6 and MCM5 mRNA and their significance in normal, dysplastic and malignant cervical cells remains to be elucidated. Using a quantitative real-time (RT) PCR assay, Murphy *et al.* (2005) compared CDC6 and MCM5 mRNA expression in normal cervical epithelium, CIN and invasive SCC of the cervix. The study cohort comprised 20 normal cervical biopsies, 20 CIN3 and eight invasive SCCs. A linear increase in MCM5 and CDC6 mRNA expression is observed in normal cervix, CIN3 and invasive cervical carcinoma. The overall difference in MCM5 mRNA expression in the normal cervix, CIN3 and invasive cohort groups is highly statistically significant ($P = 0.001$). An increase in CDC6 mRNA expression in CIN3 and invasive cervical SCC was observed.

Increased transcription of MCM5 and CDC6 occurs as a consequence of cervical neoplastic progression. This pattern of increased mRNA expression in CIN3 and invasive cervical carcinoma directly correlates with findings at the phenotypic

protein expression level. Ishimi *et al.* (2003) also showed similar results (see Fig. 28B.5).

SUMMARY: FUTURE DIRECTIONS

Although thousands of papers are published each year describing genetic mutations or alterations in expression levels that are associated with various types of cancers, very few of these are developed into reliable molecular markers that can be used routinely in the clinical setting. Professor D.P. Malinowski (personal communication, 2005) has suggested that there are potentially 20 biomarkers at this time that can provide clinical samples that may be able to create characterisation of selected biomarkers, i.e. MCM2, MCM5, MCM6, MCM7 and TOP2A (Fig. 28B.6). Some of these molecular markers are used in combination with other techniques, such as imaging or histological studies, to detect, diagnose and monitor cancer. However, as assays become more sensitive and quantitative, a more thorough assessment of a patient's cancer status will be based on molecular markers alone.

The sensitivity and specificity of a molecular marker cannot be fully realised until careful testing is carried out in large numbers of tumour specimens and compared with normal control subjects — to identify markers that are truly over-represented or qualitatively different in the neoplastic cells compared with normal cells. Incorporation of molecular marker analysis into clinical trials is therefore a crucial part of marker development.

The obvious advantage of applying a neoplasia-specific biomarker to cytological triage lies in the capacity of this technology to resolve the origin and associated cancer risk of a cytological abnormality. The major theoretical advantage of this approach over a less specific test such as HPV testing is

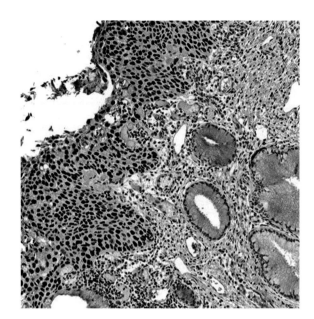

Fig. 28B.5 Overexpression of MCM6 protein in cervical high-grade dysplasia detected through immunohistochemistry.

that the cytological diagnosis can be modified based on the reclassification of the abnormal cells under scrutiny. For example, a biomarker-positive borderline smear could be reclassified as mild dyskarosis, effectively eliminating the ASCUS/ borderline category in many cases. Moreover, theoretically, this could be achieved by the simple histochemical analysis of a cytospin sample taken from the original vial. Depending upon the sensitivity and specificity of the biomarker in use, a variety of screening strategies would be possible, including immunohistochemical analysis of liquid-based preparations or, eventually, solution-based screening tests that would be suitable for exfoliated cells obtained by self-testing.

Relatively few studies have explored biomarkers in cytological diagnosis but many are expected. A study by Weaver *et al.* (2000) examined 20 cases of CIN1, 40 cases of ASCUS and 21 normal smears for the presence of cyclin E and an HPV antibody (clone K1H8) to an antigen broadly expressed in different HPV subtypes. They found 100% of LSILs to be both cyclin E and anti-HPV positive. Thirty-five ASCUS cases were cyclin E positive, 34 of which were anti-HPV antibody positive. They reported inflammatory cells as being variably immunoreactive, and no HSIL cases were included in the study.

Another group investigated immunocytochemical expression of Ki-67 (MIB-1) on the primary Papanicolaou-stained smears and showed that absence of Ki-67 staining was a reliable indicator of atrophic cells (Ejersbo *et al.*, 1999). The authors reported that this marker reduced false-positive cytological diagnoses by 86%.

Recently, another study demonstrated that molecular analyses of not only DNA, but also RNA and protein, was possible from methanol fluid-based specimens (Lin *et al.*, 2000). DNA and RNA was extracted from cell pellets obtained from the residual fluid-based Papanicolaou specimen after clinical processing. Methylation-specific PCRs were used to determine the hypermethylation status of the p16 gene and the gene for E-cadherin. Immunohistochemical staining for protein expression was also performed on the monolayer slides. The authors concluded that multiple molecular analyses were possible at the deoxyribonucleic acid, ribonucleic acid and protein level in these specimens.

A series of liquid-based (ThinPrep®) samples have been analysed recently for p16 using cytospin preparations in an effort to determine whether this antigen was preserved in methanol-based fixatives. The strength of this marker for discriminating cytological samples of low versus high risk is currently under study. However, the potential for non-specific staining, particularly in glandular cells, may limit the value of this marker.

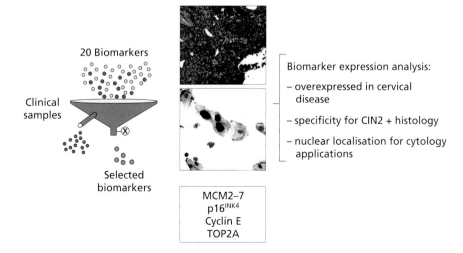

Fig. 28B.6 Characteristics of potential biomarkers of cervical neoplasia.

In conclusion, the emerging evidence strongly supports the concept that HPV induces or upregulates the expression of host genes. Depending upon the sensitivity and specificity of these biomarkers, they could be used to screen for, triage and diagnose cervical abnormalities in both cytological and histological preparations. As the field of molecular diagnosis unfolds, these markers will be used to modify and improve cytological and histological interpretation and, ultimately, for screening and triage.

ACKNOWLEDGEMENT

The authors wish to thank Professor Douglas P. Malinowski, Vice President of Research and Chief Scientific Officer, Tripath Oncology, Durham, NC, USA, for his assistance in the production of this chapter, especially in allowing the reproduction of Figures 28B.5 and 28B.6.

REFERENCES

Abati A, Jaffurs W, Wilder AM (1998) Squamous atypia in the atrophic cervical vaginal smear: a new look at an old problem. *Cancer* 84 (4): 218–225.

Altiok S (2003) Molecular markers in cervical cytology. *Clinical and Laboratory Medicine* 23 (3): 709–728.

Anderson S, Shera K, Ihle J et al. (1997) Telomerase activation in cervical cancer. *American Journal of Pathology* 151 (1): 25–31.

Bibbo M, Klump WJ, DeCecco J et al. (2002) Procedure for immunocytochemical detection of P16INK4A antigen in thin-layer, liquid-based specimens. *Acta Cytologica* 46 (1): 25–29.

Botz J, Zerfass-Thome K, Spitkovsky D et al. (1996) Cell cycle regulation of the murine cyclin E gene depends on an E2F binding site in the promoter. *Molecular and Cell Biology* 16 (7): 3401–3409.

Bravo R, Frank R, Blundell PA et al. (1987) Cyclin/PCNA is the auxiliary protein of DNA polymerase-delta. *Nature* 326 (6112): 515–517.

Cattoretti G, Becker MH, Key G et al. (1992) Monoclonal antibodies against recombinant parts of the Ki-67 antigen (MIB 1 and MIB 3) detect proliferating cells in microwave-processed formalin-fixed paraffin sections. *Journal of Pathology* 168 (4): 357–363.

Chen Y, Miller C, Mosher R et al. (2003) Identification of cervical cancer markers by cDNA and tissue microarrays. *Cancer Research* 63: 1927–1935.

Cho NH, Kim YT, Kim JW (1997) Correlation between G1 cyclins and HPV in the uterine cervix. *International Journal of Gynecological Pathology* 16 (4): 339–347.

Clavel C, Masure M, Bory J-P et al. (2001) Hybrid Capture ii-based human papillomavirus detection, a sensitive test to detect in routine high-grade cervical lesions: a preliminary study on 1518 women *British Journal of Cancer* 80: 1306–1311.

Costa S, Sideri M, Syrjanen K et al. (2000) Combined Pap smear, cervicography and HPV DNA testing in the detection of cervical intraepithelial neoplasia and cancer. *Acta Cytologica* 44 (3): 310–318.

Cotran RS, Kumar V, Collins T (1999) *Robbins Pathologic basis of disease*, 6th edn. Philadelphia: W.B. Saunders, pp. 286–294.

Cox JT, Schiffman M, Solomon D (2003) Prospective follow-up suggests similar risk of subsequent cervical intraepithelial neoplasia grade 2 or 3 among women with cervical intraepithelial neoplasia grade 1 or negative colposcopy and directed biopsy. *American Journal of Obstetrics and Gynecology* 188 (6): 1406–1412.

Cripe TC, Hangen TH, Turk JP et al. (1987) Transcriptional regulation of the human papilloma virus 16 E6–E7 promoter by a keratinocyte-dependent enhancer and by viral E2 transactivator and repressor gene products: implications for cervical carcinogenesis. *EMBO Journal* 6: 3745–3753.

Dellas A, Schultheiss E, Leivas MR et al. (1998) Association of p27Kip1, cyclin E and c-myc expression with progression and prognosis in HPV-positive cervical neoplasms. *Anticancer Research* 18 (6A): 3991–3998.

Demeter LM, Stoler MH, Broker TR et al. (1994) Induction of proliferating cell nuclear antigen in differentiated keratinocytes of human papillomavirus-infected lesions. *Human Pathology* 25 (4): 343–348.

Dent CL, McIndoe GAJ, Latchman DS (1991) The constitutively expressed octamer binding protein OTF-1 and a novel octamer binding protein expressed specifically in cervical cells bind to an octamer-related sequence in the human papillomavirus 16 enhancer. *Nucleic Acids Research* 19: 4531–4535.

Dulic V, Lees E, Reed SI (1992) Association of human cyclin E with a periodic G1–S phase protein kinase. *Science* 257 (5078): 1958–1961.

Dyson N, Howley PM, Munger K et al. (1989) The human papilloma virus-16 E7 oncoprotein is able to bind to the retinoblastoma gene product. *Science* 243 (4893): 934–937.

Ejersbo D, Jensen HA, Holund B (1999) Efficacy of Ki-67 antigen staining in Papanicolaou (Pap) smears in post-menopausal women with atypia — an audit. *Cytopathology* 10 (6): 369–374.

Fahey MT, Irwig L, Macaskill P (1995) Meta-analysis of Pap test accuracy. *American Journal of Epidemiology* 141 (7): 680–689.

Frost M, Bobak JB, Gianani R et al. (2000) Localization of telomerase hTERT protein and hTR in benign mucosa, dysplasia, and squamous cell carcinoma of the cervix. *American Journal of Clinical Pathology* 114 (5): 726–734.

Garcia RL, Coltrera MD, Gown AM (1989) Analysis of proliferative grade using anti-PCNA/cyclin monoclonal antibodies in fixed, embedded tissues. Comparison with flow cytometric analysis. *American Journal of Pathology* 134 (4): 733–739.

Geng Y, Eaton EN, Picon M et al. (1996) Regulation of cyclin E transcription by E2Fs and retinoblastoma protein. *Oncogene* 12 (6): 1173–1180.

Geng L, Connolly DC, Isacson C et al. (1999) Atypical immature metaplasia (AIM) of the cervix: is it related to high-grade squamous intraepithelial lesion (HSIL)? *Human Pathology* 30 (3): 345–351.

Gerdes J, Lemke H, Baisch H et al. (1984) Cell cycle analysis of a cell proliferation-associated human nuclear antigen defined by the monoclonal antibody Ki-67. *Journal of Immunology* 133 (4): 1710–1715.

Gerrero MR, McEvilly RJ, Turner E et al. (1993) Brn-3.0, a POU domain protein expressed in the sensory, immune and endocrine systems that functions on elements distinct from known octamer motifs. *Proceedings of the National Academy of Sciences of the USA* 90: 10841–10845.

Gloss B, Bernard HU, Seedorf K et al. (1987) The upstream regulatory region of the human papilloma virus contains an E2 protein independent enhancer which is specific for cervical carcinoma cells and regulated by glucocorticoid hormones. *EMBO Journal* 6: 3735–3743.

Hildesheim A, Wang SS (2002) Host and viral genetics and risk of cervical cancer: a review. *Virus Research* 89 (2): 229–240.

Hirama T, Miller CW, Wilczynski SP *et al.* (1996) p16 (CDKN2/cyclin-dependent kinase-4 inhibitor/multiple tumor suppressor-1) gene is not altered in uterine cervical carcinomas or cell lines. *Modern Pathology* 9 (1): 26–31.

Ishimi Y, Okayasu I, Kato C *et al.* (2003) Enhanced expression of Mcm proteins in cancer cells derived from uterine cervix. *European Journal of Biochemistry* 270 (6): 1089–1101.

Jovanovic AS, McLachlin CM, Shen L *et al.* (1995) Postmenopausal squamous atypia: a spectrum including 'pseudo-koilocytosis'. *Modern Pathology* 8 (4): 408–412.

Kadish AS, Timmins P, Wang Y *et al.* (2002) Regression of cervical intraepithelial neoplasia and loss of human papillomavirus (HPV) infection is associated with cell-mediated immune responses to an HPV type 16 E7 peptide. *Cancer Epidemiology Biomarkers and Prevention* 11 (5): 483–488.

Keating JT, Cviko A, Riethdorf S *et al.* (2001a) Ki-67, cyclin E, and p16^{INK4} are complementary surrogate biomarkers for human papilloma virus-related cervical neoplasia. *American Journal of Surgical Pathology* 25 (7): 884–891.

Keating JT, Ince T, Crum CP (2001b) Surrogate biomarkers of HPV infection in cervical neoplasia screening and diagnosis. *Advances in Anatomical Pathology* 8 (2): 83–92.

Key G, Becker MH, Baron B *et al.* (1993) New Ki-67-equivalent murine monoclonal antibodies (MIB 1–3) generated against bacterially expressed parts of the Ki-67 cDNA containing three 62 base pair repetitive elements encoding for the Ki-67 epitope. *Laboratory Investigation* 68 (6): 629–636.

Khleif SN, DeGregori J, Yee CL *et al.* (1996) Inhibition of cyclin D-CDK4/CDK6 activity is associated with an E2F-mediated induction of cyclin kinase inhibitor activity. *Proceedings of the National Academy of Sciences of the USA* 93 (9): 4350–4354.

Kim JW, Namkoong SE, Ryu SW *et al.* (1998) Absence of p15INK4B and p16INK4A gene alterations in primary cervical carcinoma tissues and cell lines with human papillomavirus infection. *Gynecologic Oncology* 70 (1): 75–79.

Klingelhutz AJ, Foster SA, McDougall JK (1996) Telomerase activation by the E6 gene product of human papillomavirus type 16. *Nature* 380 (6569): 79–82.

Knoblich JA, Sauer K, Jones L *et al.* (1994) Cyclin E controls S phase progression and its down-regulation during *Drosophila* embryogenesis is required for the arrest of cell proliferation. *Cell* 77 (1): 107–120.

Kolquist KA, Ellisen LW, Counter CM *et al.* (1998) Expression of TERT in early premalignant lesions and a subset of cells in normal tissues. *Nature Genetics* 19 (2): 182–186.

Konishi I, Fujii S, Nonogaki H *et al.* (1991) Immunohistochemical analysis of estrogen receptors, progesterone receptors, Ki-67 antigen, and human papillomavirus DNA in normal and neoplastic epithelium of the uterine cervix. *Cancer* 68 (6): 1340–1350.

Landberg G, Roos G (1991) Antibodies to proliferating cell nuclear antigen as S-phase probes in flow cytometric cell cycle analysis. *Cancer Research* 51 (17): 4570–4574.

Lees E, Faha B, Dulic V *et al.* (1992) Cyclin E/cdk2 and cyclin A/cdk2 kinases associate with p107 and E2F in a temporally distinct manner. *Genes and Development* 6 (10): 1874–1885.

Lillycrop KA, Budhram-Mahadeo VS, Lakin ND *et al.* (1992) A novel POU family transcription factor is closely related to Brn-3 but has a distinct expression pattern in neuronal cells. *Nucleic Acids Research* 20: 5093–5096.

Lin WM, Ashfaq R, Michalopulos EA *et al.* (2000) Molecular Papanicolaou tests in the twenty-first century: molecular analyses with fluid-based Papanicolaou technology. *American Journal of Obstetrics and Gynecology* 183 (1): 39–45.

Malinowski DP (2005) Molecular diagnostic assays for cervical neoplasia: emerging markers for the detection of high-grade cervical disease. *BioTechniques* 39 (Suppl.): 17–23.

Martin LG, Demers GW, Galloway DA (1998) Disruption of the G1/S transition in human papillomavirus type 16 E7-expressing human cells is associated with altered regulation of cyclin E. *Journal of Virology* 72 (2): 975–985.

Meyerson M, Counter CM, Eaton EN *et al.* (1997) hEST2, the putative human telomerase catalytic subunit gene, is up-regulated in tumor cells and during immortalization. *Cell* 90 (4): 785–795.

Mittal KR, Demopoulos RI, Goswami S (1993) Proliferating cell nuclear antigen (cyclin) expression in normal and abnormal cervical squamous epithelia. *American Journal of Surgical Pathology* 17 (2): 117–122.

Mittal K, Mesia A, Demopoulos RI (1999) MIB-1 expression is useful in distinguishing dysplasia from atrophy in elderly women. *International Journal of Gynecological Pathology* 18 (2): 122–124.

Morris PJ, Dent CL, Ring CJA *et al.* (1993) The octamer-binding site in the HPV16 regulatory region produces opposite effects on gene expression in cervical and non-cervical cells. *Nucleic Acids Research* 21: 1019–1023.

Morris PJ, Theil T, Ring CJA *et al.* (1994) The opposite and antagonistic effects of the closely related POU family transcription factors on the activity of a target promoter are dependent upon differences in the POU domain. *Molecular and Cellular Biology* 14: 6907–6914.

Murphy N, Ring M, Heffron CC *et al.* (2005) Quantitation of CDC6 and MCM5 mRNA in cervical intraepithelial neoplasia and invasive squamous cell carcinoma of the cervix. *Modern Pathology* 18 (6): 844–849.

Nakano K, Watney E, McDougall JK (1998) Telomerase activity and expression of telomerase RNA component and telomerase catalytic subunit gene in cervical cancer. *American Journal of Pathology* 153 (3): 857–864.

Ndisang D, Morris PJ, Chapman C *et al.* (1998) The HPV activating transcription factor Brn-3a is over expressed in CIN3 lesions. *Journal of Clinical Investigation* 101: 1687–1692.

Ndisang D, Budhram-Mahadeo VS, Latchman DS (1999) The Brn-3a transcription factor plays a critical role in regulating HPV gene expression and determining the growth characteristics of cervical cancer cells. *Journal of Biological Chemistry* 274: 28521–28527.

Ndisang D, Budhram-Mahadeo VS, Singer A *et al.* (2000) Widespread elevated expression of the HPV-activating cellular transcription factor Brn-3a in the cervix of women with CIN3. *Clinical Science* 98: 601–602.

Ndisang D, Budhram-Mahadeo V, Pedley B *et al.* (2001) The Brn-3a transcription factor plays a key role in regulating the growth of cervical cancer cells *in vivo*. *Oncogene* 20: 4899–4903.

Ndisang D, Faulkes DJ, Gascoyne D *et al.* (2006a) Differential regulation of different human papillomavirus variants by the POU family transcription factor Brn-3a. *Oncogene* 25: 51–60.

Ndisang D, Lorenzato F, Sindos M *et al.* (2006b) Detection of cervical abnormalities in a developing country using measurement of Brn-3a in cervical smears. *Gynecologic Oncology* 100: 89–94.

Nielsen GP, Stemmer-Rachamimov AO, Shaw J *et al.* (1999) Immunohistochemical survey of p16INK4A expression in normal human adult and infant tissues. *Laboratory Investigation* 79 (9): 1137–1143.

Quade BJ, Park JJ, Crum CP *et al.* (1998) In vivo cyclin E expression as a marker for early cervical neoplasia. *Modern Pathology* 11 (12): 1238–1246.

Raffle AE, Alden B, Quinn M *et al.* (2003) Outcomes of screening to prevent cancer: analysis of cumulative incidence of cervical abnormality and modelling of cases and deaths prevented. *British Medical Journal* 326 (7395): 901.

Raju GC (1994) Expression of the proliferating cell nuclear antigen in cervical neoplasia. *International Journal of Gynecological Pathology* 13 (4): 337–341.

Resnick M, Lester S, Tate JE *et al.* (1996) Viral and histopathologic correlates of MN and MIB-1 expression in cervical intraepithelial neoplasia. *Human Pathology* 27 (3): 234–239.

Sano T, Oyama T, Kashiwabara K *et al.* (1998a) Expression status of p16 protein is associated with human papillomavirus oncogenic potential in cervical and genital lesions. *American Journal of Pathology* 153 (6): 1741–1748.

Sano T, Oyama T, Kashiwabara K *et al.* (1998b) Immunohistochemical overexpression of p16 protein associated with intact retinoblastoma protein expression in cervical cancer and cervical intraepithelial neoplasia. *Pathology International* 48 (8): 580–585.

Shroyer KR, Thompson LC, Enomoto T *et al.* (1998) Telomerase expression in normal epithelium, reactive atypia, squamous dysplasia, and squamous cell carcinoma of the uterine cervix. *American Journal of Clinical Pathology* 109 (2): 153–162.

Shurbaji MS, Brooks SK, Thurmond TS (1993). Proliferating cell nuclear antigen immunoreactivity in cervical intraepithelial neoplasia and benign cervical epithelium. *American Journal of Clinical Pathology* 100 (1): 22–26.

Sindos M, Ndisang D, Pisal N *et al.* (2003a) Detection of cervical neoplasia using measurement of Brn-3a in cervical smears with persistent minor abnormality. *International Journal of Gynecological Cancer* 13: 515–517.

Sindos M, Ndisang D, Pisal N *et al.* (2003b) Measurement of Brn-3a levels in Pap smears provides a novel diagnostic marker for the detection of cervical neoplasia. *Gynecologic Oncology* 90: 366–371.

Tae Kim Y, Kyoung Choi E, Hoon Cho N *et al.* (2000) Expression of cyclin E and p27(KIP1) in cervical carcinoma. *Cancer Letters* 153 (1–2): 41–50.

Takakura M, Kyo S, Kanaya T *et al.* (1998) Expression of human telomerase subunits and correlation with telomerase activity in cervical cancer. *Cancer Research* 58 (7): 1558–61.

Theil T, McLean-Hunter S, Zornig M *et al.* (1993) Mouse Brn-3 family of POU transcription factors: a new amino terminal domain is crucial for the oncogenic activity of Brn-3A. *Nucleic Acids Research* 21: 5921–5929.

Turner EE, Jenne KJ, Rosenfeld MG (1994) Brn-3.2: a Brn-3-related transcription factor with distinctive central nervous system expression and regulation by retinoic acid. *Neuron* 12: 205–218.

Verrijzer CP, Van der Vliet PC (1993) POU domain transcription factors. *Biochimica et Biophysica Acta* 1173: 1–21.

Wang SS, Hildesheim A (2003) Chapter 5: Viral and host factors in human papillomavirus persistence and progression. *Journal of the National Cancer Institute Monograph* 31: 35–40.

Watt FM (1998) Epidermal stem cells: markers, patterning and the control of stem cell fate. *Philosophical Transactions of the Royal Society of London B Biological Science* 353 (1370): 831–837.

Weaver EJ, Kovatich AJ, Bibbo M (2000) Cyclin E expression and early cervical neoplasia in ThinPrep specimens. A feasibility study. *Acta Cytologica* 44 (3): 301–304.

Wegner M, Drolet DW, Rosenfeld MG (1993) POU-domain proteins. Structure and function of developmental regulators. *Current Opinion in Cell Biology* 5: 488–498.

Wright WE, Shay JW (2000) Telomere dynamics in cancer progression and prevention: fundamental differences in human and mouse telomere biology. *Nature Medicine* 6 (8): 849–851.

Yoshinouchi M, Hongo A, Takamoto N *et al.* (2000) Alteration of the CDKN2/p16 gene is not required for HPV-positive uterine cervical cancer cell lines. *International Journal of Oncology* 16 (3): 537–541.

Screening for cervical cancer in developing countries

Saloney Nazeer

INTRODUCTION: THE CHALLENGE OF CERVICAL CANCER

Cervical cancer is perhaps the most preventable and curable major form of cancer, provided it is diagnosed early enough. Raising awareness, implementing simple screening methods and standard treatments have helped reduce invasive cases by up to 80% in some industrialised countries. Yet, in developing countries cervical cancer continues to account for up to 30% of all cancers in women, the majority of whom are seen at late incurable stages, if ever. The gravity of the problem is undeniable. Technical knowledge about the prevention and cure of this disease is well documented, yet the majority of countries around the world have failed to establish control programmes. This chapter aims at understanding the issues and proposes solutions to the problem.

Cancer is currently responsible for one-tenth of all deaths in the world. According to World Health Organization (WHO) data, in the year 2000, there were 10 million new cases, 6 million deaths and 22 million people living with cancer, globally.

More than 60% of all the prevalent cancer cases in the world are found in developing countries, which have 75% of the world's population. As the proportion of elderly people increases in most countries, and tobacco use and exposure to other carcinogens grows, the burden of cancer will rise significantly. Current advances in oncology make it possible to prevent one-third of all cancers, to cure one-third and provide good palliation for the one-third that are incurable. Recent trends, however, indicate that, without rigorous control measures, cancer will become the leading cause of mortality in many countries over the next 15–25 years. An increase of 25% will occur in developed countries compared with a 100% rise in developing countries (WHO, 2002).

Cervical cancer is the most common form of cancer in women in virtually all developing countries and the second most common form of cancer in women in the world following breast cancer. It constitutes approximately 12% of all cancers in women. Globally, every year, there are approximately

Table 29A.1 Annual estimates of new cases globally of cervical cancer in comparison with other gynaecological cancers (WHO/IARC/GLOBOSCAN, 2000).

	Incidence	Mortality
Breast cancer	1 000 000	373 000
Cervical cancer	500 000	300 000
Ovarian cancer	193 000	114 000
Endometrial cancer	189 000	45 000

500 000 new cases of and 300 000 deaths from cervical cancer (Table 29A.1).

If the undiagnosed, early cases are taken into account, there would be 900 000 new cases worldwide each year. It is important to note that the estimates for incidence vary considerably in accuracy for different areas in the world, depending on the extent and accuracy of locally available data. In 1990, about 18% of the world population was covered by registries, 64% of developed countries and 5% of developing countries. In developing countries, coverage is often confined to capital cities only. Similarly for mortality data, coverage of the population is manifestly incomplete in most developing countries; hence, the mortality rates produced are implausibly low. Moreover, the information on cause-specific mortality is poor (Parkin *et al.*, 2001). Table 29A.1 gives global statistics of cervical cancer in comparison with other gynaecological cancers including breast cancer.

Developing countries harbour 80% of the global estimates of cervical cancer, representing 12% of all cancers in some countries and up to 30% in others. It is the leading cause of cancer-related deaths in women. In comparison, in industrialised countries, it accounts for 3–5% of all female cancers. There are marked regional and intraregional differences in the prevalence of cervical cancer, indicating an effect of socioeconomic and cultural influence. The highest incidences have been recorded from Cali, Colombia (52/100 000), and Madras, India (48/100 000). The lowest incidences have been recorded from Kuwait (3/100 000) and Israel (5/100 000) (Parkin *et al.*, 2001; Pisani *et al.*, 2002).

CERVICAL CANCER CONTROL IN DEVELOPING COUNTRIES

The problem

Whereas early detection and screening along with health education programmes have been successful in reducing morbidity and mortality in many developed countries by up to 80%, in most developing countries, because of lack of screening programmes, 60–80% of cases of cervical cancer are diagnosed at an advanced, incurable stage, i.e. stage III or IV. The majority of the population at risk is not covered by a screening programme or cancer care facilities, resulting in a very high burden of prevalent invasive disease. According to WHO estimates, at any given time, 40% of women are screened for cervical cancer in industrialised countries, but only 5% of women are screened in developing countries (Miller, 1992; Nazeer, 1996). Under such conditions, incidence often equates to mortality. This is evident in the marked difference in the incidence of invasive cervical cancer in developed and developing countries (Table 29A.2).

There are many factors that result in a failure either to implement an adequate screening programme or, once such a programme is initiated, to have any impact on the resultant screening programme. These factors are varied in nature and cover the whole sphere of public and social health. They are complex and vary from country to country.

Factors resulting in a failure to implement an adequate screening programme

The major factors contributing to the inability to establish screening programmes, which in turn result in the high disease burden in developing countries, include:

1 Lack of public, professional and political awareness regarding the prevention and potential curability of cervical cancer.

Table 29A.2 Estimated cases of cervical cancer in regions and selected countries (WHO, 2002).

Region/country	New cases/year
North America	15 000
Latin America	70 000
Europe + USSR	65 000
Africa	66 000
China	131 500
India	125 952
Japan	11 600
Australia/NZ	1200

There is a general fatalistic attitude towards cancer and failure to understand the benefits of screening programmes. Literacy rates are generally low, especially in rural populations and particularly among women.

2 Lack of political/national commitment. This is mainly because of unawareness of the burden of the disease. There are no population-based cancer registries in most developing countries. Most of the data are hospital based and incomplete and, therefore, current estimates of cervical cancer are underestimated because of poor data capture. This makes it difficult to convince health legislators to recognise cervical cancer as a public health priority.

3 Inadequate or total lack of health care facilities, especially in rural areas. Some 60–70% of populations reside in rural areas. The majority of them do not have access to even basic health care (WHO/SEARO/EMRO, 2000).

4 Inaccessibility of cancer care facilities. The secondary and tertiary care facilities are often concentrated in the big cities, accessible only to a small urban portion of the population. Accessibility for periurban and rural residents is impractical because of large distances and inadequate transport systems (WHO/WPRO, 2001; Robyr *et al.*, 2003).

5 Socioeconomic/cultural constraints. In developing countries, only 5% of the total world cancer resources are spent. At a national level, the health budget in these countries is limited, and the list of other competing health issues is long. In the absence of apparent disease, social and religious beliefs and taboos often restrict women from participating in health programmes such as screening, in the absence of an apparent disease (Miller, 1992; WHO, 2002).

6 Low priority for women's health issues generally and especially after reproductive age. Often, in these countries, women do not seek medical advice once they have stopped producing children.

7 Lack of quality control. In most developing countries, the concept of quality control does not exist. There is no system of monitoring and evaluation of health services, and often there is a lack of standard protocols. For example, during comparative studies evaluating alternative strategies for cervical cancer screening, the false-negative rates for cytology documented from different developing countries range from 40% to 70%. The very high prevalence of reproductive tract infections and inflammation in these countries also adds to the inaccuracies (Veena *et al.*, 1995; Chirenje *et al.*, 1999).

8 Lack of outpatient/office management facilities. Outpatient diagnostic and treatment facilities are non-existent even in urban areas because of lack of equipment and trained personnel. Currently, cervical intraepithelial neoplasia (CIN) is generally treated by cold knife conisation or hysterectomy, with or without concomitant pathology, both requiring hospitalisation and general anaesthesia.

9 HIV/AIDS and sexually transmitted disease (STD) epidemic. There has been a documented rise in the incidence of

AIDS and other STDs in recent years, especially in African and East European regions. Not only has this put a tremendous burden on the already thinly stretched national budgets, but it has complicated the debate regarding the efficacy of cervical cancer screening in AIDS-affected countries (UNAIDS/ WHO, 1997, 2002).

Factors resulting in a failure to impact on screening programmes

Although in theory most developing countries have national policies on cancer screening under the WHO-initiated National Cancer Control Programmes, they are based mainly on western textbook models and most have never been implemented practically. The few examples of attempts being made at cervical cancer screening are in Cameroon, Chile, Central American states, Costa Rica, India, Malaysia, Mexico, Mongolia, Nigeria, Pakistan, the Philippines, South Africa and Thailand. These projects are in varied stages of evolution – from pilot studies to nation-wide programmes. However, they have failed to have an impact, at local and national level, for the following reasons (WHO/PAHO, 1996; WHO/AFRO, 2000; WHO/EURO, 2000; WHO/SEARO/EMRO, 2000; WHO/WPRO, 2001):

1 Lack of organisation and monitoring. Often the projects were not tailored to the needs and resources of the locality. Baseline and process indicators were often not outlined thoughtfully at the outset. The attempts were fragmented, as were the information systems, with no real coordination or communication among the different disciplines involved.

2 Lack of motivation of staff. It was difficult to motivate already overworked staff employed at government-run health facilities, especially when incentives such as bonuses, based on examples from developed countries, could not be introduced.

3 Low coverage of screened population: coverage achieved in different countries ranged from 2% to 20%, due to disorganisation and lack of motivation of the public and professionals.

4 Limited resources. Diagnostic and treatment facilities were not equipped to take the extra load of prevalent disease detected by the screening programmes. There were long delays, up to 2 months, in reporting the results of cytology.

5 Low patient compliance. Most education campaigns, especially in illiterate societies, failed to change attitudes and practices over short periods of time. In some programmes, the loss to follow-up after a screening test was up to 50%. This was due mainly to failure to communicate, especially with women from rural areas, and the long delays between screening and management phases.

6 Affordability and availability. In most countries, in the absence of provision in the national budget for the costs of screening, the client was expected to pay for the screening and follow-up management. The costs were unaffordable in relation to the very low per capita income.

7 Lack of political support. In the absence of a sustained directive and commitment from health authorities at national level, it was difficult to sustain support at local level. Priorities change as frequently as the political appointments at the national level. Moreover, civil war outbreaks and natural disasters often create large displaced population groups in these countries.

8 Sustainability. The above factors were deterrents to establishing a sound basis for such initiatives or to sustain and expand them.

Figure 29A.1 gives the age-standardised rates of cervical cancer across the globe highlighting the differences among countries with and without successful screening programmes.

The solution

In the face of the increasing burden of the disease in these countries, there is an urgent need to look for a realistic, pragmatic approach to cervical cancer control, coupled with

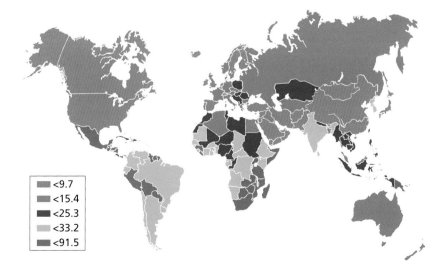

Fig. 29A.1 Incidence of cancer of the uterine cervix. Age standardised (world) rate per 100 000.

parallel provision of curative therapy for the curable, and palliative care and pain relief for the incurable. In the last decade, major advances have been made in our understanding of approaches to cervical cancer control by screening. It has been proven that screening for cervical cancer reduces the incidence of invasive disease and is applicable as a public health policy. The best results have been documented from the Nordic countries (Hristova and Hakama, 1997), British Columbia (Miller *et al.*, 1990) and England (Quinn *et al.*, 1999) where well-organised screening programmes have helped to reduce the incidence of and mortality from cervical cancer by about 80%. One factor, however, often not taken into account in evaluating these programmes, is that, at that time, there was greater health awareness among women, greater knowledge of the early symptoms of cervical cancer and availability of free standard treatment (Laara *et al.*, 1987).

Based on such documented experiences, it is recommended that countries should implement information education and communication programmes, coupled with organised screening programmes as opposed to opportunistic screening. In most developing countries, however, a meaningful coverage of all at-risk women through cytological screening will not be possible for decades to come, because of the paucity of economic and technical manpower resources. The problem is compounded in developing countries because the laboratory services are inadequate in terms of capacity, technical training and experience, information systems and quality control mechanisms (Nazeer, 1996; Miller *et al.*, 2000). Under the auspices of the WHO Study Group on Control of Cervical Cancer in Developing Countries, several studies were initiated in different countries to evaluate alternative methods to cytology for screening precancerous lesions. The criteria for the search were low cost, low expertise required and immediate diagnosis and assessment sensitivity and specificity. Affordability and immediate diagnosis and assessment were held to be of particular importance (Nazeer, 1996). Out of the two promising alternatives to Pap smear, namely visual inspection with acetic acid (VIA) and human papillomavirus (HPV) detection, VIA was considered to be ideal for developing countries because of expected low costs. However, the feasibility of these two methods has not been evaluated in an actual screening programme (Miller *et al.*, 2000).

Independent of WHO, various other attempts are being made around the world to find solutions for developing countries. In order to pool all this experience and knowledge to be able to formulate guidelines for practical implementation into appropriate screening programmes, the WHO Study Group was expanded to form the International Network on Control of Gynaecological Cancers (INCGC). It is a multidisciplinary group, comprising governmental and non-governmental organisations and institutes, which helps developing countries find collaborative solutions to their challenges in an interdependent world (Miller *et al.*, 2000).

The discussion that follows is based on analysis of the situational and scientific data concerning cervical cancer control with experts at international, regional and national levels. And the proposed solutions represent the decisions of experts and legislators from individual developing countries as they deem fit for their communities.

Logistics of health economics: background to solutions

Much of the current situation in developing countries has to do with the logistics of health economics. Hence, it warrants a brief mention in order to understand the realities in these countries and to put global advocacy regarding cancer screening into perspective.

The United Nations Development Fund's Human Development Index, which measures the overall achievements of a country using three basic dimensions of human development, i.e. longevity, knowledge and a decent standard of living, has shown considerable narrowing in the north/south gap over the past 20 years or so. However, serious deprivations still remain. Of the 4.6 billion people living in developing countries, about 900 million adults cannot read or write, 1.5 billion people do not have access to primary health care, 1.75 billion people are without safe water, approximately 100 million are homeless, some 800 million go hungry every day and more than a billion survive in absolute poverty (living on less than a $1 per day) (UNDP, 2002).

The fact that poor countries can achieve improvements in health care and life expectancy comparable to industrialised countries has tremendous policy implications. Differences among regions and countries are particularly marked in economic growth, and this affects the generation of public resources to invest in education and health services. This opens the debate on the 'growth-mediated' process, which operates through rapid economic growth, compared with a 'support-led' process, which operates through skilful social support of health care and education and other social programmes (Sen, 1993).

The basic question is how one defines development and how health relates to development. It is important to understand the relationship between economic prosperity and good health. Often, misleading conclusions are drawn taking income growth to be the basic determinant of improved health and longevity and dismissing the relevance of social arrangements. Hence, economic growth cannot be treated as an end in itself. In fact, much depends on how the economic growth is used and, in particular, whether it is used to expand public services adequately and to alleviate poverty. For example, moderate economic growth countries, such as Costa Rica, Jamaica and Sri Lanka, have achieved rapid reductions in mortality rates and better living conditions than high economic growth countries such as Brazil, Oman and Saudi Arabia (Sen and Dreze, 1995; UNDP, 2002) (Table 29A.3).

Table 29A.3 GNP per capita and selected social factors.

Country	GNP per capita ($)	Life expectancy (years)	Adult literacy (%)	Infant mortality (per 1000 live births)
Modest GNP with high human development				
Sri Lanka	400	71	87	32
Jamaica	940	74	82	18
Costa Rica	1510	75	93	18
High GNP with modest human development				
Brazil	2020	65	78	62
Oman	5810	57	30	40
Saudi Arabia	6200	64	55	70

Possible screening solutions

Over the last few years, much time and many resources have been spent on debate and research surrounding the issue of an appropriate screening test for cervical cancer, especially for developing countries. It may be an important but a very small part of the whole problem. The issues regarding implementation of a cervical cancer screening programme are much broader and complex, especially in developing countries, where the majority of the population do not have access to basic health care facilities (Nazeer, 2001).

Organisations concerned with cervical screening programmes are unanimous in their belief that a programme based on a western model will not be feasible in developing countries. Promotion of a dogmatic non-effective screening strategy should be avoided as the only relevant solution because very different situations prevail in the resource-constrained countries.

Exfoliative cytology

The Pap smear remains the only proven method over the last 50 years to be an effective screening tool. Moreover, there exist well-established quality control criteria for the test. It has been successful in reducing incidence of and mortality from cervical cancer when implemented through organised screening programmes in different countries. However, the impact on the disease has been directly propotional to the population screened in individual countries. In view of the resource constraints in developing countries, WHO and the INCGC International Consensus from Tunis 1999 recommend a 'step-up' approach using Pap smears for different resource settings, as follows (Miller, 1992; Miller *et al.*, 2000):
- screen every woman once between the ages of 40 and 45 years;
- when resources permit, screen 10-yearly at ages 35, 45 and 55 years;
- if resources are available, screen 5-yearly between the ages of 35 and 59 years;
- once coverage is achieved (80%), expand to start screening at age 25 years (if resources are available).

When devising a cytology-based programme, one should, however, be aware of the limitations of the conventional Pap smear alone as an effective screening tool. False-negative rates for the Pap smear can range from 5% to 55% in different settings (Koss, 1989; Fahey *et al.*, 1995). This is particularly relevant for settings where adequate training and quality control mechanisms are not monitored. In these settings, such a screening programme might do more harm than good.

Visual inspection techniques

Various alternatives to cytology have been suggested and evaluated in different research trials for detection of high-grade cervical neoplastic disease. Based on the analysis of data from studies around the world, visual inspection with acetic acid (VIA) holds promise based on initial studies, either as an adjunct or as an alternative to cytology. These techniques are considered in Chapter 29B.

HPV DNA testing

HPV DNA testing with molecular methods for the high-risk HPV types also holds much promise as a screening modality, and its employment is described in detail in Chapters 20 and 26. This method has been shown to have similar or higher sensitivity to detect high-grade disease than that of cytology. Sensitivity of 70–90% has been quoted in different studies for detecting high-grade squamous intraepithelial lesions (HSIL) compared with cytology. However, the specificity is lower than that of cervical cytology, as the prevalence of HPV DNA positivity in women without cervical neoplasia varies markedly and may be particularly high in young women. Moreover, the negative predictive value of HPV DNA is a major asset in respect of screening (Cuzick *et al.*, 1999; Nazeer and Shafi, 2001).

Other techniques

The place of other techniques such as cervicography, speculoscopy, gynoscopy, real-time probes (Truscreen) and automated cytology, infrared spectroscopy and laser-induced fluoroscopy remains to be evaluated further. Some of these techniques are described elsewhere (Chapter 28). Moreover, a cost–benefit advantage of these techniques is debatable (Higgins *et al.*, 1994; Miller *et al.*, 2000).

Combination of test procedures

A combination of tests has been suggested as perhaps the most effective way of screening for the future, as is being tried in Central American countries. However, whenever two techniques are combined, with abnormal results on either test leading to an overall positive result, the sensitivity of screening will increase (Ferreccio *et al.*, 2003). With this increase in sensitivity, the question remains as to whether it is sufficiently greater than random to merit consideration. Increased sensitivity will typically lead to an offsetting decrease in specificity, and it must be recognised that the trade-off has to be examined to determine the overall effect of the combination on screening accuracy. A two-stage screening process or triage, using a low-cost, simpler test such as acetic acid visual inspection, followed by an expensive, sophisticated test such as cytology only on subgroups of women who test positive with VIA, is a possibility. This sequential screening could help to save resources by selective screening and perhaps also improve specificity with little compromise on sensitivity. A conclusive recommendation cannot be made to this effect in view of insufficient data. Moreover, although programmatic issues with alternative screening approaches are assumed to be the same as those for cervical cytology, further research may provide additional leads with reference to the alternative approaches (Nazeer, 1996; Miller *et al.*, 2000).

Vaccines

HPV vaccines could in theory help to prevent and treat cervical cancer, and are being voiced as a possible solution to the problem in developing countries. This subject is covered in detail in Chapter 45. The vaccines, especially the prophylactic ones, are scheduled to be available for population use in Switzerland by the autumn of 2006. It is proposed that they will be administered to children and adolescents who have not yet engaged in sex. However, it will take up to 30 years to evaluate the exact efficacy of the vaccines. The currently available vaccines are type-specific and designed to target the two most common types of HPV, namely 16 and 18. The questions regarding quality and sustianabilty of immune response and of cross-protection against other HPV types, which may be discovered in different populations, will also be answered over time. It is also not yet clear how effective administration of vaccines will be and, as yet, there are no estimates available for compliance (Samuel, 1997; Adams *et al.*, 2001; Bosch *et al.*, 2001; Koutsky *et al.*, 2002; Harper *et al.*, 2004).

Awareness of the specific needs of developing countries

A screening programme is a multidisciplinary entity where awareness is a vital discipline for success. The provision of services alone will not solve the problem in developing countries, unless health awareness is increased to ensure that women will avail themselves of these services of their own will. A one-off education campaign will not achieve this (Nazeer, 2001). A comprehensive, community-based health education programme for public and health providers needs to be put in place.

Ignorance of screening concepts

Greater knowledge would help in communication skills and improved compliance. A demonstration project in periurban populations in Pakistan showed a total lack of awareness about cervical cancer or the benefit of a Pap smear among women with none of the 15 000 women of reproductive age in the area having ever had a smear (WHO/SEARO/EMRO, 2000) In Mexico, 60% of rural women were found to be unaware of the Pap smear, resulting in only 30% of women ever having had a smear (Lazcano-Ponce *et al.*, 1999). A survey on Vietnamese women in the United States revealed that the majority of them had not had a Pap smear, despite the availability of services, because 75% of them did not know the purpose of a Pap smear (Schulmeister and Lifsey, 1999). Similar experiences have been documented from South Africa (Wellensiek *et al.*, 2002). Thus, a woman's own initiative is vital to the success of a control programme, especially in countries where there are no officially organised screening programmes.

Lack of data concerning local facilities

One cannot underestimate the importance of accurate statistical data as they are the first step towards appreciating appropriate control measures in a global context. They form the basis of successfully devising a hypothesis about causation and help to quantify the potential for preventive activities. They play a critical role in the development and implementation of health policies and the surveillance of programmes. They are imperative to ensure the availability of standard treatment facilities for CIN and invasive cancer before embarking upon a screening project. Screening should not be carried out in isolation; other clinical aspects should also be addressed simultaneously, such as appropriate patient referral protocols and availability of treatment services including palliative care.

Programmes tailored for local settings (sociocultural and religious backgrounds)

A screening programme will have to be tailored for each individual resource setting with consideration given to the sociocultural and religious background of the population. Different algorithms will be required for different countries, perhaps for different regions in the same country, depending on available resources. Each design would then have to be tested in a demonstration project and gradually phased into a national programme. Screening means balancing the effect on the length and quality of life saved and the cost to the health service.

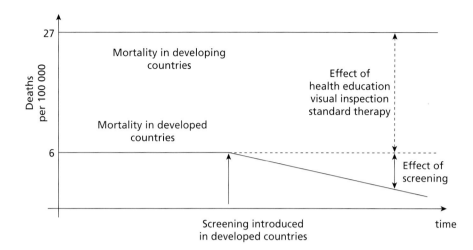

Fig. 29A.2 Cervical cancer control in developed and developing countries.

Economic inequality

The issue is not only one of economic growth or the political commitment alone. The issue at all stages of the screening agenda is invariably the question of economic inequity. Unfortunately, the Human Development Index only measures the average national achievement, not how well it is distributed in a country. This inequality is hampering the overall development process in these countries. Concentration of income at the top is undermining public policies. However, even when the economy is poor, major health improvements can be achieved if available resources are used in a productive way. The important question often raised is where will the poor countries get the money to spend on social parameters such as health. The answer is equally important and lies in the concept of the economics of relative costs. Poor economies may have less money to spend on health and education services as they are labour intensive but, in the cheap labour economies in the developing countries, it also costs less to provide these services compared with richer countries. A social commitment is vital to the whole process, and this can be achieved through informed public discussion. A major difference can be achieved by the public determination to do something about these deprivations (Sen and Dreze, 1995).

Figure 29A.2 is a schematic comparison of the situation analysis between developed and developing countries regarding cervical cancer; it also highlights the relative effect of screening on mortality. It is based on historical data from Nordic countries, namely Finland and Sweden. Experience from these countries shows that mortality from cervical cancer had fallen significantly prior to the introduction of a formal screening programme in the 1960s, presumably due to better health awareness among women, which in turn led to earlier presentation and was combined with free treatment. The subsequent contribution of screening to a decrease in mortality from cervical cancer was much less. This has an important message for developing countries where public and profes-

sional health awareness and education programmes should be the priority (Miller, 1992; Nazeer, 1996).

The way forward for cervical cancer screening and control in developing countries

The technical knowledge about the prevention and cure of this disease is well documented. Now, this knowledge needs to be translated into actual programmes in different resource settings. There is an urgent need to intensify efforts at international and national level to increase awareness and endorse politico-economical commitment to acknowledge and invest in cervical cancer screening programmes. Developing countries have failed to join the race of cancer control so far, mainly due to the lack of public and professional awareness coupled with lack of political will. This will require a collaborative effort like the International Network (INCGC). This initiative has helped increase awareness in all regions of the world and assisted local experts in India, China and United Arab Emirates to convince their governments to include cervical cancer in the national health priority list.

At the same time, preparation of public and professionals through educational programmes and organisation of basic infrastructure are imperative. Vaccines certainly would be the ideal solution for the future. The vital question, however, remains: what will come first, a highly effective screening test or a preventive vaccine. Furthermore, would the availability of a vaccine obviate the need for a screening test.

REFERENCES

Adams M, Borysiewicz L, Fiander A *et al.* (2001) Clinical studies of human papilloma vaccines in preinvasive and invasive cancer. *Vaccine* 19 (17–19): 2549–2556.

Akinremi TO, Nazeer S, Totsch M (2005) Reduced alcohol use in the staining of Pap smears: a satisfactory low-cost protocol for cervical cancer screening. *Acta Cytologica* 49: 169–172.

Bosch FX, Rohan T, Schneider A *et al.* (2001) Papillomavirus research update: highlights of the Barcelona HPV 2000 international papillomavirus conference. *Journal of Clinical Pathology* 54: 163–175.

Chirenje ZM *et al.* (1999) for the University of Zimbabwe/JHPIEGO Cervical Cancer Project. Visual inspection with acetic acid for cervical-cancer screening: test qualities in a primary-care setting. *Lancet* 353: 869–873.

Cronje HS, Cooreman BF, Beyer E *et al.* (2001) Screening for cervical neoplasia in a developing country utilizing cytology, cervicography and acetic acid test. *International Journal of Gynaecology and Obstetrics* 72 (2): 151–157.

Cuzick J, Saseini P, Davies P *et al.* (1999) A systematic review of the role of human papillomavirus testing within a cervical screening programme. *Health Technology Assessment* 3: 95–122.

Fahey MT, Irwig L, Macaskill P (1995) Meta-analysis of Pap-test accuracy. *American Journal of Epidemiology* 141 (7): 680–689.

Ferreccio C, Bratti MC, Sherman ME *et al.* (2003) The comparison of single and combined visual, cytologic and virologic tests and screening strategies in a region at high risk of cervical cancer. *Cancer Epidemiology Biomarkers and Prevention* 12: 815–823.

Harper DM, Franco EL, Wheeler C *et al.* (2004) Efficacy of a bivalent L1 virus-like particle vaccine in prevention of infection with human papillomavirus type 16 and 18 in young women; a randomised controlled trial. *Lancet* 364: 1757–1765.

Higgins RV, Hall JB, McGee JA *et al.* (1994) Appraisal of the modalities used to evaluate an initial abnormal papanicolaou smear. *Obstetrics and Gynecology* 84: 174–178.

Hristova L, Hakama M (1997) Effect of screening for cancer in the Nordic countries on deaths, cost and quality of life up to the year 2017. *Acta Oncologica* 36 (Suppl. 9): 1–60.

IARC (2005) *Cervix Cancer Screening.* Handbooks of Cancer Prevention, Vol. 10. Lyon: International Agency for Research on Cancer, IARC Press.

Koss LG (1989) The Papanicolaou test for cervical cancer detection, a triumph and a tragedy. *Journal of the American Medical Association* 261: 737–743.

Koutsky LA, Ault KA, Wheeler CM *et al.* (2002) A controlled trial of a human papillomavirus type 16 vaccine. *New England Journal of Medicine* 347 (21): 1645–1651.

Laara E, Day N, Hakama M (1987) Trends in mortality from cervical cancer in Nordic countries: association with organised screening programmes. *Lancet* 1: 1247–1249.

Lazcano-Ponce EC, Moss S, Alonso de Ruiz P *et al.* (1999) Cervical cancer screening in developing countries. Why is it ineffective? The case of Mexico. *Archives in Medical Research* 30: 240–250.

Miller AB (ed.) (1992) *Cervical Cancer Screening: Managerial Guidelines.* Geneva: World Health Organization, pp. 1–50.

Miller AB, Chamberlain J, Day NE *et al.* (1990) Report on a workshop of the UICC project on evaluation of screening for cancer. *International Journal of Cancer* 46: 761–769.

Miller AB, Nazeer S, Fonn S *et al.* (2000) Report on Consensus Conference on cervical cancer screening and management. *International Journal of Cancer* 86: 440–447.

Nazeer S (1996) Cervical Cancer Control in Developing Countries: Memorandum from a WHO Meeting. *Bulletin of the World Health Organization* 74 (4): 345–351.

Nazeer S (2001) Alternatives to cytology: new perspectives for screening and management of cervical dysplasia. Thesis, Faculty of Medicine, University of Geneva.

Nazeer S, Shafi MI (2001) Intraepithelial neoplasia, wart virus and colposcopy. *Current Obstetrics and Gynaecology* 11: 164–171.

Ottaviano M, La Torre P (1982) Examination of the cervix with the naked eye using acetic acid test. *American Journal of Obstetrics and Gynecology* 143: 139–142.

Parkin DM, Bray F, Pisani P *et al.* (2001) Estimating the world cancer burden: GLOBOCAN 2000. *International Journal of Cancer* 94: 153–156.

Pisani P, Bray F, Parkin DM (2002) Estimates of the world-wide prevalence of cancer for 25 sites in the adult population. *International Journal of Cancer* 97 (1): 72–81.

Quinn M, Babb P, Jones J *et al.* (1999) Effect of screening on incidence of and mortality from cancer of cervix in England: evaluation based on routinely collected statistics. *British Medical Journal* 318: 904–908.

Robyr R, Nazeer S, Vasilakos P *et al.* (2003) Feasibility of cytology-based cervical cancer screening programme in rural Cameroon. *Acta Cytologica* 47: 948–949.

Samuel LK (1997) Vaccine series: future vaccines and a global perspective. *Lancet* 350: 1767–1770.

Sen A (1993) The economics of life and death. *Scientific American* 5: 40–47.

Sen A, Dreze J (1995) *Economic Development and Social Opportunity,* 1st edn. Oxford: Oxford University Press.

Singh V, Sehgal A, Luthra UK (1992) Screening for cervical cancer by direct inspection. *British Medical Journal* 304: 534–535.

Slawson DC, Bennett JH, Herman JM *et al.* (1992) Are Papanicolaou smears enough? Acetic acid washes of the cervix as adjunctive therapy: a HARNET study: Harrisburg Area Research Network. *Journal of Family Practice* 35: 271–277.

Schulmeister L, Lifsey DS (1999) Cervical cancer screening knowledge, behaviours and beliefs of Vietnamese women. *Oncology Nursing Forum* 26: 879–887.

Stjernsward J, Eddy D, Luthra UK *et al.* (1987) Plotting a new course for cervical cancer screening in developing countries. *World Health Forum* 8: 42–45.

United Nations AIDS Programme (1997) *Sexually Transmitted Diseases: Policies and Principles for Prevention and Care.* Geneva: World Health Organization (UNAIDS/WHO), pp. 5–8.

United Nations AIDS Programme (2002) *World AIDS Report.* Geneva: World Health Organization (UNAIDS/WHO).

United Nations Development Programme (UNDP) (2002) *Human Development—Past, Present and Future. Human Development Report.* New York: UNDP, Chapter 1, pp. 9–25.

Veena S, Madan MG, Satayanarayana L *et al.* (1995) Association between reproductive tract infections and cervical inflammatory changes. *Sexually Transmitted Diseases* 22: 25–30.

Wellensiek N, Moodley M, Moodley J *et al.* (2002) Knowledge of cervical cancer screening and use of cervical screening facilities among women from various socioeconomic backgrounds in Durban, Kwazulu Natal, South Africa. *International Journal of Gynaecological Cancer* 12 (4): 376–382.

WHO/AFRO (2000) World Health Organization Report of Regional Technical Workshop on Cervical Cancer Control in African Region. The World Health Organization Regional Office for Africa. WHO/AFRO, Congo, April 2000.

WHO/EURO (2000) World Health Organization Report of Regional Technical Workshop on Cervical Cancer Control in Eastern European/

Central Asian Region. The World Health Organization Regional Office for Europe. WHO/EURO, Copenhagen, June 2000.

WHO/PAHO (1996) Trends in cervical cancer mortality in the Americas. Bulletin of the Pan American Health Organization. The World Health Organization Regional Office for the Americas/ Pan American Health Organization (WHO/PAHO), Washington, Vol. 30 (4): 290–301.

WHO/SEARO/EMRO (2000) World Health Organization Report of Regional Technical Workshop on Cervical Cancer: Eastern Mediterranean/Southeast Asian Regions. The World Health Organization Regional Offices for South East Asia and Eastern Mediterranean. WHO/SEARO/EMRO, New Delhi/Alexandria, 2000.

WHO/WPRO (2001) World Health Organisation. Report of Regional Technical Workshop on Cervical Cancer Control in Western Pacific Region. WHO/WPRO, Manila, March 2001.

World Health Organization (2002) *National Cancer Control Programmes: Policies and Managerial Guidelines.* World Health Organization monograph, 2nd edn. Geneva: WHO.

Visual screening for cervical neoplasia in developing countries

Rengaswamy Sankaranarayanan, Thara Somanathan and Twalib Ngoma

INTRODUCTION

The difficulties and challenges in implementing quality-assured cytology screening in low- and medium-resource countries have prompted the evaluation of visual screening tests, such as visual inspection with acetic acid and Lugol's iodine, in recent years. The accuracy of visual screening has been addressed in many cross-sectional studies now (level of evidence 3) and its effectiveness in reducing disease burden is being addressed in at least three randomised trials (level of evidence 1). This chapter discusses the findings of these trials and the utility of these tests in screening programmes, as well as for early clinical detection.

The availability of an accurate, affordable, simple, and acceptable screening test is one of the critical factors for successful cervical screening programmes; the other important factors include high coverage of target women with screening and of screen-positive women with diagnostic investigations, treatment and follow-up care (IARC, 2005). The objective of cervical screening is to prevent deaths from invasive cervical cancer by detecting and treating women with high-grade cervical intraepithelial neoplasia (CIN2 and CIN3 lesions) and preclinical, early invasive cancers. The effectiveness of screening is evaluated by the extent of reduction in cervical cancer incidence and mortality following screening.

Although cytology screening has largely been responsible for the impressive reduction in the burden of cervical cancer in developed countries over the last five decades, it has yet to be effectively implemented in many developing countries, or has failed to reduce cervical cancer burden to an appreciable extent in some developing countries as a result of resource constraints and several programmatic challenges in implementing good quality cytology screening with optimal accuracy in low-resource countries (Sankaranarayanan *et al.*, 2001; IARC, 2005). This has prompted the evaluation of various simple visual screening methods such as unaided visual inspection ('downstaging'), naked eye visual inspection after application of 3–5% dilute acetic acid (VIA; syn: direct visual inspection, acetic acid test, cervicoscopy), magnified visual inspection after application of acetic acid (VIAM) and visual inspection after

application of Lugol's iodine (VILI). The technique in each case involves visualisation of the cervix with a speculum and bright light source. Visual inspection methods to screen for cervical neoplasia essentially stemmed from the observation that acetowhite changes after application of acetic acid on the cervix can be recognised by the naked eye (Ottoviano and La Torre, 1982).

EVALUATION OF SCREENING TESTS

The important aspects of evaluating the suitability of a screening test include its accuracy in detecting the disease of interest, the reproducibility, simplicity and ease with which it can be applied in mass programmes, its safety and acceptability to the target population, the training needs, availability of quality assurance procedures and costs, and, ultimately, its ability to reduce the burden of disease (incidence or mortality, costs incurred) and improve quality of life at an affordable cost (cost-effectiveness) when implemented in mass programmes. The currently available evidence for these different parameters and further research needs for visual screening for cervical neoplasia are discussed in this chapter. It is important to remember here that the estimates of accuracy from cross-sectional studies will suffer from verification bias if the reference standard for the establishment of final disease status is applied in different proportions of screen-positive and screen-negative participants. Verification bias leads to inflated estimates of sensitivity and may be minimised by applying the reference standard to all participants irrespective of screening test results or by statistical adjustment.

Unaided visual inspection ('downstaging')

This technique involves naked eye visualisation of the cervix to detect the early stages of cervical cancer. It suffers from low sensitivity and specificity in detecting cervical neoplasia, particularly precancerous and preclinical lesions and hence it is not a sufficiently accurate screening test (Sankaranarayanan *et al.*, 1997; Basu *et al.*, 2002). It is likely that detecting the magnitude of stage shift by unaided visual inspection could be improved by a programme of health education and improving professional awareness. However, it is no longer recommended as a primary screening test for cervical neoplasia.

Visual inspection with acetic acid (VIA)

VIA is the most widely evaluated visual screening test. It involves naked eye inspection of the cervix, using a bright torch light or a halogen focus lamp, 1–2 minutes after the application of 3–5% acetic acid using a cotton swab or a spray. Test results are mostly reported as negative or positive or invasive cancer. Although a range of definitions have been used for the different test result categories in different studies, a positive test is usually characterised by well-defined acetowhite areas close to the squamocolumnar junction (SCJ) or the external os or by the entire cervix or a cervical growth turning acetowhite after application of acetic acid. The test definitions used in the studies coordinated by the International Agency for Research on Cancer (IARC) of the World Health

Table 29B.1 Visual inspection with acetic acid (VIA) test result categories and definitions.

VIA negative (−ve)
VIA is reported as negative if any of the following are observed:
  No acetowhite lesions on the cervix
  Cervical polyp with bluish-white acetowhite areas
  Nabothian cysts appearing as button-like areas
  Dot-like areas in the endocervix, due to grape-like columnar
    epithelium staining with acetic acid
  Shiny, pinkish white, cloudy white, bluish white, faint patchy, or
    doubtful lesions with ill-defined, indefinite margins, blending with
    the rest of the cervix
  Angular, irregular, digitating acetowhite lesions, resembling
    geographical regions, far away (detached) from the SCJ
    (satellite lesions)
  Faint line-like acetowhitening of the SCJ
  Streak-like acetowhitening in the columnar epithelium

VIA positive (+ve)
VIA is reported as positive if any of the following are observed:
  Distinct, well-defined, dense or dull acetowhite areas, close to or
    touching the SCJ in the transformation zone or close to the
    external os if the SCJ is not visible
  Strikingly dense acetowhite areas on the columnar epithelium
  The entire cervix becomes densely white after the application of
    acetic acid
  Condyloma and leukoplakia close to the SCJ, turning intensely white
    after application of acetic acid

VIA positive, invasive cancer
The test outcome is scored as invasive cancer if:
  A clinically visible ulceroproliferative growth on the cervix turns
    densely white after application of acetic acid and bleeds on touch

---

SCJ, squamocolumnar junction.

Organization are given in Table 29B.1 (Sankaranarayanan and Wesley, 2003).

This is a simple, inexpensive test that can be easily learned and yields real-time results allowing diagnostic investigations and treatment to be linked in the same session as screening. A range of personnel including doctors, nurses, midwives, and paramedical health workers can be rapidly trained in providing VIA in short training courses of 4–10 days duration (Blumenthal *et al.*, 2005). A wide range of teaching materials is now available for training personnel in carrying out VIA competently (McIntosh *et al.*, 2001; Sankaranarayanan and Wesley, 2003). It is possible for interested and motivated service providers to teach themselves the practice of VIA with the help of manuals and atlases. Figure 29B.1 shows a clinical chart used for interpretation of VIA results by test providers (Sankaranarayanan and Wesley, 2003).

The accuracy of VIA in detecting CIN2 and CIN3 lesions and invasive cancer has been evaluated in several cross-sectional studies in developing countries (Table 29B.2). These studies together involve more than 100 000 women. Verification bias was minimised in some of these studies. The sensitivity of VIA in detecting CIN2 and CIN3 lesions and invasive cervical cancer varied from 29% to 95% and the specificity varied from 49% to 97% (Slawson *et al.*, 1992; Cecchini *et al.*, 1993; Megavand *et al.*, 1996; Londhe *et al.*, 1997; Sankaranarayanan *et al.*, 1998; 1999; University of Zimbabwe/JHPIEGO 1999; Denny *et al.*, 2000; Cronjé *et al.*, 2001; Belinson *et al.*, 2001; Denny *et al.*, 2002; Rodrigues-Reyes *et al.*, 2002; Basu *et al.*, 2003; Cronjé *et al.*, 2003; Ngelangel *et al.*, 2003; Tayyeb *et al.*, 2003; El Shalakany *et al.*, 2004; Sankaranarayanan *et al.*, 2004a; Denny *et al.*, 2005; De Vuyst *et al.*, 2005; Doh *et al.*, 2005; Sankaranarayanan *et al.*, 2005a; Shastri *et al.*, 2005; Sarian *et al.*, 2005; Sangwa-Lugoma *et al.*, 2006). The wide range in the accuracy parameters of VIA seem to be due to the subjective nature of the test interpretation, a lack of standardised test result definitions, the heterogeneity of test providers and provider training methods, skills and experience, and the quality and accuracy of reference standards for final diagnosis, as well as a lack of standardised quality assurance procedures in various studies. Findings from studies indicate that low-level ($\times 2$–4) magnification does not improve the test performance of visual inspection with acetic acid (Denny *et al.*, 2002; Basu *et al.*, 2003; Sankaranarayanan *et al.*, 2004b; Shastri *et al.*, 2005). The pooled sensitivity, specificity and positive predictive value of VIA in detecting CIN2 and CIN3 lesions is 79%, 83% and 12%, respectively. The pooled negative predictive value of a negative VIA test is higher than 99%. Whenever conventional cytology was concurrently evaluated in studies, VIA had a similar or higher sensitivity but lower specificity than that of cytology.

A major logistic advantage of VIA is the immediate availability of test results, which allows the possibility of linking diagnosis and treatment in the same session as screening. This

VIA negative

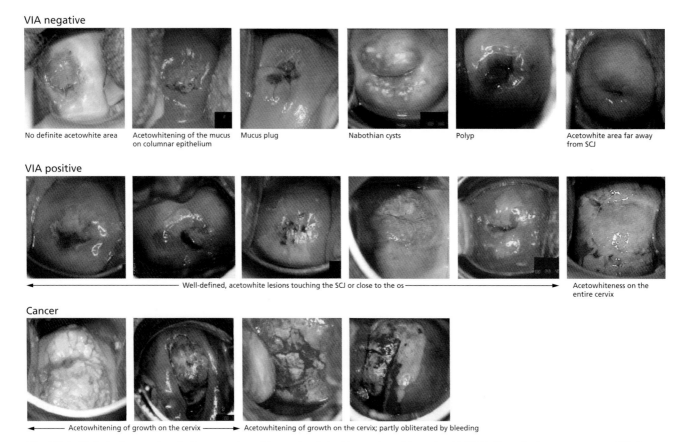

| No definite acetowhite area | Acetowhitening of the mucus on columnar epithelium | Mucus plug | Nabothian cysts | Polyp | Acetowhite area far away from SCJ |

VIA positive

◄———————— Well-defined, acetowhite lesions touching the SCJ or close to the os ————————► Acetowhiteness on the entire cervix

Cancer

◄——— Acetowhitening of growth on the cervix ———► Acetowhitening of growth on the cervix; partly obliterated by bleeding

Fig. 29B.1 Clinical reference chart for interpretation of the results of visual inspection with acetic acid (VIA). From Sankaranarayanan and Wesley (2003). SCJ, squamocolumnar junction.

has opened up the option of a 'screen-and-treat' or 'single-visit' approach, in which screen-positive women without clinical evidence of invasive cancer and satisfying the criteria for ablative therapy are immediately treated with cryotherapy, without confirmatory investigations such as colposcopy or histology, thus ensuring a high compliance with treatment. The safety, acceptability and feasibility of combining VIA and cryotherapy in a single-visit approach have been demonstrated in rural Thailand (RTCOG/JHPIEGO, 2003) and Guatemala (Mathers *et al.*, 2005).

In Roi-et Province, Thailand, 12 trained nurses screened 5999 women with VIA over 7 months (RTCOG/JHPIEGO, 2003). Test-positive women were offered cryotherapy after counselling on the benefits, potential risks and probable side-effects. The VIA test-positive rate was 13.3% (798/5999), and 98.5% (609/618) of those eligible accepted immediate treatment. Overall, 756 women received cryotherapy, 629 (83.2%) of whom returned for their first follow-up visit. No major complications were recorded, and 33 (4.4%) of those treated returned for a perceived problem. Only 17 (2.2%) of the treated women needed clinical management other than reassurance about side-effects. Both VIA and cryotherapy were highly acceptable to the women. At their 1-year visit, the

SCJ was visible to the nurses, and the VIA test-negative rate was 94.3%. This programme has been expanded in several Thai provinces.

A group of 954 women was screened with VIA in rural Guatemala and those with acetowhite changes consistent with CIN were offered immediate cryotherapy. Of the 125 VIA-positive women, 121 received immediate cryotherapy (Mathers *et al.*, 2005) and this approach was well accepted in rural Guatemala.

Recently a randomised controlled trial involving 6550 women in South Africa reported on the safety and efficacy of two types of screen-and-treat approaches for cervical cancer prevention: VIA followed by cryotherapy or human papillomavirus (HPV) testing followed by cryotherapy (Denny *et al.*, 2005). This study provides the first randomised trial evidence for the comparative efficacy of the two screen-and-treat approaches. All women were screened using HPV testing and VIA and were subsequently randomised to one of the three groups: cryotherapy if the woman had a positive HPV test, cryotherapy if she had a positive VIA, or delayed evaluation after 6 months. At 6 months, all women were investigated with colposcopy and directed biopsy depending on colposcopic findings: CIN2 and advanced lesions were diagnosed in

Table 29B.2 Accuracy of visual inspection with acetic acid (VIA) in detecting CIN2+ lesions in cross-sectional studies.

Author/country	Sample	Target population (age group)	Test provider	Reference diagnosis	Sensitivity (%)	Sensitivity (%)	Verification bias
Slawson *et al.*, 1992, United States	2690	15–45	Doctor	Colposcopy/biopsy	29	97	Yes
Cecchini *et al.*, 1993, Italy	2036	17–85	Smear taker	Colposcopy/biopsy	88	75	Yes
Megavand *et al.*, 1996, South Africa	2426	20–85	Nurse	Colposcopy/biopsy	65	98	Yes
Londhe *et al.*, 1997, India	372	25–75	Gynaecologist	Colposcopy	78	49	Yes
Sankaranarayanan *et al.*, 1998, India	2935	20–85	Cytotechnicians	Colposcopy/biopsy	87	91	Yes
Univ. Zimbabwe/JHPIEGO, 1999, Zimbabwe	2148	25–55	Midwife	Colposcopy/biopsy	77	64	Minimal
Sankaranarayanan *et al.*, 1999, India	1268	22–70	Nurse	Colposcopy/biopsy	95	68	Yes
Denny *et al.*, 2000, South Africa	2944	35–65	Nurse	Colposcopy/biopsy	67	83	Yes
Cronje *et al.*, 2001, South Africa	6298	Not known	Nurse	Biopsy	51	84	Yes
Belinson *et al.*, 2001, China	1997	35–45	Gynaecologist	Four-quadrant biopsy + ECC	71	74	Minimal
Denny *et al.*, 2002, South Africa	2754	35–65	Nurse	Colposcopy/biopsy	74	77	Yes
Rodrigues-Reyes *et al.*, 2002, Mexico	378	20–45	Doctor	Biopsy	92	59	Minimal
Cronje *et al.*, 2003, South Africa	1093	21–65	Nurse	Biopsy	79	49	Minimal
Ngelangel *et al.*, 2003, Philippines	3316	25–65	Nurse	Colposcopy/biopsy	37	91	Minimal
Basu *et al.*, 2003, India	5881	30–64	Trained college graduates	Colposcopy/biopsy	56	82	Minimal
Tayyeb *et al.*, 2003, Pakistan	501	30–60	Not known	Colposcopy/biopsy	94	78	Yes
Sankaranarayanan *et al.*, 2004a, India, Burkina Faso, Congo, Guinea, Mali, Niger	54 981	25–65	Midwife/nurse/ cytotechnician/ high-school graduates	Colposcopy/biopsy	77	86	Minimal
El Shalakany *et al.*, 2004, Egypt	2049	Not known	Not known	Colposcopy/biopsy	86	97	Yes
Shastri *et al.*, 2005, India	4039	25–65	Trained high-school graduates	Colposcopy/biopsy	60	88	Minimal
Doh *et al.*, 2005, Cameroon	4813	30–60	Nurse	Colposcopy/biopsy	70	78	Yes
Du Vuyst *et al.*, 2005, Kenya	653	25–65	Nurse	Colposcopy/biopsy	73	80	Yes
Denny *et al.*, 2005, South Africa	2165	35–65	Nurse	Colposcopy/biopsy	55	77	Minimal
Sarian *et al.*, 2005, Argentina, Brazil	11 834	18–60	Doctors and nurses	Colposcopy/biopsy	50	90	Yes
Sangwa-Lugoma *et al.*, 2006, Congo	1528	30+	Nurse	Colposcopy/biopsy	56	65	Yes
Sangwa-Lugoma *et al.*, 2006, Congo	1528	30+	Doctors	Colposcopy/biopsy	71	71	Yes

0.8% of the women in the HPV testing group and in 2.2% in the VIA group, compared with 3.6% in the delayed evaluation group ($P < 0.001$ and $P = 0.02$ for the HPV and VIA groups, respectively). A subset of women underwent a second colposcopy examination at 12 months after enrolment, when the cumulative detection of CIN2+ lesions among women in the HPV testing group was 1.4%, 2.9% in the VIA group, and 5.4% in the delayed evaluation group. The prevalence of CIN2–3 lesions was significantly lower in the two screen-and-treat groups than in the delayed evaluation group.

The efficacy of the screen-and-treat approach depends on both the sensitivity of the screening test and the efficacy of the treatment. The lower prevalence of CIN2+ in the HPV DNA group compared with the VIA group in the South African study was attributable to initial HPV DNA testing correctly identifying more women with CIN2+ at enrolment, as the efficacy of cryotherapy was similar in both groups. This interpretation is further supported by the findings among women in the delayed evaluation group: at enrolment, 84 (90%) of the 93 women subsequently identified with CIN2+ lesions at 12 months had positive HPV DNA test results whereas only 51 (55%) had positive VIA test results. One can conclude that the longitudinal sensitivity of VIA over 1 year in this study was 55% as opposed to 84% with HPV testing.

The efficacy of a single round of VIA screening (once in a lifetime) in reducing incidence of and mortality from cervical cancer in women aged 30–59 years at entry is being assessed in two large cluster randomised clinical trials in India (Sankaranarayanan *et al.*, 2004c; Sankaranarayanan *et al.*, 2005b). In the trial in Dindigul District, south India, women in 113 clusters were randomised to VIA screening by nurses (57 clusters, 48 225 women) and to a control group (56 clusters, 30 167 women) providing the existing usual care and health education (Sankaranarayanan *et al.*, 2004c). Of the 30 577 eligible women screened, 2939 (9.6%) were VIA-positive and 1% of the screened women were diagnosed with CIN2+ lesions. In a cluster randomised controlled trial in Osmanabad district, India, the comparative efficacy of a single round of VIA screening, cytology and HPV testing in reducing cervical cancer incidence and mortality in a high-risk population is being investigated (Sankaranarayanan *et al.*, 2005b). A total of 142 701 women in 52 clusters were randomised into four groups for a single round of screening by trained midwives: VIA, cytology or HPV testing or a control group receiving existing usual care. Of the eligible women, 72–74% were screened in the various groups. Test positivity rates were 14.0% for VIA, 7.0% for cytology and 10.3% for HPV. Test-positive women underwent investigations (colposcopy/biopsy) and treatment. The detection rate of CIN2 and CIN3 lesions was similar in all intervention arms (0.7% for VIA, 1.0% for cytology, and 0.9% for HPV testing; $P = 0.06$, Mann–Whitney test). Over 85% of women with high-grade lesions received treatment with cryotherapy or the loop electrosurgical excision procedure (LEEP). Follow-up is continuing in both the above studies to establish the extent of mortality reduction associated with the different screening approaches and their cost-effectiveness, and final results are expected in 2007.

Visual inspection with Lugol's iodine (VILI)

VILI involves naked eye examination of the cervix to detect mustard-yellow lesions in the transformation zone of the cervix, following application of Lugol's iodine. The VILI test results are reported immediately after application of iodine. A positive result is based on the appearance of a definite mustard-yellow area on the cervix close to the SCJ or the os or on the entire cervix or on a cervical growth (Sankaranarayanan and Wesley 2003) (Table 29B.3). It is possible to teach oneself the practice of VILI with the help of manuals and atlases. Figure 29B.2 shows a clinical chart used for interpretation of VILI results by test providers (Sankaranarayanan and Wesley, 2003). The sensitivity of VILI varied between 44 and 92% and specificity between 50 and 90% in recent cross-sectional studies (Table 29B.4) (Sankaranarayanan *et al.*, 2004a; Sarian *et al.*, 2005; Shastri *et al.*, 2005; Sangwa-Lugoma *et al.*, 2006).

LIMITATIONS OF VISUAL SCREENING

Visual screening tests are inherently subjective and provider dependent. This leads to a high false-positivity and low specificity. At best they have a moderate sensitivity but one which is higher than cytology in many low-resource settings. The subjective nature of visual testing is very much reflected by the wide range in test performance characteristics in various settings and limited reproducibility (Sellors *et al.*, 2002; Sankaranarayanan *et al.*, 2004a). In most studies, more than 12% of women were VIA- or VILI-positive. This leads to a large number of women requiring diagnosis and treatment in a programmatic setting, so the costs involved in diagnosis and

Table 29B.3 Visual inspection with Lugol's iodine (VILI) test result categories and definitions.

VILI negative (–ve)

VILI is reported as negative if any of the following are observed:

A normal cervix: the squamous epithelium turns mahogany brown or black and the columnar epithelium does not change colour

Patchy, indistinct, ill-defined, colourless or partially brown areas

Pale areas of no or partial iodine uptake are present on polyps

A leopard skin-like appearance (associated with *Trichomonas vaginalis* infection)

Pepper-like non-iodine uptake areas in the squamous epithelium, far away from the SCJ

Satellite thin, yellow, non-iodine uptake areas with angular or digitating margins, resembling geographical areas, far away from the SCJ

VILI positive (+ve)

VILI is reported as positive if any of the following are observed:

Dense, thick, bright, mustard-yellow or saffron-yellow iodine non-uptake areas in the transformation zone, close to or touching the SCJ or close to the os if the SCJ is not seen or when the entire cervix turns densely yellow

VILI positive, invasive cancer

The test outcome is scored as invasive cancer if:

A frank, nodular, irregular, ulceroproliferative growth on the cervix turns densely yellow on application of iodine

---

SCJ, squamocolumnar junction.

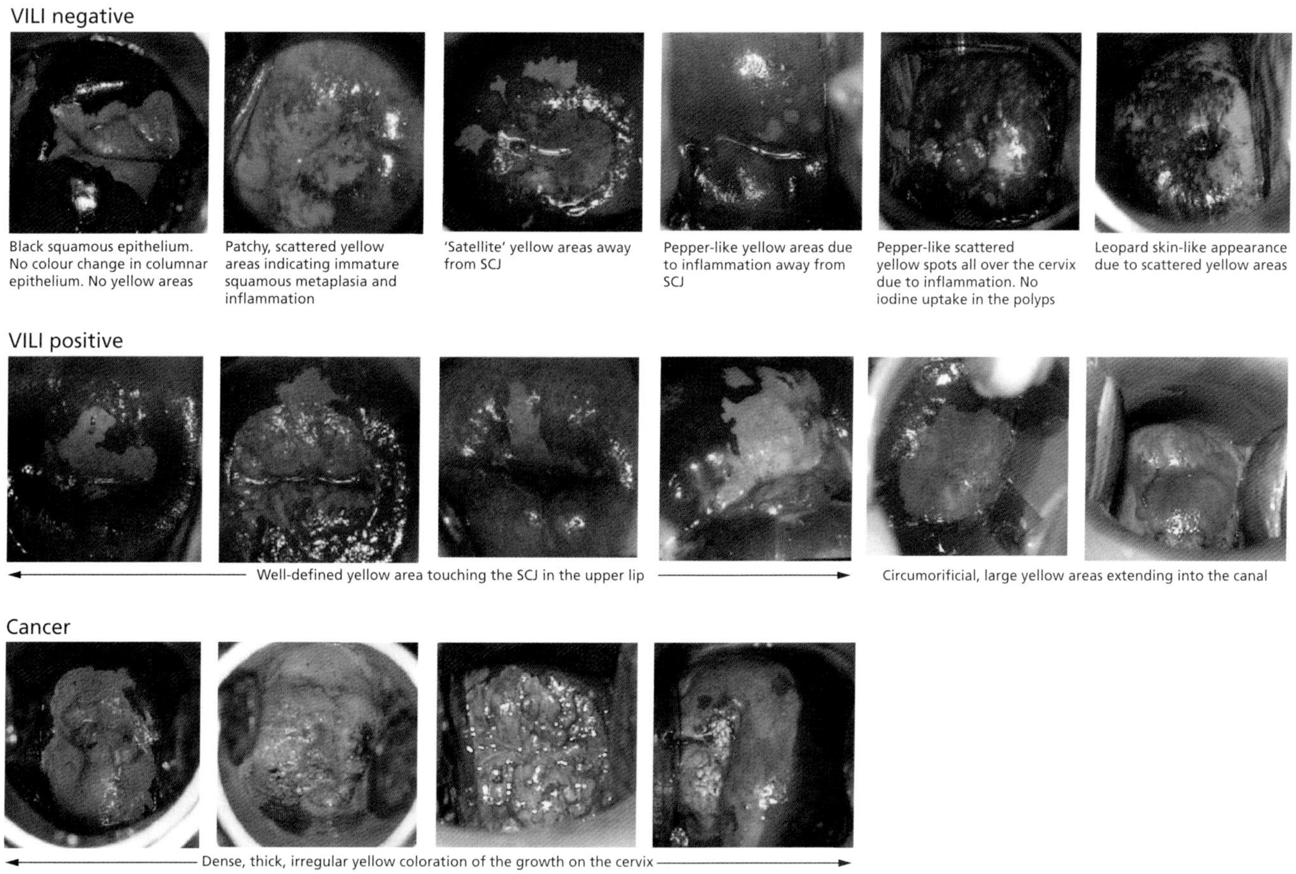

VILI negative

Black squamous epithelium. No colour change in columnar epithelium. No yellow areas

Patchy, scattered yellow areas indicating immature squamous metaplasia and inflammation

'Satellite' yellow areas away from SCJ

Pepper-like yellow areas due to inflammation away from SCJ

Pepper-like scattered yellow spots all over the cervix due to inflammation. No iodine uptake in the polyps

Leopard skin-like appearance due to scattered yellow areas

VILI positive

◄──────── Well-defined yellow area touching the SCJ in the upper lip ────────►

Circumorificial, large yellow areas extending into the canal

Cancer

◄─────── Dense, thick, irregular yellow coloration of the growth on the cervix ───────►

Fig. 29B.2 Clinical reference chart for the interpretation of the results of visual inspection with Lugol's iodine (VILI). From Sankaranarayanan and Wesley (2003). SCJ, squamocolumnar junction.

Table 29B.4 Accuracy of visual inspection with Lugol's iodine (VILI) in detecting CIN2+ lesions in cross-sectional studies

Author/Country	Sample	Target population (age group)	Test provider	Reference diagnosis	Sensitivity (%)	Sensitivity (%)	Verification bias
Sankaranarayanan *et al.*, 2004a, India, Burkina Faso, Congo, Guinea, Mali, Niger	49 089	25–65	Midwife/nurse/ cytotechnician/ high-school graduates	Colposcopy/biopsy	92	85	Minimal
Sarian *et al.*, 2005, Latin America	2944	18–60	Doctors and nurses	Colposcopy/biopsy	57	78	Yes
Shastri *et al.*, 2005, India	4039	25–65	Trained high-school graduates	Colposcopy/biopsy	75	84	Minimal
Sangwa-Lugoma *et al.*, 2006, Congo	1528	30+	Nurses	Colposcopy/biopsy	44	75	Yes

treatment need to be taken into account when introducing visual screening programmes. It is important to wait for at least 1 minute after application of acetic acid to achieve satisfactory interpretation of results, but there are no standardised quality assurance procedures yet for visual screening. Adequate train-

ing and retraining and continuing on-site monitoring of test-positive rates, disease detection rates and positive predictive values are important to ensure high-quality visual testing in field conditions (Sankaranarayanan and Wesley, 2003; IARC, 2005; Sankaranarayanan *et al.*, 2005b). Interpretation is difficult in postmenopausal women because of atrophy of the epithelium and because the transformation zone is no longer fully visible in the ectocervix. Thus, visual tests are of somewhat limited value in women over the age of 50 years.

COST-EFFECTIVENESS OF VISUAL SCREENING

The cost-effectiveness of a variety of cervical cancer screening strategies in India, Kenya, Peru, South Africa and Thailand was assessed in a recent study which reported that screening women once in their lifetime, at the age of 35, with a one- or two-visit screening strategy involving VIA, reduced the lifetime risk of cancer by approximately 25–36% and cost less than US$500 per year of life saved (Goldie *et al.*, 2005). Relative cancer risk declined by an additional 40% with two screenings at 35 and 40 years of age, resulting in a cost per year of life saved that was less than each country's per capita gross domestic product.

CONCLUSION

The major advantages of visual screening include the inexpensive nature of the test, its ability to perform in low-resource settings, safety, the fact that there is no need for a laboratory infrastructure for reporting and test results are available immediately, its moderately high sensitivity in detecting high-grade lesions if providers are well trained, and the possibility of integrating the test readily in single- or two-visit approaches. Evidence from several studies indicates that both VIA and VILI are acceptable to women and providers can be rapidly trained and provider competency can be maintained by close monitoring and periodic retraining.

Both VIA and VILI are readily used tests in low-resource settings, where cytology and HPV testing may seldom be possible, and are useful early detection tests in clinical settings. With adequate training, both are suitable tests for detecting CIN in women aged 30–50 years and thus they are useful clinical early detection tools. As a single visual test, many prefer VIA; however one can judiciously combine VIA and VILI for early detection in situations where VIA results are equivocal or doubtful. In this context, education of health workers, nurses, medical students and doctors is essential for their widespread use and diffusion in clinical practice. Results from completed and on-going studies will further clarify the scope and cost-effectiveness of large-scale implementation of VIA and VILI in organised public health screening programmes. The work carried out by the Alliance for Cervical Cancer Prevention, supported by the Bill & Melinda Gates Foundation, is instructive for cervical cancer prevention in low- and medium-resource countries (ACCP, 2004). Evidence on the extent of the reduction in disease burden associated with visual screening, as compared with other screening approaches from on-going randomised trials, will be important for the development of rational public health policies for using visual screening in organised programmes.

REFERENCES

Alliance for Cervical Cancer Prevention (ACCP) (2004) *Planning and Implementing Cervical Cancer Prevention and Control Programs: A Manual for Managers.* Seattle, WA: ACCP.

Basu PS, Sankaranarayanan R, Mandal R *et al.* (2002) Evaluation of downstaging in the detection of cervical neoplasia in Kolkata, India. *International Journal of Cancer* 100: 92–96.

Basu PS, Sankaranarayanan R, Mandal R *et al.* (2003) Calcutta Cervical Cancer Early Detection Group. Visual inspection with acetic acid and cytology in the early detection of cervical neoplasia in Kolkata, India. *International Journal of Gynecological Cancer* 13: 626–632.

Belinson JL, Pretorius RG, Zhang WH *et al.* (2001) Cervical cancer screening by simple visual inspection after acetic acid. *Obstetrics and Gynecology* 98: 441–444.

Blumenthal P, Lauterbach J, Sellors J *et al.* (2005) Training for cervical cancer prevention programs in low-resource settings: focus on visual inspection with acetic acid and cryotherapy. *International Journal of Gynecology and Obstetrics* 89 (Suppl. 2): S4–S12.

Cecchini S, Bonardi R, Mazzotta A *et al.* (1993) Testing cervicography and cervicoscopy as screening tests for cervical cancer. *Tumori* 79: 22–25.

Cronjé HS, Cooreman BF, Beyer E *et al.* (2001) Screening for cervical neoplasia in a developing country utilizing cytology, cervicography and the acetic acid test. *International Journal of Gynecology and Obstetrics* 72: 151–157.

Cronjé HS, Parham GP, Cooreman BF *et al.* (2003) A comparison of four screening methods for cervical neoplasia in a developing country. *American Journal of Obstetrics and Gynecology* 188: 395–400.

Denny L, Kuhn L, Pollack A *et al.* (2000) Evaluation of alternative methods of cervical cancer screening in resource poor settings. *Cancer* 89: 826–833.

Denny L, Kuhn L, Pollack A *et al.* (2002) Direct visual inspection for cervical cancer screening: an analysis of factors influencing test performance. *Cancer* 94: 1699–1707.

Denny L, Kuhn L, De Souza M *et al.* (2005) Screen-and-treat approaches for cervical cancer prevention in low-resource settings: a randomized controlled trial. *Journal of the American Medical Association* 294: 2173–2181.

De Vuyst H, Claeys P, Njiru S *et al.* (2005) Comparison of pap smear, visual inspection with acetic acid, human papillomavirus DNA-PCR testing and cervicography. *International Journal of Gynecology and Obstetrics* 89: 120–126.

Doh AS, Nkele NN, Achu P *et al.* (2005) Visual inspection with acetic acid and cytology as screening methods for cervical lesions in Cameroon. *International Journal of Gynecology and Obstetrics* 89: 167–173.

El Shalakany A, Hassan SS, Ammar E *et al.* (2004) Direct visual inspection of the cervix for the detection of premalignant lesions. *Journal of Lower Genital Tract Diseases* 8: 16–20.

Goldie S, Gaffikin L, Goldhaber-Fiebert J *et al.* (2005) Cost effectiveness of cervical screening in five developing countries, *New England Journal of Medicine* 353: 2158–2168.

IARC (2005) *IARC Handbooks on Cancer Prevention*, Vol. 10, *Cervix Cancer Screening.* Lyon: IARC Press.

Londhe M, George SS, Seshadri L (1997) Detection of CIN by naked eye visualization after application of acetic acid. *Indian Journal of Cancer* 1997; 34: 88–91.

McIntosh N, Blumenthal PD, Blouse A (eds) (2001) *Cervical Cancer Prevention Guidelines for Low-resource Settings*, JHPIEGO Technical Manual. Baltimore, MD: JHPIEGO.

Mathers LJ, Wigton TR, Leonhardt JG (2005) Screening for cervical neoplasia in an unselected rural Guatemalan population using direct visual inspection after acetic acid application: a pilot study. *Journal of Lower Genital Tract Diseases* 9: 232–235.

Megavand E, Denny L, Dehaeck K *et al.* Acetic acid visualization of the cervix: an alternative to cytologic screening. *Obstetrics and Gynecology* 88: 383–386.

Ngelangel CA, Limson GM, Cordero CP *et al.* (2003) Acetic-acid guided visual inspection vs. cytology-based screening for cervical cancer in the Philippines. *International Journal of Gynecology and Obstetrics* 83: 141–150.

Ottoviano M, La Torre P (1982) Examination of the cervix with the naked eye using acetic acid test. *American Journal of Obstetrics and Gynecology* 143: 139–142

Rodriguez-Reyes ER, Cerdes-Flores RM *et al.* (2002) Acetic acid test: a promising screening test for early detection of cervical cancer. *Analysis and Quantification of Cytological Histology* 24: 134–136.

Royal Thai College of Obstetricians and Gynaecologists (RTCOG)/ JHPIEGO Corporation Cervical Cancer Prevention Group (2003) Safety, acceptability, and feasibility of a single-visit approach to cervical-cancer prevention in rural Thailand: a demonstration project. *Lancet* 361: 814–820.

Sangwa-Lugoma G, Mahmud S, Nasr SH *et al.* (2006) Visual inspection as a cervical cancer screening method in a primary health care setting in Africa. *International Journal of Cancer* [epub ahead of print].

Sankaranarayanan R, Syamalakumari B, Wesley R *et al.* (1997) Visual inspection as a screening test for cervical cancer control in developing countries. In: Franco E, Monsonego J (eds) *New Developments in Cervical Cancer Screening and Prevention*. Oxford: Blackwell Science.

Sankaranarayanan R, Wesley R, Somanathan T *et al.* (1998) Visual inspection of the uterine cervix after the application of acetic acid in the detection of cervical carcinoma and its precursors. *Cancer* 83: 2150–2156.

Sankaranarayanan R, Shyamalakumari B, Wesley R *et al.* (1991) Visual inspection with acetic acid in the early detection of cervical cancer and precancers. *International Journal of Cancer* 80: 161–163.

Sankaranarayanan R, Budukh A, Rajkumar R (2001) Effective screening programs for cervical cancer in low- and middle-income developing countries. *Bulletin of the World Health Organization* 79: 954–962.

Sankaranarayanan R, Wesley R (2003) *A Practical Manual on Visual Screening for Cervical Neoplasia*, IARC Technical Publication No. 41. Lyon: IARC Press.

Sankaranarayanan R, Basu P, Wesley R *et al.* (2004a) Accuracy of visual screening for cervical neoplasia: results from an IARC multicentre study in India and Africa. *International Journal of Cancer* 110: 907–913.

Sankaranarayanan R, Shastri SS, Basu P *et al.* (2004b) The role of low-level magnification in visual inspection with acetic acid for the early detection of cervical neoplasia. *Cancer Detection and Prevention* 28: 345–351.

Sankaranarayanan R, Rajkumar R, Theresa R *et al.* (2004c) Initial results from a randomized trial of cervical visual screening in rural south India. *International Journal of Cancer* 109: 461–467.

Sankaranarayanan R, Gaffikin L, Jacob M *et al.* (2005a) A critical assessment of screening methods for cervical neoplasia. *International Journal of Gynecology and Obstetrics* 89 (Suppl. 2): S4–S12.

Sankaranarayanan R, Nene BN, Dinshaw KA *et al.* on behalf of the Osmanabad District Cervical Screening Study Group (2005b) A cluster randomised controlled trial of visual, cytology and HPV screening for cancer of the cervix in rural India. *International Journal of Cancer* 116: 617–623.

Sarian L, Derchain S, Naud P *et al.* (2005) Evaluation of visual inspection with acetic acid (VIA), Lugol's iodine (VILI), cervical cytology and HPV testing as cervical screening tools in Latin America. *Journal of Medical Screening* 12: 142–149.

Sellors JW, Jeronimo J, Sankaranarayanan R *et al.* (2002) Assessment of the cervix after acetic acid wash: inter-rater agreement using photographs. *Obstetrics and Gynecology* 99: 635–640.

Shastri SS, Dinshaw K, Amin G *et al.* (2005) Concurrent evaluation of visual, cytological and HPV testing as screening methods for the early detection of cervical neoplasia in Mumbai, India. *Bulletin of the World Health Organization* 83: 186–194.

Slawson DC, Bennett JH, Herman JM (1992) Are Papanicolaou smears enough? Acetic acid washes of the cervix as adjunctive therapy: A HARNET study. *Journal of Family Practice* 35: 271–277.

Tayyeb R, Khawaja NP, Malik N (2003) Comparison of visual inspection of cervix and Pap smear for cervical cancer screening. *Journal of the College of Physicians and Surgeons of Pakistan* 13: 201–203.

University of Zimbabwe/JHPIEGO Cervical Cancer Project (1999) Visual inspection with acetic acid for cervical cancer screening: test qualities in a primary-care setting. *Lancet* 353: 869–873.

Cervical neoplasia: management of premalignant and malignant disease

CHAPTER 30

Colposcopy

Joseph A. Jordan and Albert Singer

Hinselmann published his first paper about colposcopy in 1925 — he designed the first colposcope and described the colposcopic features of almost every benign and malignant lesion seen on the cervix. Although his work was not recognised fully during his lifetime, in the late 1940s and 1950s, clinicians and investigators in Germany, central and eastern Europe and South America gave him due credit for his contribution to the understanding of the pattern and the morphogenesis of cervical premalignant disease and early malignancy. It was not until the 1960s and 1970s that colposcopy became established in the English-speaking countries.

THE COLPOSCOPE

The binocular colposcopes in use today give a stereoscopic magnification of between 6 and 40 times and provide a transition from macroscopic to microscopic vision. The different epithelial abnormalities (benign, premalignant and malignant) can be studied *in vivo* and, with experience, it is possible to forecast the histological diagnosis with reasonable accuracy. The most common magnifications used are × 10 and × 16. The patient should be placed in a modified lithotomy position and, for the comfort of the patient and the colposcopist, it is important to have an examination table that has been designed for colposcopic use.

METHODS OF TISSUE RECOGNITION

The acetic acid technique

The traditional method of colposcopy relies on the application of 3–5% acetic acid, after which premalignant disease appears white (referred to as acetowhite) and the subepithelial angioarchitecture becomes more prominent. Unfortunately, not everything that is acetowhite is premalignant!

Acetic acid causes the tissue, especially columnar and abnormal epithelia, to become oedematous, with the former adopting a white or opaque appearance, which is then quite easily distinguishable from normal epithelium, which appears pink.

Why the atypical transformation zone epithelium appears white after the application of 3–5% aqueous acetic acid is still debatable. One explanation could be that the acetic acid is a frequent component of tissue fixatives and will thereby rapidly penetrate through the tissue with an effect upon the nucleus of a cell. In this situation, it may precipitate nucleoproteins. Maclean (2003) has shown that this process exists and that not only the nucleus but also the cytoplasm is affected, undergoing vacuolation with the cells becoming swollen and the desmosomes separating. When acetic acid is applied to normal squamous epithelium, the penetration through the sparsely nucleated surface and intermediate layers produces little precipitation. However, the basal and parabasal layers contain more nucleoproteins, but this is not sufficient to obscure the colour of the underlying cervical stroma with its rich network of subepithelial vessels and, therefore, the epithelium will appear pink. The application of acetic acid to areas of atypical epithelium containing cervical intraepithelial neoplasia (CIN) causes the precipitated nucleoproteins within the neoplastic cells to be affected and therefore obscures the underlying vessels. The light is therefore reflected and the epithelium appears white/acetowhite. In low-grade CIN, the acetic acid must penetrate into the lower half of the epithelium, and the onset of white is delayed but, in high-grade or full-thickness CIN, acetic acid will elicit an almost instant response and the tissue will appear markedly white. The effect is slowly reversed because the acid is buffered, and nucleoprotein is no longer precipitated.

Another mechanism that produces swelling of the tissues is described by Maddox *et al.* (1994), who showed that there is an increase in the keratin filament protein in epithelium which stains white with acetic acid. These filament proteins, called cytokeratins, seem to be increased in association with the cellular swelling caused by the acetic acid acting on the epithelium. Twenty different cytokeratin polypeptides exist (Smedts *et al.*, 1993), and Maddox and his group (1994) have shown that there is a significant increase in cytokeratin 10; they insist that this is an essential requirement for the formation of the so-called acetowhite epithelial change.

The appearances are not unique to neoplasia but will be seen on other occasions where there is increased nucleoprotein present, as occurs during the process of immature metaplasia formation, healing of the epithelium and with the presence of virus or viral products, such as in clinical human papillomavirus (HPV) changes in the cervical epithelium and/or the presence of condyloma.

The saline technique

The use of saline rather than acetic acid was popularised by Koller (1963) and Kolstad (1970) — this technique relies on studying the subepithelial angioarchitecture, as a result of which both authors showed that the degree of premalignant disease could be diagnosed with much more accuracy than with the technique using acetic acid. However, the saline technique is more difficult to learn, and the novice colposcopist should always use the acetic acid technique.

Schiller's iodine or Lugol's solution

Application of Schiller's or Lugol's solution as advocated by the German school is largely unnecessary but, on the other hand, does occasionally show areas of abnormality, particularly low-grade abnormality, which would otherwise not be apparent — for this reason, novice colposcopists may find it valuable. The technique relies on Schiller's observation that normal squamous epithelium is rich in glycogen, whereas squamous intraepithelial neoplasia is deficient in glycogen: glycogen absorbs iodine and so normal glycogen-containing squamous epithelium takes up the glycogen and stains dark brown/black, whereas the glycogen-free abnormal epithelium does not stain. The Schiller test is designed to detect CIN and, therefore, a positive Schiller test identifies an area of the cervix that is non-staining with iodine, and a negative Schiller test identifies an area of normal squamous epithelium. Unfortunately, although the test is sensitive, its specificity is low as some non-premalignant disease, especially metaplasia, may be Schiller positive (non-staining).

DIAGNOSTIC PROCEDURES

Colposcopic biopsy

Colposcopic vision allows biopsies to be taken from the location within the transformation zone with the most severe changes in order that histological confirmation of the degree of severity of the neoplastic process can be obtained to aid the diagnosis. As colposcopy is a procedure during which cancer must be ruled out, it is standard practice by most colposcopists to obtain a histological sample not only from the ectocervix, but also from tissue existing within the endocervical canal (if the new squamocolumnar junction cannot be seen). If

the entire transformation zone cannot be examined, the colposcopy is deemed to be unsatisfactory.

A recent study by Pretorius *et al.* (2004) assessed the relative importance of colposcopically directed biopsy in comparison with random biopsy and endocervical curettage in diagnosing high-grade CIN (CIN2–3). A total of 364 women with satisfactory colposcopy and the diagnosis of high-grade CIN were sampled. All colposcopically detected lesions were biopsied. If colposcopy showed no lesion in the cervical quadrant, a random biopsy was obtained at the squamocolumnar junction and in that quadrant. Endocervical curettage was then performed. Results were most revealing in that the diagnosis of high-grade CIN was made on a colposcopically directed biopsy in only 57.1% of cases, a random biopsy confirming these findings in 37.4% and the endocervical curettage in 5.5%. The authors found that the yield of high-grade disease for random biopsy when the cytology was of a high-grade nature but with no obvious colposcopic abnormality was 17.6% and when cytology was of a low-grade nature yield was only 2.8%. One of 20 women diagnosed solely by endocervical curettage had invasive cancer. They concluded that, even when colposcopy is satisfactory, endocervical curettage should be performed and, if cytology is of a high-grade nature, then random biopsy should be considered. These views are contentious and will be discussed below.

Endocervical curettage: its value

Whether histological sampling of the endocervical canal by endocervical curettage should be done is an ongoing debate. Most clinicians in the United States routinely undertake sampling of the endocervical canal in most women undergoing colposcopic examinations, while others prefer to use it only when the new squamocolumnar junction cannot be seen and the colposcopic examination is unsatisfactory. It is also suggested that it should be employed when the colposcopic examination is satisfactory but the cytology is of a higher grade (Spirtos *et al.*, 1987; Fine *et al.*, 1998; Pretorius *et al.*, 2004).

However, a number of authors, especially those in Europe, are averse to the use of the sharp spoon-shaped or curved curette for endocervical curettage, arguing that, in many studies, unsatisfactory material has been obtained from the canal, making an accurate diagnosis impossible. No indication of the depth of involvement of the neoplastic tissue within the stroma such as occurs with microinvasive cancer can therefore be given. A second objection is that it is a painful procedure, being carried out without anaesthetic (Singer and Monaghan, 2000). Furthermore, the accuracy of endocervical sampling as described above has been questioned. Most studies have either examined too few subjects (Sesti *et al.*, 1990) or been retrospective in that women who have had both satisfactory and unsatisfactory colposcopy have had the final histology confirmed by a punch biopsy or cone biopsy. In others, the diagnosis was made on punch biopsy material before local destructive therapy was given (Patch *et al.*, 1985; Krebs *et al.*, 1987). In many of these studies, no significant pathology was available, and there was no information on the value of the negative endocervical sampling or on whether a negative result would indeed influence treatment when colposcopy is unsatisfactory.

Anderson *et al.* (1992) examined 100 women with abnormal cervical smears who were selected for cone biopsy. They randomly underwent endocervical sampling with either a Kevorkian curette or the endocervical brush. They found that the overall sensitivity of endocervical sampling was 56% with a false-negative rate of 44% and a negative predictive value of only 26%. The breakdown of these figures showed that the sensitivity of curettage and brush cytology samples was 57% and 53%, respectively, with a specificity of 69%, but the small number of cases meant that the accuracy of this last figure is doubtful. Although the overall false-negative rate was 43%, the rate for curettage was 46% and for the brush sampling was 45%. The authors concluded that the two recognised sampling methods both have high false-negative rates and a correspondingly low ability to predict freedom from disease (26% negative predictive value).

These sampling methods certainly miss significant CIN and early invasive lesions, and their value in, for instance, avoiding negative cone biopsy when the endocervical sample is negative was seriously questioned by Lopez *et al.* (1989). In their study,

it would seem that endocervical sampling did not influence the management when colposcopy was unsatisfactory.

DIAGNOSTIC CRITERIA

There is a widely held perception that colposcopy is nothing more than the recognition of acetowhite epithelium or epithelium that is non-staining following the application of Schiller's iodine. However, this misconception leads to poor colposcopy, poor assessment of women with abnormal cervical cytology and both overtreatment and undertreatment. There is more to colposcopy than this — the colposcopist should learn to recognise and identify easily observable features (Kolstad and Stafl, 1972). These are:

1 vascular pattern;
2 intercapillary distance;
3 colour tone at the junction of normal and abnormal tissue;
4 surface contour;
5 a sharp line of demarcation between different types of epithelium.

The terminology used in describing the various morphological changes within the cervical epithelium has evolved over many years. Many of these qualitative descriptions have been quantified as to the degree of abnormality, and such a scoring system as described by Reid (Table 30.1) is used by many colposcopists to grade abnormal squamous epithelial areas. Ferris *et al.* (2006) reported the employment of an abbreviated Reid colposcopic scoring index during the National

Table 30.1 This combined colposcopic index is commonly used to score and document abnormal areas seen on colposcopic examination (Reid and Scalzi, 1985; Reid, 1993).

Colposcopic sign	Zero points	One point	Two points
Colour	Less intense acetowhitening (not completely opaque). Indistinct, semi-transparent acetowhitening. Acetowhitening beyond the margin of the transformation zone. Snow-white colour with intense surface shine	Intermediate, shiny, grey–white shade	Dull, oyster white
Lesion margin and surface configuration	Feathery, indistinct or finely scalloped edges. Angular, irregularly shaped, geographical margins. Satellite lesions with margins well removed from the new squamocolumnar junction. Lesion with a condylomatous or micropapillary contour	Regularly shaped lesion with sharp, straight edges	Rolled, peeling edges. Internal margins separating lesions with differing scores, the more central one with the higher score tending to be nearest to the new squamocolumnar junction
Blood vessels	Fine punctation or mosaic pattern	Absent vessels (after application of acetic acid)	Coarse punctation or mosaic pattern
Iodine staining	Positive iodine staining (mahogany-brown colour). Negative iodine staining in an area that scores 3 or less on the first three criteria	Partial iodine uptake, giving a variegated pattern	Negative for uptake, giving a mustard yellow appearance in area that is significant (4 or more points) by the other three criteria

A score of 0–2 is compatible with CIN1; 3–5 with CIN1 or 2; and 6–8 with CIN2 or 3.

Table 30.2 International Federation for Cervical Pathology and Colposcopy: colposcopic classification.

I.   Normal colposcopic findings
    Original squamous epithelium
    Columnar epithelium
    Transformation zone
II. Abnormal colposcopic findings
    Flat acetowhite epithelium
    Dense acetowhite epithelium*
    Fine mosaic
    Coarse mosaic*
    Fine punctation
    Coarse punctation*
    Iodine partial positivity
    Iodine negativity*
    Atypical vessels*
III. Colposcopic features suggestive of invasive cancer
IV. Unsatisfactory colposcopy
    Squamocolumnar junction not visible
    Severe inflammation, severe atrophy, trauma
    Cervix not visible
V.   Miscellaneous findings
    Condylomata
    Keratosis
    Erosion
    Inflammation
    Atrophy
    Deciduosis
    Polyps

*Indicates the characteristics of high-grade changes.
Reproduced with permission of The American College of Obstetricians and Gynaecologists (Walker *et al.*, 2003).

Cancer Institute (NCI) ASCUS, LSIL Triage Study (ALTS) to detect CIN2/3. They found that colposcopists using this abbreviated system failed to detect CIN2/3 at the levels expected. The poor correlation was not altered by colposcopic expertise. Although raising concerns about current colposcopic practice based on this system, the authors concluded that it should be used until a better alternative is available. Recently, the International Federation for Cervical Pathology and Colposcopy recommended a revised nomenclature for colposcopic findings which will be described below and is featured in Table 30.2.

Vascular patterns

The vascular pattern is best observed at magnifications of × 10–25. Following the use of either normal saline or acetic acid, a green filter will allow a very accurate assessment and evaluation of the vascular changes and of the colour tone between normal and abnormal tissue. The arrangement and the distance between the terminal vessels observed within an abnormal colposcopic area can best be assessed by comparing these vessels with those of the adjacent normal squamous epithelium.

Intercapillary distance

The capillaries of the original squamous epithelium are characterised by a regular and dense pattern, while those of preinvasive and frank invasive lesions show striking irregularities and variation in their spatial distribution, frequently with an increased distance between adjacent terminal vessels. The more the lesion moves from low- to high-grade premalignant disease to early invasive or frank invasive carcinoma, the more widely spaced the terminal vessels become.

Colour tone

Different lesions may show different colours varying from white, light yellow, yellow red to deep red. For a correct interpretation of the colposcopic image, the most important single factor is the contrast in tone of the abnormal epithelium relative to the adjacent normal epithelium, best seen when the tissues are viewed with a green filter following the application of normal saline. The contrast is also seen clearly following the application of acetic acid.

Following the application of saline, the CIN, particularly high-grade CIN, appears darker than the original squamous epithelium. Metaplastic epithelium, on the other hand, is whiter and somewhat opaque. Invasive cancer is also whitish, often with a glazed or gelatinous appearance. Following the application of acetic acid, CIN appears white and, although the vessels are more prominent, they are not as prominent or as easy to assess as they are following the use of saline and a green filter.

Surface contour

The stereoscopic view provided by the colposcope makes it easier to study the surface contours of the different lesions. Original squamous epithelium has a smooth surface, while columnar epithelium is easier to recognise, having the appearance of grape-like villi. Preinvasive lesions often have an uneven slightly elevated surface, while invasive cancer is characterised by a nodular or polypoid surface with an exophytic or ulcerated growth pattern.

Epithelial borders

The last criterion which can easily be studied with the colposcope is the border between lesions and the adjacent normal tissue. The demarcation between CIN and the original squamous epithelium is usually sharp. In contrast, the borderline between normal (original squamous epithelium) and inflammatory lesions or CIN1 may be diffuse.

COLPOSCOPIC TERMINOLOGY

The International Federation for Cervical Pathology and Colposcopy approved a revised colposcopic classification (Table 30.2) and basic colposcopic terminology in 2002 (Walker *et al.*, 2003). The new terminology has the following features:

1 It is descriptive, thereby allowing colposcopists throughout the world to be able to describe lesions to each other and to undertake important collaborative research.

2 The nomenclature was written in such a way that it can guide a colposcopist in training but can also aid the established colposcopist during the diagnostic process.

3 The terminology is pragmatic and includes a description of the three types of transformation zone — it was felt that this would lead to a more rational triage for the most appropriate treatment for women with abnormal transformation zones.

COLPOSCOPIC FINDINGS

Normal (see Chapter 2)

Original squamous epithelium

Original squamous epithelium is a smooth, pink featureless epithelium, originally established at organogenesis, on the cervix and vagina. No remnants of columnar epithelium such as columnar epithelium, cleft openings or Nabothian cysts are present in original squamous epithelium. The epithelium does not stain white after the application of a dilute solution of acetic acid; it will stain brown after the application of Lugol's iodine. Close examination of original squamous epithelium using a green filter will, in most cases, disclose two types of underlying capillaries, either so-called network capillaries or hairpin capillaries (Fig. 30.1).

Original columnar epithelium

Columnar epithelium is a single-layer, mucus-producing epithelium that extends between the endometrium cranially and either the original squamous epithelium or the transformation zone caudally. At colposcopy, after the application of acetic acid, the area has a typical grape-like structure. Columnar epithelium is normally present in the endocervix and may be present on the ectocervix (ectopy) or, on rare occasions, in the vagina (vaginal adenosis). The areas covered with columnar epithelium have an irregular surface with long stromal papillae and deep clefts. Following the application of acetic acid, the typical grape-like appearance of the columnar epithelium villi will stand out clearly (Fig. 30.2). Within the villi of columnar epithelium. a loosely coiled fine capillary system of vessels can be seen — it is this that makes the columnar epithelium appear more red than squamous epithelium (Fig. 30.3).

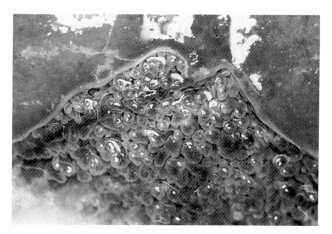

Fig. 30.2 Original columnar epithelial villi. The junction of the original columnar epithelium and the original squamous epithelium is referred to as the squamocolumnar junction (SCJ).

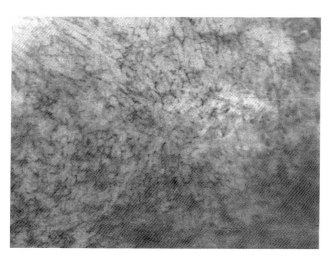

Fig. 30.1 Original squamous epithelium with dense subepithelial network capillaries. Tiny hairpin capillaries can be seen as small dots.

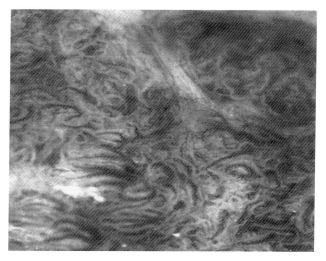

Fig. 30.3 Villi of original columnar epithelium — within each villus is a densely coiled capillary network.

The transformation zone

The transformation zone is that part of the cervix which, in fetal life, began as an area occupied by native or original columnar epithelium which now has a component of squamous epithelium within its boundary; the junction of the original squamous and the original columnar epithelium is the original squamocolumnar junction.

The original (native) columnar epithelium found on the ectocervix is a 'temporary' phenomenon. After the menarche, this epithelium exposed to the vaginal environment (pH) will sooner or later be changed to squamous epithelium. The process by which this columnar epithelium is transformed to squamous epithelium is referred to as metaplasia. The area that has been transformed from columnar epithelium to squamous epithelium by the process of metaplasia is referred to as the transformation zone, i.e. the transformation zone is that part of the cervix that was originally composed of columnar epithelium and by the process of metaplasia has been transformed to predominantly squamous epithelium. The first stage of metaplasia involves the fusion of the villi, as a result of which the surface appears flat rather than villous. Squamous metaplasia starts on the top of the single villus and little by little develops in between the clefts of columnar epithelium, which eventually become replaced by a multilayered squamous epithelium. In a normal or physiological transformation zone, metaplastic squamous epithelium can be identified in varying degrees of maturity. The components of a normal (physiological) mature transformation zone consist of islands of columnar epithelium surrounded by mature metaplastic squamous epithelium, gland openings and Nabothian cysts or follicles (Fig. 30.4). When metaplasia is taking place (immature metaplasia), the columnar epithelium undergoing the metaplastic change appears densely acetowhite and can easily be confused with CIN (Fig. 30.5a and b). Fully mature metaplastic squamous

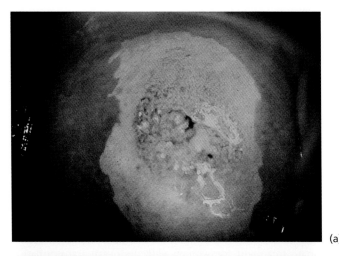

(a)

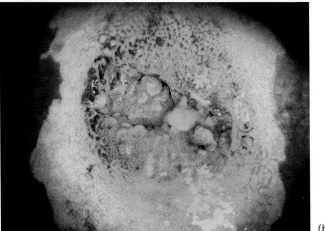

(b)

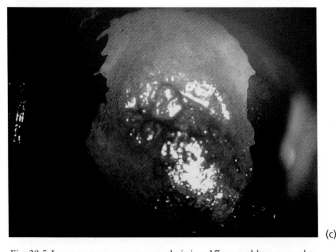

(c)

Fig. 30.5 Immature squamous metaplasia in a 17-year-old woman who presented with abnormal cytology. The cervix is seen before (a) and after (b) the application of acetic acid. The acetowhite epithelium was shown to be immature squamous metaplasia and not CIN. This area is non-staining with iodine (c).

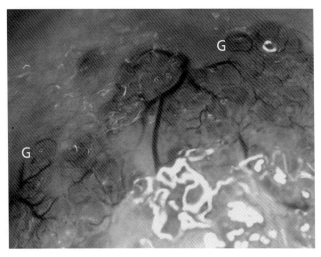

Fig. 30.4 A mature normal transformation zone with large but regularly branching (normal) vessels with gland openings (G).

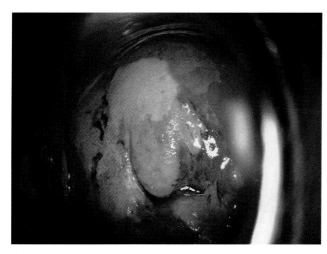

Fig. 30.6 Acetowhite squamous (abnormal) epithelium due to CIN.

epithelium is not acetowhite. This process is described in more detail in Chapter 2.

Three types of transformation zone are recognised (morphologically). A type 1 transformation zone is completely ectocervical and fully visible, and may be small or large. A type 2 transformation zone has an endocervical component, is fully visible and may have an ectocervical component that may be small or large. A type 3 transformation zone has an endocervical component that is not fully visible and may have an ectocervical component that may be small or large (Prendiville, 2003; Walker *et al.*, 2003). The relevance of these three types of transformation zone to treatment of CIN is discussed in Chapter 31.

In a small percentage of women, the transformation zone may extend caudally onto the upper vagina, usually with an anterior and posterior triangle or tongue; it may contain a fine regular mosaic pattern of blood vessels and stain partially or wholly negative after the application of Lugol's iodine.

Abnormal

Acetowhite epithelium

After the application of a dilute solution of acetic acid, areas of high nuclear density appear white. Although this may occur in cases of immature metaplasia, generally, the denser the acetowhite change, the faster the change becomes apparent, and the increased length of time the epithelium holds the change, the more severe the lesion may be (Fig. 30.6). Dense acetowhite change within columnar epithelium may indicate glandular disease.

Punctation

The term punctation describes a focal colposcopic pattern in which capillaries appear in a stippled pattern. The finer the punctation appearance, the more likely the lesion is to be of

low grade or metaplasia. The coarser the punctation, the more likely the lesion is to be of major grade (Fig. 30.7a–e).

Mosaic

This term describes a focal colposcopic appearance in which the new vessel formation appears as a rectangular pattern like a mosaic. The smaller the mosaic, the more likely the lesion is to be of low grade or metaplasia. The coarser, wider and more irregular the mosaic, the more likely the lesion is to be of major grade (Fig. 30.8).

Iodine negativity

After the application of Lugol's or Schiller's iodine (Fig. 30.7e), mature squamous epithelium, which contains glycogen, will stain a deep brown. Iodine-negative areas may represent immature metaplasia, CIN (Fig. 30.7e) or low-estrogen states (i.e. atrophy). A speckled appearance in an area with slight acetowhite change may represent immature metaplasia or low-grade intraepithelial neoplasia. Complete iodine negativity, a yellow staining in an area that has appeared strongly aceto-white, is highly suggestive of high-grade intraepithelial neoplasia. Just as not all acetowhite epithelium signifies the presence of CIN, colposcopists should realise that iodine-negative areas do not necessarily represent CIN. The original test was referred to as Schiller's test — the colposcopist should remember that a Schiller positive area is an area that is iodine negative, i.e. non-staining with iodine.

Atypical vessels

Abnormal cervical tissue may exhibit a focal abnormal colposcopic pattern in which the blood vessel pattern appears not as punctation or mosaic or as finely branching capillaries of a normal epithelium, but rather as irregular vessels with an abrupt and interrupted course appearing as commas, corkscrew capillaries or spaghetti-like forms (Figs 30.9 and 30.10).

Colposcopic features suggestive of low-grade disease (minor change)

Incorporating features described above:
1 a smooth surface with an irregular outer border;
2 slight acetowhite change, slow to appear and quick to disappear;
3 fine punctation and fine regular mosaic;
4 mild, often speckled iodine partial positivity.

Colposcopic features suggestive of high-grade disease (major change)

In addition to the features described above, these include:
1 a generally smooth surface with a sharp outer border;
2 dense acetowhite change that appears early and is slow to resolve; it may be oyster white;
3 coarse punctation and wide irregular mosaics of differing size;

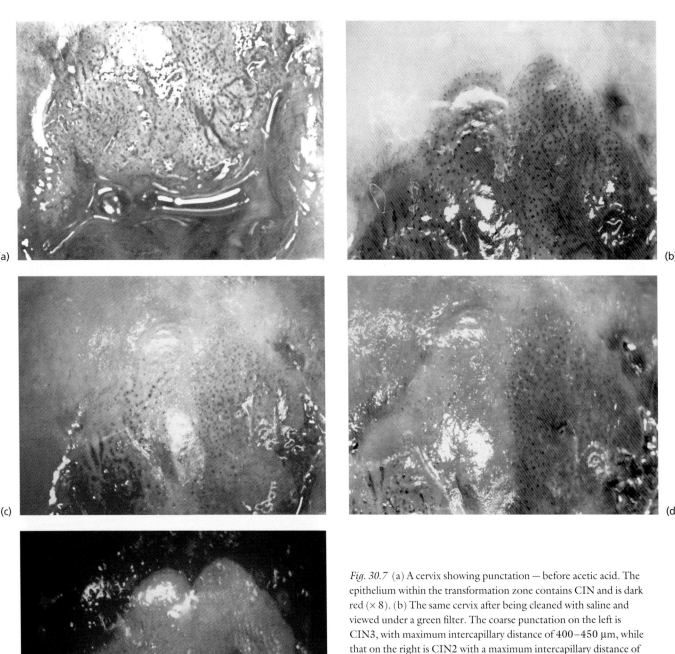

Fig. 30.7 (a) A cervix showing punctation — before acetic acid. The epithelium within the transformation zone contains CIN and is dark red (× 8). (b) The same cervix after being cleaned with saline and viewed under a green filter. The coarse punctation on the left is CIN3, with maximum intercapillary distance of 400–450 μm, while that on the right is CIN2 with a maximum intercapillary distance of 300–350 μm. The dark CIN epithelium contrasts with the light normal original squamous epithelium giving a sharp line of demarcation. Compare with Figure 30.7a, the same cervix but viewed without a green filter. (c) Area shown in Figure 30.7b but after the application of acetic acid. (d) The same area following acetic acid application but viewed through a green filter. Much of the capillary detail has been lost, especially that of the CIN3 on the left. (e) Schiller's test. The Schiller-positive (non-staining) area corresponds exactly with the CIN.

4 iodine negativity, a yellow or yellow/white appearance in a previously densely white epithelium, i.e. Schiller's positive;
5 dense acetowhite change within columnar epithelium may indicate glandular disease (Fig. 30.11a and b).

Colposcopic features suggestive of invasive cancer
These include features described above as well as:
1 irregular surface, erosion or ulceration;
2 dense acetowhite change;

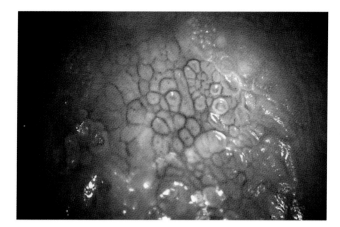

Fig. 30.8 Coarse mosaic suggestive of high-grade lesion.

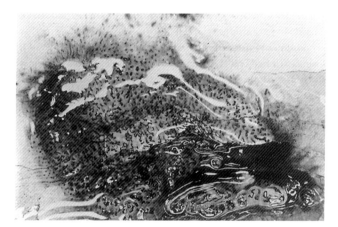

Fig. 30.9 Atypical vessels, comma-like.

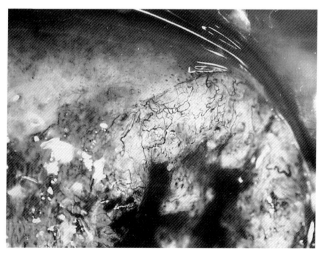

Fig. 30.10 Atypical vessels, corkscrew capilliaries.

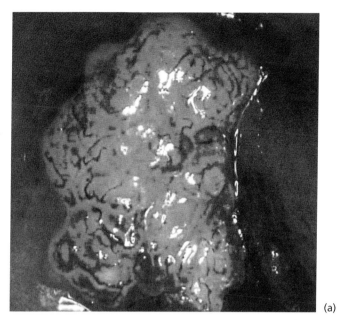

(a)

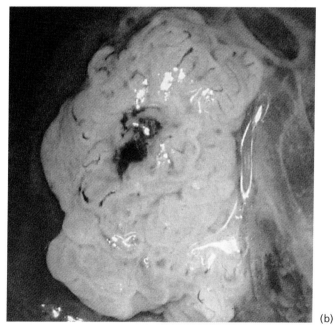

(b)

Fig. 30.11 (a) Cervical adenocarcinoma before acetic acid. (b) Cervical adenocarcinoma after acetic acid. Note the raised appearance with atypical vessels — very similar to the condylomata seen in Figure 30.12a and b.

3 wide irregular punctation and mosaic;
4 atypical vessels.

Unsatisfactory colposcopy

An unsatisfactory colposcopy examination occurs when the squamocolumnar junction cannot be visualised. It may also

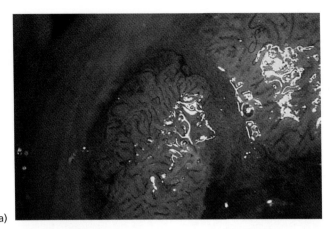

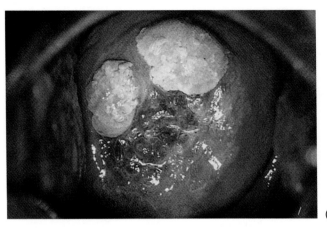

(a)   (b)

Fig. 30.12 (a) Condylomata before acetic acid. (b) Condylomata after acetic acid — note that some vessels appear atypical. Compare with Figure 30.11a and b.

occur if associated trauma, inflammation or atrophy precludes a full colposcopic assessment, or when the cervix is not visible.

Miscellaneous findings

Condylomata

These may occur within or without the transformation zone and indicate infection with human papillomavirus (Fig. 30.12a and b).

Keratosis

This term describes a focal colposcopic pattern in which hyperkeratosis is present and which appears as an elevated white plaque. The white change is present before the application of acetic acid and may preclude adequate visualisation of the underlying transformation zone.

Erosion

A true erosion represents an area of denuded epithelium. It may have been caused by trauma and may be an indication that the surface epithelium is vulnerable and possibly abnormal.

Inflammation

Atrophy

An epithelial change due to a low-estrogen state.

Deciduosis

A change identified in pregnancy.

Polyps

USES OF COLPOSCOPY

Colposcopy can be used in two circumstances, namely for primary screening and for the diagnosis of women with abnormal cytology and/or clinical suspicion of malignancy.

In a primary screening system

Many clinicians in Latin American countries and Europe use colposcopy routinely as part of the standard gynaecological examination (Jordan, 1985; Dexeus *et al.*, 2002). Cytology usually accompanies colposcopy in these circumstances, and the argument behind this is that the combined testing procedure will decrease the false-negative and -positive cytology, thereby reducing the number of women recalled for cytology. Collection of a cytology specimen is also helped by colposcopy.

However, in a number of countries, e.g. Germany, there does not seem to be any advantage in using the colposcope to increase the accuracy of cytology. This has been shown to be the case in the recent HART study (Hilgarth and Menton, 1996; Cuzick *et al.*, 2003), in which the sensitivity of cytology taken by German clinicians was only 39%. Also, recent studies have shown an inability to detect with colposcopy endocervical lesions in this screening capacity (Van Niekerk *et al.*, 1998; Bellinson *et al.*, 2001).

With abnormal cytology and/or suspected malignancy

Colposcopy is used mainly in the English-speaking world to diagnose those women who have been referred with abnormal cytology or those in whom there is a clinical suspicion of malignancy (Jordan, 1985; Dexeus *et al.*, 2002).

HOW ACCURATE IS COLPOSCOPY AND HOW REPRODUCIBLE ARE ITS FINDINGS?

The assessment of colposcopy — how accurate?

Assessing the sensitivity and specificity of colposcopy and directed biopsies is extremely susceptible to bias. The major problem is that the colposcopist's impression is usually verified by using the reference standards, which are essentially based on histology. It is obvious that the colposcopic impression dictates where the biopsy and subsequent histology is obtained. This leads to an inflated estimate of the accuracy of colposcopy. Compared with studies in which colposcopy is employed for primary screening (with or without cytology), studies that assess colposcopy done as a diagnostic procedure are on women who are referred with abnormal cytology (as found at screening) and thus have a higher probably of and possibly a more severe spectrum of cervical pathology. Also, women with more pronounced findings and disease are detected more readily by screening, and the performance of colposcopy in a diagnostic capacity may exceed its accuracy and reproducibility when it is used as a screening tool.

If possible, all women evaluated with a test under assessment should have the reference standard applied to avoid verification bias and, where this is not possible, statistical correlation should be made. When colposcopic findings are compared with pathology, both the pathologist and the colposcopist should be blinded to corresponding information from the other test (Sellors, 2005).

Belinson *et al.* (2001) conducted a large multidisciplinary study of precancerous lesions in China, in which they assessed the accuracy of colposcopy. They concluded that increasing technology alone did not determine whether detection of lesions was improved. They used not only colposcopy but also real-time devices in association with cytology. They concluded that the important factors were whether the quality of light used optimised perception, the adequacy of the trainee and the characteristics of the cervix of the population studied, i.e. the presence of cervical inflammation. They concluded that the definition of abnormality and diagnostic 'thresholds' used by colposcopists were important, as these determine replication of findings and test cut-off points. Obviously, the expertise of the colposcopist improves the ability to assess more correctly the morphological findings present at colposcopy.

Studies of diagnostic colposcopy

Mitchell *et al.* (1998) undertook a meta-analysis of the accuracy of diagnostic colposcopy in those women referred with abnormal cytology in a review of 86 articles published over a 26-year period beginning in 1960. Strict inclusion criteria were invoked, and only eight were eligible for consideration in this meta-analysis. Compared with histology (more than CIN2), the cut-off of normal versus neoplasia on colposcopy had an average weighted sensitivity, specificity and area under the receiver operating characteristic (ROC) curve of 96%, 48% and 80% respectively. The cut-off of normal and low-grade versus high-grade and cancer on colposcopy is associated with values of 85%, 69% and 82% respectively. Mitchell *et al.* (1998) suggested that, independent of prevalence and compared with low-grade lesions, high-grade lesions and cancer were more accurately diagnosed.

A second study, by Olaniyan (2002), looked at eight studies, seven of which had been included in the previous

meta-analysis by Mitchell *et al.* (1998). The results were similar in both studies.

In a final study, Kirkegaard *et al.* (1995), examining the association between colposcopic findings and histology in cervical lesions with an emphasis on the significance of size, found that, when normal versus neoplasia and normal low-grade versus high-grade cut-offs were examined, sensitivities of 96% and 38% and specificities of 52.6% and 94.7% were found respectively.

Belinson *et al.*'s (2001) Chinese study included methodological design features intended to reduce selection bias and to assess the degree to which colposcopic biopsy is confounded with a particular colposcopic impression as the reference standard. Over 8000 women between 27 and 56 years of age were screened with vaginal and cervical cytological specimens being obtained; 13 oncogenic human papillomaviruses and liquid cytology were also used. Colposcopy was performed on 3000 women who had an abnormality on screening, and a directed biopsy was obtained from any visible abnormality. If colposcopy showed no lesion in a quadrant of the transformation zone, a biopsy was obtained at the original squamocolumnar junction in that quadrant, with an endocervical curette also being performed. Based on all the women who had colposcopy — and that included 11 with unsatisfactory colposcopy — the sensitivity and specificity of colposcopy for detection of lesions more than CIN2 was 62.4% and 93.7% respectively. Among the women with satisfactory cytology in this study, directed biopsy detected 57.1% of high-grade lesions and cancers; if colposcopy showed no abnormality, four-quadrant biopsies and endocervical curettage (EC) detected 37.4 and 5.5% respectively (prevalence 4.4%). In women who were referred with a cytological abnormality, directed biopsies were 4.8 times more likely to show a high-grade lesion or cancer than four-quadrant biopsies (26.5% vs. 5.5%). The yields (more than CIN2) of four-quadrant biopsies for women referred because of an abnormal smear (ASCUS — low-/high-grade lesion who had a positive HPV DNA test) were 17.6%, 3.6% and 1.7% respectively. Only 1 of 20 women in whom diagnosis of CIN2 or more was made on EC had cancer despite satisfactory colposcopy.

In another study reported by Milne *et al.* (1999), 255 colposcopically negative women with abnormal cytology and 726 control subjects with normal cytology were followed for up to 5 years to assess the probability of false-negative colposcopy. Subsequent neoplasia was found in 19% vs. 3% of control subjects, the difference being highly significant.

Studies of screening colposcopy

In the Belinson *et al.* (2001) study described above, cross-sectional analysis of nearly 2000 unscreened Chinese women between 35 and 45 years of age was undertaken. All the women were first assessed by visual inspection with acetic acid (VIA) performed by a gynaecologist, and then a second gynaecologist who was blinded to VIA results performed colposcopy with biopsy in all abnormal areas. All women in whom no lesion was seen colposcopically had a biopsy from each of the four quadrants with an EC in order to estimate the performance of colposcopy in a screening setting. The sensitivity and specificity of colposcopy and directed biopsy for high-grade CIN or cancer were 81% and 77% in comparison with the combined histological findings from the directed four-quadrant and EC specimens (37.4% and 5.5% respectively).

In a study undertaken by Schneider *et al.* (2000) in Germany, 4700 women between 18 and 70 years of age were screened by conventional cytology obtained under colposcopic vision with associated HPV DNA testing. Endocervical curettage and biopsy were done where appropriate. The sensitivity and specificity of screening colposcopy for the detection of CIN2 or worse, which was also corrected for verification bias, were only 13.3% and 99.3% respectively.

Five other studies of a simultaneous use of colposcopy and cytology to detect cervical cancer performed over 30 years showed that the combined sensitivity of the two methods for cervical cancer detection varied from 95% to 99.4% (Dexeus *et al.*, 1977).

Recently, Hillgarth and Menton (1996) used colposcopy and cytology for primary screening and showed that the sensitivity of colposcopy for the detection of CIN2 or more was nearly 91% based on directed biopsy.

A study in the US, based on only 196 women, who were screened opportunistically in a gynaecological practice, used the Bayes predictive value theory to estimate the sensitivity of screening colposcopy, cytology and the combination. This resulted in figures of 48%, 76% and 91%, respectively, for all three modalities and specificities of 100%, 96% and 96% respectively (Davison and Marty, 1994).

Validity of visual signs

Although signs of abnormal epithelium within the transformation zone have been defined for a number of years, there are very few studies quantifying the validity of such signs. Reid and Scalzi (1985) published a scoring system (Table 30.1) that quantified the degrees of difference within certain morphological parameters including reference to the colour of the cervical epithelia, blood vessels, structure and surface configuration of the atypical transformation zone epithelium and also staining. However, there have been few major studies that have incorporated any scoring system within colposcopic management regimes as Reid and Scalzi (1985) have done.

Carriero *et al.* (1990) performed a retrospective study on 134 women with biopsy-proven lesions, using the modified Reid index score (Table 30.1) (Reid and Scalzi, 1985). They showed it to be more accurate in predicting low-grade lesions than high-grade lesions; they used the 1976 international nomenclature for colposcopy classification.

A further prospective study by Shaw *et al.* (2003), looking at the predictive validity of the visual signs in 425 women with abnormal cytology, showed that, among the three morphological characteristics routinely evaluated within the abnormal transformation zone, i.e. borders, degree of acetowhitening and abnormal blood vessels, acetowhitening performed as well as when all three signs were combined.

Massad and Collins (2003), looking for the strength of correlation between colposcopic impressions and biopsy histology in a prospective study of 2000 women in Chicago, were able to show an association between histology and colposcopic impression that was highly significant, but agreement was poor (kappa, 0.20). They did not use standardised grading criteria in this study.

It would seem that the size of the lesion (assessed on the number of quadrants with positive cytology) affects the sensitivity of colposcopy for lesions more than CIN2 when lesion grade on referral cytology or histology is controlled. In a study by Pretorius *et al.* (2001), colposcopy had a sensitivity of 65% if the lesion involved only one quadrant of the transformation zone and 100% if more surface was involved.

Shafi *et al.* (1991) showed that, when they excised the entire transformation zone by loop electrosurgical excision procedure (LEEP), they were able to confirm an association between increasing lesion size and histological grade.

Barton *et al.* (1989), when studying cervicograms of women with abnormal cytology, concluded that the lesion size affected the sensitivity of the colposcopy. Pretorius *et al.* (2004) showed that colposcopically inapparent high-grade lesions remaining after a directed biopsy had been taken are evenly distributed among the four quadrants at 2, 4, 8 and 10 o'clock. This study has been referred to above.

Interestingly, when HIV-positive women with abnormal cytology were studied in respect of a colposcopically directed biopsy, it was apparent that the rate of underestimation among these women was substantially higher than in most studies where biopsy was shown to be less than perfect in respect of sensitivity (del Priore *et al.*, 1996).

Reproducibility of colposcopy

Problems have always existed in respect of observer agreement using colposcopy. Three expert colposcopists described in a study by Li *et al.* (2003) showed poor to good intraobserver and interobserver agreement at assessing two major characteristics, namely borders and colour of acetowhitening. They showed that, in respect of border characteristics, the range of interobserver kappa values was 0.13–0.41, with the intraobserver kappa being 0.26–0.58. In relation to the colour of acetowhitening, interobserver kappa range was from 0.21 to 0.47 and the intraobserver kappa from 0.34 to 0.75. There was excellent agreement as to the site of the lesion from where a biopsy should have been obtained (raw agreement 95.3%, 143–150).

Ferris and his group (2000) studied the interobserver agreement within pairs of colposcopists using both optical and video colposcopes and found that colposcopic impression agreement with histopathology, biopsy intent agreement and biopsy site agreement by quadrant were not significantly different despite the use of different colposcopes. Similar agreement was obtained when telecolposcopy was used by an expert colposcopist at a remote location and compared with the video colposcopy performed by an expert on site (Sellors *et al.*, 1990). The kappa value for colposcopic impression and histopathology agreement varied between 0.16 and 0.27; for the biopsy intent, kappa was 0.32.

Assuming that colposcopists use the same definitions, reproducibility of colposcopic assessment depends in part on colposcopists using similar thresholds for categorising findings as to normal versus abnormality and grade.

QUALITY CONTROL

Like other medical services, colposcopy services can be audited and compared with national standards, such as those established for the British National Health Service, for process and outcome (Luesley, 1996, 2004). Indicators recommended for periodic audit include: waiting time for colposcopy by grade of referral smear; adequacy of communication between primary and secondary level; provider level and frequency of procedures; agreement between colposcopy diagnosis, referral cytology and histology; treatment method by histological diagnosis; efficacy of treatment (e.g. whether histological evidence of CIN is present in $\geq$ 90% of women undergoing 'see and treat'); and follow-up rates at 1 year (Luesley, 1996, 2004).

Cervical imaging using colpophotography, video colpography and telecolposcopy has been studied in respect of their use in a quality control role. All methods give a true representation of what is seen at colposcopy and have been recommended for teaching and audit as well as for patient care (Sellors *et al.*, 1990; Etherington *et al.*, 1997; Milne *et al.*, 1999; Harper *et al.*, 2000; Li *et al.*, 2003). Harper *et al.* (2000) showed that a telecolposcopy network among providers that allows transmission and sharing of static colposcopic images for consultation and teaching purposes on a regular basis was technically feasible, acceptable to women and providers living in remote areas and gave good interobserver agreement among the on-site colposcopists and the off-site review colposcopists as to degree of abnormality (kappa = 0.684; 95% CI 0.544–0.825). Ferris *et al.* (2002) and Ferris and Litaker (2004) showed that network telecolposcopy using high-speed telecommunications lines and computer telecolposcopy using modems and telephone lines to transmit static images were superior to cervicography as measured by the number of confirmed CIN lesions detected and timeliness of results. On-site colposcopy had the highest sensitivity to detect CIN because of the stereoscopic vision, the ability to manipulate the cervix and view the acetowhite reaction as it occurs and the ability to resolve vascular and epithelial features. Compared with telecolposcopy, the ability to assess whether a colposcopic examination is satisfactory appears to be better with on-site colposcopy (Sellors *et al.*, 1990).

The ability to document colposcopic images and data using the latest digital photographic and documentation system allows not only recording and comparison of colposcopic findings with subsequent examinations but also the retention of data for audit, post-treatment follow-up procedure and comparison of data between units and quality control to be instigated.

POTENTIAL SIDE-EFFECTS OF COLPOSCOPY

The actual colposcopic examination is associated with some discomfort during the insertion of a vaginal speculum, and this can be increased if a punch biopsy is performed, especially if local anaesthetic is not used. Psychological morbidity has to be considered. It would seem that anxiety is elevated, especially prior to surgery and also at the immediate postoperative visit (Campion *et al.*, 1988; Jones *et al.*, 1996; Wilkinson *et al.*, 1990). The subject is covered in more detail in Chapter 23. Educational booklets and counselling are highly effective in reducing anxiety (Howard *et al.*, 2002; Rogstad, 2002; Ferris *et al.*, 2003).

HOW CAN COLPOSCOPY BE IMPROVED?

Mention has already been made of quality control aspects of the colposcopy programme. Likewise, adherence to guidelines laid down by various societies (Luesley, 1996, 2004; Redman *et al.*, 2004) can also lead to improvement in the service delivered. However, it would seem that teaching of colposcopy is also important, and this is discussed in Chapter 47. As well as this, a recently described dynamic spectral imaging system has been developed which may dramatically improve the accuracy of colposcopy.

Improved training and teaching

Many centres and countries have their own defined training programmes, but these vary enormously. To help to standardise the quality of colposcopy training, the European Federation for Colposcopy (EFC) has agreed with all 26 member countries 51 core components which form the basis of basic colposcopy (Table 30.3; Redman *et al.*, 2004).

A number of studies have been undertaken to improve the colposcopic diagnostic accuracy. Sideri *et al.* (2000), in an Italian prospective study, supervised 56 colposcopists in a structured slide course based on 470 cases over 2 days. The course was structured so that distinction of normal from abnormal colposcopy was examined in various classes. After the preliminary examination, review of the cases was undertaken with a teacher. The results were analysed, comparing results for

Table 30.3 Minimum standards of training for colposcopy.

A Preliminary/preparatory	27 Recognise high-grade precancerous cervical abnormality
1 Understand the development of cervical pre-cancer and cancer	28 Recognise features suggestive of invasion
2 Take a relevant history	29 Recognise and assess vaginal intraepithelial neoplasia
3 Correctly position patient	30 Recognise and assess vulval intraepithelial neoplasia
4 Insert a speculum and visualise the cervix	31 Be able to determine extent of abnormal epithelium
5 Perform a smear including with a cytobrush	32 Recognise acute inflammatory cervical changes
6 Perform bacteriological swabs	33 Recognise HPV infection
7 Perform samples for HPV sampling	34 Recognise condylomata acuminata
8 Practice complies with health and safety recommendations	35 Recognise condylomata plana
9 Understand National Cervical Screening guidelines	36 Recognise the changes associated with treatment

B Colposcopic examination	**E Practical procedures**
10 Use and adjust the colposcope	37 Recognise benign cervical polyps
11 Determine whether or not the TZ is visible	38 Administer local analgesia
12 Determine whether or not colposcopy is satisfactory	39 Determine where to take directed biopsies
13 Examine the TZ with saline and green filter	40 Perform a directed cervical biopsy
14 Examine the TZ using acetic acid	41 Perform a directed vaginal biopsy
15 Quantify and describe acetic acid changes	42 Perform a directed vulval biopsy
16 Use an endocervical speculum	43 Control bleeding from biopsy sites
17 Recognise abnormal vascular patterns	
18 Examine the cervix and the vaginal vault using iodine solution	**F Administration**
19 Examine the vagina using acetic acid	44 Document cervical findings satisfactorily
	45 Formulate and action appropriate management plans according to guidelines
C Normal colposcopic features	
20 Recognise original squamous epithelium	**G Communication**
21 Recognise columnar epithelium	46 Adequately answer patients' questions about abnormal smears and their management
22 Recognise metaplastic epithelium	47 Counsel patients prior to colposcopy
23 Recognise a congenital TZ	48 Obtain informed consent correctly
24 Recognise the effects of pregnancy	49 Counsel patients after colposcopy
25 Recognise the normal features of a postmenopausal cervix	50 Break bad news
	51 Communicate well with other health professionals
D Abnormal colposcopic features	
26 Recognise low-grade precancerous cervical abnormality	

HPV, human papillomavirus; TZ, transformation zone.

pre- and post-tests with a gold standard (teachers' classification) using case statistics. The overall kappa (concordance with the gold standard) for slide classification in the precourse tests was 0.52 but improved to 0.67 in the post-course test. Percentage of agreement with the gold standard improved from 73% to 85% in the negative smear category, from 64% to 71% in the low-grade atypical transformation zone analysis and from 68% to 81% in the high-grade atypical transformation zone grouping. The conclusion of this unpublished study was that teaching results in objective diagnostic improvement and that the recognition of the atypical transformation zone and grading is feasible in a reproducible fashion under standardised, well-controlled conditions (Sideri *et al.*, 2000).

A further study by Sideri *et al.* (2004) evaluated the inter-observer reliability of colposcopy and the prediction of final histology by examining the visibility of the squamocolumnar junction and the presence of and grading of the atypical transformation zone, and of any associated CIN detected. In this study, nine expert colposcopists examined and assessed 100 cervicograms. The results showed that the medium pairwise kappa and the group kappa values were excellent for atypical transformation zone detection; they were acceptable for the recognition of the squamocolumnar junction but poor in respect of the other variables. The detection of the atypical transformation zone had a sensitivity for CIN of 90.2% and a specificity of 48.6%; the correct colposcopic 'impression' of high-grade CIN had a sensitivity of 54.4% and a specificity of 88%. Sideri and his group concluded that some colposcopic predictions are reproducible between observers, but felt that the prediction of a histology could be integrated into an algorithm for the management of patients with an abnormal Pap smear. Chapter 47 discusses the subject of the training and accreditation of colposcopists in more detail.

Advances in imaging techniques

There are certain limitations to the employment of colposcopy, which is an essentially subjective observational technique.

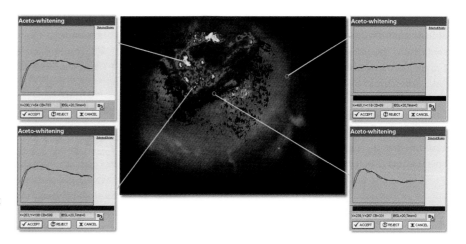

Fig. 30.13 Acetowhitening kinetic curve patterns (diffuse reflectance vs. time) corresponding to normal areas and low-grade lesions (upper and bottom right windows respectively) and to high-grade neoplasia (left windows). Diffuse reflectance vs. time curves are measured for every image pixel and quantitative parameters are calculated from each curve (CB), the values of which are displayed in the form of pseudocolours with blue–green representing low-grade lesion and red–yellow high-grade lesions (middle window).

It relies upon skilled and experienced personnel with adequate teaching and training necessarily. Recently, a new technique, albeit still experimental, has been developed with the aim of improving the accuracy of colposcopy. It depends on dynamic spectral imaging of the cervix (Mahadevan-Jansen *et al.*, 1998). In addition, other interesting methods relying on the assessment of the physical characteristics such as the electro-optical (Brown *et al.*, 2000) and the polarised light scattering properties of the tissue (Backman *et al.*, 1999) have been investigated. These new approaches rely on the fact that changes in tissue from normal to pathological alter both structure and function in ways that can be detected *in vivo*, by exploiting the light/tissue interaction phenomena. These provide a means for the *in vivo* identification and grading of the lesion. Other real-time devices with similar aims have been described in Chapter 27. Balas (2001) developed a new optical imaging technology named dynamic spectral imaging (DySIS) in an attempt to improve the diagnostic accuracy of colposcopy. It is said to provide both a higher resolution colour and spectral imaging of the cervix and, by employing this technology, it has enabled special optics to be developed that eliminate glare and enhance the visualisation of features of diagnostic importance, such as atypical vessels and acetowhitening. These features result in a substantial enhancement of the contrast between normal and abnormal areas, facilitating the *in vivo* detection of early-stage disease. Essentially, the acetowhitening of the tissues is calculated and displayed, and the spatial distribution of various parameters, previously determined, makes up the acetowhitening map of the lesion, which is visualised with the aid of a pseudocolour scale. The resultant pseudocolour kinetic map, as seen in Figure 30.13, can be overlaid onto the real-time displayed colour image of the tissue.

The technology is novel and still experimental, and long-term studies have not been forthcoming. However, it holds the potential for improving the accuracy of colposcopy.

CONCLUSION

Colposcopy is simply a means of examining the cervix and upper vagina with low-power magnification ($\times$ 6–40). In most countries, it is used to assess women who have been found to have abnormal cervical cytology while, in other countries, it is used as part of a routine gynaecological examination. In current times, its main use is in the assessment of abnormal cervical cytology, thereby allowing the colposcopist to identify and confirm the extent and characteristic of the abnormal (atypical) epithelium. Once the abnormality has been identified, then the possibility exists for its removal, which is usually quite simple using a diathermy loop. In other cases, particularly in young women with low-grade cytological abnormality, the colposcope will allow the colposcopist to identify the source of the low-grade cytological abnormality and will be able to recognise that, in many instances, the abnormality is due to 'nothing more' than immature squamous metaplasia, usually in association with human papillomavirus change; under these circumstances, the colposcopist will be able to advise as to whether conservative management without surgery is suitable.

The main purpose of colposcopy is to reduce deaths from cervical cancer by identifying premalignant disease detected during the cervical screening programme, either by cytology or by primary HPV DNA testing.

Quality of training is all important, and all colposcopists should be trained adequately. They should regularly audit their work to confirm that they are delivering a recognised high-quality standard of service and, finally, should be willing to undergo reaccreditation of their competence to practise colposcopy.

ACKNOWLEDGEMENTS

The authors wish to thank Dr J.W. Sellors of the Programme for Appropriate Technology in Health, Seattle, WA, USA, for his assistance in the preparation of this chapter. He allowed us access to data relating to a review of colposcopy that was presented to the IARC–WHO meeting of experts in Lyon, France, in April 2004. Some of these data are published and have appeared in the monograph resulting from that meeting (IARC, 2005).

The authors also wish to thank Professor C. Balas and Emmanuel Diakomanolis of Athens and Mr P. Soutter of London for their permission to describe the new dynamic spectral imaging technology.

REFERENCES

Anderson DJM, Strachan F, Parkin D (1992) Cone biopsy: has endocervical sampling a role? *British Journal of Obstetrics and Gynaecology* 99: 668.

Backman V, Gurjar R, Badizadegan K et al. (1999) Polarized light scattering spectroscopy for quantitative measurement of epithelial cellular structure in situ. *IEEE Journal of Selected Topics in Quantum Electronics* 5 (4): 1019–1025.

Balas C (2001) A novel optical imaging method for the early detection, quantitative grading and mapping of cancerous and precancerous lesions of the cervix. *IEEE Transactions on Biomedical Engineering* 48: 96–104.

Barton SE, Jenkins D, Hollingworth A et al. (1989) An explanation for the problem of false-negative cervical smears. *British Journal of Obstetrics and Gynaecology* 96: 482–485.

Belinson JL, Pretorius RG, Zhang W-H et al. (2001) Cervical cancer screening by simple visual inspection after acetic acid. *Obstetrics and Gynecology* 98: 441–444.

Brown B, Tidy J, Boston K et al. (2000) Relation between tissue structure and imposed electrical current flow in cervical neoplasia. *Lancet* 355: 892–895.

Campion MJ, Brown JR, McCance DJ et al. (1988) Psychosexual trauma of an abnormal cervical smear. *British Journal of Obstetrics and Gynaecology* 95 (2): 175–181.

Carriero C, Di Gesu A, Conte R et al. (1990) Grading colposcopic appearance: paired comparison between two methods for differentiating benign papillomaviral infection from high-grade dysplasia of the uterine cervix. *International Journal of Gynecology and Obstetrics* 34: 139–144.

Cuzick J, Szarewski A, Cubie H et al. (2003) Management of women who test positive for high risk types of human papilloma virus; The Hart Study. *Lancet* 362: 1871–1876.

Davison JM, Marty JJ (1994) Detecting premalignant cervical lesions. Contribution of screening colposcopy to cytology. *Journal of Reproductive Medicine* 39: 388–392.

del Priore G, Gilmore PR, Maag T et al. (1996) Colposcopic biopsies versus loop electrosurgical excision procedure cone histology in human immunodeficiency virus-positive women. *Journal of Reproductive Medicine* 41: 653–657.

Dexeus S, Carrera JM, Coupez F (1977) *Colposcopy*. Philadelphia: W.B. Saunders Co.

Dexeus S, Cararach M, Dexeus D (2002) The role of colposcopy in modern gynecology. *European Journal of Gynaecological Oncology* 23: 269–277.

Etherington IJ, Dunn J, Shafi MI et al. (1997) Video colpography: a new technique for secondary cervical screening. *British Journal of Obstetrics and Gynaecology* 104: 150–153.

Ferris DG, Litaker MS (2004) Colposcopy quality control by remote review of digitalised colposcopic images *American Journal of Obstetrics and Gynecology* 191: 1934–1941.

Ferris DG, Ho TH, Guijon F et al. (2000) A comparison of colposcopy using optical and video colposcopes. *Journal of Lower Genital Tract Disease* 4: 65–71.

Ferris DG, Macfee MS, Miller JA et al. (2002) The efficacy of telecolposcopy compared with traditional colposcopy. *Obstetrics and Gynecology* 99: 248–254.

Ferris DG, Litaker MS, Macfee MS et al. (2003) Remote diagnosis of cervical neoplasia: 2 types of telecolposcopy compared with cervicography. *Journal of Family Practice* 52: 298–304.

Ferris DG, Litaker MS and the ALTS Group (2006) Prediction of cervical histological results using an abbreviated Reid Colposcopic Index during ALTS. *American Journal of Obstetrics and Gynecology* 194: 704–710.

Fine BA, Feinstein GL, Sabella V (1998) The pre- and postoperative value of endocervical curettage in the detection of cervical intraepithelial neoplasia and invasive cervical cancer. *Gynecologic Oncology* 71: 48–49.

Harper DM, Moncur MM, Harper WH et al. (2000) The technical performance and clinical feasibility of telecolposcopy. *Journal of Family Practice* 49: 623–627.

Hilgarth M, Menton M (1996) The colposcopic screening. *European Journal of Obstetrics and Gynecology* 65: 65–69.

Hinselmann H (1925) Verbesserung der Inspektionsmoglichkeit von Vulva, Vagina and Portio. *Münchner Medizinische Wochenschrift* 77: 1733.

Howard M, Sellors J, Lytwyn A (2002) Cervical intraepithelial neoplasia in women presenting with external genital warts. *Journal of the American Medical Association* 166 (5): 598–599.

IARC (2005) *Cervix Cancer Screening*. Lyon: IARC Press.

Jones MH, Singer A, Jenkins D (1996) The mildly abnormal cervical smears: patient anxiety and choice of management associated with colposcopic examination. *Journal of the Royal Society of Medicine* 89 (5): 257–260.

Jordan JA (1985) Colposcopy in the diagnosis of cervical cancer and precancer. *Clinics in Obstetrics and Gynecology* 12: 67–76.

Kierkegaard O, Byrjalsen C, Hansen KC et al. (1995) Association between colposcopic findings and histology in cervical lesions: the significance of the size of the lesion. *Gynecologic Oncology* 57: 66–71.

Koller O (1963) *The Vascular Patterns of the Uterine Cervix*. Oslo: Universitets Forlaget.

Kolstad P (1970) Diagnosis and management of precancerous lesions of the cervix uteri. *International Journal of Obstetrics and Gynaecology* 8: 551–560.

Kolstad P, Stafl A (1972) *Atlas of Colposcopy*. Oslo: Universitets Forlaget.

Krebs HB, Wheelock JB, Hurt WG (1987) Positive endocervical curettage in patients with satisfactory and unsatisfactory colposcopy: clinical implications. *Obstetrics and Gynecology* 69: 601–605.

Li J, Rousseau M-C, Franco EL et al. (2003) Is colposcopy warranted in women with external anogenital warts? *American Society for Colposcopy and Cervical Pathology Journal of Lower Genital Tract Disease* 7: 22–28.

Lopez A, Pierson S, Moi R et al. (1989) Is it time for a reconsideration of the criteria for a cone biopsy? *British Journal of Obstetrics and Gynaecology* 96: 1345.

Luesley D (1996) *Standards and Quality in Colposcopy.* Sheffield: NHS Cervical Screening Programme (NHSCSP) publication no. 2, January 1996.

Luesley D (2004) *Standards and Quality in Colposcopy.* Sheffield: NHS Cervical Screening Programme (NHSCSP) publication no. 3, April 2004.

Maclean A (2003) The use of acetic action in the diagnosis of cervical neoplasia. In: Maclean A, Singer A, Critchley H (eds) *Lower Genital Tract Neoplasia.* London: RCOG Press, pp. 146–154.

Maddox P, Szarewski A, Dyson J *et al.* (1994) Cytokeratin expression and acetowhite change in cervical epithelium. *Journal of Clinical Pathology* 47 (1): 15–17.

Mahdevan-Jansen A, Mitchell MF, Ramanujam N *et al.* (1998) Near infrared Raman spectroscopy for *in vitro* detection of cervical precancers. *Photochemistry and Photobiology* 68 (1): 123–132.

Massad LS, Collins YC (2003) Strength of correlations between colposcopic impression and biopsy histology. *Gynecologic Oncology* 89: 424–428.

Milne DA, Wadehra V, Mennim D *et al.* (1999) A prospective follow up study of women with colposcopically unconfirmed positive cervical smears. *British Journal of Obstetrics and Gynaecology* 106: 38–41.

Mitchell MF, Schottenfeld D, Tortolero-Luna G *et al.* (1998) Colposcopy for the diagnosis of squamous intraepithelial lesions: a meta-analysis. *Obstetrics and Gynecology* 91: 626–631.

Olaniyan OB (2002) Validity of colposcopy in the diagnosis of early cervical neoplasia — a review. *American Journal of Reproductive Health* 6: 59–69.

Patch K, Shingleton H, Orr J *et al.* (1985) The role of endocervical curettage in colposcopy. *Obstetrics and Gynecology* 63: 403.

Prendiville W (2003) Treatment of grade 3 cervical intraepithelial neoplasia. In: Prendiville W (ed.) *Colposcopy Management Options.* London: W.B. Saunders, pp. 129–135.

Pretorius RG, Belinson JL, Zhang W-H *et al.* (2001) The colposcopic impression. Is it influenced by the colposcopist's knowledge of the findings on the referral Papanicolaou smear? *Journal of Reproductive Medicine* 46: 724–728.

Pretorius RG, Zhang W-H., Belinson JL *et al.* (2004) Colposcopically directed biopsy, random cervical biopsy, and endocervical curettage in the diagnosis of cervical intraepithelial neoplasia II or worse. *American Journal of Obstetrics and Gynecology* 191: 430–434.

Redman C, Dollery E, Jordan JA (2004) Development of the European Colposcopy Core Curriculum: use of the Delphi technique. *Journal of Obstetrics and Gynaecology* 24 (7): 780–784.

Reid R (1993) Biology and colposcopic features of human papillomavirus-associated cervical disease. *Obstetrics and Gynecology Clinics of North America* 20: 123–151.

Reid R, Scalzi P (1985) Genital warts and cervical cancer: an improved colposcopic index for differentiating benign papillomaviral infections from high-grade cervical intraepithelial neoplasia. *Obstetrics and Gynecology* 15: 611–618.

Rogstad KE (2002) The psychological impact of abnormal cytology and colposcopy. *British Journal of Obstetrics and Gynaecology* 109: 364–368.

Schneider A, Hoyer H, Lotz B *et al.* (2000) Screening for high-grade cervical intraepithelial neoplasia and cancer by testing for high-risk HPV, routine cytology or colposcopy. *International Journal of Cancer* 89: 529–534.

Sellors J (2005) Colposcopy. In: *IARC Handbooks of Cancer Prevention*, Vol. 10. *Cervical Cancer Screening.* Lyon: International Agency for Research on Cancer, IARC Press, pp. 89–90.

Sellors JW, Nieminen P, Vesterinen E *et al.* (1990) Observer variability in the scoring of colpophotographs. *Obstetrics and Gynecology* 76: 1006–1008.

Sesti F, Farne C, Mattei M *et al.* (1990) Role of endocervical curettage in the diagnostic workup of preinvasive cervical lesions. *International Journal of Gynaecology and Obstetrics* 31 (2): 153–156.

Shafi MI, Finn CB, Luesley DM *et al.* (1991) Lesion size and histology of the atypical transformation zone. *British Journal of Obstetrics and Gynaecology* 948: 490–492.

Shaw E, Sellors J, Kaczorowski J (2003) Prospective evaluation of colposcopic features in predicting cervical intraepithelial neoplasia. Degree of acetowhitening most important. *Journal of Lower Genital Tract Disease* 7: 6–10.

Sideri M, Pasquale D, Sassoli P *et al.* (2000) Teaching colposcopy: improvement of colposcopic diagnostic accuracy after a slide seminar course. CDS Regione Emilia Romagna, Cervical Cancer Screening Project. Milan: European Institute of Oncology. Presented orally at the 2000 ASCCP meeting, Orlando, FL.

Sideri M, Spolti N, Spinaci L *et al.* (2004) Interobserver variability of colposcopic interpretations and consistency with final histology. *Journal of Lower Female Genital Tract Disease* 8 (2): 212.

Singer A, Monaghan J (2000) Endocervical curettage. In: Singer A, Monaghan J (eds) *Lower Genital Tract Precancer*, 2nd edn. Oxford: Blackwell Publishing, p. 124.

Smedts F, Ramaekers FC, Vooijs GP (1993) The dynamics of keratin expression in malignant transformation of cervical epithelium: a review. *Obstetrics and Gynecology* 82 (3): 465.

Spirtos NM, Schlaerth JB, D'Ablaing G, III *et al.* (1987) A critical evaluation of the endocervical curettage. *Obstetrics and Gynecology* 70: 729–733.

Van Niekerk WA, Dunton CJ, Richart RM *et al.* (1998) Colposcopy, cervicography, speculoscopy and endoscopy. IAC Task Force Summary. *Acta Cytologica* 42: 33–49.

Walker P, Dexeus S, De Palo G *et al.* (2003) International terminology of colposcopy: an updated report from the International Federation for Cervical Pathology and Colposcopy. *Obstetrics and Gynecology* 101: 175–177.

Wilkinson C, Jones JM, McBride J (1990) Anxiety caused by abnormal result of cervical smear test: a controlled trial. *British Medical Journal* 300: 440–444.

FURTHER READING

Anderson M, Jordan JA, Sharpe F *et al.* (1996) *A Text and Atlas of Integrated Colposcopy.* London: Chapman & Hall Medical.

Luesley D, Shafi M, Jordan JA (2002) *Handbook of Colposcopy.* London: Arnold.

Singer A, Monaghan J (2000) *Lower Genital Tract Pre-cancer. Colposcopy, Pathology and Treatment.* Oxford: Blackwell Publishing.

Colposcopy and Programme Management: Guidelines for the NHS Cervical Screening Programme (NHSCSP) (www.cancerscreening.nhs.uk/cervical/publications/nhscsp20.html).

CHAPTER 31

The management of cervical intraepithelial neoplasia (squamous)

Mahmood I. Shafi, Joseph A. Jordan and Albert Singer

INTRODUCTION

The recognition of cervical intraepithelial neoplasia (CIN), being a preclinical condition, is based primarily on the detection of an abnormal cytological smear with secondary confirmation being obtained by histological examination of the cervical epithelium (see also Chapter 25). Recognition of an abnormal smear will not in itself achieve a reduction in risk or affect the incidence or the mortality rate of cervical cancer. It is, however, the recognition and subsequent treatment of the cytological abnormality that in turn will provide protection against the ultimate development of cervical cancer by the elimination of the high-grade precancerous epithelial changes of CIN2–3. It is well known and accepted that lesions histologically confirmed as CIN3 have an average likelihood of progression to cancer of 12–20%, while those with CIN2 changes have an average rate of progression to CIN3 of 22% (Ostor, 1993). However, estimates of the progression of premalignant lesions vary substantially as Mitchell *et al.* (1996) and Melnikow *et al.* (1998) have shown, but it is accepted that treatment is indicated for both CIN2 and CIN3 lesions.

RATIONALE FOR TREATMENT

Rationale for treatment (general)

Exfoliative cytology, as mentioned above, is the most common way of diagnosing the preinvasive and precancerous lesions of CIN, but other methods are also employed, and these include human papillomavirus (HPV) DNA testing, visual inspection with acetic acid (VIA), visual inspection with Lugol's iodine (VILI), screening with colposcopy and the new and still experimental methods based on real-time imaging (Chapter 27) and tumour markers (Chapters 28A and 28B).

Recent revision of the cytological classification criteria for cervical precancer, the so-called Bethesda 2001 system (Solomon *et al.*, 2002), has retained the classifications of LSIL and HSIL, referring to the low- and high-grade intraepithelial stages or lesions of these precursors, respectively, but has subdivided the lower degrees of abnormality, the so-called

atypical squamous cells (ASCs), into two categories, i.e. atypical squamous cells of undetermined significance (ASCUS) and atypical squamous cells that cannot exclude HSIL (ASC-H). It would seem that the classification of ASC-H was made because there is a recognition that a high risk of underlying high-grade disease is associated with these apparently minor cytological abnormalities.

In general, the rationale for treatment depends on women being referred with abnormal cytological findings. These women would normally then be seen for colposcopic evaluation as described in Chapter 30. The referral criteria vary from country to country. As part of the National Health Service Cervical Screening Programme in the United Kingdom, women having a high-grade smear on only one occasion are referred, whereas those with a low-grade smear are usually referred after two smears separated by 6 months; with ASCUS/borderline cellular changes, women are usually referred after two or even three such cytological abnormalities over an 18-month to 2-year period. However, recent changes in this referral system dictate that women with ASCUS/ borderline or similar low-grade smears are referred after one such diagnosis (Luesley and Leeson, 2004), thereby recognising the enormous emotional stress that women with even minor cytological abnormalities undergo. The psychological trauma associated with the findings of an abnormal smear have been considered in Chapter 23. During the colposcopic examination, a punch biopsy may be done to confirm the histological diagnosis or, as occasionally happens in some units, immediate treatment is instituted without prior histological confirmation of the disease, the so-called 'see and treat' approach.

Rationale for treatment (specific)

Low-grade lesions

The ASC classifications described above and defined as ASCUS and ASC-H are both associated with a relatively low risk of discovering underlying high-grade disease (5–17% in the former group, while the latter group has a much higher risk) (Wright *et al.*, 1995; Manos *et al.*, 1999; Solomon *et al.*, 2001). The ASCUS-LSIL triage trial (Stoler and Schiffman,

2001) confirmed that HPV DNA testing was also helpful in identifying and triaging those women with underlying high-grade disease in both groups. With a negative predictive value of HPV DNA testing of 98–99% (Chapter 28A), the immediate and virtual exclusion of the risk of any underlying high-grade disease being present in these women with negative results is achieved. In those with positive results, referral to colposcopy is encouraged, with the alternative being to employ similar viral testing with repeat cytology at 6- to 12-month intervals. Analysis by Wright *et al.* in 2002 indicated that all the diagnostic modalities involved in such management, which included cytology, HPV DNA analysis and colposcopy, were equivalent in respect of the satisfactory and safe management of women with atypical squamous cells.

When a histological confirmation of CIN1 is made, it would seem as though there are problems in respect of consistency of diagnosis. This being so, and in view of the morbidity associated with the therapy (Kyrgiou *et al.*, 2006) that will be discussed below, it is important to confirm findings of CIN1 before such therapy is instigated. Stoler and Schiffman (2001), in a triage study of low-grade disease biopsies that were originally classified as CIN1 in the ASCUS-LSIL triage study referred to above, when re-examining the biopsies initially classified as CIN1 were only able to find a repeat diagnosis of CIN1 in 43% of cases, with a downgrading of this condition in 45% of cases and in only 12% an upgrading to CIN2 and 3. Another problem has been the well-known finding of high-grade disease existing in women who present with minor cytological abnormalities such as mild dyskaryosis or LSIL (Massad *et al.*, 1996). Over 20 years ago, Singer *et al.* (1984) and, since then, others have confirmed that between 25% and 50% of women with low-grade smears will have underlying CIN2 to 3 (Walker *et al.*, 1986; Flannelly *et al.*, 1994; Massad *et al.*, 1996). Therefore, this means that women with low-grade disease need to be fully evaluated to discover those in whom there are underlying high-grade epithelial changes.

To confuse the matter further, it is well known that there is a regression of CIN1 in up to 60% with progression rates as low as 10% (Ostor, 1993; Melnikow *et al.*, 1998), and it is not clear whether these lesions (CIN1) should be treated or not. In two large British studies by Flanelly *et al.* (1994) and Shafi *et al.* (1997) in which women were monitored by cytological follow-up rather than the commonly employed practice of immediate excision when the colposcopist assumed that underlying high-grade intraepithelial disease (CIN2 or 3) existed, the findings indicated that it (regular cytological observation) was a safe procedure. Luesley *et al.* (1990) found that the rate of confirmed CIN2 to 3 in excised specimens from this group of women was low and, at the Bethesda Consensus Conference of Experts in 2001, Wright *et al.* (2003) recommended that women could be followed by regular cytological surveillance with no increased risk of severe preinvasive disease remaining undetected. With the introduction of HPV DNA testing with

its inherent high negative predictive value, i.e. 98–99%, it is possible to implant a certain amount of objectivity into the management algorithm (see Chapter 28A). When a finding of a high-risk HPV type is made, especially in a woman over 30 years of age, then referral for colposcopy would be recommended. Likewise, after two negative cytological tests over 1 year and a negative HPV DNA result, a confident return to routine 3-yearly screening can be recommended.

High-grade disease

There is universal agreement that women with a histological diagnosis of CIN3 have lesions that are most likely to persist or progress rather than regress. Review of the published medical literature, in respect of CIN2 and/or CIN3, as summarised by Ostor (1993), indicated that 43% of untreated CIN2 lesions will regress in the absence of treatment, whereas 35% will persist and 22% will progress to CIN3 (carcinoma *in situ*) or invasive cancer (Mitchell *et al.*, 1996). The study also found that 32% of CIN3 lesions regressed spontaneously, whereas 55% persisted and 14% progressed.

Trimble *et al.* (2005) have shown that, in a small observation study of CIN2/3 biopsy-proven lesions, 28% of them underwent regression. HPV 16 lesions were less likely to regress as well as non-HPV lesions with an HLA*A201 allele. This suggests that MHC class I immune responses are important in clearing CIN2/3 lesions. In the classical and historic but unethical study of Professor Green from New Zealand where women with CIN3 were left over many years, after a minimal biopsy, the risk of developing cervical cancer from untreated CIN3 was 36% over 20 years (McIndoe *et al.*, 1984; Jones, 2003). There have been no observational comparative trials that might reveal the exact risk of leaving untreated CIN3, but it is highly unlikely that such a study would receive ethical approval.

METHODS OF DIAGNOSIS

The role of biopsy

Diagnosis of CIN requires either a colposcopically directed or an excisional form of biopsy. The directed biopsy taken using as a guide the colposcopic characteristics of CIN enables sampling of the most abnormal area of the cervical transformation zone (TZ) wherein the potential preinvasive lesion may reside. The sampling of the whole cervical transformation zone area rather than of a limited area necessitates an excisional biopsy which, since the introduction of the electrodiathermy loop, has become a simple, rapid and direct method of sampling the transformation zone.

Colposcopically directed punch biopsy

To perform a directed colposcopic biopsy requires the colposcopist to identify the characteristics of the most abnormal

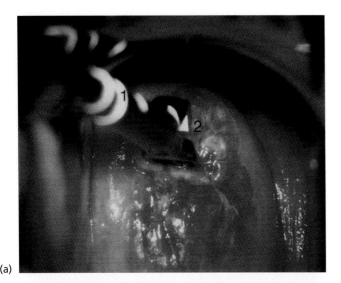

(a)

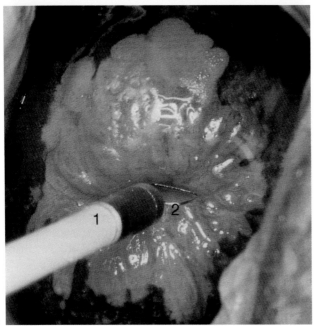

(b)

Fig. 31.1 (a) Eppendorfer forceps (1) with a rotating 25-cm shaft have been used to biopsy an area of abnormal (atypical) epithelium (2) on the anterior cervical lip. (b) A small diathermy loop biopsy device (1), developed by Dr René Cartier, is used to take a biopsy from minor-grade abnormal (atypical) epithelium at (2).

epithelial area of the transformation zone (Singer and Monaghan, 2000a) (Fig. 31.1). Colposcopic features suggestive of CIN are well defined and necessitate the recognition of different coloured surface changes and vascular patterns within the cervical epithelium. Examination also involves the recognition of the limits of the abnormal tissue within the transformation zone.

The colposcopist must appreciate the differences between high- and low-grade disease and must be able to exclude early invasive (microinvasive) disease. Colposcopy suffers from

being a subjective technique, as discussed in Chapter 30, which lacks a certain degree of sensitivity and specificity in respect of predicting the corresponding histological nature of the abnormal epithelium. It is more sensitive than cytology in the presence of high-grade lesions, but this is at the cost of reduced specificity (Kierkegaard *et al.*, 1995). This is primarily due to the fact that the immature stages of the common physiological squamous metaplastic process, and also of any associated virally induced changes, can easily be mistaken for CIN3. Furthermore, small lesions of a low-grade nature and those within the endocervix can be overlooked. The assessment of the surface of the lesion can also be used as a predictor of the histological grade of CIN (Shafi *et al.*, 1993). However, these factors are not independent of each other, and the final opinion of the examining colposcopist is usually highly influenced by knowledge of the referring cytology and the lesion's size; this has profound implications when managing the mildly abnormal smears when, for example, there is a tendency for the colposcopist to downgrade the severity of the underlying epithelial lesion. Etherington *et al.* (1997) undertook a study of pattern recognition using a selection of video clips of different case material and showed the poor correlation between the different grades of CIN predicted by trained colposcopists when CIN1 was present. The kappa score was 0.25, which rose to 0.35 if the cytology report was revealed prior to diagnostic opinion. Further studies have shown that recognition of microinvasive disease, a condition that should be obvious to an experienced colposcopist, also proved to be extremely difficult. Reiss *et al.* (1999) showed that colposcopy had a sensitivity of only 50% (CI 40.1–59.04) in recognising early invasive disease where the ultimate diagnosis was made at conisation or hysterectomy. Colposcopically directed punch biopsies also are associated with both over- and underdiagnosis with only a 54% concordance when compared with the eventual excisional biopsy specimens.

There is also a high intraobserver variability among colposcopists in the diagnosis of CIN (Buxton *et al.*, 1991). The positive predictive value is low when low-grade disease is compared with high-grade disease. More importantly, the histopathologist's ability to interpret correctly the diagnosis of the removed directed biopsy, especially those of a low-grade nature, is also limited. For instance, a false-positive rate when diagnosing viral (HPV) infection histologically is 75%, and the positive predictive value was 56% in the study by Robertson *et al.* (1989). Even when uniform and stringent histopathological criteria were applied to biopsy specimens, an overdiagnosis of HPV still occurred with a false-positive rate of 34%. Notwithstanding these problems of colposcopy, the directed biopsy using colposcopy still remains the major diagnostic tool, especially when examining women with minor cellular abnormalities. Assessment of a woman whose smear shows cellular abnormalities must include colposcopy, which will allow recognition of any abnormal features within the transformation zone.

Once visualised, the directed punch biopsy or biopsies are taken with the resultant diagnosis then considered in relation to the referral cytology and the colposcopic findings.

Excisional biopsies

The role of the excisional biopsy in enabling a diagnosis of the preinvasive lesion is linked to the role of this technique in the treatment of CIN. It will be discussed in this context below.

METHODS OF TREATMENT

The object of treating CIN must be that, whatever technique is employed, it is as efficient as possible in eradicating the lesion and also that it is associated with minimal morbidity to the patient. There are two broad sets of treatment methods available. These are firstly destruction or ablation of the abnormal transformation zone or secondly its excision. These two sets of treatment methods are listed in Table 31.1. Chemoprevention using retinoids in the management of CIN has been used in limited trials (Ruffin *et al.*, 2004; Abu *et al.*, 2005) with encouraging results and may have a role to play in the future. However, the two main modes of treatment as described above are the most commonly employed.

Destructive or ablative techniques

These techniques as listed in Table 31.1 were primarily developed in the 1970s and 1980s. Usually they can be performed under local anaesthesia in an outpatient setting. An inherent problem with these treatment methods is in the recognition of early invasive disease (microinvasion). Because of this concern, various criteria must be considered before any of these destructive techniques are involved. In examining the cervix through the colposcope:

1 the entire transformation zone must be fully visible;
2 there must be concurrence between cytology and histology;
3 there must be no cytological, colposcopic or histologically evident glandular disease or invasive cancer;

Table 31.1 Treatment methods.

Destructive
    CO_2 laser ablation (vaporisation)
    Cryocautery
    Radical electrodiathermy
    Cold (thermal) coagulation

Excisional
    CO_2 laser conisation
    Cone biopsy (various techniques)
    LLETZ
    Straight wire device
    Hysterectomy

4 there must be agreement between cytology and the histological diagnosis of the lesion (prior colposcopic directed biopsy);
5 there must be no previous treatment for CIN.

CO_2 laser vaporisation

This technique was extremely popular in the 1980s and 1990s because of the precision of control that the technique allowed (Fig. 31.2). However, the equipment was expensive. Treatment involves the destruction of tissue to a depth of 7 mm as it has been shown that, when CIN exists, it can involve gland crypts to at least a 4-mm level (Anderson and Hartley, 1980). By taking the treatment to 7 mm, this allows a suitable safety margin to be obtained. The technique is ideally suited for patients who are being treated using local anaesthesia in the outpatient department. Success rates are over 90% (Singer and Monaghan, 2000b).

Laser is an acronym for light amplification by stimulated emission of radiation. The laser converts energy such as heat, light or electricity into radiant energy at a specific wavelength. In gynaecological surgery, the carbon dioxide laser is most widely used, and this produces energy at a wavelength of 10.6 μm, which is the infrared portion of the spectrum and is invisible to the naked eye. In order to facilitate its use, the presence of the CO_2 laser beam is demonstrated by having a visible helium–neon (HeNe) laser focused on the same spot. Using mirrors and lenses, the laser energy is focused to a specific spot 0.2–2 mm diameter. The radiation is non-ionising, and its biological effect is primarily thermal as the laser beam energy is entirely absorbed by water or water-containing material; thus, it vaporises cervical tissue, which

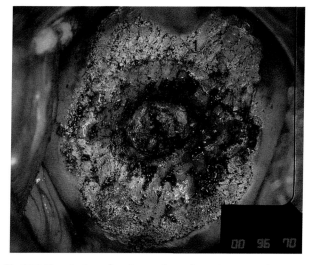

Fig. 31.2 Vaporisation of an abnormal transformation zone using the CO_2 laser. The central area of the transformation zone has been ablated to a depth of 10 mm and the more peripheral areas to a depth of 7 mm.

contains over 90% water. Tissue at the focal point of the laser is vaporised at the speed of light. The greater the absorptive capacity of the tissue, the greater the precision with which the beam may be used, minimising thermal damage to the surrounding tissue. The vaporised material (the plume) is a mixture of water vapour and carbon fragments. A micro-manipulator attached to the colposcope is used to manipulate the laser, and treatment is conducted under direct vision. As the technique is precise, it allows good control of the depth of destruction, good haemostasis and excellent healing, as there is minimal thermal damage to the adjacent tissue (Jordan *et al.*, 1985). If the destruction is adequate, cure rates are in the region of 94% of selected patients. Destruction has to be of the entire transformation zone and the deepest crypts that may harbour CIN (Monaghan, 1995). The technique is particularly useful for treating premalignant disease with vaginal involvement. As there are no gland crypts in the vaginal epithelium, destruction to 2–3 mm depth is adequate. The major disadvantage is the initial cost of equipment and the maintenance of these machines.

Cryotherapy

This technique, also developed in the early 1970s, relies on the ability to freeze the surface epithelium and stroma to a depth of about 3–4 mm (Fig. 31.3). Although initially popular, it tended to lose its appeal when a number of invasive cancers developed soon after treatment, most probably because of the shallow depth of destruction of the freezing process and because of poor patient selection. The technique has largely been replaced for the treatment of CIN by excisional techniques.

Cryocautery destroys tissues by freezing using probes of various shapes and sizes and was first described as a treatment for CIN by Crisp *et al.* in 1967. It is probably best reserved for small lesions and LSIL. The destruction of tissue relies on crystallisation of intracellular water. This crystallisation in the nucleus disrupts the cell membrane, causing cell death. While lesion size is important in determining success or failure using any of the treatment modalities (Shafi *et al.*, 1993), it is especially important when using cryocautery (Richart *et al.*, 1980). A double freeze–thaw–freeze technique is advocated to minimise failure rates (Creasman *et al.*, 1984; Schantz and Thormann, 1984). With larger lesions, multiple applications may be necessary. Cryoprobes are cheap and widely available. They can be used in the office setting without recourse to analgesia. The depth of destruction is approximately 4 mm, and this may be inadequate for some of the CIN lesions. Depth of destruction cannot be gauged accurately, and incomplete eradication of disease may lead to regenerating epithelium covering the residual disease. The type of probe and the anatomical clock position are two independent factors in relation to the cryolesion (Boonstra *et al.*, 1990). The largest cryolesions are obtained with large-cone probes, and there was a higher risk of undertreatment at the 3 and

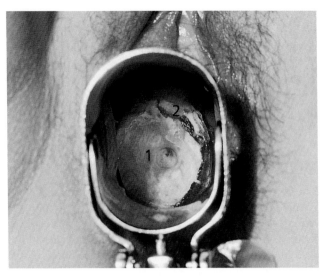

Fig. 31.3 The cervix after the application of cryotherapy using the freeze–thaw–freeze process (1). The peripheral 'iceball' of approximately 4 mm is seen (2).

9 o'clock positions on the cervix. This may be due to the profuse vascular supply at these positions. Certain parameters have been described (Benedet *et al.*, 1987) that are necessary to increase success rates in eradicating CIN:

1 minimal endocervical extension of the transformation zone;
2 fully visible lesion margins;
3 excellent probe–epithelium contact;
4 satisfactory iceball formation extending 3–4 mm beyond the lesion margins;
5 adequate cryotherapy gas pressure.

In view of the data, cryocautery is worthy of consideration as a cheap office procedure, especially for small lesions and LSIL. Healing after cryocautery is rapid, the endocervical canal is not compromised and fertility is unaffected (Ostergard, 1980; Cox, 1999).

Cold coagulation

This technique, like other ablative techniques, depends on the destruction of epithelium and stroma to a certain depth within the cervix. Although easy to use, it has never been widely employed. Its success rate, like electrodiathermy and CO_2 vaporisation, is above 90%.

Cold coagulation uses heat that is applied to tissue using a Teflon-coated thermosound. It was originally described as a treatment for benign cervical disease (Semm, 1966). The term was devised to distinguish it from electrocoagulation diathermy, which uses much higher temperatures and destroys tissue by burning. With 'cold coagulation', any temperature between 50 and 120°C can be selected. The thermosounds can easily be cleaned and sterilised at 140°C by simply pressing a button on the machine. The technique causes superficial epithelium to blister off, and the underlying stroma and glandular crypts are destroyed by desiccation. Depth of destruction varies according to the temperature selected and the time for which the thermosound is in contact with the tissue. Treatment areas are overlapped to ensure uniform coagulation. Following treatment, there is no need to place any restriction on sexual intercourse or the use of menstrual tampons. The procedure does not usually require analgesia. Some women may complain of pelvic cramp for the duration of the treatment. Operation of the apparatus is silent and does not produce charring at 100°C. The absence of smoke and smell make the procedure highly acceptable to both patient and doctor. Depth of destruction is approximately 2.5–4 mm or more after treatment at 100°C for 30 seconds and always exceeds 4 mm after treatment at 120°C for 30 seconds (De Cristofaro *et al.*, 1988). This technique has been used at the woman's first visit but with a policy of taking a directed biopsy at the same time for diagnostic purposes. However, extreme caution must be used if adopting a policy of see, biopsy and treat at the first visit and, ideally, the criteria to be met prior to ablative therapy, as described above, should be adhered to. In primary treatment for CIN3, the success rate was 95% at 1 year and 92% at 5 years (Gordon and Duncan, 1991). Repeat cold coagulation for residual or recurrent disease was less successful and is not advised. Fertility and the outcome for pregnancy are not adversely affected by treatment. Studies comparing cold coagulation and laser for the treatment of CIN2–3 showed no difference in success rates between either modality (Smart, 1987).

Electrodiathermy

This technique, popularised by Chanen *et al.* in the 1970s, required the use of general anaesthesia in most cases. The destructive current of the diathermy coagulation extended well past the 7-mm mark, and its high success rate, i.e. 97% in obliterating evidence of CIN, was due to this phenomenon (Chanen, 1989).

Electrodiathermy destroys tissue more effectively than cryocautery, but the patient is usually subjected to a general or regional anaesthetic or, in some units, the employment of just local anaesthesia. Under colposcopic control, it is possible to destroy up to 1-cm depth using a combination of needle and ball electrodes with eradication rates of 98.3% for patients with confirmed CIN (Chanen, 1989) (Fig. 31.4). The needle is inserted repeatedly to a depth of 10 mm at 1- to 2-mm intervals until the whole transformation zone has been covered. The ball achieves destruction of surface epithelium by a process of fulguration and coagulation. The apparatus is available in most operating theatres and is cheap and easy to maintain. There may be considerably more thermal necrosis than anticipated, leading to discharge and slough following therapy. While fibrosis is more common than with other forms of ablation, it was originally thought that this technique did not affect subsequent fertility or obstetric outcome (Hammond

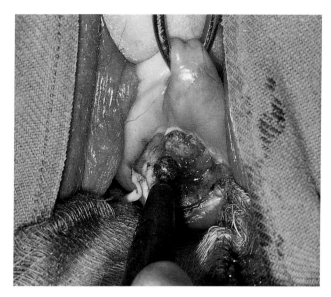

Fig. 31.4 A ball electrodiathermy device is being used to coagulate the abnormal (atypical) epithelium. Immediately prior to this the endocervix and part of the ectocervix have been destroyed by needle diathermy to a depth of at least 10 mm beyond the lateral extent of the lesion. Pressure must be maintained on the diathermy probe because mucus exudation will insulate the tissue from the heat.

and Edmonds, 1990). Data from recent studies show that there is a minimal rise in morbidity using this technique, with the risk for parameters such as premature delivery, low birth-weight, caesarean section delivery and perinatal mortality showing a relative risk below 1 with a corresponding low perinatal mortality (0.67) (Paraskevaidis *et al.*, 2005). An extension of this technique using a wire loop allows electrodiathermy to be used in an excisional mode.

All these ablative techniques can be employed for all grades of CIN. The principles of treating CIN1 do not vary from those applied to CIN3 with the whole of the transformation zone regarded as suspicious and therefore the target of treatment. The depth, however, in many of the techniques is difficult to judge, but all must produce destruction to at least 7 mm. Pretreatment biopsy is mandatory and the criteria listed above must be followed.

Excisional techniques

Surgical cone biopsy (various techniques)

Not only the CO_2 laser can be employed to undertake cone biopsy but also, traditionally, a cold knife. A wide and deep excisional defect is produced within the cervix that usually requires the insertion of a number of haemostatic sutures (Fig. 31.5). Alternatively, the defect can be left and just packed, or the base of the defect can be treated by diathermy or Monsel's solution so as to produce haemostasis. The technique is performed under general anaesthesia and is associated

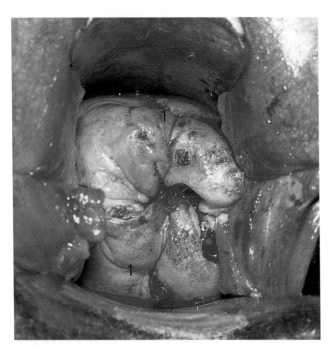

Fig. 31.5 The cervix has been fully reconstituted after the central portion has been removed by cone biopsy during the cone biopsy procedure. Sturmdorf sutures have been inserted, and both have been tied anteriorly at the 12 o'clock and 6 o'clock position (1).

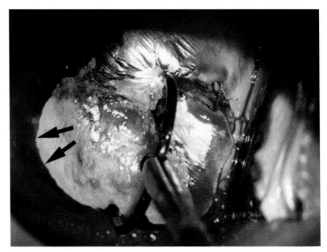

Fig. 31.6 An electrosurgical loop is seen progressing through the cervical tissue from right to left. The atypical (abnormal) transformation zone is clearly seen with its lateral margins arrowed. The loop has been laid over the area to be removed so as to encompass the lesion completely, slight pressure being put on it so that it adopts the curved attitude to the cervix. The cutting movement of the cutting direction can be either horizontally, as in this case, or in a vertical plane.

with well-described short- and long-term morbidity. Not only primary and secondary haemorrhage but fertility-related damage to the internal os with associated pelvic infection were not uncommon. Cervical stenosis may also be a consequence. The technique is popular in developing countries, and a success rate for effective treatment of CIN is again over 90% (Larson, 1983).

Hysterectomy

This technique would rarely be used in the primary treatment of CIN. It is reserved for those women who have had treatment and in whom there is still evidence of recurrent disease. It is also offered for those women who have associated gynaecological conditions that are symptomatic such as endometriosis, fibroids and uterovaginal prolapse. However, all these women must be assessed colposcopically before hysterectomy is undertaken. About 4% of women with preinvasive squamous epithelium may have it extending to the vaginal fornix, and so this area must be recognised colposcopically and removed as part of the hysterectomy procedure.

Electrosurgical excision of the transformation zone

Originally developed by a French gynaecologist, Renee Cartier, in the 1970s, it very quickly replaced ablative techniques. The technique was further popularised by Prendiville in Bristol in the mid-1980s, who developed the technique by using a larger and thinner wire loop than Cartier's original device and also by using an electrosurgical unit that produced a constant

low voltage with the ability to blend and combine both the cutting and the coagulation characteristics of the current. In the majority of cases it is performed under local anaesthesia and is now the most popular technique for the treatment of CIN in most western countries (Fig. 31.6).

The technique is relatively easy to undertake, but three basic principles need to be considered before use (Prendiville, 2003a). Firstly, it should be performed only after a comprehensive colposcopic examination by an experienced colposcopist. Secondly, its intention is to remove the entire transformation zone with an adequate margin of normal squamous epithelium surrounding the abnormal process. Thirdly, the amount of artefactual damage to the biopsy specimen to the cervix must be minimal. After the lesion has been removed, the base of the defect is coagulated (Fig. 31.7) and/or Monsel's solution applied.

Prendiville (2003b) has defined three types of excisional procedures in respect of the various morphological representations of the preinvasive lesion within the abnormal transformation zone. The recognition of these types of transformation zone is based on three indices, namely the size of the ectocervical component of the transformation zone, the position of the upper limit of the transformation zone and the visibility of the upper limit of the transformation zone. Prendiville hopes that this will enable a more rational approach to treatment to be made. These three types are as follows (Fig. 31.8 and Table 31.2):

1 when the lesion is completely ectocervical, fully visible and may be either small or large (type 1);

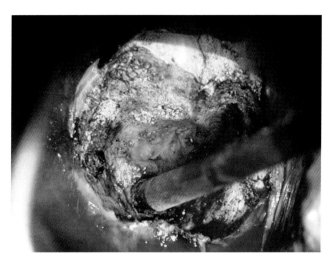

Fig. 31.7 A diathermy ball electrode is being passed across the base of the excised portion of the cervix following its removal as seen in Figure 31.6.

Transformation zone

Type 1
• Completely ectocervical
• Fully visible
• Small or large

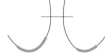

Type 2
• Has endocervical component
• Fully visible
• May have ectocervical component which may be small or large

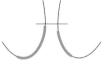

Type 3
• Has endocervical component
• Is not fully visible
• May have ectocervical component which may be small or large

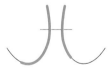

Fig. 31.8 Classifications of the transformation zone (after Prendiville, 2003b).

2 when the lesion has an endocervical component and is fully visible; there may be a small or large ectocervical component (type 2);

3 when the lesion is an entirely endocervical component and is not fully visible; there may be a small or large (type 3) ectocervical component.

The advantage of this classification is that the system is designed to be simple and acceptable to practising colposcopists as well as being able to accommodate every treatment circumstance that will arise in routine practice. It also enables the colposcopist to choose the type of diathermy loop that

Table 31.2 Transformation zone — geographical classification (after Prendiville, 2003b).

Type	Size	Site	Visibility
Type 1s	Small	Completely ectocervical	Fully visible
Type 1l	Large	Completely ectocervical	Fully visible
Type 2s	Small	Partially endocervical	Fully visible
Type 2l	Large	Partially endocervical	Fully visible
Type 3s	Small	Partially endocervical	Not fully visible
Type 3l	Large	Partially endocervical	Not fully visible

s, small; l, large.

Table 31.3 Choice of wire electrodes and alternative treatment according to the type of transformation zone (after Prendiville, 2003a).

TZ classification	LLETZ electrode choice	Alternative
Type 1s	20×15 mm loop	Any destructive treatment
Type 1l	Wider loop or a combination electrode treatment	Any destructive treatment
Type 2s Type 2l	20×20 mm or bigger loop or a straight wire or combination electrode treatment	Laser excision
Type 3s Type 3l	A longer loop or a straight wire or combination electrode treatment	Laser excision Cold knife long cone

TZ, transformation zone; s, small; l, large.

can be adapted for each one of the morphological types. For type 1, a 2×1.5 cm loop would be suitable with a 2×2 cm or bigger loop used for the type 2 cervix. A larger loop may be necessary for the type 3 (Prendiville, 2003b). In Table 31.3, various choices of wire electrodes and alternative treatments are listed according to the type of transformation zone.

In simple terms, it can be seen that, for a type 1 transformation zone, any choice of techniques is likely to be successful and associated with a low morbidity, whereas for a type 2 transformation zone, although it may be possible to use a less destructive method, an excisional technique is preferable. However, when dealing with a type 3 transformation zone, it is mandatory to use an excisional technique: type 3 also has a higher risk of incomplete excision, and it is in this circumstance that it is also wise to consider alternatives to the loop, such as the straight wire knife cone or CO_2 laser cone (Mor-Yosef *et al.*, 1990; Prendiville, 1993; Panoskaltsis *et al.*, 2004). The optimum method of performing excision of the transformation zone is still to be determined but that will be possible only with appropriately designed randomised controlled trials (RCTs). Prendiville (2003b) insists that, if the inclusion criteria of these studies contain only type 3 transformation zone and the exclusion criteria proscribe types 1 and 2, then it may be possible to discover the optimum method of management for these difficult and complex cases.

The electrosurgical use of a loop device has been modified by the introduction of a straight wire incisional device (Mor-Yosef *et al.*, 1990; Panoskaltsis *et al.*, 2004). This device is of value when treating the type 2 or type 3 cervix described above. There are yet to be any significant studies evaluating this technique.

Which technique to be employed for preinvasive lesions?

Even though a large number of RCTs have been performed comparing different treatments and techniques for CIN, there is no single method that has supplanted all the others on a universal level. All the techniques available enjoy relative popularity. A review examining 28 individual trials of various treatment alternatives for CIN has been published (Martin-Hirsch *et al.*, 2002). Data from studies and trials were extracted by two of the reviewers independently analysing seven different surgical treatment techniques. Not all the trials were purely randomised or controlled, with the main conclusion being that there was no significant difference in respect of success rates between the studies. However, the authors concluded that the LLETZ procedure (large loop excision of transformation zone) produced the least morbidity and the most favourable surgical specimen for histological analysis. When the ablative techniques were compared, there was no technique superior to any other, except that cryosurgery was less successful than CO_2 laser ablation for the treatment of high-grade CIN.

When differences between the excisional techniques were examined, there was no difference in the incidence of residual disease when the cone biopsy technique used either cold knife or the CO_2 laser. There was likewise no difference in haemorrhage rates between cold knife and CO_2 laser cones, although laser cones were associated with a higher rate of satisfactory colposcopy in the postoperative period. Likewise, with this latter technique, there was less cervical stenosis.

When the CO_2 laser cone was compared with the LLETZ in respect of residual disease, there was an odds ratio in favour of LLETZ of 1.22 (Prendiville, 2003c). However, the 95% confidence limit crossed unity and, as such, no inference could be drawn from the results. LLETZ was shown to be much quicker than the CO_2 laser cone and less painful, but there was no difference in secondary haemorrhage, nor was there any apparent difference in either cervical stenosis or the adequacy of the colposcopic examination at the follow-up between these two techniques.

When cold knife was compared with LLETZ therapy, there appeared to be a higher residual disease rate after LLETZ in these studies, but the difference was only just significant, and

the confidence limit reached did not cross unity. There was no difference, surprisingly, between the methods in terms of haemorrhage or cervical stenosis, but LLETZ was associated with a lower rate of unsatisfactory colposcopy at follow-up; again, the confidence intervals just passed zero.

In summary, when the differences between excisional technique and ablative technique were compared, it was found that there were very few comparative studies. When CO_2 laser ablation was compared with LLETZ, there were three studies in the Cochrane meta-analysis of Martin-Hirsch *et al.* (2002) and, in all of these studies, there was no difference in residual disease or in haemorrhage rates. Prendiville (2003c) has questioned the validity of some of the results emanating from the Martin-Hirsch *et al.* (2002) study. Although accepting that the meta-analysis showed that there was very little difference between the methods in terms of success and morbidity, he highlighted the difficulties in deriving evidence from pooled data from random or quasi-random trials. He made the point that nomenclature was a problem, with, for instance, the term cone biopsy not being universally agreed. Notwithstanding these comments, review of the literature outside the Martin-Hirsch *et al.* (2002) study shows that the technique of LLETZ would seem to be the ideal method for treating CIN.

Success rates in treatment

The efficacy of LLETZ as the most popular technique in the treatment of CIN has now been established in several short-term observational studies over the last 15 years. More recently, longer term studies in which LLETZ was employed have reported cure rates that compare favourably with the other excisional and even ablative techniques (Prendiville, 2003b). In Flannelly *et al.*'s (1997) study of 1000 women, 317 were followed up for over 4 years with the residual dyskaryosis rate being only 4.4% during the first 12 months. A further study by Flannelly's (2001) group showed that 346 women were followed up after LLETZ for a mean of 35 months; of 417 women, 12.2% had dyskaryosis at the same time during follow-up. Age and a histological report of incomplete incision were found to be independent risk factors for residual/recurrent disease. Flannelly *et al.* (2001) were able to categorise groups in respect of risk of recurrence. These groups were: women less than 50 years of age without margin involvement of the excised specimen, resulting in 92% of them having a normal smear at follow-up; women aged 50 years or over with margin involvement have a 57% chance of a normal smear; and women aged less than 50 years with margin involvement have an 86% chance of a normal smear.

Factors influencing cure rates — the role of incomplete excision

Dobbs *et al.* (2000) followed 394 women over 10 years for a mean of 73 months with an average of six smears and found,

Table 31.4 Incomplete excision in cone biopsy; involvement of margins.

Series and reference	Date	Margins (% endocervical)	Method	Disease	Patients (n)
Cullimore *et al.*	1992	15.6[a]	Cold knife	CIGN	51
Mathevet *et al.*	1994	14.0	Cold knife	CIN, microinvasion	37
Jansen *et al.*	1994	22.0[a]	Cold knife	CIN	316
Wolf *et al.*	1996	43.0[a]	Cold knife	CIGN, CIN	42
Guerra *et al.*	1996	5.4	Cold knife	CIN, microinvasion	73
Gurgel *et al.*	1997	46.6*	Cold knife	Microinvasion	163
Partington *et al.*	1998	18.0*	Laser	CIN	50
Mor-Yosef *et al.*	1990	20.0	Laser	—	550
Lopes *et al.*	1993	24.0	Laser	CIN, microinvasion	313
Mathevet *et al.*	1994	51.0[b]	Laser	CIN, microinvasion	37
Andersen *et al.*	1994	6.6	Laser	CIN, CIGN	473
Guerra *et al.*	1996	5.4	Laser	CIN, microinvasion	275
Mor-Yosef *et al.*	1990	10.0	Loop diathermy	CIN3, microinvasion	50
Byrne *et al.*	1991	22.0	LLETZ	CIN, invasion	50
Montz *et al.*	1993	48.0[b]	LLETZ	CIN	25
Naumann *et al.*	1994	25.8[b]	LLETZ	CIN, microinvasion	120
Mathevet *et al.*	1994	53.0[b]	LEEP	CIN	36
Felix *et al.*	1994	28.0	LEEP	CIN, microinvasion	57
Houghton *et al.*	1998	42.1[a]	LLETZ	CIGN	19

[a]Not defined margin; [b]thermal artefact; CIN, cervical intraepithelial neoplasia; LEEP, loop electrosurgical excision procedure; LLETZ, large loop excision of the transformation zone.
From Prendiville (2003c) with kind permission.

after examining the complete records of 343 patients, that only 4% had a proven histological recurrence. Two patients had invasive disease, but both were microinvasive (IA) and were treated by simple hysterectomy. In both cases, incomplete excision had been recognised at the time of the LLETZ. The role of incomplete excision in histological specimen has also been examined, with its not uncommon prevalence seen in Table 31.4. Prendiville (2003c) asserts that this does not equate with residual disease as cytological and colposcopic follow-up shows that many revert to normal even though there has been doubt about the complete excision assessed by histology. The failure rate for this technique in respect of recurrences within 12 months is between 3% and 6.9% (Table 31.5), notwithstanding the higher rate of incomplete removals as seen in the initial excised specimen. There are other important predictors of residual disease after LLETZ apart from histologically incomplete excision, and these, as Flannelly *et al.* (2001) showed, are in respect of patients' age and severity of the disease. However, in Dobbs *et al.*'s (2000) long-tem follow-up study of LLETZ-treated women, it was obvious that incomplete excision was an important factor in predicting residual disease. Theoretically, it should be possible to excise the entire transformation zone completely by simply using a bigger loop, although this would be at an increased risk of morbidity. In Table 31.4, the reported published

Table 31.5 Failure rates (recurrence within 1 year).

Reference and year	No. of patients	Rate of residual disease (%)
Prendiville *et al.* (1989)	102	3.0
Murdoch *et al.* (1992)	721	4.6
Bigrigg *et al.* (1994)	1000	5.0
Gardell *et al.* (1997)	225	8.5
Flannelly *et al.* (1997)	1000	8.0
Baldouf *et al.* (1998)	288	6.9
Paraskevaides *et al.* (2000)	635	4.9
Dobbs *et al.* (2000)	322	4.3
Narducci *et al.* (2000)	505	3.7

From Prendiville (2003b), with kind permission.

rates for incomplete excision in cone biopsies range between 5% and 51% for all methods of excision, and the reasons for these figures would tend to be multifaceted. It is likely that performing excision of the transformation zone using inappropriately sized electrodes is a major cause of incomplete removal. Reference to the new specification of transformation zone excision, as listed by Prendiville (2003c), may assist colposcopists in obtaining more satisfactory clearance of the transformation zone. Development of a straight wire device

Table 31.6 Findings of unexpected microinvasion or invasion.

Series	Unexpected invasion	Cytology or punch biopsy findings (when known)
Prendiville *et al.* (1989)	1/102 (1%)	CIN3
Bigrigg *et al.* (1990)	5/1000 (0.5%)	CIN1–2, CIN2–3
Gunaskera *et al.* (1990)	1/91 (1%)	CIN3
Luesley *et al.* (1990)	4/616 (0.6%)	—
Whiteley and Olah (1990)	0/9 (0%)	—
Murdoch *et al.* (1991)	11/1143 (1%)	—
Hallam *et al.* (1991)	8/1000 (0.8%)	—
Wright *et al.* (1991)	1/157 (9.6%)	CIN2

From Prendiville (2003b), with kind permission.

may also help (Mor-Yosef *et al.*, 1990; Prendiville, 2003c; Panoskaltsis *et al.*, 2004).

If CIN has been identified in the margins of the diagnostic excisional biopsy or in the immediate post-treatment endocervical sampling, it is recommended that the 4- to 6-month follow-up include a colposcopic examination with a further endocervical sample. If CIN2–3 is identified at the endocervical margins or in the endocervical sampling at follow-up, then an excisional procedure must be performed. Hysterectomy can be considered acceptable for treatment of recurrent or persistent biopsy-proven CIN2–3 (Wright *et al.*, 2003).

Factors influencing cure rates — the role of undiagnosed microinvasive carcinoma

In line with the incomplete excision margin involvement is the risk of finding undiagnosed microinvasive carcinoma. This can be seen from Table 31.6 for, in every study listed in respect of incomplete excision, there is a high proportion where microinvasion is found unexpectedly with rates ranging from 0.6% to 1%. It could be argued that this is one of the advantages of an excisional technique over an ablative method. However, most undiagnosed microinvasions were of a very early nature (early stromal invasion) and found in women treated by local ablation and excisional techniques. The ablation group have unwittingly been treated resulting in a cure in most cases. Unexpected invasive cancer is also revealed in LLETZ procedures in 1–5% of cases (Prendiville, 2003c).

MANAGEMENT OF DIFFERENT CIN LESIONS

Which treatment should be employed for low-grade (LSIL/CIN1) lesions?

In the section dealing with techniques, it has already been mentioned that there was no discernible difference in cure rates for CIN between either ablative or excisional techniques.

The Consensus Grouping of Experts gathered in Bethesda in 2001 and reported by Wright *et al.* (2003) concluded that 'if treatment is selected, the choice of treatment should be determined by the judgement of the clinician and should be guided by experience, resources and clinical value for the specific patient'.

Women in the uncommon situation of having an unsatisfactory colposcopic examination in which CIN1 has been diagnosed are advised to have an excision procedure. However, exceptions can also be made where the woman is pregnant, immunosuppressed or when an adolescent is seen by a colposcopist with limited experience. An endocervical curettage or endocervical cytology sample is also recommended in such procedures in association with unsatisfactory colposcopy. However, the use of endocervical curettage when colposcopy is satisfactory is not considered necessary by most European authors (Singer and Monaghan, 2000a).

Which treatment for high-grade (HSIL/CIN2–3) lesions?

There is general agreement that either ablation or excision of CIN2–3 will reduce the incidence of mortality caused by invasive cancer in women with these lesions. To be effective, the treatment must remove the entire transformation zone rather than selectively targeting colposcopically identified lesions. As already discussed, in clinical trials comparing different treatment modalities significant differences in cure rates are generally not found (Prendiville, 2003c). However, as also mentioned above, the excisional procedures allow pathological assessment of the excised tissue and also the detection of microinvasion or occult invasive cancer that has inadvertently been treated as a preinvasive lesion (Table 31.6). It would seem that the excisional procedures would be favoured if there is a risk of microinvasive or occult invasive cancers in those women who colposcopically have a large-volume lesion, i.e. existing in three out of four quadrants of the transformation zone (Tidbury and Singer, 1992; Wright *et al.*, 1992; Andersen *et al.*, 1995; Singer and Monaghan, 2000a).

Women in whom the colposcopic examination is unsatisfactory in the presence of high-grade epithelial disease have a significant risk of having underlying microinvasive or occult invasive lesions. Diagnostic (excisional) conisation procedures must be employed. There is no place for destructive therapy. The 2001 consensus document (Wright *et al.*, 2003) recommends that, where CIN2–3 has been discovered on biopsy, then the choice of treatment technique depends purely on whether the colposcopy is satisfactory or unsatisfactory. If the upper limit of the transformation zone cannot be seen and the colposcopy is deemed to be unsatisfactory, then an excisional procedure is performed; if there is satisfactory colposcopy, then an ablative or excisional procedure can be undertaken except, as mentioned above, where a large-volume lesion exists and there is an increased risk of underlying early cancer.

'See and treat' protocol

This philosophy dictates that a patient can be seen and treated at the initial visit. If the cytological suspicion of high-grade disease is present, then many authors (Luesley *et al.*, 1990; Prendiville, 2003a) have advocated that women be treated at the first visit. In Luesley's (1990) study, all women with an abnormal smear of all grades were treated, with an increased number of negative histological specimens being found. Prendiville (2003c) has been more selective and has shown that, over a 7-year period, by using a 'selective see and treat' policy, the rate of normal histology has remained consistently low; concerns that the 'see and treat' policy would inevitably lead to overtreatment in a high proportion of women have not been confirmed in his analysis. It would seem that there are four groups of women who would benefit from a 'see and treat' policy. They are:

1 women in whom the smear report indicates high-grade disease in the presence of a colposcopically visible transformation zone indicating high-grade disease;

2 women in whom colposcopically directed biopsy taken elsewhere supports cytological and colposcopic suspicion of CIN3;

3 women in whom a biopsy a reveals a lesser grade of abnormality but in whom an experienced colposcopist diagnoses high-grade disease;

4 women in whom colposcopic impressions are those of early invasive disease, i.e. large-volume lesion.

MORBIDITY ASSOCIATED WITH THE TREATMENT METHODS

Every treatment technique is associated with immediate complications and long-term morbidity. The former subject has been dealt with above with a review of the individual techniques employed. However, long-term morbidity has been assessed, but all techniques have, in the past, been shown to have very little long-term effect on the woman. Indeed, Murdoch *et al.* (1991) quoted morbidity for excisional procedures of 2–4% with immediate discomfort and bleeding or subsequent cervical stenosis leading to dysmenorrhoea. Bigrigg *et al.* (1991, 1994), in a study of 1000 women, found that, in 250 in whom a LLETZ procedure had been performed, details of the subsequent menstrual and fertility problems were assessed using a questionnaire protocol. No differences between them and a matched control group, who had a negative smear, were found, and LLETZ, from that study, would seem to have no effect on menstruation and fertility. It has been known for a number of years that there is an increased risk of obstetric complications following cervical conisation

(Jones, 1979; Kristensen, 1993; El-Bastawissi, 1999; Sadler *et al.*, 2004; Samson *et al.*, 2005). Also, studies have shown that a cone length of more than 2 cm is associated with low birthweight and second-trimester pregnancy loss (Leiman, 1980) and a cone biopsy greater than 1 cm in depth has been reported to be an independent risk factor for preterm delivery (Raio *et al.*, 1997). Recently Klaritsch *et al.* (2005) have again examined the risk for preterm delivery and maternal complications after cold knife conisation. They showed that cold knife conisation is associated with a higher risk of preterm delivery, premature rupture of membranes, low birthweight and cervical tears.

Crane *et al.* (2006) recently observed that pregnant women who had an excisional procedure previously had a shortened cervix which could be diagnosed by ultrasonography between 24 and 30 weeks. They had an increased risk of preterm labour, which was associated with an odds ratio of 3.45 (95% CI 1.28–10.0). For previous loop excisional procedures or for prior cold-knife conisation, the risk was 2.63 (95% CI 1.28–5.56). Highly significant differences existed between them and a matched control group.

However, a recent unpublished study from the Cochrane Gynaecological Cancer Collaborative Review Group (Kyrgiou *et al.*, 2006) casts serious doubt on the previously held notion that the less traumatic techniques of excision and ablation are associated with minimal morbidity. Using MedLine and other retrieval systems and looking at only case–control studies between 1960 and 2005 of women with CIN who were treated by local ablation, laser cone biopsy and LLETZ, the authors found disturbing outcomes in respect of maternal and neonatal morbidity. In their meta-analysis, they looked at duration of pregnancy in weeks, modes of delivery, the duration of labour and the premature rupture of membranes. Considering the neonatal aspects, they reviewed birthweight, neonatal intensive care unit admissions and perinatal mortality.

They found, in considering cold knife conisation, that there was a relative risk (RR) of 2.59 [1.00, 3.72] for preterm delivery; for low birthweight under 2500 g, the RR was 2.53 [1.19, 5.36]; for caesarean section, there was a RR of 3.17 [1.07, 9.40]; and for the important factor of perinatal mortality, the RR was 1.89 [0.77, 4.65].

When considering CO_2 laser conisation, not too dissimilar findings appeared for, when premature delivery under 37 weeks was calculated, the RR was 1.97 [0.05, 4.07]; for low birthweight, the RR was 2.17 [1.05, 4.48]; for caesarean section 1.30 [0.55, 3.07]; for premature rupture of membranes, the RR was 2.18 [0.77, 6.16] and for perinatal mortality, it was 8.00 [0.91, 70.14].

The results for the most popular excisional technique of LLETZ were not much better and showed for premature delivery under 37 weeks a RR of 1.70 [1.24, 2.35]; for low birthweight, the RR was 1.82 [1.09, 3.06]; and for premature rupture of membranes, the RR was 2.769 [1.62, 4.46]. The caesarean section rate, surprisingly, was below 1 at 0.88 [0.71, 1.09]. However, for premature labour, perinatal mortality and neonatal unit admissions, the rates were all above 1, with premature labour having a RR of 1.26 [0.75, 2.11], for perinatal mortality a very serious rise at 3.40 [0.62, 18.63] and, finally, for neonatal unit admissions 1.25 [0.93, 1.67] in respect of the relative risk.

Local ablation, by carbon dioxide laser vaporisation, cryosurgery or diathermy, was associated with only a minimal rise in morbidity, and that was seen in relation to premature rupture of membranes where the RR was 1.23 [0.56, 2.70]. For the other parameters of premature delivery, low birthweight, caesarean section delivery and perinatal mortality, the RR was below 1, and for the most important, perinatal mortality, it was only 0.67 [0.11, 3.96].

These very detailed results, summarising the literature for over four decades, clearly show that excisional procedures, be they in the form of cold knife cone biopsy or cone biopsy by CO$_2$ laser or the now common diathermy LLETZ excisional procedures, are associated with a significant increase in morbidity for the woman and her infant. These results will obviously have significant effects on the management of premalignant cervical disease. It may be necessary to review indications for treatment of minor lesions, i.e. LSIL/CIN1 (and even possibly for HSIL/CIN2 lesions in very young women where the risk of invasive cancer is extremely low), but where the resultant morbidity of the procedure is now recognised to be significant.

FOLLOW-UP AFTER TREATMENT OF CIN

The risk of recurrence of CIN is well recognised, and it is well appreciated that invasive cancer rarely follows ablative or excisional treatment. Table 31.5 clearly shows the failure rate following loop excision at the end of 1 year. Follow-up of women who have had treatment for CIN2–3 dictates the use of cervical cytology and possibly colposcopy at 4- to 6-month intervals until at least three cytological results negative for squamous intraepithelial lesions or malignancy are obtained (Wright *et al.*, 2003). Annual cytological follow-up after that is recommended in the consensus document. During the follow-up period, the recommended threshold for referral to colposcopy is the result of ASC (atypical squamous cells) or greater. The HPV DNA testing at least 6 months after treatment is acceptable and with the high negative predictive value, i.e. 99%, the finding of a negative HPV DNA result would indicate that the patient could be absolved of rigorous annual follow-ups and be converted to a 3-yearly follow-up (Crum and Berkowitz, 2002) (see Chapter 28A).

It is usual at the first postoperative visit to use colposcopy to evaluate the healing process that has gone on in the cervix after the technique and to determine the mode of follow-up. In a small number of women there is significant cervical con-

striction and, for these women, an endocervical brush for smear testing is recommended. Very rarely, complete stenosis ensues, in which case the consequences of endometriosis and of severe dysmenorrhoea must be recognised immediately. The efficacy of postoperative surveillance using the smear will certainly be determined by the structure of the cervix and the techniques employed in the collection of specimens.

The use of an adjunctive technique to cytology in the follow-up of women having undergone treatment for CIN has recently involved the employment of HPV DNA. As already mentioned, the high negative predictive value of this technique makes it invaluable in excluding the presence of residual neoplastic tissue. Zielinski *et al.* (2004) monitored women after treatment of CIN3 using HPV DNA testing in association with cytology and showed that there was an increased sensitivity to detecting persistent or recurrent CIN. The combination proved more effective than using cytology or HPV DNA testing alone, and it was concluded that women treated for CIN3 should have the combined test after 6 months. If it was positive on either one of these two tests, then colposcopy and close surveillance was indicated, but women with a double negative test, i.e. cytology and HPV DNA both negative, could be safely seen at 24 months and, if negative at that stage, could be referred back to routine screening. The Zielinski *et al.* (2004) review examined 20 studies published between 1996 and 2003, and 11 of these were used in the meta-analysis.

Paraskevaidis *et al.* (2004) have also produced two systematic reviews of the follow-up after treatment for CIN2 and 3 and, within these reviews, there was a meta-analysis of data from the relevant literature. Their findings were similar to those of Zielinski *et al.* (2004). They reviewed the studies of post-treatment follow-up using both HPV DNA and cytology. Twelve studies were examined, of which 10 were prospective and two were case–control. Their conclusions were that HPV DNA testing after treatment predicted residual or recurrent CIN with higher sensitivity than cytology or histological assessment of the resection margins of the removed specimen. They also showed that the specificity of HPV DNA did not differ significantly from the other methods, but the caveat was that these studies were very heterogeneous in composition and the methods of timing of the follow-up visits varied. They also stressed that a positive HPV test, even in the presence of a normal cytological result, could indicate treatment failures more quickly and accurately. For the future, they recommended that the role of HPV typing and viral load should be examined further.

ACKNOWLEDGEMENTS

Figures 31.1 to 31.7 are from Singer A. and Monaghan J.M., *Lower Genital Tract Precancer: Colposcopy, Pathology and Treatment*, 2nd edition, Blackwell Publishing, Oxford, 2000. The authors wish to thank Professor W. Prendiville of Dublin for his kind permission to reproduce Figure 31.8 and Tables 31.1 to 31.6 as they appear in the text.

FURTHER READING

Following its sixth congress in Paris in April 2006, the European Research Organization on Genital Infection and Neoplasia (EUROGIN) issued an expert consensus report entitled *Innovations in Cervical Cancer Prevention: Science, Practice and Actions*. This document covers four major topics, each of which was considered by a committee of experts, and their findings are a critical up-to-date review of the subject.

The four topics covered and the chairpersons of the individual expert committees are as below:

1 HPV DNA Testing in Cervical Cancer Screening: From Evidence to Policies, chaired by T. Cox and J. Cuzick.
2 Clinical Utility of HPV Genotyping, chaired by P. Castle and C.J.L.M. Meijer.
3 Molecular Markers: How to Apply in Practice, chaired by K. Syrjanen and M. Von Knebel Doeberitz.
4 Prevention Strategies of Cervical Cancer in the HPV Vaccine Era, chaired by X. Bosch and D. Harper.

The key message that runs throughout the document is the on-going need for information, training, communication and coordination of resources to ensure that the best-practice solutions for the prevention, control and treatment of cervical cancer are implemented worldwide. As the Chairman of the Scientific Committee of EUROGIN, Dr Joseph Monsonego, commented, 'this report has been published as part of EUROGIN's mission to provide up-to-date information from basic and clinical research, as well as to encourage and facilitate the transfer of high-quality evidence-based information and results into clinical practice.'

The document can be downloaded from the EUROGIN website (http://www.eurogin.com) and is highly recommended for further reading on this and other subjects related to cervical cancer management.

REFERENCES

Abu J, Batuwangala M, Herbert K *et al.* (2005) Retinoic acid and retinoid receptors: potential chemopreventive and therapeutic role in cervical cancer. *Lancet Oncology* 6: 712–720.

Andersen ES, Nielsen K, Paterson B (1995) The reliability of preconisation diagnostic evaluation in patients with cervical intraepithelial neoplasia and microinvasive carcinoma. *Gynecologic Oncology* 59: 143–147.

Anderson M, Hartley R (1980) Cervical crypt involvement by intraepithelial neoplasia. *Obstetrics and Gynecology* 55: 546–550.

Benedet JL, Miller DM, Nickerson KG *et al.* (1987) The results of cryosurgery treatment for cervical intraepithelial neoplasia at 1, 5 and 10 years. *American Journal of Obstetrics and Gynecology* 157: 268–273.

Bigrigg A, Codling BW, Pearson P *et al.* (1991) Description of long term complications after treatment of cervical intraepithelial neoplasia (CIN) with low voltage loop diathermy *International Journal of Obstetrics and Gynecology* 5: 43–47.

Bigrigg MA, Codling BW, Pearson P *et al.* (1994) Efficacy and safety of large loop excision of the transformation zone. *Lancet* 343: 32–34.

Boonstra H, Koudstal J, Oosterhuis JW *et al.* (1990) Analysis of cryolesions in the uterine cervix: application techniques, extension and failures. *Obstetrics and Gynecology* 75: 232–239.

Buxton EJ, Luesley SM, Shafi MI *et al.* (1991) Colposcopically directed punch biopsy: a potentially misleading investigation. *British Journal of Obstetrics and Gynaecology* 98: 1273–1276.

Chanen W (1989) The efficacy of electrocoagulation diathermy performed under local anaesthesia for the eradication of precancerous lesions of the cervix. *Australian and New Zealand Journal of Obstetrics and Gynaecology* 29: 189–193.

Cox JT (1999) Management of cervical intraepithelial neoplasia. *Lancet* 353: 857–889.

Crane JMC (2006) Transvaginal ultrasonography in the prediction of preterm birth after treatment for cervical intraepithelial neoplasia. *Obstetrics and Gynecology* 107: 37–44.

Creasman WT, Hinshaw WM, Clarke-Pearson DL (1984) Cryosurgery in the management of cervical intraepithelial neoplasia. *Obstetrics and Gynecology* 63: 145–149.

Crisp WE, Asadourian L, Romberger W (1967) Application of cryosurgery to gynaecological malignancy. *Obstetrics and Gynecology* 30: 668–670.

Crum CP, Berkowitz RS (2002) Human papillomaviruses, applications, caveats and prevention. *Journal of Reproductive Medicine* 47: 519–529.

De Cristofaro D, Fontana P, Pizzoli C (1988) Pathological study of the cervix after cold coagulation. *American Journal of Obstetrics and Gynecology* 159: 1053–1054.

Dobbs P, Asmussen TM, Nunns D *et al.* (2000) Does histological incomplete excision of CIN following LLETZ increase recurrence rates? A six-year cytological follow-up. *British Journal of Obstetrics and Gynaecology* 107: 1298–1301.

El-Bastawissi AY, Becker TM, Daling JR (1999) Effect of cervical carcinoma in situ and its management on pregnancy outcome. *Obstetrics and Gynecology* 93: 207–212.

Etherington IJ, Luesley DM, Shafi MI *et al.* (1997) Observer variability amongst colposcopists from the West Midlands region. *British Journal of Obstetrics and Gynaecology* 104: 1380–1384.

Flannelly G, Anderson D, Kitchener HC *et al.* (1994) Management of women with mild and moderate cervical dyskaryosis. *British Medical Journal* 308: 1399–1403.

Flannelly G, Langham H, Jandial L *et al.* (1997) A study of treatment failures following large loop excision of the transformation zone for the treatment of cervical intraepithelial neoplasia. *British Journal of Obstetrics and Gynaecology* 104: 718–722.

Flannelly G, Bolger B, Fawzi HD *et al.* (2001) Follow-up after LLETZ: could schedules be modified according to risk of recurrence. *British Journal of Obstetrics and Gynaecology* 108: 1025–1030.

Gordon HK, Duncan ID (1991) Effective destruction of cervical intraepithelial neoplasia (CIN3) at 100°C, using the Semm cold coagulator: 14 years experience. *British Journal of Obstetrics and Gynaecology* 98: 14–20.

Hammond RH, Edmonds DK (1990) Does treatment for cervical intraepithelial neoplasia affect fertility and pregnancy? *British Medical Journal* 301: 1344–45.

Jones JM, Sweetnam P, Hibbard BM (1979) The outcome of pregnancy after cone biopsy of the cervix: a case-controlled study. *British Journal of Obstetrics and Gynaecology* 86: 913–916.

Jones RW (2003) The natural history of lower genital tract precancer: historical perspective. In: Maclean A, Singer A, Critchley H (eds) *Lower Genital Tract Neoplasia*. London: RCOG Press, pp. 69–81.

Jordan JA, Woodman CBJ, Mylotte MJ *et al.* (1985) The treatment of cervical intraepithelial neoplasia by laser vaporization. *British Journal of Obstetrics and Gynaecology* 92: 394–398.

Kierkegaard O, Byrjalsen C, Hansen KC *et al.* (1995) Association between colposcopic findings and histology in cervical lesions: significance of the size of the lesion. *Gynecologic Oncology* 57: 66–71.

Klaritsch P, Reich A, Giuliani J *et al.* (2005) Pregnancy outcome after cold knife conisation of the uterine cervix. *International Journal of Gynaecological Cancer* 15 (Suppl. 2): 127.

Kristensen J, Langhoff-Roos J, Kristensen FB (1993) Increased risk of pre-term birth in women with cervical conisation. *Obstetrics and Gynecology* 81: 1005–1008.

Kyrgiou M, Koliopoulos G, Martin-Hirsch P *et al.* (2006) Obstetric outcomes after conservative treatment for intraepithelial or early invasive cervical lesions: systematic review and meta-analysis. *Lancet* 367: 489–498.

Larson G (1983) Conisation for pre-invasive and invasive carcinoma. *Acta Obstetrica et Gynecologica Scandinavica Supplementary Issue* 114: 1–40.

Leiman G, Harrison NA, Rubin A (1980) Pregnancy following conisation of the cervix, complications related to cone size. *American Journal of Obstetrics and Gynecology* 136: 14–18.

Luesley D, Leeson S (eds) (2004) *Colposcopy and Programme Management: Guidelines for the NHS Cervical Screening Programme.* NHSCSP publication no. 20. London: NHSCSP, April 2004 (available online at http://www.cancerscreening.nhs.uk/cervical/publications/nhscsp20.html).

Luesley DM, Cullimore EJ, Redman CW *et al.* (1990) Loop diathermy excision of the cervical transformation zone in patients with abnormal cervical smears. *British Medical Journal* 300: 1690–1693.

Manos MM, Kinney WK, Hurley LB *et al.* (1999) Identifying women with cervical neoplasia: using human papillomavirus DNA testing for equivocal papanicolaou results. *Journal of the American Medical Association* 281: 1605–1610.

Martin-Hirsch PL, Paraskevaidis E, Kitchener H (2002) Surgery for cervical intraepithelial neoplasia. *Cochrane Database Systematic Review* 3.

Massad LS, Halperin CJ, Bitterman P (1996) Correlation between colposcopically directed biopsy and cervical loop excision. *Gynecologic Oncology* 60: 400–403.

McIndoe WA, McLean MA, Jones RW *et al.* (1984) The invasive potential of carcinoma in situ of the cervix. *Obstetrics and Gynecology* 64: 451–454.

Melnikow J, Nuovo J, Willan AR *et al.* (1998) Natural history of cervical squamous intraepithelial lesions: a meta-analysis. *Obstetrics and Gynecology* 92: 727–735.

Mitchell MF, Tortolero-Luna G, Wright T *et al.* (1996) Cervical human papillomavirus infection and intraepithelial neoplasia: a review. *Journal of the National Cancer Institute Monograph* 21: 17–25.

Monaghan JM (1995) Laser vaporization and excisional techniques in the treatment of cervical intraepithelial neoplasia. *Bailliere's Clinical Obstetrics and Gynaecology* 9: 173–187.

Mor-Yosef S, Lopez A, Pearson S *et al.* (1990) Loop diathermy cone biopsy. *Obstetrics and Gynecology* 75: 884–886.

Murdoch JB, Crimshaw RN, Morgan RP *et al.* (1991) The impact of loop diathermy on management of early invasive cervical cancer. *International Journal of Gynecological Cancer* 2: 129–132.

Ostergard DR (1980) Cryosurgery treatment of cervical intraepithelial neoplasia. *Obstetrics and Gynecology* 56: 231–233.

Ostor AG (1993) Natural history of cervical intraepithelial neoplasia: critical review. *International Journal of Gynecological Pathology* 12: 186–192.

Panoskaltsis T, Ind TE, Perryman K *et al.* (2004) Needle versus loop diathermy excision of the transformation zone for the treatment of cervical intraepithelial neoplasia: a randomised controlled trial. *British Journal of Obstetrics and Gynaecology* 111: 748–753.

Paraskevaidis E, Arbyn M, Sotiriadis A *et al.* (2004) The role of HPV testing in the follow-up period after treatment of CIN: a systematic review of the literature. *Cancer Treatment Review* 30: 205–211.

Prendiville W (ed.) (1993) *Large Loop Excision of the Transformation Zone. A Practical Guide to LLETZ.* London: Chapman & Hall Medical.

Prendiville W (2003a) LLETZ: theoretical rationale, practical aspects, clinical experience, optimising the technique. In: Prendiville W (ed.) *Colposcopy Management Options*. London: W. Saunders, pp. 75–89.

Prendiville W (2003b) Treatment of grade 3 cervical intraepithelial neoplasia. In: Prendiville W (ed.) *Colposcopy Management Options*. London: W. Saunders, pp. 129–135.

Prendiville W (2003c) Excision of the transformation zone. In: Maclean A, Singer A, Critchley H (eds) *Lower Genital Tract Neoplasia*. London: RCOG Press, pp. 179–188.

Raio L, Ghezzi F, DiNaro E *et al.* (1997) Duration of pregnancy after CO_2 laser conisation of the cervix: influence of cone height. *Obstetrics and Gynecology* 90: 978–982.

Reiss M *et al.* (1999) Validity of cytological and colposcopically guided biopsy for the diagnosis of preclinical cervical cancer 1992. *Revista Bras Ginecol Obstet* 24: 193–200.

Richart RM, Townsend D, Crisp W *et al.* (1980) An analysis of long term follow-up results in patients with cervical intraepithelial neoplasia treated by cryotherapy. *American Journal of Obstetrics and Gynecology* 137: 823–826.

Robertson HA, Anderson JM, Swanson Beck J *et al.* (1989) Observer variability in histopathological reporting of cervical biopsy specimens. *Journal of Clinical Pathology* 42: 231–238.

Ruffin MT, Bailey JM, Normolle DP *et al.* (2004) Low dose topical delivery of all-trans retinoic acid for cervical intraepithelial neoplasia II and III. *Cancer Epidemiology Biomarkers and Prevention* 13: 2148–2152.

Sadler L, Saftlas A, Wang W *et al.* (2004) Treatment of cervical intraepithelial neoplasia and risk of pre-term delivery. *Journal of the American Medical Association* 291: 2100–2106.

Samson SL, Bentley JR, Fahey TJ *et al.* (2005) The effect of loop electrosurgical excision procedure on future pregnancy outcome. *Obstetrics and Gynecology* 105: 325–332.

Schantz A, Thormann L (1984) Cryosurgery for dysplasia of the uterine ectocervix. A randomised study of the efficacy of a single and double-freeze techniques. *Acta Obstetrica et Gynecologica Scandinavica* 63: 417–420.

Semm K (1966) New apparatus for the 'cold coagulation' of benign cervical lesions. *American Journal of Obstetrics and Gynecology* 95: 963–966.

Shafi MI, Dunn JA, Buxton EJ *et al.* (1993) Abnormal cervical cytology following large loop excision of the transformation zone, a case-controlled study. *British Journal of Obstetrics and Gynaecology* 100: 145–148.

Shafi MI, Luesley DM, Jordan JA *et al.* (1997) Randomised trial of immediate versus deferred treatment strategies for the management of minor cervical cytological abnormalities. *British Journal of Obstetrics and Gynaecology* 104: 590–594.

Singer A, Monaghan J (2000a) Diagnosis of cervical precancer: cytology colposcopy and pathology. In: Singer A, Monaghan J (eds) *Lower Genital Tract Precancer.* Oxford: Blackwell Publishing, pp. 47–101.

Singer A, Monaghan J (2000b) Diagnosis of cervical precancer: cytology colposcopy and pathology. In: Singer A, Monaghan J (eds) *Lower Genital Tract Precancer.* Oxford: Blackwell Publishing, pp. 115–117.

Singer A, Walker P, Tay SK *et al.* (1984) Impact of introduction of colposcopy to a district general hospital. *British Medical Journal* 289: 1049–1051.

Smart GE (1987) Randomised trial to compare laser with cold coagulation therapy in the treatment of CIN2 and 3. *Colposcopy and Gynaecology Laser Surgery* 3: 48–50.

Solomon D, Schiffman M, Tarraone R (2001) Comparison of three management strategies for patients with atypical squamous cells. *Journal of the National Cancer Institute* 93: 293–299.

Solomon D, Davey D, Kurman R *et al.* (2002) The 2001 Bethesda System: determination for reporting results of cervical cytology. *Journal of the American Medical Association* 287: 2114–2119.

Stoler MH, Schiffman M (2001) Inter-observer reproducibility of cervical cytology and histological interpretation: realistic estimates from the ASCUS-LSIL triage study. *Journal of the American Medical Association* 285: 1500–1505.

Tidbury P, Singer A (1992) CIN 3: the role of lesion size in invasion. *British Journal of Obstetrics and Gynaecology* 99: 583–586.

Trimble CL, Prantadosi S, Gravitt P *et al.* (2005) Spontaneous regression of high grade cervical dysplasia: effects of HPV and HLA phenotype. *Clinical Cancer Research* 11: 4717–4723.

Walker EM, Dodgson J, Duncan ID (1986) Does mild atypia on a cervical smear warrant further investigation? *Lancet* 2: 672–675.

Wright TC, Gagnon MD, Richart RM *et al.* (1992) Treatment of cervical intraepithelial neoplasia using the loop electrosurgical excision procedure. *Obstetrics and Gynecology* 79: 173–178.

Wright TC, Sun XW, Koulos J (1995) Comparison of management algorithms for the evaluation of women with low grade cytological abnormalities. *Obstetrics and Gynecology* 85: 202–210.

Wright TC, Cox TJ, Massad SL *et al.* (2002) 2001 Consensus guidelines for the management of women with cervical cytological abnormalities *Journal of the American Medical Association* 287 (16): 2122–2129.

Wright TC, Cox TJ, Massad S *et al.* (2003) 2001 Consensus guidelines for the management of women with cervical intraepithelial neoplasias. *American Journal of Obstetrics and Gynecology* 189 (1): 295–304.

Zielinski GD, Bais AG, Helmerhorst TJ *et al.* (2004) HPV testing and monitoring of women after treatment of CIN 3: review of the literature and meta-analysis. *Obstetrics and Gynaecology Surveys* 59: 543–553.

CHAPTER 32

The management of cervical intraepithelial neoplasia (glandular)

David M. Luesley and Richard W. Todd

INTRODUCTION

The introduction of screening programmes for cervical intraepithelial neoplasia (CIN) has seen a dramatic fall in the incidence of and deaths from invasive squamous carcinoma. Unfortunately, the same cannot be said for glandular neoplasia of the cervix. Over the last 30 years, there has been a relative and absolute increase in the incidence of invasive cervical adenocarcinoma and its precursors (Peters *et al.*, 1986; Schwartz and Weiss, 1986; Vesterinen *et al.*, 1989). This is explained in part by an increased awareness of the condition leading to more frequent diagnosis. Increasing exposure to certain oncogenic human papillomavirus (HPV) types has also been implicated in the observed rise.

The last decade has seen a move away from radical treatments for preinvasive glandular lesions to a more conservative approach (Muntz, 1996; Shin *et al.*, 2000; McHale *et al.*, 2001) as more has become known about their natural history. For women wishing to conserve their fertility, this is a welcome development although, obviously, it is important not to expose women to unacceptable risks in the pursuit of conservatism. This chapter discusses the concept of preinvasive glandular lesions in terms of their definition, detection and treatment.

CLASSIFICATION OF LESIONS

The terms that have been used to describe glandular abnormalities of the cervix are numerous, reflecting the difficulties in classifying this heterogeneous group of disorders. The temptation has been to invent a classification that is comparable to that used for preinvasive squamous lesions. In reality, this is difficult to do, particularly as lesions at the lower end of the spectrum may be difficult to distinguish from benign, inflammatory lesions and tubal metaplasia (Zaino, 2002). One would also need to distinguish different grades of abnormality in the middle of the spectrum as well as defining criteria for invasion. Unfortunately, because of a lack of definite pathognomonic histological characteristics of glandular lesions, this is

not entirely possible. As a result, many definitions have been presented. These include:

- glandular dysplasia;
- endocervical glandular dysplasia;
- endocervical glandular atypia;
- cervical glandular atypia (CGA);
- cervical glandular intraepithelial neoplasia (CGIN);
- glandular intraepithelial neoplasia (GIN).

The result is that there has been no widespread acceptance of any of these terms.

Adenocarcinoma *in situ* (AIS)

In 1953, Friedell and McKay described AIS (Friedell and McKay, 1953). This lesion has been characterised by certain histological features. These include:

- preservation of normal glandular architecture coupled with an alteration involving part or all of the surface epithelium
- nuclear enlargement;
- coarse chromatin;
- single or multiple nucleoli;
- increased mitotic activity;
- variable stratification of nuclei.

Cytoplasmic mucin may be scant or abundant. Moritani *et al.* (2002) described the use of the mitotic index as a way of differentiating benign from neoplastic lesions. A variety of subtypes of AIS have been described based on their cytoplasmic characteristics, including endocervical, intestinal, endometrioid and adenosquamous. No biological significance has been linked to these different types.

Glandular dysplasia and lesions of lesser severity than AIS

The significant heterogeneity in the exhibition of atypia in biopsies of cervical glandular lesions would be in keeping with the concept of a progressive process to invasive adenocarcinoma (Zaino, 2002). With this in mind, the term glandular dysplasia has been proposed as a diagnostic term to describe glandular lesions of lesser severity than AIS. Suggested definitions have included:

- glands lined by cells with atypical nuclei that are not fully malignant and with fewer mitoses than AIS;
- the presence of only one gland with features of AIS;
- nuclear atypia and evidence of cell turnover and two or fewer mitoses per gland;
- nuclear enlargement, hyperchromasia, stratification, pleomorphism, abnormal chromatin, increased mitoses, mucin depletion and abnormal gland architecture;
- moderate nuclear enlargement, hyperchromasia, atypia, with fewer mitoses than AIS;
- architectural and cytological features less marked than AIS.

In 1986, Brown and Wells further distinguished low-grade and high-grade dysplasia based on the absence of mitoses, paucity of vesicular nuclei and restriction of stratification of the nuclei to the basal two-thirds of the epithelium in low-grade lesions (Brown and Wells, 1986). Gloor and Hurlimann (1986) also divided dysplasia into three grades of cervical intraglandular neoplasia (CIGN) based on hyperchromasia, nuclear stratification, number of mitoses and amount of mucin. CIGN3 most closely correlated with AIS.

The problem remains that glandular lesions of lesser severity than AIS represent a heterogeneous group of uncertain biological behaviour. The ability to recognise these lesions in a reproducible fashion is also questionable. Therefore, it has been argued that, irrespective of the number of glands involved, lesions containing columnar cells with enlarged nuclei, coarse chromatin, increased nuclear cytoplasmic ratio and mitotic activity are probably best classified and treated as AIS (Zaino, 2000).

IS AIS A PREMALIGNANT CONDITION?

There is good evidence to support the concept that AIS is a premalignant condition.

Age of onset

The average age of women found to have AIS is approximately 35 years. This is 10–20 years younger than women with invasive adenocarcinoma. This would be consistent with AIS being a precursor lesion. Plaxe and Saltzstein *et al.* (1999) estimated that the average time for progression of AIS to invasive cancer was 13 years based on information in the SEER database. This figure is similar to that suggested by Hitchcock *et al.* (1993).

Co-location

Adenocarcinomas frequently have adjacent areas of AIS (Boon *et al.*, 1981).

Viral types

Similar HPV types have been found in AIS and invasive adenocarcinoma. HPV 18 DNA has been identified in up to 90% of cases of AIS (Pirog *et al.*, 2000).

Observed progression

Some cases of untreated AIS progressing to invasive cancer have been reported (Kashimura *et al.*, 1990; Poynor *et al.*, 1995; Hocking *et al.*, 1996).

Retrospective pathology review

Archived specimens predating the diagnosis of adenocarcinoma have been studied. Boon *et al.* (1981) studied cervical biopsies from patients who subsequently developed adenocarcinoma. With the benefit of hindsight, evidence of AIS was found that had not previously been identified. Retrospective review of smears taken from patients going on to develop adenocarcinoma has also revealed glandular atypia (Boddington *et al.*, 1976).

INCIDENCE AND AETIOLOGY OF GLANDULAR LESIONS

While the average annual age-adjusted incidence of invasive squamous cancer is decreasing, the rate for adenocarcinoma is increasing at a rate of 1.4% per year (Plaxe and Saltzstein, 1999).

Plaxe and Saltzstein (1999) reported an increase from 11% to 23% of adenocarcinomas among newly diagnosed invasive cervical cancers over a 23-year period. These figures are in keeping with those quoted by other authors and have been confirmed in 25 countries (Vizcaino *et al.*, 1998). The increasing incidence of adenocarcinomas is not fully understood. Proposed factors to explain this increase include a birth cohort effect associated with changing sexual behaviour, leading to greater exposure to certain HPV types, particularly type 18 (Gordon *et al.*, 1989). Pirog *et al.* (2000) studied 105 adenocarcinomas and adenosquamous carcinomas using polymerase chain reaction (PCR) to detect the HPV type. For adenocarcinomas, the most frequent HPV types were HPV 16 (50%), HPV 18 (40%), HPV 52 (2%) and HPV 35 (1%) (Pirog *et al.*, 2000). These results were similar to those described by other authors (Duggan *et al.*, 1995; Anciaux *et al.*, 1997). These results differ from squamous carcinomas, in which HPV 16 occurs with a much greater frequency than HPV 18 (Bosch *et al.*, 1995). A number of authors have found combined oral contraceptive (COC) pill users to be at greater risk of cervical adenocarcinomas (Brinton *et al.*, 1990; Ursin *et al.*, 1994; Thomas and Ray, 1996). A study by Lacey *et al.* (1999) found current use of COC to be associated with AIS but not invasive adenocarcinomas. Whether this association reflected detection bias, selection bias or confounding by HPV was not established.

DETECTION OF GLANDULAR LESIONS

Cytology (see also Chapter 24)

As preinvasive glandular lesions are asymptomatic, detection occurs either by cytology or by chance following biopsy for different reasons. A significant proportion of cases of AIS are detected by chance following treatment for squamous intra-epithelial lesions. Cytology has a poor sensitivity for detection of glandular lesions. Östör *et al.* (2000) describe how only 56% (55/98) of patients in their series had glandular lesions detected by cytology. This figure is in keeping with most other series, with cytology predicting glandular disease in between 23% and 72% (Casper *et al.*, 1997; Azodi *et al.*, 1999; Soutter *et al.*, 2001; Andersen and Nielsen, 2002). The possible reasons for this poor detection rate are varied. One explanation may be inadequate sampling of endocervical cells. Alternatively, the relative infrequency with which glandular lesions are encountered may leave cytologists and screeners less familiar with the relevant feature. The frequency with which glandular and squamous abnormalities co-exist may also be a factor. In a smear with predominantly squamous abnormalities, glandular abnormalities may be overlooked (Ayer *et al.*, 1987; Luesley *et al.*, 1987).

Endocervical curettage (ECC)

Because of the location of glandular disease (see below), the attraction of endocervical curettage as a diagnostic tool is obvious. In reality, its use is questionable. Azodi *et al.* (1999) described ECC in 27 cases of AIS preconisation; only 11 (41%) reported positive. In a similar study by Poynor *et al.* (1995), only 43% (9/21) of patients had ECC positive for AIS and 35% (15/43) in the study by Wolf *et al.* (1996). Denehy *et al.* (1997) reported on the use of ECC as a predictor for residual disease after treatment for AIS. Forty ECCs taken either at colposcopy or immediately after conisation in 32 patients with AIS were compared with the pathology findings in 28 cones and 12 hysterectomy specimens in the same group of patients. They found that, of 28 ECCs with a subsequent conisation, 18 showed no significant pathology. Nine of 12 patients subsequently undergoing hysterectomy also had negative results. Of these 27 negative ECCs, 18 (66.7%) were found to have residual disease. Therefore, even in a highly selected group of patients, some of whom had already had the diagnosis of AIS made, the false-negative rate was unacceptably high.

Colposcopy

Colposcopy is poor at detecting glandular disease for two

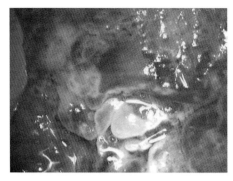

Fig. 32.1 Acetowhite fused columnar villi. Biopsy showed high-grade CGIN.

reasons. First, the location of the disease is likely to be within the endocervical canal and therefore out of view of the examiner. Secondly, even if within view, there are no generally accepted colposcopic features of preinvasive glandular disease. It has been suggested (Andersen and Arffmann, 1989) that AIS is associated with dense acetowhite villi (Fig. 32.1) or epithelium that is dense acetowhite, fragile and easily stripped, although these features are by no means pathognomonic.

In a study by Östör *et al.* (2000), although 67/90 (74%) patients with AIS had an abnormal colposcopy, only 19 (28%) were predicted to have had glandular disease. One might also argue that the examiner had been alerted to the possibility of AIS by an abnormal glandular smear. In the report by Maini *et al.* (1998), of 50 patients diagnosed with AIS, none was diagnosed on the basis of colposcopic findings.

Co-existence with squamous lesions

Adenocarcinoma *in situ* frequently co-exists with squamous intraepithelial lesions. A number of series have addressed the frequency with which this occurs, quoting an average of approximately 50% (range 25–100%) (Table 32.1).

TOPOGRAPHY OF AIS

Previously, concerns over the location of disease within the endocervical canal and the fear of 'skip lesions' have led some authors to recommend hysterectomy for AIS. For effective diagnostic and treatment strategies to be determined, a clear understanding of the topography of disease is needed. Many authors have now shown that AIS begins at the squamo-columnar junction (SCJ) in the majority of cases (Bertrand *et al.*, 1987; Jaworski *et al.*, 1988; Tobon and Dave, 1988; Andersen and Arffmann, 1989). Nicklin *et al.* (1991) demonstrated how the extent of lesions ranged up to 25 mm within the canal (mean 8.4 mm). Similarly, Bertrand *et al.* (1987) also noted that the disease extended at least 2 cm up the endocervical canal in four out of 19 cases. Consequently, it

Table 32.1 Co-existent squamous and glandular disease rates.

Author	Number of cases	Percentage with co-existent squamous lesion
Andersen	25/36	69
Andersen	18/60	30
Azodi	26/51	51
Bertrand	11/23	48
Cullimore	26/51	51
Denehy	27/42	64
Im	9/18	50
Jaworski	32/72	45
Maini	35/50	70
Muntz	25/40	63
Östör	15/21	71
Östör	65/100	65
Poynor	14/28	50
Qizilbash	7/7	100
Shin	74/132	56
Tobon	3/12	25
Widrich	19/46	41
Wolf	19/55	35
Total	412/833	49

has been suggested that an adequate cone should encompass the entire transformation zone and extend parallel to the canal for a length of at least 25 mm. Having said that, Andersen and Nielsen (2002) in their prospective study found that only 16.7% of their cones were greater than 25 mm in length and suggested that no benefit was seen for cones greater than 20 mm in length. The caveat is made, however, that the patient numbers involved were small and no firm conclusions can be made.

Reports concerning the focality or multifocality of AIS are scanty and conflicting, but are obviously important if rational decisions are to be made regarding management after local excision. Several studies have described the number of quadrants involved in specimens, with some authors describing how the likelihood of involved cone margins increases the more quadrants are involved (Shin *et al.*, 2000). Qizilbash (1975) found AIS limited to one quadrant in six out of seven cases, and Andersen and Arffmann (1989) also noted unifocal involvement in almost all cases. Östör *et al.* (1984), in a study of 17 cases, found AIS to be focal in two, multicentric in three and diffuse in 12 (diffuse defined as involving a whole microscopic field). Disease averaged 7 mm in length and 12 mm in width. Shin *et al.* (2000) reported that, in 50 of 94 cone specimens for AIS, multiple quadrants were involved, whereas disease was confined to one quadrant in 44. Bertrand *et al.* (1987) described AIS in one quadrant in two cases, two quadrants in four cases, three quadrants in four cases and four quadrants in three cases. In the study by Östör *et al.* (2000),

only 13% were multicentric, defined as foci separated by more than 2 mm of normal mucosa. It seems likely that AIS frequently begins as a single focus but, by the time of diagnosis, as a consequence of lateral or horizontal spread, it often involves multiple quadrants and may extend high up in the endocervical canal. It has been suggested that the length of the lesion may correlate with the age of the patient, suggesting progressive development of the lesion over time (Nicklin *et al.*, 1991). Widrich *et al.* (1996), however, failed to demonstrate such a correlation in their series. It would seem that true skip lesions, in which several millimetres of normal glands intervene between foci of AIS, are relatively rare, occurring in < 15% of cases.

Equally significant are observations about the location of involvement within the endocervical mucosa. Jaworski *et al.* (1988), in a study of 72 cases of AIS, described involvement primarily centred in the neck of glands with surface or deep gland extension in some cases. Andersen and Arffmann (1989) found AIS along the mucosal surface in 34 out of 36 cases, with gland extension limited to within 2 mm of the surface in two-thirds of cases. In general, most cases seem to involve the surface epithelium and superficial glands near the transformation zone. This would suggests that AIS is usually accessible to diagnosis by endocervical cytological sampling if correctly performed.

MANAGEMENT OF AIS

The recommended treatments for preinvasive glandular lesions of the cervix have ranged from radical hysterectomy with lymphadenectomy through to simple hysterectomy, cone biopsy and transformation zone excision. The poor understanding of the natural history of the condition, concerns over multifocality and reports of invasive disease developing after conservative treatment have led many authors to recommend hysterectomy as the definitive treatment for AIS. However, taking into account the mean age of women with the condition, the desire to retain fertility and the wish to be more conservative if possible, many series have reported the probable safety of a more conservative approach to management using local excisional methods with good follow-up. This seems very pertinent now, when conservative techniques are considered in selected cases of frank invasion.

What is the role of conservative management?

Demonstration of residual disease in subsequent hysterectomy specimens after local excision and reports of invasive carcinoma developing after conservative treatment are two of the main concerns with regard to conservative management.

Residual AIS has been demonstrated in up to 75% of patients if the excision margins of the initial biopsy/treatment were involved. Even if the margins were uninvolved, the residual disease rate can be as high as 44% (Cullimore *et al.*, 1992;

Table 32.2 Residual disease in hysterectomy specimens after conisation depending on margin status.

Author	Margins negative	Margins positive
Azodi	5/16 (31%)	9/16 (56%)
Cullimore	0/4 (0%)	1/8 (13%)
Denehy	2/7 (29%)	7/10 (70%)
McHale	1/6 (17%)	10/14 (71%)
Im	4/9 (44%)	4/6 (66%)
Kennedy	0/6 (0%)	14/21 (67%)
Muntz	1/12 (8%)	7/10 (70%)
Östör	2/8 (25%)	9/12 (75%)
Poynor	4/10 (40%)	3/8 (38%)
Shin	1/16 (6%)	13/21 (62%)
Widrich	0/3 (0%)	9/14 (64%)
Wolf	7/21 (33%)	10/19 (53%)
Total	27/118 (23%)	96/159 (60%)

Muntz *et al.*, 1992; Im *et al.*, 1995; Poynor *et al.*, 1995; Widrich *et al.*, 1996; Wolf *et al.*, 1996; Denehy *et al.*, 1997; Azodi *et al.*, 1999; Östör *et al.*, 2000; Shin *et al.*, 2000; McHale *et al.*, 2001; Kennedy and Biscotti, 2002) (Table 32.2).

There are also concerns about patients treated conservatively either developing or having co-existent invasive disease. Poynor *et al.* (1995) reported the largest number of such patients. This has resulted in many being wary of conservative management. To date, there have been at least eight reported cases of conservatively managed patients developing invasive adenocarcinoma, five of whom had margins free of disease and three involved margins. Because the interval from initial conisation to diagnosis of invasive cancer ranged from 4 months to 6 years, it is likely that this represented both residual disease progression and *de novo* disease.

With time, a growing number of authors have reported on their experiences with a more conservative approach when cone margins are uninvolved. One of the largest of these, by Shin *et al.* (2000), reported on the conservative management of 95 patients, 92 of whom had negative margins. During a median follow-up period of 30 months, nine women required evaluation for cytological abnormality, but none was shown to have recurrent AIS. Twenty-three live births were recorded in this group. Another large retrospective study by Östör *et al.* (2000) describes the experience with 100 cases of AIS over a 22-year period. Fifty-three patients, having been found to have uninvolved margins, were treated by conisation alone. Follow-up ranged from 1 to 16 years (median 8 years). Over this time period, none was found to have recurrent disease.

Only two prospective studies of conservative management have been published to date. In the first, by Cullimore *et al.* (1992), 51 patients were identified as having CIGN by cone biopsy. Patients with negative cone biopsy margins were treated conservatively and followed up with cytology and colposcopy.

Those with positive margins were offered a hysterectomy. Of the 42 patients with negative margins, 35 were managed by cone biopsy alone. After a median follow-up of 12 months, all remained disease free. Seven of those with uninvolved margins underwent further surgery, two for unrelated gynaecological disorders and the remaining five for cytological abnormalities. None of these was found to have residual glandular disease. Eight patients were found to have involved margins and underwent hysterectomy. Of these, only one was shown to have residual glandular disease. This patient had also had an abnormal glandular smear preoperatively. The conclusions from this study were that conservative management is acceptable providing the excision margins of the initial cone biopsy were negative and adequate colposcopic and cytological follow-up is available.

More recently, Andersen and Nielsen (2002) took things a step further and reported a larger prospective study of conservative management. This study differed from the above in that conisation was proposed as a definitive treatment irrespective of cone margins. Fifty-eight out of 60 patients identified as having AIS were treated by conisation alone and followed up for a mean of 49 months. Follow-up involved colposcopy and cytology 3-monthly for the first year, 6-monthly for the second year and annually thereafter. Abnormal cytology was evaluated with colposcopy, biopsies and endocervical sampling. Positive histology was required before recording a treatment failure. Of the 58 patients, 15 (26%) had involved cone margins, a proportion of whom would therefore be expected to have residual disease. In total, four recurrences were observed. One of these was diagnosed after 4 months in a patient with involved cone margins. The subsequent hysterectomy specimen showed residual AIS (a recurrence rate of 6.7% if margins are involved). Three other patients with uninvolved margins developed further intraepithelial neoplasia; only one of these had AIS, the other two having squamous lesions. The point is made that, if hysterectomy was performed for involved margins, then 14 'unnecessary' procedures would have been performed.

Impressive as these data are, they are not entirely in keeping with what would be expected. The retrospective and prospective studies described above demonstrate an interesting point. Given the data describing residual disease rates in hysterectomy specimens according to margin status (23% if uninvolved, 60% if involved), much higher recurrence rates would be expected than described in those patients managed conservatively. One explanation may be that, although residual disease may have been present in those patients treated conservatively, irrespective of margin status, the inflammation and local immune responses that result from local excisional treatments may lead to spontaneous resolution of residual disease. The study by Andersen and Nielsen (2002) would certainly suggest that this is the case, as a significant proportion of those women managed conservatively with involved margins would have been expected to have residual disease that would display itself at a later stage. Of concern is that a review of the literature reveals at least another 29 patients with AIS conservatively managed after conisation with involved margins. Three of these developed invasive adenocarcinoma, between 4 months and 5 years after diagnosis, and six developed further *in situ* disease between 4 and 45 months after initial diagnosis (Brown *et al.*, 1991; Hitchcock *et al.*, 1993; Poynor *et al.*, 1995; Widrich *et al.*, 1996; Wolf *et al.*, 1996; Östör *et al.*, 2000; Shin *et al.*, 2000; McHale *et al.*, 2001).

Although the study by Andersen and Nielsen (2002) may suggest that the situation with AIS is more comparable with CIN than previously thought, i.e. that conservative management of AIS is safe irrespective of margin status, further studies are needed to confirm that this is the case. Until then, conservative management assuming negative margins is probably a more appropriate treatment.

What is the best method of local excision?

Assuming that an adequately sized cone biopsy is performed, it should not matter which method is used. The reality would appear to be somewhat different, with some authors questioning the safety of diathermy loop excision (LLETZ or LEEP) in the management of patients with AIS. Numerous authors have described the apparent superiority of cold knife cone (CKC) excision compared with other methods, particularly diathermy loop excision, in terms of both likelihood of residual disease and excision margin status. Widrich *et al.* (1996) described 33% of patients having positive margins after cold knife excision compared with 50% after loop excision and a recurrence rate of 29% among LLETZ patients compared with 6% among CKC patients. Azodi *et al.* (1999) reported positive margins in 75% after LLETZ compared with 24% for CKC and laser cone (57%). Wolf *et al.* (1996) reported 38% positive margins in CKC compared with 71% in LLETZ specimens. Denehy *et al.* (1997) also reported 33% margin positivity after CKC compared with 69% for LLETZ. What is the reason for this apparent inferiority of LLETZ in obtaining adequate excision? Mathevet *et al.* (1994) showed that CKC specimens were of larger volume and more adequate for histological evaluation than specimens obtained with LLETZ. Similarly, Girardi *et al.* (1994) in a prospective study showed that specimens obtained by LLETZ were likely to be lighter and shorter. Another concern is that LLETZ specimens are frequently fragmented due to multiple 'passes' being made with the loop. The effects of diathermy artefact may also make histological interpretation of the nature of the lesion and its margins difficult. Based on these data, it would appear that knife cone excision is the method of choice. There are no data as yet available on straight wire excision. Some preliminary data comparing it with loop excision for squamous lesions suggest that it may be associated with a lower incomplete excision rate (Soutter *et al.*, 2001).

CONCLUSION

Both preinvasive and invasive glandular disease of the cervix appear to be increasing in incidence. Despite this, the relative infrequency with which these lesions are seen and the lack of large prospective studies means that the natural history of preinvasive glandular lesions is poorly understood. Similarly, the optimum management for such lesions remains unclear. At the time of writing, it would seem that management should be adapted to the individual with scope for conservative management by cone biopsy assuming that margins are clear and appropriate follow-up is available. Despite reports that margin status may not be as important as previously thought, it is too early to introduce a change in practice until further large prospective studies of such management have been performed.

REFERENCES

Anciaux D, Lawrence WD, Gregoire L (1997) Glandular lesions of the uterine cervix: prognostic implications of human papillomavirus status. *International Journal of Gynecological Pathology* 16 (2): 103–110.

Andersen ES, Arffmann E (1989) Adenocarcinoma in situ of the uterine cervix: a clinico-pathologic study of 36 cases. *Gynecologic Oncology* 35 (1): 1–7.

Andersen ES, Nielsen K (2002) Adenocarcinoma in situ of the cervix: a prospective study of conization as definitive treatment. *Gynecologic Oncology* 86 (3): 365–369.

Ayer B, Pacey F, Greenberg M *et al.* (1987) The cytologic diagnosis of adenocarcinoma in situ of the cervix uteri and related lesions. I. Adenocarcinoma in situ. *Acta Cytologica* 31 (4): 397–411.

Azodi M, Chambers SK, Rutherford TJ *et al.* (1999) Adenocarcinoma in situ of the cervix: management and outcome. *Gynecologic Oncology* 73 (3): 348–353.

Bertrand M, Lickrish GM, Colgan TJ (1987) The anatomic distribution of cervical adenocarcinoma in situ: implications for treatment. *American Journal of Obstetrics and Gynecology* 157 (1): 21–25.

Boddington MM, Spriggs AI, Cowdell RH (1976) Adenocarcinoma of the uterine cervix: cytological evidence of a long preclinical evolution. *British Journal of Obstetrics and Gynaecology* 83 (11): 900–903.

Boon ME, Baak JP, Kurver PJ *et al.* (1981) Adenocarcinoma in situ of the cervix: an underdiagnosed lesion. *Cancer* 48 (3): 768–773.

Bosch FX, Manos MM, Muñoz N *et al.* (1995) Prevalence of human papillomavirus in cervical cancer: a worldwide perspective. International Biological Study on Cervical Cancer (IBSCC) Study Group. *Journal of the National Cancer Institute* 87 (11): 796–802.

Brinton LA, Reeves WC, Brenes MM *et al.* (1990) Oral contraceptive use and risk of invasive cervical cancer. *International Journal of Epidemiology* 19 (1): 4–11.

Brown LJ, Wells M (1986) Cervical glandular atypia associated with squamous intraepithelial neoplasia: a premalignant lesion? *Journal of Clinical Pathology* 39 (1): 22–28.

Brown JV, Peters WA, Corwin DJ (1991) Invasive carcinoma after cone biopsy for cervical intraepithelial neoplasia. *Gynecologic Oncology* 40 (1): 25–28.

Casper GR, Östör AG, Quinn MA (1997) A clinicopathologic study of glandular dysplasia of the cervix. *Gynecologic Oncology* 64 (1): 166–170.

Cullimore JE, Luesley DM, Rollason TP *et al.* (1992) A prospective study of conization of the cervix in the management of cervical intraepithelial glandular neoplasia (CIGN) — a preliminary report. *British Journal of Obstetrics and Gynaecology* 99 (4): 314–318.

Denehy TR, Gregori CA, Breen JL (1997) Endocervical curettage, cone margins, and residual adenocarcinoma in situ of the cervix. *Obstetrics and Gynecology* 90 (1): 1–6.

Duggan MA, McGregor SE, Benoit JL *et al.* (1995) The human papillomavirus status of invasive cervical adenocarcinoma: a clinicopathological and outcome analysis. *Human Pathology* 26 (3): 319–325.

Friedell G, McKay D (1953) Adenocarcinoma in situ of the endocervix. *Cancer* 6: 887–897.

Girardi F, Heydarfadai M, Koroschetz F *et al.* (1994) Cold-knife conization versus loop excision: histopathologic and clinical results of a randomized trial. *Gynecologic Oncology* 55 (3 Pt 1): 368–370.

Gloor E, Hurlimann J (1986) Cervical intraepithelial glandular neoplasia (adenocarcinoma in situ and glandular dysplasia). A correlative study of 23 cases with histologic grading, histochemical analysis of mucins, and immunohistochemical determination of the affinity for four lectins. *Cancer* 58 (6): 1272–1280.

Gordon AN, Bornstein J, Kaufman RH *et al.* (1989) Human papillomavirus associated with adenocarcinoma and adenosquamous carcinoma of the cervix: analysis by in situ hybridization. *Gynecologic Oncology* 35 (3): 345–348.

Hitchcock A, Johnson J, McDowell K *et al.* (1993) A retrospective study into the occurrence of cervical glandular atypia in cone biopsy specimens from 1977–1978 with clinical follow-up. *International Journal of Gynecological Cancer* 3 (3): 164–168.

Hocking GR, Hayman JA, Östör AG (1996) Adenocarcinoma in situ of the uterine cervix progressing to invasive adenocarcinoma. *Australian and New Zealand Journal of Obstetrics and Gynaecology* 36 (2): 218–220.

Im DD, Duska LR, Rosenshein NB (1995) Adequacy of conization margins in adenocarcinoma in situ of the cervix as a predictor of residual disease. *Gynecologic Oncology* 59 (2): 179–182.

Jaworski RC, Pacey NF, Greenberg ML *et al.* (1988) The histologic diagnosis of adenocarcinoma in situ and related lesions of the cervix uteri. Adenocarcinoma in situ. *Cancer* 61 (6): 1171–1181.

Kashimura M, Shinohara M, Oikawa K *et al.* (1990) An adenocarcinoma in situ of the uterine cervix that developed into invasive adenocarcinoma after 5 years. *Gynecologic Oncology* 36 (1): 128–133.

Kennedy AW, Biscotti CV (2002) Further study of the management of cervical adenocarcinoma in situ. *Gynecologic Oncology* 86 (3): 361–364.

Lacey JV, Jr, Brinton LA, Abbas FM *et al.* (1999) Oral contraceptives as risk factors for cervical adenocarcinomas and squamous cell carcinomas. *Cancer Epidemiology Biomarkers and Prevention* 8 (12): 1079–1085.

Luesley DM, Jordan JA, Woodman CB *et al.* (1987) A retrospective review of adenocarcinoma-in-situ and glandular atypia of the uterine cervix. *British Journal of Obstetrics and Gynaecology* 94 (7): 699–703.

McHale MT, Le TD, Burger RA *et al.* (2001) Fertility sparing treatment for in situ and early invasive adenocarcinoma of the cervix. *Obstetrics and Gynecology* 98 (5 Pt 1): 726–731.

Maini M, Lavie O, Comerci G *et al.* (1998) The management and follow-up of patients with high-grade cervicalglandular intraepithelial neoplasia. *International Journal of Gynecological Cancer* 8: 287–291.

Mathevet P, Dargent D, Roy M *et al.* (1994) A randomized prospective study comparing three techniques of conization: cold knife, laser, and LEEP. *Gynecologic Oncology* 54 (2): 175–179.

Moritani S, Ioffe OB, Sagae S *et al.* (2002) Mitotic activity and apoptosis in endocervical glandular lesions. *International Journal of Gynecological Pathology* 21 (2): 125–133.

Muntz HG (1996) Can cervical adenocarcinoma in situ be safely managed by conization alone? *Gynecologic Oncology* 61 (3): 301–303.

Muntz HG, Bell DA, Lage JM *et al.* (1992) Adenocarcinoma in situ of the uterine cervix. *Obstetrics and Gynecology* 80 (6): 935–939.

Nicklin JL, Wright RG, Bell JR *et al.* (1991) A clinicopathological study of adenocarcinoma in situ of the cervix. The influence of cervical HPV infection and other factors, and the role of conservative surgery. *Australian and New Zealand Journal of Obstetrics and Gynaecology* 31 (2): 179–183.

Östör AG, Pagano R, Davoren RA *et al.* (1984) Adenocarcinoma in situ of the cervix. *International Journal of Gynecological Pathology* 3 (2): 179–190.

Östör AG, Duncan A, Quinn M *et al.* (2000) Adenocarcinoma in situ of the uterine cervix: an experience with 100 cases. *Gynecologic Oncology* 79 (2): 207–210.

Peters RK, Chao A, Mack TM *et al.* (1986) Increased frequency of adenocarcinoma of the uterine cervix in young women in Los Angeles County. *Journal of the National Cancer Institute* 76 (3): 423–428.

Pirog EC, Kleter B, Olgac S *et al.* (2000) Prevalence of human papillomavirus DNA in different histological subtypes of cervical adenocarcinoma. *American Journal of Pathology* 157 (4): 1055–1062.

Plaxe SC, Saltzstein SL (1999) Estimation of the duration of the preclinical phase of cervical adenocarcinoma suggests that there is ample opportunity for screening. *Gynecologic Oncology* 75 (1): 55–61.

Poynor EA, Barakat RR, Hoskins WJ (1995) Management and follow-up of patients with adenocarcinoma in situ of the uterine cervix. *Gynecologic Oncology* 57 (2): 158–164.

Qizilbash AH (1975) In-situ and microinvasive adenocarcinoma of the uterine cervix. A clinical, cytologic and histologic study of 14 cases. *American Journal of Clinical Pathology* 64 (2): 155–170.

Schwartz SM, Weiss NS (1986) Increased incidence of adenocarcinoma of the cervix in young women in the United States. *American Journal of Epidemiology* 124 (6): 1045–1047.

Shin CH, Schorge JO, Lee KR *et al.* (2000) Conservative management of adenocarcinoma in situ of the cervix. *Gynecologic Oncology* 79 (1): 6–10.

Soutter WP, Haidopoulos D, Gornall RJ *et al.* (2001) Is conservative treatment for adenocarcinoma in situ of the cervix safe? *British Journal of Obstetrics and Gynaecology* 108 (11): 1184–1189.

Thomas DB, Ray RM (1996) Oral contraceptives and invasive adenocarcinomas and adenosquamous carcinomas of the uterine cervix. The World Health Organization Collaborative Study of Neoplasia and Steroid Contraceptives. *American Journal of Epidemiology* 144 (3): 281–289.

Tobon H, Dave H (1988) Adenocarcinoma in situ of the cervix. Clinicopathologic observations of 11 cases. *International Journal of Gynecological Pathology* 7 (2): 139–151.

Ursin G, Peters RK, Henderson BE *et al.* (1994) Oral contraceptive use and adenocarcinoma of cervix. *Lancet* 344 (8934): 1390–1394.

Vesterinen E, Forss M, Nieminen U (1989) Increase of cervical adeno-carcinoma: a report of 520 cases of cervical carcinoma including 112 tumors with glandular elements. *Gynecologic Oncology* 33 (1): 49–53.

Vizcaino AP, Moreno V, Bosch FX *et al.* (1998) International trends in the incidence of cervical cancer: I. Adenocarcinoma and adenosquamous cell carcinomas. *International Journal of Cancer* 75 (4): 536–545.

Widrich T, Kennedy AW, Myers TM *et al.* (1996) Adenocarcinoma in situ of the uterine cervix: management and outcome. *Gynecologic Oncology* 61 (3): 304–308.

Wolf JK, Levenback C, Malpica A *et al.* (1996) Adenocarcinoma in situ of the cervix: significance of cone biopsy margins. *Obstetrics and Gynecology* 88 (1): 82–86.

Zaino RJ (2000) Glandular lesions of the uterine cervix. *Modern Pathology* 13 (3): 261–274.

Zaino RJ (2002) Symposium part I: adenocarcinoma in situ, glandular dysplasia, and early invasive adenocarcinoma of the uterine cervix. *International Journal of Gynecological Pathology* 21 (4): 314–326.

CHAPTER 33

The role of HPV in the management of cervical neoplasia

Chris J.L.M. Meijer, Peter J.F. Snijders and René H.M. Verheijen

PRESENT SITUATION

Women with histologically proven cervical intraepithelial neoplasia (CIN)2/CIN3 are treated by removal or destruction of the abnormal epithelium of the transformation zone, the area of the cervix uteri where most of these lesions are localised. Treatment modalities include large loop excision of the transformation zone (LLETZ), loop electrosurgical excision procedure (LEEP), cryocoagulation, laser evaporation or laser or cold knife conisation. In many European countries, women are then monitored by cytology at 6, 12 and 24 months post treatment and, if necessary, yearly thereafter until three consecutive smears are read as normal. In the case of abnormal smears, retreatment follows according to standard procedures. Treatment failures between 5% and 25% have been reported (Alvarez *et al.*, 1994; Bigrigg *et al.*, 1994; Mitchell *et al.*, 1998; Bollen *et al.*, 1999; Nuovo *et al.*, 2000; Nobbenhuis *et al.*, 2001). In the United States, the American Society for Colposcopy and Cervical Pathology (ASCCP) published guidelines in 2001 (Wright *et al.*, 2003). Although the ASCCP confirmed that no prospective randomised trials evaluating different follow-up protocols have been performed, their guidelines suggest repeat cytology at 4- to 6-month intervals up to 2 years and yearly follow-up thereafter. Prolonged follow-up was recommended as late recurrences of CIN lesions have been reported. The guidelines also recognised that simultaneous colposcopy combined with cytology adds very minimally to the detection rate of recurrent or persistent CIN.

Another parameter used in the past to monitor women for post-treatment CIN2/CIN3 is the presence of positive resection margin at operation. Several studies have shown that a positive resection margin status is associated with 20–25% recurrent or persistent CIN3.

However, although this originally seemed to be a useful indicator, the results of several studies show that its sensitivity and specificity for recurrent CIN3 is highly variable and depends heavily on the operation technique, operation setting and the gynaecologist performing the operation (Chua and Hjerpe, 1997; Jain *et al.*, 2001; Paraskevaidis *et al.*, 2001).

Therefore, follow-up procedures cannot be tailored according to the involvement of the resection margins.

HPV TESTING FOR CLINICAL USE

Infection with high-risk human papillomavirus (hrHPV) has been implicated as the major cause of cervical cancer (Walboomers *et al.*, 1999). It is now well accepted that hrHPV is necessary for the development, maintenance and progression of CIN lesions to cervical cancer (Bosch *et al.*, 2002). It exerts its oncogenic actions through the oncoproteins E6 and E7, which interact with the cell cycle control proteins p53 and pRB, respectively, leading to uncontrolled cell proliferation, immortalisation and genetic instability. This results in additional changes in the cellular genome necessary for transformation of cervical epithelial cells and progression to cervical cancer. Based on this knowledge, the conclusion is justified that the true precursor lesion for cervical cancer is the hrHPV-positive CIN lesion of which hrHPV-positive CIN3 is the most advanced. Hence, it follows that the presence of hrHPV can be used for several clinical purposes including the management of CIN lesions.

Based on epidemiological and phylogenetic data, 15 hrHPV types have now been recognised (Muñoz *et al.*, 2003). The question can be posed whether these all carry a similar risk for CIN3/cervical carcinoma. A recent meta-analysis performed by the IARC comparing CIN2/CIN3 with cervical squamous cell carcinoma (SCC) indicates that this is not the case (Clifford *et al.*, 2003). Given a CIN2/CIN3 lesion, the risk of cervical carcinoma is (in decreasing order of magnitude) increased in the case of an infection with HPV 16, 18 or 45. Interestingly, population-based data from the POBASCAM study (prospective POpulation-BAsed cervical cancer SCreening trial in AMsterdam) for implementation of DNA-based hrHPV testing by consensus primer GP5+/6+ polymerase chain reaction (PCR) (Bulkmans *et al.*, 2004) revealed that the risk of CIN3 is increased for HPV 16 and 33, but not for HPV 18 and HPV 45 (Bulkmans *et al.*, 2005). Combined, these data imply that, during different morphological phases of the oncogenic process, different HPV types have different oncogenic potential. Thus, HPV 33 might have a lower oncogenic potential, in terms of progression from CIN3 to cervical carcinoma, than HPV 18 and 45. On the contrary, the risk posed by HPV 33 in inducing CIN3 seems higher than that of HPV 18 and 45. HPV 16 exerts the highest risk for both CIN3 and cervical carcinoma. However, long-term follow-up studies should be awaited to further strengthen the conclusions based on cross-sectional data.

Tests that detect hrHPV types as a pool can easily be used in clinical settings and, consequently, pooled hrHPV detection is the clinical practice today. The tests that detect all relevant hrHPV types by consensus PCR include GP 5+/6+ PCR (Jacobs *et al.*, 1995), PGMY09/11 (Gravitt *et al.*, 1998), SPF10 (Kleter *et al.*, 1998, 1999) and MWAmplicor (Roche). Another assay, based on hybridisation of target DNA with RNA probes followed by signal amplification, is the Hybrid Capture 2 (i.e. HC2; Digene) test (Terry *et al.*, 2001). This method detects the 13 most common hrHPV types. These tests are referred to here as general hrHPV tests (ghrHPV). Before these ghrHPV tests can be used in a clinical setting, they should have been validated in clinical studies (Snijders *et al.*, 2003). Ultrasensitive tests with a very high analytical sensitivity such as the SPF10 system and methods with equal sensitivities are likely to have a low clinical specificity for detecting CIN3, because they detect too many hrHPV infections in normal smears that are clinically irrelevant. Tests with a lower analytical sensitivity such as GP5+/6+ PCR, PGMY09/11 and HC2 have a much better clinical specificity and are presently used in clinical settings (Lorincz and Richart, 1999; Bulkmans *et al.*, 2004). The lower number of hrHPV-positive test results detected by these systems, while not missing CIN3, makes these tests useful for monitoring women with recurrent or persistent CIN2/CIN3.

GHRHPV TESTING FOR RISK ASSESSMENT OF POST-TREATMENT CIN3

Presently, most countries follow the strategy of ending the follow-up of women treated for CIN3 when three consecutive normal smears are found at 6, 12 and 24 months. Several studies have addressed the question whether ghrHPV testing can be of help in detecting recurrent or persistent CIN2/CIN3 (reviewed by Paraskevaidis *et al.*, 2004; Zielinski *et al.*, 2004). The advantage of ghrHPV testing is its high sensitivity for detecting CIN3 and its high negative predictive value for CIN3. Evaluating the results in the literature, all meta-analyses show that hrHPV testing in combination with cytology has higher sensitivity (range 89–96%), negative predictive value (range 98–100%), specificity (range 77–84%) and positive predictive value (range 38–54%) for CIN3, than sole HPV testing, HPV testing in combination with resection margin status and cytology alone (Paraskevaidis *et al.*, 2004; Zielinski *et al.*, 2004). Thus, the combined test (ghrHPV testing in combina-

tion with cytology) increases the sensitivity of detecting persistent or recurrent CIN2/3 and increases the negative predictive value, thereby sorting out women with little or no risk for CIN3/cervical cancer. Combined cytology and ghrHPV testing proved more effective than either test alone or resection margin status (Izumi *et al.*, 2001; Nobbenhuis *et al.*, 2001; Zielinski *et al.*, 2003).

GHRHPV TESTING TO REDUCE FOLLOW-UP VISITS

Our own follow-up studies of women treated for CIN3/cervical carcinoma by either cytology or ghrHPV testing show that both tests do miss CIN3/cervical carcinoma, although very few. Combining cytology and ghrHPV testing yields the best results. Moreover, cervical cytology has the disadvantage that it is not reliable at 3 months because it may show atypical cells as part of the healing process that might be interpreted as neoplastic but will disappear in over 50% of cases (Nobbenhuis *et al.*, 2001). Conversely, ghrHPV testing does not have this disadvantage.

Also, based on meta-analysis studies (Paraskevaidis *et al.*, 2004; Zielinski *et al.*, 2004) and our own experience (Elfgren *et al.*, 1996; Nobbenhuis *et al.*, 2001; Zielinski *et al.*, 2003), we recommend monitoring women for CIN3/cervical cancer with cervical cytology in combination with ghrHPV testing at 6 months. Women who test positive by cytology and/or hrHPV should be referred for colposcopy and may need further treatment for persistent or recurrent CIN3. However, 70% of women treated for CIN3 will have both negative cytology and a negative HPV tests at 6 months' follow-up. Because these women have a risk of persistent or recurrent CIN approaching zero, they can omit the 12-month follow-up visit. We recommend a 24-month examination with both ghrHPV testing and cytology as these women are at high risk of another high-risk HPV infection in that period (Nobbenhuis *et al.*, 1999). If both tests are negative at 24 months, they may be referred to the routine screening programme.

IS HPV TYPING NECESSARY FOR MONITORING POST-TREATMENT CIN3?

In general, HPV typing of CIN3 and cervical cancer is not necessary because the treatment will always be the same. So for clinical use, a ghrHPV test is sufficient. However, additional HPV typing has some small advantages and perhaps some prognostic value. Demonstrating the same HPV type in the post-treatment specimen as in the treated CIN3 lesion may indicate recurrent HPV infection, and this indicates that the women apparently cannot cope with this particular HPV type (Carrington *et al.*, 2005) and might require more intense follow-up. In this context, differences in risk of CIN3/

cervical carcinoma by different HPV types seem important. The highest risk of CIN3/cervical carcinoma is posed by HPV 16, and it would be interesting to evaluate whether HPV 16 and perhaps also HPV 18 are more present in recurrent or persistent CIN3 than in primary CIN3 (Clifford *et al.*, 2003; Bulkmans *et al.*, 2005). However, no systematic analysis of hrHPV types in primary and post-treatment CIN3 has been published to date.

ROLE OF VIRAL LOAD

Several authors have shown that an increased viral load for HPV 16 is associated with an increased risk of high-grade CIN and cervical carcinoma (Ylitalo *et al.*, 2000; Josefsson *et al.*, 2000; Lorincz *et al.*, 2002; van Duin *et al.*, 2002). As the risk of a positive ghrHPV test for CIN3/cervical carcinoma is rather low, the question arises whether the positive predictive value of an HPV test can be improved by using viral load as an indicator for CIN3/cervical carcinoma. Previous studies on viral load are difficult to compare because of the use of different techniques. Thus, HC2, a semi-quantitative technique measuring relative light units (Lorincz *et al.*, 2002), and quantitative real-time PCR assays (Josefsson *et al.*, 2000; van Duin *et al.*, 2002) have been used to determine the viral load in the past. In contrast to quantitative techniques, semi-quantitative methods have the advantage of being less laborious and, consequently, can be used for high-volume applications and have often been used in clinical and epidemiological studies. These semi-quantitative studies suggest a relationship between the presence of cervical lesions and viral load. However, as they do not adjust for the cellular input, these results should be interpreted with caution. Quantitative type-specific real-time PCR assays are superior in viral load assessment. The results of studies using real-time PCR assays are mostly restricted to HPV type 16 and show that an increased viral load confers an increased risk for high-grade CIN lesions and cervical carcinoma (Josefsson *et al.*, 2000; Lorincz *et al.*, 2002; van Duin *et al.*, 2002). With the advent of type-specific real-time PCR assays it is now possible to assess viral load in scrapes containing hrHPV types.

We have initiated viral load analysis for six hrHPV types by type-specific real-time PCR in a cohort of 44 102 women participating in the POBASCAM study (Bulkmans *et al.*, 2004). In a first analysis, we used baseline cervical scrapings from women with normal cytology who were positive for HPV 16, 18, 31 or 33 DNA as a reference to define various viral load thresholds (25th, 33rd and 50th percentiles). The resulting viral load threshold values were subsequently validated on a large series of abnormal cervical scrapes of women with underlying CIN lesions containing one of these four hrHPV types (Snijders *et al.*, in press). All women with CIN3 had viral load levels above the 33rd percentile threshold of women with normal cytology containing the corresponding hrHPV type (sensitivity 100%). On the other hand, about 10% and 22% of women with CIN3 had viral load levels below the 50th and 67th percentile thresholds. From the data, it can be concluded that, although women with CIN3 generally display increased viral loads, there exists a substantial overlap between viral DNA load levels in women with and without CIN3. Therefore, viral load analysis will allow the distinction of at maximum 33% of women without clinically relevant hrHPV infections. Thus, it will not be practical to use viral load in monitoring recurrent/residual CIN lesions.

VALUE OF HRHPV E6/E7 MRNA DETECTION IN THE MANAGEMENT OF CIN LESIONS

It is widely established that the viral oncogenes E6 and E7 drive the oncogenic process mediated by hrHPV and that persistent expression of E6 and E7 is pivotal for the maintenance of the malignant phenotype of cervical cancer cells. Hence, viral oncogene expression may provide a valuable marker for detecting clinically relevant HPV infections, i.e. those associated with an increased relative risk of CIN3/cervical carcinoma. The recent introduction of preservation media for the collection of cervical scrapes for liquid-based cytology purposes has opened possibilities for HPV transcript analysis as these media preserve RNA sufficiently for amplification purposes (Cuschieri *et al.*, 2005). Interestingly, data from some small studies indeed suggest that hrHPV mRNA testing may distinguish clinically relevant from irrelevant hrHPV infections, and there are data suggesting that lack of E6/E7 mRNA in HPV DNA-positive cytologically normal cervical scrapes predicts future loss of HPV DNA (Cuschieri *et al.*, 2004; Molden *et al.*, 2005a,b). For the management of CIN lesions, detection of E6/E7 transcripts might be useful in the future in addition to HPV DNA testing. It may distinguish hrHPV DNA-positive infections, which are associated with CIN3/cervical cancer (E6/E7 transcript positive), and clinically regressing lesions or absence of lesions (E6/E7 transcript negative). As such, it might even better distinguish recurrent CIN3 from tissue repair as seen at 3 months after treatment of CIN3. However, the present data about the relation between HPV E6/E7 transcripts and the presence of ≥ CIN3 lesions are too limited to draw firm conclusions.

IN CONCLUSION

The detection of hrHPV is important not only for the diagnosis, but also for the follow-up of premalignant lesions of the cervix. New techniques are likely to render hrHPV testing more specific and may select patients that are at high risk of persistent or recurrent disease. At the same time, follow-up of low-risk patients may be reduced.

REFERENCES

Alvarez RD, Helm CW, Edwards RP *et al.* (1994) Prospective randomized trial of LLETZ versus laser ablation in patients with cervical intraepithelial neoplasia. *Gynecologic Oncology* 52 (2): 175–179.

Bigrigg A, Haffenden DK, Sheehan AL *et al.* (1994) Efficacy and safety of large-loop excision of the transformation zone. *Lancet* 343 (8888): 32–34.

Bollen LJ, Tjong-A-Hung SP, van der Velden J *et al.* (1999) Prediction of recurrent and residual cervical dysplasia by human papillomavirus detection among patients with abnormal cytology. *Gynecologic Oncology* 72 (2): 199–201.

Bosch FX, Lorincz A, Muñoz N *et al.* (2002) The causal relation between human papillomavirus and cervical cancer. *Journal of Clinical Pathology* 55 (4): 244–265.

Bulkmans NWJ, Rozendaal L, Snijders PJF *et al.* (2004) POBASCAM, a population-based randomised controlled trial for implementation of high-risk HPV testing in cervical screening: design, methods and baseline data of 44 102 women. *International Journal of Cancer* 110: 94–101.

Bulkmans NWJ, Bleeker MCG, Berkhof J *et al.* (2005) Prevalence of types 16 and 33 is increased in high-risk human papillomavirus positive women with cervical intraepithelial neoplasia grade 2 or worse. *International Journal of Cancer* 117: 177–181.

Carrington M, Wang S, Martin MP *et al.* (2005) Hierarchy of resistance to cervical neoplasia mediated by combinations of killer immunoglobulin-like receptor and human leukocyte antigen loci. *Journal of Experimental Medicine* 201: 1069–1075.

Chua KL, Hjerpe A (1997) Human papillomavirus analysis as a prognostic marker following conization of the cervix uteri. *Gynecologic Oncology* 66 (1): 108–113.

Clifford GM, Smith JS, Aguado T *et al.* (2003) Comparison of HPV type distribution in high-grade cervical lesions and cervical cancer: a meta-analysis. *British Journal of Cancer* 89 (1): 101–105.

Cuschieri KS, Whitley MJ, Cubie HA (2004) Human papillomavirus type specific DNA and RNA persistence — implications for cervical disease progression and monitoring. *Journal of Medical Virology* 73: 65–70.

Cuschieri KS, Beattle G, Hassan S *et al.* (2005) Assessment of human papillomavirus mRNA detection over time in cervical specimens collected in liquid based cytology medium. *Journal of Virological Methods* 124: 211–215.

Elfgren K, Bistoletti P, Dillner L *et al.* (1996) Conization for cervical intraepithelial neoplasia is followed by disappearance of human papillomavirus deoxyribonucleic acid and a decline in serum and cervical mucus antibodies against human papillomavirus antigens. *American Journal of Obstetrics and Gynecology* 174 (3): 937–942. Reviewed *British Journal of Cancer* (2001) 84 (6): 796–801.

Gravitt PE, Peyton CL, Apple RJ *et al.* (1998) Genotyping of 27 human papillomavirus types by using L1 consensus PCR products by a single-hybridization, reverse line blot detection method. *Journal of Clinical Microbiology* 36 (10): 3020–3027.

Izumi T, Kyushima N, Genda T *et al.* (2001) Margin clearance and HPV infection do not influence the cure rates of early neoplasia of the uterine cervix by laser conization. *European Journal of Gynaecological Oncology* 21 (3): 251–254.

Jacobs MV, de Roda Husman AM, van den Brule AJ *et al.* (1995) Group-specific differentiation between high- and low-risk human papillomavirus genotypes by general primer-mediated PCR and two cocktails of oligonucleotide probes. *Journal of Clinical Microbiology* 33 (4): 901–905.

Jain S, Tseng CJ, Horng SG *et al.* (2001) Negative predictive value of human papillomavirus test following conization of the cervix uteri. *Gynecologic Oncology* 82 (1): 177–180.

Josefsson AM, Magnusson PK, Ylitalo N *et al.* (2000) Viral load of human papilloma virus 16 as a determinant for development of cervical carcinoma in situ: a nested case-control study. *Lancet* 355 (9222): 2189–2193.

Kleter B, van Doorn LJ, Schrauwen L *et al.* (1999) Development and clinical evaluation of a highly sensitive PCR-reverse hybridization line probe assay for detection and identification of anogenital human papillomavirus. *Journal of Clinical Microbiology* 37 (8): 2508–2517.

Kleter B, van Doorn LJ, ter Schegget J *et al.* (1998) Novel short-fragment PCR assay for highly sensitive broad-spectrum detection of anogenital human papillomaviruses. *American Journal of Pathology* 153 (6): 1731–1739.

Lorincz AT, Richart RM (1999) Human papillomavirus DNA testing as an adjunct to cytology in cervical screening programs. *Lancet* 354 (9172): 20–25. Reviewed in *Archives of Pathology and Laboratory Medicine* 127 (8): 959–968.

Lorincz AT, Castle PE, Sherman ME *et al.* (2002) Viral load of human papillomavirus and risk of CIN3 or cervical cancer. *Lancet* 360 (9328): 228–229.

Mitchell MF, Tortolero-Luna G, Cook E *et al.* (1998) A randomized clinical trial of cryotherapy, laser vaporization, and loop electrosurgical excision for treatment of squamous intraepithelial lesions of the cervix. *Obstetrics and Gynecology* 92 (5): 737–744.

Molden T, Nygard JF, Kraus I *et al.* (2005a) Predicting CIN2+ when detecting HPV mRNA and DNA by PreTect HPV-Proofer and consensus PCR: a 2-year follow-up of women with ASCUS or LSIL Pap smear. *International Journal of Cancer* 114: 973–976.

Molden T, Kraus I, Karlsen F *et al.* (2005b) Comparison of human papillomavirus messenger RNA and DNA detection: a cross-sectional study of 4136 women > 30 years of age with a 2-year follow-up of high grade squamous intraepithelial lesion. *Cancer Epidemiology Biomarkers and Prevention* 14: 367–372.

Muñoz N, Bosch FX, de Sanjose S *et al.* (2003) Epidemiologic classification of human papillomavirus types associated with cervical cancer. *New England Journal of Medicine* 348: 518–527.

Nobbenhuis MA, Walboomers JM, Helmerhorst TJ *et al.* (1999) Relation of human papillomavirus status to cervical lesions and consequences for cervical-cancer screening: a prospective study *Lancet* 354: 20–25.

Nobbenhuis MA, Meijer CJ, van den Brule AJ *et al.* (2001) Addition of high-risk HPV testing improves the current guidelines on follow-up after treatment For cervical intraepithelial neoplasia. *British Journal of Cancer* 84: 796–801.

Nuovo J, Melnikow J, Willan AR *et al.* (2000) Treatment outcomes for squamous intraepithelial lesions. *International Journal of Gynaecological Obstetrics* 68 (1): 25–33.

Paraskevaidis E, Koliopoulos G, Alamanos Y *et al.* (2001) Human papillomavirus testing and the outcome of treatment for cervical intraepithelial neoplasia. *Obstetrics and Gynecology* 98 (5 Pt 1): 833–836.

Paraskevaidis E, Arbyn M, Sotiriadis A *et al.* (2004) The role of HPV DNA testing in the follow-up period after treatment for CIN: a systematic review of the literature. *Cancer Treatment Review* 30 (2): 205–211.

Snijders PJ, van den Brule AJ, Meijer CJ (2003) The clinical relevance of human papillomavirus testing: relationship between analytical and clinical sensitivity. *Journal of Pathology* 201: 1–6.

Snijders PJ, Hogewoning CJA, Hesselink AT *et al.* (2006) Determination of viral load thresholds in cervical scrapings to rule out CIN3 in HPV 16, 18, 31 and 33-positive women with normal cytology. *International Journal of Cancer* (in press).

Terry G, Ho L, Londesborough P *et al.* (2001) Detection of high-risk HPV types by the hybrid capture 2 test. *Journal of Medical Virology* 65 (1): 155–162.

van Duin M, Snijders PJ, Schrijnemakers HF *et al.* (2002) Human papillomavirus 16 load in normal and abnormal cervical scrapes: an indicator of CIN II/III and viral clearance. *International Journal of Cancer* 98 (4): 590–595.

Walboomers JM, Jacobs MV, Manos MM *et al.* (1999) Human papillomavirus is a necessary cause of invasive cervical cancer worldwide. *Journal of Pathology* 189 (1): 12–19.

Wright TC, Jr, Cox JT, Massad LS *et al.* (2003) American Society for Colposcopy and Cervical Pathology 2001 Consensus Guidelines for the Management of Women With Cervical Intraepithelial Neoplasia. *American Journal of Obstetrics and Gynecology* 189 (1): 295–304.

Ylitalo N, Sorensen P, Josefsson AM *et al.* (2000) Consistent high viral load of human papillomavirus 16 and risk of cervical carcinoma in situ: a nested case–control study. *Lancet* 355 (9222): 2194–2198.

Zielinski GD, Rozendaal L, Voorhorst FJ *et al.* (2003) HPV testing can reduce the number of follow-up visits in women treated for cervical intraepithelial neoplasia grade 3. *Gynecologic Oncology* 91 (1): 67–73.

Zielinski GD, Bais AG, Helmerhorst TJ *et al.* (2004) HPV testing and monitoring of women after treatment of CIN 3: review of the literature and meta-analysis. *Obstetrics and Gynecology Surveys* 59 (7): 543–553.

CHAPTER 34

The management of cervical premalignancy and malignancy in pregnancy

Theresa Freeman-Wang and Patrick G. Walker

INTRODUCTION

Pregnancy is a common physiological condition and cervical intraepithelial neoplasia (CIN) a common premalignant pathological condition, both of which may coincidentally affect women of reproductive age. There are several misconceptions about the significance of CIN in pregnancy. The risk of developing CIN is the same for pregnant and non-pregnant women. Cytological dyskaryosis suggesting CIN found in pregnancy has been reported at 1.26–2.2% (Lurain *et al.*, 1979). Most (86%) are low-grade abnormalities. Histologically diagnosed CIN is found in 0.19–0.53% of pregnant women (Yoonessi *et al.*, 1982).

While invasive cancer of the cervix is uncommon in countries with a well-organised cervical screening programme, it remains the most common gynaecological malignancy encountered in pregnancy. The reported incidence varies from 1.6 to 10.6 cases per 10 000 pregnancies (Hacker *et al.*, 1982), depending on whether women with CIN and those who are postpartum patients are included. Approximately 1% of cervical cancer patients are pregnant at the time of diagnosis.

PHYSIOLOGICAL CHANGES IN PREGNANCY

Pregnancy is one of the three occasions in life when there is a significant increase in the area and rate of squamous metaplasia of the cervical epithelium (Figs 34.1–34.6).

The other times in female life when metaplasia is active are in late fetal life and adolescence (see Chapters 5 and 6). High circulating levels of estrogen encourage eversion of the endocervical canal with its original columnar epithelium and hypertrophy of the underlying cervical stroma. This helps to explain the change in shape and consistency of the cervix that occurs as pregnancy progresses. In addition, there is an associated increase in vascularity, causing a classic bluish tinge to the cervical epithelium (Chadwick's sign). A detailed description of the epithelial changes within the pregnant cervix is given in Chapter 7.

CERVICAL CYTOLOGY IN PREGNANCY

Difficulties in interpretation

The physiological changes occurring within the cervical epithelium in pregnancy along with the increase in endocervical mucus can make cytological interpretation difficult. The cytologist has to be aware of specific cytological changes that occur in pregnancy, such as decidualisation, the Arias–Stella reaction and the predominance of an intermediate cell pattern within the smear. This may explain the lower sensitivity of exfoliative cytology at this time and, for this reason, some advocate avoiding taking a cervical smear in pregnancy. Others state that the smear taker, anxious to avoid bleeding from the more vascular pregnant cervix, may be reticent in obtaining a representative sample of transformation zone elements. In addition, depending on gestation, lax vaginal walls and the often posterior position of the cervix may make its full visualisation difficult. Sampling errors in this population account for at least 50% of false-negative smears (Shield *et al.*, 1987). These arguments, however, do not preclude a properly obtained sample being adequately assessed by an efficient cytologist. However, if a smear is taken, it is important to inform the woman that she may have a lightly blood-stained discharge afterwards. As for non-pregnant women, it is also necessary to inform her as to when and how the results will be communicated and make her aware that there is a 1 in 10 to 1 in 12 chance that the smear will be reported as other than normal. This does not mean that she has cancer or that the pregnancy is in any way threatened.

Cytology in pregnancy as part of a screening programme

In some screening programmes for cervical cancer such as in the UK, the traditional advice was that a smear should be taken opportunistically at the first antenatal visit, despite the difficulties of cytological interpretation. With the introduction

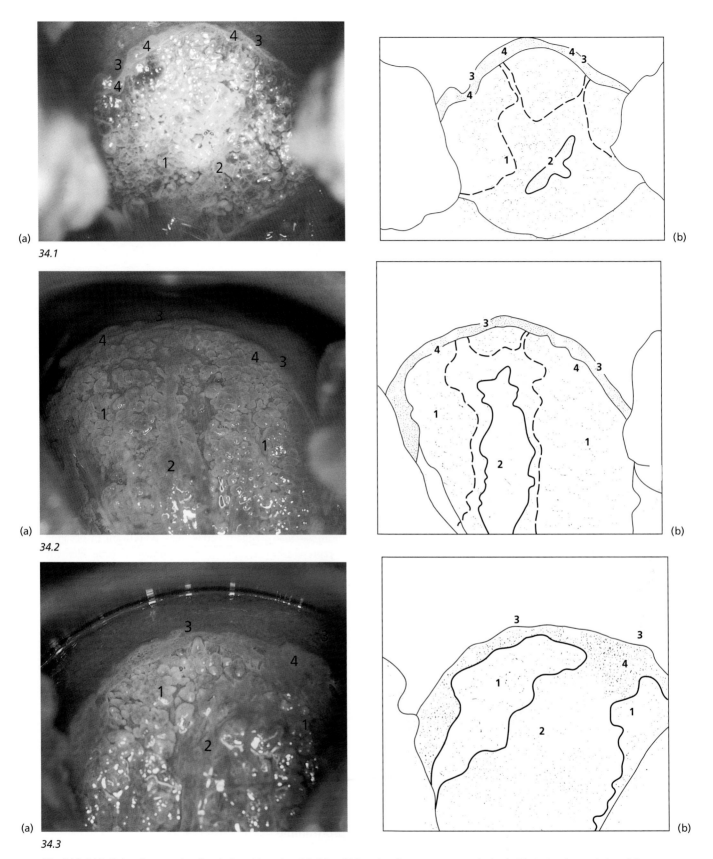

(a)

34.1

(b)

(a)

34.2

(b)

(a)

34.3

(b)

Figs 34.1–34.3 Colpophotographs of a primigravid cervix at 12, 26 and 36 weeks of pregnancy respectively. At 12 weeks, the cervix is mainly composed of original columnar epithelium (1), with a small island of metaplastic squamous epithelium (2). At 26 weeks (Fig. 34.2), this island (2) has enlarged principally by fusion of the adjacent columnar epithelium at (1) and is in the second stage of the metaplastic process where there is already fusion between the columnar villi. At 36 weeks (Fig. 34.3), the new metaplastic epithelium (2) has extended to the original squamocolumnar junction (3). Some columnar villi have not undergone complete metaplastic transformation and are seen in an arrested stage at (1). A rim of squamous metaplastic tissue (4) is already visible by 12 and 26 weeks. From Singer A. and Monaghan J.M. (2000) *Lower Genital Tract Precancer.* Oxford: Blackwell Publishing, with kind permission.

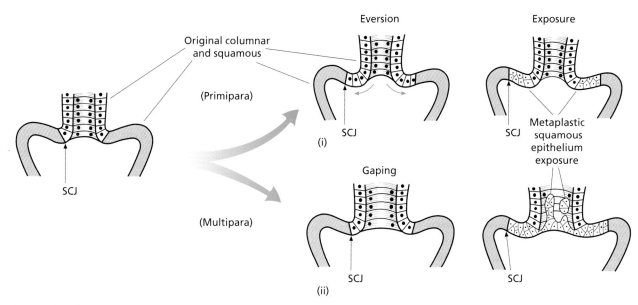

Fig. 34.4 Physiological mechanisms operating in the cervix during pregnancy.

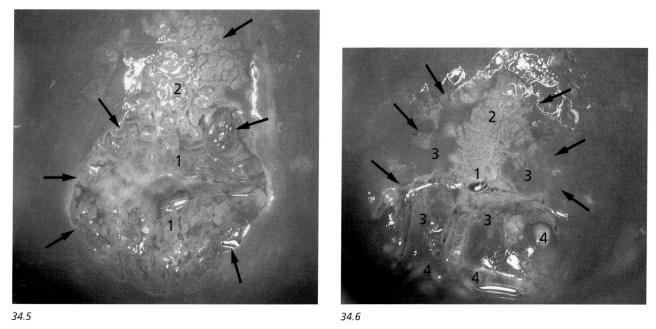

34.5

34.6

Figs 34.5 and 34.6 Colpophotographs of the primigravid cervix at 12 and 36 weeks of gestation. The original squamocolumnar junction (arrowed) has extended outwards onto the ectocervical portion as the pregnancy progresses and has resulted in the development of metaplastic squamous transformation (2 and 3) of the exposed columnar epithelium. Further, on the anterior lip, an area of fine mosaic and punctation can be seen, which could be mistaken for a neoplastic change. However, these changes are representative of active squamous metaplasia that has occurred very early in pregnancy, i.e. before the 12th gestational week, and has become accentuated as pregnancy has progressed. This tissue was confirmed to be metaplastic by biopsy of this area in the postpartum period.

of the British National Health Service Cervical Screening Programme (NHSCSP) call and recall programme in 1988, the proportion of eligible women having smears within the programme increased from 40% to 80–85%. Associated with this improved coverage, fewer women needed to have opportunistic smears as it became apparent that cytology was less sensitive in the pregnant woman.

As a consequence, the British recommend the following in relation to cervical screening in pregnancy (Luesley *et al.*, 2004):
1 Unless a pregnant woman with a negative history has gone beyond 5 years without a smear, then having a smear should be postponed until the postpartum period.
2 If a woman has been called for screening and she is pregnant, the smear should be deferred to the postpartum period.

3 If a previous smear was abnormal and, in the interim, the woman becomes pregnant, the smear should not be delayed.

Cronje *et al.* (2000) argued that, in developing countries, pregnancy may provide a unique opportunity for cervical screening. They too were concerned about the apparent low sensitivity of cytology in this group and therefore looked at a combination of cytology with either cervicography or visual inspection with acetic acid (VIA). In their study, 842 pregnant women were screened using cytology, cervicography and VIA. Cytological smears were abnormal in 1.4% of cases, cervicography in 6.3% and VIA in 14.3%. A combination of tests increased the overall sensitivity in detecting epithelial abnormalities by 30% and 52% respectively. However, cervicography is expensive and not readily available. Although VIA may lead to overdiagnosis and greater anxiety at an already vulnerable time, some suggest it may still prove a more pragmatic screening solution in low-resource settings with high rates of cervical cancer.

HPV and pregnancy

The prevalence of human papillomavirus (HPV) infection in pregnancy varies between 5.4% and 68.8%. The population with the highest risk is those under the age of 26 years (Arena *et al.*, 2002). A number of different opinions emerge from the literature regarding the possibility of vertical maternal–fetal virus transmission. The data reported in relation to the association between HPV and pregnancy are highly discordant. This discrepancy is a result of the diagnostic techniques used in various studies, the clinical history of the pregnant woman and the period of pregnancy when the sample is collected. Possible perinatal vertical HPV transmission was suspected when it was found that caesarean section delivery was not effective in protecting children from maternal–fetal transmission (Smith *et al.*, 1995, 2004; Tseng *et al.*, 1998). Armbruster-Morares *et al.* (1994) detected the presence of HPV DNA sequences in amniotic fluids obtained at different times during pregnancy by means of transabdominal amniocentesis, using the polymerase chain reaction (PCR). This confirmed the presence of HPV DNA in the amniotic fluid in 24 of 37 pregnant women with cervical lesions. Of these, 13 were HPV type 16 and five were HPV type 18. A correlation between viral DNA amplification and the grade of CIN was also noted (Malone *et al.*, 1988).

The possibility of maternal–fetal transmission of the virus is possibly important as a main factor responsible for the rare condition of juvenile laryngeal papillomatosis. A number of authors report an initial presence of HPV in newborns which often disappears within 6 months after birth (Armbruster-Morares *et al.*, 1994; Pakarian *et al.*, 1994; Cason *et al.*, 1995).

Cervical deciduosis (see Chapter 8)

This benign condition results from a decidual reaction of the stroma. Colposcopically, there may be evidence of intense acetowhite change following the application of dilute acetic acid. A mosaic surface pattern may also be evident. Coupled with the physiological changes of pregnancy, deciduosis may mimic invasive disease (Chapter 8). Making the diagnosis can pose a challenge. Cytologically oedematous superficial squames are seen. Characteristically, on histological assessment, widely expanded cells are seen beneath a single layer of cuboidal cells.

THE ABNORMAL SMEAR IN PREGNANCY

Being told of an abnormal smear result is associated with a great deal of anxiety. There is a perceived threat to one's mortality, fertility and sexuality and an associated loss of body image, as well as the added concern for the unborn fetus. Correct diagnosis as to the degree of abnormality, the exclusion of malignancy and the appropriate planning of management in relation to the abnormal result are therefore particularly important. Recently, Massad *et al.* (2005) have published specific guidelines for the management of abnormal cytology results in pregnancy which were developed at the 2001 Consensus Conference on Management of Cervical Cytological Abnormalities in CIN. CIN is not treated during pregnancy except to exclude the presence of early invasive cancer; surveillance using cytology is sufficient for most pregnant women with abnormal Pap smear tests and the management guidelines are discussed below.

Colposcopy in pregnancy

In the recent literature, Paraskevaidis *et al.* (2002) set out to investigate the evolution of CIN and to evaluate the safety of cytological and colposcopic surveillance of women with CIN during pregnancy. Ninety-eight women with antenatal cytological and/or colposcopic impression of CIN were followed up during pregnancy with cytology and colposcopy every 2 months. A cytological and colposcopic re-evaluation was performed 2 months post partum, and large loop excision of the transformation zone (LLETZ), or loop electrosurgical excision procedure (LEEP), as it is known on the North American continent, was carried out if appropriate. Punch or loop biopsies were taken only if there was suspicion of microinvasion. In 14 of 39 (35.9%) and in 25 of 52 (48.1%) women with an antenatal impression of CIN1 and CIN2–3, respectively, there was postnatal impression of regression. Seven women with findings suspicious of microinvasion underwent small loop biopsies during pregnancy, but early stromal invasion (< 1 mm) was seen in just one case. There was one more case of microinvasion (1.5 mm of stromal invasion) diagnosed postnatally in which the antenatal impression was of CIN3. Eighty-four per cent of the women with regression compared with 67.3% of the women with stable disease or

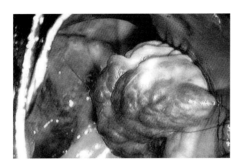

Fig. 34.7 A vaginal varicosity, not uncommon in pregnancy, making visualisation of the cervix difficult.

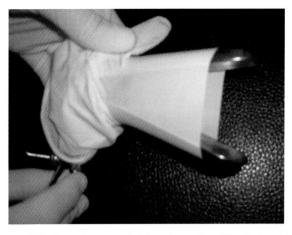

Fig. 34.8 Placing a glove over a lubricated speculum. The distal end of the finger stall is removed, enabling, when the speculum is inserted into the vagina, a clear view of the cervix. The prolapsed vaginal walls are pushed aside when the speculum blades are opened and the attached rubber of the glove acts as a protective wall.

progression had a vaginal delivery ($P = 0.057$). The authors concluded that there is a considerable regression rate of CIN after pregnancy, possibly attributable to the loss of the dysplastic cervical epithelium during cervical 'ripening' and vaginal delivery. However, without biopsy confirmation of the epithelial abnormality in pregnancy and with the possibility of an overcall of cytological features in the pregnancy smear, the true regression rates may have been overestimated by this study. The authors' conclusions were that frequent cytological and colposcopic evaluation seemed to be safe and small loop biopsies are recommended in suspected cases of possible microinvasion. This was in concordance with other earlier studies (DePetrillo *et al.*, 1975; Talebian *et al.*, 1976; Kohan *et al.*, 1980; Economos *et al.*, 1993).

The physiological changes of pregnancy (with the increased rate of squamous metaplasia, the increase in vascularity and the changes in the size and shape of the cervix) together conspire to make colposcopic assessment a particular challenge. Benign lesions may appear to be suspicious of abnormality, while active squamous metaplasia may be associated with a fine mosaic or punctate surface pattern that may be indistinguishable from a low-grade CIN (Figs 34.4 and 34.5).

Performing colposcopy in pregnancy produces particular technical challenges. The vaginal walls are often lax, and there may be vulval and vaginal varicosities (Fig. 34.7). When examining, it is recommended that a large speculum be used. To keep the vaginal walls apart, a latex glove with the tip of the finger portion removed may be used to cover the speculum blades. The speculum is then opened once inserted into the vagina. A condom instead of the finger of a glove may also be used (Fig. 34.8).

Punch biopsy or not — the evidence and the philosophy?

Economos *et al.* (1993) looked at 612 pregnant women with abnormal cytology retrospectively. Of their patients, 112 underwent surgical procedures that provided a surgical specimen to compare with the cervical smear, colposcopic impression and directed biopsies. Cytology and colposcopic impression had a

91% concordance within one degree of severity. Colposcopic impression and directed biopsies had a 95% concordance within one degree of severity. No cases of invasive carcinoma were missed. Complications of biopsies were minimal. There were three cases of delayed bleeding that resolved with the application of pressure. The authors concluded that directed biopsies (Figs 34.9 and 34.10) are a safe and reliable method of evaluating pregnant women referred with abnormal smears.

In their series of 117 pregnant women and 234 control subjects, Baldauf *et al.* (1995) also looked at the reliability of colposcopy and directed biopsies in pregnancy. They found the sensitivity of cytology to be similar in both groups and that colposcopy was significantly less frequently unsatisfactory than in the control group (12.8% vs. 23.1%, $P = 0.023$); directed biopsies were equally reliable in both groups. Other authors have all found similar results (Ortiz *et al.*, 1971; Benedet *et al.*, 1977; Hellberg *et al.*, 1987; Kashimura *et al.*, 1991; Campion *et al.*, 1993; Baldauf *et al.*, 1996; Madej *et al.*, 1996; Vlahos *et al.*, 2002). Importantly, they all stressed the necessity of the colposcopist being familiar with the physiological changes of pregnancy. A lack of experience can lead to overestimation of the severity of the lesion and a mistaken diagnosis of invasive disease for pregnancy-associated changes.

However, while several studies point to the relative safety of directed biopsies, the value of this in pregnancy remains open to debate. In the UK, there has remained a reticence to incorporate directed biopsies as a standard part of the management algorithm.

The evidence suggests that CIN does not as a rule progress during pregnancy (Bertini-Oliveira *et al.*, 1982; Kaminski *et al.*, 1992; Nahhas *et al.*, 1993; Mikhail *et al.*, 1995; Shivvers *et al.*, 1997; Guerra *et al.*, 1998; Yost *et al.*, 1999; Murta *et al.*, 2002). When considering the natural history of the development

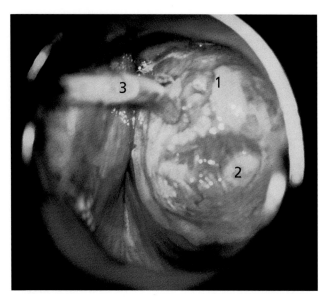

Fig. 34.9 A punch biopsy (3) about to remove an area of atypical epithelium at (1) and (2). The cervix was that of a woman at 24 weeks' gestation with a severely dyskaryotic smear.

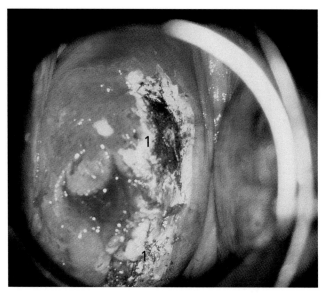

Fig. 34.10 Haemostasis after the biopsy has been achieved by the application of two silver nitrate applicators for a minimum of 3 minutes to both biopsy sites (1) and (1).

of cervical cancer (see Chapter 19), delaying treatment for CIN to the postpartum period is safe and the preferred option. If there is serious concern of the presence of early or frankly invasive disease, a substantial biopsy will be required. Thus, there is no obvious advantage to the liberal use of usually small directed punch biopsies, which may miss the invasive carcinoma or fail to give a representative sample of the most severe lesion. Multiple punch biopsies may also cause trauma and significant bleeding.

When malignancy is suspected, a possibly better option is to perform a knife wedge biopsy of the worst-affected area of epithelium identified colposcopically. This is usually performed under general anaesthesia with the use of suture material for the wedge area and local infiltration with a solution of xylocaine and dilute adrenaline (1:80 000) to aid haemostasis (Figs 34.11–34.14). However, this technique also suffers from the fact that, if microinvasive disease is ruled out on the wedge specimen, there remains the possibility of it being present in the remaining cervical tissue. All this adds weight to the importance of colposcopy in pregnancy being performed by expert colposcopists and consideration being given to some form of conisation.

Endocervical curettage is not routinely practised in the UK, but is contraindicated in pregnancy because of the risk of premature rupture of membranes, preterm labour and haemorrhage (Ostergard, 1979).

Cone biopsy in pregnancy

The indication for cervical conisation during pregnancy is the exclusion of invasive cancer. In the past, cold knife cone biopsy

was the only available excisional treatment modality. It was shown to be associated with high complication rates and high rates of residual disease, even when performed in the first trimester (Hannigan *et al.*, 1982; Coppola *et al.*, 1997).

Many practitioners prefer to continue using a standard cold knife cone biopsy technique with two laterally placed haemostatic sutures and intracervical xylocaine and adrenaline prior to knife cone, with diathermy to the base and a vaginal pack. Cold knife cone biopsy offers a high diagnostic accuracy, but also significant complications for mother and fetus. Excess haemorrhage has been reported in 8.9% of cases (range 5.2–13.9%). The reported spontaneous miscarriage rate is up to 33% (Hacker *et al.*, 1982; Hannigan *et al.*, 1982). Hannigan *et al.* (1982) reported a high complication rate for cone biopsy undertaken during pregnancy in a large study of 82 pregnant women. Some authors advocate deferring treatment to the second trimester to reduce this rate (Coppola *et al.*, 1997; Robinson *et al.*, 1997; Penna *et al.*, 1998; Demeter *et al.*, 2002). To decrease the amount of bleeding, cervical cerclage at the time of conisation has also been tried (Dunn *et al.*, 2003).

Laser cone biopsy allows a more precise excision of the transformation zone with less anatomical distortion to the cone base and the cervix itself. It is therefore less likely to be associated with medium- and long-term complications and, in expert hands, should be as effective as a cold knife cone biopsy for effecting simultaneous diagnosis and treatment of suspected microinvasion. However, the technique does appear to be associated with increased intraoperative blood loss, particularly with high-grade lesions, and this may be compounded by the increased vascularity of pregnancy. For this reason, some

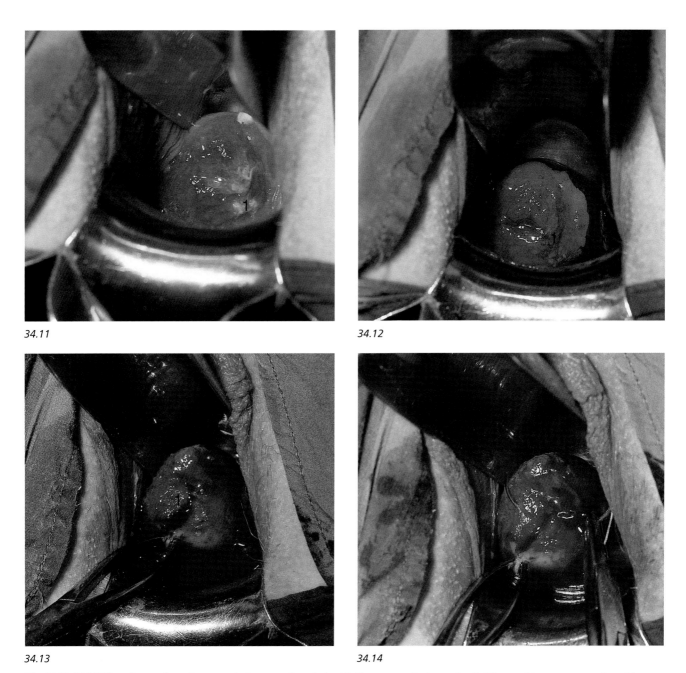

34.11

34.12

34.13

34.14

Figs 34.11–34.14 These figures show the removal of an area of atypical epithelium present in the cervix of a 32-year-old woman presenting with severe dyskaryosis in a smear in early pregnancy. In Figure 34.11 is the anterior lip, which was suspicious of invasive cancer and warranted a wedge biopsy. In Figure 34.12, Schiller's iodine solution has been applied, so that the full extent of the atypical epithelium can be seen (representing the area of major concern). In Figure 34.13, two elliptical incisions have been made to encompass the whole of the atypical area; the incisions have been carried down to at least 10 mm into the stroma to ensure adequate removal of the lesion. Figure 34.14 shows an interrupted suture, using 3/0 material and, if bleeding is excessive, then a haemostatic 'figure of eight' suture can be inserted.

may prefer to use an electrical method of excision (Robinson *et al.*, 1997; Penna *et al.*, 1998; Mitsuhashi *et al.*, 2000; Palle *et al.*, 2000; Dunn *et al.*, 2003).

LLETZ/LEEP has become the popular treatment modality for CIN in the last 15 years. The advantages of the technique include its low cost, the ease of the procedure, high curative rates, little evidence as yet of an adverse effect on subsequent pregnancy outcome and a lower complication rate.

There are only three studies in the literature evaluating LLETZ/LEEP during the index pregnancy (Robinson *et al.*, 1997; Mitsuhashi *et al.*, 2000; Paraskevaidis *et al.*, 2002). Robinson *et al.* (1997) reported on the outcome of 20 women who underwent loop excision between 8 and 34 weeks of gestation. All but two of their procedures were carried out under general or regional anaesthesia, and cervical sutures were placed in the cervix at 12, 3, 6 and 9 o'clock. The loop excisions were performed excising the anterior lip as one specimen and the posterior lip as a second specimen. Ball-type electrodes were used for cauterisation to achieve haemostasis and a Surgicel-type membrane left in the loop bed, following which the 3 and 9 o'clock sutures were tied together in the midline. The authors reported a significant complication rate of 25%. All five women with a significant morbidity had their procedure performed between 27 and 34 weeks. Only 70% (14/20) of specimens contained CIN, and 57% (8/14) had involved margins. Residual disease was seen in nine women, including three patients whose initial loop specimen did not contain CIN (Robinson *et al.*, 1997).

In a small study of nine patients who underwent a LLETZ procedure under local anaesthesia within the first 14 weeks of pregnancy, histological assessment showed CIN1 in two, CIN3 in five and microinvasive disease in two women (Mitsuhashi *et al.*, 2000). Margins were incompletely excised in two women who went on to have a repeat procedure post partum. There were no cases of spontaneous miscarriage, preterm labour or excessive haemorrhage. One woman developed cervical incompetence at 21 weeks' gestation and required cervical cerclage. All pregnancies continued to term. Six women delivered vaginally. The reasons for three caesarean sections were previous section and breech presentation. In the retrospective study by Paraskevaidis *et al.* (2002), seven women with findings suspicious of microinvasion underwent small loop biopsies in pregnancy. Histology showed decidual reaction in five cases, CIN3 in one and early stromal invasion (< 1 mm) in one more at 26 weeks' gestation. This woman delivered at 37 weeks' gestation after induction of labour. Six weeks post partum, a LLETZ was performed. Histology confirmed stage 1aI disease with clear margins. The authors did not advocate LLETZ in pregnancy because of the high risks of bleeding and the possibility of incomplete excision. Instead, they were using the smallest loop wire to obtain a sufficient sample to examine for possible microinvasion instead of a conventional punch biopsy.

In view of the recent new classification of transformation zones, further research which comments on the type of transformation zone treated and the depth of specimen may make more meaningful comparisons of techniques possible (Walker *et al.*, 2003).

Glandular lesions

There are few data concerning the significance of glandular atypia during pregnancy and in the postpartum period. Chhieng *et al.* (2001) reported on the outcome for 35 women diagnosed with an atypical glandular cells of uncertain origin (AGUS) smear in pregnancy between 1995 and 1997. This represented 0.26% of all smears performed on pregnant women. The mean age was 29 years with a range of 17–45 years. Eleven had a concomitant minor squamous lesion [one low-grade squamous intraepithelial lesion (LSIL) and 10 atypical squamous cells of uncertain significance (ASCUS)]. Seventeen women underwent colposcopy and directed punch biopsy, while repeat cytology was performed in 10. Eight women were lost to follow-up. Of those who had a biopsy, two had evidence of a high-grade squamous intraepithelial lesion (HGSIL). There were no significant glandular lesions among these patients.

In non-pregnant women, the significance of glandular atypia is also uncertain, although in an audit of women referred with smears reported as glandular neoplasia, 50% were subsequently found to have significant disease (Drew, 1984).

Adenocarcinoma *in situ* and primary adenocarcinoma of the cervix are uncommon, accounting for up to 15% of all cervical neoplasms. There are very few reported cases occurring in pregnancy. Even in the non-pregnant state, colposcopic evaluation of glandular abnormalities is challenging and often unreliable. Usually, there is a concomitant squamous lesion. In view of the high rate of pathology in women with glandular smear abnormalities, and the difficulty of colposcopic assessment, formal conisation is necessary for the management of these women.

Until there is a better understanding of the natural history and implications of glandular atypia in pregnancy, close follow-up with colposcopy during pregnancy and post partum with directed biopsy of suspicious areas remains important.

Pregnancy outcome after LLETZ/LEEP

Between 1980 and 2002, there were 36 studies in the literature with reference to pregnancy following a LLETZ/LEEP procedure (Crane *et al.*, 2003). Three performed LLETZ/LEEP during the index pregnancy and have been discussed. Of the remainder, only five cohort studies were included in a recent meta-analysis. All studies matched for age and parity. Only three matched for smoking, a potential confounder. The obstetric outcomes following LLETZ/LEEP showed a higher rate of preterm birth (12.6% vs. 7%; OR = 1.81, 95% CI 1.18–2.76, $P = 0.006$) and a higher rate of neonates with a birthweight less than 2500 g (10.9% vs. 6.2%; OR = 1.60, 95% CI 1.01–2.52, $P = 0.04$). However, these studies were retrospective, four were carried out in the UK and one in Greece (Blomfield *et al.*, 1993; Haffenden *et al.*, 1993; Braet *et al.*, 1994; Cruickshank *et al.*, 1995). There may be other confounders, including socioeconomic status and previous obstetric history, that were not taken into account. In addition, the mean depth of the tissue specimen was not mentioned in three of the studies. Thus, the authors were not able to evaluate depth of specimen in relation to preterm labour, neither was it possible to assess any risk of cervical incompetence after LLETZ/LEEP.

A recent paper by Sadler *et al.* (2004) looked at the risks of preterm labour in those treated by LLETZ/LEEP or laser treatment. Again, it was a retrospective cohort study. The overall rate of preterm delivery was 13.8%. The rate of preterm premature rupture of membranes before 37 weeks' gestation (PROM) was 6.2% and the rate of spontaneous preterm delivery was 3.8%. Analyses showed no significant increase in risk of total preterm delivery [adjusted relative risk (aRR) = 1.1; 95% CI 0.8–1.5] or spontaneous preterm delivery (aRR = 1.3; 95% CI 0.7–2.6) for any treatment. The risk of PROM was significantly increased following treatment with laser conisation (aRR = 2.7; 95% CI 1.3–5.6) or LLETZ/LEEP (aRR = 1.9; 95% CI 1.0–3.8), but not laser ablation (aRR = 1.1; 95% CI 0.5–2.4). Moreover, the risk of PROM and total preterm delivery increased significantly with increasing height of tissue removed from the cervix in conisation. Women in whom the cone height removed was ≥ 1.7 cm had a greater than three-fold increase in risk of PROM compared with untreated women (aRR = 3.6; 95% CI 1.8–7.5) (Sadler *et al.*, 2004).

A recent meta-analysis by Kyrgiou *et al.* (2006) has presented evidence that a significantly increased number of women treated by laser cone biopsy or LLETZ deliver before 37 weeks' gestation compared with control subjects and those treated by ablative techniques. In addition, those treated by LLETZ were more likely to have prelabour rupture of the membranes. However, there were no such risks associated with laser vaporisation. Happily, the analysis showed no increased admissions to neonatal intensive care and no increase in perinatal mortality. The results raise a series of interesting questions regarding the influence of the size of tissue removed compared to the cervical length, the possible influence of how the treatment is performed, i.e., if the base is desiccated or fulgurated or vaporised. The findings also suffer from having been derived from a meta-analysis. It is clear that further prospective work needs to be done. In the meantime, the findings also call into question the advisability of treating young women with low-grade abnormalities. These results and conclusions are further discussed in detail in the section on Management of different CIN lesions in Chapter 31. Crane *et al.* (2006) have also recently shown that previous cone biopsy shortens the cervix and is associated with preterm labour in later pregnancies.

Further studies are needed in this area to counsel women undergoing treatment appropriately, particularly those considering future pregnancy and having treatment for minor grade changes that are probably of low malignant potential.

Summary: management of CIN in pregnancy

Conservative management of high-grade CIN in pregnancy appears safe, although close postpartum follow-up is essential. In cases where microinvasion is suspected, colposcopically directed punch biopsies are of little value. A specimen of reasonable size and depth is required for histological evaluation. Traditionally, this has been obtained with wedge biopsies performed in an operating theatre under a general or regional anaesthetic, with close observation for 24 hours after the procedure. The study by Paraskevaidis *et al.* (2002) suggests that a small diagnostic loop specimen may be of similar value, but with a lower morbidity. However, no definite conclusions can be drawn from the small numbers discussed in the available literature.

CERVICAL CANCER AND PREGNANCY

Cervical cancer remains the most commonly diagnosed malignancy in pregnancy, presenting at a mean age of 31.6 years (range 31–36 years). It is, however, a rare situation. For this reason and because of the added concern for both mother and fetus, it is essential that each case be managed by a multidisciplinary team including the mother's obstetrician and paediatrician in addition to the gynaecological oncology and pathology teams (Figs 34.14 and 34.15).

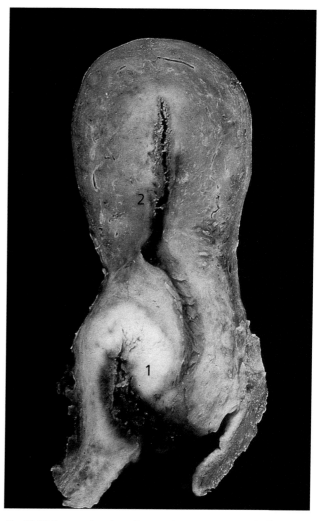

Fig. 34.15 A coronal section of a recently pregnant uterus. It shows a large stage 1B cancer of the anterior lip of the cervix (1). The decidua in the upper cavity can be seen at (2).

The management of cervical cancer in pregnancy will depend on: (i) the gestational age at presentation; (ii) the stage of disease; and (iii) the mother's wishes regarding continuation or termination of the pregnancy and future childbearing desires.

As already discussed, for women with a suspected micro-invasive or, more accurately, an early invasive disease stage IA1 lesion, a cone biopsy is sufficient. The pregnancy can continue to term, and there is no contraindication to vaginal delivery. A repeat colposcopy examination should be arranged about 3 months post partum (Oehler *et al.*, 2003).

In situations where invasive disease is suspected, again as discussed previously, an adequate specimen is required to confirm the diagnosis (Hacker *et al.*, 1982; Hannigan *et al.*, 1982; van der Vange *et al.*, 1995). A wedge biopsy or small loop cone biopsy may provide sufficient tissue for assessment.

Once diagnosed, staging of invasive cervical cancer is clinical in accordance with the International Federation of Gynaecology and Obstetrics (FIGO) classification. Radiological assessment with magnetic resonance imaging (MRI) of the abdomen–pelvis and chest is generally performed in preference to a chest X-ray or computerised tomography (CT) scan, because MRI does not involve radiation and gives a clearer assessment of spread and lymph node involvement.

In general, for stage IA2 cervical cancer, the pregnancy has traditionally been allowed to continue to term. Delivery by classical caesarean section, followed by a radical hysterectomy at the same time has been the management of choice.

For women presenting with stage IB–IIA disease (where the tumour is confined to the cervix or extends only to the upper third of the vagina), in the first and early second trimester, chemoradiation or a radical hysterectomy with the fetus *in utero* are options. However, radical surgery has the advantage of ovarian preservation and the avoidance of the complications of radiotherapy (Saunders and Landon, 1988; Greer *et al.*, 1989; Allen *et al.*, 1995; van Vliet *et al.*, 1998; Siddiqui *et al.*, 2001).

Between 24 and 32 weeks, the advice might be to await viability, give maternal steroids to enhance fetal lung function and deliver by classical caesarean section followed by a radical hysterectomy, while beyond 32 weeks, delivery and definitive treatment would be advised (Nisker *et al.*, 1983; Baltzer *et al.*, 1990; Hopkins and Morley, 1992; Nevin *et al.*, 1995; Sorosky *et al.*, 1995; Magrina, 1996; Norstrom *et al.*, 1997; Nguyen *et al.*, 2000; McDonald *et al.*, 2002). Sood *et al.* (1998) did not observe an adverse maternal outcome for women with stage I disease who had a treatment delay after 20 weeks' gestation.

Although all the evidence comes from retrospective case-control studies, a classical caesarean section appears to be the method of choice for delivery. The risks of vaginal delivery with invasive cervical cancer have been reported to include implantation of malignant cells in the episiotomy site, dissemination of disease into the lymphovascular channels,

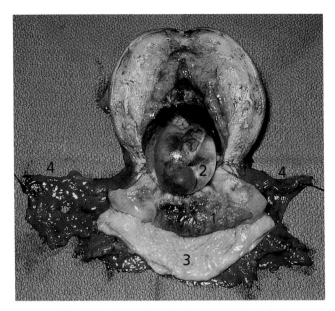

Fig. 34.16 A sagittal section of a radical hysterectomy specimen showing an exophytic stage 1B posterior lip cancer (1), with a small pregnancy sac (2). The large cuff of the vagina (3) and the paracolpos dissection (4) are also shown.

haemorrhage, sepsis, obstructed labour and cervical laceration (Cliby *et al.*, 1994). A classical incision allows the lower uterine segment and cervix to be left undisturbed for subsequent detailed pathological assessment.

The uterine incision should be repaired with the placenta left *in situ* before performing the radical hysterectomy, in an effort to reduce blood loss and dissemination of the disease if present in the placenta (Zemlickis *et al.*, 1991; Jones *et al.*, 1996; Manuel-Limson *et al.*, 1997; Sood *et al.*, 1998; Takushi *et al.*, 2002; Charkviani *et al.*, 2003).

Usually, if a woman presents with higher stage disease at less than 20 weeks' gestation, the advice is to sacrifice the pregnancy and proceed with either radical surgery or chemoradiation with the fetus *in situ* (Fig. 34.16). Radiotherapy will usually induce a spontaneous miscarriage after a dose of 34–40 Gy.

Should the diagnosis be made after 20 weeks' gestation, a formal termination prior to definitive treatment may be advised to avoid a protracted miscarriage after radiation. Some women may prefer to defer any treatment until delivery of a viable fetus. However, there are currently insufficient data regarding the safety of delaying treatment for late-stage cervical cancer in pregnant women.

Tewari *et al.* (1998) published an experimental approach in a report of two women, one with stage IIa and one with bulky stage Ib2 cervical cancer, who refused to interrupt their pregnancies. In both cases, the intent of chemotherapy was to stabilise the malignant disease process until fetal viability was achieved. One woman with a poorly differentiated, non-keratinising, papillary squamous cell carcinoma underwent three cycles of vincristine and cisplatin followed by three cycles of cisplatin between 21 and 30 weeks' gestation. She underwent a caesarean section at 34 weeks and delivered a viable female infant of 2.16 kg. A radical hysterectomy was performed. The tumour extended into the lower uterine segment and vaginal cuff. As there was microscopic parametrial involvement, she received external beam radiotherapy, but developed widespread recurrence within 5 months of surgery. The other patient, with a moderately differentiated tumour, had four cycles of vincristine and cisplatin. She was delivered and underwent a radical hysterectomy at 32 weeks' gestation. Disease was confined to the cervix, and she remains disease free. Few other such case reports are as yet to be found in the literature. Overall, the prognosis for pregnant women presenting with cervical cancer appears to be similar to that of non-pregnant patients.

CONCLUSIONS

Recently, the NHSCSP has issued guidelines for the management of women with abnormal cytology in relation to pregnancy as well as recommendations in respect of invasive cervical cancer. These are:

• A woman who meets the criteria for colposcopy in respect of an abnormal smear still needs colposcopy even if she is pregnant. The primary aim of colposcopy for pregnant women is to exclude invasive disease and to defer biopsy/treatment until the woman has delivered.

• If a colposcopy has been performed during pregnancy, postpartum assessment of women with an abnormal smear or biopsy-proven CIN is essential. Excision biopsy in pregnancy cannot be considered therapeutic, and these women should be seen for colposcopy post partum. This requires a system to ensure that women are given an appointment after delivery.

• If invasive disease is suspected clinically or colposcopically, a biopsy adequate to make the diagnosis is essential. Punch biopsy suggesting only CIN cannot reliably exclude invasion. Cone, wedge or diathermy loop biopsies are all associated with a risk of haemorrhage, and such biopsies should be taken where appropriate facilities to deal with haemorrhage are available.

ACKNOWLEDGEMENTS

The authors wish to thank Professor A. Singer and Mr J.M. Monaghan for permission to use all the colour illustrations in this chapter except Figures 34.6 and 34.7. The former have all appeared in *Lower Genital Tract Precancer*, Oxford: Blackwell Publishing, 2000.

REFERENCES

Allen DG, Planner RS, Tang PT *et al.* (1995) Invasive cervical cancer in pregnancy. *Australian and New Zealand Journal of Obstetrics and Gynaecology* 35 (4): 408–412.

Arena S, Marconi M, Ubertosi M *et al.* (2002) HPV and pregnancy: diagnostic methods, transmission and evolution. *Minerva Ginecology* 54 (3): 225–237.

Armbruster-Morares E, Ioshimoto LM, Leao E *et al.* (1994) Presence of human papillomavirus DNA in amniotic fluids of pregnant women with cervical lesions. *Gynecologic Oncology* 54 (2): 152–158.

Baldauf JJ, Dreyfus M, Ritter J *et al.* (1995) Colposcopy and directed biopsy reliability during pregnancy: a cohort study. *European Journal of Obstetrics, Gynecology and Reproductive Biology* 62 (1): 31–36.

Baldauf JJ, Dreyfus M, Gao J *et al.* (1996) Management of pregnant women with abnormal cervical smears. A series of 146 patients. *Journal of Gynecology Obstetrics and the Biology of Reproduction* (Paris) 25 (6): 582–587.

Baltzer J, Regenbrecht ME, Kopcke W *et al.* (1990) Carcinoma of the cervix and pregnancy. *International Journal of Gynaecology and Obstetrics* 31 (4): 317–323.

Benedet JL, Boyes DA, Nichols TM *et al.* (1977) Colposcopic evaluation of pregnant patients with abnormal cervical smears. *British Journal of Obstetrics and Gynaecology* 84 (7): 517–521.

Bertini-Oliveira AM, Keppler MM, Luisi A *et al.* (1982) Comparative evaluation of abnormal cytology, colposcopy and histopathology in preclinical cervical malignancy during pregnancy. *Acta Cytologica* 26 (5): 636–644.

Blomfield PI, Buxton J, Dunn J *et al.* (1993) Pregnancy outcome after large loop excision of the cervical transformation zone. *American Journal of Obstetrics and Gynaecology* 169 (3): 620–625.

Braet PG, Peel JM, Fenton DW (1994) A case controlled study of the outcome of pregnancy following loop diathermy excision of the transformation zone. *Journal of Obstetrics and Gynaecology* 14: 79–82.

Campion MJ, Sedlacek TV (1993) Colposcopy in pregnancy. *Obstetrics and Gynecology Clinics of North America* 20 (1): 153–163.

Cason J, Kaye JN, Jewers RJ *et al.* (1995) Perinatal infection and persistence of human papillomavirus types 16 and 18 in infants. *Journal of Medical Virology* 47 (3): 209–218.

Charkviani L, Charkviani T, Natenadze N *et al.* (2003) Cervical carcinoma and pregnancy. *Clinical Experiments in Obstetrics and Gynecology* 30 (1): 19–22.

Chhieng DC, Elgert P, Cangiarella JF *et al.* (2001) Significance of AGUS Pap smears in pregnant and postpartum women. *Acta Cytologica* 45 (3): 294–299.

Cliby WA, Dodson MK, Podratz KC (1994) Cervical cancer complicated by pregnancy: episiotomy site recurrences following vaginal delivery. *Obstetrics and Gynecology* 84 (2): 179–182.

Coppola A, Sorosky J, Casper R *et al.* (1997) The clinical course of cervical carcinoma in situ diagnosed during pregnancy. *Gynecologic Oncology* 67 (2): 162–165.

Crane JM (2003) Pregnancy outcome after loop electrosurgical excision procedure: a systematic review. *Obstetrics and Gynecology* 102 (5 Pt 1): 1058–1062.

Crane JM, Delaney T, Hutchens D (2006) Transvaginal ultrasonography in the prediction of preterm birth after treatment for cervical intraepithelial neoplasia. *Obstetrics and Gynecology* 107: 37–44.

Cronje HS, van Rensburg E, Niemand I *et al.* (2000) Screening for cervical neoplasia during pregnancy. *International Journal of Gynaecology and Obstetrics* 68 (1): 19–23.

Cruickshank ME, Flannely G, Campbell DM *et al.* (1995) Fertility and pregnancy outcome following large loop excision of the transformation zone. *British Journal of Obstetrics and Gynaecology* 102: 467–470.

Demeter A, Sziller I, Csapo Z *et al.* (2002) Outcome of pregnancies after cold-knife conization of the uterine cervix during pregnancy. *European Journal of Gynecologic Oncology* 23 (3): 207–210.

DePetrillo AD, Townsend DE, Morrow CP *et al.* (1975) Colposcopic evaluation of the abnormal Papanicolaou test in pregnancy. *American Journal of Obstetrics and Gynecology* 121 (4): 441–445.

Drew NC (1984) Adenocarcinoma-in-situ of the cervix uteri associated with cervical intraepithelial neoplasia in pregnancy. Case report. *British Journal of Obstetrics and Gynaecology* 91 (5): 498–502.

Dunn TS, Ginsburg V, Wolf D (2003) Loop-cone cerclage in pregnancy: a 5-year review. *Gynecologic Oncology* 90 (3): 577–580.

Economos K, Perez Veridiano N, Delke I *et al.* (1993) Abnormal cervical cytology in pregnancy: a 17-year experience. *Obstetrics and Gynecology* 81 (6): 915–918.

Greer BE, Easterling TR, McLennan DA *et al.* (1989) Fetal and maternal considerations in the management of stage I-B cervical cancer during pregnancy. *Gynecologic Oncology* 34 (1): 61–65.

Guerra B, De Simone P, Gabrielli S *et al.* (1998) Combined cytology and colposcopy to screen for cervical cancer in pregnancy. *Journal of Reproductive Medicine* 43 (8): 647–653.

Hacker NF, Berek JS, Lagasse LD *et al.* (1982) Carcinoma of the cervix associated with pregnancy. *Obstetrics and Gynecology* 59 (6): 735–746.

Haffenden DK, Biggrigg A, Codling BW *et al.* (1993) Pregnancy following large loop excision of the transformation zone. *American Journal of Obstetrics and Gynecology* 100: 1059–1060.

Hannigan EV, Whitehouse HH 3rd, Atkinson WD *et al.* (1982) Cone biopsy during pregnancy. *Obstetrics and Gynecology* 60 (4): 450–455.

Hellberg D, Axelsson O, Gad A *et al.* (1987) Conservative management of the abnormal smear during pregnancy. A long-term follow-up. *Acta Obstetrica et Gynecologica Scandinavica* 66 (3): 195–199.

Hopkins MP, Morley GW (1992) The prognosis and management of cervical cancer associated with pregnancy. *Obstetrics and Gynecology* 80 (1): 9–13.

Jones WB, Shingleton HM, Russell A *et al.* (1996) Cervical carcinoma and pregnancy. A national patterns of care study of the American College of Surgeons. *Cancer* 77 (8): 1479–1488.

Kaminski PF, Lyon DS, Sorosky JI *et al.* (1992) Significance of atypical cervical cytology in pregnancy. *American Journal of Perinatology* 9 (5–6): 340–343.

Kashimura M, Matsuura Y, Shinohara M *et al.* (1991) Comparative study of cytology and punch biopsy in cervical intraepithelial neoplasia during pregnancy. A preliminary report. *Acta Cytologica* 35 (1): 100–104.

Kohan S, Beckman EM, Bigelow B *et al.* (1980) The role of colposcopy in the management of cervical intraepithelial neoplasia during pregnancy and postpartum. *Journal of Reproductive Medicine* 25 (5): 279–284.

Kyrgiou M, Koliopoulos G, Martin-Hirsch P *et al.* (2006) Obstetric outcome after conservative treatment for intraepithelial and early invasive cervical lesions: systematic review and meta-analysis. *Lancet* 367: 489–498.

Luesley D, Leeson S (eds) (2004) *Colposcopy and Programme Management: Guidelines for the NHS Cervical Screening Programme*. NHSCSP publication no. 20, Chap. 10. London: NHSCSP.

Lurain JR, Gallup DG (1979) Management of abnormal Papanicolaou smears in pregnancy. *Obstetrics and Gynecology* 53 (4): 484–488.

McDonald SD, Faught W, Gruslin A (2002) Cervical cancer during pregnancy. *Journal of Obstetrics and Gynaecology of Canada* 24 (6): 491–498.

Madej JG, Jr (1996) Colposcopy monitoring in pregnancy complicated by CIN and early cervical cancer. *European Journal of Gynaecological Oncology* 17 (1): 59–65.

Magrina JF (1996) Primary surgery for stage IB–IIA cervical cancer, including short-term and long-term morbidity and treatment in pregnancy. *Journal of the National Cancer Institute Monograph* 21: 53–59.

Malone JM, Jr, Sokol RJ, Ager JW (1988) Pregnancy, human papillomavirus and cervical intraepithelial neoplasia. *European Journal of Gynaecological Oncology* 9 (2): 120–124.

Manuel-Limson GA, Ladines-Llave CA, Sotto LS *et al.* (1997) Cancer of the cervix in pregnancy: a 31-year experience at the Philippine General Hospital. *Journal of Obstetrics and Gynaecological Research* 23 (6): 503–509.

Massad SL, Wright TC, Cox T *et al.* (2005) Managing abnormal cytology results in pregnancy. *Journal of Lower Genital Tract Diseases* 9: 146–148.

Mikhail MS, Anyaegbunam A, Romney SL (1995) Computerized colposcopy and conservative management of cervical intraepithelial neoplasia in pregnancy. *Acta Obstetrica et Gynecologica Scandinavica* 74 (5): 376–378.

Mitsuhashi A, Sekiya S (2000) Loop electrosurgical excision procedure (LEEP) during first trimester of pregnancy. *International Journal of Gynaecological Obstetrics* 71 (3): 237–239.

Murta EF, de Souza FH, de Souza MA *et al.* (2002) High-grade cervical squamous intraepithelial lesion during pregnancy. *Tumori* 88 (3): 246–250.

Nahhas WA, Clark MA, Brown M (1993) 'Abnormal' Papanicolaou smears and colposcopy in pregnancy: ante- and post-partum findings. *International Journal of Gynecological Cancer* 3 (4): 239–244.

Nevin J, Soeters R, Dehaeck K *et al.* (1995) Cervical carcinoma associated with pregnancy. *Obstetric and Gynecology Survey* 50 (3): 228–239.

Nguyen C, Montz FJ, Bristow RE (2000) Management of stage I cervical cancer in pregnancy. *Obstetric and Gynecology Survey* 55 (10): 633–643.

Nisker JA, Shubat M (1983) Stage IB cervical carcinoma and pregnancy: report of 49 cases. *American Journal of Obstetrics and Gynecology* 145 (2): 203–206.

Norstrom A, Jansson I, Andersson H (1997) Carcinoma of the uterine cervix in pregnancy. A study of the incidence and treatment in the western region of Sweden 1973 to 1992. *Acta Obstetrica et Gynecologica Scandinavica* 76 (6): 583–589.

Oehler MK, Wain GV, Brand A (2003) Gynaecological malignancies in pregnancy: a review. *Australian and New Zealand Journal of Obstetrics and Gynaecology* 43 (6): 414–420.

Ortiz R, Newton M (1971) Colposcopy in the management of abnormal cervical smears in pregnancy. *American Journal of Obstetrics and Gynecology* 109 (1): 46–49.

Ostergard DR (1979) The effect of pregnancy on the cervical squamo-columnar junction in patients with abnormal cervical cytology. *American Journal of Obstetrics and Gynecology* 134: 759.

Pakarian F, Kaye J, Cason J *et al.* (1994) Cancer associated human papillomaviruses: perinatal transmission and persistence. *British Journal of Obstetrics and Gynaecology* 101 (6): 514–517.

Palle C, Bangsboll S, Andreasson B (2000) Cervical intraepithelial neoplasia in pregnancy. *Acta Obstetrica et Gynecologica Scandinavica* 79 (4): 306–310.

Paraskevaidis E, Koliopoulos G, Kalantaridou S *et al.* (2002) Management and evolution of cervical intraepithelial neoplasia during pregnancy and postpartum. *European Journal of Obstetrics Gynecology and Reproductive Biology* 104 (1): 67–69.

Penna C, Fallani MG, Maggiorelli M *et al.* (1998) High-grade cervical intraepithelial neoplasia (CIN) in pregnancy: clinicotherapeutic management. *Tumori* 84 (5): 567–570.

Robinson WR, Webb S, Tirpack J *et al.* (1997) Management of cervical intraepithelial neoplasia during pregnancy with loop excision. *Gynecologic Oncology* 64: 153–155.

Sadler L, Saftlas A, Wang W *et al.* (2004) Treatment for cervical intraepithelial neoplasia and risk of preterm delivery. *Journal of the American Medical Association* 291 (17): 2100–2106.

Saunders N, Landon CR (1988) Management problems associated with carcinoma of the cervix diagnosed in the second trimester of pregnancy. *Gynecologic Oncology* 30 (1): 120–122.

Shield PW, Daunter B, Wright RG (1987) The Pap smear revisited. *Australian and New Zealand Journal of Obstetrics and Gynaecology* 27: 269–282.

Shivvers SA, Miller DS (1997) Preinvasive and invasive breast and cervical cancer prior to or during pregnancy. *Clinical Perinatology* 24 (2): 369–389.

Siddiqui G, Kurzel RB, Lampley EC *et al.* (2001) Cervical dysplasia in pregnancy: progression versus regression post-partum. *International Journal of Fertility and Women's Medicine* 46 (5): 278–280.

Smith EM, Johnson SR, Cripe T *et al.* (1995) Perinatal transmission and maternal risks of human papillomavirus infection. *Cancer Detection and Prevention* 19 (2): 196–205.

Smith EM, Ritchie JM, Yankowitz J *et al.* (2004) Human papillomavirus prevalence and types in newborns and parents: concordance and modes of transmission. *Sexually Transmitted Diseases* 31 (1): 57–62.

Sood AK, Sorosky JI (1998) Invasive cervical cancer complicating pregnancy. How to manage the dilemma. *Obstetrics and Gynecology Clinics of North America* 25 (2): 343–352.

Sorosky JI, Squatrito R, Ndubisi BU *et al.* (1995) Stage I squamous cell cervical carcinoma in pregnancy: planned delay in therapy awaiting fetal maturity. *Gynecologic Oncology* 59 (2): 207–210.

Takushi M, Moromizato H, Sakumoto K *et al.* (2002) Management of invasive carcinoma of the uterine cervix associated with pregnancy: outcome of intentional delay in treatment. *Gynecologic Oncology* 87 (2): 185–189.

Talebian F, Krumholz BA, Shayan A *et al.* (1976) Colposcopic evaluation of patients with abnormal cytologic smears during pregnancy. *Obstetrics and Gynecology* 47 (6): 693–696.

Tewari K, Cappuccini F, Gambino A *et al.* (1998) Neoadjuvant chemotherapy in the treatment of locally advanced cervical carcinoma in pregnancy: a report of two cases and review of issues specific to the management of cervical carcinoma in pregnancy including planned delay of therapy. *Cancer* 82 (8): 1529–1534.

Tseng CJ, Liang CC, Soong YK *et al.* (1998) Perinatal transmission of human papillomavirus in infants: relationship between infection rate and mode of delivery. *Obstetrics and Gynecology* 91 (1): 92–96.

van der Vange N, Weverling GJ, Ketting BW *et al.* (1995) The prognosis of cervical cancer associated with pregnancy: a matched cohort study. *Obstetrics and Gynecology* 85 (6): 1022–1026.

van Vliet W, van Loon AJ, ten Hoor KA *et al.* (1998) Cervical carcinoma during pregnancy: outcome of planned delay in treatment. *European Journal of Obstetrics Gynecology and Reproductive Biology* 79 (2): 153–157.

Vlahos G, Rodolakis A, Diakomanolis E *et al.* (2002) Conservative management of cervical intraepithelial neoplasia (CIN(2–3)) in pregnant women. *Gynecology and Obstetric Investigations* 54 (2): 78–81.

Walker P, Dexeus S, De Palo G *et al.* (2003) Nomenclature Committee of the International Federation for Cervical Pathology and Colposcopy. International terminology of colposcopy: an updated report from the International Federation for Cervical Pathology and Colposcopy. *Obstetrics and Gynecology* 101 (1): 175–177.

Yoonessi M, Wieckowska W, Mariniello D *et al.* (1982) Cervical intra-epithelial neoplasia in pregnancy. *International Journal of Gynaecology and Obstetrics* 20 (2): 111–118.

Yost NP, Santoso JT, McIntire DD *et al.* (1999) Postpartum regression rates of antepartum cervical intraepithelial neoplasia II and III lesions. *Obstetrics and Gynecology* 93 (3): 359–362.

Zemlickis D, Lishner M, Degendorfer P *et al.* (1991) Maternal and fetal outcome after invasive cervical cancer in pregnancy. *Journal of Clinical Oncology* 9 (11): 1956–1961.

Immunosuppression and the cervix: human immunodeficiency virus (HIV)

Thomas C. Wright Jr

INTRODUCTION

Over the last two decades, infection with human immuno-deficiency virus (HIV) has emerged as one of the most devastating epidemics of all time. According to estimates from the United Nations Programme for AIDS (UNAIDS), as of December 2003, there were 40 million adults and children living with AIDS worldwide (UNAIDS Statistical Summary, 2003). This represents 1.1% of all adults aged 15–45 years living around the world. In 2003 alone, there were 5 million newly acquired infections with HIV and 3 million deaths. In many regions of the globe, such as sub-Saharan Africa, the impact of this epidemic is simply astonishing (Fig. 35A.1).

In 2003, UNAIDS estimated that 26.6 million people in sub-Saharan Africa were infected with HIV, including 3.2 million who became infected during 2003. Southern Africa is home to only about 2% of the world's population, yet it has about 30% of all people infected with HIV/AIDS worldwide. The change in HIV prevalence that has occurred over the last 15 years in this region is dramatic. In 1988, there were no sub-Saharan African countries where the prevalence of HIV seropositivity in adults was over 20% and only one where 10% of the adult population was infected (UNAIDS Statistical Summary, 2003). By 1998, there were four countries where over 20% of adults were HIV seropositive and an additional five where 10% of adults were infected. By 2003, an additional two countries, Angola and South Africa, had reached the point where 20% of all adults are infected with HIV.

Women are particularly devastated by the HIV/AIDS epidemic in sub-Saharan Africa. Women aged 15–45 years living in sub-Saharan Africa are 2.5 times more likely to be HIV infected than are their male counterparts, and up to 75% of young people infected with HIV in this region of the world are women and girls (UNAIDS Statistical Summary, 2003). Currently, more than one in five pregnant women is HIV infected in most countries in southern Africa and, in selected urban areas, up to 40% of women attending prenatal clinics are infected.

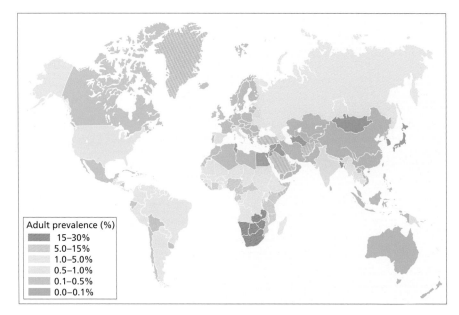

Adult prevalence (%)
15–30%
5.0–15%
1.0–5.0%
0.5–1.0%
0.1–0.5%
0.0–0.1%

Fig. 35A.1 Distribution of HIV infections globally. The prevalence of HIV infections in adults is shown on this map. UNAIDS Statistical Summary (2003) (http://www.unaids.org).

HIV/AIDS is having a dramatic impact on our efforts to control cervical cancer. Cervical cancer is the leading cause of cancer death among women living in many of the countries hit hardest by the HIV/AIDS epidemic (Parkin *et al.*, 1999a). Not only has the HIV/AIDS epidemic adversely impacted on the ability of the public health sector to provide preventative health services, such as cervical cancer screening, to women in these areas, but there also appears to be a synergistic effect between HIV infection and human papillomavirus (HPV) infection that results in particularly high rates of intraepithelial neoplasia in HIV-infected men and women (Wright and Sun, 1996). To date, the HIV/AIDS epidemic has not resulted in a dramatic increase in HPV-associated invasive cancers in those regions of the world hit hardest by the epidemic. In large part, this reflects the fact that most women who are infected with HIV in these areas of the world die relatively quickly of other opportunistic infections such as *Pneumocystis carinii* pneumonia or tuberculosis. As cervical cancer has a very long development phase, it is likely that HIV-infected women in these regions of the world are simply not living long enough to develop cervical cancer.

Over the next decade, it is expected that HIV infection will be converted globally to more of a chronic disease through the widespread introduction of highly active antiretroviral therapies (HAART) via initiatives such as the Global Fund for AIDS, Tuberculosis, and Malaria. As an unwanted consequence of this effort, it is possible that the rates of invasive cervical cancer will increase in parts of the world where effective cervical cancer screening and prevention programmes are not in place. Therefore, it is imperative that we develop a comprehensive understanding of the relationships between human papillomavirus (HPV), HIV and cervical cancer.

IMPACT OF IMMUNOSUPPRESSION IN GENERAL ON CERVICAL NEOPLASIA

Multiple studies have demonstrated that both men and women who are immunosuppressed are at increased risk of developing precancerous and invasive squamous lesions of the lower anogenital tract. The increased risk was best documented in older studies of women who had relatively profound immunosuppression, such as those who had undergone an organ transplant and were taking high dosages of immunosuppressive medications prior to the introduction of drugs such as ciclosporin (Penn, 1986, 1988). Increases in cervical intraepithelial neoplasia (CIN) have also been documented for women with less profound immunosuppression, such as those with Hodgkin's disease or systemic lupus erythematosus (Cibere *et al.*, 2001). Because both HIV and HPV are sexually transmitted agents, there was considerable concern when the AIDS epidemic first extended to women that HIV-infected women might be at especially increased risk of developing HPV-associated invasive cancers of the lower genital tract (CDC, 1990).

PREVALENCE OF ANOGENITAL HPV INFECTIONS IN HIV-INFECTED WOMEN

It is now accepted that there are strong and consistent associations between infection with HIV and anogenital tract HPV infections in both women and men. This review will focus on the results of three large multicentre studies from the United States. The first large study was conducted in the New York City area. This study, referred to as the New York Cervical Disease Study or NYCDS, enrolled a cohort of HIV-infected women together with a control group of high-risk HIV-uninfected women from methadone maintenance programmes, sexually transmitted disease (STD) clinics and heterosexual transmission studies of HIV-discordant couples. Those enrolled were followed prospectively at 6-monthly intervals for up to 5 years (Wright *et al.*, 1994). At each examination, women were tested using cervical cytology and HPV DNA testing and underwent colposcopy. HPV DNA was detected and typed using a polymerase chain reaction (PCR)-based assay incorporating the MY09/11 HPV L1 'consensus' primers that amplify most of the known anogenital types of HPV. The specific types of HPV present in a sample were determined using a restriction fragment length polymorphism (RFLP) assay. At the enrolment visit, HPV DNA was detected in 208 (60%) of the 344 HIV-infected women compared with 116 (36%) of the 325 HIV-uninfected control women (Sun *et al.*, 1995). Because a colposcopic examination, with biopsy when indicated, was performed at each visit during this study, it was possible to determine the prevalence of HPV infections in women with and without CIN. Among HIV-infected women with no evidence of CIN, 50% were HPV DNA positive compared with 32% of the control HIV-uninfected women ($P < 0.001$). After approximately 2 years of follow-up, the cumulative prevalence of HPV infection was 83% in the HIV-infected group compared with 62% in HIV-uninfected women (Sun *et al.*, 1997).

There were no significant differences in the distribution of HPV types found in HIV-infected and uninfected women enrolled in the NYCDS. 'Novel' or unknown HPV types were the most commonly detected HPV types in women who had no evidence of CIN, regardless of their HIV serostatus. HPV 16 was the single most commonly identified HPV type found in both HIV-infected and uninfected women with no evidence of CIN. HPV 16 accounted for 18% and 15% of all HPV infections identified at the enrolment visit in HIV-infected and uninfected women respectively. HPV 16-associated types (including HPV 16, 31, 33, 35 and 58) were identified in 15% of the HIV-infected women (Fig. 35A.2).

HPV 18 was also common and accounted for 13% and 8% of HPV infections in HIV-infected and uninfected women without CIN respectively. The NYCDS was prospective, and women were followed for up to 5 years. After 2 years of follow-up, the cumulative detection rate for HPV 16-associated types in the HIV-infected cohort was almost 45% and, of HPV

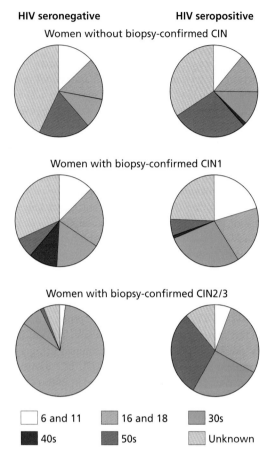

HIV seronegative   **HIV seropositive**

Women without biopsy-confirmed CIN

Women with biopsy-confirmed CIN1

Women with biopsy-confirmed CIN2/3

☐ 6 and 11   ▨ 16 and 18   ▤ 30s
■ 40s   ▦ 50s   ▨ Unknown

Fig. 35A.2 Distribution of specific HPV types in HIV-infected and uninfected women. The distribution of specific types of HPV in HPV-positive women stratified by cervical disease status and HIV serostatus. Modified from Sun *et al.* (1995).

18-associated types (HPV 18 and 45), the cumulative detection rate was almost 30% (Fig. 35A.3).

Infections with multiple types of HPV were very common in HIV-infected women. At their enrolment visit, multiple types of HPV were identified in 51% of the HIV-infected women with HPV infections compared with 36% of HIV-uninfected women. Two other even larger prospective multi-centre studies from the United States, as well as numerous smaller studies from around the world, subsequently confirmed and expanded on the above findings from the NYCDS. The largest of these studies is the Women's Interagency HIV Study (WIHS), which enrolled a total of 1778 HIV-infected and 500 uninfected women from six different clinical sites across the United States (Barkan *et al.*, 1998). Data from WIHS confirmed that HIV-infected women have a higher prevalence of HPV infections than age- and risk-matched HIV-uninfected women (Palefsky *et al.*, 1999). In addition, a high prevalence of infection with multiple types of HPV in HIV-infected women was confirmed. In WIHS, a large number of 'novel' HPV types were identified among the HIV-infected women. These were mostly from the A3 clade, which includes a number of HPV types not generally considered to be oncogenic. The other large US multicentre study is the HIV Epidemiology Research Study (HERS) (Smith, 1998). HERS enrolled 767 HIV-infected women and 390 HIV-uninfected women from four cities from around the US. HERS also confirmed an increased prevalence of HPV infections, as well as increased number of infections with multiple HPV types in HIV-infected compared with uninfected women (Ahdieh *et al.*, 2001; Jamieson *et al.*, 2002). Overall, 64% of HIV-infected women in HERS were HPV DNA positive at the enrolment examination compared with 27% of the HIV-uninfected women. A wide variety of HPV types was identified in both HIV-infected and uninfected women. HIV-infected

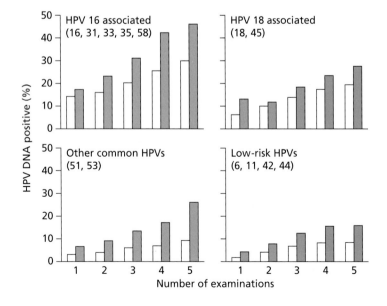

Fig. 35A.3 Cumulative detection of specific HPV types in HIV-infected and uninfected women. The cumulative detection of HPV 16-associated types, HPV 18-associated types, low-risk types and other common HPV types during 2.5 years of follow-up in HIV-infected (white bars) and HIV-uninfected women (green bars). Modified from Sun *et al.* (1997).

women were more likely to have any of the HPV risk groups than were HIV-seronegative women. This includes HPV types considered to be 'high-risk' types (16, 18, 31, 45), which had a prevalence ratio (PR) of 2.5 between HIV-infected and uninfected women (95% CI 1.7–3.6); types considered to be 'intermediate risk' (33, 35, 39, 51, 52, 56, 58, 59, 68, 73, 82), which had a PR of 2.9 (95% CI 2.1–4.4), as well as 'low-risk' HPV types, which had a PR of 4 (95% CI 2.8–5.7) (Jamieson *et al.*, 2002). However, unlike the NYCDS and the WIHS, in which HPV 16 was found to be the single most common HPV type in HIV-infected women, in HERS, HPV 53 was the single most common HPV type. HPV 53 was identified in 11% of the HPV-positive women. HPV 18 and 31 were also identified more frequently than HPV 16.

Several of the early studies investigating relationships between HIV and HPV found indications that HIV-infected women shed higher levels of HPV DNA than HIV-uninfected women (Feingold *et al.*, 1990). However, other studies reported that the quantity of HPV DNA detected in HIV-infected and uninfected women was similar (Vernon *et al.*, 1994). These early studies were hampered by relatively small numbers of HPV DNA-positive samples and the fact that the presence of CIN was often not controlled for. In HERS, quantitative assessment of HPV viral load was made by estimating the signal intensity on dot-blot probing. Using this method, higher HPV viral loads were identified in HIV-infected, than in uninfected, women (Jamieson *et al.*, 2002). Recently, Weissenborn *et al.* (2003) used real-time PCR to quantify HPV DNA loads of six oncogenic HPV types in cervical scrapes from HIV-infected and uninfected women. HPV DNA viral load increased in both HIV-infected and uninfected women with increasing grade of referral cytology. However, in women without high-grade squamous epithelial lesion (HSIL) referral cytology, there was no difference in the viral load for HPV types 16, 18, 31, 33, 45 and 56 between HIV-infected and uninfected women.

RELATIONSHIPS BETWEEN IMMUNOSUPPRESSION AND HPV DNA DETECTIONS

Associations between the degree or level of immunosuppression and the detection of HPV DNA have been investigated in the three large prospective follow-up studies of HIV-infected women. The relationships between immunosuppression and HPV DNA detection appear to be complex, but highly consistent results were observed in the three studies. In general, it appears that the detection of HPV DNA increases with decreasing CD4+ lymphocyte counts. In the NYCDS, decreasing absolute CD4+ T-lymphocyte counts were associated with an increased prevalence of HPV DNA positivity (Fig. 35A.4).

An almost identical relationship was also observed in both the WIHS and the HERS clinical trials (Fig. 35A.4). HERS

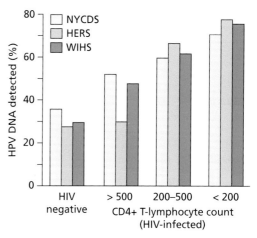

Fig. 35A.4 Impact of immunosuppression on detection of HPV DNA. In all three of the large multicentre studies from the US, there was a consistent association between relative level of immunosuppression as determined by CD4+ T-lymphocyte count and detection of HPV DNA by PCR-based assays. Solid bars, NYHPV; stippled bars, HERS; diagonally striped, WIHS.

found that, at the enrolment examination, approximately 54% of HIV-infected women with CD4+ T-cell counts of > 500 cells/mm^3 were HPV DNA positive compared with 75% of HIV-infected women with CD4+ T-cell counts of 0–200 cells/mm^3 (Ahdieh *et al.*, 2001). Heard *et al.* (2000) also compared the relative HPV DNA 'viral loads' in HIV-infected women with differing levels of immunosuppression in a group of 307 HIV-seropositive women from France. HPV DNA was detected using two techniques: Southern blot hybridisation, which has a relatively low sensitivity, and PCR, which has a high sensitivity for HPV DNA. High-load HPV infection was twice as frequent in the severely immuno-suppressed women (CD4+ T-lymphocyte count of less than 200 cells/mm^3) than among those women with higher CD4+ T-lymphocyte counts ($P = 0.002$).

In WIHS, the association between detection of HPV and lower CD4+ lymphocyte count was found for all HPV types including low-risk types such as HPV 6 or 11 as well as for high-risk types such as HPV 16 or 18 (Palefsky *et al.*, 1999). Similarly, the mean number of HPV types identified per specimen increased progressively with decreasing CD4+ lymphocyte count. Although all HPV types were more commonly detected among women with lower CD4+ T-cell counts, the relationship between immunosuppression and detection of HPV was less marked for HPV 16 and phylogenetically related types than for other HPV types. This was interpreted as indicating that HPV 16 infections are less influenced by immunosuppression than other types of HPV infections, and it was postulated that this might explain why HPV 16 is the most common oncogenic type identified among women in the general population.

In a follow-up analysis that combined the results of both the WIHS and the HERS clinical trials, Strickler *et al.* (2003)

Table 35A.1 Impact of HIV viral load and CD4+ T-cell count on HPV DNA positivity.

	% HPV DNA positive by CD4+ T-cell count		
Plasma viral load	*< 200 cells/mm³*	*200–499 cells/mm³*	*> 500 cells/mm³*
< 4000	44%	59%	78%
4000–20 000	49%	55%	83%
20 001–100 000	64%	67%	78%
> 100 000	71%	64%	71%

Modified from Palefsky *et al.* (1999).

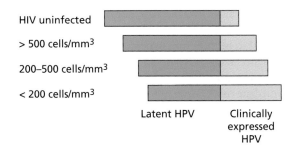

Fig. 35A.5 Impact of immunosuppression on relationship between latent and clinically expressed HPV infections.

used prevalence ratios to compare the prevalence of each HPV type in HIV-infected women with the lowest CD4+ T-cell counts (< 200 cells/mm³) and those with the highest (> 500 cells/mm³). This analysis included information from approximately 2900 HIV-infected women and confirmed that HPV 16 is somewhat less influenced by immune status than other HPV types.

In both the HERS and the WIHS, there was an association between HIV viral load and HPV DNA detection. Only 31% of HIV-infected women with HIV viral loads of less than 200 copies/mL were HPV DNA positive in HERS compared with 79% of those with HIV viral loads of greater than 30 000 copies/mL (Jamieson *et al.*, 2002). Demonstration of the complex relationship between relative levels of immunosuppression, as measured by CD4+ T-cell counts, HIV viral load and HPV, comes from an analysis of data from WIHS that was done by Palefsky *et al.* (1999). High rates of HPV DNA positivity were identified among all women with low CD4+ T-cell counts (< 200 cells/mm³) irrespective of HIV viral load (Table 35A.1). However, among women with higher CD4+ T-cell counts, the prevalence of HPV DNA positivity was dependent on HIV viral load. For example, among women with > 500 CD4+T cells/mm³, the prevalence of HPV DNA positivity was 44% among those with HIV viral loads of less than 4000 copies/µL compared with 71% in women with HIV viral loads of over 100 000 copies/µL.

One of the advantages of the NYCDS compared with HERS and WIHS is that all women enrolled in NYCDS underwent colposcopy with biopsy if indicated at every clinical examination. This allowed a determination of the relationships between HPV and cervical disease status in individual women. Level of immunosuppression was found to affect the relative proportion of women with latent HPV infections (i.e. HPV DNA positivity without cytological or colposcopic evidence of CIN) as opposed to clinically expressed HPV infections (i.e. HPV DNA positivity associated with cytological or histological evidence of a lesion). In women in the general population, latent HPV infection occurs much more commonly

than clinically expressed infection. In the HIV-seronegative women enrolled in NYCDS, there were 8.7 times more latent HPV infections than there were clinically expressed infections (Fig. 35A.5) (Wright and Sun, 1996).

In contrast, there were only 1.9 times as many latent HPV infections as clinically expressed infections in HIV-seropositive women. When the impact of the degree of immunosuppression was evaluated on the relative relationship between latent and clinically expressed HPV infections, it is clear that. with increasing levels of immunosuppression. there are more marked alterations in the relationship.

NATURAL HISTORY OF HPV INFECTIONS IN HIV-INFECTED WOMEN

In HIV-uninfected individuals, the majority of HPV infections are transient and self-limited (Wright and Schiffman, 2003). HIV seropositivity is associated with increased rates of HPV persistence and lower rates of HPV clearance. In the NYCDS, persistent detection of HPV DNA was found in 24% of the HIV-infected women compared with only 4% of the HIV-uninfected women (Sun *et al.*, 1995). Persistent detection of HPV DNA of HPV 16 or 18-associated types was also much more common in HIV-infected women (20% overall) than in HIV-uninfected women (3% overall). In another longitudinal study of HIV-infected and uninfected women from New York City, Minkoff *et al.* (1998) found similar elevated rates of persistent high-risk HPV infections in HIV-infected women (18.5% had persistent infections) compared with HIV-uninfected women (1.5% had persistent infections). Subsequent prospective data from HERS have confirmed these findings (Ahdieh *et al.*, 2001). In HERS, persistent HPV infection was defined as finding the same type of HPV at the follow-up visit as was identified at the preceding visit. Persistence was greater in HIV-infected than in uninfected women and increased with increasing degree of immunosuppression. Among HIV-infected women, high viral load as well as infection with multiple types of HPV was strongly associated with viral persistence.

There is also increased detection of new types of HPV during prospective follow-up of HIV-infected compared with uninfected women. In HERS, the risk of an incident new detection of a previously undetected type of HPV was significantly higher for many types of HPV in HIV-infected than in uninfected women. For example, the incidence rate for HPV 16 infections was 1.67 among HIV-uninfected women compared with 2.59 in HIV-infected women [relative risk (RR) = 1.5, 95% CI 0.8–3.0]. For any high-risk HPV, defined as HPV 16, 18, 31 or 45, the comparative incidence rates were 4.42 and 8.05 (RR = 1.8, 95% CI 1.3–2.7) in HIV-uninfected and infected women (Ahdieh *et al.*, 2001). Detection of HPV DNA among women with previously negative test results was not associated with sexual activity in the intervening period between visits in either of these two studies (Sun *et al.*, 1997; Minkoff *et al.*, 1998). Similarly, in both the WIHS and the HERS, the number of male sexual partners during the preceding 6 months was not associated with detection of HPV DNA at the enrolment examination.

The clear relationship identified in all three large follow-up studies between detection of HPV DNA, CD4+ T-lymphocyte count and HIV viral load suggests that the increase in apparent HPV infections observed in HIV-infected women is due to reactivation of HPV infections that had been contracted at some point in the past. This hypothesis is strengthened by the finding that the detection of a 'new' HPV type during follow-up in these older, HIV-infected women is unrelated to recent sexual activity. This has important implications for understanding the natural history of HPV infections in older women in the general population, as it suggests that previously acquired HPV infections can exist for considerable periods of time while shedding insufficient amounts of HPV DNA to be detected with currently available diagnostic tests.

RELATIONSHIPS BETWEEN HIV INFECTION AND CIN

Cross-sectional studies

There is a considerable amount of highly consistent information from countries around the globe demonstrating that the prevalence of CIN is increased among HIV-infected women. When considering the impact of HIV on cervical neoplasia, it is important to separate studies that have used cervical cytology to determine the presence or absence of disease from those that have used colposcopy and cervical biopsy. This distinction is important because cytology is a screening as opposed to a diagnostic test, and considerable numbers of women with a given cytological diagnosis will have either less severe or more severe disease.

One of the first controlled studies of cervical disease in HIV-infected women was conducted in 1988 and compared cytological findings in 201 HIV-infected and 213 HIV-uninfected

women presenting to the outpatient clinics at the University of Miami for HIV serotesting (Provencher *et al.*, 1988). The prevalence of cytological abnormalities was 63% in the HIV-infected women versus 5% in the HIV-uninfected women (Table 35A.2). Numerous other studies subsequently confirmed higher rates of cytological abnormalities in HIV-infected women compared with HIV-uninfected women. For example, in a study that recruited HIV-infected and uninfected women from France and French Guyana, Six *et al.* (1998) found that 26.5% of 253 HIV-infected women had SIL on cytology compared with 7.5% of 160 HIV-uninfected control women. Overall, it appears that between 20% and 40% of HIV-infected women will have cytological abnormalities on a given cervical cytology specimen compared with 5–10% of HIV-uninfected control women. A cytological result of HSIL occurs less commonly, but also appears to be increased in HIV-infected women. HSIL was identified in 18% of HIV-infected compared with 5% of the HIV-uninfected women attending family planning clinics in Zimbabwe (Temmerman *et al.*, 1999).

The three large multicentre prospective studies from the United States (NYCDS, HERS and WIHS) as well as the DIANAIDS study from Italy all incorporated blinded, expert cytology review (Table 35A.3). In the HERS, WIHS and DIANAIDS studies, colposcopy was not routinely performed at enrolment or during follow-up. In these studies, women were serially screened using cervical cytology, and only women with abnormal screening cytology examinations were referred for colposcopy. At enrolment, 18.9% of the 774 HIV-seropositive women in HERS had a SIL on cytology compared with 5.3% of the 391 HIV-seronegative women (Duerr *et al.*, 2001; Schuman *et al.*, 2003). Similar results were reported from WIHS. At enrolment, 17.4% of the 1713 HIV-seropositive women in WIHS had cytological diagnosis of SIL compared with 3.5% of the 482 HIV-seronegative women (Massad *et al.*, 1999). In the DIANAIDS cooperative study from Italy, cytological SIL of any grade was identified at enrolment in 29.5% of 266 HIV-infected women compared with 10% of the 193 HIV-uninfected control women (Branca *et al.*, 2000).

Fewer studies have used colposcopy to identify biopsy-confirmed CIN in comparable groups of HIV-infected and uninfected women. One of the few studies to use this approach in a large cohort of HIV-infected and uninfected women was the NYCDS. In the NYCDS, biopsy-confirmed CIN1 was detected at the enrolment visit in 13% of the HIV-infected women compared with 4% of the high-risk HIV-uninfected women (*P* < 0.001) (Wright *et al.*, 1994). Biopsy-confirmed CIN2/3 was detected in 7% of the HIV-infected group at enrolment compared with 1% of the HIV-uninfected group (*P* < 0.001). Another study with a similar study design to the NYCDS, in that all women underwent a colposcopic examination at enrolment, was published from Italy (Conti *et al.*,

Table 35A.2 Prevalence of cytological abnormalities in HIV-seropositive and HIV-seronegative women.

Reference	Location	Population studied	HIV-seropositive women		HIV-seronegative women	
			No.	% Abnormal*	No.	% Abnormal*
Provencher *et al.* (1988)	Miami/USA	Requesting screening	201	63	213	5
Feingold *et al.* (1990)	Bronx/USA	Methadone clinic	35	40	32	9
Vermund *et al.* (1991)	Bronx/USA	Methadone clinic	51	33	49	13
Marte *et al.* (1992)	Chicago and NYC/USA	HIV clinics	135	26	Clinics†	6
Laga *et al.* (1992)	Kinshasa/Zaire	Prostitutes	41	27	41	3
Kreiss *et al.* (1992)	Nairobi/Kenya	Prostitutes	42	26	21	24
Maggwa *et al.* (1993)	Kenya	Family planning	205	5	3853	2
Smith *et al.* (1993)	London/UK	HIV and methadone clinics	43	35	43	19
Conti *et al.* (1993)	Milan/Italy	IVDU	273	42	161	8
Wright *et al.* (1994)	New York/USA	Methadone/STD/HIV clinic	398	30	357	8
Johnstone *et al.* (1994)	Edinburgh/Scotland	IVDU and IVDU partners	92	38	157	22
Seck *et al.* (1994)	Senegal	ID clinic and HIV partners	14	43	50	6
Branca *et al.* (1995)	Italy	IVDU and STD clinic	121	23	100	11
Six *et al.* (1998)	France/French Guyana	Various clinics	253	26	160	7
Massad *et al.* (1999)	United States	Multicentre study	1713	38	482	16
Minkoff *et al.* (1999)	Bronx/USA	Community based clinics	262	23	646	5
Branca *et al.* (2000)	Italy	Multicentre study	266	32	193	11
Hawes *et al.* (2003)	Senegal	Outpatient clinics	338	38	3552	16

*Differing criteria and cut-offs for defining what constitutes a cytological 'abnormality' were used in the different studies.
†Used prevalence of cytological abnormalities in general outpatient clinic.
IVDU, intravenous drugusers; NYC, New York City.

1993). In the Italian study, an even higher rate of CIN was identified in the HIV-infected group. In the study from Italy, 42% of the HIV-infected women had biopsy-confirmed CIN of any grade compared with 8% of the HIV-uninfected women, and 51% of the CIN that was detected was CIN2/3 in the HIV-infected group. Heard *et al.* (2000) examined 307 HIV-infected French women using a combination of cervical cytology and a colposcopic examination. Biopsy-confirmed CIN3 was identified in 11.7% of the women and biopsy-confirmed CIN3 in 11.4%.

HIV infection in women in developed countries, where most of the studies listed above were conducted, often occurs in conjunction with other behavioural and biological risk factors that are associated with the development of CIN. These include multiple sexual partners, young age of first intercourse, sex with males who have multiple partners, low socioeconomic status, cigarette smoking and poor compliance with recommended Pap smear screening programmes. These conditions are all common in HIV-infected women in developed countries and, as a result, these women are likely to be

Table 35A.3 Prevalence of cytological abnormalities in HIV-seropositive and HIV-seronegative women in large, multicentre studies.

Reference	Location	Population studied	HIV-seropositive women		HIV-seronegative women	
			No.	% Abnormal*	No.	% Abnormal*
Wright *et al.* (1994)	US NYCDS	Multisite in NYC	398	30	357	8
Massad *et al.* (1999)	US WIHS	Multicentre study	1713	38	482	16
Branca *et al.* (2000)	Italy DIANAIDS	Multicentre study	266	32	193	11
Duerr *et al.* (2001)	US HERS	Multicentre study	701	40	336	20

*Differing criteria and cut-offs for defining what constitutes a cytological 'abnormality' were used in the different studies.
†Used prevalence of cytological abnormalities in general outpatient clinic.
NYC, New York City.

at increased risk of developing anogenital tract lesions on the basis of these non-HIV-related risk factors alone. In order to determine the relative contributions of these factors compared with that of HIV infection to the high prevalence of CIN in HIV-infected women, it is necessary to study well-matched groups of HIV-infected and uninfected women. In the NYCDS, demographic information and CIN risk factor information were analysed to determine whether behavioural and biological factors, other than HIV infection, explain the increased risk of CIN in this population. Using various multiple logistic regression models, it was shown that HIV infection is a strong risk factor for biopsy-confirmed CIN that is independent of other risk factors (Wright, 1995). Moreover, HIV-infected women with higher levels of immunosuppression (CD4+ T-lymphocyte counts < 200 cells/mm^3) are at greater risk of CIN than HIV-infected women with less profound immunosuppression. However, even HIV-infected women with relatively intact immune function (defined by relatively high CD4+ counts) are at greater risk than uninfected women. These analyses indicate that both HIV infection and HIV-associated immunosuppression appear to be risk factors for CIN.

Prospective studies

There is now a considerable number of data indicating that the incidence of both cervical cytological abnormalities as well as biopsy-confirmed CIN is increased in HIV-infected women. The NYCDS was the first prospective study to report the incidence of CIN in HIV-infected women. In this study, a total of 328 HIV-infected and 325 HIV-uninfected women with no evidence of CIN on either cervical cytology or colposcopy were prospectively followed for up to 5 years (Ellerbrock *et al.*, 2000). The median length of follow-up of the HIV-infected women was 29.5 months, compared with 33.3 months for the HIV-uninfected group. Sixty-seven (20%) of the HIV-infected women and 16 (5%) of the HIV-uninfected control women developed biopsy-confirmed CIN during follow-up (Fig. 35A.6, left).

The incidence of CIN was 8.3 and 1.8 cases per 100 years of follow-up in HIV-infected and uninfected women respect-

ively. Most of the incident CIN was low grade (CIN1). In the HIV-infected women, 91% of the incident cases of CIN were first diagnosed as CIN1. In the HIV-uninfected group, 75% of the incident cases of CIN were first diagnosed as CIN1. No invasive cervical cancers were identified on follow-up in either group.

CD4+ T-lymphocyte count at enrolment had a non-significant impact on the incidence of CIN in HIV-infected women ($P = 0.08$) (Fig. 35A.6, right). At 36 months of follow-up, 37% of the HIV-infected women with CD4+ T-lymphocyte counts of less than 200 cells/mm^3 at entry had developed biopsy-confirmed CIN compared with 13% of those with greater than 500 cells/mm^3. As expected, HPV DNA status at enrolment had a major impact on the incidence of CIN in HIV-infected women (Fig. 35A.7, left).

At 36 months of follow-up, 48% of the HIV-infected women who had HPV 16 or 18 identified at enrolment had developed biopsy-confirmed CIN. The incidence of CIN at 36 months was 26% in women who had an HPV type other than 16 or 18 identified at enrolment, and only 4% in women who were HPV DNA negative. Enrolment cytology result also had a significant impact. Women with a cytological finding of LSIL or HSIL at enrolment were excluded from the follow-up analysis, but women with an enrolment cytology result of ASCUS (atypical squamous cells of undetermined significance) who did not have biopsy-confirmed CIN were included. A cytology result of ASCUS at enrolment, in the absence of a colposcopically identified lesion, had a significant impact on incident CIN (Fig. 35A.7, right). Among HIV-infected women, incident CIN was identified by 36 months of follow-up in 48% of those with an ASCUS enrolment cytology result compared with 16% of those with a within-normal limits enrolment cytology result.

Other follow-up studies that have used cytology to determine the incidence of CIN have reported similar findings. For example, Six *et al.* (1998) reported that, during a median follow-up of 13 months, there was an incidence of cytological SIL of 20.5% for HIV-infected vs. 4.9% for HIV-uninfected women. In WIHS, there were 2864 women–years of follow-up in HIV-infected women with a normal enrolment cytology

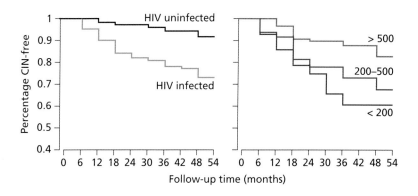

Fig. 35A.6 Impact of HIV infection and immunosuppression on the incidence of biopsy-confirmed CIN. Modified from Ellerbrock *et al.* (2000).

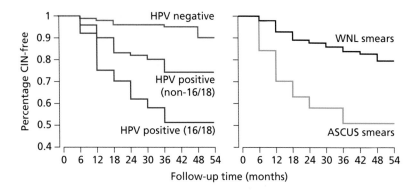

Fig. 35A.7 Impact of HPV DNA status and enrolment cytology result on the incidence of biopsy-confirmed CIN in HIV-infected women. Modified from Ellerbrock *et al.* (2000).

who were followed 6-monthly for up to 5 years (Massad *et al.*, 2001). The incidence of a cytological result of LSIL or greater was 8.9 per 100 women–years of follow-up in this cohort of HIV-infected women vs. 2.2 per 100 women–years of follow-up among the HIV-uninfected cohort. As in the NYCDS, HPV status and CD4+ T-lymphocyte count were predictive of the development of a cytological abnormality on follow-up among HIV-infected women in WIHS. Similar results have also been reported from HERS (Schuman *et al.*, 2003). In HERS, women were followed semi-annually for up to 5.5 years. During follow-up, 35% of the HIV-infected women and 9% of the HIV-uninfected women had incident SIL detected cytologically. The incidence of SIL was 11.5 per 100 women–years of follow-up among the HIV-infected cohort vs. 2.6 in the HIV-uninfected group. Again, risk of incident SIL was increased among women with lower CD4+ T-lymphocyte counts and those who had HPV infections, with risk ordering from low- to high-risk HPV type (Schuman *et al.*, 2003).

IMPACT OF HIGHLY ACTIVE ANTIRETROVIRAL THERAPY (HAART) ON HPV INFECTIONS AND CIN

The introduction of highly active antiretroviral therapy (HAART) in 1995 dramatically changed the natural history of HIV infections. Prior to the introduction of HAART, the major causes of death in HIV-infected individuals were opportunistic infections such as *Pneumocystis carinii* pneumonia, *Mycobacterium avium* complex and toxoplasmosis. Because HAART is very effective in reducing HIV levels and can restore immune function and produce improvements in CD4+ T-cell counts, the spectrum of disease in the AIDS epidemic has been shifting since its introduction (MMWR Guidelines, 2002). Death from opportunistic infections has become much less common in HIV-infected individuals, and the overall morbidity and mortality of HIV infection have been reduced. It is now projected that 20–40% of HIV-infected individuals will live long enough to be diagnosed with a malignancy (Goedert *et al.*, 1998). The associations between HPV and level of immunosuppression described above indicate that a high rate of reactivation of previously acquired HPV infections occurs in HIV-infected women and that this reactivation can occur even at relatively minor levels of immunosuppression (Palefsky *et al.*, 1999). Moreover, immunosuppression favours the development of lesions in women with detectable levels of HPV DNA. Understanding the impact that reconstitution of immune function through the use of HAART has on the reactivation of HPV infections or the preferential development of HPV-associated lesions is essential to understanding the impact that changes in therapy will have on HPV-associated disease.

The impact that HAART is having on either the shedding of HPV DNA or CIN is currently unclear because different studies have observed discordant results. Studies by Heard *et al.* from France have reported quite encouraging results with the use of HAART. In an initial study, 49 HIV-infected women who started HAART were followed for 5 months after initiation of therapy (Heard *et al.*, 1998). The prevalence of SIL decreased from 69% to 53% during follow-up, and cytology returned to normal in nine out of 21 women who had a LSIL cytology result at the initiation of HAART. Despite the impact of HAART on cytologically detected SIL, there was no impact on the detection of HPV DNA. In a subsequent study from the same group, 168 HIV-infected women with evidence of CIN (based on either cytology or colposcopy with biopsy) were followed. Ninety-six of these women received HAART, and the rates of regression were twice as high in women receiving HAART as in those not receiving HAART (Heard *et al.*, 2002). In contrast to these encouraging results, Lillo *et al.* (2001) found less of an effect of HAART in 163 HIV-infected Italian women who were followed for a median of 15.4 months (Uberti-Foppa *et al.*, 2003). During follow-up, women receiving HAART showed a significant increase in CD4+ T-lymphocyte counts relative to baseline values. However, the use of HAART was not associated with a reduction in the persistence of HPV DNA detection, nor was it associated with an improvement in existing cytological lesions or reduction in the incidence of new cytological abnormalities. In a subsequent study from the same group, 154 HIV-infected women were followed for 36 months (Uberti-Foppa *et al.*, 2003). In that study, they reported that time-based analyses found no relationship between the type of anti-HIV treatment and cytological results. None of the treatments was associated with a changed cytological diagnosis. There was, however, a significant reduction in the number of biopsy-confirmed CIN lesions in women undergoing long-term, stable HAART. Analysis of the data from HERS indicates that women receiving HAART were 0.68 times (95% CI 0.52–0.8) less likely to show cytological progression and 1.5 times (95% CI 1.3–1.9) more likely to show cytological regression than HIV-infected women not receiving HAART (Minkoff *et al.*, 2001).

INVASIVE CERVICAL CANCER IN HIV-INFECTED WOMEN

Developed countries

On 1 January 1993, invasive cervical cancer was included among the AIDS-defining conditions in the Centers for Disease Control and Prevention (CDC) expanded AIDS surveillance case definition (CDC, 1993). During the first year after the CDC included invasive cervical cancer in the AIDS case definition, 1.3% of women who were diagnosed with AIDS had invasive cervical cancer as their AIDS-defining illness (Klevens *et al.*, 1996). Among women with AIDS at a Brooklyn, NY, inner city teaching hospital, invasive cervical cancer was the sixth most common AIDS-defining illness (Maiman *et al.*, 1997). During the 6-year period from 1993 to 1998, 23 561 women were diagnosed with AIDS in the World Health Organization European region. Invasive cervical cancer was the AIDS-defining illness in 2.3% of these women, and the proportion of women that had invasive cervical cancer was relatively stable during this time period (Dal Maso *et al.*, 2001). The three European countries most affected by HIV are Spain, Italy and France and, in these three countries, a greater proportion of intravenous drug users presented with invasive cervical cancer as their AIDS-defining illness than did non-intravenous drug users (3.2% vs. 1.8%) (Dal Maso *et al.*, 2001).

In 1993, when the CDC made invasive cervical cancer an AIDS-defining condition, the linkage between AIDS and cervical cancer was poorly quantified. Numerous small cases series had indicated the possibility of a linkage between invasive cervical cancer and HIV infection, and increases in the prevalence of CIN lesions in HIV-infected women were well documented. However, there were few data to indicate that the prevalence of invasive cervical cancer was actually increased in this population. In the decade since invasive cervical cancer was designated as an AIDS-defining condition, considerable evidence has accumulated clearly linking HIV infection with cervical cancer. There are now data from the United States that clearly indicate a higher prevalence of cervical cancer in HIV-infected than in uninfected women. In 1998, a report from the CDC's Sentinel Hospital Surveillance System for

HIV Infection found that the prevalence of invasive cervical cancer was modestly higher for HIV-infected women (10.4 cases per 1000 women) than for HIV-uninfected women (6.2 cases per 1000 women) (RR = 1.7; 95% CI 1.1–2.5) (Chin *et al.*, 1998). Goedert *et al.* (1998) matched various AIDS registries and cancer registries in the United States and Puerto Rico and found a fivefold elevated risk of invasive cervical cancer during the early pre-AIDS period but weaker (elevated but non-significant) risks after AIDS. Similar registry matches in New York state, New York City and Texas have reported significant increases in invasive cervical cancer among HIV-infected women (Cooksley *et al.*, 1999; Fordyce *et al.*, 2000; Gallagher *et al.*, 2001). For example, in New York City, the standardised incidence ratio (SIR) for invasive cervical cancer in HIV-infected women compared with uninfected women is 9.2 (Fordyce *et al.*, 2000).

Frisch *et al.* (2000), from the National Cancer Institutes, studied *in situ* and invasive HPV-associated lesions among 51 760 HIV-infected women using registry information. They found significant increases for a variety of HPV-associated non-invasive neoplasms including *in situ* cervical (RR = 4.6), vulvovaginal (RR = 3.9) and anal (RR = 7.8) lesions. For invasive cancer, there were significant increases for cervical (RR = 5.4), vulva/vagina (RR = 5.8) and anus (RR = 6.8). Among the invasive cancers, relative risks changed little during the 10 years spanning AIDS onset. This suggests that HPV persistence, but not late-stage cancer invasion, is strongly influenced by immune status. Moreover, the 'dose–response' relationship between degree of immunosuppression and development of invasive cancer is substantially different for HPV-associated cancers than for other common cancers such as Kaposi's sarcoma and non-Hodgkin's lymphoma (Frisch *et al.*, 2000).

Even greater increases in risk of cervical cancer have been reported in a registry matching study from Italy (Franceschi *et al.*, 1998). The Italian study linked the National AIDS Registry and 13 population-based Italian cancer registries and found a relative risk of 15.5 (95% CI 4.0–40.1) for invasive cervical cancer in women with HIV/AIDS. Differences in the magnitude of risk for invasive cervical cancer associated with HIV between the United States and southern Europe may be attributed to the more aggressive screening for and treatment of precancerous lesions in HIV-infected women under intense medical scrutiny in the United States. This may mask associations between HIV infection and invasive cervical cancer, particularly as HIV-related disease progresses.

A prospective follow-up study of HIV-infected and control uninfected women in the US, HERS, reported a relatively low invasive cervical cancer incidence among HIV-infected women that was not significantly increased compared with that of the HIV-uninfected control women (Phelps *et al.*, 2001). This study followed 871 HIV-infected women between 1993 and 2000 and identified five invasive cervical carcinomas. No cervical cancers were identified in the HIV-uninfected control group. The rate of invasive cervical cancer was 1.2 per 1000 person–years in the HIV-infected group compared with 0 per 1000 patient–years in control, HIV-uninfected group ($P =$ 017). The cancers that were identified in HIV-infected women were all relatively early stage (four stage 1B and one stage 1A) and were identified in women with a mean age of 36 years and a mean CD4 T-cell count of 443 cells/mm^3. In the larger Women's Interagency HIV Study (WIHS), which followed 1661 HIV-infected women for a total of 8260 women–years of observation, only a single case of incident invasive cervical cancer was identified, yielding an incidence rate of 1.2/10 000 women–years (95% CI 0.3–6.7/10 000 women–years) (Massad *et al.*, 2004). In contrast, a European cohort study that included 2141 HIV-infected women from France and Italy reported a significant 13-fold increase in invasive cervical cancer in HIV-infected compared with HIV-uninfected women (Serraino *et al.*, 1999). In the European cohort study, increased risk was particularly evident among known intravenous drug users (standardised incidence ratio of 16.7 compared with 6.7 for non-intravenous drug users). Additional follow-up of this cohort indicated that, during the period 1981–1995, there was an increasing trend observed in the incidence of invasive cervical cancer and other AIDS-defining diseases. After 1996, with the introduction of HAART, this trend continued for invasive cervical cancer, whereas the incidence of other AIDS-defining diseases has decreased since 1996 (Dorrucci *et al.*, 2001). Clinically, one of the most important points shown by the prospective follow-up studies is that, when regular cytological screening is combined with appropriate work-up and treatment of abnormalities, invasive cervical cancer should be an uncommon outcome in HIV-infected women.

Developing countries

Somewhat paradoxically, there are few data supporting an increase in invasive cervical cancer in sub-Saharan Africa over the last decade as the HIV/AIDS epidemic has devastated the population of women of reproductive age in entire countries. In many sub-Saharan African countries, invasive cervical cancer was one of the most common causes of cancer-associated death in women prior to the HIV/AIDS epidemic (Parkin *et al.*, 1993, 1999a). However, reports from Rwanda, Kenya and Côte d'Ivoire have not documented a clear association between cervical cancer and HIV infection (La Ruche *et al.*, 1998; Newton *et al.*, 2001; Gichangi *et al.*, 2002). In Kenya, for example, the incidence of invasive cervical cancer was estimated to be 45/100 000 women in the early 1980s. Over the next decade, there was absolutely no change in the proportion of invasive cervical cancers compared with that of other gynaecological malignancies, despite the fact that the prevalence of HIV infection in women increased threefold (Gichangi *et al.*, 2002). A case–control study from Kampala,

Uganda, found a strong association between HIV infection and non-Hodgkin's lymphoma and conjunctival squamous cell carcinoma, but not with invasive cervical cancer (Newton *et al.*, 2001). Patil *et al.* (1995) reported no change in the frequency of cervical cancer during the 1980s in Lusaka, Zambia. Case series of women with invasive cervical cancer from South Africa, Uganda and Kenya indicated that HIV-infected women present approximately 5–10 years earlier with invasive cervical cancer than do HIV-uninfected women (Lomalisa *et al.*, 2000; Gichangi *et al.*, 2002; Wabinga *et al.*, 2003). However, no change in the age distribution of women presenting with invasive cervical cancer has been observed in Kenya or Zambia over the last decade (Patil *et al.*, 1995; Gichangi *et al.*, 2002). In Uganda, Parkin *et al.* (1999b) found that a marked increase in the incidence of cervical cancer occurred in the period from 1960 to 1990 but that, after 1990, the incidence of cervical cancer stabilised. They concluded that the increases occurring prior to 1990 were unlikely to be related to increases in HIV (Parkin *et al.*, 1999b). The reason that there has not been an increase in invasive cervical cancer in sub-Saharan Africa is most likely the short survival of most HIV-infected women in these countries and the lack of cytological screening programmes to identify invasive cervical cancers should they arise. In Kenya, the mean survival time for women with HIV infection is 5 years (Gichangi *et al.*, 2002). Even if HIV markedly reduced the time required for the development of invasive cervical cancer, it is unlikely that the average HIV-infected African woman would live long enough to present with symptomatic cancer. Some support for this speculation comes from a study from Côte d'Ivoire that found no association between invasive cervical cancer and HIV-1 infection but a weak association between invasive cervical cancer and HIV-2 infection ($P =$ 0.05) (La Ruche *et al.*, 1998). HIV-2 infection typically has a considerably better prognosis than HIV-1 infection and, therefore, HIV-2-infected women may survive long enough to develop invasive cervical cancer. Further study is required to determine whether the risk of cervical cancer in HIV-infected women will increase as the women survive longer with the advent of combination treatment using HAART.

SUMMARY

Based on over a decade of work by numerous investigators, it is now clear that HIV infection has a profound impact on cervical neoplasia. There are extremely high rates of anogenital HPV infections in HIV-infected women, and these infections are significantly more likely to be persistent in this population. There is also a high prevalence of CIN in HIV-infected women, and much of the CIN is high grade (CIN2/3). In countries with relatively low endemic rates of invasive cervical cancer, where HIV-infected women live long enough to develop invasive cervical cancer, an increase in invasive cervical cancer has been documented. However, there is much that is simply not known about the mechanisms by which HIV infection impacts on HPV DNA shedding from the genital tract and the mechanism responsible for the development of CIN in HPV DNA-positive, HIV-infected women. An additional area where more studies are needed is to define better the impact that treatment with HAART has on the natural history of HPV infections and the incidence of cervical neoplasia.

REFERENCES

Ahdieh L, Klein RS, Burk R *et al.* (2001) Prevalence, incidence, and type-specific persistence of human papillomavirus in human immunodeficiency virus (HIV)-positive and HIV-negative women. *Journal of Infectious Diseases* 184 (6): 682–690.

Barkan SE, Melnick SL, Preston-Martin S *et al.* (1998) The Women's Interagency HIV Study. WIHS Collaborative Study Group. *Epidemiology* 9 (2): 117–125.

Branca M, Delfino A, Rossi E *et al.* (1995) Cervical intraepithelial neoplasia and human papillomavirus related lesions of the genital tract in HIV positive and negative women. *European Journal of Gynaecologic Oncology* 16 (5): 410–417.

Branca M, Migliore G, Giuliani ML *et al.* (2000) Squamous intraepithelial lesions (SILs) and HPV associated changes in HIV infected women or at risk of HIV. DIANAIDS Cooperative Study Group. *European Journal of Gynaecologic Oncology* 21 (2): 155–159.

CDC (1990) Risk for cervical disease in HIV-infected women — New York City. *Morbidity and Mortality Weekly Report* 39: 846–849.

CDC (1993) Revised classification system for HIV infection and expanded surveillance case definition for AIDS among adolescents and adults. *Morbidity and Mortality Weekly Review* 41: 1–20.

Chin KM, Sidhu JS, Janssen RS *et al.* (1998) Invasive cervical cancer in human immunodeficiency virus-infected and uninfected hospital patients. *Obstetrics and Gynecology* 92: 83–87.

Cibere J, Sibley J, Haga M (2001) Systemic lupus erythematosus and the risk of malignancy. *Lupus* 10 (6): 394–400.

Conti M, Agarossi A, Parazzini F *et al.* (1993) HPV, HIV infection, and risk of cervical intraepithelial neoplasia in former intravenous drug abusers. *Gynecologic Oncology* 149 (3): 344–348.

Cooksley CD, Hwang LY, Waller DK *et al.* (1999) HIV-related malignancies: community-based study using linkage of cancer registry and HIV registry data. *International Journal of STD and AIDS* 10 (12): 795–802.

Dal Maso L, Serraino D, Franceschi S (2001) Epidemiology of AIDS-related tumours in developed and developing countries. *European Journal of Cancer* 37 (10): 1188–1201.

Dorrucci M, Suligoi B, Serraino D *et al.* (2001) Incidence of invasive cervical cancer in a cohort of HIV-seropositive women before and after the introduction of highly active antiretroviral therapy. *Journal of Acquired Immune Deficiency Syndrome* 26 (4): 377–380.

Duerr A, Kieke B, Warren D *et al.* (2001) Human papillomavirus-associated cervical cytologic abnormalities among women with or at risk of infection with human immunodeficiency virus. *American Journal of Obstetrics and Gynecology* 184 (4): 584–590.

Ellerbrock TV, Chiasson MA, Bush TJ *et al.* (2000) Incidence of cervical squamous intraepithelial lesions in HIV-infected women. *Journal of the American Medical Association* 283 (8): 1031–1037.

Feingold AR, Vermund SH, Burk RD *et al.* (1990) Cervical cytologic abnormalities and papillomavirus in women infected with human immunodeficiency virus. *Journal of Acquired Immune Deficiency Syndrome* 3 (9): 896–903.

Fordyce EJ, Wang Z, Kahn AR *et al.* (2000) Risk of cancer among women with AIDS in New York City. *AIDS Public Policy Journal* 15 (3–4): 95–104.

Franceschi S, Dal Maso L, Arniani S *et al.* (1998) Risk of cancer other than Kaposi's sarcoma and non-Hodgkin's lymphoma in persons with AIDS in Italy. Cancer and AIDS Registry Linkage Study. *British Journal of Cancer* 78 (7): 966–970.

Frisch M, Biggar RJ, Goedert JJ (2000) Human papillomavirus-associated cancers in patients with human immunodeficiency virus infection and acquired immunodeficiency syndrome. *Journal of the National Cancer Institute* 92 (18): 1500–1510.

Gallagher B, Wang Z, Schymura MJ *et al.* (2001) Cancer incidence in New York State in acquired immunodeficiency syndrome patients. *American Journal of Epidemiology* 154 (6): 544–556.

Gichangi P, De Vuyst H, Estambale B *et al.* (2002) HIV and cervical cancer in Kenya. *International Journal of Gynaecology and Obstetrics* 76 (1): 55–63.

Goedert JJ, Cote TR, Virgo P *et al.* (1998) Spectrum of AIDS-associated malignant disorders. *Lancet* 351 (9119): 1833–1839.

Guidelines for preventing opportunistic infections in HIV-infected persons (2002) *Morbidity and Mortality Weekly Review* (MMWR) 51 (No. RR-8): 1–46.

Hawes SE, Critchlow CW, Faye Niang MA *et al.* (2003) Increased risk of high-grade cervical squamous intraepithelial lesions and invasive cervical cancer among African women with human immunodeficiency virus type 1 and 2 infections. *Journal of Infectious Diseases* 188 (4): 555–563.

Heard I, Schmitz V, Costagliola D *et al.* (1998) Early regression of cervical lesions in HIV-seropositive women receiving highly active antiretroviral therapy. *AIDS* 12 (12): 1459–1464.

Heard I, Tassie JM, Schmitz V *et al.* (2000) Increased risk of cervical disease among human immunodeficiency virus-infected women with severe immunosuppression and high human papillomavirus load (1). *Obstetrics and Gynecology* 96 (3): 403–409.

Heard I, Tassie JM, Kazatchkine MD *et al.* (2002) Highly active antiretroviral therapy enhances regression of cervical intraepithelial neoplasia in HIV-seropositive women. *AIDS* 16 (13): 1799–1802.

Jamieson DJ, Duerr A, Burk R *et al.* (2002) Characterization of genital human papillomavirus infection in women who have or who are at risk of having HIV infection. *American Journal of Obstetrics and Gynecology* 186 (1): 21–27.

Johnstone FD, McGoogan E, Smart GE *et al.* (1994) A population-based, controlled study of the relation between HIV infection and cervical neoplasia. *British Journal of Obstetrics and Gynaecology* 101 (11): 986–991.

Klevens MR, Fleming PL, Mays MA *et al.* (1996) Characteristics of women with AIDS and invasive cancer. *Obstetrics and Gynecology* 88: 76–80.

Kreiss JK, Kiviat NB, Plummer FA *et al.* (1992) Human immunodeficiency virus, human papillomavirus, and cervical intraepithelial neoplasia in Nairobi prostitutes. *Sexually Transmitted Diseases* 19 (1): 54–59.

La Ruche G, Ramon R, Mensah-Ado I *et al.* (1998) Squamous intraepithelial lesions of the cervix, invasive cervical carcinoma, and immunosuppression induced by human immunodeficiency virus in Africa. *Cancer* 82: 2401–2408.

Laga M, Icenogle JP, Marsella R *et al.* (1992) Genital papillomavirus infection and cervical dysplasia — opportunistic complications of HIV infection. *International Journal of Cancer* 50 (1): 45–48.

Lillo FB, Ferrari D, Veglia F *et al.* (2001) Human papillomavirus infection and associated cervical disease in human immunodeficiency virus-infected women: effect of highly active antiretroviral therapy. *Journal of Infectious Diseases* 184 (5): 547–551.

Lomalisa P, Smith T, Guidozzi F (2000) Human immunodeficiency virus infection and invasive cervical cancer in South Africa. *Gynecologic Oncology* 77 (3): 460–463.

Maggwa BN, Hunter DJ, Mbugua S *et al.* (1993) The relationship between HIV infection and cervical intraepithelial neoplasia among women attending two family planning clinics in Nairobi, Kenya. *AIDS* 7 (5): 733–738.

Maiman M, Fruchter RG, Clark M *et al.* (1997) Cervical cancer as an AIDS-defining illness. *Obstetrics and Gynecology* 89 (1): 76–80.

Marte C, Kelly P, Cohen M *et al.* (1992) Papanicolaou smear abnormalities in ambulatory care sites for women infected with the human immunodeficiency virus. *American Journal of Obstetrics and Gynecology* 166 (4): 1232–1237.

Massad LS, Riester KA, Anastos KM *et al.* (1999) Prevalence and predictors of squamous cell abnormalities in Papanicolaou smears from women infected with HIV-1. Women's Interagency HIV Study Group. *Journal of Acquired Immune Deficiency Syndrome* 21 (1): 33–41.

Massad LS, Ahdieh L, Benning L *et al.* (2001) Evolution of cervical abnormalities among women with HIV-1: evidence from surveillance cytology in the women's interagency HIV study. *Journal of Acquired Immune Deficiency Syndrome* 27 (5): 432–442.

Massad LS, Seaberg EC, Watts DH *et al.* (2004) Low incidence of invasive cervical cancer among HIV-infected US women in a prevention program. *AIDS* 18 (1): 109–113.

Minkoff H, Feldman J, DeHovitz J *et al.* (1998) A longitudinal study of human papillomavirus carriage in human immunodeficiency virus-infected and human immunodeficiency virus-uninfected women. *American Journal of Obstetrics and Gynecology* 178: 982–986.

Minkoff HL, Eisenberger-Matityahu D, Feldman J *et al.* (1999) Prevalence and incidence of gynecologic disorders among women infected with human immunodeficiency virus. *American Journal of Obstetrics and Gynecology* 180 (4): 824–836.

Minkoff H, Ahdieh L, Massad LS *et al.* (2001) The effect of highly active antiretroviral therapy on cervical cytologic changes associated with oncogenic HPV among HIV-infected women. *AIDS* 15 (16): 2157–2164.

Newton R, Ziegler J, Beral V *et al.* (2001) A case–control study of human immunodeficiency virus infection and cancer in adults and children residing in Kampala, Uganda. *International Journal of Cancer* 92 (5): 622–627.

Palefsky JM, Minkoff H, Kalish LA *et al.* (1999) Cervicovaginal human papillomavirus infection in human immunodeficiency virus-1 (HIV)-positive and high-risk HIV-negative women. *Journal of the National Cancer Institute* 91 (3): 226–236.

Parkin DM, Pisani P, Ferlay J (1993) Estimates of the worldwide incidence of eighteen major cancers in 1985. *International Journal of Cancer* 54 (4): 594–606.

Parkin DM, Wabinga H, Nambooze S *et al.* (1999a) AIDS-related cancers in Africa: maturation of the epidemic in Uganda. *AIDS* 13 (18): 2563–2570.

Parkin DM, Pisani P, Ferlay J (1999b) Estimates of the worldwide incidence of 25 major cancers in 1990. *International Journal of Cancer* 80 (6): 827–841.

Patil P, Elem B, Zumla A (1995) Pattern of adult malignancies in Zambia (1980–1989) in light of the human immunodeficiency virus type 1 epidemic. *Journal of Tropical Medicine and Hygiene* 98 (4): 281–284.

Penn I (1986) Cancers of the anogenital region in renal transplant recipients. *Cancer* 58: 611–616.

Penn I (1988) Tumors of the immunocompromised patient. *Annals of Internal Medicine* 39: 63–73.

Phelps RM, Smith DK, Heilig CM *et al.* (2001) Cancer incidence in women with or at risk for HIV. *International Journal of Cancer* 94 (5): 753–757.

Provencher D, Valme B, Averette HE *et al.* (1998) HIV status and positive Papanicolaou screening: identification of a high-risk population. *Gynecologic Oncology* 31 (1): 184–190.

Schuman P, Ohmit SE, Klein RS *et al.* (2003) Longitudinal study of cervical squamous intraepithelial lesions in human immunodeficiency virus (HIV)-seropositive and at-risk HIV-seronegative women. *Journal of Infectious Diseases* 188 (1): 128–136.

Seck AC, Faye MA, Critchlow CW *et al.* (1994) Cervical intraepithelial neoplasia and human papillomavirus infection among Senegalese women seropositive for HIV-1 or HIV-2 or seronegative for HIV. *International Journal of STD and AIDS* 5 (3): 189–193.

Serraino D, Carrieri P, Pradier C *et al.* (1999) Risk of invasive cervical cancer among women with, or at risk for, HIV infection. *International Journal of Cancer* 82 (3): 334–337.

Six C, Heard I, Bergeron C *et al.* (1998) Comparative prevalence, incidence and short-term prognosis of cervical squamous intraepithelial lesions amongst HIV-positive and HIV-negative women. *AIDS* 12 (9): 1047–1056.

Smith D (1998) The HIV Epidemiology Research Study, HIV Out-Patient Study, and the Spectrum of Disease Studies. *Journal of Acquired Immune Deficiency Syndrome Human Retrovirology* 17 (Suppl. 1): S17–19.

Smith JR, Kitchen VS, Botcherby M *et al.* (1993) Is HIV infection associated with an increase in the prevalence of cervical neoplasia? *British Journal of Obstetrics and Gynaecology* 100 (2): 149–153.

Strickler HD, Palefsky JM, Shah KV *et al.* (2003) Human papillomavirus type 16 and immune status in human immunodeficiency virus-seropositive women. *Journal of the National Cancer Institute* 95 (14): 1062–1071.

Sun XW, Ellerbrock TV, Lungu O *et al.* (1995) Human papillomavirus infection in human immunodeficiency virus-seropositive women. *Obstetrics and Gynecology* 85 (5 Pt 1): 680–686.

Sun XW, Kuhn L, Ellerbrock TV *et al.* (1997) Human papillomavirus infection in HIV-seropositive women; natural history and variability of detection. *New England Journal of Medicine* 337: 1343–1349.

Temmerman M, Tyndall MW, Kidula N *et al.* (1999) Risk factors for human papillomavirus and cervical precancerous lesions, and the role of concurrent HIV-1 infection. *International Journal of Gynaecology and Obstetrics* 65 (2): 171–181.

Uberti-Foppa C, Ferrari D, Lodini S *et al.* (2003) Long-term effect of highly active antiretroviral therapy on cervical lesions in HIV-positive women. *AIDS* 17 (14): 2136–2138.

UNAIDS Statistical Summary (2003) *2004 Report on Global AIDS Epidemic.* Geneva: UNAIDS.

Vermund SH, Kelley KF, Klein RS *et al.* (1991) High risk of human papillomavirus infection and cervical squamous intraepithelial lesions among women with symptomatic human immunodeficiency virus infection. *American Journal of Obstetrics and Gynecology* 165 (2): 392–400.

Vernon SD, Reeves WC, Clancy KA *et al.* (1994) A longitudinal study of human papillomavirus DNA detection in human immuno-deficiency virus type 1-seropositive and -seronegative women. *Journal of Infectious Diseases* 169 (5): 1108–1112.

Wabinga H, Ramanakumar AV, Banura C *et al.* (2003) Survival of cervix cancer patients in Kampala, Uganda: 1995–1997. *British Journal of Cancer* 89 (1): 65–69.

Weissenborn SJ, Funke AM, Hellmich M *et al.* (2003) Oncogenic human papillomavirus DNA loads in human immunodeficiency virus-positive women with high-grade cervical lesions are strongly elevated. *Journal of Clinical Microbiology* 41 (6): 2763–2767.

Wright TC (1995) Cervical disease in HIV-infected women: prevalence, pathogenesis, detection, and treatment. In: Luesley D, Jordan J, Richart RM (eds) *Intraepithelial Neoplasia of the Lower Genital Tract*. Edinburgh: Churchill Livingstone, pp. 263–277.

Wright TC, Schiffman M (2003) Adding a test for human papil-lomavirus DNA to cervical-cancer screening. *New England Journal of Medicine* 348 (6): 489–490.

Wright TC, Sun X-W (1996) Anogenital papillomavirus infection and neoplasia in immunodeficient women. *Obstetrics and Gynecology Clinics of North America* 23: 861–894.

Wright TC, Jr, Ellerbrock TV, Chiasson MA *et al.* (1994) Cervical intraepithelial neoplasia in women infected with human immuno-deficiency virus: prevalence, risk factors, and validity of Papanicolaou smears. New York Cervical Disease Study. *Obstetrics and Gynecology* 84 (4): 591–597.

Immunosuppression and the cervix: other immunosuppressive disorders

Adeola Olaitan and Theresa Freeman-Wang

INTRODUCTION

It has long been recognised that men and women who are immunosuppressed are at increased risk of developing precancerous and invasive squamous lesions of the lower anogenital tract (Penn, 1986a; Fruchter *et al.*, 1996). Apart from human immunodeficiency virus (HIV) infection, the commonest cause of immunosuppression in women in the western world is immunosuppressive medication to reduce the risk of organ rejection in recipients of allograft transplants. Approximately 1500 renal transplants are performed per year in the United Kingdom, and approximately 5000 patients, 50% of those undergoing dialysis, are waiting for renal transplants. Other organs or organ groups are transplanted less commonly, with 675 liver transplants, 166 heart transplants, 94 lung transplants and 32 heart and lung transplants occurring per annum. Improved therapeutic strategies have been associated with better patient and graft survival rates, with 95% of renal transplant recipients alive at 1 year and 87% alive at 5 years. However, susceptibility to neoplastic disorders is increased as a consequence of prolonged immunosuppression. Available data pertaining to cancer risks in renal transplant recipients have been inconsistent, and many of them are derived from international studies, mainly from the United States, which may not be truly representative of the UK population.

CANCERS AFTER TRANSPLANTATION

The incidence of cancers after renal transplantation is significantly higher than in populations that have not undergone transplantation (Table 35B.1). The risk of post-transplantation malignancy is as high as 80%. Interestingly, the cancers occurring most often in the general population — breast, colon, lung, cervix and prostate cancer — are not as prevalent in transplant patients. The increased risk of cancer was best documented in older studies of women who had relatively profound levels of immunosuppression, because of high dosages of immunosuppressive medication prior to the introduction of drugs such as ciclosporin (Porreco *et al.*, 1975; Penn, 1986b, 1988).

Barret *et al.* (1993) reported the clinical course of malig-

nancies in 876 renal transplant recipients. Forty-four patients had epithelial skin cancers, and 36 had non-skin cancers or melanoma. No correlations could be established between disease course and type of immunosuppressive agent, type of disease for which transplantation was required or type of renal allograft donor. The skin cancers demonstrated a propensity for multifocality: 22 of the 44 patients developed multiple separate lesions. The majority of patients had a poor outcome, and the authors concluded that the natural history of cancers developing in renal transplant patients is often more aggressive than would be expected in patients who have not undergone transplants, and that the immunosuppression induced to allow viability of the renal allograft may allow tumour cells to thrive.

Up to 42% of transplant patients develop skin cancer in one form or another within 14 years of surgery. Multiple lesions are more common than in non-transplant patients, as are nodal metastases and precursor lesions such as actinic keratoses. The prevalence of squamous cell carcinoma is increased 27-fold and that of basal cell carcinoma sixfold, which makes their relative prevalence the reverse of that in the population at large. Risk analysis studies indicate that the incidence of skin cancer correlates with the degree and duration of immunosuppression, but no one drug has been implicated as a particular risk. Although environmental factors may be involved, perhaps the most intriguing influence on carcinogenesis is viral infection. Renal transplant patients, both before and after transplantation, are particularly susceptible to viruses that have long been associated with certain types of cancer — Epstein–Barr with non-Hodgkin's lymphoma, HPV with cervical cancer, hepatitis B and C with hepatocellular cancer, and herpes with Kaposi's sarcoma (Sheil, 1999).

Tumours of the lower genital tract

Porreco *et al.* (1975) showed that, in 21 out of 224 patients with post-transplant tumours (9%), the primary site was gynaecological. The predominant lesions were cervical (18 cases), of which 16 were CIN and two were invasive. Halpert *et al.* (1986) evaluated lower genital cytopathology in 105 immunosuppressed renal transplant recipients. Evidence of

Table 35B.1 Most common *de novo* cancers in renal allograft recipients (1968–1999).

Type of neoplasm	No. of tumours
Skin and lip cancers	3897
Post-transplant proliferative disorder (PTLD)	1108
Lung carcinomas	515
Kaposi's sarcoma	422
Uterus carcinomas	406
Kidney carcinomas	393
Colon and rectum carcinomas	342
Breast carcinomas	330
Vulva/perineum/penis/scrotum carcinoma	272

HPV infection was found in 17.5% and of lower genital neoplasia in 9.5%. The rate of virus infection in the immunosuppressed was nine times greater than in a general population and 17 times greater than in a matched immunocompetent population. The rate of cervical neoplasia was 16 times greater than in a general population and nine times greater than in a matched immunocompetent population. In one-third of patients with HPV lesions and one-half of patients with neoplastic lesions, multiple lower genital sites were also involved.

More recent studies have established the relationship between lower genital tract neoplasms and HPV infection, and high-risk oncogenic subtypes have been identified (HPV 16, 18, 45 and 56). Brown *et al.* (2000) evaluated HPV subtypes present in lower genital tract neoplasms in post-renal transplant women and compared the HPV subtypes found in these patients with those found in immunocompetent patients with similar neoplasms and normal immunocompetent control subjects. Twenty specimens from lower genital tract neoplasms of 16 renal transplant patients, 13 specimens from 13 immunocompetent patients with similar histology and 13 patients with normal lower genital tract histology were analysed for the presence of HPV using polymerase chain reaction (PCR). HPV was detected in 21/46 specimens tested. Thirteen of the HPV-positive specimens were from transplant patients, and eight were from immunocompetent patients (five immunocompetent with disease and three normal patients). This difference in the total number of HPV-positive cases was statistically significant between the transplant and immunocompetent groups ($P = 0.02$). Although no difference in HPV 6 and/or 11 was detected between the two groups, HPV subtypes 16 and/or 18 approached statistically significant difference ($P = 0.06$). The authors concluded that high-risk oncogenic HPV subtypes 16 and/or 18 were found at a higher rate in transplant patients than in their immunocompetent counterparts, and that the combination of immunocompromise and increased HPV 16 and/or 18 positivity may place these patients at increased risk for aggressive lower genital tract neoplastic progression.

The aetiology of cancers in immunosuppressed allograft recipients

Managing maintenance immunosuppressive regimens after kidney transplantation is often complex, as the risks of excessive immunosuppression have to be balanced against the risk of graft rejection. Most protocols combine a primary immunosuppressant (ciclosporin or tacrolimus) with one or two adjunctive agents (azathioprine, mycophenolate mofetil, sirolimus, corticosteroids). Formation of neoplasms in post-transplant patients appears to be related not to any particular agent, but more to the cumulative intensity of immunosuppression (Denton *et al.*, 1999).

The cell-mediated immune response is the mainstay in defence against viral agents. When viruses first gain access into the human body, they are taken up by macrophages and other antigen-presenting cells, leading to the release of the soluble immune mediator interleukin 1 (IL-1). IL-1 acts via specific receptors to activate T lymphocytes. There are two distinct populations of T lymphocytes, the CD4 receptor-bearing T-helper cells, which recognise the major histocompatibility complex (MHC) class II antigens, and the CD8+ cytotoxic, suppressor T cells, which recognise MHC class I antigens. Under normal circumstances, both subsets act in synergy to eliminate virus. The CD4+ cells respond to MHC class II antigens on the surface of macrophages and release IL-2 and other soluble chemotactic agents. Cytotoxic T cells then express IL-2 receptors and, under the influence of IL-2, proliferate and acquire cytolytic cytoplasmic granules, which confer the ability to destroy virally infected cells. Other cytokines, such as interferon-γ, which inhibits viral replication, and IL-10, which suppresses CD4+ IL-2 secretion, are released, serving to enhance and regulate the cell-mediated immune response. The proliferation of T cells can lead to a 20- to 30-fold increase in the proportions of virus-specific cytotoxic T-lymphocyte precursor cells. After resolution of the viral infection, T-cell numbers return to normal levels by apoptosis of the expanded population. This T-cell homeostasis is under cytokine control and is a finely balanced mechanism. Failure in any of its steps can lead to an impairment of the cell-mediated immune response.

Immunosuppressive drugs exert their effect by modulating cell-mediated immunity. The individual properties of commonly used drugs are reviewed below.

Prednisone

The historic mainstay of immunosuppression is prednisone. By blocking the production of IL-1 and -6, it depresses the proliferation and activation of T cells, the predominant cellular mediators of organ rejection. The consequence of impaired

T-cell function is the extended persistence of oncogenic HPV, leading to an increased risk of cervical neoplasia.

Ciclosporin

The steroid-sparing drug of choice is ciclosporin, a fungus-derived cyclic polypeptide discovered in the early 1980s. It inhibits the production of IL-2, interferon and other cytokines and, like prednisone, reduces T-cell activation and proliferation. Evidence from animal models suggests that ciclosporin may promote cancer progression. Experimental administration of ciclosporin *in vitro* led to invasive growth of non-transformed cells and was associated with striking morphological changes. It has also been shown to promote tumour growth in immuno-deficient animals.

Azathioprine

Azathioprine is a derivative of 6-mercaptopurine. It functions as an antimetabolite to decrease DNA and RNA synthesis and is used for maintenance immunosuppression. Adverse effects include leucopenia and thrombocytopenia.

Tacrolimus

The macrolide antibiotic tacrolimus, like ciclosporin, is derived from a fungus and inhibits the production of IL-2. It is several times more potent than ciclosporin at the same dosage, however. The adverse effects of the two drugs are similar.

Mycophenolate mofetil

One of the newest drugs used in combination with steroids, mycophenolate mofetil, inhibits both B- and T-cell production. Blood cell counts must be monitored frequently, as one of the principal effects of daily use is bone marrow suppression.

Monoclonal antibodies

Other inhibitors of T-cell activation and proliferation, such as the monoclonal antibodies OKT3 and basiliximab, are used as induction agents under certain conditions. They are typically given for brief periods to patients with a high risk of early rejection, such as those receiving their second or third organ or with a history of multiple blood transfusions.

Screening and management of immunosuppressed women

Although an increased prevalence of cervical cancer has been observed in immunosuppressed women, controlled studies remain rare.

Because of the complexities of screening and managing immunosuppressed women, it is essential that they are managed in centres with demonstrable skill and expertise and with sufficient access to other specialties to facilitate a multidisciplinary management approach. There must be a compromise between the risk of cervical intraepithelial neoplasia (CIN) and the additional psychological and physical trauma of assessment and treatment.

TREATMENT OF CERVICAL NEOPLASIA IN TRANSPLANT RECIPIENTS

The recognition that life expectancy is increasing for recipients of organ transplants has led the National Health Service Cancer Screening Programmes (NHSCSP) to issue evidence-based guidelines for the screening and management of CIN in the immunosuppressed woman (NHSCSP, 2004). The screening and management of immunosuppressed women is complex and, thus, these women should be managed in a centre of excellence with sufficient numbers to maintain expertise.

All women aged 25–65 years with renal failure requiring dialysis are recommended to have cervical cytology performed at or shortly after diagnosis. Colposcopy is also recommended if resources permit. Any cytological abnormality should be managed as a high-grade abnormality requiring prompt referral to colposcopy.

In women iatrogenically immunosuppressed following transplantation who have no history of CIN, cervical screening should be carried out in accordance with the national guidelines. Abnormal cytology should prompt referral to colposcopy.

Women with a history of CIN should have routine follow-up in accordance with the guidelines for the immunocompetent population.

There is no indication for increased surveillance in women receiving chemotherapy for non-genital cancers, women taking steroids or women on estrogen antagonists such as tamoxifen.

CIN, once detected, should be treated with the same criteria and modalities as in the general population. It should be recognised, however, that disease may be multifocal. In addition, excisional techniques may be preferable to ablative techniques so that tissue is available for histology, and occult microinvasive disease is not overlooked.

SUMMARY

Increases in CIN have also been documented for women with less profound levels of immunosuppression, such as those with Hodgkin's disease or systemic lupus erythematosus (Cibere *et al.*, 2001). Gynaecological malignancies have also been encountered in non-transplant patients who were treated with immunosuppressive agents or cancer chemotherapy.

REFERENCES

Barrett WL, First MR, Aron BS *et al.* (1993) Clinical course of malignancies in renal transplant recipients. *Cancer* 72 (7): 2186–2189.

Brown MR, Noffsinger A, First MR *et al.* (2000) HPV subtype analysis in lower genital tract neoplasms of female renal transplant recipients. *Gynecologic Oncology* 79 (2): 220–422.

Cibere J, Sibley J, Haga M (2001) Systemic lupus erythematosus and the risk of malignancy. *Lupus* 10 (6): 394–400.

Denton MD, Magee CC, Sayegh MH (1999) Immunosuppressive strategies in transplantation. *Lancet* 353: 1083.

Fruchter RG, Maiman M, Sedlis A *et al.* (1996) Multiple recurrence of cervical intraepithelial neoplasia in women with the human immunodeficiency virus. *Obstetrics and Gynecology* 87: 338–344.

Halpert R, Fruchter RG, Sedlis A *et al.* (1986) Human papillomavirus and lower genital neoplasia in renal transplant patients. *Obstetrics and Gynecology* 68 (2): 251–258.

NHS Cervical Screening Programme (2004) *Colposcopy and Programme Management. Guidelines for the NHS Cervical Screening Programme.* NHSCSP Publication no. 20. London: NHSCSP.

Penn I (1986a) Cancer as a complication of severe immunosuppression. *Surgery in Gynecology and Obstetrics* 162: 603–610.

Penn I (1986b) Cancers of the anogenital region in renal transplant recipients. *Cancer* 58: 611–616.

Penn I (1988) Tumors of the immunocompromised patient. *Annals of Internal Medicine* 39: 63–73.

Porreco R, Penn I, Droegemueller W *et al.* (1975) Gynecologic malignancies in immunosuppressed organ homograft recipients. *Obstetrics and Gynecology* 45 (4): 359–364.

Sheil A (1999) Patterns of malignancies following renal transplantation. *Transplant Proceedings* 31: 1263.

CHAPTER 36

Staging and pretreatment evaluation of women with cervical cancer

Howard W. Jones III

INTRODUCTION

After the diagnosis of invasive cancer of the cervix has been made, the extent of disease must be determined so that treatment planning can proceed. The extent of disease or stage is also the single most important prognostic factor in cervical cancer. The extent of disease is usually classified by one of several widely accepted staging systems. These staging systems for cervical cancer and the practical techniques for evaluating the extent of disease are discussed in this chapter.

The concept of allocating patients with a similar prognosis to a defined subgroup is not new. In the early part of the twentieth century, the Radiological Subcommission of the Health Organization of the League of Nations requested that a group of radiation therapists put together a report on the results of treatment for cervical cancer. One of the first projects that this group undertook was to develop a classification system that grouped together patients with a similar anatomical extent of disease. This staging system was first published in 1929 and was referred to as the League of Nations Classification for Cervical Cancer (League of Nations, 1929). This early staging system was basically similar to the one we use today. Using this staging system, six European radium institutes published their 5-year survival statistics in an Annual Report (Heyman, 1937) and, the next year, a separate publication called the *Atlas on Cervical Cancer Staging* (Heyma and Strandqvist, 1938) was authored by Professor James Heyman from Stockholm. Cervical cancer was probably the first malignancy to have a specific, well-defined, internationally accepted staging system. The original staging system remained unchanged until 1950 when minor modifications to the early stages were made at an International Gynecological Conference in New York. In 1958, the International Federation of Gynecology and Obstetrics (FIGO) established a Cancer Committee and became a sponsor of the Annual Report, which had been published sporadically since 1937. The FIGO Cancer Committee also assumed the role of updating the staging system for cervical cancer and developing staging systems for other gynaecological malignancies (Table 36.1).

Over the years, the staging of cervical cancer has remained relatively unchanged, which has provided us with a large worldwide database of comparable patients (Boyle *et al.*, 2001).

There are several key elements to every staging system and several somewhat unique factors in the staging of cervical cancer. It is basic to all staging systems that the extent of disease be determined before any therapy can affect the tumour, and that the stage of disease cannot be changed once it has been assigned. If an early-stage cancer was upstaged 8 months later when pulmonary metastases were diagnosed, these patients with a poor outcome would be removed from the early-stage group, thus giving a falsely higher 5-year survival for early-stage patients. Because cervical cancer can be effectively treated by either radiation therapy or surgery, and the staging system should be the same for both sets of patients to provide a fair comparison of each different treatment modality, the cervical cancer staging system is clinical, and the findings at pelvic surgery should not be considered when assigning the FIGO stage. An examination under anaesthesia is permitted (and even encouraged in patients with stage IIB or IIIB disease), as is a biopsy of the cervix, vagina, vulva and superficial nodes. Cystoscopy and proctoscopy with indicated biopsy are also permitted.

In addition, the FIGO Cancer Committee has always wanted to have a universal staging system that would be equally applicable to patients in resource-poor areas of the world as well as those in the most well-equipped cancer centres. For this reason, some of the newer imaging techniques that require expensive equipment, such as computerised tomography (CT) and positron emission tomography (PET), are not yet permitted for official staging. As a result of these restrictions, cancer of the cervix is often understaged (Kupets and Covens, 2001; Martin-Loeches *et al.*, 2002). The most obvious example is the 15% of stage I patients and 35% of stage II patients with metastases to the pelvic lymph nodes. Nevertheless, FIGO staging for cervical cancer is highly correlated with survival (Fig. 36.1).

Although the FIGO staging system has a long history and is the most commonly used staging system in the world,

Table 36.1 Carcinoma of the cervix uteri: FIGO nomenclature (Montreal, 1994) (Benedet *et al.*, 2001).

Stage 0	Carcinoma *in situ*, cervical intraepithelial neoplasia grade III
Stage I	The carcinoma is strictly confined to the cervix (extension to the corpus would be disregarded)
IA	Invasive carcinoma that can be diagnosed only by microscopy
	IA1 Measured stromal invasion of not > 3.0 mm in depth and extension of not > 7.0 mm
	IA2 Measured stromal invasion of > 3.0 mm and not > 5.0 mm with an extension of not > 7.0 mm
IB	Clinically visible lesions limited to the cervix uteri or preclinical cancers greater than stage IA
	IB1 Clinically visible lesions not > 4.0 cm
	IB2 Clinically visible lesions > 4.0 cm
Stage II	Cervical carcinoma invades beyond the uterus, but not to the pelvic wall or to the lower third of the vagina
IIA	No obvious parametrial involvement
IIB	Obvious parametrial involvement
Stage III	The carcinoma has extended to the pelvic wall. On rectal examination, there is no cancer-free space between the tumour and the pelvic wall. The tumour involves the lower third of the vagina. All cases with hydronephrosis or non-functioning kidney are included, unless they are known to result from other causes
IIIA	Tumour involves the lower third of the vagina, with no extension to the pelvic wall
IIIB	Extension to the pelvic wall and/or hydronephrosis or non-functioning kidney
Stage IV	The carcinoma has extended beyond the true pelvis or has involved (biopsy-proven) the mucosa of the bladder or rectum. A bullous oedema, as such, does not permit a case to be allotted to stage IV
IVA	Spread of the growth to adjacent organs
IVB	Spread to distant organs

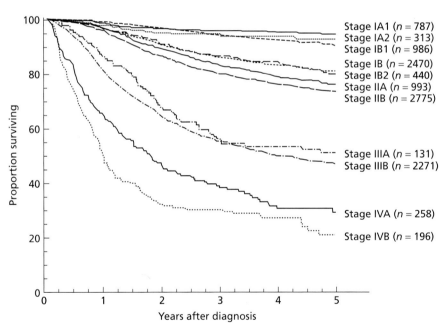

Fig. 36.1 Cervix cancer survival by FIGO stage (Benedet *et al.*, 2001).

there are several other staging classifications in use. The International Union Against Cancer (UICC for its French name) uses the TNM system, which stages cancers using: (i) the size of the untreated primary tumour (T); (ii) the presence or absence of regional lymph node metastases (N); and (iii) distant metastases (M) (Fig. 36.2).

For gynaecological cancers, this staging system is more or less a translation of the FIGO system. This TNM system is also

used by the American Joint Commission on Cancer (Greene *et al.*, 2002). Others have used a very basic classification with three stages: localised, regional and distant metastases. In the past, several surgical staging systems have been used (Onnis *et al.*, 1988). These involved a very precise surgical/anatomical classification of tumours including the diameter of the primary cervical cancer, invasion of the parametrium and lymph node metastases. Such systems required the patients to be treated

DEFINITIONS

Clinical	Pathological	Primary Tumor (T) TNM Categories	FIGO Stages	Definitions
☐	☐	TX		Primary tumour cannot be assessed
☐	☐	T0		No evidence of primary tumour
☐	☐	Tis	0	Carcinoma *in situ*
☐	☐	T1	I	Cervical carcinoma confined to uterus (extension to corpus should be disregarded)
☐	☐	T1a	IA	Invasive carcinoma diagnosed only by microscopy.[1] All macroscopically visible lesions — even with superficial invasion — are T1b/IB. Stromal invasion with a maximal depth of 5.0 mm measured from the base of the epithelium and a horizontal spread of 7.0 mm or less. Vascular space involvement, venous or lymphatic, does not affect classification
☐	☐	T1a1	IA1	Measured stromal invasion 3.0 mm or less in depth and 7.0 mm or less in horizontal spread
☐	☐	T1a2	IA2	Measured stromal invasion more than 3.0 mm and not more than 5.0 mm with a horizontal spread 7.0 mm or less
☐	☐	T1b	IB	Clinically visible lesion confined to the cervix or microscopic lesion greater than T1a2/IA2
☐	☐	T1b1	IB1	Clinically visible lesion 4.0 cm or less in greatest dimension
☐	☐	T1b2	IB2	Clinically visible lesion more than 4.0 cm in greatest dimension
☐	☐	T2	II	Cervical carcinoma invades beyond uterus but not to pelvic wall or to lower third of vagina
☐	☐	T2a	IIA	Tumour without parametrial invasion
☐	☐	T2b	IIB	Tumour with parametrial invasion
☐	☐	T3	III	Tumour extends to pelvic wall and/or involves lower third of vagina and/or causes hydronephrosis or non-functioning kidney
☐	☐	T3a	IIIA	Tumour involves lower third of vagina, no extension to pelvic wall
☐	☐	T3b	IIIB	Tumour extends to pelvic wall and/or causes hydronephrosis or non-functioning kidney
☐	☐	T4	IVA	Tumour invades mucosa of bladder or rectum and/or extends beyond true pelvis (bullous oedema is not sufficient evidence to classify a tumour as T4)

Notes

1. The depth of invasion is defined as the measurement of the tumour from the epithelial–stromal junction of the adjacent most superficial dermal papilla to the deepest point of invasion.

Regional lymph nodes (N)

Clinical	Pathological			
☐	☐	NX		Regional lymph nodes cannot be assessed
☐	☐	N0		No regional lymph node metastasis
☐	☐	N1		Regional lymph node metastasis

Distant metastasis (M)

Clinical	Pathological			
☐	☐	MX		Distant metastasis cannot be assessed
☐	☐	M0		No distant metastasis
☐	☐	M1	IVB	Distant metastasis

Biopsy of metastatic site performed.......... ☐Y .... ☐N
Source of pathological metastatic specimen _____

Fig. 36.2 TNM staging for cervix cancer. From Greene *et al.*, 2002, with permission from Springer–Verlag.

by radical surgery and a careful histopathological study of the surgical specimen. The TNM system can be used for surgically or clinically staged patients. The prefix 'p' is added to the TNM designation to indicate that surgical/pathological staging has been used. Surgical staging has allowed us to learn much about the prognostic importance of various factors in cervical cancer, but such surgical staging systems are not applicable to the majority of patients who are treated with radiation therapy; thus, they are not widely used.

THE FIGO STAGING SYSTEM

The 2003 FIGO staging system for cervical cancer is shown in Figure 36.3. In its simplest form, stage I disease is localised to the cervix while stage II tumours involve the adjacent upper vagina or invade the parametrium lateral to the cervix. In stage III cervical cancer, the tumour extends to involve the distal vagina or the pelvic sidewall on one or both sides and/or causes ureteral obstruction. Patients with stage IV disease have

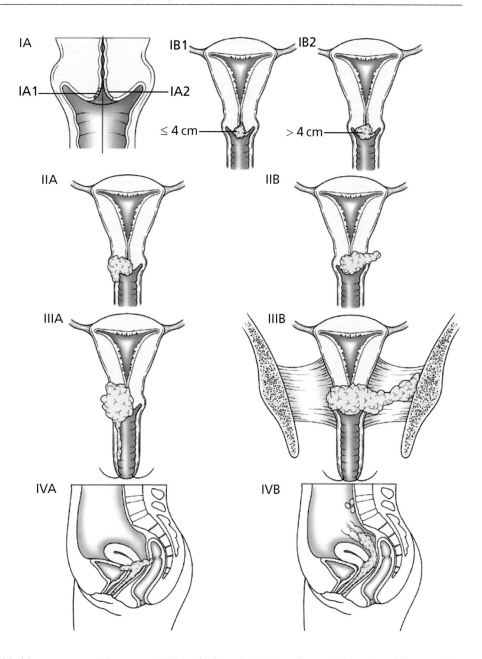

Fig. 36.3 Carcinoma of the cervix uteri: staging cervical cancer (primary tumour and metastases) (Benedet *et al.*, 2001).

distant metastases or invasion of the bladder or rectum. There is also a stage 0 that is defined as carcinoma *in situ* or cervical intraepithelial neoplasia (CIN) grade III. These intraepithelial lesions are discussed elsewhere in this book and will not be covered in this chapter.

Stage IA

Most of the changes in staging have occurred in stage I as improved understanding of the concept of 'microinvasive' cancer has increased the specificity of this classification (Table 36.2).

The idea of a minimally invasive cancer with little or no risk of lymph node metastasis or recurrence was introduced in 1961 with the subdivision of stage I into A and B. stage IA disease was originally defined as 'cases of early stromal invasion (preclinical carcinoma)'. Through the work of Burghardt *et al.* (1991) and others, a great deal of data have been accumulated on the relationship of depth of invasion, tumour volume and the risk of metastatic disease. This information has led to a series of modifications so that stage IA is now very specifically defined and subdivided into stage IA1 (stromal invasion of less than or equal to 3.0 mm) and IA2 (stromal invasion of 3.1–5.0 mm). All stage IA lesions must be no greater than 7.0 mm in diameter as measured by the width of the invasive tumour in any one section. Invasion of lymphatic or vascular spaces does not affect FIGO staging, although several studies have shown that lymph/vascular space invasion increases the

Table 36.2 Substages of FIGO stage 1 (Benedet *et al.*, 2001).

Stage I	The carcinoma is strictly confined to the cervix (extension to the corpus should be disregarded)
IA	Invasive carcinoma that can be diagnosed only by microscopy. All macroscopically visible lesions — even with superficial invasion — are allotted to stage IB. Invasion is limited to a measured stromal invasion with a maximal depth of 5.0 mm and a horizontal extension of not > 7.0 mm. Depth of invasion should not be > 5.0 mm taken from the base of the epithelium of the original tissue — superficial or glandular. The involvement of vascular spaces — venous or lymphatic — should not change the stage allotment
	IA1 Measured stromal invasion of not > 3.0 mm in depth and extension of not > 7.0 mm
	IA2 Measured stromal invasion of > 3.0 mm and not > 5.0 mm with an extension of not > 7.0 mm
IB	Clinically visible lesions limited to the cervix uteri or preclinical cancers greater than stage IA
	IB1 Clinically visible lesions not > 4.0 cm
	IB2 Clinically visible lesions > 4.0 cm

risk of nodal metastasis (Grisaru *et al.*, 2003). The Society of Gynecologic Oncologists has favoured upstaging of patients with lymphatic or vascular space invasion and has recommended that patients with this finding should be treated as if lymph node metastases are definitely possible. Lesions that are clinically visible to the naked eye should be classified as stage IB even if only superficial microscopic invasion is present.

In order adequately to evaluate the depth of stromal invasion and the lateral extent of the lesion, it is necessary to provide the pathologist with a large biopsy — in most cases, a traditional cone biopsy is preferred. When early invasive cancer is suspected, many experts recommend a classic cold knife cone biopsy as it is difficult to obtain a large, well-oriented, single cone specimen by large loop electrosurgical excision of the transformation zone (LLETZ). Careful orientation and processing of the cone specimen and examination of multiple sections are important if accurate staging is to be expected.

Stage IB

Cervical cancer confined to the cervix that is clinically visible and/or microscopically more invasive than stage IA is defined as stage IB. In most areas of the world with well-developed screening programmes, more patients with stage IB cancers are diagnosed than any other stage. Because of the significantly worse prognosis of women with large stage I lesions, in 1994, FIGO subdivided stage IB into IB1, which included lesions 4.0 cm or less in diameter, and IB2 for lesions greater than 4.0 cm (Fig. 36.4). Once again, staging is officially performed by physical examination The results of ultrasound, CT and/or magnetic resonance imaging (MRI) are not permitted to influence official staging, although they may be clinically useful for treatment planning purposes. If two clinicians disagree about the stage of the lesion, by convention, the lower stage is selected. (This is to prevent improving the reported results of treatment due to overstaging.)

It is very difficult to evaluate invasion of the uterine corpus as an extension of a primary cervical cancer so that involvement of the corpus is not considered in staging.

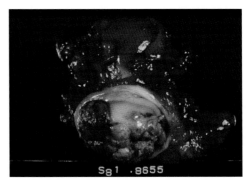

Fig. 36.4 Large, 5.0 cm diameter stage IB2 cervical cancer. Radical hysterectomy specimen.

Stage IIA

Patients with cervical cancer extending from the cervix to involve the vagina are stage IIA. If the lesion is so extensive that it involves the lower one-third of the vagina, the patient is advanced to stage IIIA. Because cervical cancer is so much more common than vaginal cancer, if both the cervix and the vagina are involved, the lesion should be officially staged as a cervical primary. Despite this rule, the author recommends good common sense by the clinician in defining the origin of the tumour.

Stage IIB

When the cancer has spread laterally from the cervix to invade the paracervical or parametrial tissues, it is classified as stage IIB. One or both sides may be involved. This is also a very common stage in many countries. Rectal examination will usually allow the clinician to evaluate lateral parametrial extension.

Stage IIIA

Extension of the cervical cancer to involve the lower one-third of the vagina without pelvic sidewall involvement is defined as stage IIIA. This is an uncommon clinical presentation.

Stage IIIB

When a tumour extends laterally from the cervix to involve one or both pelvic sidewalls, the patient is classified as stage IIIB. This is a relatively common finding in areas where advanced cervical cancer is seen. Women with ureteral obstruction due to cancer (unilateral or bilateral) are also stage IIIB.

Rectal examination is most useful to evaluate the extent of parametrial involvement. For stage IIIB, the tumour must be fixed to the pelvic sidewall with no tumour-free space between the parametrial tumour and the musculofascial sidewall of the pelvis.

Stage IVA

Patients with stage IVA disease have biopsy-proven extension of the primary cervical cancer invading the mucosa of the bladder or rectum. A clinical impression of involvement is not sufficient for this diagnosis — a biopsy must be done to confirm invasion. Bullous oedema of the bladder is also not enough to warrant classification of a patient as stage IVA. Even malignant urine cytology must be confirmed by biopsy.

Stage IVB

When distant metastases are present, then the patient is classified as stage IVB. This would include women with pulmonary metastases on a chest radiograph or those with inguinal or supraclavicular lymph node metastases. As the findings of advanced imaging techniques are not permitted to influence official staging, the results of CT, MRI and PET cannot be used to identify extracervical metastatic disease for staging (although they can be used for treatment planning). Histological confirmation of distant metastases is not required, but biopsy confirmation of superficial nodal metastases is recommended, and other lesions should be sampled if possible.

PATHOLOGY

All histopathological types of primary cervical cancer are suitable for staging. The FIGO classification specifically recognises:
- squamous cell carcinoma, keratinising, non-keratinising and verrucous;
- endometrioid adenocarcinoma;
- clear cell adenocarcinoma;
- adenosquamous carcinoma;
- adenoid cystic carcinoma;
- small cell carcinoma.

Both squamous cell carcinoma *in situ* (or CIN3) and adenocarcinoma *in situ* are also recognised. While histopathological grading is briefly discussed in the FIGO staging classification and grade 1 (well differentiated), grade 2 (moderately differentiated) and grade 3 (poorly or undifferentiated)

are listed, these grades are not defined further, and there is little evidence that grading of cervical cancer is of prognostic significance (Alfsen *et al.*, 2001; Grisaru *et al.*, 2001; Graflund *et al.*, 2002a). Tumour grade is rarely recorded in squamous cell carcinoma of the cervix (Graflund *et al.*, 2002b).

STAGING WORK-UP

The work-up of patients with cancer of the cervix is dependent on the findings on physical examination and the resources available. Although official FIGO staging limits the studies that can be performed to allow uniform staging in various circumstances throughout the world, most clinicians proceed with as thorough a pretreatment evaluation as is clinically indicated and available to them. As with all cancers, a careful history and complete physical examination is the best way to start an evaluation of the extent of disease. In addition to questions about the amount of bleeding and the length of time vaginal bleeding or discharge has been going on, questions about any changes in bladder or bowel function should be asked. Haematuria and rectal bleeding are especially significant. Weight loss, back or hip pain, leg oedema and cough or shortness of breath are all worrisome symptoms of advanced disease. A history of other medical illness may also be very significant. A previous history of renal disease or stones may explain ureteral obstruction or decreased renal function. Serious medical problems may compromise the patient's ability to tolerate surgery, radiation or chemotherapy. A history of medications that may inhibit blood clotting or reduce haematopoietic function is significant. A family history of someone who died from cancer, or was cured, may be important in helping to understand how the patient reacts to her diagnosis.

While the pelvic examination is crucial in staging the patient with cervical cancer, a complete physical examination is also important. Leg oedema, sacroiliac tenderness and enlarged inguinal or supraclavicular nodes may be signs of metastatic cancer. Many patients may not have had regular medical care, and a thorough history and physical examination may identify other medical conditions with no connection to the diagnosis of cervical cancer. Such co-morbidities may influence treatment planning and overall prognosis.

In women with more advanced disease, an examination under anaesthesia is often very helpful in evaluating the extent of pelvic involvement. This examination can be combined with cystoscopy and sigmoidoscopy to complete a thorough staging evaluation in one step. However, in the United States, insurance companies will often refuse to cover these staging examinations as they are not 'therapeutic'. Nevertheless, an examination under anaesthesia is very useful in the pretreatment evaluation and staging of women with suspected stage IIB, IIIB or IV cervical cancer.

While we no longer routinely do a cystoscopy or sigmoidoscopy on all women with cervical cancer, patients with clinical stage III lesions and those with any anterior or posterior extension of tumour should probably undergo cystoscopy and/or sigmoidoscopy.

Biopsy

A biopsy of the primary cancer is, of course, needed to confirm the diagnosis but, in women with large tumours and significant bleeding, many clinicians may be reluctant to do a biopsy as it may initiate further bleeding. Such patients should be referred to a gynaecological oncologist who is trained and experienced in dealing with such problems. A cervical biopsy to diagnose cancer should sample viable tumour and should be large enough to allow identification of the cell type and differentiation if indicated. A small biopsy of necrotic tissue at the tip of an exophytic cervical tumour will not be satisfactory. As noted previously, women with suspected stage IA tumours (microinvasive) should have a large, traditional cold knife cone biopsy to provide an adequate, well-oriented specimen to allow the pathologist to measure depth and width of invasion adequately.

If bleeding occurs following biopsy, it can almost always be controlled by pressure. A large swab or a gauze sponge in a ring forceps can be used immediately after the biopsy to put pressure on the biopsy site. A thick paste of Monsel's solution (ferric subsulphate) applied directly to the biopsy site is also useful, and a combination of pressure and Monsel's solution will control most post-biopsy bleeding. If bleeding persists, the cervix and upper vagina can be packed with a gauze roll. This can be left in place for several hours, overnight or even several days if necessary. The upper vagina can be packed tightly and, if the packing does not extend down the vagina more than halfway, the patient can usually void without difficulty.

It is difficult to control bleeding from a large necrotic cervical cancer with sutures. They usually cut through and may cause even more bleeding. Cryotherapy has been used successfully in some cases. An acetone-soaked pack is painful but can be used as a last resort to control difficult bleeding. Radiation therapy is the definitive treatment for bleeding from cervical cancer. It should be initiated immediately when bleeding is a problem. In most cases, bleeding from the tumour will stop after three to five treatments of 200 cGy each.

Laboratory tests

Relatively few blood studies are required for patients with cervical cancer. A haemoglobin measurement or haematocrit to evaluate the patient for possible anaemia is probably the most important. Recent studies have shown increased effectiveness of radiation therapy in patients who are not anaemic (Grogan *et al.*, 1999). Measurement of serum creatinine and/or blood urea nitrogen is helpful to evaluate renal function, and liver function tests may be useful for a baseline if anaesthesia or

chemotherapy is planned. Other studies may be indicated to evaluate any associated medical conditions. There are no serum tumour markers that have been shown to be clinically useful in cervical cancer.

Imaging studies

Traditionally, the staging work-up of a woman with cervical cancer consisted of an examination under anaesthesia with cystoscopy and proctoscopy and a chest radiograph, intravenous pyelogram (IVP) and barium enema. Even today, these radiological studies are the only ones permitted for official staging, although most patients with advanced disease are evaluated with a CT scan of the abdomen and pelvis (Scheidler and Heuck, 2002).

An IVP is used to identify any ureteral obstruction (advancing the patient to stage IIIB) and can identify the occasional patient with a duplicated ureter (which might be good to know if surgery is planned). It also serves as a baseline study, alerting the clinician to any pre-existing abnormalities of the urinary tract and providing a study for later comparison with any post-treatment abnormalities that may be diagnosed on subsequent studies.

A barium enema is rarely useful, although it has been part of the traditional pretreatment evaluation of the woman with cervical cancer. Direct extension of the tumour posteriorly with rectal involvement is not well visualised on a barium enema because it is so low and often minimal. Occasionally, diverticulosis will be diagnosed, and this may alert the radiation oncologist to an increased risk of bowel complications from pelvic radiation. A pretreatment barium enema may also prove to be a useful baseline study for comparison with a later study done to evaluate rectal bleeding months or years after treatment.

Similar comments could be made about a staging chest radiograph . Rarely will it show metastatic disease or malignant effusions. Most pulmonary nodularity diagnosed in the asymptomatic patient proves to be benign inflammatory granuloma, and these findings on a routine staging work-up usually initiate a costly and eventually negative evaluation. However, an argument can be made that chest radiography is inexpensive, simple and non-invasive so it should be included in the staging work-up.

Today, most women with bulky cervical cancers, stage IIB or greater, will be evaluated with a CT scan or MRI (Nicolet *et al.*, 2000; Scheidler and Heuck, 2002). These studies provide detailed imaging of the soft tissues of the pelvis and abdomen and can be helpful in identifying lymph node metastases as well as ureteral obstruction or other metastatic disease. Usually one technique or the other is used — not both. Some authors have suggested that these studies can replace cystoscopy (Chung *et al.*, 2001), but remember that biopsy confirmation of bladder invasion is necessary for allocation of a patient to stage IV. We have also tried to obtain tissue confirmation of suspicious, enlarged retroperitoneal lymph nodes identified by

CT or MRI. This can usually be done by fine needle aspiration (FNA) of the node using CT guidance. Both CT and MRI have been useful in evaluating the lateral extension of the primary cervical tumour. The results have been shown to correlate well with surgical–pathological staging (Kodaira *et al.*, 2003; Okamoto *et al.*, 2003; Ozsarlak *et al.*, 2003).

Lymphangiography has also been used by some centres to identify lymph node metastasis from primary cervical cancer. A large study from the M.D. Anderson Cancer Center reported a positive predictive value of about 75% and a negative predictive value of 76–77% (Munkarah *et al.*, 2002). While these are reasonable numbers, they demonstrate that lymphangiography is not a terribly sensitive or specific test for identifying lymph node metastases in patients with cervical cancer. The procedure is also technically difficult to perform and, thus, is little used today. Indeed, the sensitivity and specificity of all imaging studies for lymph node metastases in cervical cancer have been unsatisfactory as it has proved difficult to identify small metastatic deposits. These are precisely the ones that need to be identified because they have the greatest potential for cure.

Other imaging studies such as a bone scan or pelvic ultrasound are not recommended as a routine for cervical cancer staging as they are rarely positive. They may be indicated in specific patients with symptoms or signs of bone metastases or adnexal masses.

PET scans are relatively new. They demonstrate areas of increased metabolic activity and so may be particularly useful in identifying small-volume metastatic cancer. Recently, Singh *et al.* (2003) published a report of 47 patients with stage IIIB cervical cancer that suggested a good correlation between PET scan evidence of metastases and survival. PET scanning may also be useful in the diagnosis of metastatic, recurrent disease (Havrilesky *et al.*, 2003), but there have been only a limited number of patients studied.

SURGICAL STAGING

In the past, surgical staging has been done as part of the radical surgical treatment of cervical cancer. However, some have suggested that pretreatment surgical staging may be useful for evaluating the presence of extrapelvic disease, especially para-aortic lymph node metastases, before giving pelvic radiation therapy (Holcomb *et al.*, 1999; Odunsi *et al.*, 2001). This has been done by laparotomy, extraperitoneal dissection and, more recently, by laparoscopy (Vergote *et al.*, 2002).

All these approaches increase the morbidity of radiation therapy. Radiation bowel injury as a result of postoperative adhesions and lymphoedema of the lower extremities associated with an extensive lymph node dissection followed by pelvic radiation are two of the most significant. Some clinicians have attempted to limit the extent of nodal dissection by identifying and removing 'sentinel nodes'. These nodes are felt to represent the first potential site of lymph node mestastasis and, if negative, indicate that there are no nodal metastases. Several investigators have reported the identification of sentinel pelvic nodes in women with cervical cancer, but the clinical significance of this finding remains to be seen (Ramirez and Levenback, 2001; van Dam *et al.*, 2003).

While surgical staging may be able accurately to identify most patients with nodal or extrapelvic metastases, it may have little or no impact on survival, as present treatment modalities are largely ineffective in curing metastatic cervical cancer, especially when the disease has spread beyond the pelvis (Ramirez and Levenback, 2001). Nevertheless, improvements in staging techniques that allow us to identify metastatic disease may reduce morbidity from unnecessary, ineffective treatments and provide a stimulus to develop new, more effective, therapies.

STAGING IN THE FUTURE

To this point, the staging of cervical cancer has remained entirely anatomical. Patients are grouped together in this stage or that based on the anatomical extent of disease. But new developments in the field of tumour markers and genetics may provide us with new and very specific prognostic characteristics that will allow us to define more accurately groups of patients with similar prognoses. Even these factors are all tumour related, and we know that prognosis is also dependent upon host factors. Women with human immunodeficiency virus (HIV) infection are well known to have a very poor prognosis, regardless of stage, because of their lack of immunological defence. There are other less dramatic influences of various medical conditions or lifestyle characteristics on the prognosis of a patient with cervical cancer. These patient characteristics have been termed 'co-morbidities', and several attempts have been made to incorporate them into a more comprehensive staging system. These factors could include not only HIV status but the presence of anaemia, diabetes with vascular disease, diverticulitis, obesity, smoking and other medical or lifestyle characteristics known to affect cervical cancer survival specifically or overall life expectancy in general.

The idea of 'superstaging' using many different factors, both tumour specific and host related, requires large, accurate databases to be useful. Fortunately, with the increased use of computers and worldwide instant connectivity of the internet, it is possible to imagine a clinician in Manchester, UK, accessing a worldwide FIGO database and entering 10 or 20 patient and tumour characteristics, and the database would be able to provide a very specific 5-year survival estimate for that patient. It might even provide different survivals if the patient were to be treated surgically or with radiation therapy. The patient could then be entered in the database, regular follow-up would be requested by the database from the clinician and, over time, a very large, very detailed superstaging system would be developed.

REFERENCES

Alfsen GC, Kristensen GB, Skovlund E *et al.* (2001) Histologic subtype has minor importance for overall survival in patients with adenocarcinoma of the uterine cervix: a population-based study of prognostic factors in 505 patients with nonsquamous cell carcinomas of the cervix. *Cancer* 92: 2471–2483.

Benedet JL, Odicino F, Maisonneuve P *et al.* (2001) Carcinoma of the cervix uteri. In: Boyle P, la Vecchia C, Walker A (eds) *Annual Report on the Results of Treatment in Gynaecological Cancer*, Vol. 24. *Journal of Epidemiology Biostatistics* 6: 24.

Boyle P, la Vecchia C, Walker A (eds) (2001) Annual report on the results of treatment in gynaecological cancer, Vol. 24. *Journal of Epidemiology and Biostatistics* 6: 24.

Burghardt E, Girardi F, Lahousen M *et al.* (1991) Microinvasive carcinoma of the uterine cervix (International Federation of Gynecology and Obstetrics Stage IA). *Cancer* 67: 1037–1045.

Chung H, Ahn HS, Kim YS *et al.* (2001) The value of cystoscopy and intravenous urography after magnetic resonance imaging or computed tomography in the staging of cervical carcinoma. *Yonsei Medical Journal* 42: 527–531.

Graflund M, Sorbe B, Hussein A *et al.* (2002a) The prognostic value of histopathologic grading parameters and microvessel density in patients with early squamous cell carcinoma of the uterine cervix. *International Journal of Gynecological Cancer* 12: 32–41.

Graflund M, Sorbe B, Bryne M *et al.* (2002b) The prognostic value of a histologic grading system, DNA profile, and MIB-1 expression in early stages of cervical squamous cell carcinomas. *International Journal of Gynecological Cancer* 12: 149–157.

Greene FL, Page DL, Fleming ID *et al.* (eds) (2002) *AJCC Cancer Staging Manual*, 6th edn. New York: Springer-Verlag.

Grisaru D, Covens A, Chapman B *et al.* (2001) Does histology influence prognosis in patients with early-stage cervical carcinoma? *Cancer* 92: 2999–3004.

Grisaru DA, Covens A, Franssen E *et al.* (2003) Histopathologic score predicts recurrence free survival after radical surgery in patients with stage IA2–IB1–2 cervical carcinoma. *Cancer* 97: 1904–1908.

Grogan M, Thomas GM, Melamed I *et al.* (1999) The importance of hemoglobin levels during radiotherapy for carcinoma of the cervix. *Cancer* 86: 1528–1536.

Havrilesky J, Wong TZ, Secord AA *et al.* (2003) The role of PET scanning in the detection of recurrent cervical cancer. *Gynecologic Oncology* 90: 186–190.

Heyman J (ed.) (1937) *Annual Report on the Results of Radiotherapy in Carcinoma of the Uterine Cervix*, vol. 1. Stockholm: League of Nations Health Organization.

Heyman J, Strandqvist M (1938) *Atlas Illustrating the Division of Cancer of the Uterine Cervix into Four Stages*. Stockholm: League of Nations.

Holcomb K, Abulafia O, Matthews RP *et al.* (1999) The impact of pretreatment staging laparotomy on survival in locally advanced cervical carcinoma. *European Journal of Gynaecological Oncology* 20: 90–93.

Kodaira T, Fuwa N, Toita T *et al.* (2003) Comparison of prognostic value of MRI and FIGO stage among patients with cervical carcinoma treated with radiotherapy. *International Journal of Radiation Oncology and Biological Physics* 56: 769–777.

Kupets R, Covens A (2001) Is the International Federation of Gynecology and Obstetrics Staging System for cervical carcinoma able to predict survival in patients with cervical carcinoma? *Cancer* 92: 796–804.

League of Nations (1929) *Document CH 788, series III, no. 5.* Stockholm: League of Nations Publications.

Martin-Loeches M, Orti M, Aznar I *et al.* (2002) Does FIGO clinical stage influence the survival of patients with early stages of uterine cervix carcinoma? *European Journal of Gynaecological Oncology* 23: 501–504.

Munkarah AR, Jhingran A, Iyer RB *et al.* (2002) Utility of lymphangiography in the prediction of lymph node metastases in patients with cervical cancer. *International Journal of Gynecological Cancer* 12: 755–759.

Nicolet V, Carignan L, Bourdon F *et al.* (2000) MR imaging of cervical carcinoma: a practical staging approach. *Radiographics* 20: 1539–1549.

Odunsi KO, Lele S, Ghamande S *et al.* (2001) The impact of pretherapy extraperitoneal surgical staging on the evaluation and treatment of patients with locally advanced cervical cancer. *European Journal of Gynaecological Oncology* 22: 325–330.

Okamoto Y, Tanaka YO, Nishida M *et al.* (2003) MR imaging of the uterine cervix: imaging-pathologic correlation. *Radiographics* 23: 425–445.

Onnis A, Marchetti M, Maggino T *et al.* (1988) Management of cervical cancer and surgical–pathological staging (SPS). Report of our clinical case series. *European Journal of Gynaecological Oncology* 9: 115–119.

Ozsarlak O, Tjalma W, Schepens E *et al.* (2003) The correlation of preoperative CT, MR imaging, and clinical staging (FIGO) with histopathology findings in primary cervical carcinoma. *European Radiology* 13: 2338–2345.

Ramirez PT, Levenback C (2001) Sentinel nodes in gynecologic malignancies. *Current Opinion in Oncology* 13: 403–407.

Scheidler J, Heuck AF (2002) Imaging of cancer of the cervix. *Radiology Clinics of North America* 40: 577–590.

Singh AK, Grigsby PW, Dehdashti F *et al.* (2003) FDG-PET lymph node staging and survival of patients with FIGO stage IIIb cervical carcinoma. *International Journal of Radiation Oncology and Biological Physics* 56: 489–493.

van Dam PA, Hauspy J, Vanderheyden T *et al.* (2003) Intraoperative sentinel node identification with technetium-99m-labeled nanocolloid in patients with cancer of the uterine cervix: a feasibility study. *International Journal of Gynecological Cancer* 13: 182–186.

Vergote I, Amant F, Berteloot P *et al.* (2002) Laparoscopic lower para-aortic staging lymphadenectomy in stage IB2, II, and III cervical cancer. *International Journal of Gynecological Cancer* 12: 22–26.

CHAPTER 37

The management of microinvasive carcinoma of the cervix

Donald E. Marsden, Neville F. Hacker and Lyndal Edwards

INTRODUCTION

Since the concept of microinvasive cancer of the cervix was first suggested in 1947 (Mestwerdt, 1947), it has been one of the most controversial topics in gynaecological oncology. As Maimon and colleagues (1988) state:

> Superficially invasive squamous cell carcinoma of the cervix is a subject associated with decades of confusion, a multiplicity of definitions, and a variety of therapeutic approaches.

The aim is to identify a group of patients with 'early' invasive cancer who may safely be treated with procedures carrying lower morbidity and mortality than radical surgery or radiotherapy. More recently, the additional aim of allowing the possibility of pregnancy for women with this disease has become a major issue. As the rate of cervical screening in the community increases, the proportion of early-stage cancers should increase, as most of the patients present with abnormal smears (Östör and Rome, 1994).

An important issue in all considerations of microinvasive cancer of the cervix is 'an unrealistic expectation that the definition should guarantee the safety of conservative therapy' when in fact 'biological phenomena . . . form a spectrum, and do not lend themselves easily to rigid categorisation' (Östör, 1995). Notwithstanding this, there has been considerable progress in our understanding of the nature and management of this condition.

Despite areas of ongoing debate, microinvasive squamous carcinoma of the cervix is a well-accepted entity, whereas the concept of microinvasive adenocarcinoma is more controversial, partly because of a paucity of data on its behaviour, but also because of the difficulty in determining the true extent of such lesions.

MICROINVASIVE SQUAMOUS CELL CARCINOMA OF THE CERVIX

Definitions and staging

One of the fundamental problems in any discussion of this entity is the range of different definitions over the years. Overall, there have been over 20 different definitions of microinvasion! The definition proposed by Mestwerdt in 1953 (Mestwerdt, 1953) was any tumour invading the cervical stroma to a depth of less than 5 mm, and most likely was an arbitrary choice rather than being based on proven outcome measures (Östör, 1995). In the face of this definition, other authors proposed that a depth of invasion of less than 1 mm was more appropriate in order to prevent undertreatment and the possible death of patients (Friedell et al., 1959; Averette et al., 1976).

The International Federation of Gynecology and Obstetrics (FIGO) made its first attempt at defining microinvasion in 1961. It divided stage 1 disease into stage 1A and 1B, with stage 1A being defined as preclinical cancer with 'early stromal invasion' but no defined measurements. This definition was of little help in either informing treatment or researching the behaviour of the disease. FIGO added 'occult invasion' to the definition of stage 1A in 1971, but this was changed again in 1974 with occult cancer being classified as 'stage 1B occult'.

It was the Society of Gynecologic Oncologists (SGO) that provided the first rigorous definition of microinvasive cancer when, in 1974, it defined it as a cancer with a depth of invasion of 3 mm or less from the basement membrane without evidence of lymphatic or vascular invasion. In 1978, the Japanese Society of Obstetrics and Gynecology accepted the SGO criteria with the exception that it excluded cases with a confluent growth pattern.

FIGO redefined stage 1A cervical cancer again in 1985: it was preclinical cancer, only recognised by microscopy, with stage 1A1 having 'minimal' stromal invasion and stage 1A2 having invasion not exceeding 5 mm and a lateral extent of no more than 7 mm. The addition of a lateral dimension recognised the fact that tumours were multidimensional. This definition was again modified in 1994, with stage 1A1 consisting of tumours invading no more than 3 mm, with a lateral dimension of no more than 7 mm, while stage 1A2 tumours invaded to depths between 3 and 5 mm, again with a maximum lateral dimension of 7 mm. Details of the morphological characteristics are presented in Figures 37.1 and 37.2 and are considered in more detail in Chapter 21.

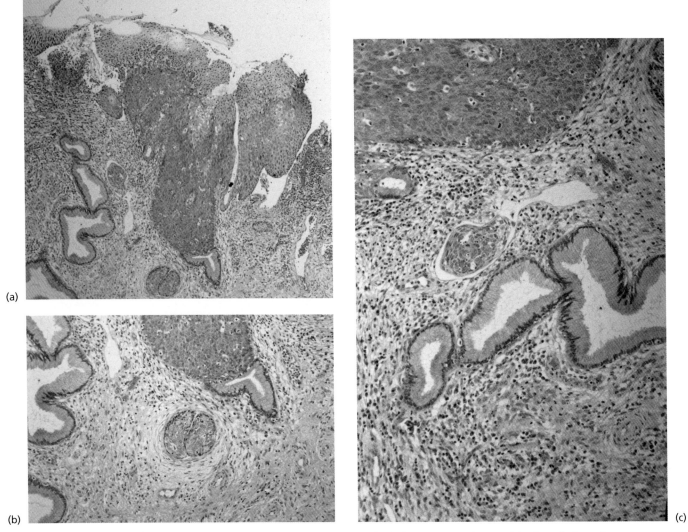

Fig. 37.1 Case 1: Microinvasive squamous cell carcinoma of the cervix. (a) A tiny bud of invasive cancer is seen arising from the base of an endocervical gland involved by CIN3. (b) Focal lymphatic space invasion is seen between the CIN3-affected gland and the adjacent normal endocervical gland. The focus of invasive cancer elicits a stromal response characterised by oedema and fibrosis. (c) A high-power view of the lymphatic space involvement seen on the low-power view.

In the interests of research into microinvasive cervical cancer, it is to be hoped that the current definitions can be maintained for long enough to allow adequate series of patients to accrue to allow outcomes to be determined with various treatments.

Possible prognostic factors

Tumour volume

Definitions of microinvasion originally considered only the depth of invasion, because this was a relatively simple measurement to make. But it is obvious that the depth and lateral extent of tumours are related (Sedlis *et al.*, 1979) and that even tumours that are only superficially invasive may have

extensive lateral spread, so tumour volume may be much greater than indicated by depth alone (Burghardt *et al.*, 1991). Using extensive step sectioning of cone biopsy specimens to calculate the volume of microinvasive cancers, Burghardt and Holzer (1977) concluded that tumours with a volume of less than 500 mm^3 were 'in general, incapable of metastatic spread' regardless of their FIGO stage, although they cautioned that, in the presence of lymph–vascular permeation, rather smaller volumes might, on rare occasions, be associated with recurrence and even death. It was this and similar information that led to the introduction of the lateral dimension, as a surrogate for volume, into the criteria of the 1985 FIGO staging system (Benedet and Anderson, 1996).

Measurement of tumour volume by pathological examination of cone biopsy specimens is not feasible except in a research environment, so is of little relevance to clinical practice, On the other hand, newer non-invasive imaging techniques may well allow tumour volume to be assessed preoperatively. Magnetic resonance imaging (MRI) shows great promise in this respect. Peppercorn *et al.* (1999) used MRI with a special pelvic coil to assess tumour dimension and the presence of residual disease after cone biopsy and, in a series of 30 patients, claimed a sensitivity of 100%, a specificity of 96% and a positive predictive value of 83%. While the use of MRI will clearly be limited because of the availability of the equipment and the expense of the examination, it is an entirely feasible technique for estimating tumour volumes and helping to provide further information on their prognostic significance.

Lymph–vascular space involvement

In its definition framed in 1974, the Society of Gynecologic Oncologists excluded cases with lymph–vascular space permeation from the category of microinvasion. The prognostic significance of lymph–vascular space involvement in frankly invasive cervical carcinoma was demonstrated by Barber *et al.* (1978), who reported that the 5-year survival rate for stage 1B disease was 90% when no lymph–vascular space involvement was seen and 59% when it was present.

The significance of this finding in microinvasive lesions is less clear. Roche and Norris (1975) made multiple step sections of cone biopsy specimens from 30 patients with microinvasive carcinoma in whom radical hysterectomy had subsequently been performed. Lymph–vascular permeation had been reported in nine cases following the initial examination of the cones, but step sectioning demonstrated it in a further eight cases, bringing the total incidence to 57%, but in no case were positive lymph nodes found. Lymph–vascular permeation was found to be related to both the depth of invasion and the number of sites of invasion. Leman *et al.* (1976) demonstrated lymph–vascular permeation in 24% of their patients, but none had lymph node involvement.

While these and many other authors minimise the significance of lymph–vascular space permeation, others consider the finding to be highly significant. Averette (1983) described a patient with only 0.2 mm invasion, but obvious lymph–vascular permeation, who had massive lymph node metastases. Seski *et al.* (1977) found no positive nodes among 37 women without lymph–vascular permeation, but one of four patients with this feature had positive nodes. In a study of lesions invading to a maximum depth of 5 mm, Iverson *et al.* (1979) found a 38% recurrence rate for women with lymph–vascular permeation, and only 1% when this was absent. Larsson *et al.* (1983) performed a multivariate analysis to determine the prognostic factors in 343 cases of early cervical cancer and concluded that lymph–vascular permeation was an important

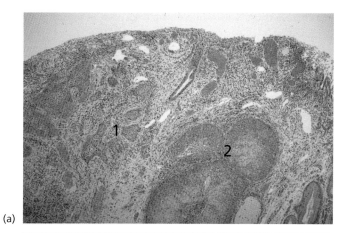

(a)

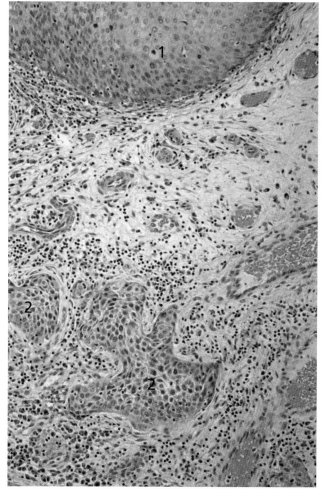

(b)

Fig. 37.2 Case 2: Microinvasive squamous cell carcinoma of the cervix. (a) More extensive microinvasive squamous cell carcinoma (1) adjacent to a gland (2) containing CIN3. (b) CIN3 within the gland (1) contrasts with the irregular islands of microinvasive squamous cell carcinoma (2), which are surrounded by chronic inflammatory cells and stromal oedema.

risk factor. It should be noted that, in their series, 23% of patients had invasion between 3 and 5 mm.

Östör (1995) has reviewed the significance of lymph–vascular permeation in microinvasive cancer and believes that, as it is related to tumour size and a very difficult feature to characterise and quantify accurately, it should not be considered an independent prognostic factor.

Growth pattern

In the Society of Gynecologic Oncologists' original definition, the pattern of invasion was considered to be an important prognostic factor. Fidler and Boyes (1959) distinguished between 'intraepithelial carcinoma with discrete microinvasive foci' and 'occult carcinoma where there are confluent, frankly invasive foci', which they considered to be much more ominous. Subsequently, Lohe (1978) distinguished 'early stromal invasion' from 'microcarcinoma': the former consisted of isolated foci of invasion originating from a field of carcinoma *in situ*, while the latter was defined as a confluent mass of microinvasive carcinoma. In a clinical study of the significance of the pattern of invasion, Lohe *et al.* (1978) showed that the latter lesion carried a poorer prognosis than the former. On the other hand, Roche and Norris (1975) dismissed the confluent pattern as 'ill defined and vague' and of doubtful significance, as did Seski *et al.* (1977). In a multivariate analysis performed by Larsson *et al.* (1983), confluent invasive patterns carried no increased risk of recurrence or death. Leman *et al.* (1976) found no correlation between confluence, depth of invasion, lymph–vascular permeation or nodal metastases.

Burghardt *et al.* (1991) pointed out that both lymph–vascular space involvement and confluent growth patterns had a high sensitivity in predicting invasive recurrence, but a very low specificity. On the basis of his extensive review of the literature, Östör (1995) agreed with that conclusion.

Lymph node metastasis

In any discussion of the management of cervical malignancy, the issue of the rate of lymph node metastasis is crucial. The many changes in terminology, staging and treatment of early cervical cancer over the years make the exact likelihood of nodal involvement difficult to ascertain.

In a review of 41 publications reporting over 2100 cases of early cervical cancer, Benson and Norris (1977) found only four reports, encompassing a total of 98 cases, that were free from factors that could markedly alter the apparent frequency of nodal metastases. The incidence of positive nodes will be higher if preclinical or occult invasive disease, rather than true microinvasive lesions, is studied, if the diagnosis is by punch biopsy, wedge biopsy or a small cone or if only the more advanced cases are selected for lymphadenectomy. On the other hand, lymph node involvement will be apparently less common if cases of questionable invasion are included or, possibly, if those with lymph–vascular space permeation or confluent growth patterns are excluded.

Van Nagell *et al.* (1983) combined the cases considered suitable for evaluation by Benson and Norris with their own experience and that of other authors, and estimated that the incidence of lymph node metastasis with stromal invasion of 3 mm or less is of the order of 0.25%, while for invasion between 3.1 mm and 5 mm, it was estimated to be about 8%.

On the other hand, in an attempt to exclude confounding variables, Creasman *et al.* (1998) analysed those patients from a Gynecologic Oncology Group study of early invasive cervical cancer who had 3–5 mm of invasion on cone biopsy with a maximum lateral dimension of 7 mm and who, at definitive surgery, had no residual disease in the cervix. It was felt that this group would represent true microinvasive cancer. Of 51 patients meeting these criteria, none had lymph node metastases.

Östör (1995) conducted an exhaustive literature review of 48 papers on early invasive cancers of the cervix published between 1976 and 1993 in an effort to determine prognostic factors. He found that, of 2274 cases where the depth of invasion was less than 1 mm, only three patients were reported to have lymph node metastases. Of the patients in this group, only 267 were noted to have had lymph node dissection, although it was assumed that many more did. Among the 2274 patients, there were 13 recurrences and five cancer-related deaths. Among 1324 cases where there was invasion between 1 and 3 mm, there were seven said to have lymph node metastases. A total of 333 patients in this group definitely had lymph node dissection, giving a maximum rate of nodal involvement of 1%, but, assuming that many more patients actually had node dissection, it is likely to be considerably less than this. There were 26 recurrences and nine deaths among the 1324 cases. It should be emphasised that these figures will overestimate the incidence of nodal metastases for stage 1A disease as currently defined because they do not take lateral dimensions into account. On the basis of these findings, Östör (1995) concluded that there is no place for lymph node dissection in women with adequately assessed cone biopsies with clear surgical margins and depth of invasion of less than 3 mm. Where invasion was between 3 and 5 mm, 221 of 674 patients were known to have lymph node dissections and, of these, 6% had demonstrated metastases. Tables 37.1–37.3 present the reported incidence of lymph node metastasis, recurrence and death. It can reasonably be assumed that the number having node dissections is considerably higher than this, and so the actual incidence of node metastases is likely to be of the order of 2%, according to Östör (1995). The invasive recurrence rate in this group was 4%, and 2% died of disease.

These tables all reported the above findings for various depths of invasion but, because the current FIGO definitions are recent, it has not been possible, in some cases in each of the groups, to assess the lateral dimensions of the invasive lesions where they have been greater than 7 mm.

Table 37.1 Incidence of nodal metastasis, recurrence and death from tumour in women with invasive squamous cell carcinoma of the cervix invading less than 1 mm (it should be noted that these cases may have had lateral extension greater than 7 mm).

First author (date)	Cases	Node dissections	Positive nodes	Invasive recurrence	Deaths from disease
Seski (1977)	26	14	0	0	0
Lohe (1978)	285	29	0	0	0
Burghardt (1991)	369	6	0	2	1
Copeland (1992)	37	8	0	0	0
Jones (1993)	36	8	0	0	0
Östör (1993)	119	6	0	2	0
Totals	872	71	0	4	1

Table 37.3 Incidence of nodal metastasis, recurrence and death from tumour in women with invasive squamous cell carcinoma of the cervix invading between 3 and 5 mm (it should be noted that these cases may have had lateral extension greater than 7 mm).

First author (date)	Cases	Node dissections	Positive nodes	Invasive recurrence	Deaths from disease
Van Nagell (1983)	32	32	3	3	2
Bremond (1985)	26	26	0	0	0
Maiman (1988)	30	30	4	0	0
Copeland (1992)	59	29	1	2	0
Jones (1993)	24	18	0	1	1
Östör (1993)	31	21	0	1	1
Totals	202	156	8	7	4

Table 37.2 Incidence of nodal metastasis, recurrence and death from tumour in women with invasive squamous cell carcinoma of the cervix invading between 1 and 3 mm (it should be noted that these cases may have had lateral extension greater than 7 mm).

First author (date)	Cases	Node dissections	Positive nodes	Invasive recurrence	Deaths from disease
Bohm (1976)	56	56	4	2	2
Seski (1977)	28	23	0	0	0
Maiman (1988)	47	41	1	0	0
Copeland (1992)	84	43	0	2	0
Sevin (1992)	74	74	0	0	0
Östör (1993)	50	31	0	4	1
Totals	339	268	5	8	3

DIAGNOSIS OF MICROINVASIVE CANCER

A definitive diagnosis of microinvasive cancer can only be made on either a cone biopsy with clear surgical margins or examination of the entire cervix after trachelectomy or hysterectomy if the diagnosis has been missed preoperatively. But, even when stringent criteria are specified, the diagnosis is not necessarily reliable. Of 265 patients entered into a Gynecologic Oncology Group study after being diagnosed as having microinvasive carcinoma by pathologists at their own institution, 132 were rejected by the reviewing board on the grounds that their condition did not constitute microinvasion. Specifically, 99 cases showed no invasion and 18 had invasion greater than 5 mm, while the cone was considered inadequate in nine (Sedlis *et al.*, 1979). Such a rate of errors among a group of institutions committed to the study of gynaecological cancer indicates the extreme importance of careful patho-

logical review of all specimens in which microinvasion is suspected.

Directed biopsy, even in the most experienced hands, is not adequate to exclude invasive disease elsewhere in the cervix. Larsson *et al.* (1983) showed that the depth of invasion and the incidence of lymph–vascular permeation were both significantly underestimated when assessed from wedge biopsies rather than from cone biopsies or excised uteri.

Seski *et al.* (1977) demonstrated that cone biopsy had a diagnostic accuracy of 83% for microinvasive carcinoma, but that the most significant area was not detected in 5% of cases, and the presence of microinvasion was missed in 13% of cases in which it was subsequently found in the excised uterus. They also claimed that cone biopsy failed to eliminate all intra-epithelial and invasive disease in 78% of cases. It is therefore essential that there is a thorough colposcopic evaluation of both the cervix and the vagina preoperatively.

Proper histological evaluation of the cone is essential. Cursory examination may over- or underestimate the depth of invasion and may miss such features as lymph–vascular permeation. Burghardt and Holzer (1977) stated that 60–70 sections were required for an adequate evaluation. They believed that each section should be examined using a microscope with an ocular micrometer to accurately assess the depth of invasion. Östör and Rome (1994) also advocated a 'whole embedding method' of processing cone biopsies: this technique results in 60–80 individual sections on which to base a diagnosis. They point out that the detection rate of early disease and features such as lymph–vascular space involvement increase with the number of sections taken.

It is particularly important to assess the margins of excision of the cone for, if they are positive, there is a high chance that residual disease, possibly more severe than that in the cone, remains behind. Residual disease in the uterus is more common when the cone margins are involved and in tumours with large surface areas. Cold knife cone biopsies are preferable for diagnosing the presence of microinvasive carcinoma because thermal artefact from either laser or diathermy loops may prevent adequate assessment of margins.

Burghardt and Holzer (1977) found involved cone margins in almost half their cases and, of patients having a hysterectomy following a cone with involved margins, 38% had residual neoplasia, one-quarter of which was invasive carcinoma.

Greer *et al.* (1990) reviewed 50 patients they had treated for early carcinoma of the cervix by radical hysterectomy and lymphadenectomy, after cone biopsy had been performed by referring gynaecologists in the community. Positive margins were present on the cone biopsy in 33 of the 50 cases: in six of these patients, there was no residual disease at definitive surgery, in six there was carcinoma *in situ*, and in the remaining 21 cases, there was residual invasive cancer present. Among the 17 women with reportedly negative margins on cone biopsy, four had residual invasive cancer and two had carcinoma *in situ* in the surgical specimen. These results stress the importance of adequate sectioning of cone specimens, and of performing cone biopsies in facilities where there are experienced gynaecological pathologists.

In another study, Roman *et al.* (1997) reported on 87 cases of microinvasive carcinoma reported on cone biopsy, and subsequently followed by either a further cone biopsy or a hysterectomy. Where cone margins were negative for dysplasia or cancer, only 3% of women had residual invasion, whereas if the margin was positive for either, residual invasion was found in 22%. Both the status of the cone margin and the endocervical curettage were important, with residual disease found in 13% if one was positive and 33% if both were positive.

It is readily apparent that the diagnosis of microinvasive carcinoma is dependent on both the clinical skills and acumen of the gynaecologist and the knowledge and expertise of an experienced gynaecological pathologist. In an exhaustive review of papers discussing the diagnosis and management of microinvasive carcinoma of the cervix undertaken by Östör (1995), it is notable that only about half had a pathologist among the authors. It is hardly surprising that there is confusion regarding the salient clinical and pathological features influencing the prognosis of this condition.

TREATMENT OPTIONS FOR MICROINVASIVE SQUAMOUS CARCINOMA

For stage 1A1 disease diagnosed by cone biopsy with clear margins and a negative endocervical curettage, the treatment options are either careful follow-up with cytology and colposcopy or an extrafascial hysterectomy (Table 37.4). Hysterectomy does not rule out the possibility of the patient developing intraepithelial or even invasive lesions in the vagina, so careful follow-up with vault smears and colposcopy is important, even when this option has been chosen.

Table 37.4 Treatment options for microinvasive cervical cancer.

Stage 1A1	
If fertility desired:	Large cone biopsy with clear margins (if no lymph–vascular space invasion)*
If childbearing completed:	Extrafascial hysterectomy, either abdominal or vaginal
Stage 1A2	
If fertility desired:	Large cone biopsy with clear margins plus pelvic node dissection Radical trachelectomy, either abdominal or vaginal, plus pelvic node dissection
If childbearing completed:	Type 2 radical hysterectomy plus pelvic node dissection

*The possibility of 'skip' lesions must be kept in mind when dealing with adenocarcinoma.

For stage 1A2 lesions, we believe that the preferred option for treatment is a modified radical hysterectomy with pelvic node dissection. In women who have a strong desire to retain fertility, and who understand the risks of conservative treatment, we would accept either a large cone with clear margins or a radical trachelectomy, combined with extraperitoneal or laparoscopic pelvic node dissection. Radical trachelectomy (see Chapter 38) may be performed vaginally (Roy and Plante, 1998) or abdominally (Rodriguez *et al.*, 2001; Shepherd *et al.*, 2001) with good prospects for future childbearing. These more conservative treatments are still experimental and should only be used in specialised units.

MICROINVASIVE ADENOCARCINOMA OF THE CERVIX

The concept of microinvasive adenocarcinoma of the cervix is far more controversial than that of its squamous counterpart. There is a relative paucity of data, and this is further compounded by the problem of accurately determining the true extent of glandular lesions. Data on microinvasion, as currently defined by FIGO, are sparse.

The majority of cases of early cervical adenocarcinoma arise adjacent to the transformation zone. Teshima *et al.* (1985) reported that 90% of cases arose in this region. The morphological characteristics of these lesions are seen in Figure 37.3.

Estimating the depth of invasion for adenocarcinomas of the cervix is somewhat more difficult than with their squamous counterparts. In some reports, the depth of invasion has been measured from the overlying mucosal surface (Berek *et al.*, 1985; Östör *et al.*, 1997), while others have measured from the base of the surface epithelium (Kaku *et al.*, 1997). Teshima *et al.* (1985) reported that normal endocervical glands vary in depth from 2 to 9 mm and that, in their series of

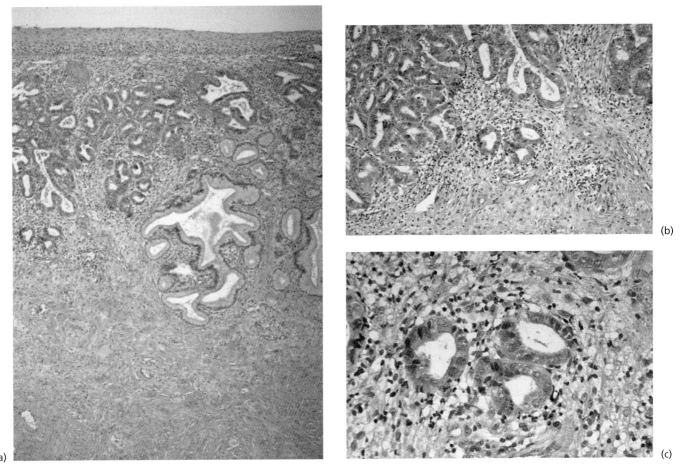

Fig. 37.3 Case 3: Microinvasive adenocarcinoma of the cervix. (a) Microinvasive adenocarcinoma of the cervix with normal endocervical glands deep to the tumour. (b) A chronic inflammatory cell infiltrate and oedema surround the infiltrating glands. (c) The malignant glands show a high nuclear to cytoplasmic ratio and nuclear pleomorphism.

microinvasive cancers, almost half invaded deeper than the level of the deepest normal endocervical gland.

An important consideration with early adenocarcinoma of the cervix is its propensity to be multifocal in origin. Östör *et al.* (1997) reported that 27% of their 77 cases had lesions involving both anterior and posterior cervical lips, without any connecting lesion. On the other hand, they did not find any cases with 'skip' lesions which, for the sake of the article, they defined as separation of discrete invasive foci in the same lip of the cervix of more than 3 mm. This finding clearly has relevance in the conservative treatment of microinvasive glandular lesions.

There has only been one report of positive lymph nodes in a woman with true FIGO stage 1A1 adenocarcinoma (Nagarsheth *et al.*, 2000). In this case, a 62-year-old woman underwent total abdominal hysterectomy and pelvic lymphadenectomy for what was thought to be an endometrial cancer. She was actually found to have an endometrioid adenocarcinoma of the cervix invading to a depth of 2.5 mm, with a width of

4 mm and an estimated tumour volume of 40 mm³. There was one microscopic positive lymph node on each side of the pelvis.

In a study of 51 surgically treated cases of adenocarcinoma of the cervix, Berek *et al.* (1985) found that no patients with tumours of maximum diameter of less than 2 cm had positive nodes, although, among 18 patients with a depth of invasion between 2 and 5 mm, there were two with positive nodes. While this study indicates a relationship between tumour size, depth of invasion and nodal metastases, most of the patients included had stage 1B disease, as the width of the invasive tumour was not taken into account.

Recurrent adenocarcinoma occurred in 7% of patients with less than 5 mm invasion in the series of Kaku *et al.* (1997), although one of these was in a woman with an estimated tumour volume in excess of 1000 mm³. In the series reported by Östör *et al.* (1997), there was only one recurrence among 77 patients, and that was in a woman with a tumour invading only 3.2 mm, but with a length of 21 mm.

Covens *et al.* (1999) reviewed 68 women with adenocarcinoma of the cervix with a depth of invasion of less than 1 cm who underwent either radical hysterectomy or radical trachelectomy with pelvic lymph node dissection. Once again, many of the patients would not have had true stage 1A disease. The authors demonstrated a clear relationship between tumour volume and nodal metastases and recurrent disease. Of 46 patients with tumour volumes of less than 600 mm^3, none had either nodal involvement or recurrence, whereas of 22 patients with tumour volumes over 600 mm^3, positive pelvic nodes were found in two, and three who were node negative developed recurrent disease.

In an attempt to understand better the natural history of early invasive adenocarcinoma, Östör (2000) combined the results of his own studies with those in the literature. He was able to collect a total 436 cases in which depth of invasion was less than 5 mm. There were 126 patients who had been treated by radical hysterectomy, none of whom was reported to have parametrial involvement. A total of 219 patients underwent pelvic node dissection, and five of these (2%) had nodal metastases. A total of 155 patients had one or both ovaries removed, none of which showed evidence of malignancy. Recurrent disease occurred in 3.5% of patients, and 1.4% of the patients died of tumour. Of the 21 patients who had cone biopsy alone, none recurred. It appears likely that recurrence or death was associated with stage 1B disease, because many of the studies did not differentiate between cancers diagnosed clinically and those found only on microscopy, and few took the lateral dimension into account. Despite the limitations of a study such as this, it offers support for a more conservative approach to early invasive adenocarcinoma.

Smith *et al.* (2002) conducted a retrospective review of 560 cases of adenocarcinoma of the cervix with depth of invasion of 5 mm or less and lateral extent of 7 mm or less in Surveillance, Epidemiology and End Results (SEER) databases in the United States. It must be pointed out that this group is not strictly FIGO stage 1A, as a proportion of patients would have had clinically detectable (stage 1B) lesions; the wide range of treatments that the patients received indicates that there was a considerable degree of heterogeneity in the study group. Furthermore, the cases were not subjected to pathological review. Nevertheless, the censored 5-year survival rates for stage 1A1 and stage 1A2 of 98.5% and 98.6%, respectively, were not significantly different. Combining their cases with 610 others reported in the literature, the authors found no difference in the rate of nodal metastases, recurrence or death between stage 1A1 and 1A2 adenocarcinomas.

TREATMENT OF MICROINVASIVE ADENOCARCINOMA OF THE CERVIX

It would appear that microinvasive adenocarcinoma of the cervix can be managed in much the same way as its squamous counterpart, although more studies need to be undertaken to confirm this. One should be particularly cautious in women with stage 1A1 lesions treated by cone biopsy alone, because the cytological and colposcopic recognition of glandular lesions in the cervix, both primary and recurrent, is less reliable than for squamous cancer. Furthermore, in one series (Poynor *et al.*, 1995), only 43% of women had positive endocervical curettings before cone biopsy revealed the presence of adenocarcinoma.

CONCLUSIONS

While much has been written on the subject of microinvasive carcinoma of the cervix, it still remains a controversial area that demands further study, mainly because of the ever-changing definition. This is particularly so as women become more aware of the possibility of fertility preservation in the treatment of cervical malignancy. It is to be hoped that the current staging system remains unchanged for long enough to allow adequate data to be collected to adequately assess the effectiveness and safety of the various treatment options.

REFERENCES

Averette HE (1983) In: Discussion of Van Nagell *et al.* (1983) *American Journal of Obstetrics and Gynecology* 145: 989.

Averette HE, Nelson JH, Ng AB *et al.* (1976) Diagnosis and management of microinvasive (Stage 1A) carcinoma of the uterine cervix. *Cancer* 38: 414–425.

Barber HR, Somers SC, Rotterdam H *et al.* (1978) Vascular invasion as a prognostic factor in stage 1B cancer of the cervix. *Obstetrics and Gynecology* 52: 343–350.

Benedet JL, Anderson GH (1996) Stage 1A carcinoma of the cervix revisited. *Obstetrics and Gynecology* 87: 1052–1059.

Benson WL, Norris HJ (1977) A critical review of the frequency of lymph node metastasis and death from microinvasive carcinoma of the cervix. *Obstetrics and Gynecology* 49: 632–638.

Berek JS, Hacker NF, Fu YS *et al.* (1985) Adenocarcinoma of the uterine cervix: histologic variables associated with lymph node metastasis and survival. *Obstetrics and Gynecology* 65: 46–52.

Bohm JW, Krup PJ, Lee FY *et al.* (1976) Lymph node metastasis in microinvasive epidermoid cancer of the cervix. *Obstetrics and Gynecology* 48: 65–67.

Bremond A, Frappart L, Miguard C (1985) Etude de 68 carcinomes microinvasifs du col uterin. *Journal of Gynecology Obstetrics and the Biology of Reproduction* 14: 1025–1031.

Burghardt E, Holzer E (1977) Diagnosis and treatment of microinvasive carcinoma of the cervix uteri. *Obstetrics and Gynecology* 49: 641–652.

Burghardt E, Girardi F, Lahousen M *et al.* (1991) Microinvasive carcinoma of the uterine cervix (International Federation of Gynecology and Obstetrics Stage 1A). *Obstetrics and Gynecology* 67: 1037–1045.

Copeland LJ, Silva EG, Gershenson DM *et al.* (1992) Superficially invasive squamous cell carcinoma of the cervix. *Gynecologic Oncology* 45: 307–312.

Covens A, Kirby J, Shaw P *et al.* (1999) Prognostic factors for relapse and pelvic lymph node metastases in early stage 1 adenocarcinoma of the cervix. *Gynecologic Oncology* 74: 423–427.

Creasman WT, Zaino RJ, Major FJ *et al.* (1998) Early invasive carcinoma of the cervix (3 to 5 mm invasion): risk factors and prognosis. *American Journal of Obstetrics and Gynecology* 178: 62–65.

Fidler HK, Boyes DA (1959) Patterns of early invasion from intraepithelial carcinoma of the cervix. *Cancer* 12: 673–684.

Friedell GH, Graham JB (1959) Regional lymph node involvement in small carcinoma of the cervix. *Surgery in Gynecology and Obstetrics* 108: 513–517.

Greer BE, Figge DC, Tamimi HK *et al.* (1990) Stage 1A2 squamous carcinoma of the cervix: difficult diagnosis and therapeutic dilemma. *American Journal of Obstetrics and Gynecology* 162: 1406–1411.

Iverson T, Abeler V, Kjorstad KE (1979) Factors influencing the treatment of patients with stage 1A carcinoma of the cervix. *British Journal of Obstetrics and Gynaecology* 86: 593–597.

Jones WB, Mercer GO. Lewis JL, Jr *et al.* (1993) Early invasive carcinoma of the cervix. *Gynecologic Oncology* 51: 26–32.

Kaku T, Kamura T, Sakai K *et al.* (1997) Early adenocarcinoma of the uterine cervix. *Gynecologic Oncology* 65: 281–285.

Larsson G, Alm P, Gullberg B *et al.* (1983) Prognostic factors in early carcinoma of the uterine cervix. A clinical, histopathological and statistical analysis of 343 cases. *American Journal of Obstetrics and Gynecology* 146: 145–153.

Leman MH, Benson WL, Kurman RJ *et al.* (1976) Microinvasive carcinoma of the cervix. *Obstetrics and Gynecology* 48: 571–578.

Lohe KJ (1978) Early squamous cell carcinoma of the uterine cervix. 1. Definition and histology. *Gynecologic Oncology* 6: 10–30.

Lohe KJ, Burghardt E, Hillemanns HG *et al.* (1978) Early squamous cell carcinoma of the uterine cervix. II. Clinical results of a cooperative study in the management of 419 patients with early stromal invasion and microcarcinoma. *Gynecologic Oncology* 6: 31–50.

Maimon MA, Fruchter RG, DiMaio TM *et al.* (1988) Superficially invasive squamous cell carcinoma of the cervix. *Obstetrics and Gynecology* 72: 399–403.

Mestwerdt G (1947) Die Fruhdiagnose des Kollumkarzinoms. *Zentralblatt für Gynäkologie* 69: 198–202.

Mestwerdt G (1953) *Atlas der Kolposkopie.* Jena: Fischer.

Maimon MA, Fruchter RG, DiMaio TM *et al.* (1988) Superficially invasive squamous cell carcinoma of the cervix. *Obstetrics and Gynaecology* 72: 399–403.

Nagarsheth NP, Maxwell GL, Bentley RC *et al.* (2000) Bilateral pelvic lymph node metastases in a case of FIGO Stage 1A1 adenocarcinoma of the cervix. *Gynecologic Oncology* 77: 467–470.

Östör AG (1995) Pandora's box or Ariadne's thread? Definition and prognostic significance of microinvasion in the uterine cervix. Squamous lesions. In: *Pathology Annual,* Part 2. Melbourne: Department of Pathology. pp. 103–136.

Östör AG (2000) Early invasive adenocarcinoma of the uterine cervix. *International Journal of Gynecologic Pathology* 19: 29–38.

Östör AG, Rome RM (1994) Micro-invasive squamous cell carcinoma of the cervix: a clinicopathologic study of 200 cases with long term follow up. *International Journal of Gynecologic Cancer* 4: 257–264.

Östör AG, Rome RM, Quinn MA (1997) Microinvasive adenocarcinoma of the cervix: a clinicopathologic study of 77 women. *Obstetrics and Gynecology* 89: 88–93.

Peppercorn PD, Jeyarajah AR, Woolas R *et al.* (1999) Role of MR imaging in the selection of patients with early cervical carcinoma for fertility preserving surgery: initial experience. *Radiology* 212: 395–399.

Poynor EA, Barakat RR, Hoskins WJ (1995) Management and follow up of patients with adenocarcinoma in situ of the uterine cervix. *Gynecologic Oncology* 57: 158–164.

Roche WD, Norris HJ (1975) Microinvasive carcinoma of the cervix. The significance of lymphatic invasion and confluent patterns of stromal growth. *Cancer* 36: 180–186.

Rodriguez M, Guimares O, Rose PG (2001) Radical abdominal trachelectomy and pelvic lymphadenectomy with uterine conservation and subsequent pregnancy in the treatment of early invasive cervical cancer. *American Journal of Obstetrics and Gynecology* 185: 370–374.

Roman LD, Felix JC, Muderspach LI *et al.* (1997) Risk of residual disease in women with microinvasive squamous cancer in a conization specimen. *Obstetrics and Gynecology* 90: 759–764.

Roy M, Plante M (1998) Pregnancies following vaginal radical trachelectomy for early stage cervical cancer. *American Journal of Obstetrics and Gynecology* 179: 1491–1496.

Sedlis A, Sall S, Tsukada Y *et al.* (1979) Microinvasive carcinoma of the uterine cervix. A clinicopathologic study. *American Journal of Obstetrics and Gynecology* 133: 64–74.

Seski JC, Abell MR, Morley GW (1977) Microinvasive squamous carcinoma of the cervix. Definition, histologic analysis, late results of treatment. *Obstetrics and Gynecology* 50: 410–414.

Sevin BU, Nadji M, Averette HE *et al.* (1992) Microinvasive carcinoma of the cervix. *Cancer* 70: 2121–2128.

Shepherd JH, Mould T, Oram DH (2001) Radical trachelectomy in early stage carcinoma of the cervix: outcome as judged by recurrence and fertility rates. *British Journal of Obstetrics and Gynaecology* 108: 882–885.

Smith HO, Qualls, CR, Romero AA *et al.* (2002) Is there a difference in survival for 1A1 and 1A2 adenocarcinoma of the uterine cervix? *Gynecologic Oncology* 85: 229–241.

Teshima S, Shimosata Y, Kishi K *et al.* (1985) Early stage adenocarcinoma of the cervix. *Cancer* 56: 167–172.

Van Nagell JR, Greenwell N, Powell DF *et al.* (1983) Microinvasive carcinoma of the cervix. *American Journal of Obstetrics and Gynecology* 145: 981–991.

CHAPTER 38

Management of early-stage cervical cancer by surgery

John H. Shepherd

Invasive cancer peaks between the ages of 35 and 44 years in most developed countries, but these ages are different from those expected in underdeveloped countries with an unscreened population where invasive lesions continue to rise in incidence after the age of 45 years. The emphasis for treatment, therefore, will be different in the developed and underdeveloped world, with more early-stage invasive cancers being detected in the younger age group in a screened population in the developed world, while more advanced tumours will present in an older age group in the underdeveloped world. The regrettable irony is that it is the more advanced group of patients who require treatment by radiotherapy with or without chemotherapy, and these facilities are rarely available in the underdeveloped world.

Surgery remains the mainstay of treatment for early-stage disease, although recent evidence has demonstrated that an improvement in survival can be expected with combination chemo/radiotherapy when compared with radiotherapy alone in patients treated with that modality primarily (Keyes *et al.*, 1999; Morris *et al.*, 1999; Rose *et al.*, 1999a; Whitney *et al.*, 1999; Peters *et al.*, 2000; Green *et al.*, 2001).

MANAGEMENT SELECTION

Early carcinomas of the cervix can be treated either surgically or by radiation therapy. Early-stage disease has similar results in terms of survival and cure rates; however, the morbidity of surgery is clearly different from that of radiotherapy. The long-term consequences of radiotherapy, especially in younger women, have a major effect on tissues surrounding the cervix, with a resulting enforced menopause due to ovarian ablation and therefore failure, difficulties with sexual function resulting from the effect of the radiotherapy on the vaginal epithelium as well as effects on the bladder mucosa and gastrointestinal tract. Radiation cystitis and enterocolitis can result. Surgery may prevent this, although a certain number of patients may require combination treatment. As a general rule, this should be avoided unless there are particularly adverse prognostic factors making postoperative radiotherapy an important adjunct

to treatment. The risks of combined treatment include all those consequences mentioned above as well as an increased risk of fistula and lymphoedema.

Traditional surgical treatment for invasive cancer has been a radical hysterectomy, performed either abdominally as a Wertheim's procedure or, alternatively, vaginally as the Schauta procedure. Both of these will compromise fertility as the uterus is removed. A bilateral pelvic node dissection is performed at the same time with a bilateral salpingo-oophorectomy depending upon the age of the patient. This topic is covered in Chapter 37.

Staging procedures

Early-stage disease, however, may offer an option for a more conservative approach. This will depend upon the overall size and therefore stage of the tumour. The most commonly used staging system is as described by FIGO (Benedet *et al.*, 2001; see also Table 36.1 in Chapter 36). Other staging systems include those proposed by the American Joint Committee on Cancer and the International Union against Cancer. Most scientific literature reports gynaecological oncology statistics using the FIGO system, however. Traditionally, FIGO staging and reporting has been used to compare international data, and guidelines for clinical staging of invasive cancers have necessitated a non-surgical staging to include inspection and examination with palpation, colposcopy, endocervical curettage, hysteroscopy, cystoscopy, proctoscopy, intravenous pyelography and radiographic examination of the lungs and skeleton. Conisation of the cervix is considered a clinical examination and, if there is a question about the most appropriate stage, the earlier stage should be assigned. Clearly, however, this staging has its limitations, although it may be generally applied across the underdeveloped world where more sophisticated studies are not available.

Much work has recently been carried out on the value of the more sophisticated techniques, such as computerised axial tomography (CT scans), magnetic resonance imaging (MRI) and positron emission tomography (PET scanning). Staging allows not only a management plan to be performed, but also a realistic view on prognosis to be given. This also will enable a decision to be made regarding the extent of treatment and especially surgery that may be necessary. If there is any prospect of reducing the morbidity of radical treatment and especially surgery, then careful and precise imaging is essential. CT of the abdomen and pelvis is the most widely used imaging study and is useful in detecting para-aortic lymphadenopathy with a high specificity and low sensitivity (Heller *et al.*, 1990). Accuracy of CT scanning has improved with better imaging resolution (Scheidler *et al.*, 1997). MRI has been shown to be as accurate as CT in assessing pelvic nodal involvement, but is better at assessing the primary tumour itself within the cervix and surrounding pelvic tissues. Using different planes, sagittal, axial and oblique, will accurately assess the parametrial tumour extension with different weighted spin echo images (Baumgartner and Bernardino, 1989). Contrast media may be useful to assess bladder and rectal invasion (Sironi *et al.*, 1993), and dynamic enhancement may give a further advantage (Yamashita *et al.*, 1992). PET scanning adds a further dimension for increasing non-invasive staging with initial encouraging reports of a sensitivity of 75% but a specificity of 92% (Rose *et al.*, 1999b).

With an increasing demand for fertility-sparing surgery, MRI has been shown to be useful in the selection of patients for this new technique (Peppercorn *et al.*, 1999).

Lymph node evaluation (see also Chapters 4 and 36)

Much work has been carried out in trying to assess lymph node involvement. Quite apart from CT scans and MRI, lymphangiography was used for many years but has now been largely superseded. Sentinel node detection has been described (Dargent *et al.*, 2000; Malur *et al.*, 2001). Initial studies using lymphazurin dye, isosulfan blue dye, patent blue or technitium-99m colloidal albumin in patients with cervical cancer showed sensitivity with a negative predicted value of accuracy of 100% (Echt *et al.*, 1999; Dargent *et al.*, 2000). The localisation of the sentinel nodes and highest detection rate appear to occur using a combination of radioactively labelled albumin with blue dye. However, the value of the detection of circulating tumour cells or micrometastases in sentinel nodes and, indeed, more proximal nodes by immunohistochemistry is not clear, but does raise doubt as to the value of the sentinel node concept (Van Trappen *et al.*, 2001). Laparoscopic staging of both retroperitoneal lymph nodes and intraperitoneal disease is feasible with a relatively low morbidity (Querleu, 1993; Possover *et al.*, 1998). Sentinel node mapping by laparoscopy with combined blue dye and lymphoscintigraphy have been shown to be feasible and accurate (Plante *et al.*, 2003) but, in the future, it is hoped that improved imaging with developing PET CT will avoid the need for such intervention and improve the accuracy of assessment and staging by non-invasive methods.

SURGICAL MANAGEMENT OF EARLY-STAGE DISEASE

Management of microinvasive (stage IA1 and 2) disease (see also Chapter 37)

Microinvasive carcinoma of the cervix was first recognised in 1947 (Mestwerdt, 1947). The fact that the definition of microinvasive carcinoma has been altered by FIGO seven times between 1961 and 1994 shows the difficulty in gaining universal acceptance of this entity and, as a result, agreement over the correct surgical management. Volume was shown to be an important concept, in that a tumour with a volume of < 500 m^3 was not associated with metastases (Burghardt and Holzer, 1977). In 1994, the current staging definitions were introduced with a concept of superficially invasive carcinoma being divided into stage IA1 with a depth of invasion no greater than 3 mm and no wider than 7 mm, and stage IA2 with a depth of invasion > 3 mm but < 5 mm but still no wider than 7 mm. Cone biopsy is clearly essential to assess accurately the depth of invasion and overall size of the tumour. It is generally carried out by cold knife (Figs 38.1 and 38.2), and this is accepted as being more accurate than the more newly introduced electrosurgical excision procedures or laser excision, which may result in artefacts. However, the biopsy will remove part of the lesion and therefore alter the apparent depth of invasion (Greer *et al.*, 1990).

Nodal involvement with minimally invasive lesions, stage IA1, occurs in 1% of patients, with a death rate of < 1%. However, stage IA2 lesions have a 7.8% rate of nodal metastases with a death rate of 2.4%. Lesions of < 5 mm have higher incidence of nodal metastases when the lateral spread is > 7 mm (Sevin *et al.*, 1992).

It is generally accepted that, using FIGO staging, those patients with a stage IA1 carcinoma of the cervix may be treated adequately by either simple hysterectomy without node dissection or, alternatively, by conisation in selected cases where uterine-sparing surgery is required or requested especially for fertility conservation. Stage IA2 patients, however, require more extensive treatment with surgical excision, and general teaching is still that these patients should undergo a radical hysterectomy and pelvic lymphadenectomy (Benedet and Anderson, 1996; National Comprehensive Cancer Network, 2000).

Lymphovascular space invasion (LVSI) does not alter FIGO staging, but it may be an important factor when determining treatment. The prevalence of LVSI involvement is 3.1% in stage IA1 disease, but this increases to 15.7% with stage IA2. The inference is that LVSI indicates the need for more radical surgery to improve survival. Whether or not the presence of LVSI in patients who have undergone radical hysterectomy and pelvic node dissection is an indication for adjunctive radiotherapy, however, appears questionable (Creasman and Kohler, 2004). What is clear, however, is that the risk of

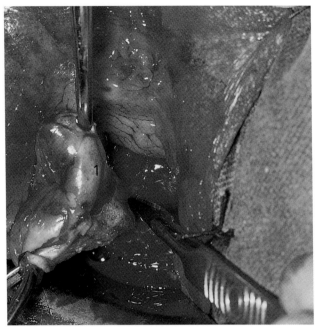

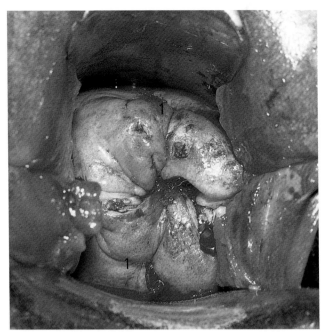

38.1

38.2

Figs 38.1 and 38.2 A cone biopsy using the cold knife technique. A 2- to 2.5-cm cone-shaped specimen is obtained, and the defect within the lower cervix is covered by vaginal and lateral cervical tissues using Sturmdorf sutures as seen in Figure 38.2.

recurrence does increase with the density of LVSI, which does affect the prognosis in patients with stage Ib and IIA node-negative disease (Sykes *et al.*, 2003). This topic is covered in more detail in Chapter 35.

Fertility-sparing surgery: radical trachelectomy

With postponement of childbearing, the desire to preserve fertility potential has become an increasingly important issue in the western world and developed countries. A significant number of younger women will be diagnosed with early-stage cervical cancer as a result of better medical care and earlier presentation of symptoms. Screening programmes will inevitably detect some small invasive cancers as well as precancerous intraepithelial neoplasia. While superficially invasive disease (stage IA1) may be treated by cone biopsy, deeper invasive lesions as well as some stage IA2 tumours may require more extensive surgery that would traditionally entail a radical hysterectomy and pelvic node dissection. Individualisation may lead to some patients with stage IA2 tumours being treated by cone biopsy and pelvic node dissection. These would need careful selection and precise follow-up.

Others with more high-risk prognostic factors will require more than even a large cone biopsy, and wide local excision of the primary tumour would entail complete excision of the cervix with adequate clear margins including a cuff of vagina and paracervical tissue. Hence, the concept of a radical trachelectomy, removing the whole of the cervix up to the isthmus

giving a clear margin of at least 1 cm beyond the tumour with 1-cm margins all around including the paracervical tissue and an adequate cuff, usually 2 cm, of vagina (Fig. 38.3).

At the same time, a pelvic node dissection may be performed, either by extraperitoneal open surgery (as described by Meigs) or, alternatively, laparoscopically and transperitoneally. This procedure is therefore the bottom part of a radical vaginal hysterectomy which conserves the corpus uteri so that a vagino-isthmic anastomosis may be performed (Shepherd *et al.*, 1998). This procedure is a modification of the technique described by Dargent *et al.* in 1994. He in turn had applied a laparoscopic approach with node dissection after Novak in 1948 described trachelectomy as a modification of the Schauta procedure for patients who might be able to conserve the corpus uteri. Schauta's radical vaginal hysterectomy was commonly carried out in Europe as an alternative to the abdominal approach. However, poor selection of cases, ranging from invasive lesions that were too large to premalignant cases that did not require such extensive surgery, led to the procedure being abandoned. Abrumil introduced the concept in Romania in 1956 but with little success. Interest has developed, however, in Canada, in Toronto (Covens *et al.*, 1999) and Montreal (Roy and Plante, 1998), as well as in Lyons, France (Dargent *et al.*, 2000), and England (Shepherd *et al.*, 2001), with over 400 cases being reported. A smaller number have also been reported from Jena (A. Schneider, personal communication, 2004) and California (Burnett, 2004) with sporadic smaller numbers also (see Table 38.1).

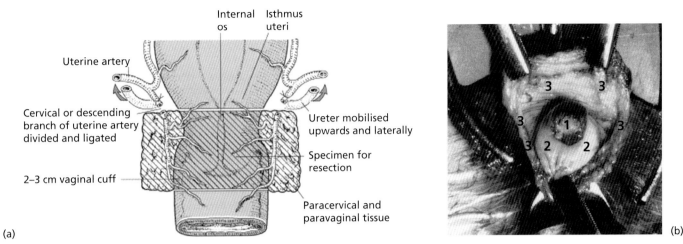

(a)   (b)

Fig. 38.3 (a) A diagrammatic representation of the area that is removed during a radical trachelectomy procedure. This area is shaded. Ligation of the cervical or descending branch of the uterine artery has taken place with removal of a corresponding paracervical and paravaginal portion of tissue as well as a 2- to 3-cm vaginal cuff. (b) The excised area can be seen with the early cervical cancer (Stage IB1) at (1), ectocervix at (2) and vaginal vault at (3).

Table 38.1 Radical vaginal trachelectomy (worldwide data 1994–2004).

Centre (author)	Number	Pregnancies	No. of women	No. of births	Less than 32 weeks	Recurrence	Deaths
Lyon (Dargent)	96	55	36	36	1	4	3
London (Shepherd)	91	43	28	26	6	3	0
Toronto (Covens)	80	22	18	12	2	7	0
Quebec (Roy)	66	37	22	24	4	2	1
Jena (Schneider)	36	7	7	4	1	1	0
Los Angeles USC (Burnett)	21	3	3	3	1	1	0
Los Angeles PAS (Schlaerth)	12	4	4	4	2	0	0
Total	402	171	118	109	17	18	4

Although at first it was thought that only squamous cell lesions confined to the ectocervix would be suitable for such treatment, it was quickly realised that certain glandular tumours arising from the lower endocervical canal would also be appropriate for such treatment providing that the whole of the cervix up to the isthmus could be removed. Careful selection with preoperative MRI allows careful selection to ensure that a clear margin is feasible. Imaging of the lymph nodes can be enhanced by the use of ultrasmall iron oxide particles (Rockall *et al.*, 2003). Such techniques with MRI will allow a more careful selection of patients when a desire for fertility preservation is clearly a prerequisite, although as the procedure gains more acceptance, it will become more difficult to deny women who are suitable by all other criteria a chance of undergoing the procedure. However, as the technique remains as yet new and under careful scrutiny and investigation in controlled circumstances, clearly a realistic chance and desire for fertility should remain a prerequisite. Having said this, the author's oldest patient in his series was aged 46 years, and she subsequently gave birth 2 years later following successful reimplantation on a planned *in vitro* fertilisation (IVF) programme that had in fact been arranged prior to the trachelectomy procedure being carried out.

The technique

The technique is well described. It does require adequate laparoscopic skills with pelvic wall dissection and transperitoneal lymphadenectomy, although a perfectly reasonable alternative approach to lymphadenectomy would be via an extraperitoneal approach. Experience with radical vaginal surgery is necessary. If there is doubt about surgical clearance, then it is wise to obtain frozen section analysis of the isthmic end of the specimen prior to reanastomosing the vagina to the isthmus having inserted an isthmic cerclage of non-absorbable suture material (such as no. 1 nylon) tied around a no. 6 Hegar dilator. This, on the one hand, acts as a cerclage to prevent opening of the isthmus and miscarriage, while on the other hand, it allows exit for the menses as well as an early first-trimester miscarriage. The main problem with removing the cervix is not in fact conceiving but premature rupture of the membranes due to ascending infection and presumed chorioamnionitis. Delivery has to be by a caesarean section performed via a low vertical incision, i.e. classical section, as trachelectomy itself would have removed the majority of the lower segment, or at least shortened it, by resecting the cervix up to and including the isthmus. The risk of a lower segment and transverse incision extending out into the parametria and tearing the uterine vessels is high and indeed has happened in one case where this advice was not followed.

Fertility rates appear to be satisfactory with the suture holding and not rupturing, allowing viability to be reached with a satisfactory delivery rate (see Table 38.1). Over 100 deliveries have occurred to the approximately 400 women who have undergone the procedure. Recurrence rates appear to be low, in the region of 4%, and have been described between 7 months and 7 years following the procedure. These recurrence rates are less than would be expected stage for stage with patients who have a stage IB1 disease, indicating that careful selection is possible but the procedure should be confined to lesions of less than 2 cm in diameter as a general rule.

Radical hysterectomy and bilateral pelvic node dissection: the traditional surgical treatment for invasive carcinoma of the cervix and other procedures

It was Ernst Wertheim who in 1898 first described his surgical procedure for an abdominal radical approach to treating invasive cervical carcinoma. He had been a pupil in Vienna of Schauta who, 2 years previously, had described his radical vaginal approach to deal with the same lesion. Schauta's procedure fell into disfavour while Wertheim's operation found supporters who championed it both in Europe and across the Atlantic in the United States. At the same time, radiotherapy was developed with the discovery of X-rays by Wilhelm Roentgen and subsequently radium by Pierre and Marie Curie in the 1890s in Paris. Margaret Cleaves first described the use of radium to treat cervical cancer in 1912. Radiotherapy to the pelvis and radical surgery thus developed in parallel, with proponents of each modality strongly voicing their opinions. Combined treatment was strongly advocated through the twentieth century, but the inevitable increased morbidity, with fistulae, lymphoedema and significant radiation cystitis, enterocolitis, as well as an impairment of sexual function, led to a better rationalisation of individual patient care. Studies have shown that chemo/radiotherapy improves survival and is replacing radiotherapy alone. However, the majority of specialists still favour treating early-stage disease by surgery in order to avoid the inevitable consequences of radiotherapy. This topic is also covered in detail in Chapter 37.

A role for the vaginal approach

Of late, the vaginal approach has found favour once more (Dargent, 1987). The laparoscope has been used to undertake virtually any intra-abdominal surgical procedure and, inevitably, radical hysterectomy is no exception, proving that almost any procedure that can be performed by open surgery may also be performed laparoscopically with magnification providing adequate instrumentation is available (Spiritos *et al.*, 2002). A more rational approach is to undertake a laparoscopically assisted radical vaginal hysterectomy (Hertel *et al.*, 2003). Bladder complications with the vaginal approach do appear to be higher than with the traditional radical abdominal procedure, but the radicality of surgery is responsible for this, being related to the extent of sympathetic and parasympathetic denervation during the pelvic dissection (Chen *et al.*, 2002). This nerve-sparing procedure has been described in Chapter 3 in relation to the technique of Sakaragi *et al.* (2005).

Nerve-sparing procedures

Nerve-sparing procedures have been described in an attempt to reduce morbidity (Trimbos *et al.*, 2001; Sakaragi *et al.*, 2005). A significant reduction in long-term bladder disturbance and sexual dysfunction has been claimed (Havenga *et al.*, 2000). This appears to be feasible in the case of patients undergoing radical surgery for rectal cancer or radical hysterectomy for cervical cancer (Maas, 2003).

Individualisation of the radical hysterectomy

It was Piver *et al.* (1974) who first described five classes of radical hysterectomy but, in the literature, differences in classification between class 2 (modified radical) and class 3 (radical) hysterectomy are imprecise. Although some studies have shown a difference in blood loss and operating time as well as fistula rate and rectal function (Photopulos and Zwaagrv, 1991; Magrina *et al.*, 1995), others have shown that there is a lower morbidity in carrying out the lesser procedure with adjuvant radiotherapy as opposed to the class 3 radical hysterectomy without giving adjuvant treatment (Sartori *et al.*, 1995; Landoni *et al.*, 2001).

Place of parametrial resection

Much of the reasoning behind advocating resection of the parametria has been based on giant section histopathology indicating occult parametrial involvement in up to 39% of patients (Girardi *et al.*, 1993; Benedetti-Panici *et al.*, 2000). As a result of this, complete *en bloc* resection with radical hysterectomy and complete parametrectomy has been advocated (Burghardt *et al.*, 1987). However, the mitigating argument against this approach is that patients who are at high risk of metastatic disease have a significant risk of micrometastases not only in the parametria but beyond, locoregionally and distally. There is a lack of demonstrable data showing improved survival with complete parametrectomy (Hayes and Eremin, 1992; Caddy, 1997; Page *et al.*, 1999).

Individualisation of techniques

What becomes clearly evident is that individualisation of care in ideal circumstances will allow good imaging, which at present is by MRI but may become more accurate in the future with PET CT in conjunction with an assessment of the histopathology. Clearly, it is advisable to try and avoid combination treatment and, therefore, early-stage disease that is unlikely to require adjuvant radiotherapy should be treated by radical hysterectomy. What is also becoming obvious is that, with the advent of laparoscopic approaches, lessons have been learnt for open surgery so that smaller incisions, shorter operating times and better handling of tissues have allowed patients to mobilise more quickly and be discharged home earlier. The laparoscopic approach may take longer and not be as aesthetically satisfying in some traditionalists' eyes but, undoubtedly, these techniques will become more popular and successful. There will always be a need for open surgery, especially with larger lesions and also when particular potential complications may be present due to previous surgery or co-existing co-incidental pathology such as inflammatory bowel disease, which may make the minimalistic approach hazardous. As a general rule, larger lesions are better tackled by open surgery as well as those in which it is anticipated that there may be significant blood loss due to increased vascularity for whatever reason. Open surgery will allow a better control and view with detection of large bleeding vessels and sinuses. This may not be straightforward when dealing with a case laparoscopically or by a limited vaginal approach with little in the way of descent.

Place of adjuvant therapy

Women who have a high likelihood of requiring adjuvant therapy would be better treated initially by chemo/radiotherapy in order to avoid the increased morbidity of adding a radical surgical procedure to an already morbid and difficult combined treatment that the woman has to undergo. Under these circumstances, surgery would be confined to those patients who fail to respond to chemo/radiotherapy and may require either salvage central radical hysterectomy for persistent central disease or, alternatively, pelvic exenteration for more extensive advanced disease involving the bladder or rectum.

While surgical treatment for lymph node metastases in early-stage cancer may undoubtedly cure some patients, it is entirely more logical to treat these women who have a high risk of micrometastases in hitherto undetected nodes not resected or beyond the field of surgical extirpation by radiotherapy with or without chemotherapy. The advocates of a

more extensive and lateral parametrectomy (Ungar and Palfalvi, 2003) are to be commended, but it is wiser to confine such surgery to those centres that do not have adequate adjunctive modalities. This may be applicable especially to underprivileged and Third World countries, but randomised studies would be required before advocating such surgical approaches in lieu of adjunctive chemo/radiotherapy. This applies especially when one is considering nerve-sparing techniques.

OPTIONS FOR SURGICAL AND NON-SURGICAL TREATMENT OF EARLY CERVICAL CANCER

Stages IB and IIA cervical cancer may be treated by either radical surgery or radical radiotherapy to the pelvis. As a general rule, if it is felt that adjunctive radiotherapy can be avoided, then primary surgery is the treatment of choice in order to avoid the long-term effects and consequences of radiotherapy. Primary surgery involves a radical hysterectomy with a bilateral pelvic lymphadenectomy. Although the abdominal route has been favoured using the Wertheim–Meigs procedure, a resurgence with the Schauta radical vaginal approach is occurring, especially with smaller lesions when there is some degree of vaginal prolapse and descent.

Role of radiation and chemotherapy

The alternative of primary radiation therapy has now been superseded by concomitant chemotherapy used as a sensitiser for radiotherapy, given by both external beam treatment and then either high- or low-dose rate intracavity brachytherapy. Reviews of collective retrospective studies show a 5-year survival in excess of 85%, and up to 90% may be expected with either modality (Averette *et al.*, 1996).

Although no studies have been carried out prospectively comparing surgery with chemo/radiotherapy, an Italian study (Landoni *et al.*, 1997) compared radical hysterectomy with adjuvant radiotherapy in high-risk cases and primary radiotherapy. This is the only randomised study to have been performed in what would be an extremely difficult area to recruit patients prospectively when individualisation of care becomes increasingly important. This study included stage IB1 and IB2 patients. Survival rates were similar at 5 years in both groups. Morbidity, however, was greatly increased in the combined surgery and postoperative radiation group (28%) than in the radiation-only group (12%). However, in this study, adjuvant radiotherapy after surgery was used in 54% of stage IB1 tumours and in 84% of patients with stage IB2 tumours. Prognostic factors that were of significance were overall tumour diameter, the presence of positive lymphadenopathy and adenocarcinoma tumours. These results confirm that it is possible to individualise patients to either surgery or radiotherapy in an attempt to reduce the morbidity of combination therapy. Other factors that need to be considered are the patient's age, overall health and associated co-morbidity factors.

The other argument in favour of radical surgery is that the vagina remains unaffected by radiotherapy and, therefore, sexual function is less likely to be compromised. Ovarian function may be preserved in younger women premenopausally although, if oophorectomy is necessary, hormone replacement may be given depending on the patient's wishes. The other argument in favour of surgery is that a full surgical staging may be carried out. Other strong indications are in women who have had significant pelvic sepsis related to either pelvic inflammatory disease or inflammatory bowel disorders such as diverticular disease, Crohn's disease or ulcerative colitis.

ADJUVANT TREATMENT FOLLOWING SURGERY

It is accepted that certain high-risk factors, including lymph node metastases and involved margins of resection, will increase the risk of recurrence, while other factors, such as lymphovascular space invasion, grade of tumour and overall size, may also put patients into a higher risk group. Adjuvant treatment has consisted of postoperative radiotherapy to the pelvis and, if there has been a high risk or evidence of distal spread, giving chemotherapy (Koh *et al.*, 2000).

With the recent demonstration that combination chemo/radiotherapy using cisplatin-based chemotherapy as a sensitising agent is more effective than radiotherapy alone, it is only logical to assume that this combination approach will be beneficial in an adjuvant setting. This has been confirmed in two studies in patients with pelvic lymph node involvement and positive margins at primary surgery (Sedlis *et al.*, 1999; Peters *et al.*, 2000).

What is unclear is whether those patients who have intermediate or relative risk factors (such as large tumour size, lymphovascular space involvement and deep stromal infiltration) benefit from postoperative radiotherapy. There is a suggestion that relapse-free survival may improve, but overall survival has not yet been demonstrated (Sedlis *et al.*, 1999).

LOCALLY ADVANCED CERVICAL CANCER

The overall increase in survival that has been demonstrated using combination chemo/radiotherapy over radiotherapy alone indicates that this modality should be used when treating patients with either bulky or locally advanced primary cervical cancer (Morris *et al.*, 1999; Rose *et al.*, 1999a; Keyes *et al.*, 1999; Whitney *et al.*, 1999; Peters *et al.*, 2000). These studies have shown that patients with locally advanced tumours in whom chemo/radiotherapy has been given as primary treatment, those with bulky early-stage disease in whom chemo/radiotherapy was given prior to adjuvant hysterectomy and pati-

ents undergoing radical hysterectomy and then found to have high-risk pathological factors and in whom postoperative adjuvant chemo/radiotherapy was to be given all had a better outcome when treated with combination chemo/radiotherapy rather than with radiotherapy alone. Cisplatin appears to be the chemotherapeutic agent of choice used as a sensitising agent. A dramatic 30% reduction in the relative risk of death in these five trials was demonstrated, and this gave rise to the National Cancer Institute issuing a statement that 'strong consideration' should be given to the incorporation of concurrent cisplatin-based chemotherapy with radiation therapy in women who require radiation therapy for the treatment of cervical cancer (National Cancer Institute, 2002).

SQUAMOUS CELL CARCINOMA VERSUS ADENOCARCINOMA

It is generally agreed that both glandular and squamous cell tumours should be treated stage for stage in the same way. It is, however, unclear whether the two lesions share the same aetiological cause and also whether outcome and survival are similar. While it is now generally agreed that the aetiology may well be similar, it is also accepted that screening for glandular tumours is not as straightforward as for squamous cell lesions to which the Papanicolaou smear and therefore most screening programmes are directed. There is no evidence or reason to differentiate in the treatment of these two morphological entities. Survival rates appear to be similar for patients with adenocarcinoma of the cervix and squamous cell carcinoma after associated risk factors have been taken into account. However, adenosquamous cell tumours do appear to be associated with a significant reduction in overall survival, although relapse-free survival rate is similar to that of the other tumours (Look *et al.*, 1996). It does appear that adenosquamous histology is predictive of disease recurrence and decreased survival in otherwise low-risk stage IB1 cervical adenocarcinoma. Further studies will therefore need to show whether adjuvant therapy in this subgroup of patients is of benefit (Lea *et al.*, 2003).

VILLO-GLANDULAR PAPILLARY ADENOCARCINOMA

Villo-glandular papillary adenocarcinoma was initially reported in 1989 (Young and Scully, 1989). It has now been included as a histopathological entity in the WHO histological typing of cervical cancers (Scully *et al.*, 1994). This entity is generally thought to be morphologically distinct from the more commonly recognised glandular adenocarcinoma with an extreme villous and papillary growth. It is therefore regarded as being at one end of the glandular spectrum, much as a verrucous carcinoma might be thought to be at the benign end of the spectrum of squamous cell carcinoma of either the cervix or the vulva. However, the biological behaviour of villo-glandular cancers does not appear to be as benign or indolent. Capillary space involvement and lymph node metastases may occur and, in the small studies reported, this appears to be at a similar incidence to other cervical cancers. Although studies are small, in a combined series of three reports, 5 out of 35 patients had positive lymph nodes (Kaku *et al.*, 1999; Khunamornpong *et al.*, 2001; Utsugi *et al.*, 2004).

These tumours may be heterologous and, therefore, a small biopsy specimen may not be representative. With the demonstrated incidence of lymph node involvement, consideration does need to be given to standard treatment for cervical cancer including pelvic lymph node dissection. This is a rare disease and therefore further studies are required before deciding if more conservative treatment is possible. Again, individualisation of patient care appears to be of great importance.

PREGNANCY ASSOCIATED WITH CERVICAL CARCINOMA (SEE ALSO CHAPTER 34)

Cervical cancer being a disease that affects younger women of childbearing years, it is inevitable that a certain number of cases will occur during or shortly after pregnancy. Approximately 3% of patients will have a diagnosis made during pregnancy, and this presents a major therapeutic dilemma (Donegan, 1983). Cervical cancer does not appear to be a major cause of maternal mortality as shown by confidential enquiry into maternal death reports over the last few decades with no such cases reported recently. The survival of patients with early-stage disease appears to be good regardless of when the diagnosis is made, and survival rates appear to be similar to those cases occurring outside pregnancy (Hopkins and Morley, 1992; Monk and Montz, 1992).

The clinical dilemma that occurs requires careful multidisciplinary discussion and review between not only the obstetricians but also the neonatologists and gynaecological oncologists. Histopathological confirmation of invasive disease and the depth of invasion is crucial and, if necessary, conisation of the cervix should be performed to obtain an overall impression of depth of invasion. This may be possible with a large wedge biopsy. Consideration would therefore need to be given to cervical cerclage if the pregnancy is to be continued. Imaging is possible to help with staging using MRI. Full counselling is important taking into account not only ethical but also religious and cultural issues, with the patient making the final decision after as much information as possible can be given to her and her partner. It is individualisation of this situation that will lead to a final decision regarding treatment. Cancer during pregnancy is three times more likely to be early stage at diagnosis than in the non-pregnant state, most probably due to the occurrence of more regular clinical examinations (Zemlickis *et al.*, 1991). Not only do the majority of patients present with stage IB carcinoma, but squamous

cell lesions appear to have the same incidence as in the non-pregnant state.

Those patients in whom the diagnosis is made following cone biopsy of superficially invasive carcinoma of stage IA1 or IA2 may be reasonably expected to deliver vaginally and then be re-evaluated and treated at 6 weeks post partum. Full staging with MRI can be performed and the decision made regarding definitive treatment. This will depend upon the future fertility wishes as well as other prognostic factors. Women with a truly invasive stage IB lesion will have to decide between termination, on the one hand, and continuation of the pregnancy with an elective delivery early once the fetus is mature enough to survive with appropriate neonatal care but without delaying treatment too much, on the other. Hence, if the diagnosis is made in the first trimester of pregnancy, treatment by radical hysterectomy may be carried out providing the patient so wishes. Diagnosis during the middle trimester is more problematic, but delay of 3 months up to a fetal viability time of 28–32 weeks is probably reasonable without worsening the overall prognosis. This has been shown in a retrospective series where a delay of 6–15 weeks did not appear to have made any significant difference to overall outcome (Takushi *et al.*, 2002). Clearly, patients should be made aware that delaying treatment does carry a risk of disease progression. However, the benefits of fetal maturity outweigh the risks of the tumour itself progressing significantly in the great majority of cases. There does not appear to be a significant increased maternal risk in that the overall recurrence rate of 5% appears to be similar to that of women in the non-pregnant state (Goff *et al.*, 2000). With regard to mode of delivery, although patients with small lesions may be considered for vaginal delivery, it is generally preferred that birth should be by caesarean section as a planned procedure when radical surgery including radical caesarean hysterectomy may be performed. There is a theoretical risk that large lesions might bleed with cervical dilatation and tearing. It is clearly not practical to contemplate randomised studies into this subject. There are anecdotal reports of implantation at episiotomy sites following vaginal delivery (Copeland *et al.*, 1987; Cliby *et al.*, 1994) and, indeed, the author has also experienced such cases.

When radical caesarean hysterectomy is decided upon, this should be carried out at a planned and elective time either at 32–34 weeks with a stage IB lesion or at 37–38 weeks if the lesion is stage IA2. The operation is carried out as a combined procedure by the gynaecological oncologist and the obstetrician. A classical caesarean section is undertaken with a lower midline incision into the uterus. Having removed the fetus, syntocinon and prostaglandins may be given intravenously. The uterus is closed in layers, and three may be necessary. The contracted uterus is then removed with parametria prior to performing the pelvic node dissection. Although haemorrhage is potentially a major risk, the oedematous planes allow highly satisfactory definition of tissue spaces. With careful planning, there does not appear to be a significant increase in operative morbidity or major complications (Sood *et al.*, 1996).

Patients with more advanced disease who require radiotherapy will need careful planning in order to take into account the inevitable anatomical changes caused by the pregnancy. In fact, radiotherapy given during pregnancy does cause spontaneous abortion in most cases, but subsequent surgical evacuation is necessary when spontaneous abortion does not occur. This does risk additional morbidity. Evacuation of the uterus prior to commencing radiotherapy is therefore preferable, and this is possible using misoprostol as an alternative to surgical evacuation (Ostrom *et al.*, 2003).

CONCLUSIONS

Early-stage cancer of the cervix can be treated by surgery or radiotherapy. Superficially invasive disease with good prognostic factors can be treated adequately by cone biopsy, but more advanced invasive tumours, either stage IA2 with poor prognostic factors or stage IB1 or selected stage IB2 and stage IIA tumours, may be treated surgically by radical hysterectomy and pelvic node dissection.

Carefully selected young patients with small stage IB1 lesions may be suitable for fertility-sparing surgery by radical vaginal trachelectomy and laparoscopic pelvic lymphadenectomy.

Patients who are likely to require adjuvant therapy as shown by preoperative assessment should be treated initially by chemo/radiotherapy rather than by surgery in order to avoid increased morbidity. This applies especially to patients with stage IB2 tumours.

Stage IIB and greater tumours should initially be treated by external beam therapy and brachytherapy with concurrent cisplatin-based chemotherapy.

It should be realised that these recommendations may be applicable to ideal circumstances in the developed world. However, where expensive predominantly non-surgical facilities are not available, then these may not be practical and, under those circumstances, a pragmatic approach to management will be necessary on an individualised basis depending on the limited resources available as well as the needs of the patient and her supporting community. Political and health economic arguments will clearly determine the short-term outcomes while, in the longer term, it is hoped that advances in screening and prevention will become available to those most in need as well as those fortunate enough to be born and live where these facilities exist.

REFERENCES

Averette HE, Method MW, Sevin B-U *et al.* (1996) Radical abdominal hysterectomy in the primary management of invasive cervical cancer. In: Rubin SC, Hoskins WJ (eds) *Cervical Cancer and Pre-invasive Neoplasia*. Philadelphia: Lippincott-Raven Publishers, pp. 189–206.

Baumgartner BR, Bernardino ME (1989) MR imaging of the cervix: off axis scan to improve visualisation as a zonal anatomy. *American Journal of Roentgenology* 153: 1001–1002.

Benedet JL, Anderson GH (1996) Stage Ia carcinoma of the cervix revisited. *Obstetrics and Gynecology* 87: 1052–1059.

Benedet JL, Odicino F, Maisonneuve P *et al.* (2001) Carcinoma of the cervix uteri. *Journal of Epidemiology and Biostatistics* 6: 7–43.

Benedetti-Panici P, Maneschi F, D'Andrea G *et al.* (2000) Early cervical carcinoma: the natural history of lymph node involvement redefined on the basis of thorough parametrectomy and giant section study. *Cancer* 88: 2267–2274.

Burghardt E, Holzer E (1977) Diagnosis and treatment of microinvasive carcinoma of the cervix uteri. *Obstetrics and Gynecology* 49: 641–653.

Burghardt E, Pickle H, Haas J *et al.* (1987) Prognostic factors and operative treatment of stages Ib to IIb cervical cancer. *American Journal of Obstetrics and Gynecology* 156: 988–996.

Burnett AF, Roman L, O'Meara AT *et al.* (2003) Radical vaginal trachelectomy and pelvic lymphadenectomy: preservation of fertility in early cervical cancer. *Gynecologic Oncology* 3: 419–423.

Caddy B (1997) Basic principles in surgical oncology. *Archives of Surgery* 132: 338–346.

Chen G-D, Lin L-Y, Wang P-H *et al.* (2002) Urinary tract dysfunction after radical hysterectomy in cervical cancer. *Gynecologic Oncology* 85: 292–297.

Cliby WA, Dodson MK, Podratz KC (1994) Cervical cancer complicated by pregnancy: episiotomy site recurrences following vaginal delivery. *Obstetrics and Gynecology* 84: 1979–1982.

Copeland LJ, Saul PV, Sneige N (1987) Cervical adenocarcinoma: tumour implantation in episiotomy sites of two patients. *Gynecologic Oncology* 28: 230–235.

Covens A, Shaw P, Murphy J *et al.* (1999) Is radical trachelectomy a safe alternative to radical hysterectomy for patients with stage Ia–b carcinoma of the cervix? *Cancer* 86: 2273–2279.

Creasman WT, Kohler MF (2004) Is lymphovascular space involvement an independent prognostic factor in early cervical cancer? *Gynecologic Oncology* 92: 525–529.

Dargent D (1987) A new future for Schauta operation through presurgical retroperitoneal pelviscopy. *European Journal of Gynecologic Oncology* 8: 2912–2916.

Dargent D, Brun JL, Roy M *et al.* (1994) La trachelectomie elargie (TE). Une alternative à l'hysterectomie radicale dans le traitement des cancers infiltrantes developpés sur la face externe du col uterin. *Journal of Obstetrics and Gynaecology* 2: 285–292.

Dargent D, Martin X, Mathevet P (2000) Laparoscopic assessment of the sentinel lymph node in early stage cervical cancer. *Gynecologic Oncology* 79: 411–415.

Donegan WL (1983) Cancer in pregnancy. *Californian Cancer Clinics* 33: 194–214.

Echt MLO, Finan MA, Hoffman MS *et al.* (1999) Detection of sentinel lymph nodes with lymphazuria in cervical, uterine and vulvar malignancies. *Southern Medical Journal* 92: 204–208.

Girardi F, Pickle H, Winter R (1993) Pelvic and parametrial lymph nodes in the quality control of the surgical treatment of cervical cancer. *Gynecologic Oncology* 50: 330–333.

Goff BA, Paley PJ, Koh WJ *et al.* (2000) Cancer in the pregnant patient. In: Hoskins WJ, Perez CA, Young RC (eds) *Principles and Practice of Gynecologic Oncology*. Philadelphia: Lippincott Williams and Wilkins, pp. 501–528.

Green JA, Kirwan JM, Tierney JF *et al.* (2001) Survival and recurrence after concomitant chemotherapy and radiotherapy for cancer of the uterine cervix: a systematic review and meta-analysis. *Lancet* 358: 781–786.

Greer BE, Figge DC, Timimi HK *et al.* (1990) Stage Iaii squamous carcinoma of the cervix: difficult diagnosis and therapeutic dilemma. *American Journal of Obstetrics and Gynecology* 162: 1406–1409.

Havenga K, Maas CP, DeRuiter MC *et al.* (2000) Avoiding long-term disturbance to bladder and sexual dysfunction in pelvic surgery, particularly with rectal cancer. *Seminars in Surgical Oncology* 18: 235–243.

Hayes SD, Eremin O (1992) The relevance of tumour draining lymph nodes in cancer. *Surgery in Gynecology and Obstetrics* 174: 533–540.

Heller PB, Maletano JH, Bundy BN *et al.* (1990) Clinical pathologic study of stage IIB, III and IVA carcinoma of the cervix: extended diagnostic evaluation for para-aortic node metastasis — a gynaecological oncology group study. *Gynecologic Oncology* 38: 425–430.

Hertel H, Kohler C, Michels W *et al.* (2003) Laparoscopic-assisted radical vaginal hysterectomy (LARVH): prospective evaluation of 200 patients with cervical cancer *Gynecologic Oncology* 90: 505–511.

Hopkins MP, Morley JW (1992) The prognosis and management of cervical cancer associated with pregnancy. *Obstetrics and Gynecology* 80: 9–13.

Kaku T, Kamura T, Shigematsu T *et al.* (1999) Adenocarcinoma of the uterine cervix with predominantly villoglandular papillary growth pattern. *Gynecologic Oncology* 64: 147–152.

Keyes HM, Bundy BN, Stehman FB *et al.* (1999) Cisplatin, radiation and adjuvant hysterectomy compared with radiation and adjuvant hysterectomy for bulky stage Ib cervical carcinoma. *New England Journal of Medicine* 340: 1198–2000.

Khunamornpong S, Maleemonkol S, Siriankgul S *et al.* (2001) Well-differentiated villoglandular adenocarcinoma of the uterine cervix: a report of 15 cases including two with lymph node metastasis. *Journal of the Medical Association of Thailand* 84: 882–888.

Koh WJ, Panwala K, Greer D (2000) Adjuvant therapy for high-risk early stage cervical cancer. *Seminars in Radiation Oncology* 10: 51–60.

Landoni F, Maneo A, Colombo A *et al.* (1997) Randomised study of radical surgery versus radiotherapy for stage Ib–IIa cervical cancer. *Lancet* 350: 535–540.

Landoni F, Maneo A, Cormio G *et al.* (2001) Class 2 versus class 3 radical hysterectomy in stage Ib–IIa cervical cancer: a prospective randomised study. *Gynecologic Oncology* 80: 3–12.

Lea JS, Coleman RL, Garner EO *et al.* (2003) Adenosquamous histology with its poor outcome in low risk stage Ibi cervical adenocarcinoma. *Gynecologic Oncology* 91: 558–562.

Look KY, Brunetto VL, Clarke-Pearson DL *et al.* (1996) An analysis of cell type in patients with surgically staged Ib carcinoma of the cervix: a gynecologic oncology group study. *Gynecologic Oncology* 63: 304–311.

Maas CP (2003) Nerve-sparing radical surgery. Thesis. Leiden, The Netherlands.

Magrina JF, Goodrich MA, Weaver AL *et al.* (1995) Modified radical hysterectomy: morbidity and mortality. *Gynecologic Oncology* 59: 277–282.

Malur S, Krause N, Köhler C *et al.* (2001) Sentinel lymph node detection in patients with cervical cancer. *Gynecologic Oncology* 80: 254–257.

Mestwerdt G (1947) Probe-excizision und Kolposkopie Fruhdiagnose des Portokarzinomas. *Zentralblatt der Gynaekologie* 67: 326–332.

Monk BJ, Montz FJ (1992) Invasive cervical cancer complicating intra-uterine pregnancy: treatment with radical hysterectomy. *Obstetrics and Gynecology* 80: 199–203.

Morris M, Eifel P, Lu J *et al.* (1999) Pelvic irradiation with concurrent chemotherapy compared with pelvic and para-aortic radiation for high-risk cervical cancer. *New England Journal of Medicine* 340: 1137–1143.

National Cancer Institute PDQ treatment summary for health professionals (2002) *Cervical Cancer.* Bethesda, MD: National Institutes of Health.

National Comprehensive Cancer Network (2000) Practice guidelines for cervical cancer. In: *The Complete Library of NCCN Oncology Practice Guidelines,* Version 2000 (CD-ROM).

Ostrom K, Ben-Arie A, Edwards C *et al.* (2003) Uterine evacuation with misoprostol during radiotherapy for cervical cancer in pregnancy. *International Journal of Gynecological Cancer* 13: 340–343.

Page DL, Anderson TJ, Carter BA (1999) Minimal solid tumour involvement of regional and distal sites: when is a metastasis not a metastasis? *Cancer* 86: 2589–2592.

Peppercorn DP, Reznek RH, Jeyarajah AR *et al.* (1999) MRI in the selection of patients with early cervical carcinoma for fertility-preserving surgery: initial experience. *Radiology* 212: 395–399.

Peters WA, Liu PW, Barrett RJ, III *et al.* (2000) Concurrent chemotherapy and pelvic radiation therapy compared with pelvic radiation therapy alone as adjuvant therapy after radical surgery in high-risk early stage cancer of the cervix. *Journal of Clinical Oncology* 18: 1606–1613.

Photopulos GJ, Zwaag RV (1991) Class 2 radical hysterectomy shows less morbidity and good treatment efficacy compared to class 3. *Gynecologic Oncology* 40: 21–24.

Piver MS, Rutledge F, Smith JP (1974) Five classes of extended hysterectomy for women with cervical cancer. *Obstetrics and Gynecology* 44: 265–272.

Plante M, Renaud M-C, Tetu B *et al.* (2003) Laparoscopic sentinel node mapping in early stage cervical cancer. *Gynecologic Oncology* 91: 494–503.

Possover M, Krause N, Plaul K *et al.* (1998). Laparoscopic para-aortic and pelvic lymphadenectomy: experience with 150 patients and a review of the literature. *Gynecologic Oncology* 78: 19–28.

Querleu D (1993) Laparoscopic para-aortic node sampling in gynaecologic oncology: a preliminary experience. *Gynecologic Oncology* 49: 24–29.

Rockall AG, Sohaib SA, Harisinghani M *et al.* (2003) Diagnostic performance of MRI with ultrasmall particles of iron oxide in the diagnosis of lymph node metastases in patients with endometrial and cervical cancer. *European Radiology* 1: 636.

Rose PG, Bundy BN, Watkins EB *et al.* (1999a) Concurrent cisplatin-based radiotherapy and chemotherapy for locally advanced cervical cancer. *New England Journal of Medicine* 340: 1144–1153.

Rose PG, Adler LP, Rodriguez M *et al.* (1999b) Positron emission tomography for evaluating para-aortic nodal metastases in locally advanced cervical cancer before surgical staging: a surgico-pathologic study. *Journal of Clinical Oncology* 17: 41–45.

Roy M, Plante M (1998) Pregnancies after radical vaginal trachelectomy for early stage cervical cancer. *American Journal of Obstetrics and Gynecology* 179: 1491–1496.

Sakaragi K, Todo Y, Kudo M *et al.* (2005) A systematic nerve-sparing radical hysterectomy technique in invasive cervical cancer for preserving post-surgical bladder function. *International Journal of Gynecological Cancer* 15, 389–397.

Sartori E, Fallow L, Laface B *et al.* (1995) Extended radical hysterectomy in early stage carcinoma of the uterine cervix: tailoring the radicality. *International Journal of Gynecological Cancer* 5: 143–147.

Sasieni P, Adams J (1999) Effect of screening on cervical cancer mortality in England and Wales: analysis of trends with an age period cohort model. *British Medical Journal* 318: 1244–1255.

Scheidler J, Hricak H, Yu KK *et al.* (1997) Radiological evaluation of lymph node metastases in patients with cervical cancer. A meta-analysis. *Journal of the American Medical Association* 278: 1096–1101.

Schlaerth MD, Spirtos NM, Schlaerth AC (2003) Radical trachelectomy and pelvic lymphadenectomy with uterine preservation. *American Journal of Obstetrics and Gynecology* 188: 29–34.

Scully RE, Bonfiglio TA, Coleman RJ *et al.* (1994) Histological typing of female genital tract lesions. In: *World Health Organization Internal Histology Classification of Tumours*, 2nd edn. New York: Springer-Verlag, p. 44.

Sedlis A, Bundy BN, Rotman MZ *et al.* (1999) A randomised trial of pelvic radiation therapy versus no further therapy in selected patients with stage Ib carcinoma of the cervix after radical hysterectomy and pelvic lymphadenectomy: a gynecologic oncology study group study. *Gynecologic Oncology* 73: 177–183.

Sevin BU, Nadji M, Averette HE *et al.* (1992) Microinvasive carcinoma of the cervix. *Cancer* 70: 2121–2128.

Shepherd JH, Crawford RAF, Oram D (1998) Radical trachelectomy: a way to preserve fertility in the treatment of early cervical cancer. *British Journal of Obstetrics and Gynaecology* 105: 912–916.

Shepherd JH, Mould T, Oram DH (2001) Radical trachelectomy in early stage carcinoma of the cervix: outcome as judged by recurrence and fertility rates. *British Journal of Obstetrics and Gynaecology* 108: 882–885.

Sironi S, DeCobelli F, Scarfone G *et al.* (1993) Carcinoma of the cervix: value of plain and gadolinium-enhanced MR imaging in assessing degree of its invasiveness. *Radiology* 188: 797–801.

Sood AK, Sorosky JI, Krogman S *et al.* (1996) Surgical management of cervical cancer complicating pregnancy: a case–control study. *Gynecologic Oncology* 63: 294–298.

Spirtos NM, Eisenkop SM, Schlaerth JB *et al.* (2002) Laparoscopic radical hysterectomy (type 3) with aortic and pelvic lymphadenectomy in patients with stage I cervical cancer. Surgical morbidity and intermediate follow-up. *American Journal of Obstetrics and Gynecology* 187 (2): 340–348.

Sykes P, Allen D, Cohen C *et al.* (2003) Does the density of lymphatic vascular space invasion affect the prognosis of stage Ib and IIa node negative carcinoma of the cervix? *International Journal of Gynecological Cancer* 13: 313–316.

Takushi M, Moromizato H, Sakumoto K *et al.* (2002) Management of invasive carcinoma of the uterine cervix associated with pregnancy: outcome of intentional delay in treatment. *Gynecologic Oncology* 87: 185–189.

Trimbos JB, Maas CP, DeRuiter MC *et al.* (2001) Nerve-sparing radical hysterectomy; guidelines and feasibility in western patients. *International Journal of Gynecological Cancer* 11: 180–186.

Ungar L, Palfalvi L (2003) Surgical treatment of lymph node metastases in stage Ib cervical cancer: the laterally extended parametrectomy (LEP) procedure. *International Journal of Gynecological Cancer* 13: 647–651.

Utsugi K, Shimizu Y, Akiyama F *et al.* (2004) Clinicopathologic features of villoglandular papillary adenocarcinoma of the uterine cervix. *Gynecologic Oncology* 92: 64–70.

Van Trappen P, Gyselman VG, Lowe DG *et al.* (2001) Molecular quantification and mapping of lymph node micrometastases in cervical cancer. *Lancet* 357: 15–20.

Whitney CW, Sause W, Bundy BM *et al.* (1999) Randomised comparison of fluorouracil plus cisplatin versus hydroxyurea as an adjunct to radiation therapy in stage IIIB to IVA carcinoma of the cervix with negative para-aortic lymph nodes: a Gynaecologic Oncology Group and South West Oncology Group study. *Journal of Clinical Oncology* 17: 1339–1348.

Yamashita Y, Takahashi M, Sawada T *et al.* (1992) Carcinoma of the cervix: dynamic MR imaging. *Radiology* 182: 643–648.

Young RH, Scully RE (1989) Villoglandular papillary adenocarcinoma of the uterine cervix. *Cancer* 63: 1773–1779.

Zemlickis D, Lishner M, Degendorfer P *et al.* (1991) Maternal and foetal outcome after invasive cervical cancer in pregnancy. *Journal of Clinical Oncology* 9: 1956–1961.

CHAPTER 39

The surgical techniques employed for treating early-stage cervical cancer

Joseph Hanoch and G. Angus McIndoe

WHICH SURGICAL TECHNIQUE TO USE?

On 16 November 1898, Ernst Wertheim performed the first radical abdominal hysterectomy for cervical cancer. This operation bears his name and gives him a place of honour in surgical history. The primary mortality was 30% with his first hundred patients, but it must be remembered that there was no alternative treatment at that time. In an effort to reduce the mortality, Schauta (1904) developed the radical vaginal operation for primary treatment of cervical cancer, which has remained popular in many centres, particularly in Europe and India. Since the turn of the last century, when Schauta developed his radical vaginal hysterectomy, the operation has been modified by Amreich (1943) and by Stoeckel (1956). In fact, it is these techniques that are practised today.

In 1934, Bonney (1935) presented his interpretation of the Wertheim technique in London and, in the same year, Taussig (1934) from the US published his pelvic lymphadenectomy technique. The next development was by Meigs in Boston in 1944, who published his experience with the Wertheim operation for cervical carcinoma (Meigs, 1944a,b). He also

Table 39.1 The Piver–Rutledge classification.

Type I	Extrafascial hysterectomy
Type II	Modified radical hysterectomy
Type III	Radical hysterectomy
Type IV	Extended radical hysterectomy
Type V	Partial exenteration

introduced a term for this operation that is commonly used today: 'radical hysterectomy with bilateral pelvic lymph node dissection'. The enormous importance of his series of publications in those years was that he showed that the procedure carried a mortality rate of 1%.

In 1974, Piver *et al.* classified the surgical treatment of cervical cancer into five types of surgical procedures (Table 39.1); the extent of the section of the pelvic ligaments and spaces is represented diagrammatically in Figure 39.1.

The type I procedure is in fact what is widely known as a simple hysterectomy and is suitable for microinvasive cervical carcinoma.

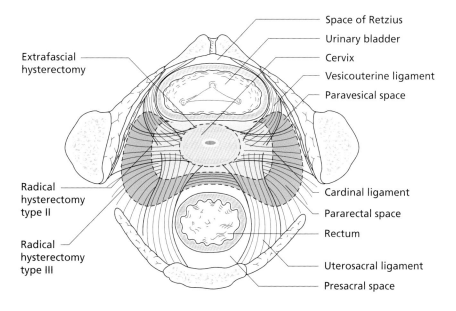

Fig. 39.1 An outline (dotted line) of the extent of dissection of the pelvic ligaments and spaces involved in the type II and III radical hysterectomies classified by Piver and Rutledge (1974). The extent of cardinal ligament removal and the extension of the procedures into both the paravesical and pararectal spaces can be clearly seen. Modified from Berek and Hacker (2000).

The type II or modified radical hysterectomy is the original Wertheim operation (Meigs, 1944a), in which the medial halves of the cardinal and proximal uterosacral ligaments are resected. Along with the uterus, the upper one inch of vagina is also removed. Wertheim's original operation included selective removal of enlarged nodes: however, nowadays, it is customary to perform a systematic pelvic lymphadenectomy as a therapeutic module. The type II hysterectomy is appropriate for stage IA2 cervical cancer.

The type III radical hysterectomy was described by Meigs in 1944. In this operation, the entire width of the cardinal ligaments is resected, with the uterosacrals being excised close to their sacral origin, and the upper half of the vagina removed *en bloc*. This type of radical hysterectomy is commonly performed for stage IB cervical cancer.

The type IV extended radical hysterectomy involves the ureter being completely dissected from the vesicouterine web, with the superior vesicle artery sacrificed and three-quarters of the vagina excised. Piver *et al.* (1974) suggested that this operation is suitable for selected small central recurrences after radiation therapy.

The type V procedure is indeed a partial exenteration. If the disease is found to involve a portion of the distal ureter or bladder, then the relevant organ is partially excised and the ureter reimplanted. The indication for this procedure is usually a central recurrence of cervical cancer.

In the last 100 years, the radical abdominal operation with standardised pelvic lymphadenectomy has become the method of choice for cervical cancer. The vaginal radical operation in its various forms plays a very restricted role, being abandoned by many because of the discontinuous spreading of disease into the regional pelvic lymph nodes (Raatz and Borner, 2000). Owing to its simplicity, the vaginal radical procedure may still be useful today in aged or high-risk patients. Since 1989, attempts have been made to combine the vaginal radical operation with laparoscopic pelvic and/or para-aortic lymphadenectomy. The development has passed the following stages: the development of laparoscopic pelvic and para-aortic lymphadenectomy based on staging criteria, followed by the combination of laparoscopic lymphadenectomy with vaginal radical operation and, recently, reports of complete laparoscopic radical hysterectomy and lymphadenectomy (Canis *et al.*, 1992; Nezhat *et al.*, 1994; Spirtos *et al.*, 1996).

The place of a fertility-sparing procedure (i.e. radical trachelectomy) for locally invasive cervical cancer is discussed in detail in Chapter 38.

PREOPERATIVE ASSESSMENT

Prior to surgery, and once a tissue diagnosis of invasive carcinoma has been established, the patient must undergo a staging procedure (also discussed in Chapter 36). Stage is determined at the time of initial diagnosis and should never be changed, even on the discovery of more extensive disease during surgery. Currently, stage is determined clinically, on the basis mainly of the size of the tumour in the cervix or its extension into the pelvis. The staging procedure includes an examination under anaesthesia, with or without a cystoscopy or rectosigmoidoscopy. Our experience of clinical staging and that of others has shown that this form of assessment is often inaccurate. The patient may then be evaluated with pertinent diagnostic tests, although in developing countries, computerised tomography (CT) and magnetic resonance imaging (MRI) techniques may not be readily available. These tests include: chest radiography, CT scan of abdomen and pelvis, pelvic MRI, cystoscopy, proctoscopy and assessment of the nutritional status, hepatic and urinary function. Although the results of CT, MRI or positron emission tomography (PET) cannot be used for FIGO staging, the information obtained from such studies has been used to assess more accurately the extent of pelvic disease and lymph node metastasis, which might affect treatment recommendations.

PREOPERATIVE PREPARATION

Perioperative thromboembolism prevention is attained with an injection of a low-molecular-weight heparin (e.g. Enoxaparine 40 mg daily) starting the night before the operation. Pressure stockings are also used. Prophylactic treatment with a broad-spectrum antibiotic is routine, and it would be prudent to cross-match at least 2 units of blood to be available for the operation.

EXTENT OF SURGICAL PROCEDURE

The procedure is intended to remove the uterus with or without the adnexae, part of the vaginal canal, all of the parametrium and a significant part of the uterosacral and vesicouterine ligaments; the pelvic lymph nodes, dissected from the lower aorta, common iliacs, external and internal iliacs and obturator fossae are removed as well. The parametrial lymph tissue will be removed, along with the cardinal ligament.

RADICAL HYSTERECTOMY AND LYMPHADENECTOMY

Incision

The abdomen may be opened via a midline incision or through one of the following transverse incisions: Maylard — a transverse incision from one anterior superior iliac spine to the opposite one (Fig. 39.2).

The fascia is incised transversely. The deep inferior epigastric vessels are located, sectioned and tied. The rectus muscles are then incised, preferably with a diathermy needle. The Cherney incision is another option, although less commonly

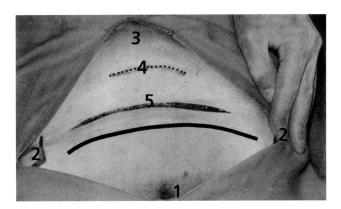

Fig. 39.2 Skin markings showing the site of the Maylard incision at the level of the thick black line. This is shown in relation to the usual gynaecological incision to emphasise the fact that the ends can be extended laterally above the anterior superior iliac spines to give width and access if required. Skin markings are numbered as follows: umbilicus (1), anterior superior iliac spines (2), symphysis pubis (3), low incision for lesser pelvic surgery (4), normal gynaecological incision (5).

used. The abdomen is opened in the same manner as in a Pfannenstiel incision, but the rectus muscles and the pyramidalis are dissected from their insertion at the symphysis by a Bovie electrodiathermy knife.

The transverse incisions provide excellent exposure of the pelvis and comfortable access to the pelvic sidewalls. However, midline incision allows good access to the para-aortic region; nevertheless, this is seldom necessary with early-stage cervical cancer.

Exploration

The inevitable exploration stage is at least as important as in any other gynaecological oncology operation. It needs to be systematic, and any evidence of metastatic disease should be confirmed with a frozen section. Specific locations in which to look for extrauterine spread are the vesicouterine fold and the pouch of Douglas. Another area that deserves special attention is the para-aortic lymph chain. If any suspicious para-aortic lymph node is palpated, it should be dissected for a frozen section. The importance of this exploration cannot be stressed enough, as the detection (and confirmation) of metastatic spread, unlike in debulking surgery for ovarian cancer for instance, has an immediate practical consequence: the option to abort the procedure and treat the patient with primary chemo/radiotherapy becomes relevant.

The dilemma whether to abort is not rare and, because staging for cervical cancer is a clinical one, 'undercalling' is frequent. However, recent studies have shown that the MRI scan can be useful in making the staging procedure more accurate and in helping to define better the extent of the disease and the volume of the primary tumour (Russell *et al.*, 1992; Kim *et al.*, 1993; deSouza *et al.*, 2000).

Most gynaecological oncologists would abandon the planned radical hysterectomy upon finding evidence of extrauterine spread. In a recent prospective Gynecological Oncology Group (GOG) study (Whitney and Stehman, 2000) evaluating the frequency with which intended radical hysterectomy for cervical cancer was abandoned, it was found that 98 out of 992 patients did not have the proposed radical operation completed. No preoperative characteristics that clearly and distinctly separated patients whose surgery was abandoned from those whose operation was completed were identified. The only required imaging studies were chest radiography and intravenous urography. Even though it is tempting to hypothesise that 'debulking' of metastatic nodes could improve outcomes, this large GOG study could offer no data to suggest that completion of the radical hysterectomy followed by radiation with or without chemotherapy would have produced superior results. The patient and her gynaecological oncologist therefore have to be aware of the risk (9% according to this study) that the operative procedure will be abandoned.

Lymphadenectomy

The round ligaments are clamped and divided bilaterally, providing access into the retroperitoneum (Fig. 39.3). The ureters are identified as they cross the pelvic brim.

The pararectal and paravesical spaces (Fig. 39.4) are developed by a combination of sharp and blunt dissection. Long diathermy forceps serve as a useful instrument in developing these spaces, with dissection beginning medial and slightly inferior to the external iliac vein. The paravesical space is bordered by the obliterated umbilical artery running along the bladder medially, with the obturator internus muscle laterally, the cardinal ligament posteriorly and the pubic symphysis anteriorly. The pararectal space is then opened, using a similar technique. This space is bounded by the rectum medially, the hypogastric artery laterally, the cardinal ligament anteriorly and the sacrum posteriorly.

The pelvic lymph node dissection can then be done in either the extra- or the intraperitoneal approach. The lymphadenectomy can begin at the bifurcation of the common iliac vessels, excising the loose lymphatic tissue overlying the external and internal iliac arteries and veins. This is performed in a caudal direction, having first identified the psoas muscle and the genitofemoral and lateral cutaneous nerve of the thigh. The dissection of the external iliac vessels continues caudally until the circumflex iliac vessels are encountered. Dissection in a cephalad direction allows clearance of common iliac and para-aortic nodes. Presacral nodes are also removed.

Once the external iliac vessels are exposed, they can be separated from the underlying tissue laterally. With gentle lateral and/or medial traction on the external iliac vessels, the obturator fossa is now entered. It is often helpful to sweep the external iliac vessels off the pelvic sidewall and approach

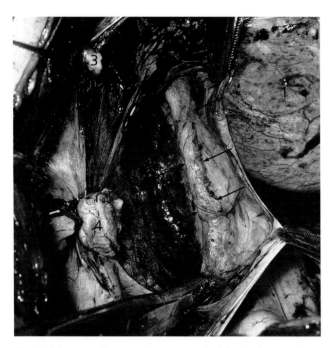

Fig. 39.3 Access to the retroperitoneum on the left side, showing the ureter (arrowed) with the left round ligament pedicle at (1) and left ovarian pedicle at (2). These have been ligated and are held laterally by the uncut sutures. The peritoneum of the posterior layer of the broad ligament is held medially by dissecting forceps (3), and the left ureter is clearly seen lying on it extraperitoneally.

the obturator fossa from the lateral side. The obturator nerve should be identified and preserved (Figs 39.5 and 39.6).

On the other hand, the obturator artery and vein are occasionally sacrificed to allow adequate dissection of the tissues lateral and posterior to the nerve.

The removal of the uterus

The uterine arteries are ligated and severed at their origin from the hypogastric or superior vesicle arteries.

The peritoneum across the vesicouterine fold is opened, and the bladder is then deflected to expose the anterior cervix and the portion of vagina that is to be excised (Figs 39.7 and 39.8). The ureters are taped, exposed and dissected laterally all the way down to their insertion into the bladder, taking care to preserve some blood supply and peritoneal attachments to them. This exposes the posterior vesicouterine ligament, which is also divided in a type III hysterectomy.

The peritoneum across the pouch of Douglas is incised to enter the rectovaginal space (Figs 39.9 and 39.10). This gives access that will allow isolation of the uterosacral ligaments, which are then removed along with the uterus and upper vagina, parametrial, paracervical and paracolpeal tissues (Figs 39.11 and 39.12).

The vaginal cuff is closed with interrupted sutures, and it is our experience as well as that of others (Jensen *et al.*, 1993) that there is no need for drains to be left *in situ*, unless there is concern about haemostasis.

Complications

Bladder injuries

Performing Wertheim's hysterectomy causes damage to the innervation and anatomical structures of the lower urinary tract, resulting from the ureteral and bladder dissection described above. Most patients who undergo type III radical hysterectomies will develop various degrees of neurogenic bladder after surgery. This form of bladder dysfunction may vary from a minimal change to a complete loss of any sensation in the bladder. Often, some recovery can be expected during the first year postoperatively but, after this period, no improvement

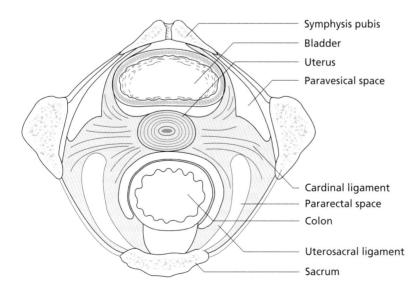

Symphysis pubis
Bladder
Uterus
Paravesical space

Cardinal ligament
Pararectal space
Colon

Uterosacral ligament

Sacrum

Fig. 39.4 Relations of the paravesical and pararectal spaces in the pelvis: cross-section of the pelvis showing the paravesical and pararectal spaces. The base of the broad ligament (cardinal ligament) extends to the lateral pelvic wall and contains the major lymphatics draining the cervix.

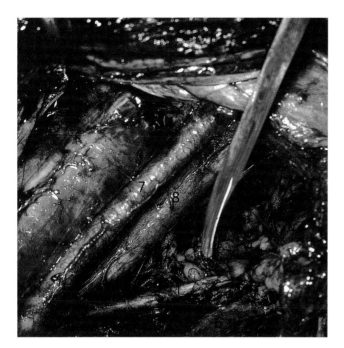

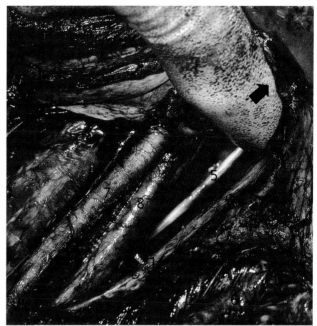

Fig. 39.5 Dissection of the left internal iliac (hypogastric) and obturator gland is taking place with sharp dissection of the gland groups except where they have to be separated from the obturator nerve digitally. The glands are removed off the obturator nerve (1), which is elevated and held in forceps while separation towards the obturator foramen continues, until eventually the gland mass has been separated from the sidewall (2). It is dissected *en bloc* with the external iliac glands that sometimes have a slight attachment to the bladder angle. The same numbering is used in Figure 39.6.

Fig. 39.6 The angle between the external iliac (3) and the internal iliac artery (4) is held open with the forefinger and is seen to be quite clear of glands and fat. The external iliac artery is at (5) and the ureter at (6). The same numbering is used in Figure 39.5.

can be expected. It is important to avoid overdistension of the bladder because it can result in bladder atony and a permanent inability to void. It is therefore prudent to keep an indwelling bladder catheter for 3–5 days and 'exercise' the bladder before removing it. Although the majority of patients recover, some continue to have a neurogenic bladder, whereas others might develop bladder instability. Prolonged bladder dysfunction has been found in 0.8–5.2% of patients after radical hysterectomy for cervical cancer (Powell *et al.*, 1981; Sivanesaratnam *et al.*, 1993; Samlal *et al.*, 1996). Urinary stress incontinence as a sequel of radical hysterectomy is rarely severe enough to warrant surgical repair. It is important to delay any consideration of surgical correction of stress incontinence for at least 12 months after the operation, because bladder function can improve during the first postoperative year.

In a recent study (Gulati *et al.*, 2001), urodynamic assessment was done in 20 patients with histopathologically proven cancer of the cervix who were about to undergo Wertheim's hysterectomy. The study was performed preoperatively, in the immediate postoperative period and 6 weeks after surgery. Urinary symptoms were also correlated with the urodynamic profile. It was concluded that the bladder was hypertonic in the immediate postoperative period, and urethral closure

pressures were low. Some regeneration of damaged nerve fibres was found to occur during the 6–8 weeks after surgery, resulting in some improvement in sensory and motor functions of the bladder. Postoperatively, continuous catheter drainage appeared to be the most important part of the management of hypertonic bladder.

Ureteric strictures and fistulae
These injuries occur if the blood supply to the distal ureter is compromised, or if the dissection is carried too close to the ureter.

Too vigorous dissection of the bladder base may also weaken its wall, and fistula formation may result. Ureterovaginal fistulas may occur in 1.8% (Powell *et al.*, 1981) and vesicovaginal fistulas occurred in 0.7% in a recent study. Important factors in the prevention of ureteric fistula formation are: preservation of the longitudinal blood supply in the ureteral adventitia; minimal handling of the ureter; using sharp dissection during mobilisation; and avoidance of skeletonising of the lower 2 cm of the ureter just before it enters the bladder. If a ureteric fistula develops, an attempt should be made to stent the ureter, preferably via a percutaneous nephrostomy. If this is not successful in healing the fistula or if the stent cannot be passed along the ureter, 3 months is allowed for the pelvic inflammation and induration to resolve before repair is attempted. Surgical repair usually entails ureteroneocystostomy, possibly with a psoas muscle hitch (Podratz *et al.*, 1982; Webb, 1997).

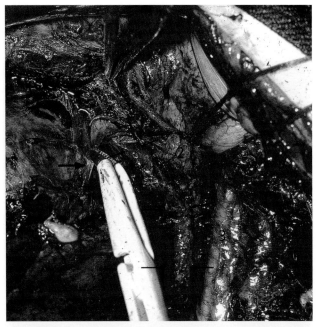

39.7

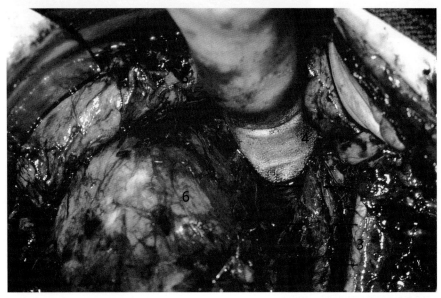

39.8

Figs 39.7 and 39.8 Further separation of
the bladder from the uterus is taking place
(Fig. 39.7). Once the rectum has been freed
posteriorly, it is possible to elevate the uterus
into the wound, allowing separation of the
bladder to a deeper level anterior. Vascular
attachment (arrowed) just medial to the
right ureter (1) is touched with diathermy
before division. The uterine pedicle, already
ligated, is seen at (2), and the external iliacs
are seen in (3). After further bladder
separation in the midline by the division of
adhesions with scissors, the finger displaces
the area of the right uterovesical junction
(Fig. 39.8), and this displacement is
downwards so as to expose the vagina (5),
which has been distended by the placement
of a gauze pack. The bladder is at (5) and
the vagina at (6).

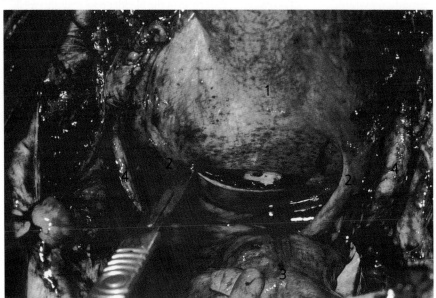

Fig. 39.9 The opening of the rectovaginal
space with a scalpel incising the peritoneum
between and deep to the attachment of the
uterosacral ligament. The uterus (1) is held
upwards, and the uterosacral ligaments are
therefore exposed (2) with the rectum lying
posteriorly at (3). The ureters are seen
laterally at (4). The level of incision has been
carefully chosen so that the firmly attached
uterine peritoneum becomes more loosely
applied and is just mobile on the posterior
cervical surface.

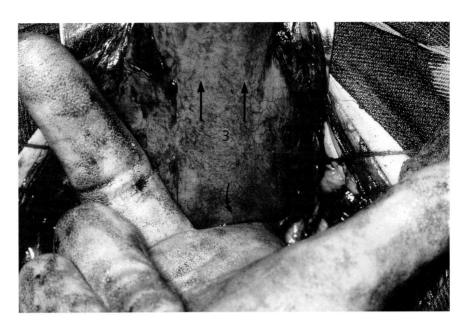

Fig. 39.10 The upper vagina is being separated from the rectum. That has been facilitated by a firm gauze pack placed in the vagina preoperatively, thereby forming a column which the finger follows downward, and it is a simple matter to free the vagina posteriorly and separate the rectum from it. The separation is carried well laterally so that there is no question of the rectum being caught up and damaged when the parametrium is divided during hysterectomy. The uterus is held upwards in the direction of the arrows, and the right forefinger acts as a blunt dissector.

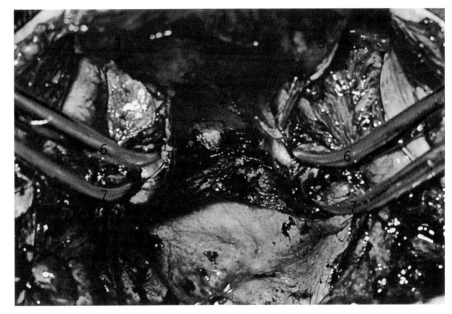

Fig. 39.11 The uterus, cervix, parametrium and upper vagina have been freed from the lower uterine attachments. This is obviously a posterior view. The uterus is labelled at (1), the cervix at (2) and the parametrium at (3) with the upper vagina at (4). These four structures have been divided from their lateral attachments, and it only remains to separate them from the rest of the vagina at (5). Two forceps on each side have divided the cardinal (6) and the uterosacral ligaments at (7). These two forceps on each side secure the two portions of the parametrium.

Vesicovaginal fistulae are seen mainly in patients who have previously had irradiation. Again, after establishing that the upper tracts have not been injured, repair is not attempted for 3 months. Simple fistulae may be repaired vaginally, but more complex fistulae are best managed by an abdominal approach.

Blood vessel injury

This can occur during dissection of the pelvic lymph nodes. This scenario includes perforations, cuts, abrasions and tears to the abundant vascular system of the pelvis. Smaller branches can be sacrificed for haemostasis, and major vessels should be repaired, usually with a vascular stitch. If a large vein is damaged, it may be necessary to repair the damage with a venous patch.

Lymphocysts

After excision of the pelvic lymph system, the lymph from the lower extremities flows through the collateral lymph system; later, new routes of lymph flow form. When collateral lymph routes are excised and new ones have not yet developed, the lymph continues to flow into the cavity and, with the precipitated fibrin, the result is a lymph fluid collection, encapsulated in a connective tissue sheath. Lymphocysts are usually asymptomatic with an incidence of 1.5% (Powell *et al.*, 1981). Correlation between lymph node metastasis and development of lymphocysts has not been found. Unilateral lymphocysts develop more frequently than bilateral ones (Charkviani *et al.*, 2000). Lymphocysts usually arise 11–12 days after surgery.

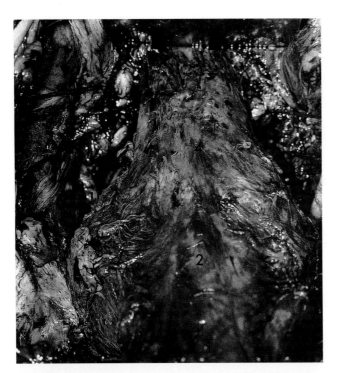

Fig. 39.12 The upper vagina prior to transection has been defined by the dotted line. The retractor held in the direction of the arrows has displaced the bladder to show the considerable length of upper vagina available for removal (4). The uterus (1), cervix (2) and parametrium (3) are clearly seen.

Ultrasonography is a highly informative diagnostic method to detect this condition. Most of them will disappear with time, mostly over several months. They should be treated only when they cause pain and pressure, ureteric obstruction or when they become infected or result in lymphoedema. Treatment can be by percutaneous drainage, sometimes with the addition of sclerosing agents, or by surgery (laparotomy or laparoscopy), with marsupialisation of the lymphocyst into the peritoneal cavity.

Thromboembolism

Clotting occurring in the veins of the lower limb and pelvis is a relatively common complication. The causes of clotting were described many years ago by Virchow in his classical triad of stasis, hypercoagulable state and endothelial damage. Stasis is the major cause of venous clotting and occurs with intra- and postoperative bed rest. A hypercoagulable state can occur in the postoperative period when there is an elevation of platelet count and a change in clotting factors. It also accompanies polycythaemia and thrombocytosis. Endothelial damage occurs secondary to pressure on veins during the surgical procedures adjacent to the pelvic veins. Various measures can then be used to keep the risk as low as possible. These include anticoagulant medicines, compression stockings and an intermittent compression pump. In one very large series, Sivanesaratnam *et al.* (1993) reported a venous thrombosis rate of 2.3% in 397 patients after radical hysterectomy and a 0.5% pulmonary embolism rate.

Obturator nerve injury

The nerve may be avulsed at the time of pelvic node dissection or be incorporated in a paravaginal suture. The injury may result in thigh adduction disability. However, if the nerve is not transected, then there is recovery of function with time. If the nerve is transected, the patient will compensate by using other thigh muscles for adduction, with little residual disability.

OVARIAN CONSERVATION

Ovarian management during radical hysterectomy is still controversial. In young women, premature cessation of ovarian function may lead to serious short-term and long-term complications, with impairment of their quality of life.

Ovaries are seldom subject to metastases, so their preservation would be plausible in radical cervical cancer surgery. Preservation would guarantee natural estrogen production for young patients with early-stage disease. Hence, retention of the ovaries is recommended, except when postoperative irradiation is necessary. The latter inevitably leads to castration. Thus, when postoperative irradiation therapy is necessary, the ovaries can be preserved only when placed outside the radiation field during the operation.

Sipos *et al.* (2002) published a study of 422 radical hysterectomies performed for early-stage (IA2 or IB) cervical cancer. In 21 cases, at least one of the ovaries was conserved and suspended. After a minimum follow-up period of 2 years, only one woman required hormone replacement. The ovaries removed in this study showed no metastasis.

In another study, a 7-year retrospective review at the University of South Florida College of Medicine (USA) found 99 patients who had their ovaries removed during surgery (Owens *et al.*, 1989). None of the ovaries contained metastatic disease, including those from 22 patients with adenocarcinoma or adenosquamous carcinoma. All patients had early-stage cancer except three who had stage IIB disease. Of the 17 patients with retained ovaries, 14 had transposition into the paracolic gutters. Only one of the 14 patients with transposed ovaries developed symptoms of ovarian failure. No patients with retained ovaries developed metastatic disease or required reoperation for ovarian recurrence.

In a more recent study from the US, the records of 200 consecutive women with stage I–IIA cervical cancer treated primarily with radical hysterectomy and pelvic lymphadenectomy were reviewed (van Beurden *et al.*, 1990). Lateral ovarian transposition was performed at the time of radical hysterectomy in 132 (66%) patients, and 28 (21%) received postoperative pelvic radiation therapy. Only 3/104 (2.9%) patients who underwent lateral ovarian transposition without postoperative pelvic radiotherapy experienced menopausal symptoms; nevertheless, follicle-stimulating hormone (FSH) levels in all three cases suggested continued ovarian function. In 14/28 (50%) patients who received postoperative pelvic radiation therapy, ovarian failure occurred, making the risk of ovarian failure with pelvic radiation therapy after lateral ovarian transposition significant (relative risk = 17.3). Moreover, the incidence of adnexal disease in transposed ovaries requiring further surgery was 3%.

In a study from the Netherlands, a different aspect of the issue was examined. This study looked into the practicality of the transposition, in terms of whether the transposed ovaries are entirely out of the radiation field. A series of 126 patients with cervical cancer was critically analysed (Samlal *et al.*, 1996). The ovaries were transposed in 44 of the 64 women. At least one ovary was placed outside the radiation field in only 68% of the women. Their results showed that, because of scattered radiation, i.e. 5% of the total radiation dose at a distance of 4 cm outside the radiation field, a substantial loss of ovarian function might occur.

In one of the few prospective studies looking into this issue, Morice *et al.* (2000) studied 107 patients treated for cervical cancer who underwent ovarian transposition with radical hysterectomy and lymphadenectomy. Preservation of ovarian function was achieved in 83% of the patients. The rates of ovarian preservation were 100% for patients treated exclusively with surgery, 90% for patients treated by postoperative vaginal brachytherapy and 60% for patients treated by postoperative external radiation therapy and vaginal brachytherapy. This French study concluded that ovarian transposition was a safe and effective procedure for preserving ovarian function in patients treated with a radiosurgical combination.

In conclusion, ovarian management at the time of radical hysterectomy is still under investigation. It seems that, according to the data from the international literature, transposition of ovaries during radical hysterectomy could be applied for well-selected younger patients with early stage cervical cancer, thus harbouring a small risk, but with a much better quality of life for the patients.

SENTINEL LYMPH NODES IN CERVICAL CANCER SURGICAL MANAGEMENT

Carcinoma of the uterine cervix spreads predominantly by local extension and via the pelvic lymph nodes. Pelvic lymph node metastases are demonstrated in 10–35% of stage I–II cervical cancer patients, and this is an important prognostic factor.

The sentinel node is the first node in the lymphatic system that drains the primary tumour site through specific lymphatic channels (see Chapter 4). If the sentinel node does not contain tumour metastasis, all other nodes should be free of disease as well. Sentinel nodes can be identified either using peritumoral

injection of blue dye (Fig. 39.13), which will visually colour the first draining node, or by peritumoral injection of a radioactive tracer that spreads to the sentinel node and can be detected with a gamma probe.

Buist *et al.* (2003) from Amsterdam have recently published their work designed to investigate the feasibility of sentinel node detection through laparoscopy in patients with early cervical cancer. Twenty-five patients with early-stage cervical cancer in whom radical hysterectomy and pelvic lymph node dissection was planned received an intracervical injection of technetium–99m colloidal albumin as well as blue dye. With a laparoscopic gamma probe and with visual detection of blue nodes, the sentinel nodes were identified and separately removed via laparoscopy. One or more sentinel nodes could be detected via laparoscopy in 25/25 patients (100%). A sentinel node was found bilaterally in 22/25 patients (88%). Histologically positive nodes were detected in 10/25 patients (40%). One patient (11%) had two false-negative sentinel nodes in the obturator fossa, whereas a positive lymph node was found in the parametrium removed together with the primary tumour. In seven patients (28%), the planned laparotomy and radical hysterectomy were abandoned because of a positive sentinel node. In two patients, a micrometastasis in the sentinel node was demonstrated after surgery. They concluded that laparoscopic removal of sentinel nodes in cervical cancer was a feasible technique. If radical hysterectomy is aborted in the case of positive lymph nodes, sentinel node detection via laparoscopy, followed by laparoscopic lymph node dissection, could prevent potentially unnecessary surgery.

In the same month, Lambaudie *et al.* (2003), from France, published their work aimed at determining the feasibility of intraoperative radioisotopic mapping using an endoscopic gamma probe associated with patent blue dye injection in patients with early-stage cervical cancer. Twelve patients took part in that study. A total of 35 sentinel lymph nodes were detected. Eight sentinel lymph nodes were detected only by colour, eight were detected by endoscopic gamma probe

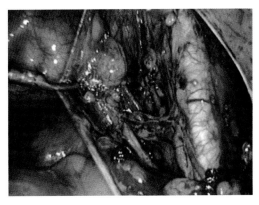

Fig. 39.13 Blue nodes clearly visible in the obturator fossa after injection of peritumoral blue dye. The first draining nodes are thereby coloured. From Buist *et al.* (2003), with permission from Elsevier.

and 19 sentinel lymph nodes were 'hot and dyed'. The authors found three metastatic lymph nodes. In one case, bilateral positive sentinel nodes were detected only by the endoscopic gamma probe. Paraffin sections identified one submillimetric micrometastasis in a lymph node that was neither blue nor hot intraoperatively. They showed that the identification of the sentinel lymph node with blue dye and radioisotope using an endoscopic gamma probe is feasible and improves the detection rate. False negatives did occur, but the proportion was relatively low.

Another recent French study (Barranger *et al.*, 2003) also set out to evaluate the feasibility of a laparoscopic sentinel lymph node procedure with combined radioisotopic and patent blue labelling in patients with cervical carcinoma. Thirteen women with cervical carcinoma underwent a laparoscopic sentinel lymph node procedure using an endoscopic gamma probe after both radioactive isotope and patent blue injections. Sentinel lymph nodes were identified in 12 out of 13 patients. No lymph node involvement was detected in sentinel lymph nodes with haematoxylin and eosin staining. Immunohistochemical studies identified four metastatic sentinel lymph nodes in two patients, with micrometastases in two sentinel lymph nodes from the first patient and isolated tumour cells in two sentinel lymph nodes from the second patient. No false-negative sentinel lymph node results were obtained. The results of this study and a more recent one by Lin *et al.* (2005) examining sentinel node detection with radiocolloid lymphatic mapping suggest that sentinel lymph node detection with a combination of radiocolloid and patent blue is feasible in patients with cervical carcinoma. The combination of laparoscopy and the sentinel lymph node procedure could permit minimally invasive management of early-stage disease.

This novel and experimental technique still needs time and large-scale studies to validate its place in clinical management. Nevertheless, if the sentinel node concept is valid in cervical cancer and if the sentinel node can be identified easily through laparoscopy, a less radical procedure for cervical cancer can be performed, and the surgical morbidity would be significantly reduced. This is a promising approach that could minimise major and maybe unnecessary surgical interventions.

Schauta radical vaginal hysterectomy

Radical vaginal hysterectomy has been performed in surgical treatment of cervical cancer for over 100 years. After a period of decreasing popularity, we can observe a gradual return to its previous status. The possibility of association of laparoscopic lymphadenectomy with this vaginal operation has changed the approach to the surgical treatment of cervical cancer. The aim of this section is to present the method of vaginal radical hysterectomy based on the Schauta–Amreich technique. This involves the following stages:

• The routine lithotomy position is usually adequate so long as the buttocks are well over the end of the table, but improved access is achieved if the thighs are hyperflexed by advancing the poles towards the head of the table, while care is taken that the calves are not compressed.

• Clamps are used to demarcate the amount of vagina to be removed, and then pulled towards the introitus, enclosing the cervix in the base of this 'pocket', thus forming the vaginal cuff (Fig. 39.14). An anterior incision is made on the cuff, and the bladder is dissected from the vagina (Fig. 39.15). Posteriorly, the plane of cleavage between vaginal wall and rectum is found and entered, and the dissection is carried up as far as the peritoneum of the pouch of Douglas.

• Now is the time for the Schuchardt incision. Although the authors use this as a standard procedure, other surgeons (Monaghan *et al.*, 2004) feel it is unnecessary because it causes significant postoperative discomfort and scarring. Monaghan *et al.* (2004) believe that, when the incision is made, it is a large left lateral episiotomy incision (Fig. 39.16), which allows widening of the entrance to the vagina to give greater access. If the Schuchardt incision is made, then it is usually made on the patient's left side. The incision is best made with a diathermy needle through vaginal and perineal skin. Extending from the cut edge of the vagina above, well out on to the lateral perineum, the subcutaneous tissues are divided, so that the incision reaches as high and deep as the levator ani, while the rectum is protected by the surgeon's finger. Once the pararectal fossa is opened up, both the pararectal space posteriorly and the paravesical space above can be developed with the surgeon's

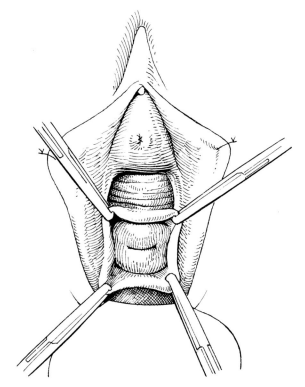

Fig. 39.14 Formation of the vaginal cuff (see text).

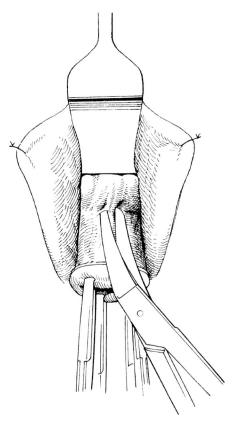

Fig. 39.15 Dissection of the bladder from the vagina (see text).

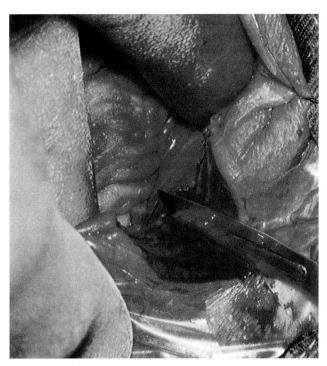

Fig. 39.16 Preparation for vaginal part of operation. An episiotomy-type relief incision is made posteromedially on the left side to improve access still further.

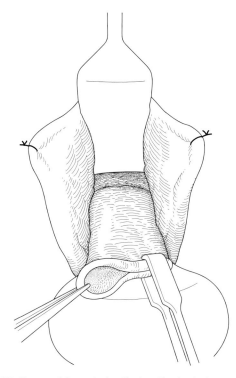

Fig. 39.17 Closure of the vaginal cuff using Chrobach clamps.

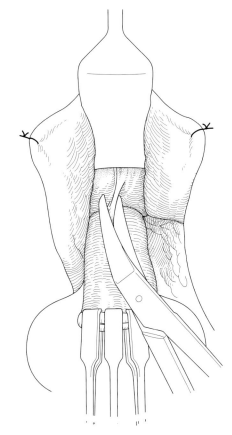

Fig. 39.18 Division of the cervicovesical ligament.

fingers so that they are continuous. During the procedure, the top few fibres of the levator ani muscle must be recognised and should not be resected as they will be used as a guide both to develop the paravesical fossa and to reconstruct the muscle at the end of the Schuchardt incision.

• The next step involves enclosure of the vaginal cuff (Fig. 39.17) and moving back to the anterior surface of this cuff with subsequent dissection between the bladder and vagina until the cervicovesical ligament presents itself for division (Fig. 39.18). Subsequently the vesicocervical space is opened, leading to the uterocervical pouch of peritoneum. Once the bladder edge has been defined, it can be gently elevated upwards, with this procedure having been made easier by division of the cervicovesical ligament. At this point, the medial side of a broad pillar of tissue is defined; within this bladder pillar lies the base of the ureteric tunnel, just demonstrable on either side of the midline. The cervix is then drawn to one side, and the proximal lateral edge of the incised vagina is grasped with a straight forceps. At this point, the angled Monaghan scissors can be inserted at right angles to the edge of this vaginal skin, being placed upwards and laterally and thereby gently having their opening seen towards the paravesical fossa, which can be simply and accurately assessed (Fig. 39.19), then developed further by placing the narrow curved Wertheim retractor into the space. This retractor fits neatly around the pubic

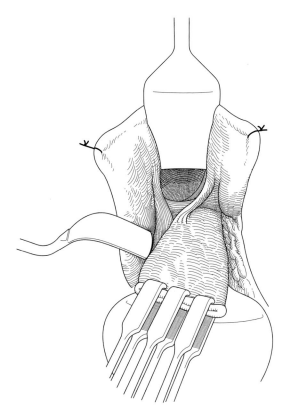

Fig. 39.20 Both the paravesical and the pararectal spaces have been joined and the horizontal fascia is exposed.

ramus, thereby opening up the space completely (Fig. 39.20). On the medial side of this space, which has been developed, there is situated a pillar of tissue that is bordered on its lateral side by the Wertheim retractor in the paravesical space and on its medial side by the open area that has been separated as the central part of the bladder has been drawn upwards. With this retractor in place, the index finger is placed below the bladder and lying on the cervix, at which stage the ureter can be palpated within the ureteric tunnel and a 'click' can be felt as the firm ureter is rotated against the retractor, and this allows the surgeon to identify the ureter and to see how far up the pillar it is situated. The pillar is then divided in order to demonstrate the ureter (Fig. 39.21). Within the bladder pillars, the ureter has now been identified and is exposed, as it curves downwards and then upwards to enter the bladder (Fig. 39.22).

The bladder and ureters having been retracted upwards, the bladder pillars can now be ligated and divided, after which the uterine vessels become obvious and can be isolated and ligated.

• The uterovesical pouch of the peritoneal opening is now enlarged laterally to the origins of the round ligaments. If the ovaries are to be removed, the adnexae are then grasped and the vessels contained in the infundibulopelvic ligament are ligated and divided. In the next step, the uterosacrals are divided (Fig. 39.23), followed by the cardinal ligaments (Fig. 39.24).

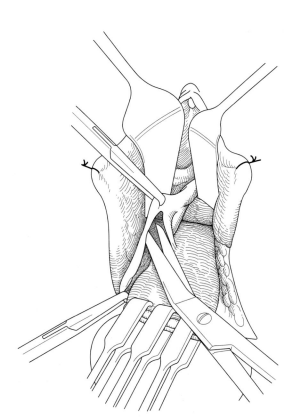

Fig. 39.19 The right paravesical space is seen being opened with the angled Monaghan scissors.

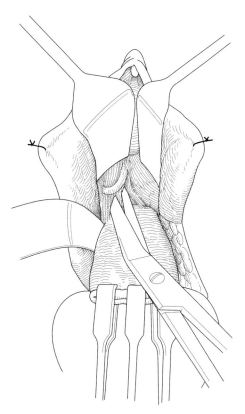

Fig. 39.21 The right ureter is now displayed by separation of the bladder pillar, which connects the bladder to the cervix.

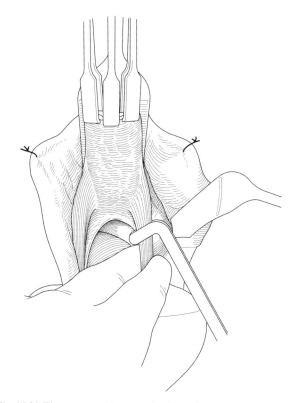

Fig. 39.23 The uterosacral ligament has been clamped and is about to be divided.

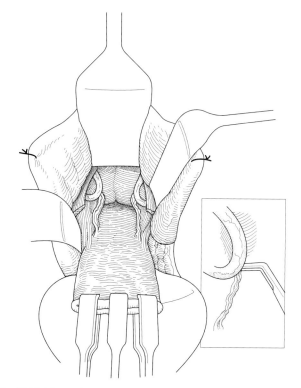

Fig. 39.22 The medial walls of the bladder pillars are now divided with the scissors having been close to the ureters, and together with the bladder are deflected upwards, thereby displaying the uterine vessels. A series of ligatures which 'creep upwards' are applied to these vessels until the displaced ureters are reached and the vessels are then divided as high as possible.

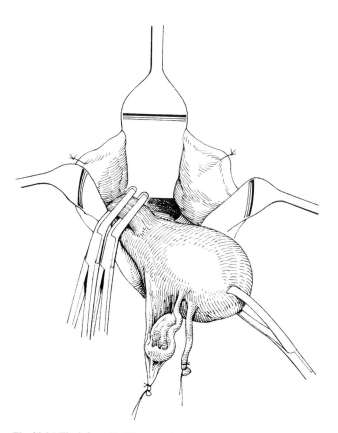

Fig. 39.24 The left cardinal ligament has been clamped and is also about to be divided.

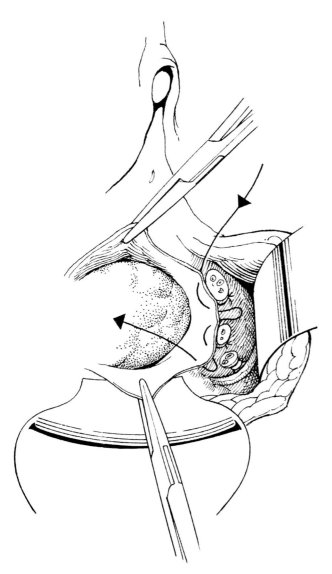

Fig. 39.25 Purse-string suture closes the peritoneum with the extraperitonalisation of the ligated pedicles.

Table 39.2 Comparison of treatment modalities in the management of cervical cancer (after Waggoner, 2003).

Stage	Treatment	Comments
IA1	Conisation (fertility desired) or a simple hysterectomy	If lymphovascular space invasion, hysterectomy with or without pelvic lymphadenectomy
1A2	Radical hysterectomy with pelvic lymphadenectomy	Or radiotherapy
1B1	Radical hysterectomy with pelvic lymphadenectomy (or radiotherapy) Radical trachelectomy (fertility desired) (see Chapter 38)	Plus chemoradiotherapy for poor prognostic surgical–pathological factors*
1B2	Radical hysterectomy with pelvic lymphadenectomy, plus chemoradiotherapy for poor prognostic surgical–pathological factors* or chemoradiotherapy	Chemoradiotherapy can be followed by adjuvant hysterectomy
IIA	Radical hysterectomy with pelvic lymphadenectomy or chemoradiotherapy	
IIB	Chemoradiotherapy	
IIIA	Chemoradiotherapy	
IVA	Chemoradiotherapy	Or primary pelvic exenteration
IVB	Palliative chemotherapy or chemoradiotherapy	

*Pelvic lymph node metastasis; large tumour; deep cervical stromal invasion; lymphovascular space invasion; positive vaginal or parametrial margins.

To conclude the operation, the peritoneum is stitched back, leaving all the stumps extraperitoneal (Fig. 39.25).

TREATMENT OPTIONS – THE DILEMMA

The controversy between surgery and radiotherapy has existed for decades and essentially surrounds the treatment of the early stages. Three large, and now considered classic, studies by Currie (1971), Zander *et al.* (1981) and Fletcher and Rutledge (1972) have shown that both treatment techniques result in similar survival rates and, as seen in Table 39.2, both techniques are equally acceptable in management.

Radical hysterectomy is a procedure that must be performed by a skilled gynaecological oncologist with sufficient experience to make the morbidity acceptable (1–5%). Following this imperative, primary surgery has the advantage of removing the primary disease and allowing accurate surgical staging, as well as avoiding the chronic radiation damage to the bladder, small and large bowel and vagina. Sexual dysfunction can be a major problem for many, especially following both external beam therapy and brachytherapy, with its attendant vaginal atrophy, fibrosis and stenosis. Although the vagina is shortened after radical hysterectomy, it is more elastic and, in premenopausal patients, ovarian function can be preserved. In postmenopausal patients, the non-irradiated vagina responds much better to estrogen therapy (Hacker, 2000). This topic is discussed further in Chapter 42.

The Schauta radical vaginal hysterectomy has never had the popularity among British and American gynaecological oncologists that it has among the European and, in particular, the German school of surgeons. Unfortunately, in the leading American gynaecological oncology textbooks, this procedure is seldom mentioned as an alternative. The consequences of all the above is that, today, it is probably regarded as more of historical interest than of practical use (Coppleson, 1992).

Some surgeons combine laparoscopic lymphadenectomy with a radical vaginal hysterectomy, i.e. the Schauta procedure. In this way, the procedure resembles the AVRUEL procedure (abdominal vaginal radical uterus extirpation with transperitoneal lymphadenectomy), as developed in 1957 by Sindram (1959), who combined the Wertheim and the Schauta procedures together with abdominal lymphadenectomy in one single operation. Because of the high complication rate in the form of voiding problems and sexual impairment caused by the Schauta part, this operation (AVRUEL) is no longer performed. In order to pay attention to the morbidity associated in the past with the combined abdominovaginal approach compared with the single abdominal approach, a large retrospective study was recently published that reassembled the data from several large Dutch centres where patients were treated either by the AVRUEL procedure or by abdominal radical hysterectomy (Kenter and Heintz, 2002). A total of 730 patients underwent an AVRUEL procedure. Fistulae occurred in 57 patients (7.8%), long-term urological complications in 233 patients (32%) and sexual dysfunction in 71 (9.7%). A total of 928 patients underwent an abdominal radical hysterectomy, the complication rates of which have been described in 511 cases. Twelve fistulae occurred (2%), long-term micturition problems in 55 (10%) and sexual problems in 11 (2%). There was no difference in 5-year survival rates in both groups. They concluded that returning to the old days in terms of a reintroduction of the Schauta procedure is not to be preferred. It is the authors' opinion that laparoscopically assisted radical vaginal hysterectomy is an improvement, but it should be carried out according to clearly defined prospective protocols in which data can be compared with those of other techniques with special attention paid to late complications such as micturition difficulties and sexual morbidity.

Dargent (1987), in an effort to resuscitate Schauta's operation, was the first to suggest that laparoscopic pelvic lymphadenectomy could be followed by a Schauta radical vaginal hysterectomy, and declared that the 3-year survival rate of 51 patients with negative pelvic lymph nodes was 95.5%.

The ability to treat the primary tumour adequately using the laparoscopically assisted Schauta procedure is an operator-dependent one. The large published series of such operations by Massi *et al.* (1993) and Dargent (1987) indicated that the Schauta procedure resulted in survival rates that were comparable with those achieved by the Wertheim–Meigs operation.

The major obstacle to gaining wide acceptance has been the lack of surgical training and experience with the Schauta procedure.

Current evidence on the safety and efficacy of laparoscopic radical hysterectomy does not appear to be adequate to support the use of this procedure without special arrangements for consent and for audit or research (NICE, 2003).

The use of laparoscopy as a technique for evaluation prior to a planned radical operation to define patients in whom the procedure would be abandoned has also been suggested (Childers *et al.*, 1992). However, it is not clear at this point whether laparoscopy should be used routinely to rule out extrauterine disease. Such a decision awaits the results of prospective evaluations in multiple institutions. At this point, open operation remains the most sensitive approach for evaluating the true extent of the disease.

Radical hysterectomy with pelvic lymphadenectomy is an effective, established and well-tolerated treatment for early-stage carcinoma of the cervix. It has the potential to preserve ovarian function and, to allow improved coital function, the ability to identify surgical pathological risk factors and outcomes comparable to radiation therapy. Cure rates in the ranges of 85–90% are commonly reported, and it would seem as though this time-honoured procedure occupies a key position as a definitive treatment option for cancer of the cervix.

ACKNOWLEDGEMENTS

The authors wish to thank Professor A. Singer for allowing reproduction of intraoperative photographs (Figs 39.2, 39.3, 39.5–39.12) that were originally published in *A Colour Atlas of Gynaecological Surgery* (D.H. Lees and A. Singer, Vol. 3: *Operations for Malignant Disease*, Wolfe Medical Publishing Limited, London, 1979). They also wish to thank Mr J.M. Monaghan for his permission to reproduce intraoperative drawings (Figs 39.14–39.25) that appeared in *Bonney's Gynaecological Surgery* (10th edn), published by Blackwell Publishing, Oxford, 2004.

REFERENCES

Amreich AI (1943) Bericht über die Gefahren und Erfolge der erweiterten vaginalen Total extirpation auf Gund von 1505 Operationen. *Wiener Klinische Wochenschrift* 56: 162.

Barranger E, Grahek D, Cortez A *et al.* (2003) Laparoscopic sentinel lymph node procedure using a combination of patent blue and radioisotope in women with cervical carcinoma. *Cancer* 97 (12): 3003–3009.

Berek JS, Hacker NF (eds) (2000) *Practical Gynecologic Oncology*, 3e. Philadelphia: Lippincott Williams & Wilkins.

Bonney MS (1935) The treatment of carcinoma of the cervix by Wertheim's operation. *American Journal of Obstetrics and Gynecology* 30: 815.

Buist MR, Pijpers RJ, van Lingen A *et al.* (2003) Laparoscopic detection of sentinel lymph nodes followed by lymph node dissection in patients with early stage cervical cancer. *Gynecologic Oncology* 90 (2): 290–296.

Canis M, Mage G, Wattiez A *et al.* (1992) Vaginally assisted laparoscopic radical hysterectomy. *Journal of Gynecological Surgery* 8: 103–104.

Charkviani L, Kekelidze N, Charkviani T (2000) Management of lymphocysts after cervical carcinoma surgery. *European Journal of Gynaecologic Oncology* 21 (5): 487–490.

Childers JM, Hatch K, Surwit EA (1992) The role of laparoscopic lymphadenectomy in the management of cervical carcinoma. *Gynecologic Oncology* 47 (1): 38–43.

Coppleson M (ed.) (1992) *Gynecologic Oncology*, 2nd edn. Edinburgh: Churchill Livingstone, p. 1191.

Currie DW (1971) Operative treatment of carcinoma of the cervix. *Journal of Obstetrics and Gynaecology of the British Commonwealth* 78 (5): 385–405.

Dargent D (1987) A new future for Schauta's operation through a presurgical retroperitoneal pelviscopy. *European Journal of Gynaecologic Oncology* 8: 292–296.

deSouza NM, Whittle M, Williams AD *et al.* (2000) Magnetic resonance imaging of the primary site in stage I cervical carcinoma: a comparison of endovaginal coil with external phased array coil techniques at 0.5T. *Journal of Magnetic Resonance Imaging* 12 (6): 1020–1026.

Fletcher GH, Rutledge FN (1972) Extended field technique in the management of the cancers of the uterine cervix. *American Journal of Roentgenology Radium Therapy and Nuclear Medicine* 114 (1): 116–122.

Gulati N, Kumar VJ, Barsaul M *et al.* (2001) Urodynamic profile after Wertheim's hysterectomy. *Indian Journal of Cancer* 38 (2–4): 96–102.

Hacker NF (2000) Cervical cancer. In: Berek JS, Hacker NF (ed.) *Practical Gynecologic Oncology*. Philadelphia: Lippincott Williams & Wilkins.

Jensen JK, Lucci JA, 3rd, DiSaia PJ *et al.* (1993) To drain or not to drain: a retrospective study of closed-suction drainage following radical hysterectomy with pelvic lymphadenectomy. *Gynecologic Oncology* 51 (1): 46–49.

Kenter GG, Heintz AP (2002) Surgical treatment of low stage cervical carcinoma: back to the old days? *International Journal of Gynecological Cancer* 12 (5): 429–434.

Kim SH, Choi BI, Han JK *et al.* (1993) Preoperative staging of uterine cervical carcinoma: comparison of CT and MRI in 99 patients. *Journal of Computer Assisted Tomography* 17 (4): 633–640.

Lambaudie E, Collinet P, Narducci F *et al.* (2003) Laparoscopic identification of sentinel lymph nodes in early stage cervical cancer: prospective study using a combination of patent blue dye injection and technetium radiocolloid injection. *Gynecologic Oncology* 89 (1): 84–87.

Lin YS, Tzeng CC, Huang KF *et al.* (2005) Sentinel node detection with radiocolloid lymphatic mapping in early invasive cancer. *International Journal of Gynaecological Cancer* 15 (2): 273–277.

Massi G, Savino L, Susini T (1993) Schauta–Amreich vaginal hysterectomy and Wertheim–Meigs abdominal hysterectomy in the treatment of cervical cancer: a retrospective analysis. *American Journal of Obstetrics and Gynecology* 168 (3 Pt 1): 928–934.

Meigs JV (1944a) Carcinoma of the cervix. The Wertheim operation. *Surgery in Gynecology and Obstetrics* 78: 195–199.

Meigs JV (1944b) Gynecology: carcinoma of the cervix. *New England Journal of Medicine* 230: 577.

Monaghan JM, Lopes T, Naik R (2004) *Bonney's Gynaecological Surgery*, 10th edn. Oxford: Blackwell Publishing.

Morice P, Juncker L, Rey A *et al.* (2000) Ovarian transposition for patients with cervical carcinoma treated by radiosurgical combination. *Fertility and Sterility* 74 (4): 743–748.

Nezhat C, Nezhat F, Burrell MO *et al.* (1994) Laparoscopic radical hysterectomy with paraaortic and pelvic node dissection. *American Journal of Obstetrics and Gynecology* 170 (2): 699.

NICE (2003) *Laparoscopic Radical Hysterectomy for Early Stage Cervical Cancer*. London: NICE.

Owens S, Roberts WS, Fiorica JV *et al.* (1989) Ovarian management at the time of radical hysterectomy for cancer of the cervix. *Gynecologic Oncology* 35 (3): 349–351.

Piver M, Rutledge F, Smith J (1974) Five classes of extended hysterectomy for women with cervical cancer. *Obstetrics and Gynecology* 44: 265–272.

Podratz KC *et al.* (1982) Complications of ureteral surgery in the nonirradiated patient. In: Delgado G, Smith JP (eds) *Management of Complications in Gynecologic Oncology*. New York: John Wiley & Sons, pp. 113–149.

Powell JL, Burrell MO, Franklin EW, 3rd (1981) Radical hysterectomy and pelvic lymphadenectomy. *Gynecologic Oncology* 12 (1): 23–32.

Raatz D, Borner P (2000) Renaissance of vaginal hysterectomy for cervical carcinoma. 100th anniversary of the first abdominal radical surgery of cervical carcinoma by Ernst Wertheim on November 16, 1898. *Wiener Klinische Wochenschrift* 112 (7): 299–309.

Russell AH, Anderson M, Walter J *et al.* (1992) The integration of computed tomography and magnetic resonance imaging in treatment planning for gynecologic cancer. *Clinics in Obstetrics and Gynecology* 35 (1): 55–72.

Samlal RAK, van der Velden J, Hart AAM *et al.* (1996) Disease-free interval and recurrence pattern after the Okabayashi variant of Wertheim's radical hysterectomy for stage Ib and IIa cervical carcinoma. *International Journal of Gynecological Cancer* 6: 120–127.

Sindram DI (1959) A new combined approach in the treatment of cancer of the uterine cervix. *Acta Unio International Contra Cancrum* 15 (2): 403–405.

Sipos N, Szantho A, Csapo Z *et al.* (2002) Transposition of ovaries during radical hysterectomy for cervical cancer. *Orv Hetil* 143 (4): 189–192.

Sivanesaratnam V, Sen DK, Jayalakshmi P *et al.* (1993) Radical hysterectomy and pelvic lymphadenectomy for early invasive cancer of the cervix — 14-year experience. *International Journal of Gynecological Cancer* 3 (4): 231–238.

Spirtos NM, Schlaerth JB, Kimball RE *et al.* (1996) Laparoscopic radical hysterectomy (type III) with aortic and pelvic lymphadenectomy. *American Journal of Obstetrics and Gynecology* 174 (6): 1763–1767; discussion 1767–1768.

Stoeckel W (1956) *Typische Gynacologischen Operationen*. München: Urban und Schwarzenberg.

Taussig FJ (1934) Iliac lymphadenectomy with irradiation in the treatment of cancer of the cervix. *American Journal of Obstetrics and Gynecology* 28: 650.

van Beurden M, Schuster-Uitterhoeve AL, Lammes FB (1990) Feasibility of transposition of the ovaries in the surgical and radiotherapeutical treatment of cervical cancer. *European Journal of Surgical Oncology* 16 (2): 141–146.

Waggoner SE (2003) Cervical cancer. *Lancet* 361 (9376): 2217–2225.

Webb MJ (1997) Radical hysterectomy. *Baillière's Clinical Obstetrics and Gynaecology* 11 (1): 149–166.

Whitney CW, Stehman FB (2000) The abandoned radical hysterectomy: Oncology Group Study. *Gynecologic Oncology* 79: 350–356.

Zander J, Baltzer J, Lohe KJ *et al.* (1981) Carcinoma of the cervix: an attempt to individualize treatment. Results of a 20-year cooperative study. *American Journal of Obstetrics and Gynecology* 139 (7): 752–759.

CHAPTER 40

The management of advanced cervical cancer by surgery

John M. Monaghan

INTRODUCTION

In most parts of the world, cervical cancer is treated by surgery, radiotherapy or chemo/radiotherapy. Surgery is predominantly preserved for the primary management of early-stage disease. The usual limits for the use of surgery are stage IB1/stage IB2. In some centres where surgery is the major skill technique available, surgery may extend its role into the management of stage IIA and stage IIB. Very rarely, in some centres, primary surgery has been used in the management of stage IIIB disease, usually as a combination with neoadjuvant chemotherapy.

Surgery for advanced cancer of the cervix is predominantly preserved for the management of recurrent cancer and, until recently, surgery was confined to the treatment of central recurrences in the pelvis generating the procedure of pelvic exenteration. In more recent times, the management of pelvic sidewall recurrence has been investigated extensively, particularly by Hockel *et al.* (1996), working in Germany. They demonstrated that, for a highly selected group of patients who have already been treated with primary radiotherapy or chemo/radiotherapy, surgical excision of pelvic sidewall recurrences may be technically feasible and can give surprisingly good results. This new procedure, described as the LEER/CORT procedure, has been shown to be a feasible and realistic option for this small select group of patients.

The procedure of pelvic exenteration was first described in its present form by Brunschwig in 1948. Over the years, it has been used mainly in the treatment of advanced and recurrent carcinoma of the cervix. Its primary role at the present time is the management of that relatively large number of patients who will develop recurrent cancer of the cervix following primary radiotherapeutic treatment. It has been estimated that between one-third and one-half of patients with invasive carcinoma of the cervix will have residual or recurrent disease after treatment (Disaia and Creasman, 1981; Shingleton and Orr, 1983). Approximately one-quarter of these cases will develop a central recurrence, which may be amenable to exenterative surgery. However, pelvic exenteration as a therapy for recurrent cancer of the cervix has not been widely accepted, and many patients will succumb to their disease having been through the process of radiotherapy followed by chemotherapy and other experimental therapies without being given the formal opportunity of a curative procedure. In the early years, high operative mortalities and relatively low overall survival (20% 5-year survival in Brunschwig's series) resulted in few centres taking up the surgery. The more recently published results of exenterative procedures show an acceptable primary mortality of approximately 3–4% (Symmonds and Webb, 1981, 1992) and an overall survival/cure rate of between 30% and 60% (Robertson *et al.*, 1994). The procedures may also be applicable to a wide range of other pelvic cancers, including cancer of the vagina, vulva and rectum, for both primary and secondary disease. It is relatively rarely applicable to ovarian epithelial cancers and melanomas and sarcomas because of their tendency for widespread metastases.

The surgery involved is extensive and postoperative care complex; as a consequence, the operation has become part of the repertoire of the advanced gynaecological oncologist working in a centre with a wide experience of radical surgery. It is now clear that a large team of individuals is necessary, firstly to make the important decisions about selection of patients for exenteration but, secondly, skills in plastic surgery, urology and bowel surgery may be needed to complement the skills of the advanced gynaecological oncologist. The procedure demands of the surgeon considerable expertise and flexibility as virtually no two exenterations are identical. Also, considerable judgement and ingenuity are required during the procedure in order to achieve a comprehensive removal of all tumour. A degree of tailoring of surgery can be carried out as it may well be that with small recurrences a more limited procedure can be carried out with a degree of conservation of structures in and around the pelvis. Where extensive radiotherapy has been carried out, complete clearance of all organs from the pelvis (total exenteration) together with widespread lymphadenectomy may be essential in order to achieve a cure. There is now considerable evidence that, even in those patients with pelvic node metastases at the time of exenteration, a significant salvage rate can be achieved.

SELECTION OF PATIENTS FOR EXENTERATIVE SURGERY

Exenterative surgery should be considered for advanced primary pelvic carcinoma as well as recurrent disease. Many patients will be eliminated from the possibility of surgery at an early stage because of complete fixity of the cancer to the bony structures of the pelvis. The only exception to this rule is the rare circumstance where a vulva or vaginal cancer is attached to one of the pubic rami, when the ramus can be resected and a clear margin around the cancer obtained.

Palliative exenteration

In general terms, exenterative surgery should not be used as a palliative except perhaps in the presence of malignant fistulae in the pelvis, when it may significantly improve the quality of the patient's life without any significant extension to that life. The patient and her relatives must be made fully aware that the surgery is not being carried out with a curative intent.

PREOPERATIVE PREPARATION

It is important that the surgeon and his/her team of nurses and ancillary workers are confident in their ability to manage not only the extensive surgery involved, but also the difficult, testing and sometimes bizarre complications that can sometimes occur after exenteration.

Patient assessment

The average age of patients who are subject to exenteration lies between 50 and 60 years, but the age range is wide from early childhood through to the eighth or ninth decade. Advanced age is not a bar to success in exenterative surgery. It is frequently difficult following radiotherapeutic treatment to be certain that the mass palpable in the pelvis is due to recurrent disease and not to radiation reaction or persistent scarring associated with infection or the effects of adhesion of bowel to the irradiated areas.

In recent years, computerised tomography (CT) scan and magnetic resonance imaging (MRI) have been used extensively in the preoperative assessment of patients for many oncological procedures. The considerable difficulties and uncertainties that are generated for the radiologist assessing the CT or MRI scan where patients have had preceding surgery or radiotherapy is rarely more problematic than when patients are being assessed for exenteration. Some clinicians (Crawford *et al.*, 1996) feel that the scan is an integral part of preoperative assessment, whereas the author has not found the level of reliability of CT scan in particular to be acceptable. A tissue diagnosis is essential prior to embarking on exenterative surgery, and needle biopsy, aspiration cytology or frequently open biopsy at laparotomy will need to be performed. As distant metastases tend to occur with recurrent and residual disease, it is sometimes helpful to perform scalene node biopsies and radiological assessments of the pelvic and para-aortic lymph nodes together with fine needle aspiration in order to assist with the assessment. The mental state of the patient is also vital, but should not in itself be a bar to the performance of such surgery.

ABSOLUTE CONTRAINDICATIONS TO THE PERFORMANCE OF AN EXENTERATION

If there are metastases in extrapelvic lymph nodes, upper abdominal viscera, lungs or bones, there appears to be little value in performing such major surgery. However, there is evidence that a small but significant percentage of patients with pelvic lymph node metastases may well survive and have a high quality of life (Stanhope and Symmonds, 1985; Symmonds and Webb, 1992).

RELATIVE CONTRAINDICATIONS

Pelvic sidewall spread

If the tumour has extended to the pelvic sidewall in the form of either direct extension or nodal metastases, the prospects of a cure are extremely small, and the surgeon must decide whether the procedure will materially improve the patient's quality of life. The triad of unilateral uropathy, renal non-function or ureteric obstruction together with unilateral leg oedema and sciatic leg pain is an ominous sign. The prospects of a cure are poor. Perineural lymphatic spread is not visible on CT and can be a major source of pain and eventual death. The work of Hockel *et al.* (1996) has demonstrated that, in a highly selected group of patients, the laterally extended endopelvic resection (LEER procedure) may be performed and, in appropriate circumstances, this is followed up by further treatment of the tumour bed with a combined operative and radiotherapeutic treatment (CORT).

Obesity is a problem with all surgical procedures, producing many technical difficulties as well as postoperative respiratory and mobilisation problems. The more massive the surgery, the greater are these problems. Barber in 1969 noted the very high risk associated with obesity in their series.

TYPES OF EXENTERATION

In North America, the majority of exenterations performed are total (Fig. 40.1); in the author's series, approximately half of his exenterations have been of the anterior type (Fig. 40.1), removing the bladder, uterus, cervix and vagina, but preserving the rectum. For small, high lesions around the cervix, lower uterus and bladder, it may be possible to carry out a more limited procedure (a supralevator exenteration) retaining considerable parts of the pelvic floor. Posterior exenteration

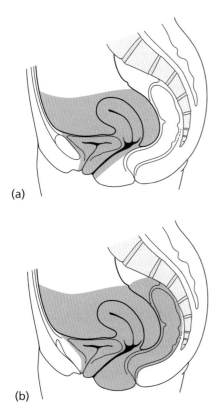

Fig. 40.1 The limits of resection for an anterior (a) and a total (b) exenteration.

(abdomino-perineal procedure) is relatively rarely performed by gynaecological oncologists as these operations tend to be the area of activity of the general surgeon.

PREOPERATIVE PREPARATION

Probably the most important part of the preoperative preparation is the extensive counselling which must be carried out to make certain that the patient and her relatives, particularly her partner, understand fully the extent of the surgery and the marked effect it will have upon normal lifestyle, particularly discussion about the removal of normal sexual function when the vagina has been taken out. It is important to discuss the possibility of reconstructive surgery of the vagina and bladder and the necessary transference of urinary and bowel function to the chosen type of diversionary procedure that will be performed and to communicate honestly the significant risks of such extensive surgery. During the course of this counselling, the patient should be seen by a stomatherapist. The senior nurse specialist will arrange for psychosexual counsellors skilled in cancer treatment to make preliminary contact with the patient.

At this very traumatic time, it is important not to completely overwhelm the patient and her family with too much information. A fine judgement has to be made about the pace and volume of information imparted. To aid this communication,

the author finds it ideal for the patient to meet with other patients who have had the procedure to discuss on a woman-to-woman basis the real problems and feelings of the exenteration patient.

Most preoperative investigations are now performed in the outpatient setting and will include a full blood analysis, heart and lung assessments, including chest radiography, electrocardiogram (ECG) and echocardiography, CT scan and MRI of the pelvis and periaortic regions and appropriate tests dependent on the patient's fundamental condition.

The patient is usually admitted to hospital 2 or 3 days prior to the planned procedure in order to obtain high-quality bowel preparation. With the modern alternative liquid diets and antibiotic therapy, complete cleaning of the small and large bowel can be achieved very rapidly. The anaesthetist responsible for the patient's care will see the patient and explain the process of anaesthesia. The author prefers to carry out all radical surgery under a combination of epidural or spinal analgesia together with general anaesthetic. Cardiac and blood gas monitoring is essential. Although the majority of patients do not require intensive care therapy, its availability must be identified prior to the surgical procedure. Prophylaxis against deep venous thrombosis is usually organised by the ward team using a combination of modern elastic stockings and low-dose heparin, which is initiated immediately following surgery. High-risk patients may require fractionated heparin.

THE OPERATION

The final intraoperative assessment

The final decision to proceed with the extenteration will not be made until the abdomen has been opened and assessment of the pelvic sidewall and posterior abdominal wall has been made using frozen sections where necessary. In the author's practice, the procedure is performed by a single team. If the patient has decided that a plastic surgical procedure such as the formation of a neovagina is to be carried out, then a second plastic surgical team will carry out any necessary operation at the same time as the diversionary procedures are being performed by the primary team, which may require input from a urologist or a bowel surgeon, depending on the expertise of the gynaecological oncologist.

Once the patient has been anaesthetised and placed in the lithotomy position in the operating theatre, the final assessment can begin with pelvic examination followed by catheterisation of the bladder with an indwelling size 14 Foley catheter. If it thought likely that an anterior exenteration will be performed, it is useful to pack the vagina firmly with a long gauze roll (Fig. 40.2).

The patient is returned to the supine position, and the abdomen is opened using either a longitudinal midline incision extending above the umbilicus or a high transverse (Maylard)

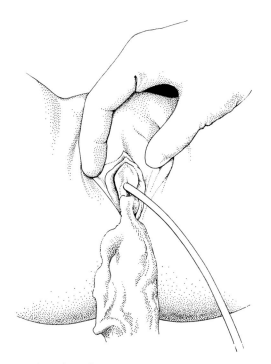

Fig. 40.2 Packing the vagina.

incision (Fig. 40.3) cutting through muscles at the interspinous level.

Exploration of the abdomen will confirm the mobility of the central tumour mass and, thereafter, dissection of para-aortic lymph nodes and pelvic sidewall nodes will be carried out (Fig. 40.4) and sent for frozen section.

At the time of this initial intraoperative assessment, the experienced exenterative surgeon will have assessed the pelvic sidewall by dividing the round ligament, drawing back the infundibulopelvic ligament and opening up the pelvic sidewall (Fig. 40.5).

This manoeuvre will have opened tissue planes, including the paravesical, pararectal and presacral spaces, to a deep level (Fig. 40.6), allowing the surgeon to become familiar with the full extent of the tumour.

These dissections can be carried out without any significant blood loss. If it is not considered possible to proceed with the operation due to fixity of the tumour, the abdomen may be closed at this stage as no significant trauma has been carried out by the surgeon. Considerable experience and judgement are required in order to make this decision. It is sometimes helpful to remove any suspicious tissue from the pelvic sidewall and obtain further frozen sections. Time spent here may really mean 'life or death' for the patient. Often the most difficult decision is actually to stop operating. Very occasionally with some vulval cancers, resection of pubic bones may be necessary but, in general terms, if there is bony involvement by tumour, the procedure should be abandoned.

After the comprehensive manual and visual assessment of the pelvis and abdominal cavity has been made, a line of incision for removal of the entire pelvic organs will begin at the pelvic sidewall, over the internal iliac artery and will pass forward through the peritoneum of the upper part of the bladder meeting with the similar lateral pelvic sidewall incision at the opposite side.

The sigmoid colon will be elevated and will be transected at a suitable point; the peritoneal incision will be carried along around the brim of the pelvis identifying the ureter as it passes over the common iliac artery and meeting up with the similar incision on the opposite side. Having divided and tied

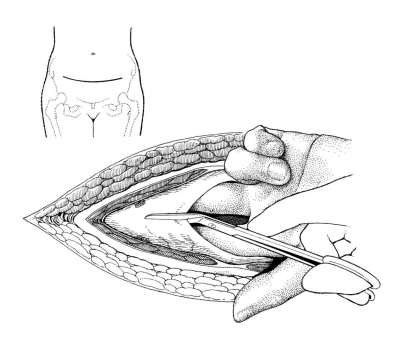

Fig. 40.3 A Maylard or high transverse incision.

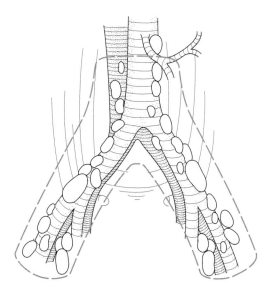

Fig. 40.4 Pelvic and para-aortic node assessment.

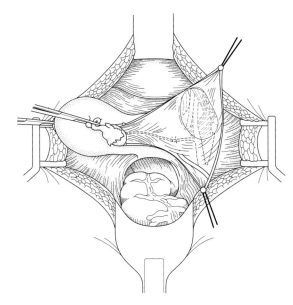

Fig. 40.6 Deepening the lateral pelvic dissection to reveal the pelvic spaces.

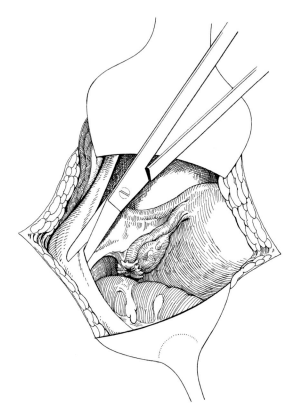

Fig. 40.5 Division of the round and infundibulopelvic ligaments and the beginning of the lateral pelvic dissection.

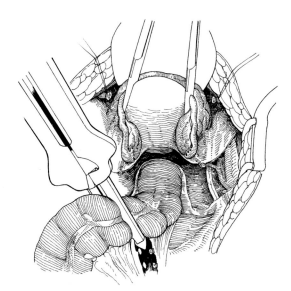

Fig. 40.7 Dividing the sigmoid colon in a total exenteration.

the round ligaments, opening the pelvic sidewall space, the infundibulopelvic ligament can also be identified, divided and tied. The incision is continued posteriorly and the ureters separated and identified. If an anterior exenteration is to be performed, the peritoneal dissection will be brought down into the pelvis to run across the anterior part of the rectum,

just above the pouch of Douglas. This will then allow a dissection from the anterior part of the rectum passing posteriorly around the uterosacral ligaments to the sacrum releasing the entire anterior contents of the pelvis. For a total exenteration, the dissection is even simpler: the mesentery of the sigmoid colon is opened and individual vessels clamped, divided and tied. The colon is divided usually using a GIA stapling device, which allows the sealed ends of the colon to lie without interfering with the operation (Fig. 40.7). A dissection posterior to the rectum is then carried out from the sacral promontory, deep behind the pelvis; this dissection is rapid and simple, and complete separation of the rectum from the sacrum will be

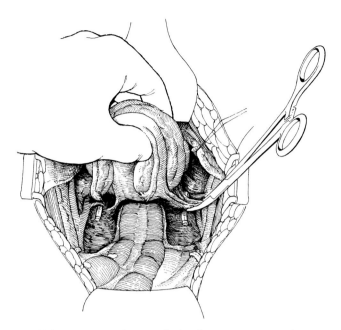

Fig. 40.8 Exenteration clamps applied to the anterior division of the internal iliac arteries.

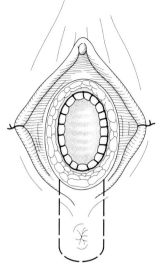

Fig. 40.9 The perineal incisions for anterior and total exenterations and closure of the pelvic floor musculature (see also Figure 40.10 for view of the pelvic floor from the inside).

allowed. This allows complete and usually bloodless removal of the rectal mesentery including lymph nodes. Anteriorly, the bladder is dissected with blunt dissection from the cave of Retzius, resulting in the entire bladder with its peritoneal covering falling posteriorly. This dissection is carried right down to the pelvic floor, isolating the urethra as it passes through the pelvic floor (perineal diaphragm). As dissection is carried posteriorly into the paravesical spaces, the uterine artery and the terminal part of the internal iliac artery will become clearly visible. By steadily deepening this dissection, the anterior division of the internal iliac will be isolated, the tissues of the lower obdurator fossa identified and, at this point, large exenteration clamps may be placed over the anterior division of the internal iliac artery and its veins (Fig. 40.8). The ureter by this time will have been divided a short distance beyond the pelvic brim. The pelvic phase of the procedure is completed at this point, and the perineal phase is now to be carried out.

The patient is placed in extended lithotomy position and an incision made to remove the lower vagina for an anterior exenteration and the lower vagina and rectum in a total exenteration (Fig. 40.9). Anteriorly, the incision is carried through above the urethra just below the pubic arch to enter the space of the cave of Retzius, which has been dissected in the pelvic procedure. The dissection is carried laterally and posteriorly dividing the pelvic floor musculature, and the entire block of tissue is then removed through the inferior pelvic opening. Small amounts of bleeding will occur at this point, usually arising from the edge of the pelvic floor musculature. These can be picked up by either isolated or running suture which will act as a haemostat.

Once the perineal dissection has been completed and haemostasis achieved, the surgeon has choices available to him/her depending on the preoperative arrangements that have been made with the patient. If, in the preoperative assessment period, it has been decided by the clinician and the patient that a neovagina should be formed then, at this point, either the surgeon or his/her plastic surgery colleague will initiate the development of a neovagina. This may be in the form of a myocutaneous graft, such as the vagina formed using the gracilis muscle, or a Singapore graft may be used from alongside the vulva, or techniques that revolve around the development of a skin graft placed within an omental pad or the technique of transposition of a segment of sigmoid colon in order to form a sigmoid neovagina. For many patients, however, the desire to have a new vagina is a very low priority, and it is surprising how frequently the patients will put off these decisions until well after the time of exenteration. Survival of the cancer appears to be their uppermost desire and they are determined to achieve this. To this end, the careful closure of the posterior parts of the pelvic musculature, a drawing together of the fat (Fig. 40.9) anterior to that and a careful closure of the skin is all that is required. It is usually possible to preserve the clitoris, the clitoral fold and significant proportions of the anterior parts of the labia minora and labia majora so that, when recovery is finally made, the anterior part of the genitalia has a completely normal appearance. On some occasions, patients will be able to have a neovagina formed some significant period of time following the exenteration. This is now becoming the predominant pattern in the author's experience of some 89 cases.

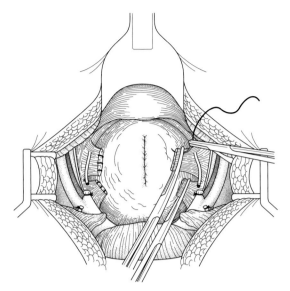

Fig. 40.10 Suture of the internal iliac arteries and lateral pelvic pedicle.

Once the perineal phase is finished, the legs can then be lowered so the patient is once more lying supine, and attention can be addressed to dealing with the pedicles deep in the pelvis.

All that remains following a total exenteration will be the two exenteration clamps on either side of the pelvis and a completely clean and clear pelvis. The pelvic sidewall dissection of lymph nodes can be completed before dealing with the clamps, and any tiny blood vessels that require haemostasis are ligated. As the exenteration clamps are attached to the distal part of the internal iliac arteries, it is important that comprehensive suture fixation is carried out (Fig. 40.10). This is usually readily and easily done, although occasionally the large veins of the pelvic wall can provide difficulties, and the use of mattress sutures may be necessary in order to deal with these complex vascular patterns. Having completed the dissection of the pelvis, the clinician now moves to produce either a continent urinary conduit or a Wallace- or Bricker-type ileal conduit and, if the procedure has been a total exenteration, as the majority are, a left iliac fossa stoma will be formed; the individual techniques of these procedures are dealt with elsewhere.

Dealing with the empty pelvis

A problem that must be avoided is that of small bowel adhesion to the tissues of a denuded pelvis. This is particularly important when patients have had preceding radiotherapy, as the risk of fistula formation in these circumstances is extremely high.

There have been a variety of techniques used to attempt to deal with this potentially life-threatening complication including the placing in the pelvis of artificial materials such as

Merselene sacs, Dacron and Gortex sacs, or even using bull's pericardium. Stanley Way (1974) described a sac technique in which he manufactured a bag of peritoneum that allowed the entire abdominal contents to be kept above the pelvis. This resulted in an empty pelvis, which from time to time became infected and generated a new problem, that of the empty pelvis syndrome. Intermittently, over the years, patching with the peritoneum has been used, but the most successful technique appears to be the mobilisation of the omentum from its attachment to the transverse colon, leaving a significant blood supply from the left side of the transverse colon and allowing the formation of a complete covering of the pelvis forming a soft 'trampoline of omentum', which will then stretch and completely cover and bring a new blood supply into the pelvis. From time to time, procedures such as bringing gracilis muscle flaps into the empty pelvis have been carried out in order to try to deal with the difficulty of a devitalised epithelium due to previous radiation. It is the author's current preference to use an omental graft mobilising the omentum from the transverse colon using a powered PLDS stapler; this allows a broad pedicle to be left at the left-hand end of the transverse colon maintaining an excellent blood supply to the omentum. This is brought down to the right side of the large bowel, dropping into the pelvis immediately to the left side of the ileal conduit, which is anchored just above the sacral promontory. By careful individual suturing around the edge of the pelvis and sometimes by refolding the peritoneum upon itself, a complete covering of the true pelvis with a soft central trampoline area can be generated (Fig. 40.11). A Redivac drain is inserted below the omentum which, when activated, will draw the omentum down into soft contact with the pelvic floor.

The small bowel can thus come into contact with an area with a good blood supply, obviating the risk of adherence and subsequent fistula formation. At the end of the procedure, the bowel is carefully orientated to make sure that no hernia can develop, and the abdomen is closed with a mass closure. The stomas are dressed in theatre and their appliances put in place. The patient leaves the operating theatre and is then transferred back to the ward at the appropriate time.

POSTOPERATIVE CARE

The postoperative care of exenterations is straightforward. It is essentially a matter of maintaining good fluid balance, good haemoglobin levels and, ideally, a significant flow of urine between 2.5 and 3.5 L/day. Bowel function often returns at the usual time of 2–4 days following the procedure, and a nasogastric tube, which is the author's preference, can be removed at 3–4 days and the patient returned to oral intake beginning with simple fluid on the third day. During and following the procedure, prophylactic antibiotic cover is maintained, as is subcutaneous heparin cover as a deep venous thrombosis prophylaxis.

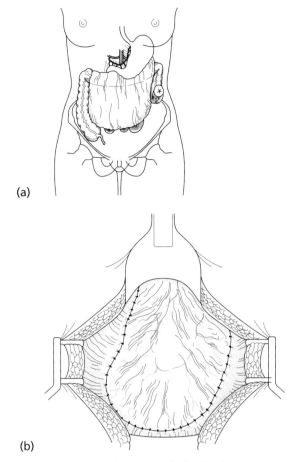

(a)

(b)

Fig. 40.11 Development of the 'omental pelvic floor'.

Mobilisation should be rapid, and the patient is most often discharged between 10 and 15 days postoperatively once she is used to dealing with her stomas and the ileal conduit tubes have been removed.

RESULTS OF EXENTERATION

Most series show that the 5-year survival following exenteration is of the order of 40–60%; these figures depend very largely upon selection of patients (Robertson *et al.*, 1994).

A figure that is rather more difficult to obtain is to determine the exact number who have been assessed for exenteration but have then failed at one of the many hurdles that the patient must pass before finally having the procedure carried out. It is therefore likely that the final, truly salvageable figure is an extremely low percentage. In more recent times, the value of carrying out exenterations in patients who have positive lymph nodes has been shown to be low but significant, and it is now many clinicians' practice to carry on with an exenterative procedure even in the circumstances where one or two lymph nodes are involved by tumour.

THE LEER/CORT PROCEDURE

I am indebted to Michael Hockel for information concerning this important innovative procedure, which he developed during the 1990s.

Introduction

As noted in the section on exenteration, pelvic sidewall recurrences are usually considered to be a contraindication for attempts at surgical management. This means that most of the patients who have had stage IIIB carcinoma of the cervix treated by radiotherapy or chemoradiation, because of the nature of the disease extending to the pelvic sidewall, are highly unlikely to be suitable for the performance of an exenterative procedure. In recent times, the LEER/CORT procedure has redefined our concept of pelvic sidewall recurrence. Michael Hockel has demonstrated the possibility in selected patients of carrying out extensive resection of the pelvic sidewall recurrence, particularly in the posterolateral part of the pelvis, and following up this procedure by further radiotherapy, usually by means of intraoperatively replaced implants, which will add further treatment to this affected area.

Selection of patients

The LEER/CORT procedure is appropriate only for histologically confirmed unifocal pelvic sidewall recurrence. Such patients must be free from tumour dissemination to other sites, and tumours should be limited to a maximum diameter of less than 5 cm. The patient has to accept the need for diversion of both bladder and bowel function. The identification of the size and position of the recurrence on the pelvic sidewall is made by detailed MRI investigation, and the patient will be primarily selected but will also understand, as with exenteration, that the final extent of surgery will be determined only once the procedure has begun and intraoperative findings have been assessed.

The operative procedure

The patient is prepared very much as for an exenteration with stoma sites being developed prior to the procedure.

A longitudinal midline incision is used. Often, it needs to be extended well above the umbilicus. The rectus abdominis muscle on the side of the lesion may be separated without severing the inferior epigastric vessels.

Once the abdomen has been opened, biopsies are taken from any suspected sites, and the dissection of the pelvic sidewall begins after mobilisation and resection of the large bowel.

The internal iliac artery is ligated and, thereafter, a resection of the internal iliac artery and vein between surgical clips is performed after retracting the common and external iliac blood vessels medially.

Once the pelvic sidewall has been opened, the obturator internus muscle is incised having retracted the obturator nerve and, at this point, the nerves of the sciatic plexus will become visible. The whole obturator internus muscle is removed after dividing its distal end following separation of the muscle from the acetabulum. The muscle mass, together with any tumour overlying it, is removed entirely, having identified the lateral vaginal wall in the lower part of the incision.

Assessment of the pelvic sidewall recurrence is necessary through frozen sections. If the margins are clear, it is not necessary to follow up the surgical procedure with the CORT radiotherapy procedure. The denuded pelvis is covered over with an omental flap developed in the standard manner, mobilising the omentum from the right side of the transverse colon and retaining its left-sided blood supply. This is drawn down into the pelvis and covers over any defects, allowing rapid reperitonealisation.

For patients in whom the margins are uncertain, the CORT procedure, which involves the implantation of tubes that are anchored in place over the site of the previous LEER procedure, will complete the whole process. These tubes are brought out into the abdominal wall, so that, using a Selectron type of procedure, the radiotherapy can be guided to the site of recurrence and a further treatment field developed. These tube-guided brachytherapy systems are possible even where previous radiotherapy has been applied in the primary treatment of the patient.

The LEER/CORT procedure is suitable for a highly selected group of patients. The skills at the present time are limited to a small number of individuals around the world, although primary results are currently showing a significant cure rate, albeit with a high primary morbidity.

REFERENCES

Barber HRK (1969) Relative prognostic significance of preoperative and operative findings in pelvic exenteration. *Surgical Clinics of North America* 49 (2): 431–437.

Brunschwig A (1948) Complete excision of the pelvic viscera for advanced carcinoma. *Cancer* 1: 177.

Crawford RAF, Richards PJ, Reznek RH *et al.* (1996) The role of CT in predicting the surgical feasibility of exenteration in recurrent carcinoma of the cervix. *International Journal of Gynaecological Cancer* 6 (3): 231.

Disaia PJ, Creasman WT (1981) *Clinical Gynaecologic Oncology; Cancer of the Cervix, Pelvic Exenteration*, Chapters 2–8. New York: Mosby, pp. 82–88.

Hockel M, Schlenger K, Hamm H *et al.* (1996) Five year experience with combined operative and radiotherapeutic treatment of recurrent gynaecologic tumors infiltrating the pelvic wall. *Cancer* 77: 1918–1933.

Robertson G, Lopes A, Beynon G *et al.* (1994) Pelvic exenteration: a review of the Gateshead Experience 1974–1992. *British Journal of Obstetrics and Gynaecology* 101: 529–531.

Shingleton HM, Orr JW (1983) Transmission electron microscopy of the physiological epithelium. In: Singer A, Jordan J (eds) *Cancer of the Cervix, Diagnosis and Treatment*. Edinburgh: Churchill Livingstone, p. 170.

Stanhope CR, Symmonds RE (1985) Palliative exenteration — what, when and why? *American Journal of Obstetrics and Gynecology* 152: 12–16.

Symmonds RE, Webb MJ (1981) Pelvic exenteration. In Coppleson M (ed.) *Gynecologic Oncology*. Edinburgh: Churchill Livingstone, Chapter 71, pp. 896–922.

Symmonds RE, Webb MJ (1992) Pelvic exenteration. In Coppleson M (ed.) *Gynecologic Oncology*. Edinburgh: Churchill Livingstone, Chapter 81, pp. 1283–1312.

Way S (1974) The use of the sac technique in pelvic exenteration. *Gynecologic Oncology* 2: 476–481.

CHAPTER 41

The management of multifocal precancer of the lower genital tract

Nigel Acheson and Richard W. Todd

INTRODUCTION

Descriptions of intraepithelial neoplasia affecting various sites in the lower genital tract have led to the development of management strategies for each site over the last 50 years. Intraepithelial disease of the cervix in association with similar disease in other sites, such as vagina, vulva, perineum, anal canal and natal cleft, has been described; multifocal intraepithelial neoplasia (MIN) exists when any combination of these sites is involved.

Chenoy and Luesley (1995) have defined MIN of the lower genital tract as intraepithelial change in squamous epithelium occurring either simultaneously or at intervals. The lesions should be separated by normal squamous epithelium. Whether MIN actually exists as a disease in itself, or whether it is simply an extension of intraepithelial neoplasia occurring in one part of the lower genital tract, is unknown.

In recent years, there has been an increase in the number of women diagnosed with MIN. This could be due to increased surveillance of the lower genital tract as a result of either screening or follow-up for premalignant/malignant conditions. The alternative explanation, that there is a true increase in the incidence of MIN, is also possible, but the true incidence is impossible to assess. For patients with immune deficiency, there has certainly been an increase in the number of cases, but differentiating between increased detection and increased incidence is difficult.

The management of patients with multifocal disease of the lower genital tract is challenging, with many factors to be considered (Shafi et al., 1989). These include the balance between the risk of malignant change and the effect on normal anatomical structure and function resulting from treatment. In some patients, the control of symptoms, e.g. in patients with pruritus secondary to vulval intraepithelial neoplasia, is also required.

AETIOLOGY

The aetiology of MIN is not clearly understood — as yet, there is uncertainty as to the existence of the condition as a separate disease entity. Although much research has been forthcoming on the aetiology of cervical intraepithelial neoplasia (CIN), vulval, vaginal and perineal intraepithelial disease have not been so intensively studied.

A number of aetiological factors have been forthcoming and they will be discussed. These are:
- human papillomavirus (HPV);
- smoking;
- oral contraceptive use;
- immune suppression;
- human immunodeficiency virus (HIV) infection.

It seems probable that MIN shares at least some of the aetiological factors involved in the development of intra-epithelial neoplasia involving other sites in the lower genital tract. These are discussed below.

RISK FACTORS FOR MIN

Sexual behaviour

The link between sexual activity and cervical cancer is well documented. Several studies have also attempted to examine the association between sexual activity and vulval intraepithelial neoplasia (VIN). Two large studies have demonstrated a positive association between the number of sexual partners and VIN (Brinton et al., 1990). The relative risk (RR) associated with between five and nine sexual partners was 5.1 (95% CI 1.7–14.8) compared with zero with one partner. A second large study (Sherman et al., 1991) determined that women with 15 or more sexual partners had up to an eightfold risk of VIN.

The role of HPV

HPV has been intimately involved in the aetiology of lower genital tract pre-cancer. Hording et al. (1993), using polymerase chain reaction (PCR), detected HPV types 16, 18 and 33 in 31% of 62 vulval cancers and none of 101 normal vulval specimens. Although there is a significant association between HPV infection and vulval cancer, the relationship is less strong than that which exists for cervical cancer, and the majority of vulval cancers do not seem to be associated with HPV. However, the same does not apply to the precancerous stage of VIN. It is suggested that vulval cancer consists of two distinct diseases, with HPV-related types primarily affecting women under the age of 65 years and a second type with unknown pathogenesis affecting the older woman (Lee *et al.*, 1994). In this latter group, keratinising squamous cell cancers arise in the background of non-neoplastic epithelial disorders such as lichen sclerosus that are not HPV related. Commonly, however, invasive vulval cancer arises from an area of HPV-related warty vulval VIN lesions, particularly in the younger woman.

In view of this proposed involvement of HPV in the development of VIN, it is not surprising that the association between HPV seropositivity and the risk of developing VIN has been studied. Seropositivity to HPV 16 has been shown to be associated with a RR of between 3.6 and 13 (Hildesheim *et al.*, 1997; Madeleine *et al.*, 1997).

In respect of vaginal intraepithelial neoplasia (VaIN), it has been suggested that the lack of metaplastic squamous epithelium in the vagina is an explanation for the lower incidence of VaIN compared with CIN. The true incidence of VaIN is unknown, but is less than for CIN (Lopes *et al.*, 1995). One report found VaIN to be 100 times less common than CIN, and an incidence of between 0.2 and 0.42 per 100 000 women has been suggested in the USA (Sillman *et al.*, 1997).

The role of HPV subtypes, and HPV 16 in particular, in this process is poorly understood. The association of HPV 16 infection with cancers of the vagina (and cervix, vulva and penis) has been demonstrated using serological reactivity to HPV 16 virus-like particles (Strickler *et al.*, 1998)

Squamous cell carcinomas of the anus and perianal region are associated with high-risk HPVs, as are high-grade anal and/or perianal intraepithelial neoplasia (Frisch *et al.*, 1999).

For all the conditions listed above, other factors are thought to play a role in the development of these intraepithelial neoplasias, possibly by their interaction with the immune response to infection by high-risk HPV subtypes.

Smoking

The association between smoking and cervical cancer and CIN has been thoroughly investigated. Smoking seems to be an important associated risk factor for the development of MIN. Although studied most extensively in CIN, smoking has also been shown to be associated with the development of cancers affecting the lower genital tract (Hildesheim *et al.*, 1997; Ylitalo *et al.*, 1999). The mechanism for this effect of smoking has not been clearly defined, but an effect upon the immune response to HPV seems likely. Similarly, an association between smoking and vulval cancer and pre-cancer has been seen. A number of studies (Newcomb *et al.*, 1984; Brinton

et al., 1990; Daling *et al.*, 1992) have shown an increased risk of VIN in smokers. RR ranges from 1.5 to 4.8. These studies may be flawed by not considering HPV status. The two studies that adjusted for HPV serology (Hildesheim *et al.*, 1997; Madeleine *et al.*, 1997) showed relative risks for VIN3 of 1.7 and 6.4 respectively. In the case of CIN, smoking has been shown to affect local immunity by reducing the numbers of Langerhans cells within the epithelium (Barton *et al.*, 1988). It is likely that a similar mechanism is involved in the vulva.

Oral contraceptive use

In a recent study, Moreno and colleagues (2002) have suggested that long-term use of oral contraceptives could be a cofactor that increases the risk of cervical carcinoma by up to fourfold in women who are positive for cervical HPV DNA. Newcomb *et al.* (1984) reported a fourfold increase in risk of VIN associated with previous oral contraceptive use. This study corrected only for age, education and obesity. Sherman *et al.* (1994) also demonstrated an increased risk of VIN3 associated with contraceptive use of 5 years or more (RR 1.3). They corrected for age, number of sexual partners, smoking and education.

Immune suppression

The association between patients with immune suppression and neoplasia of the lower genital tract is well established. In addition to women immunosuppressed following organ transplantation, patients on high-dose steroids for severe asthma and systemic lupus erythematosus have an increased risk of developing MIN (Sillman *et al.*, 1984; Penn, 1986a,b). It has been known for some time that invasive vulval cancer is significantly more common in women with renal transplants (Blohme and Brynger, 1985), and the incidence of both vulval cancer and its precancerous state of VIN is increased in HIV-seropositive women (Chiasson *et al.*, 1997; Frisch *et al.*, 2000).

Human immunodeficiency virus (HIV) infection
(see also Chapter 35A)

In recent years, it has become apparent that women with HIV infection are at increased risk of developing anogenital neoplasia (Kadish, 2001). A prospective cohort study of 925 women found that 6% of HIV-positive women had vulvovaginal and perianal condylomata acuminata at enrolment, compared with 1% of HIV-negative women. During the course of the study (median follow-up 3.2 years), 9% of HIV-positive women and 1% of HIV-negative women developed vulvovaginal or perianal intraepithelial lesions (Conley *et al.*, 2002). One of the striking features of this study was the fact that the majority of the HIV-positive patients in the study were under the age of 35 years at enrolment, and this will inevitably have consequences for the long-term follow-up of these women.

CLINICAL FEATURES

Vulval intraepithelial neoplasia (VIN)

Presentation and clinical examination of the vulva

Between 10% and 60% of women with VIN may be asymptomatic (Friedrich *et al.*, 1980; Wolcott and Gallup, 1984; Husseinzadeh *et al.*, 1989). Diagnosis may be made during the course of gynaecological examination for reasons such as colposcopy, taking cervical cytology or screening for sexually transmitted disease. Broen and Ostergard (1971) claimed that up to 1 in 200 asymptomatic women have VIN. This followed the examination of 1071 women using toluidine blue and colposcopy to delineate VIN. This may have represented an overdiagnosis as the methods used have since been shown to be unreliable (Anon., 1982). However, a significant number of women will present to a gynaecologist, dermatologist or genitourinary physician because of either symptoms or the appearance of a vulval lesion. Pruritus has been described in up to 60% of cases (Campion and Hacker, 1998) and vulval pain and burning are well described (Buscema *et al.*, 1980a). Dyspareunia may be the presenting complaint and may be severe enough to lead to apareunia (Planner and Hobbs, 1988).

With the naked eye

There is no typical appearance of VIN on macroscopic examination (Collins *et al.*, 1970). The clinical appearance may vary from flat erythematous areas to raised white warty lesions (Fig. 41.1). Herod and colleagues (1996) described raised, hyperkeratotic lesions in 41% of cases in their series (Fig. 41.2). VIN can affect hair-bearing and non-hair-bearing areas of the vulva. Although it has been suggested that the posterior vulval skin is most commonly involved (Di Saia and Rich, 1981), the labia are more frequently affected (Husseinzadeh *et al.*, 1989) and, in the series reported by Crum and colleagues (1984), 81% had gross involvement of the labia, 5% of the clitoris and 14% of the perineum. A number of reported series have described the multifocality of the disease (Barbero *et al.*, 1990; Anon., 1996; Herod *et al.*, 1996; Kuppers *et al.*, 1997).

With the colposcope

The use of a colposcope is helpful when performing assessment of the vulva. The extra magnification and adequate lighting allow a more detailed examination. Although diagnoses based on vulvoscopic appearances have a poor correlation with histology, colposcopy facilitates the identification of abnormal areas and directed biopsy. Acetic acid has a well-established role in colposcopy in helping to identify abnormal epithelium on the cervical transformation zone. A solution of 3–5% acetic acid is sprayed on or applied to the cervix on a cotton wool

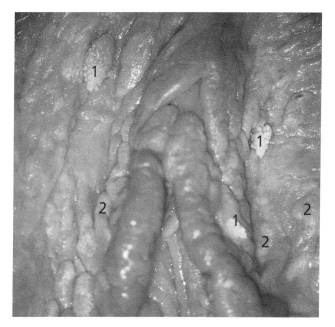

Fig. 41.1 Colposcopic appearance of VIN (vulval intraepithelial neoplasia). In this photograph, a condyloma acuminata is seen at (1) with thickened white epithelium (2) extending over the larger part of the vulva including the labia minora and majora, clitoris and periurethral area. Biopsy of the area at (2) showed it to contain a VIN3 lesion with uniform neoplastic cell population within the epithelium, with hyperkeratosis and acanthotic rete pegs, with numerous mitoses.

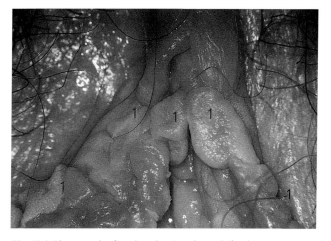

Fig. 41.2 Photograph of a vulva, showing the multifocal nature of a VIN lesion, again with a thickened and granular surface. A hyperkeratotic layer of epithelium exists at (1), which overlies an epithelium that, on biopsy, was revealed to have had disturbed maturation with pleiomorphic and hyperchromatic nuclei and abnormal mitotic figures.

ball. Areas of CIN turn white. The reason for this 'acetowhite' change is obscure. It has been suggested that a reversible coagulation of intracellular proteins reduces the light reflection from the pink subepithelial vasculature. Therefore, the greater the

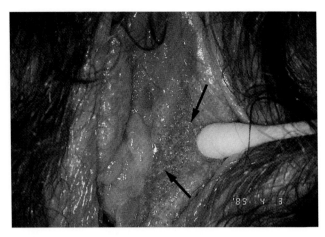

Fig. 41.3 Filamentous lesions (vestibular papillae) shown on the inside of a labia minora (arrowed) that has been exposed with a cotton tip swab.

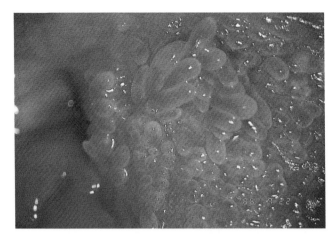

Fig. 41.4 High-power view of the filamentous lesion (vestibular papillae). Histology of these lesions shows them to be composed of a central capillary core surmounted by a thickened layer of squamous cells that give rise to the intense acetowhiteness found when acetic acid is applied.

nuclear density within an area, for example in atypia, the greater the acetowhite change. In fact, not all white areas represent atypia, and 'normal acetowhiteness' can appear in metaplastic epithelium for example.

As in using colposcopy for examining the cervical epithelium, caution should be used when interpreting the changes seen on the vulva following the application of acetic acid as acetowhite change is not necessarily associated with abnormality. In order to address the question of what can be regarded as a normal examination finding, van Beurden *et al.* (1997) recruited 40 healthy volunteers without vulval complaints via a newspaper advertisement. Gross examination and vulvoscopy was performed before and after the application of 5% acetic acid followed by HPV PCR of vulval swabs. Naked eye vulval examination showed vestibular papillomatosis in 13 women (33%) and vestibular erythema in 17 women (43%). The former comprised filamentous lesions that may be found around the introital area and can occasionally be confused with condyloma or even VIN. Such lesions may be multipapillary or villiform and can be found in virginal females, and they are called vestibular papillae or micropapilloma labialis (Figs 41.3 and 41.4). Vulvoscopy (examination of the vulva using the colposcope) after the application of 5% acetic acid showed an acetowhite vestibule in all women. Twelve women (30%) had acetowhite lesions outside the vestibule. Six women (15%) were positive for HPV DNA. The presence of HPV DNA did not correlate with vestibular erythema or vestibular papillomatosis. There was a weak association between HPV DNA and acetowhite lesions outside the vestibule. They concluded that vestibular erythema, vestibular papillomatosis and acetowhite lesions are common in healthy women without vulval complaints. Foulques *et al.* (1991) demonstrated HPV negativity in 78% of subclinical acetowhite lesions. Jonsson *et al.* (1997) evaluated acetowhite changes of the cervix and vulva as a predictor of HPV infection. In a group of 535 women, the

sensitivity of detection of HPV infection by acetowhitening was 22% and the specificity was 90%.

With toluidine blue

The Collins toluidine blue test is another method previously used to facilitate the identification of abnormal areas. Toluidine blue (1%) is a nuclear dye used to identify areas of parakeratosis and abnormal maturation with nuclear atypia (Fig. 41.5). Joura *et al.* (1998) attempted to determine the effectiveness of the toluidine blue test in the differentiation of VIN and non-neoplastic epithelial disorders (NNEDs). Vulvar epithelium demonstrated toluidine blue staining in 100% of the patients with VIN3, in 83% of women with VIN1–2, in 50% of the women with squamous cell hyperplasia and in 10% of the women with lichen sclerosus. In view of the high false-positive results experienced, the toluidine blue test is no longer recommended (Anon., 1982).

Natural history of VIN

Classification

Classification of squamous VIN between the years 1986 and 2003 was similar to that which existed for CIN. However, the International Society for the Study of Vulvo-vaginal Disease (ISSVD) has recently recommended (2003) a change to the current classification (Sideri *et al.*, 2005). Lesions will be divided into two types, both related/referred to as high-grade VIN, namely:
• VIN usual type;
• VIN differentiated type.

VIN usual type (Bowenoid or basaloid) is associated with HPV infections, occurs predominantly in young women and tends to be multifocal and pigmented. It is related to other neoplasms of the lower genital tract (generally CIN3 in more than 30% of cases).

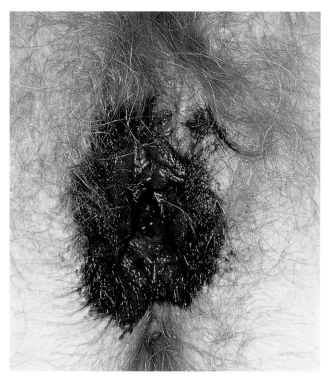

Fig. 41.5 Application of toluidine blue to the vulva shows it to contain, in this picture, multiple condylomata acuminata and some areas of VIN, which are present around the vaginal introitus and fourchette. This shows the problems encountered with the application of toluidine blue.

VIN differentiated type is not so associated with HPV and is related to the non-neoplastic vulval epithelial disorders such as lichen sclerosus and squamous hyperplasia. Postmenopausal women tend to have these lesions, which are predominantly focal and leukoplastic. They are not connected with other types of epithelial neoplasia of the lower genital tract. It would seem that VIN1 is an uncommon histological diagnosis and usually represents an HPV effect or reactive change alone. Most VIN lesions present as high grade (VIN3). There is no evidence that the VIN1–3 histological spectrum represents a biological continuum. Jones (2003), in discussing the natural history of VIN, believes that the subject has been confused by failure to differentiate clearly between the outcome of treated and untreated VIN. He believes that the VIN rating system should be seen as a convenient histological description of a spectrum of intraepithelial changes, and it should not be inferred that it is a biological continuum. The term VIN should therefore apply only to histologically high-grade squamous lesions (former terms VIN2 and VIN3, and differentiated VIN3; Sideri *et al.*, 2005).

Progression to invasive cancer

Despite the use of the VIN1–3 grading system, it must be emphasised that this does not imply a disease continuum.

Only rarely has the progression of VIN1 through to VIN3 been seen (Clark *et al.*, 1998). For the true 'natural' history of VIN to be understood, we would need the long-term follow-up of a large cohort of untreated women with VIN. This is unlikely to happen as not only is the process of diagnosis (i.e. biopsy) likely to alter the biology of the disease, but a significant proportion of women will undergo treatment for symptom control. Also, in this litigious era, it would take considerable bravery on the part of the physician to avoid any interference even if the evidence to support it is weak. Another factor making analysis of the natural history difficult is the variation in what has been defined as VIN in the past. There is no doubt that, although convenient from the point of view of classification, the different disease entities behave differently. Jones (Luesley, 2000) performed a thorough review of the literature with regard to the natural history. Despite the obvious limitations of a retrospective review such as this, certain generalisations can be made. Overall, a total of 22 series were reviewed (1378 cases of VIN). Between 2% and 5% of cases progressed to invasive cancer. This represents the progression of treated disease rather than untreated [the largest series of untreated cases (Jones and Rowan, 1994) reports a progression rate in seven out of eight cases including three women in their 30s]. Progression to invasive cancer occurred within 10 years in 93% (25/27) of cases. This was similar to the time for progression in the untreated series, suggesting that progression in the treated may reflect inadequate treatment.

Two mechanisms may exist for the development of vulval cancer in women with VIN. Firstly, the cancer may arise as a result of a progression of existing VIN and, secondly, the appearance could be the result of a *de novo* development of cancer in the field of risk. Iverson and Tretli (1998), in a large Norwegian study, reported that 8 out of 16 (50%) women who later developed vulval cancer had negative resection margins at the time of the primary surgery for VIN. Further evidence of these mechanisms is presented by Jones and Rowan (1994) when reviewing the data from 113 women with VIN3 in New Zealand. Twenty-one women developed invasive cancer and 10 of these were untreated, having received inadequate sampling. The transit time for invasion was a mean of 3.5 years. Eleven (3.2%) of the treated patients subsequently developed vulval cancer between 1.8 and 17 years later (mean 7.7 years). Jones (2003) and his group estimate that at least half the cancers that arose in previously treated VIN represented new disease and not progression from pre-existing disease. Only 3 of the 15 cases presenting with progression since 1980 have been in patients over 50 years of age. He also showed that, in 32 of the original group of 370 women studied, there was evidence of regression of the disease.

A disproportionate number of cancers occurred adjacent to the anal margin and urethra. This is likely to reflect inadequate primary excision. Immunosuppression is known to be associated with an increased risk of lower genital tract intraepithelial neoplasia (Penn, 1986b). It is thought that immunosuppression is also a risk factor for progression to invasive cancer (Korn *et al.*, 1996).

Spontaneous regression of VIN

It has long been recognised that a particular group of women exists in whom spontaneous regression can occur (Friedrich, 1972). This demonstrates the danger of grouping all disease under the title 'VIN'. Bowenoid papulosis is a well-described variant of VIN that typically occurs in young sexually active women who may be pregnant. Lesions are typically pigmented, multifocal and papular. Histologically, they have the features of high-grade VIN and are usually positive for HPV 16. Jones and Rowan (2000) reviewed 14 such cases to determine the background and clinical features of a group of women who experienced spontaneous regression of VIN2–3 before treatment was undertaken. The women were 15–27 years of age (median 19.5 years). Ninety-three per cent were non-white and, with one exception, all had been treated previously for genital condyloma acuminata. Four of the 14 cases were pregnancy associated. Half of the women were asymptomatic. The transit time to regression of VIN2–3 was 3–30 months (median 9.5 months). All lesions were multiple and pigmented. However, caution should be exercised in such cases as progression to invasive cancer has also been reported (Bergeron *et al.*, 1987).

Vaginal intraepithelial neoplasia (VaIN)

Presentation and clinical features

VaIN is asymptomatic and is usually detected as a result of examination of the vagina using a colposcope as a result of abnormal cytology.

Examination of the vaginal vault using a colposcope entails a colposcopic examination similar to that used on the cervix, and the changes in the epithelium can be seen and are similar following the application of acetic acid with acetowhite areas with or without punctation observed (Fig. 41.6). If suspected, the application of aqueous iodine is very useful in defining the distribution of VaIN on the vagina, as the areas of VaIN do not stain brown following the application of the aqueous iodine (Fig. 41.7).

VaIN is most commonly situated in the upper third of the vagina, although extension to the lower third of the vagina and multifocal lesions can occur (Gallup and Morley, 1975).

VaIN is more commonly diagnosed in patients who have previously undergone a hysterectomy (Rome and England, 2000). In these patients, it is important to assess all the vault suture line for areas of VaIN. This involves the horns of the vaginal vault. The examination of the whole vaginal vault is important in planning diagnostic biopsies and subsequent treatment (Figs 41.8–41.10). Sometimes, examination under anaesthetic is required for accurate mapping of high-grade

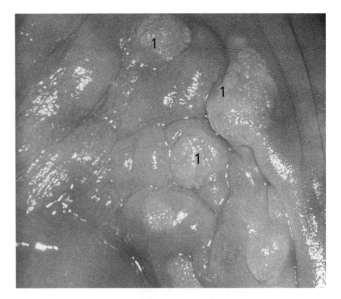

Fig. 41.6 Colpophotograph of the upper vagina, showing the multifocal nature of VaIN. Lesions labelled (1) have a typical appearance of condylomata, making diagnosis impossible without a biopsy.

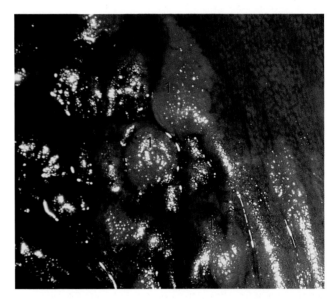

Fig. 41.7 Application of Lugol's iodine solution to the lesions as seen in Figure 41.6 shows partial uptake of iodine.

VaIN in order to assess the extent of the disease prior to treatment.

Natural history of VaIN

Classification

The natural history of VaIN is poorly understood, but the histological grading of VaIN into VaIN1, VaIN2 and VaIN3

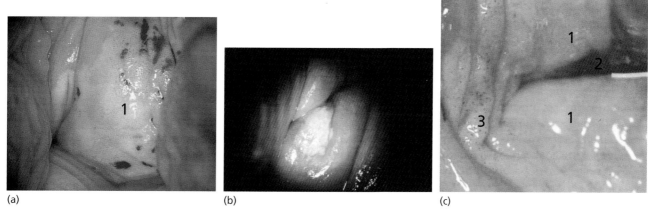

(a)   (b)   (c)

Fig. 41.8 (a) Vaginal vault of a 48-year-old woman who underwent an abdominal hysterectomy some 4 years previously, in which microinvasive disease of the cervix was found (stage IA1). Dense acetowhite epithelium extends onto the anterior and posterior aspects of the upper third of the vagina (1). Excision biopsy of this area revealed the presence of early invasive cancer with infiltration to a depth of 2.5 mm. (b) A view of the vaginal fornix in a woman who had previously undergone abdominal hysterectomy. CIN showing a hyperkeratotic white lesion which on biopsy shows VaIN3. The lesion extends into the recess of the vault horn. (c) Dense acetowhite area (1) involving the vault of a woman who had previously had an abdominal hysterectomy. The dense acetowhite lesion extends to the suture line (2). An area of punctation is seen at the entrance to the right vaginal fornix (3).

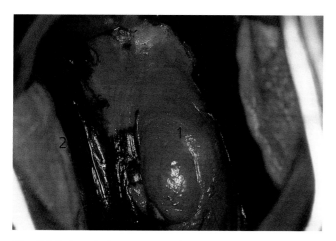

Fig. 41.9 Early vaginal cancer appeared as a superficial ulcerative lesion in a woman who had had a hysterectomy for CIN3 some 8 years before. Lugol's iodine has been applied and delineates the abnormal (atypical) epithelium. Excision biopsy was necessary to confirm the diagnosis. Occasionally, in a premenopausal woman, a tampon-induced ulcer may be confused with a very early ulcerative vaginal carcinoma. At (1), the central malignant area may be seen. The vaginal fornix is at (2).

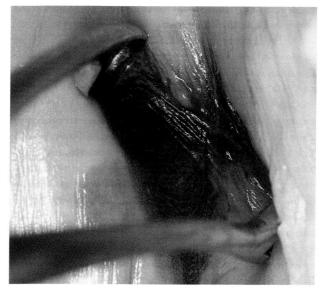

Fig. 41.10 Desjardin's forceps have been gently inserted into the recess in the vaginal vault to determine the presence of any abnormal (atypical) epithelium. These forceps have been opened wide, and the base of the recess has been painted with Lugol's iodine solution. Complete uptake of the iodine has occurred and therefore no abnormality exists at the apex of the recess.

bears similarities to the grading of CIN. The situation may be similar to the vulva, where the VIN1–3 grading system represents a morphological spectrum of intraepithelial change but does not represent a biological continuum. VIN3 is without doubt a cancer precursor. VaIN is frequently seen as part of an HPV effect. It was shown nearly 20 years ago that

two-thirds of cases of VaIN were associated with prior, concomitant or subsequent intraepithelial or invasive cancer in the vulva, including the urethra and cervix (Benedet and Sanders, 1984). Rome and England (2000) likewise noted that 55

(42.5%) women had previously undergone history for CIN or invasive cancer, and occult invasion has been noted in between 13% and 28% of surgically excised specimens in Rome and England's (2000) and Ireland and Monaghan's (1988) studies.

Progression and regression

Quantifying the risk of malignant transformation of VaIN is difficult because the incidence of the condition is unknown, but progression from VaIN3 to vaginal cancer may occur in between 8% and 20% of cases (Lenehan *et al.*, 1986; Rome and England, 2000). However, it is difficult to assess these progression rates because of the rarity of this condition. Also, in many cases, histological diagnosis has been obscured and includes any minor lesions (i.e. VaIN1) that may represent only HPV effects and should not be regarded as cancer precursors. Aho *et al.* (1991) reported that 14 out of 18 (78%) VaIN1–2 lesions regressed spontaneously, and this is what one would expect from the natural history of CIN1/HPV lesions. In their study, only one VIN lesion progressed to invasion in 5 years and one VaIN3 to invasion in 4 years. However, in those studies in which persistent VaIN3 disease existed in the vaginal vault after hysterectomy for this condition, a form of natural history can be inferred. They found that, of 29 women with persistent abnormal vaginal cytology, nine developed cancer in the vaginal vault. They showed that VaIN3 can slowly extend over a wide area of the vagina before progression to invasion (Fig. 41.8c). In Rome and England's (2000) study, 8 out of 132 women with VaIN3 developed invasive cancer over 1–7 years, and five of these were deemed to be treatment failures with two progressing without treatment and the remainder probably representing new disease. In Benedet and Sanders's (1984) series, 4 out of 136 cases progressed to malignancy.

Perianal intraepithelial neoplasia (PAIN)

Presentation and clinical features

Examination of the perianal area (Fig. 41.11) and anal canal (Fig. 41.12) is essential in patients with suspected MIN. The appearance of the perianal skin can be similar to, and may be in continuity with, vulval lesions — this ranges from erythematous, flat lesions to raised warty lesions.

These lesions may be asymptomatic, but may give rise to perianal pruritus. It is the practice in our unit to manage such patients in a multidisciplinary team along with a colorectal surgeon with whom we perform joint examinations, either in the clinic or under a general anaesthetic.

When suspected, we routinely perform clockface perianal mapping biopsies initially to confirm the diagnosis of PaIN and exclude invasive disease. Such examination and mapping includes proctoscopy to allow adequate investigation of the anal canal.

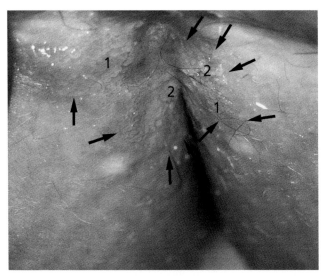

Fig. 41.11 Photograph showing the extension of acetowhite covering of the perianal area extending into the natal cleft (arrows outline extent). Histological confirmation showed it to be a grade 3 intraepithelial neoplasia. However, the pattern of disease posteriorly in the natal cleft was that of condyloma acuminata presenting as acetowhite patches with hyperkeratosis. Punch biopsies at points (1) and (1) revealed the presence of a clinical papillomavirus infection, and biopsies at (2) showed the presence of grade 2 intraepithelial neoplasia. However, a wider local excision revealed the grade 3 nature of the lesion and illustrates the need for meticulous biopsy excision to ascertain the exact nature of the lesion.

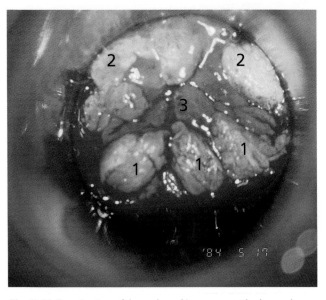

Fig. 41.12 Examination of the anal canal in a woman who has anal intraepithelial neoplasia grade 3 shows typical condylomata acuminata at (1) with a dense acetowhite area present at (2). Normal mucosa is present at (3). The biopsy from area (2) showed the presence of intraepithelial neoplasia grade 2. This again shows the multifocal nature of perianal and anal intraepithelial disease.

Natural history of PaIN

The true incidence of perianal intraepithelial disease is difficult to establish, especially as the terminology is variable. Bowen's disease of the perianal region is, in many texts, separated from anal intraepithelial neoplasia (AIN). Both conditions share similar features with VIN and CIN and, indeed, AIN can be graded following the same criteria as CIN. However, there are no specific histopathological features that would allow VIN to be separated from AIN. Therefore, without strict criteria for the point at which VIN ends and AIN begins, there remains a possibility of error in assessing the incidence of AIN (Tidy, 2003).

As in other lower genital tract precancer, HPV is a major aetiological agent, with HPV 16 being found in approximately 56–80% of cases of squamous cancer of the anus and AIN, with a higher incidence in AIN III than in AIN I (Scholefield *et al.*, 1992). Woodman *et al.* (2001) believe that the acquisition of HPV infection occurs soon after the onset of sexual activity, mirroring other genital neoplasias in this respect. Hildesheim *et al.* (1997) have also shown that variant forms of HPV 16 would seem to be linked to an increased risk of developing both intraepithelial and invasive neoplasia of the cervix, and such variant forms of HPV 16 have now been linked to the development of anal neoplasia (Da Costa, 2002).

Immunosuppression, discussed elsewhere (Chapter 35), is associated with an increased risk of developing neoplastic change, with approximately 5–6% risk after transplantation due to suppression of T-cell response consequent upon the use of immunosuppressive drugs (Penn, 1986a,b). AIN was found to exist in renal transplantation in approximately 24% of cases in Ogunbiyi *et al.*'s (1994) study. The risk associated with HIV infection in respect of AIN is increased, with Holly *et al.* (2001) studying the prevalence of AIN in 317 women. AIN III was present in 6% of women who were HIV positive and in 2% who were HIV negative. In the former group, 28% had either abnormal anal cytology or biopsy-proven disease. Recently, Scholefield *et al.* (2005) reviewed their 10-year experience with conservative management of high-grade AIN and were able to formulate some opinions as to the natural history of this lesion. They concluded that AIN III appears to have a relatively low potential for malignant transformation in the immunocompetent patient but that, in the immunosuppressed patient, there are more likely to be extensive AIN III lesions and there is a much greater risk of malignant change within them.

MANAGEMENT OF VIN

Management of VIN is tailored on an individual basis. Faced with a disease whose natural history is poorly understood, subjecting women to radical, disfiguring treatments can no longer be justified in the majority of cases. Having made the

initial diagnosis, treatment should be offered if symptoms are intolerable or if invasion is suspected. Factors to be considered when planning treatment should include:

1 the age and fitness of the patient;
2 symptoms experienced;
3 focality of the lesions;
4 involvement of skin appendages;
5 malignant potential;
6 preservation of the structure and function of the vulvo-perineal unit;
7 psychological issues;
8 likely recurrence rates.

Treatments can be broadly divided into surgical and medical.

Surgical treatments for VIN

These can be further subdivided into excisional and ablative or destructive methods.

Excisional treatments

Vulvectomy

In the past, the aim of excisional methods was to achieve complete disease clearance. This was based on the multifocality of the disease and an overly pessimistic view of the risk of progression to invasive disease. Vulvectomy gained initial popularity in both its radical and simple forms. Recurrence rates after radical surgery were reportedly 7% (Collins *et al.*, 1970). Over time, there was a move to less mutilating surgery and simple vulvectomy gained in popularity. Boutselis (1972) reported recurrence rates of 4% in a small series over 10 years. The quest for further conservatism continued with the introduction of the skinning vulvectomy by Rutledge and Sinclair (1968). Indicated in women with large areas of disease (Fig. 41.13), it was claimed that this procedure provided the opportunity to excise the disease with wide margins, produce satisfactory cosmesis, minimise the effect on function and produce a specimen for histological analysis. The need for a split skin graft (Fig. 41.14) from a donor site was felt to be an acceptable trade-off. Ayhan *et al.* (1998) claimed no recurrences in a series of 21 patients treated by skinning vulvectomy, although only three of the patients had multifocal disease. This success has not been matched by other authors, with recurrence rates of between 8% and 39% more usually reported (Di Saia and Rich, 1981; Caglar *et al.*, 1986). Recurrence may occur in grafted and ungrafted skin (Cox *et al.*, 1986).

A report by Buscema *et al.* (1980b) claimed no difference in recurrence rates between patients treated with vulvectomy and those treated with wide local excision. The morbidity associated with vulvectomy is significant. The physical sequelae include vaginal stenosis, problems with micturition, difficulty with vaginal delivery, dyspareunia and altered self-image. A significant number of patients report psychosexual problems after these procedures. The complications are of particular

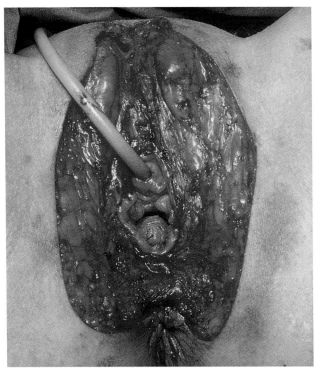

41.13

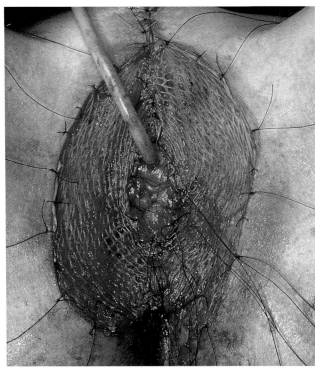

41.14

Figs 41.13 and 41.14 View of the vulva after the excision using the skinning technique in a woman with extensive large areas of multifocal intraepithelial disease grade 3. In Figure 41.13, the area removed is seen and, in Figure 41.14, the area has been covered with meshed split skin grafts.

significance in younger women. In view of this, there has been a concerted effort to move towards local excisional procedures.

Wide local excision

The aim of this technique is to remove the affected skin by dissecting deep to the dermis and with a lateral disease-free margin of 5–10 mm. A wider excision is obviously needed in respect of the presence of early microinvasive disease, as seen in Figure 41.15. Primary skin closure is used. This may not always be possible, particularly when lesions are adjacent to structures such as the urethra and anus. Margin status is thought to be important in predicting disease recurrence, although many recurrences occurred with apparently complete primary excision. Recurrence rates of between 28% and 54% have been reported (Buscema *et al.*, 1980b; Di Saia and Rich, 1981; Leuchter *et al.*, 1984; Wolcott and Gallup, 1984; Andreasson and Bock, 1985). Recurrences can be treated by repeat excision if necessary.

Destructive techniques
Laser destruction (Fig. 41.16)
The aim of treatment by laser is to destroy the affected epithelium to a depth sufficient to remove the affected epithelium but to allow regeneration from residual keratinocytes in

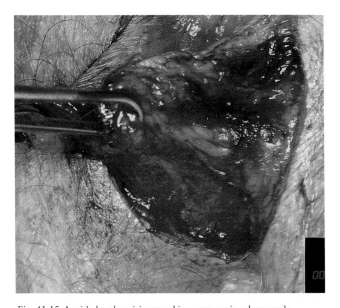

Fig. 41.15 A wide local excision used in a woman in whom early microinvasive carcinoma had been found. Biopsy had confirmed the presence of early invasion, and the incision was carried to the deep fascia with the inclusion of at least a 1-cm margin of normal skin around the area. Frozen sections were taken to confirm these clear margins. In this photograph, the lateral margin is the labiocrural fold, and the medial margin is just within the introitus.

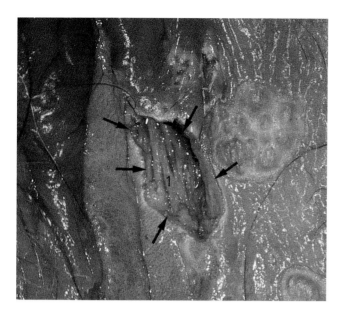

Fig. 41.16 View after removal of a VIN3 lesion using the carbon dioxide laser on the superpulse mode (area removed arrowed). Dense collagen of the mid-reticular dermis is seen at (1), and this is the layer to which the resection is taken, measuring no more than 2–3 mm below the surface. This layer is below the dermal papillae in the immediate subepithelial dermis.

the pilosebaceous units (Reid *et al.*, 1985). The proposed advantages are that it provides a non-mutilating treatment that can be performed with the aid of a colposcope to allow great accuracy over the areas destroyed. Healing is usually cosmetically acceptable and interferes little with function. Treatment can often be performed after preoperative use of local anaesthetic creams, avoiding the need for general anaesthesia (Barrasso, 1997; Monsonego and Semaille, 2000). Baggish and Dorsey (1981) suggested destruction to a depth of 3 mm as being adequate. Wright and Davies (1987) have since proposed that destruction to 1 mm may be adequate in areas such as the labia minora and clitoris. Shatz *et al.* (1989) suggested that, on the basis of measurement of skin appendage involvement, destroying tissue to a depth of 2.5 mm would remove 98% of VIN in hair-bearing areas. Results after laser ablation are variable, with reported recurrences of 9–88% (Townsend *et al.*, 1982; Ferenczy, 1983; Leuchter *et al.*, 1984; Riva *et al.*, 1989). These apparently high recurrence rates may reflect the failure of laser to remove the underlying reservoir of HPV. Postoperative complications are common with frequent reports of pain and febrile reactions. The failure of treatment with laser to provide a specimen for histological analysis makes thorough examination and possibly biopsy mandatory to rule out invasive foci of disease. Combinations of excisional and destructive treatments have been reported (Bornstein and Kaufman, 1988; Ferenczy *et al.*, 1994). Again, recurrence rates are disappointing. However, the simultaneous use of laser ablation of surgical margins after excisional partial vulvectomy

for VIN seems to be a promising combination of both modalities. Brown *et al.* (2005) have reported a significantly reduced recurrence rate in those patients having a combination of excisional and CO_2 ablative therapy.

Medical treatments

A variety of chemotherapeutic agents have been used in the treatment of VIN.

5-Fluorouracil

5-Fluorouracil (5-FU) exerts its effects mainly by preventing DNA synthesis. The usual method of use is topical application directly to the lesions. Side-effects include erythema, oedema, ulceration, blistering and necrosis. The use of 5-FU to treat VIN has been reported by a number of authors (Carson *et al.*, 1976; Krupp and Bohm, 1978; Krebs, 1986) and reviewed by Sillman *et al.* (1985). The reported series usually involve small numbers of patients. A variety of treatment regimens are described. Usually, the length of treatment is determined by the ability of the patient to tolerate side-effects. Response rates vary widely but, overall, the failure rate is approximately 60%. Factors influencing the chance of success include lesion size, the presence of lesions on hair-bearing skin and the degree of keratinisation. Reid *et al.* (1990) described the use of 5-FU as an adjuvant treatment to laser vaporisation. They claimed improved success rates in women with adverse prognostic features.

Dinitrochlorobenzene

Dinitrochlorobenzene (DNCB) uses the delayed hypersensitivity reaction to exert its effects. The individual is initially sensitised with an application of DNCB followed by a later application of DNCB to the vulva. The resulting inflammatory reaction leads to erythema and ulceration. The effects of DNCB appear to be due to crude tissue destruction rather than any immunological effect. Two series relating to DNCB use for vulval lesions are reported (Weintraub and Lagasse, 1973; Foster and Woodruff, 1981). Responses range from 33% to 83%. Side-effects limited treatment. A combination of 5-FU and DNCB may be more efficacious (Raaf *et al.*, 1976).

Interferon

Interferons are an important component of the antiviral defence mechanism with wide-ranging effects particularly related to cell-mediated immunity. A number of groups have published their experiences of treating VIN with interferon (De Palo *et al.*, 1985; Slotman *et al.*, 1988; Gross *et al.*, 1990; Spirtos *et al.*, 1990; Lebbe *et al.*, 1993). A variety of treatment regimens are described using a combination of topical and intralesional applications. Complete response rates vary from 25% to 50%. Overall, treatment was well tolerated with only influenza-like symptoms described.

Topical corticosteroids

Although used to treat the inflammatory component of VIN, no good data exist to support the use of topical corticosteroids. In view of the link between VIN and HPV infection, the effects of local immunosuppression and disease response warrant further investigation.

Cidofovir

Koonsaeng *et al.* (2001) report the use of this deoxycytidine monophosphate analogue to treat a patient with high-grade VIN. Complete eradication of the lesion was seen. Further work is needed to establish the true efficacy of this compound.

Imiquimod (5% cream)

Imiquimod is an immune response modulator with its major mechanism of action being used for the active treatment of external genital warts (Tyring *et al.*, 1998). It is one of the imidazoquinoline compounds, of which imiquimod, formulated as Aldara™, is the best characterised to date. It and its homologues are agonists of TLR7 and TLR8, thereby inducing secretion of the proinflammatory cytokines, predominantly interferon (IFN)-α, tumour necrosis factor (TNF)-α and interleukin (IL)-12. This locally generated cytokine milieu is biased to a Th1 cell-mediated immune response with the generation of cytotoxic effectors, and this has been exploited clinically in the treatment of both benign and neoplastic HPV-associated disease. The mechanism of action in neoplasms seems to relate to this powerful proapoptotic property of imiquimod, which, in conjunction with its cytokine-mediated proinflammatory effect, makes it a most novel and exciting anti-tumour therapy (Stanley, 2005).

A number of studies have testified to the effectiveness and safety of the 5% cream for the treatment of the undifferentiated or classical VIN (Bowenoid/basaloid VIN2/3). They have shown that recurrence rates after treatment are substantially reduced. The study described recently by Marchitelli *et al.* (2004) followed eight patients with undifferentiated biopsy-proven VIN. The cream was applied three times a week until total clearance of the lesion or up to a maximum of 16 weeks, and response was assessed by lesion size regression. The follow-up was carried out monthly for 30 months. They showed total clearance of the lesion in six subjects after 10–16 weeks, with a further two having a partial response. Post-treatment biopsy showed no precancerous lesions in seven patients (87.5%). They concluded that this preparation was effective for treating undifferentiated VIN2/3 in young women, in whom it was well tolerated, causing minimal local reaction. In a larger series, van Seters *et al.* (2004) carried out a prospective, randomised, placebo-controlled, double-blind trial in 50 patients with histologically proven multifocal high-grade disease. Each patient received either imiquimod cream containing 12.5 mg of imiquimod or a placebo and the treatment period was 16 weeks with a dose frequency of twice a week. Of the patients, who ranged in age from 22 to 59 years (mean 42 years), 37 had previously been treated with a surgical procedure and 34 (69%) had symptoms of vulval pain or pruritus at baseline. The vast majority were smokers. To date, half the patients (50%) have noted reduction of symptoms, whereas four patients (11%) have mentioned a progression of symptoms. Some 45% have had a histological regression, with complete response evident in eight patients and partial response in a further nine. Thirty patients have been followed for 1 year, and recurrences were seen in only one patient. However, caution must be used when treating women with VIN3 using this therapy. Jayne and Kaufman (2002) noted 2 out of 13 cases of invasion occurring in fields of regressing VIN in women who were treated with imiquimod. It would seem as though the place for imiquimod in the treatment of VIN can be assessed only when the results of properly controlled studies with long-term follow-up are published (Jones, 2003). Le *et al.* (2006) have recently shown significant regression of VIN2/3 lesions using a slow dose-escalating regime.

Vaccines

The use of vaccines for treating multifocal multicentric disease of the lower genital tract has recently been reviewed by Fiander and Man (2003). The rationale for this therapy depends on the expression of HPV antigens that distinguish neoplastic from normal epithelia. Specific approaches to date have been derived from animal models aided by a knowledge of the natural history of HPV infections and the process of HPV carcinogenesis. Vaccines rely on the induction of a strong cell-mediated response, with most vaccine development, especially in the case of therapeutic vaccines, directed at strategies designed to induce CD8+ T-cell effectors. However, it would seem that an optimum therapeutic immune response would also include cytotoxic T lymphocytes (CTL) and T-helper cells. Fiander and Man, who analysed a number of trials, particularly for high-grade CIN and VIN, describe both partial and complete responses. Quoting the results of Davidson *et al.* (2001), when 18 women with HPV 16-positive VIN3 received one dose of the vaccine TA-HPV and were followed for 24 weeks, lesion shrinkage, classified as 50% reduction in the longest lesion diameter, occurred in eight women and one had complete regression of all vulval lesions. Histological improvement occurred in a further 5 out of 18. In a further study, using the vaccine TA-HPV in high-grade anogenital intraepithelial neoplasia (AGIN) of up to 15 years' duration, 12 HPV-positive women with these lesions received one dose of this vaccine and were followed for 24 weeks. Five of the patients showed at least a 50% reduction in total lesion diameter, of whom one patient showed complete regression of the lesion. Overall, there was an average decrease in lesion size of 40%, with 83% of women showing some improvement (Baldwin *et al.*, 2002).

Although these two trials and many others are in a preliminary state, the future for vaccines looks extremely promising. They may well find a place in the therapy of HPV-related lower genital tract neoplasia. Fiander and Man (2003) believe that, while the approach of a vaccine relies on antigen-specific responses, it is possible that optimum treatment will combine non-specific responses based on the innate immune response with strong systemic immunity against HPV. They suggest in this regard that the application of immune modifiers such as cidofovir or imiquimod, together with specific vaccination using current vaccines, may well be the ideal combination (Fiander and Man, 2003).

Photodynamic therapy

Photodynamic therapy (PDT) involves sensitising the skin with topical 5-aminolaevulinic acid followed by exposure to laser light, usually at 635 nm. Animal studies have suggested that a PDT response involves an immune reaction in which cytotoxic T cells play a role. Of those series reported (Hillemanns *et al.*, 2000; Kurwa *et al.*, 2000; Abdel-Hady *et al.*, 2001; Fehr *et al.*, 2001), response rates range from 0 to 73%. The procedure can be performed without general anaesthetic and is usually well tolerated. After healing, cosmesis is usually good. Factors shown to be associated with poor response include multifocality, hyperkeratosis, reduced CTL infiltration into treated tissue and class 1 major histocompatibility complex (MHC) downregulation.

Summary of treatment options

The fact that so many treatments have been used for VIN suggests that no one approach is ideal. Treatment certainly needs to be tailored to the individual patient. Overall, the available medical treatments have produced disappointing results, and many are associated with high levels of morbidity.

MANAGEMENT OF VAIN

A number of treatment modalities have been employed in the management of VaIN. There is a significant risk of recurrent VaIN with all treatment modalities for VaIN, and the method chosen is sometimes a balance between the effectiveness and the morbidity of the treatment chosen.

In a review of 104 patients with VaIN, Sillman *et al.* (1997) reported that, despite satisfactory treatment and follow-up, there was a progression rate to invasive vaginal cancer of 5%. Dodge *et al.* (2001) reported only a 2% progression rate to invasive vaginal cancer in a review of 121 patients, but a 33% recurrence of VaIN after primary treatment.

Excision

Surgical excision of VaIN may involve removing small discrete lesions on the vagina, an upper vaginectomy or a total vaginectomy.

Success rates of 70–80% are reported for excisional methods (Curtis *et al.*, 1992; Hoffman *et al.*, 1992; Rome and England, 2000).

Patient selection for excisional management of VaIN is important, and accurate mapping of the lesions is required so that the potential morbidity of the procedure can be discussed with the patient. The approach to surgery, i.e. vaginal, abdominal or combined, must be planned. Excision of the upper vagina, and certainly the whole vagina, carries risks of damage to the bladder, ureters and bowel, and may have profound psychosexual sequelae. Patients must be in full possession of the facts necessary for them to make an informed decision.

Radiotherapy

Both intravaginal brachytherapy and external beam radiotherapy have been used as first-line treatments for VaIN III. Morbidity from vaginal radiotherapy can include vaginal stenosis and atrophy of the vaginal mucosa. Woodman *et al.* (1988) reported that the use of vaginal dilators could prevent the vaginal stenosis following vaginal radiotherapy and, in our cancer centre, we have a dedicated clinic run by nurse specialists for all women undergoing pelvic radiotherapy to advise on the prevention of stenosis using vaginal dilators.

Apart from the morbidity associated with vaginal radiotherapy, both recurrence of VaIN and progression to invasive carcinoma have been described (MacLeod *et al.*, 1997; Sillman, 2003). In many cancer centres, including our own, radiotherapy is now seldom used as a first-line treatment for VaIN, with excisional methods preferred in the majority of situations.

Expectant

A strong case can be made for a policy of careful follow-up for some patients with VaIN, in whom the disease is low grade (VaIN1 or 2) or in whom the morbidity of treatment may be high. An example of this may be a young woman with VaIN throughout the vagina in whom a vaginectomy may be contemplated.

Other treatment modalities

Laser, cryotherapy and topical 5-FU are examples of destructive treatments that have been used in the treatment of VaIN but, for the majority of patients, excisional treatment is now the treatment of choice in the first instance (Woodruff *et al.*, 1975; Jobson and Homesley, 1983; Townsend, 1992).

Because of the relatively low incidence of VaIN, and the significant recurrence rate of the condition over a long time course, the management of VaIN is probably best carried out in specialist centres with multidisciplinary expertise in managing the condition.

MANAGEMENT OF PAIN

The management of patients with PaIN should involve a multidisciplinary team approach.

Excision of small areas of PaIN may allow diagnosis and treatment as for areas of VIN.

For patients with widespread PaIN, a policy of close follow-up is often appropriate, with rebiopsy of any suspicious lesions that may develop. Should excision of large areas of PaIN become necessary, skin grafting may be required and, as for patients with VIN, recurrence remains a possibility.

SUMMARY

Whether MIN exists as a separate entity remains a subject of debate.

What is not in doubt is the challenge of managing patients with lower genital tract intraepithelial neoplasia affecting multiple sites. The primary aim of management in these patients is to provide symptom control, surveillance to detect invasive change and retention of function of the lower genital tract.

To achieve these aims requires long-term follow-up and careful monitoring, assessment, biopsy and treatment where indicated.

ACKNOWLEDGEMENTS

The authors wish to thank Professor A. Singer and Mr J.M. Monaghan for the contribution of Figures 41.1 to 41.16, excluding Figures 41.8b and c. These figures appeared previously in *Lower Genital Tract Precancer: Colposcopy, Pathology and Treatment* published by Blackwell Publishing, Oxford, 2000. Figures 41.13 and 41.14 were also published in the above text and were originally contributed to it by Mr J.A. Jordan with his surgical colleagues, Mr M.I. Shafi and Professor D. Luesley, Birmingham, UK. The authors would also like to thank Professor M. Sideri, Milan, Italy, for his comments on the new classification of VIN.

REFERENCES

Abdel-Hady ES, Martin-Hirsch P, Duggan-Keen M *et al.* (2001) Immunological and viral factors associated with the response of vulval intraepithelial neoplasia to photodynamic therapy. *Cancer Research* 61 (1): 192–196.

Aho M, Vesterinen E, Myer B *et al.* (1991) National history of vaginal intraepithelial neoplasia. *Cancer* 63: 195–197.

Andreasson B, Bock JE (1985) Intraepithelial neoplasia in the vulvar region. *Gynecologic Oncology* 21 (3): 300–305.

Anon (1982) Clinical stains for cancer. *Lancet* 1 (8267): 320–321.

Anon (1996) Clinicopathologic analysis of 370 cases of vulvar intraepithelial neoplasia. Italian Study Group on Vulvar Disease. *Journal of Reproductive Medicine* 41 (9): 665–670.

Ayhan A, Tuncer ZS, Dogan L *et al.* (1998) Skinning vulvectomy for the treatment of vulvar intraepithelial neoplasia 2–3: a study of 21 cases. *European Journal of Gynaecological Oncology* 19 (5): 508–510.

Baggish MS, Dorsey JH (1981) CO_2 laser for the treatment of vulvar carcinoma in situ. *Obstetrics and Gynecology* 57 (3): 371–375.

Baldwin P, van Der Burgh SH, Coleman, N *et al.* (2002) Vaccination for anogenital intraepithelial neoplasia with recombinant vaccinia virus expressing HPV-16 and 18E6 and E7. Posted abstract presented at the 20th International Human Papillomavirus Conference, 4–9 October 2002, Paris.

Barbero M, Micheletti L, Preti M *et al.* (1990) Vulvar intraepithelial neoplasia. A clinicopathologic study of 60 cases. *Journal of Reproductive Medicine* 35 (11): 1023–1028.

Barrasso R (1997) Effectiveness of local anesthesia using EMLA cream for laser treatment of cervical and vulvar lesions. *Contraception, Fertility and Sexuality* 25 (11): 861–864.

Barton SE, Maddox PH, Jenkins D *et al.* (1988) Effect of cigarette smoking on cervical epithelial immunity: a mechanism for neoplastic change? *Lancet* 2 (8612): 652–654.

Benedet JL, Sanders BH (1984) Carcinoma in situ of the vagina. *American Journal of Obstetrics and Gynecology* 148: 695–670.

Bergeron C, Naghashfar Z, Canaan C *et al.* (1987) Human papillomavirus type 16 in intraepithelial neoplasia (bowenoid papulosis) and coexistent invasive carcinoma of the vulva. *International Journal of Gynecological Pathology* 6 (1): 1–11.

Blohme I, Brynger H (1985) Malignant disease and renal transplantations. *Transplantation* 39: 23–25.

Bornstein J, Kaufman RH (1988) Combination of surgical excision and carbon dioxide laser vaporization for multifocal vulvar intraepithelial neoplasia. *American Journal of Obstetrics and Gynecology* 158 (3 Pt 1): 459–464.

Boutselis JG (1972) Intraepithelial carcinoma of the vulva. *American Journal of Obstetrics and Gynecology* 113 (6): 733–738.

Brinton LA, Nasca PC, Mallin K *et al.* (1990) Case–control study of cancer of the vulva. *Obstetrics and Gynecology* 75 (5): 859–866.

Broen EM, Ostergard DR (1971) Toluidine blue and colposcopy for screening and delineating vulvar neoplasia. *Obstetrics and Gynecology* 38 (5): 775–778.

Brown JV, Goldstein BH, Rettenmaier MA *et al.* (2005) Laser ablation of surgical margins after excisional partial vulvectomy for VIN: effect on recurrence. *Journal of Reproductive Medicine* 50 (5): 345–350.

Buscema J, Stern J, Woodruff JD (1980a) The significance of the histologic alterations adjacent to invasive vulvar carcinoma. *American Journal of Obstetrics and Gynecology* 137 (8): 902–909.

Buscema J, Woodruff JD, Parmley TH *et al.* (1980b) Carcinoma in situ of the vulva. *Obstetrics and Gynecology* 55 (2): 225–230.

Caglar H, Delgado G, Hreshchyshyn MM (1986) Partial and total skinning vulvectomy in treatment of carcinoma in situ of the vulva. *Obstetrics and Gynecology* 68 (4): 504–507.

Campion MJ, Hacker NF (1998) Vulvar intraepithelial neoplasia and car-cinoma. *Seminars in Cutaneous Medicine and Surgery* 17 (3): 205–212.

Carson TE, Hoskins WJ, Wurzel JF (1976) Topical 5-fluorouracil in the treatment of carcinoma in situ of the vulva. *Obstetrics and Gynecology* 47 (1): 59S–62S.

Chenoy R, Luesley DM (1995) Vulvar and multifocal intraepithelial neoplasia. In: Luesley DM, Jordan JA, Richart RM (eds) *Intraepithelial Neoplasia of the Lower Genital Tract*. London: Churchill Livingstone, pp. 121–132.

Chiasson MALO, Brock TV, Bush DJ *et al.* (1997) Increased prevalence of vulvo-vaginal condyloma and vulval intraepithelial neoplasia in women infected with human immunodeficiency virus. *Obstetrics and Gynecology* 89: 690–640.

Clark TJ, Herod JJ, Kehoe S *et al.* (1998) The development of invasive vulvar cancer in a patient with Job's syndrome, a rare immunodeficient condition. *British Journal of Obstetrics and Gynaecology* 105 (4): 468–470.

Collins CG, Roman-Lopez JJ, Lee FY (1970) Intraepithelial carcinoma of the vulva. *American Journal of Obstetrics and Gynecology* 108 (8): 1187–1191.

Conley LJ, Ellerbrock TV, Bush TJ *et al.* (2002) HIV-1 infection and risk of vulvovaginal and perianal condylomata acuminata and intraepithelial neoplasia: a prospective cohort study. *Lancet* 359 (9301): 108–113.

Cox SM, Kaufman RH, Kaplan A (1986) Recurrent carcinoma in situ of the vulva in a skin graft. *American Journal of Obstetrics and Gynecology* 155 (1): 177–179.

Crum CP, Liskow A, Petras P *et al.* (1984) Vulvar intraepithelial neoplasia (severe atypia and carcinoma in situ). A clinicopathologic analysis of 41 cases. *Cancer* 54 (7): 1429–1434.

Curtis P, Shepherd JH, Lowe DG *et al.* (1992) The role of partial colpectomy in the management of persistent vaginal neoplasia after primary treatment. *British Journal of Obstetrics and Gynaecology* 99 (7): 587–589.

Da Costa MM, Hogeboom CJ, Holly EA *et al.* (2002) Increased risk of high grade anal neoplasia associated with a human papillomavirus Type 16E6 sequence variant. *Journal of Infectious Diseases* 185 (9): 1229–1237.

Daling JR, Sherman KJ, Hislop TG *et al.* (1992) Cigarette smoking and the risk of anogenital cancer. *American Journal of Epidemiology* 135 (2): 180–189.

Davidson E, Tomlinson A, Stern PS, *et al.* (2001) A phase II trial to assess the safety, immunogenicity and efficacy of TA-HPV in patients with high grade vulval intraepithelial neoplasia (VIN). Posted abstract presented at the 19th International Papillomavirus Conference, 1–7 September 2001, Brazil.

De Palo G, Stefanon B, Rilke F *et al.* (1985) Human fibroblast interferon in cervical and vulvar intraepithelial neoplasia associated with viral cytopathic effects. A pilot study. *Journal of Reproductive Medicine* 30 (5): 404–408.

Di Saia PJ, Rich WM (1981) Surgical approach to multifocal carcinoma in situ of the vulva. *American Journal of Obstetrics and Gynecology* 140 (2): 136–145.

Dodge JA, Eltabbakh GH, Mount SL *et al.* (2001) Clinical features and risk of recurrence among patients with vaginal intraepithelial neoplasia. *Gynecologic Oncology* 83 (2): 363–369.

Fehr MK, Hornung R, Schwarz VA *et al.* (2001) Photodynamic therapy of vulvar intraepithelial neoplasia III using topically applied 5-aminolevulinic acid. *Gynecologic Oncology* 80 (1): 62–66.

Ferenczy A (1983) Using the laser to treat vulvar condylomata acu-minata and intraepidermal neoplasia. *Canadian Medical Association Journal* 128 (2): 135–137.

Ferenczy A, Wright TC, Richart RM (1994) Comparison of CO_2 laser surgery and loop electrosurgical excision/fulguration procedure (LEEP) for the treatment of vulvar intraepithelial neoplasia (VIN). *International Journal of Gynecological Cancer* 4 (1): 22–28.

Fiander A, Man S (2003) Antiviral vaccination for treating intraepithelial neoplasia. In: Maclean A, Singer A, Critchley H (eds) *Lower Genital Tract Neoplasia*. London: RCOG Press, pp. 191–209.

Foster DC, Woodruff JD (1981) The use of dinitrochlorobenzene in the treatment of vulvar carcinoma in situ. *Gynecologic Oncology* 11 (3): 330–339.

Foulques H, Barrasso R, Caubel P *et al.* (1991) [Possibilities and limitations of the acetic acid test in the identification of vulvar papillomavirus lesions. A colposcopic, histologic and virologic study]. *Journal of Gynecology Obstetrics and Biology of Reproduction (Paris)* 20 (6): 791–795.

Friedrich EG, Jr (1972) Reversible vulvar atypia. A case report. *Obstetrics and Gynecology* 39 (2): 173–181.

Friedrich EG, Jr, Wilkinson EJ, Fu YS (1980) Carcinoma in situ of the vulva: a continuing challenge. *American Journal of Obstetrics and Gynecology* 136 (7): 830–843.

Frisch M, Fenger C, van den Brule AJ *et al.* (1999) Variants of squamous cell carcinoma of the anal canal and perianal skin and their relation to human papillomaviruses. *Cancer Research* 59 (3): 753–757.

Frisch M, Biggar RJ, Goedert JJ (2000) Human papillomavirus-associated cancers in patients with human immunodeficiency virus infection — an acquired immunodeficiency syndrome. *Journal of the National Cancer Institute* 92: 1500–1510.

Gallup DG, Morley GW (1975) Carcinoma in situ of the vagina. A study and review. *Obstetrics and Gynecology* 46 (3): 334–340.

Gross G, Roussaki A, Papendick U (1990) Efficacy of interferons on bowenoid papulosis and other precancerous lesions. *Journal of Investigative Dermatology* 95 (6 Suppl.): 152S–157S.

Herod JJ, Shafi MI, Rollason TP *et al.* (1996) Vulvar intraepithelial neoplasia: long term follow up of treated and untreated women. *British Journal of Obstetrics and Gynaecology* 103 (5): 446–452.

Hildesheim A, Han CL, Brinton LA *et al.* (1997) Human papillomavirus type 16 and risk of preinvasive and invasive vulvar cancer: results from a seroepidemiological case–control study. *Obstetrics and Gynecology* 90 (5): 748–754.

Hillemanns P, Untch M, Dannecker C *et al.* (2000) Photodynamic therapy of vulvar intraepithelial neoplasia using 5-aminolevulinic acid. *International Journal of Cancer* 85 (5): 649–653.

Hoffman MS, DeCesare SL, Roberts WS *et al.* (1992) Upper vaginectomy for in situ and occult, superficially invasive carcinoma of the vagina. *American Journal of Obstetrics and Gynecology* 166 (1 Pt 1): 30–33.

Holly EA, Rawlston ML, Darragh TM *et al.* (2001) Prevalence and risk factors for anal squamous intraepithelial lesions in women. *Journal of the National Cancer Institute* 93: 843–849.

Hording U, Kringsholm B, Andreasson B *et al.* (1993). Human papillomavirus in vulval squamous cell cancer and in normal vulval tissue; the search for a possible impact of HPV on vulvar cancer prognosis. *International Journal of Cancer* 55: 394–396.

Husseinzadeh N, Newman NJ, Wesseler TA (1989) Vulvar intraepithelial neoplasia: a clinicopathological study of carcinoma in situ of the vulva. *Gynecologic Oncology* 33 (2): 157–163.

Ireland D, Monaghan JM (1988) The management of abnormal vaginal cytology following hysterectomy. *British Journal of Obstetrics and Gynaecology* 95: 973–975.

Iversen T, Tretli S (1998) Intraepithelial and invasive squamous cell neoplasia of the vulva: trends and incidence, recurrence and survival rates in Norway. *Obstetrics and Gynecology* 91 (6): 969–972.

Jayne CJ, Kaufman RH (2002) Treatment of vulvar intraepithelial neoplasia II/III with Imiquimod. *Journal of Reproductive Medicine* 47: 395–398.

Jobson VW, Homesley HD (1983) Treatment of vaginal intraepithelial neoplasia with the carbon dioxide laser. *Obstetrics and Gynecology* 62 (1): 90–93.

Jones RW (2003) The natural history of lower genital tract precancers; an historical perspective. In: Maclean AB, Singer A, Critchley H (eds) *Lower Genital Tract Neoplasia*. London: RCOG Press, pp. 69–80.

Jones RW, Rowan DM (1994) Vulvar intraepithelial neoplasia III: a clinical study of the outcome in 113 cases with relation to the later development of invasive vulvar carcinoma. *Obstetrics and Gynecology* 84 (5): 741–745.

Jones RW, Rowan DM (2000) Spontaneous regression of vulvar intraepithelial neoplasia 2–3. *Obstetrics and Gynecology* 96 (3): 470–472.

Jonsson M, Karlsson R, Evander M *et al.* (1997) Acetowhitening of the cervix and vulva as a predictor of subclinical human papillomavirus infection: sensitivity and specificity in a population-based study. *Obstetrics and Gynecology* 90 (5): 744–747.

Joura EA, Zeisler H, Losch A *et al.* (1998) Differentiating vulvar intraepithelial neoplasia from nonneoplastic epithelial disorders. The toluidine blue test. *Journal of Reproductive Medicine* 43 (8): 671–674.

Kadish AS (2001) Biology of anogenital neoplasia. *Cancer Treatment Research* 104: 267–286.

Koonsaeng S, Verschraegen C, Freedman R *et al.* (2001) Successful treatment of recurrent vulvar intraepithelial neoplasia resistant to interferon and isotretinoin with cidofovir. *Journal of Medical Virology* 64 (2): 195–198.

Korn AP, Abercrombie PD, Foster A (1996) Vulvar intraepithelial neoplasia in women infected with human immunodeficiency virus-1. *Gynecologic Oncology* 61 (3): 384–386.

Krebs HB (1986) Prophylactic topical 5-fluorouracil following treatment of human papillomavirus-associated lesions of the vulva and vagina. *Obstetrics and Gynecology* 68 (6): 837–841.

Krupp PJ, Bohm JW (1978) 5-Fluorouracil topical treatment of in situ vulvar cancer. A preliminary report. *Obstetrics and Gynecology* 51 (6): 702–706.

Kuppers V, Stiller M, Somville T *et al.* (1997) Risk factors for recurrent VIN. Role of multifocality and grade of disease. *Journal of Reproductive Medicine* 42 (3): 140–144.

Kurwa HA, Barlow RJ, Neill S (2000) Single-episode photodynamic therapy and vulval intraepithelial neoplasia type III resistant to conventional therapy. *British Journal of Dermatology* 143 (5): 1040–1042.

Le T, Hicks W, Menard C *et al.* (2006) Preliminary results of 5% imiquimod cream in the primary treatment of vulva intraepithelial neoplasia grade 2/3. *American Journal of Obstetrics and Gynecology* 194: 377–380.

Lebbe C, Rybojad M, Ochonisky S *et al.* (1993) Extensive human papillomavirus-related disease (bowenoid papulosis, Bowen's disease, and squamous cell carcinoma) in a patient with hairy cell leukemia: clinical and immunologic evaluation after an interferon alfa trial. *Journal of the American Academy of Dermatology* 29 (4): 644–646.

Lee YY, Wilczynski SP, Chumakov A *et al.* (1994) Carcinoma of the vulva; HPV and p53 mutations. *Oncogene* 9 (6): 1655–1659.

Lenehan PM, Meffe F, Lickrish GM (1986) Vaginal intraepithelial neoplasia: biologic aspects and management. *Obstetrics and Gynecology* 68 (3): 333–337.

Leuchter RS, Townsend DE, Hacker NF *et al.* (1984) Treatment of vulvar carcinoma in situ with the CO_2 laser. *Gynecologic Oncology* 19 (3): 314–322.

Lopes A, Monaghan J, Robertson G (1995) Vaginal intraepithelial neoplasia. In: Luesley DM, Jordan JA, Richart RM (eds) *Intraepithelial Neoplasia of the Lower Genital Tract*. London: Churchill Livingstone, pp. 169–176.

Luesley DM (2000) *Cancer and Pre-cancer of the Vulva*. New York: Arnold, pp. 67–73.

MacLeod C, Fowler A, Dalrymple C *et al.* (1997) High-dose-rate brachytherapy in the management of high-grade intraepithelial neoplasia of the vagina. *Gynecologic Oncology* 65 (1): 74–77.

Madeleine MM, Daling JR, Carter JJ *et al.* (1997) Cofactors with human papillomavirus in a population-based study of vulvar cancer. *Journal of the National Cancer Institute* 89 (0): 1516–1523.

Marchitelli C, Secco G, Perrotta M *et al.* (2004) Treatment of bowenoid and basaloid vulvar intraepithelial neoplasia 2/3 with imiquimod 5% cream. *Journal of Reproductive Medicine* 49 (11): 876–882.

Monsonego J, Semaille C (2000) Local anesthesia of genital mucosa with a lidocaine/prilocaine combination cream before laser therapy of human papillomavirus lesions. *European Journal of Dermatology* 10 (8): 607–610.

Moreno V, Bosch FX, Muñoz N *et al.* (2002) Effect of oral contraceptives on risk of cervical cancer in women with human papillomavirus infection: the IARC multicentric case–control study. *Lancet* 359 (9312): 1085–1092.

Newcomb PA, Weiss NS, Daling JR (1984) Incidence of vulvar carcinoma in relation to menstrual, reproductive, and medical factors. *Journal of the National Cancer Institute* 73 (2): 391–396.

Ogunbiyi OA, Scholefield JH, Robertson G *et al.* (1994) Anal human papillomavirus infection and squamous neoplasia in patients with invasive vulvar cancer. *Obstetrics and Gynecology* 83: 212–216.

Penn I (1986a) Cancers of the anogenital region in renal transplant recipients. Analysis of 65 cases. *Cancer* 58 (3): 611–616.

Penn I (1986b) Cancer as a complication of immunosuppression. *Surgery in Gynecology and Obstetrics* 162: 603–610.

Planner RS, Hobbs JB (1988) Intraepithelial and invasive neoplasia of the vulva in association with human papillomavirus infection. *Journal of Reproductive Medicine* 33 (6): 503–509.

Raaf JH, Krown SE, Pinsky CM *et al.* (1976) Treatment of Bowen's disease with topical dinitrochlorobenzene and 5-fluorouracil. *Cancer* 37 (4): 1633–1642.

Reid R, Elfont EA, Zirkin RM *et al.* (1985) Superficial laser vulvectomy. II. The anatomic and biophysical principles permitting accurate control over the depth of dermal destruction with the carbon dioxide laser. *American Journal of Obstetrics and Gynecology* 152 (3): 261–271.

Reid R, Greenberg MD, Lorincz AT *et al.* (1990) Superficial laser vulvectomy. IV. Extended laser vaporization and adjunctive 5-fluorouracil therapy of human papillomavirus-associated vulvar disease. *Obstetrics and Gynecology* 76 (3 Pt 1): 439–448.

Riva JM, Sedlacek TV, Cunnane MF *et al.* (1989) Extended carbon dioxide laser vaporization in the treatment of subclinical papillomavirus infection of the lower genital tract. *Obstetrics and Gynecology* 73 (1): 25–30.

Rome RM, England PG (2000) Management of vaginal intraepithelial neoplasia: a series of 132 cases with long-term follow-up. *International Journal of Gynecological Cancer* 10 (5): 382–390.

Rutledge F, Sinclair M (1968) Treatment of intraepithelial carcinoma of the vulva by skin excision and graft. *American Journal of Obstetrics and Gynecology* 102 (6): 807–818.

Scholefield JH, Hickson JG, Smith JH *et al.* (1992) Anal intraepithelial neoplasia: part of a multifocal disease process. *Lancet* 340: 1271–1273.

Scholefield JH, Castle MT, Watson NFS (2005) Malignant transformation of high-grade anal intraepithelial neoplasia. *British Journal of Surgery* 92: 1133–1136.

Shafi MI, Luesley DM, Byrne P *et al.* (1989) Vulval intraepithelial neoplasia — management and outcome. *British Journal of Obstetrics and Gynaecology* 96 (11): 1339–1344.

Shatz P, Bergeron C, Wilkinson EJ *et al.* (1989) Vulvar intraepithelial neoplasia and skin appendage involvement. *Obstetrics and Gynecology* 74 (5): 769–774.

Sherman KJ, Daling JR, Chu J *et al.* (1991) Genital warts, other sexually transmitted diseases, and vulvar cancer. *Epidemiology* 2 (4); 257–262.

Sherman KJ, Daling JR, McKnight B *et al.* (1994) Hormonal factors in vulvar cancer. A case–control study. *Journal of Reproductive Medicine* 39 (11): 857–861.

Sideri M, Jones RW, Wilkinson EJ *et al.* (2005) Squamous vulvar intraepithelial neoplasia: 2003 modified terminology. ISSVD Vulvar Oncology Subcommittee. *Journal of Reproductive Medicine* 50: 807–810.

Sillman F (2003) Vaginal intraepithelial neoplasia.; characteristics, investigation and management. In: Luesley DM (ed.) *Cancer and Pre-cancer of the Vulva*. New York: Arnold.

Sillman F, Stanek A, Sedlis A *et al.* (1984) The relationship between human papillomavirus and lower genital intraepithelial neoplasia in immunosuppressed women, *American Journal of Obstetrics and Gynecology* 150 (3): 300–308.

Sillman FH, Sedlis A, Boyce JG (1985) A review of lower genital intraepithelial neoplasia and the use of topical 5-fluorouracil. *Obstetrics and Gynecology Surveys* 40 (4): 190–220.

Sillman FH, Fruchter RG, Chen YS *et al.* (1997) Vaginal intraepithelial neoplasia: risk factors for persistence, recurrence, and invasion and its management. *American Journal of Obstetrics and Gynecology* 176 (1 Pt 1): 93–99.

Slotman BJ, Helmerhorst TJ, Wijermans PW *et al.* (1988) Interferon-alpha in treatment of intraepithelial neoplasia of the lower genital tract: a case report. *European Journal of Obstetrics Gynecology and Reproductive Biology* 27 (4): 327–333.

Spirtos NM, Smith LH, Teng NN (1990) Prospective randomized trial of topical alpha-interferon (alpha-interferon gels) for the treatment of vulvar intraepithelial neoplasia III. *Gynecologic Oncology* 37 (1): 34–38.

Stanley MA (2005) The Imidazoquinolines — mechanism of action and therapeutic potential in HPV-associated disease. *Papillomavirus Report* 16 (3): 141–146.

Strickler HD, Schiffman MH, Shah KV *et al.* (1998) A survey of human papillomavirus 16 antibodies in patients with epithelial cancers. *European Journal of Cancer Prevention* 7 (4): 305–313.

Tidy J (2003) Management of perianal intraepithelial and invasive neoplasia. In: Maclean A, Singer A, Critchley H (eds) *Lower Genital Tract Neoplasia*. London: RCOG Press, p. 326.

Townsend DE (1992) Cryosurgery. In: Coppleson M (ed.) *Gynecologic Oncology*. Edinburgh: Churchill Livingstone, pp. 1139–1146.

Townsend DE, Levine RU, Richart RM *et al.* (1982) Management of vulvar intraepithelial neoplasia by carbon dioxide laser. *Obstetrics and Gynecology* 60 (1): 49–52.

Tyring SK, Arany I, Stanley MA (1998) A randomised, controlled molecular study of condyloma acuminata clearance during treatment with Imiquimod. *Journal of Infectious Diseases* 178: 551–555.

van Beurden M, van der Vange N, de Craen AJ *et al.* (1997) Normal findings in vulvar examination and vulvoscopy. *British Journal of Obstetrics and Gynaecology* 104 (3): 320–324.

van Seters M, van Beurden M, Burger M *et al.* (2004) Preliminary results of a randomised controlled trial of Imiquimod 5% cream in multifocal high grade vulvar intraepithelial neoplasia. *Journal of Reproductive Medicine* 49 (11): 940.

Weintraub I, Lagasse LD (1973) Reversibility of vulvar atypia by DNCB-induced delayed hypersensitivity. *Obstetrics and Gynecology* 41 (2): 195–199.

Wolcott HD, Gallup DG (1984) Wide local excision in the treatment of vulvar carcinoma in situ: a reappraisal. *American Journal of Obstetrics and Gynecology* 150 (6): 695–698.

Woodman CB, Mould JJ, Jordan JA (1988) Radiotherapy in the management of vaginal intraepithelial neoplasia after hysterectomy. *British Journal of Obstetrics and Gynaecology* 95 (10): 976–979.

Woodman CB, Colin C, Winter H *et al.* (2001) Natural history of cervical human papillomavirus infection in young women: a longitudinal cohort study. *Lancet* 357: 1831–1836.

Woodruff JD, Parmley TH, Julian CG (1975) Topical 5-fluorouracil in the treatment of vaginal carcinoma-in-situ. *Gynecologic Oncology* 3 (2): 124–132.

Wright VC, Davies E (1987) Laser surgery for vulvar intraepithelial neoplasia: principles and results. *American Journal of Obstetrics and Gynecology* 156 (2): 374–378.

Ylitalo N, Sorensen P, Josefsson A *et al.* (1999) Smoking and oral contraceptives as risk factors for cervical carcinoma in situ. *International Journal of Cancer* 81 (3): 357–365.

CHAPTER 42

Radiotherapy in the treatment of cervical cancer

Peter Blake

INTRODUCTION

Radiotherapy uses ionising radiation, X-rays, γ-rays or high-energy particles, to eradicate malignant cells while sparing normal tissues. Most commonly, X-rays are generated in linear accelerators (linacs) (Fig. 42.1) whereas γ-rays arise from the radioactive decay of radioisotopes, either naturally occurring, such as radium, or produced in an atomic pile, such as cobalt-60, caesium-137 or iridium-192. High-energy particles can also be emitted by radioisotopes as α-particles (helium nuclei) and β-particles (electrons) but therapeutically useful electrons are produced in linacs or betatrons. The mainstay of most radiotherapy departments treating cervical cancer is the linac, producing high-energy X-rays and electrons for external irradiation of the patient, and an afterloading system which uses a sealed radioisotope for internal irradiation (intracavitary brachytherapy). These facilities will be backed up by modern treatment simulation and planning equipment.

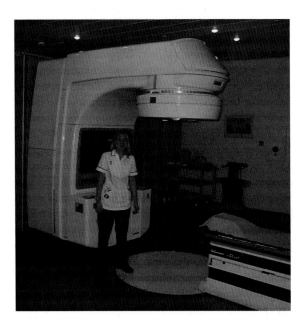

Fig. 42.1 A linear accelerator (linac) capable of producing two energies of X-rays and high-energy electrons.

The therapeutic ratio between radiation damage done to tumour and to normal tissues is maximised by a number of strategies. In treating cervical cancer, the first is to target accurately the radiation to the primary tumour and sites of possible metastases, the regional lymph nodes and upper vagina. This 'targeting' uses information from clinical examination, findings at examination under anaesthetic (EUA) and imaging. Radiation beams are shaped and oriented to deliver the maximum dose to the tumour but the minimum to normal tissues, particularly the rectum and bladder. Computer planning and multi-leaf collimators are used to achieve this. As a check that the beams are consistently in the correct orientation in the patient, images can be generated from the radiation passing through the patient during treatment and checked against standards set for that patient.

The second strategy is to use the relative inability of malignant cells to repair radiation damage in contrast to normal cells. By dividing the treatment into multiple small 'fractions' over several weeks this difference can be utilised to eradicate all malignant cells while allowing normal cells to repopulate. The total time over which treatment is given is then limited so as not to allow tumour cells to enter a state known as 'accelerated repopulation', which would jeopardise tumour cure. Effectively this means that all treatment should be complete within 7–8 weeks.

The third strategy is to integrate external radiotherapy, treating large volumes of tissue to a homogeneous dose, with intracavitary brachytherapy, delivering a very inhomogeneous, high dose to the cervix while relatively sparing sensitive tissues such as the rectum and the bladder. This combination is paramount for the effective use of radiotherapy to cure cervical cancer.

The fourth strategy is to add concomitant chemotherapy. There is clear evidence that this improves the results of treatment but whether this is by chemosensitisation of cells to radiotherapy or by a separate cytotoxic assault on the tumour is not yet clear (Green *et al.*, 2001). Concurrent chemoradiotherapy and the results of clinical trials (Morris *et al.*, 1999; Rose *et al.*, 1999; Peters *et al.*, 2000) are discussed in detail in another chapter.

A further method of maximising the effectiveness of radiotherapy is to ensure that the haemoglobin level is maintained above 11–12 g/dL, either by transfusion or by the use of recombinant erythropoietin. Patients with haemoglobin levels lower than this have poor outcomes, probably as a result of the protective effect of anoxia on the tumour (Grogan *et al.*, 1999).

PRIMARY TREATMENT

The treatment of invasive cervical cancer will depend on the stage of disease, the size of the tumour and the fitness of the patient. It can incorporate chemotherapy, radiotherapy and surgery, and the treatment strategy for individual patients should be arrived at after discussion between specialists in all three disciplines.

Surgery is the treatment of choice for young patients with small-volume stage IB disease. Good histological differentiation and the absence of lymphatic vessel invasion in a biopsy, small tumour volume and normal-sized nodes on imaging are indicators that lymph node metastases are unlikely and surgery should be considered. Advantages of surgery over radiotherapy, in young women, include the avoidance of an early menopause and the maintenance of pliability and lubrication of the vaginal mucosa. In addition, the very small risk of late induction of a second malignancy by radiation is avoided.

RADIOTHERAPY

For older, unfit women with stage I disease, radiotherapy is the treatment of choice as the results of treatment are equal to those of surgery and the treatment is better tolerated. Women with a high risk of nodal involvement or with more advanced disease should receive radiotherapy, usually with concomitant chemotherapy.

External radiotherapy

Carcinoma of the cervix is treated by a combination of external and intracavitary radiotherapy. The volume treated by external radiotherapy should cover the lymph nodes draining the cer-

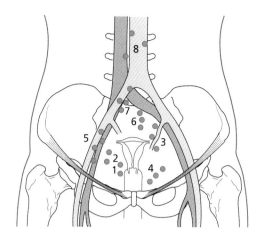

Fig. 42.2 Lymphatic drainage in the cervix. 1, paracervical; 2, parametrial; 3, internal iliac; 4, obturator; 5, external iliac; 6, presacral; 7, common iliac, 8, para-aortic nodes.

vix, which are the internal, external and common iliac nodes in addition to the parametrial, obturator and presacral nodes (Fig. 42.2). Spread to the para-aortic and supraclavicular nodes is uncommon without pelvic node involvement.

Unless imaging shows para-aortic node involvement, the volume encompassed by external radiotherapy will be from the junction of the fourth and fifth lumbar vertebrae to the bottom of the obturator foramina, and laterally to 2 cm outside the bony margin of the pelvis. In the absence of uterosacral ligament involvement, either a four-field 'box' technique or an anterior and two wedged lateral fields can be used to spare the posterior half of the rectum. If the uterosacral ligaments are involved then an antero-posterior parallel opposed pair should be used, recognising that this will deliver a higher dose to the rectum and to the skin. A 5–10-MV linac should be used, in view of the depth of the tumour volume below the surface of the lateral fields (Fig. 42.3). The volume may be more individually designed with shielding of the upper corners of the antero-posterior fields, or individualised, computerised

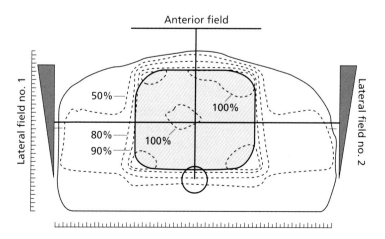

Fig. 42.3 A three-field pelvic plan showing the central high-dose volume.

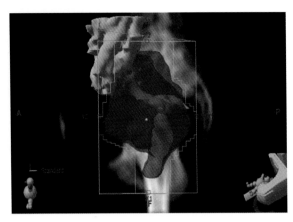

Fig. 42.4 A lateral view of a conformally planned pelvic volume with the tumour volume in red and the small bowel (to be avoided) in yellow.

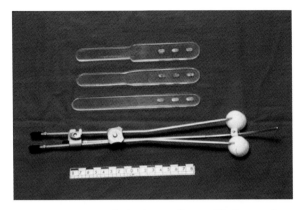

Fig. 42.5 High dose rate afterloading applicators. The intrauterine tube and two vaginal 'ovoids' are fixed together as they would be in the patient. The plastic spatulas can be used to push the rectum away from the high-dose volume.

tomography-planned (CT-planned) 'conformal' shielding, to protect normal tissues (Fig. 42.4).

Those patients with disease in the vaginal mucosa below the upper third should have the field extended to cover the full length of the vagina. This will involve marking the introitus with a lead marker inserted just inside the labia at the time of simulation. If para-aortic nodes are involved then a long, 'spade-shaped' field may be used to cover the para-aortic nodes (usually with an upper border of T12/L1) and the pelvis. This volume is treated by a parallel opposed pair to a maximum dose of 45 Gy in 1.8- to 2-Gy fractions. Unfortunately, diarrhoea and nausea are common during treatment of this large volume.

INTRACAVITARY BRACHYTHERAPY

Cervical cancer was one of the first tumours to be treated by radiotherapy, whereby radium was inserted into the endocervical canal and upper vagina to irradiate local disease. Techniques were developed in several centres, notably Paris, Stockholm and Manchester, which enabled the effectiveness and morbidity of treatment to be measured. A commonly used technique is the 'Manchester' technique, or variations on it, comprising an intrauterine tube and two 'ovoids' placed in the lateral vaginal fornices (Fig. 42.5) (Blake *et al.*, 2002).

Afterloading brachytherapy

In afterloading brachytherapy, hollow applicators are placed in the cervix and vaginal fornices and the radioisotope is introduced into these after the applicators are correctly positioned. Check that radiographs have been taken and the patient is comfortable in a radiation-protected environment. The sources are driven into the applicators remotely, either pneumatically (as in the Selectron) or on the end of cables (as in the microSelectron) when all staff are away from the area.

Low dose rate afterloading

Remote afterloading allows the dose rate of brachytherapy to be increased. With the standard Manchester radium system, the dose rate to point A, a geometrically defined prescription point, was approximately 0.5 Gy/h. Nowadays, caesium-137 pellets can be produced which will allow a dose rate of between 1.5 and 2 Gy/h. While this has the advantage of reducing treatment time by a factor of three, it does have radiobiological consequences, necessitating a small reduction in dose of 10–15% (Hunter, 1994; Fowler, 1997). Typically, the brachytherapy component of treatment will take 12–18 hours when using these increased activity sources.

High dose rate afterloading

High dose rate brachytherapy using iridium-192, delivering doses at rates in excess of 1 Gy/min to point A, allows very short treatment times of only a few minutes (Fig. 42.6). There is complete geometrical stability of the applicator during the treatment; this has advantages, in terms of normal tissue sparing, over a low dose rate insertion lasting several hours, during which time both applicators and tissues move. Short treatment times allow rapid patient throughput, which has advantages in areas of high incidence of cervical cancer but requires that there is a full and efficient infrastructure for the treatment process.

There is considerably less time for repair of sublethal radiation damage in the normal tissues in a high dose rate treatment than there is during a low dose rate brachytherapy implant. Therefore, such treatments have to be fractionated over several days or weeks to allow repair in normal tissues between fractions. As the patient needs several treatment fractions instead of one, it means that the applicators must be positioned consistently for each fraction, in order to take

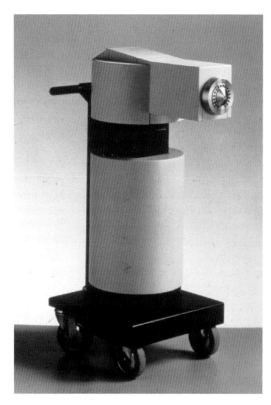

Fig. 42.6 The HDR microSelectron, which uses a moving high-activity iridium-137 source to create shaped high-dose volumes for cervical brachytherapy.

advantage of the geometrical stability. Radiobiological models of repair predict that a reduction of 35–45% from the dose that would be given at standard dose rate needs to be made in order to avoid excessive late normal tissue damage. With such a dose reduction and with fractionation, clinical results show no difference between treatment at low dose rate and high dose rate in terms of local control of disease or late normal tissue complications (Fu and Philips, 1990; Patel *et al.*, 1994; Tanaka *et al.*, 2003).

THE INTEGRATION OF EXTERNAL AND INTRACAVITARY BRACHYTHERAPY

External therapy is used prior to intracavitary brachytherapy and, typically, a dose of 45–50 Gy would be given to the pelvis over 4.5–5.5 weeks in 1.8- to 2-Gy fractions. An intracavitary insertion would then be undertaken to give the equivalent at standard dose rate of a further 25–30 Gy to point A. If higher than standard dose rates are used, then a lower dose would be delivered. Parametrial boosts may then give a further 5 Gy to bulky disease within the parametria or involved nodes on the pelvic sidewalls.

When using the Manchester system, the maximum dose to the rectal mucosa from the intracavitary insertion should not

exceed two-thirds of the dose given to point A if late radiation damage is to be avoided. Care must be taken that the uterus is not pushed against the rectum, sigmoid colon or small bowel; intrauterine applicator tubes should conform to the anteversion of the uterus by having a curvature of 20–40°.

RESULTS OF TREATMENT

It is now standard practice to use concomitant chemoradiotherapy in most patients with cervical cancer who are fit for this. This recent change in practice means that historical results of radiotherapy alone are not relevant, although an example is given in Table 42.1. Results of chemoradiotherapy are discussed in detail in Chapter 43 (Morris *et al.*, 1999; Rose *et al.*, 1999; Peters *et al.*, 2000).

Postoperative adjuvant radiotherapy for poor prognostic factors

Occasionally poor prognostic features are found when a radical hysterectomy and lymphadenectomy specimen is examined histologically. Some of these features, such as lymph node involvement, are taken as an absolute indicator for postoperative adjuvant radiotherapy. Others are only relative indicators and the presence of only one such indicator would not warrant adjuvant radiotherapy (Thomas and Dembo, 1991).

Nodal status
Patients having stage IB carcinoma of the cervix with pelvic nodal involvement have a 5-year survival only half that of those with negative nodes, the number of nodes involved being a powerful prognostic factor (Inoue and Morita, 1990). The survival value of postoperative adjuvant radiotherapy or chemoradiotherapy against no postoperative treatment has not yet been proven in a randomised controlled clinical trial. However, the local recurrence rate was reduced in several historical series (Kinney *et al.*, 1989).

Lymphovascular permeation
Lymphovascular space involvement has a prognostic significance both in being an indicator of the likelihood of pelvic nodal involvement (Kamura *et al.*, 1993) and in having a prognostic effect even in the absence of nodal disease. In association with another relative indicator, such as narrow margins of excision or high tumour grade, it is taken as indicating a need for postoperative adjuvant therapy.

Histology
In some series patients with poorly differentiated squamous tumours have fared worse than those with well or moderately differentiated tumours. However, this has not been a universal finding and differentiation alone would not normally be taken as an absolute indicator for adjuvant radiotherapy.

Narrow margins

Margins of less than 5 mm on the fixed postoperative specimen are associated with local recurrence (Creasman *et al.*, 1986). If the narrow margin is at the edge of the vaginal cuff and there are no other poor prognostic features then adjuvant radiotherapy can be limited to the vaginal vault by using brachytherapy. If the narrow margins are within the paracervical tissues then external radiotherapy will be needed.

Pelvic radiotherapy is tolerated less well after surgery than when given as primary treatment, but it is usually possible to deliver 40–50 Gy over 5–6 weeks without undue late morbidity. If there is residual disease at the vaginal vault or at the margins of excision, then a second phase of treatment is needed to take the total tumour dose to at least 60–65 Gy, accepting that there is a greater likelihood of late morbidity. This may be minimised by restricting the treatment to the smallest volume of tissue necessary by using CT-planned external radiotherapy, intracavitary or interstitial brachytherapy, depending on the site and size of residual disease.

Special situations

The incidental finding of cervical cancer

Occasionally invasive cervical cancer is found in the specimen following a simple hysterectomy. If the depth of invasion indicates a risk of lymphatic spread (stage IB or further or if there are other poor prognostic features), then postoperative pelvic radiotherapy should be prescribed. If the vaginal cuff is inadequate then vault brachytherapy should also be delivered. With this technique the results of treatment are not worse than those of radical surgery or radical radiotherapy alone in terms of tumour cure, although morbidity may be higher (Roman *et al.*, 1993).

Cervical carcinoma during pregnancy

Treatment would be similar to that for non-pregnant patients in the first and second trimester of pregnancy, with treatment preceded by abortion or hysterotomy. Caesarean section should precede treatment in the third trimester when there is the chance of producing a viable child.

Haemorrhage

Carcinoma of the cervix can present with severe haemorrhage, which should be treated by firm vaginal packing, bed rest and blood transfusion. If this is ineffective, external radiotherapy may produce haemostasis within 24–48 hours. Classically, large fractions of at least 4 Gy have been used, without evidence that this is superior to standard fractions (1.8–2 Gy). In intractable cases, embolisation or ligation of the internal iliac arteries should be considered.

Recurrent carcinoma of the cervix

Recurrence following surgery can be treated by radiotherapy with concomitant chemotherapy to a dose of at least 63–65 Gy.

This usually involves a two-phase approach with external radiotherapy followed by a CT-planned small volume boost, intracavitary brachytherapy or interstitial brachytherapy. Very occasionally the last can be combined with debulking surgery as intra-operative brachytherapy, during which sensitive structures, such as the bowel, can be packed away from the high-dose regions and be spared damage.

Complications of treatment

Reactions to radiotherapy are divided into 'acute' reactions, which occur during or immediately after a radiotherapy course, and 'late' reactions, which arise more than 3 months later. Generally, acute reactions are transitory and manageable whereas late reactions can become chronic and difficult to manage. Radiotherapy regimens are designed assuming that all patients have a similar sensitivity, but a wide range of both acute and late reactions is seen at standard doses. The prediction of individual normal tissue radiosensitivity is in its infancy but, when developed, may allow a degree of 'tailoring' of radiotherapy regimens to suit individual patients. In the meantime, only crude criteria can be used to identify those at risk of developing a severe radiation reaction, with the exception of rare patients with conditions such as telangiectasia ataxia or xeroderma pigmentosum, who are highly radiosensitive. These criteria include identifying those who sunburn and blister without tanning and those with rheumatoid arthritis or other connective tissue disorders. These last groups may contain patients who have a defect of DNA repair, who may show exaggerated radiation sensitivity (Harris *et al.*, 1985). Patients with diabetic vascular changes or diverticulitis and those with inflammatory bowel disease, such as Crohn's disease and ulcerative colitis, may also show excessive radiation reactions in the bowel. Infection with HIV is said to worsen radiation reactions and is becoming more prevalent in women with cervical cancer.

The addition of concomitant cisplatin chemotherapy to radiotherapy worsens acute fatigue, haematological depression and gastrointestinal tract toxicity. Whether this will result in worse late effects remains to be seen.

Acute effects

At the dose levels necessary to treat carcinoma of the cervix with curative intent, some degree of acute radiation reaction in the bowel is common and results in diarrhoea, which starts in the second or third week of treatment. This can usually be controlled by a low-roughage, low-fat diet and an anti-motility drug such as codeine phosphate or loperamide. Radiation cystitis occurs less commonly than bowel disturbance and must be distinguished from infection. It is not uncommon for there to be an uncomfortable moist desquamation of the skin in the natal cleft.

Late effects

Late radiation effects usually become apparent months or years after treatment and may arise gradually over time or acutely following some other pelvic event, such as a ruptured bowel diverticulum or appendicitis. Severe late effects occur in approximately 6% of patients treated with radical radiotherapy in the UK (Denton *et al.*, 2000) and most frequently affect the bowel.

Rectal bleeding may result either from ulceration of the bowel mucosa or from radiation-induced telangiectasia. Recurrent cervical cancer and primary carcinoma of the bowel should be excluded by colonoscopy. Treatment of rectal bleeding may be by the use of steroid enemas and, occasionally, tranexamic acid may help in intractable cases. Sometimes cautery of the telangiectatic vessels by argon beam is helpful. Radiation damage may also cause stenosis or obstruction of the small bowel or sigmoid colon and this may occur at more than one level.

Late damage to the bladder may result in only a small volume of urine being tolerated, because fibrosis restricts expansion and high pressure in the bladder triggers the desire to micturate. Haematuria from telangiectasia may occur and must be distinguished from recurrent tumour or primary bladder cancer. Treatment with tranexamic acid may help lesser degrees of bleeding, but severe bleeding may be treatable only by urinary diversion. Post-radiotherapy ureteric stenosis can be due to radiation fibrosis but is more often caused by recurrent tumour on the pelvic sidewall.

Necrosis of the femoral heads seldom occurs with high-energy radiotherapy but pelvic osteopenia and 'insufficiency fractures' are not uncommon and may be misdiagnosed as bony metastases, which are very rare for cervical cancer. Lower limb oedema is seldom due to radiotherapy alone and is often a symptom of recurrent tumour in the pelvis or of a deep vein thrombosis. However, the incidence is increased after combination of radiotherapy and radical surgery, especially if the latter was associated with any infection or with pelvic lymphoceles.

Intracavitary brachytherapy produces a dose distribution which falls off rapidly with distance from the sources. Small changes in the relationship of normal tissues to the applicators may produce very large changes in the dose received by those tissues. Doses may be so large as to cause necrosis of the cervix, which may become infected and produce an unpleasant discharge. Necrosis can be disastrous if it occurs in the vaginal mucosa, rectum, bladder or terminal ureter as a fistula may ensue.

Hormonal changes

Radiotherapy to the ovaries will produce sterility after only 2–3 Gy, the dose delivered in the first one or two fractions of a radiotherapy course or from radiation 'scatter' to the ovaries outside the treated volume. Doses of 8–15 Gy usually produce a menopause in 1–3 months. Unopposed estrogen hormone replacement therapy may be used safely in patients who have

undergone a hysterectomy, but those who have not should be prescribed an estrogenic/progestogenic preparation. Although radical radiotherapy ablates the endometrium in the great majority of patients, a small percentage of patients will still have active endometrium, probably in the cornua. Not only may they have withdrawal bleeds but they can develop haematometra as the cervix is, generally, sclerosed and closed after brachytherapy.

Sexuality

Radiotherapy can lead to shortening and drying of the vagina with loss of lubrication and pliability. Shortening due to the formation of adhesions in the vagina can be avoided by regular douching during treatment and using a douche or dilator for a few months after treatment. However, radiation fibrosis in the walls of the vagina will still lead to some loss of length and pliability. Continued use of a vaginal dilator, with a lubricant gel, in those patients who have not resumed sexual activity, will maintain patency of the vagina, enabling resumption of sexual activity at a later date and also examination in the follow-up clinic.

CONCLUSION

Treatment of early disease with both radiotherapy and surgery is equally effective, but for more advanced tumours radiotherapy is preferable. Radiotherapy should consist of both an external beam phase and an intracavitary brachytherapy phase if curative doses are to be delivered without major normal tissue toxicity. Concomitant chemotherapy may benefit patients and has become standard for those fit to receive it as either primary or postoperative adjuvant treatment. Brachytherapy may be at high or low dose rate and, so far, little difference has been seen between the two when the high dose rate regimen is fractionated and the total dose reduced from that given at low dose rate. Mild radiotherapy side-effects are common but a small percentage of patients develop severe chronic reactions that require management by a specialist team of gynaecologist, oncologist, urologist and gastroenterologist.

REFERENCES

Blake P, Jones CH, Steel GG (2002) Intracavitary therapy. In: Souhami R, Tannock I, Hohenberger P *et al.* (eds) *Oxford Textbook of Oncology.* 2nd edn. New York: Oxford University Press, pp. 443–458.

Creasman WT, Hill GB, Weed JC *et al.* (1986) Radical hysterectomy as therapy for early carcinoma of the cervix. *American Journal of Obstetrics and Gynecology* 155: 964.

Denton AS, Bond SJ, Mathews S *et al.* (2000) Short report: national audit of the management and outcome of carcinoma of the cervix treated with radiotherapy in 1993. *Clinical Oncology* 12: 347–353.

Fowler JF (1997) Dose reduction factors when increasing dose rate in LDR or MDR brachytherapy of carcinoma of the cervix. *Radiotherapy and Oncology* 45: 49–54.

Fu K, Philips T (1990) High dose-rate versus low dose-rate intracavitary brachytherapy for carcinoma of the cervix. *International Journal of Radiation Oncology, Biology and Physics* 19: 791–796.

Green JA, Kirwan JM, Tierney JF *et al.* (2001) Survival and recurrence after concomitant chemotherapy and radiotherapy for cancer of the uterine cervix: a systematic review and meta-analysis. *Lancet* 358: 781–786.

Grogan M, Thomas GM, Melamed I *et al.* (1999) The importance of hemoglobin levels during radiotherapy for carcinoma of the cervix. *Cancer* 86: 1528.

Harris G, Cramp WA, Edwards JC *et al.* (1985) Radiosensitivity of peripheral blood lymphocytes in autoimmune disease. *International Journal of Radiation Biology* 47: 689–699.

Hunter RD (1994) Dose rate correction in LDR intracavitary therapy. In: Mould RF, Martinez AA, Batfermann JJ *et al.* (eds) *Brachytherapy from Radium to Optimisation*. Veenendaal, the Netherlands: Nucletron International BV, pp. 55–59.

Inoue T, Morita K (1990) The prognostic significance of number of positive nodes cervical carcinoma stages Ib, IIa and IIb. *Cancer* 65: 1923.

Kamura T, Tsukamoto N, Tsuruchi N *et al.* (1993) Histopathological prognostic factors in stage IIb cervical carcinoma treated with radical hysterectomy and pelvic node dissection: an analysis with mathematical statistics. *International Journal of Gynecological Cancer* 3: 219–225.

Kinney WK, Alvarez RD, Reid GC *et al.* (1989) Value of adjuvant whole-pelvis irradiation after Wertheim hysterectomy for early-stage squamous carcinoma of the cervix with pelvic nodal metastasis: a matched-control study. *Gynecologic Oncology* 34: 258.

Morris M, Eifel PJ, Lu J *et al.* (1999) Pelvic radiation with concurrent chemotherapy compared with pelvic and para-aortic radiation for high-risk cervical cancer. *New England Journal of Medicine* 340: 1137–1143.

Patel FG, Sharma SC, Negi PS *et al.* (1994) Low dose rate vs high dose rate brachytherapy in the treatment of carcinoma of the uterine cervix: a clinical trial. *International Journal of Radiation Oncology, Biology and Physics* 28: 335–341.

Peters WA III, Liu PY Barret RJ *et al.* (2000) Concurrent chemotherapy and pelvic radiation therapy compared with pelvic radiation therapy alone as adjuvant therapy after radical surgery in high-risk early-stage cancer of the cervix. *Journal of Clinical Oncology* 18: 1606–1613.

Roman LD, Morris M, Eifel PJ *et al.* (1993) Prognostic factors for patients undergoing simple hysterectomy in the presence of invasive cancer of the cervix. *Gynecologic Oncology* 50: 179.

Rose PG, Bundy BN, Watkins EB *et al.* (1999) Concurrent cisplatin-based chemotherapy and radiotherapy for locally advanced cervical cancer. *New England Journal of Medicine* 340: 1144–1153.

Tanaka E, Ryoong-Jin O, Yamada Y *et al.* (2003) Prospective study of HDR (192Ir) versus MDR (137Cs) intracavitary brachytherapy for carcinoma of the uterine cervix. *Brachytherapy* 2: 85–90.

Thomas GM, Dembo AJ (1991) Is there a role for adjuvant pelvic radiotherapy after radical hysterectomy in early stage cervical cancer? *International Journal of Gynecological Cancer* 1: 1.

CHAPTER 43

Management of cervical cancer by radiotherapy and chemotherapy

H. Margot L. Lehman and Gillian M. Thomas

For patients who present with small volume, organ-confined cervical cancer (stages IA and IB1), surgery and radiotherapy have proven to be effective definitive therapies, resulting in 5-year survival figures of 85–95% (Alvarez *et al.*, 1991; Eifel *et al.*, 1994; Landoni *et al.*, 1997). For locally advanced disease (stages IB2–IVA), treatment with a combination of external beam radiotherapy and intracavitary brachytherapy has produced less favourable results with 5-year survival figures of 65–75% for stage IIB, 45–50% for stage IIIA, 25–30% for stage IIIB and 10–15% for stage IVA reported in the literature (Lanciano *et al.*, 1991; Lowrey *et al.*, 1992; Barillot *et al.*, 1997; Logsdon *et al.*, 1999). The major impediment to cure by the use of radiation therapy alone is persistent or recurrent local disease. Unfortunately, increasing the radiation dose would exceed the radiation tolerance of normal pelvic structures (rectum and bladder) and lead to an unacceptable incidence of late effects. Thus, alternative strategies aimed at improving the efficacy of radiation therapy have been developed. One strategy involves combining radiation with chemotherapeutic agents, either in a sequential (neoadjuvant) or concurrent fashion.

NEOADJUVANT CHEMOTHERAPY

The theoretical advantages of administering chemotherapeutic agents prior to definitive radiation are: (1) a reduction in tumour volume may facilitate the delivery of radiation therapy; (2) an intact tumour vascular supply undamaged by prior therapy may facilitate the delivery of chemotherapeutic agents; (3) less toxicity associated with the administration of a single modality may allow maximum doses of chemotherapy to be delivered; and (4) micrometastatic disease will be treated earlier.

The theoretical limitations of this approach are: (1) cross-resistance and sensitivity may develop between the chemotherapeutic agents and radiation therapy; (2) toxicity associated with initial chemotherapy may compromise the intensity of delivery of subsequent radiation therapy; and (3) prolongation of overall treatment time may result in accelerated repopulation of tumour clones, inhibiting local tumour control (Withers *et al.*, 1988).

The salient features and findings of nine phase III trials comparing neoadjuvant chemotherapy and radiation therapy to radiation therapy alone in stages IB2–IVA cervical cancer are presented in Table 43.1.

No benefit for neoadjuvant chemotherapy was found in seven studies whereas improved survival with radiation therapy alone was found in two studies. Because individual studies lacked the power to detect a survival difference, the Medical Research Council (MRC), United Kingdom, undertook a meta-analysis of the available data. No survival benefit for neoadjuvant chemotherapy at either 2 years [odds ratio (OR) = 1.09, 95% confidence interval (CI) = 0.83–1.45, $P = 0.37$] or 3 years (OR = 0.96, 95% CI = 0.73–1.25, $P = 0.45$) was evident (Tierney *et al.*, 1999). This analysis was considered inconclusive because survival data were not available for all patients. The results of a subsequent MRC meta-analysis utilising updated individual data from 2074 patients enrolled in 18 randomised controlled trials of neoadjuvant chemotherapy conducted between 1982 and 1995 are available (Tierney and Stewart, 2002). The pooled hazard ratio (HR) for death was 1.01 with a 95% confidence interval of 0.88–1.10 ($P = 0.913$).

Thus, a survival benefit for the addition of neoadjuvant chemotherapy to radical radiation therapy in the management of locally advanced cervical cancer has not been demonstrated.

CONCURRENT CHEMORADIATION

Rationale

The concurrent administration of chemotherapy and radiotherapy has theoretical advantages over the use of neoadjuvant chemotherapy. Concurrent administration avoids any delay in the initiation of the primary therapeutic modality (radiotherapy) and shortens the overall treatment duration; both are important in minimising tumour cell repopulation, which can negatively impact on local tumour control (Withers *et al.*, 1988).

Proposed mechanisms for the benefit of administering chemotherapy concurrently with radiotherapy include (1) the two modalities targeting different cell populations in the

Table 43.1 Randomised controlled trials comparing neoadjuvant chemotherapy and radiation therapy to radiation therapy alone in stages IB2–IVA cervical cancer.

Author	n	Regimen	Response CT/RT (%)	Response RT (%)	Survival CT/RT (%)	Survival RT (%)	P
Chauvergne *et al.*, 1990	138	MtxCVP	84.9	88.9	63	60	ns
Tobias *et al.*, 1990	66	BIP	75	56	–	–	ns
Souhami *et al.*, 1991	107	BOMP	47	32	23	39	0.02
Cardenas *et al.*, 1992	28	PEpCy	5	86	36	50	ns
Kumar *et al.*, 1994	177	BIP	70	69	38	43	ns
Leborgne *et al.*, 1997	130	BOP	68	65	38	49	ns
Tattersall *et al.*, 1995	260	EpP	72	92	47	70	0.02
Sundfor *et al.*, 1996	94	PF	53	57	38	40	ns
Chiara *et al.*, 1994	58	P	78	81	72	83	ns

CT, chemotherapy; RT, radiotherapy; Mtx, methotrexate; C, chlorambucil; V, vinblastine; P, cisplatin; B, bleomycin; I, ifosfamide; O, vincristine; M, mitomycin C; Ep, epirubicin; Cy, cyclophosphamide; F, 5-fluorouracil; ns, not significant.

Table 43.2 Chemotherapy agents employed in trials of concurrent chemoradiation in the management of locally advanced cervical cancer.

Agent → MOA ↓	Cisplatin	5-FU	Hydroxyurea	Mitomycin C
Inhibition of repair of SLD	+	+	+	–
Hypoxic cell sensitisation	+	–	–	–
Recruiting cells into S phase	–	+	–	–
Synchronising cells in G1–S	–	–	+	–
Cytotoxic to cells in S phase	–	–	+	–
Comments	Most active single agent; limited bone marrow toxicity; renal toxicity	Radiosensitisation time and dose dependent; diarrhoea dose-limiting	Synergistic with 5-FU; haematological toxicity	Selectively cytotoxic to hypoxic cells; increased rate of late bowel complications

SLD, sublethal damage.

target tumour leading to independent but additive cytotoxic effects (additive effects); and (2) interaction between the two modalities at the molecular or cellular level leading to enhanced tumour cell kill (supra-additive effects).

Chemotherapeutic agents — mechanism of action

The chemotherapy agents most frequently used in gynaecological oncology practice and their proposed mechanism of action are detailed in Table 43.2.

Cisplatin

Cisplatin is the most active cytotoxic agent in the management of cervical cancer. The exact mechanism by which cisplatin interacts with radiotherapy is unknown, but possible mechanisms include inhibition of repair of radiation-induced sublethal DNA damage and sensitisation of hypoxic cells (Carde and Laval, 1981). Kallman *et al.* (1991) found that combinations of cisplatin and radiation were supra-additive, yielding similar tumour regrowth delay whether the drug was given in a single dose before five fractions of radiotherapy or in divided daily doses with radiotherapy. The limited bone marrow toxicity associated with cisplatin makes it an ideal agent to combine with radiation. The most important dose-limiting toxicity of cisplatin is renal. This is relevant because renal impairment (from ureteric obstruction) is a common finding at the time of diagnosis of locally advanced cervical cancer.

5-Fluorouracil

5-Fluorouracil (5-FU) enhances radiation cytotoxicity by (1) inhibiting the repair of radiation-induced sublethal DNA damage and (2) recruiting cells into the radiation-sensitive S phase of the cell cycle. *In vitro* data suggest that 5-FU's mechanism of radiosensitisation is both time and dose dependent. Maximum tumour cell kill is observed when cells are exposed to low concentration of 5-FU for at least 24–48 hours (Byfield *et al.*, 1982). This is the rationale for the use of infusional 5-FU in combination with radiotherapy. Diarrhoea is the predominant dose-limiting toxic effect of infusional 5-FU, of concern in patients receiving pelvic radiotherapy.

Hydroxyurea

Hydroxyurea is believed to act by: (1) synchronising cells in the G1–S interphase from which they progress to the more radiation-sensitive S phase; (2) inhibiting the repair of radiation-induced sublethal DNA damage; and (3) directly killing cells in the S phase of the cell cycle (Phillips and Tolmach, 1966; Sinclair, 1968; Piver *et al.*, 1972). Hydroxyurea has been shown to be synergistic with 5-FU. Hydroxyurea inhibits ribonucleotide reductase, which decreases the formation of deoxyuridine monophosphate (dUMP). dUMP normally functions to inhibit the binding of the active form of 5-FU, fluorodeoxyuridine monophosphate (FdUMP), to thymidylate synthase. Thus, in the absence of dUMP, FdUMP binds thymidylate synthase unimpeded, leading to enhanced inhibition of DNA synthesis. This is the rationale for the combined use of 5-FU, hydroxyurea and radiotherapy. The major toxicities associated with the use of hydroxyurea are haematological.

Mitomycin C

Mitomycin C is an alkylating agent and inhibits DNA and RNA synthesis. Laboratory and animal studies have demonstrated that mitomycin C does not interact with radiation but is selectively cytotoxic to hypoxic cells. The incorporation of mitomycin C into treatment regimens was based on the effectiveness of this agent in regimens used to treat squamous cell carcinoma of the anus (Nigro *et al.*, 1983). However, a retrospective review of patients entered in a series of phase II studies demonstrated a significantly increased rate of serious late bowel complications in those who received a regimen containing mitomycin C rather than 5-FU alone (Rakovitch *et al.*, 1997).

Historical development

Early Gynaecologic Oncology Group trials

Early randomised studies of combined modality therapy were conducted by the Gynaecologic Oncology Group (GOG) and used hydroxyurea. The GOG randomised patients with stage IIIB or IVA squamous cell carcinoma of the cervix to receive either standard radiotherapy or radiotherapy and concurrent hydroxyurea. The addition of hydroxyurea resulted in a higher complete response rate (68% vs. 49%), longer median progression-free interval (13.6 months vs. 7.6 months) and a longer median survival (19.5 months vs. 10.7 months) (Hreshchyshyn *et al.*, 1979). These findings are questionable because 53% of the randomised patients were deemed ineligible or unevaluable and thus excluded from analysis and because doses of radiation lower than what are now considered optimal were used.

In a subsequent GOG protocol (GOG 56), 296 patients with surgically staged node-negative stage IIB to IVA disease were randomised to receive radiation concurrent with either hydroxyurea or the hypoxic cell sensitiser misonidazole. On subset analysis, patients with stage IIIB or IVA disease who received

hydroxyurea were found to have a statistically significant improvement in progression-free survival (42.9 months vs. 40.4 months) but not survival, compared with those who received misonidazole (Stehman *et al.*, 1993). This study was taken as confirmation of the benefit of hydroxyurea in the management of cervical cancer and the GOG subsequently adopted the combination of hydroxyurea and radiotherapy as the standard therapy against which future therapies were to be tested.

The results of a study conducted by the Radiation Therapy Oncology Group (RTOG) (RTOG 80-05) challenged the apparent benefit of hydroxyurea (Leibel *et al.*, 1987). A total of 120 patients with stage IIIB or IVA squamous cell carcinoma of the cervix were randomised to receive either standard radiotherapy or radiotherapy and misonidazole. Patients who received misonidazole had survival rates similar to or slightly worse than those patients treated with conventional radiotherapy. This raised concern that the observed difference in GOG 56 was due to a reduced survival associated with the use of misonidazole rather than additional benefit from hydroxyurea.

In the absence of positive results from well-conducted trials it can be concluded that the benefit of hydroxyurea is unproven. Indeed, outside the GOG, this agent has not been incorporated into treatment protocols.

Single-institution trials

The results of a phase III trial conducted by Wong *et al.* (1989) found no survival benefit for the use of concurrent low-dose cisplatin in patients with stage IIB and III disease. A study conducted by Thomas *et al.* (1998), which closed without having reached its target patient accrual, found no improvement in pelvic control or overall survival with the addition of infusional 5-FU in patients with bulky IB to IVA disease. A phase III trial conducted by Lorvidhaya *et al.* (2003) demonstrated a statistically significant improvement in disease-free survival but not overall survival when mitomycin C and oral 5-FU were administered concurrently with radiotherapy in patients with stages IIB and IIIB disease. These results did not have the power to impact upon patterns of practice.

Multi-institution randomised controlled trials

Patterns of practice did change with the coincident announcement in 1999 of the results of five multi-institution randomised controlled trials demonstrating a survival advantage for the use of combined modality therapy over radiotherapy alone in the management of locally advanced cervical cancer (Keys *et al.*, 1999; Morris *et al.*, 1999; Rose *et al.*, 1999; Whitney *et al.*, 1999; Peters *et al.*, 2000). While these studies differed in their inclusion criteria, radiotherapy regimens and chemotherapy protocols, their results suggested a need to redefine the standard approach to the management of cervical cancer. Indeed the NCI issued a rare clinical alert stating that 'strong consideration should be given to the incorporation of concurrent cisplatin-based chemotherapy in women who

Table 43.3 Randomised controlled trials comparing concurrent chemoradiation with radiation therapy alone in locally advanced cervical cancer.

Trial	n	Stage	Staging	Control arm	Trial arm
Keys GOG 123	369	IB	Simple TAH	XRT	XRT + C 40 mg/m^2 i.v. weekly × 6 weeks
Whitney GOG 85	368	IIB–IVA	Yes	XRT + HU 80 mg/kg p.o. 2 ×/week	XRT + C 50 mg/m^2 i.v. days 1, 29 + 5-FU infusion 1 g/m^2/day days 2–5 and 30–33
Rose GOG 120	526	IIB–IVA	Yes	XRT+HU 3 g/m^2 p.o. 2 ×/week	XRT + C 40 mg/m^2 i.v. weekly × 6 weeks vs. XRT + C 50 mg/m^2 i.v. days 1, 29 + 5-FU infusion 1 g/m^2/day days 1–4, 29–33 + HU po 2 g/m^2 2 ×/week × 6 weeks
Morris RTOG 9001	386	IIB–IVA, IB–IIA*	Yes (25%)	XRT (pelvic + PA)	XRT + C 75 mg/m^2 i.v. day 1 + 5-FU infusion 1 g/m^2/day days 1–5 (3 cycles at 3-weekly intervals)
Peters SWOG 8797	243	IA2, IB, IIA*	Yes	XRT	XRT + C 70 mg/m^2 i.v. + 5-FU 1 g/m^2 infusion days 1–5 (4 cycles at 3 weekly intervals)
Pearcey NCIC	253	IB*–IVA	No	XRT	XRT+ C 40 mg/m^2/week

TAH, total abdominal hysterectomy; XRT, radiation therapy; C, cisplatin; HU, hydroxyurea; 5-FU, 5-fluorouracil; i.v., intravenously; p.o., by mouth.

Table 43.4 Results of randomised controlled trials comparing concurrent chemoradiotherapy with radiotherapy alone in locally advanced cervical cancer.

Trial	Follow-up (months)	PFS (%) XRT XRT/CT	OS (%) XRT XRT/CT
Keys	36	63/79*	74/85*
Whitney	104	47/57*	43/55*
Rose	35	47/67*	66*
		64*	67*
Morris	43	40/67*	58/73*
	78		41/67*
Peters	42	63/80*	71/81*
Pearcey	82	58/62	58/62

*$P < 0.05$; PFS, progression-free survival; OS, overall survival; CT, chemotherapy; XRT, radiation therapy.

require radiation therapy for treatment of cervical cancer' (National Cancer Institute, 1999).

In contrast to the findings of these five studies, the results of the National Cancer Institute of Canada (NCIC) trial (Pearcey *et al.*, 2002) published later did not demonstrate a survival benefit for the concurrent administration of chemotherapy and radiotherapy.

In Table 43.3, the treatment protocols of each of the six randomised controlled trials are presented and, in Table 43.4, the results achieved in each trial are documented.

GOG 123

In the study conducted by Keys *et al.*, the concurrent administration of single-agent cisplatin (40 mg/m^2 weekly for 6 weeks) and radiotherapy in patients with bulky stage IB disease resulted in a statistically significant improvement in progression-free and overall survival compared with radiotherapy alone. The study was large enough ($n = 369$) to make the results meaningful and the overall duration of treatment (median 50 days, range 21–90 days) was acceptable. However, the total radiation dose prescribed to point A (75 Gy) was low. This was because all patients proceeded to an extrafascial hysterectomy at the completion of radiotherapy because of concern that patients with bulky stage IB disease had higher rates of pelvic failure when treated with radiotherapy alone. This decision was made before the results of a GOG study, showing no survival advantage with the addition of a completion hysterectomy, were available. However, since all study patients proceeded to a hysterectomy the benefit or lack of benefit of this procedure should be apparent in both groups. Thus the progression-free and overall survival benefit achieved with chemotherapy should be considered real.

GOG 85; GOG 120

These trials studied patients with more extensive disease (stages IIB–IVA) (Rose *et al.*, 1999; Whitney *et al.*, 1999). GOG 85 was opened first and randomised patients to receive pelvic radiotherapy given concurrently with either hydroxyurea or a combination of cisplatin and infusional 5-FU. As an early interim analysis of this trial did not demonstrate a difference between these two treatment arms, the GOG then adopted hydroxyurea as the control in its subsequent trial (GOG 120) and compared this regimen with either weekly cisplatin alone or a combination of cisplatin, 5-FU and hydroxyurea. All patients received pelvic radiotherapy. In both trials, eligible patients were subjected to surgical staging and excluded if found to be para-aortic node positive, thereby selecting a cohort of patients more likely to benefit from improved local control. The results of GOG 85 were reported at a median follow-up of 8.7 years and demonstrated statistically significant better progression-free and overall survival rates for patients randomised to the cisplatin treatment arm. The results of GOG 120 were reported with a shorter follow-up and also demonstrated superior progression-free and overall survival rates for patients enrolled in the cisplatin-containing arms compared with patients receiving hydroxyurea. An analysis of failure patterns demonstrated that those patients receiving cisplatin had lower incidences of both pelvic failure (19% and 20%) and pulmonary metastases (3% and 4%) than those receiving concurrent hydroxyurea (pelvic failure rate 30%, pulmonary metastases 10%). The highest incidence of adverse effects was observed in those patients receiving the three-drug regimen. Thus, the GOG has adopted single-agent cisplatin as the chemotherapy agent of choice to be given concurrently with radiation.

The GOG studies have been criticised because the total radiation dose delivered was comparatively low (80.8–81 Gy) and the overall treatment duration (median 63 days) was prolonged. These deficiencies in radiotherapy delivery may have magnified the apparent benefit of chemotherapy. The authors argue that, because the dose and duration of radiotherapy for each arm of these trials were nearly identical, the observed survival benefit was due to the intervention — cisplatin-based chemoradiation. Assessment of the relative risk reduction observed when patients were partitioned into those who received 'optimal' radiotherapy (defined as having received more than 85% of the prescribed dose without any substantial delay, median treatment time 57 days) and those who received 'protracted' radiation therapy confirmed the presence of a statistically significant reduction in the risk of death with the addition of cisplatin-based chemotherapy (Bundy, 2002). The results of tests looking for a differential benefit between optimal and protracted radiation subgroups were not significant. This analysis suggests that adding cisplatin-based chemotherapy to both optimal and protracted radiation therapy is beneficial.

RTOG 9001

The Morris study for the RTOG differed from the previous studies in several ways. Patients randomised to the control arm received radiation therapy alone. Radiation was delivered to both pelvic and para-aortic fields as a previous RTOG study had demonstrated a survival advantage for this approach in predominantly clinically staged IB and IIB disease (Rotman *et al.*, 1995). The experimental arm consisted of chemotherapy given concurrently with radiotherapy delivered to the pelvis only because a previous phase II trial of combined chemotherapy and extended field radiotherapy had shown unacceptable toxicity (Grigsby Petal, 2001). In both arms, the radiotherapy was delivered in an 'optimal' fashion with a higher median radiation dose delivered to point A (89 Gy) and a shorter

median duration of treatment (58 days). A more aggressive chemotherapy regimen was utilised with a higher dose of cisplatin (75 mg/m^2) given in combination with 5-FU and a third cycle of chemotherapy scheduled to coincide with one of the intracavitary procedures. Finally, while eligible patients needed to be para-aortic node negative, only 25% of patients in each arm were subjected to surgical staging. Thus, the patient cohort was less highly selected than the cohorts participating in the Rose and Whitney trials. This study was initially reported with a median follow-up of 43 months, at which time a statistically significant disease-free and overall survival advantage was apparent for chemoradiotherapy over extended field radiotherapy alone. An assessment of the patterns of failure demonstrated that chemoradiation decreased the rate of both local and distant failure and, while acute toxicity was more common with concurrent chemoradiotherapy, late complication rates were similar.

Updated results of RTOG 9001, with a median follow-up of 6.6 years, continue to show a survival advantage for chemoradiotherapy (Eifel *et al.*, 2004). The addition of chemotherapy provided an overall reduction in the risk of death or recurrence of 51% (95% CI 34–64%) and an overall reduction in the risk of locoregional recurrence of 58% (95% CI 36–72%). Furthermore, at 5 years the cumulative incidence of grade 3 or higher late complications was the same in both arms (14%).

SWOG 8797: combined modality therapy in the adjuvant setting

Peters *et al.* (2000) reported the results of a cooperative study of the Southwest Oncology Group, GOG and RTOG which evaluated the role of combined modality therapy in the adjuvant setting. Patients with stage IB or IIA disease considered at high risk of recurrence following hysterectomy and pelvic lymphadenectomy because of positive pelvic nodes, positive parametria or positive surgical margins were randomised to receive either radiotherapy alone or radiotherapy and chemotherapy. A total dose of 49.3 Gy was delivered to the pelvis via external beam therapy. If high common iliac nodes were involved, the para-aortic nodes received 45 Gy. The chemotherapy regimen consisted of cisplatin (70 mg/m^2) and a 96-hour infusion of 5-FU given every 3 weeks for four cycles. With a median follow-up of 43 months, the 3-year survival for women receiving adjuvant concurrent chemotherapy with radiation was significantly better than that achieved with adjuvant radiotherapy alone. Updated results with a median follow-up of 5.2 years continue to demonstrate a survival advantage with the addition of chemotherapy (Monk *et al.*, 2005).

An exploratory hypothesis-generating reanalysis of this study has been undertaken to determine which sub-group of patients benefited most from the addition of chemotherapy. The results suggested that the addition of adjuvant chemotherapy to radiotherapy after radical hysterectomy is beneficial regardless of patient age, histological type or tumour grade. However, the absolute benefit appeared to be smaller in women with tumours ≤ 2 cm or where only one node was positive. (Monk *et al.*, 2005). These findings need to be explored in properly designed randomised controlled trials.

The NCIC trial

In contrast to the previous studies, the NCIC trial (Pearcey *et al.*, 2002) was negative. In this trial, 253 patients with stages IB (> 5 cm) to IVA squamous cervical cancer were randomised to receive either pelvic radiotherapy alone or pelvic radiotherapy and weekly cisplatin at a dose of 40 mg/m^2. In both arms the total cumulative radiation dose prescribed to point A was acceptable at 80 Gy and the mean duration of treatment was 50.4 days for patients treated with radiation alone and 51.3 days for those receiving combined-modality therapy. At 3 years and 5 years of follow-up no significant difference in survival was observed.

However, it is possible that the NCIC trial result is not inconsistent with the findings of the other five trials due to statistical variation. The NCIC trial demonstrated a 12% lower death rate for the chemoradiation group compared with the control group, but the 95% confidence intervals around this risk reducation were wide, suggesting that the true effect could lie anywhere between a 40% and a 30% increase in the risk of death. This range incorporates the pooled relative reduction in risk of death for all six trials (36%).

Other chemoradiation trials

The results of a single institution trial from the Queen Mary Hospital, Hong Kong, published after the NCI announcement, also provided a positive result for combined chemoradiation therapy (Wong *et al.*, 1999). A total of 220 patients with clinically staged bulky stage I, II or III cervical cancer were randomised to receive either standard pelvic radiation therapy or standard pelvic radiotherapy with 60 mg/m^2 epirubicin given on the first day followed by 90 mg/m^2 given as a bolus every 4 weeks for five courses. No effort to synchronise the chemotherapy and radiation therapy was made. With a median follow-up of 77 months, patients who received radiation therapy and epirubicin demonstrated significantly longer disease-free and cumulative survival than those treated with radiation therapy alone. The addition of epirubicin decreased the incidence of distant failure whereas the incidence of central recurrence was similar.

Concurrent chemoradiation versus radiotherapy alone: meta-analysis

A Cochrane systematic review based on the results of 4921 women enrolled in 24 randomised controlled trials (21 published, 3 unpublished) of concomitant chemotherapy and radiation therapy in cervical cancer has recently been published (Green *et al.*, 2005). However, because of patient exclusion

and differential reporting the analyses were based on 61% to 75% of the total number of women randomised. The meta-analysis demonstrated a 10% absolute improvement in survival (95% CI 7–13%) and a 13% absolute improvement in progression-free survival (95% CI 10–16%) with the concurrent administration of chemoradiotherapy. A significant reduction in the rate of local recurrence was observed but in contrast to the preceding analysis (Green *et al.*, 2001) the reduction in the rate of distant metastases was not statistically significant. Acute haematological and gastrointestinal toxicity was significantly greater in the concurrent chemoradiotherapy group but late effects were not well reported so that the impact of combined modality therapy on these effects could not be determined. As the results were inconsistent across trials, the Meta-analysis Group of the UK Medical Research Council (MRC) Clinical Trials Unit has initiated an international, collaborative systematic review and meta-analysis of individual patient data to more fully define the role of concomitant chemoradiotherapy in cervical cancer, to determine whether particular sub-groups of patients benefit more or less from chemoradiotherapy, and to evaluate long-term toxicity.

While the weight of evidence presented favours the use of combined-modality therapy in the management of locally advanced cervical cancer, a number of questions remain. Firstly, the best chemotherapy regimen to use concurrently with radiation and the optimal route of administration, dose and schedule for that agent is uncertain. Cisplatin is the most active systemic agent currently available for use in metastatic or recurrent disease and its limited bone marrow toxicity makes it an ideal agent to use in combination with radiotherapy. However, a number of different cisplatin schedules were employed in the six randomised controlled trials previously discussed, making the choice of the 'ideal' regimen difficult. The results of the GOG studies would suggest the use of single-agent cisplatin, as this regimen resulted in equivalent survival figures but less toxicity than a three-drug regimen of cisplatin, 5-FU and hydroxyurea. The RTOG study employed the highest dose intensity of cisplatin in combination with 5-FU. Whether 5-FU has a role to play in the management of cervical cancer is uncertain.

The results of GOG 165, which randomised patients with stage IIB to IVA disease to either pelvic radiotherapy and concurrent weekly cisplatin (40 mg/m^2) or radiotherapy and a protracted venous infusion (PVI) of 5-FU (225 mg/m^2/day for 5 days/week for six cycles) have been published (Lanciano *et al.*, 2005). This study was closed prematurely when a planned interim futility analysis indicated that PVI FU/radiotherapy had a 35% higher treatment failure rate and would, most likely, not result in an improvement in progression-free survival compared with weekly cisplatin/radiotherapy.

Results have now been published with a median follow-up of those still alive at the time of analysis of 40.4 months. The unadjusted relative risk for recurrence was 1.29 (95% CI 0.93–1.80) and the unadjusted relative risk for recurrence was

1.37 (95% CI 0.90–1.74) in the PVI FU arm. While this result indicates that protracted venous infusion FU is not superior to weekly cisplatin in combination with radiation, the question as to whether FU given in combination with cisplatin and radiation is a superior regimen remains unanswered. There is currently no trial comparing a combination of the two drugs with either drug alone.

THE FUTURE

Clinical trials of chemoradiotherapy using new and established chemotherapeutic agents and biological response modifiers are currently being undertaken in a variety of solid tumour types. In the future, direct comparisons between cisplatin and the drug regimens found efficacious in these studies will need to be made. However, given the high incidence of advanced cervical cancer in developing nations, emphasis needs to be given to cost-effectiveness.

Future studies should also address chemotherapy scheduling issues. In particular, (1) the impact of chemotherapy administration at the time of the intracavitary insertion (when a significant component of the central pelvic dose is delivered) and (2) the impact of adjuvant chemotherapy on the incidence of distant metastases need to be studied. These studies also need to include quality of life assessments and address toxicity issues.

Finally, further analysis may allow us to determine whether the effect of treatment differs between sub-groups of patients.

CONCLUSION

In conclusion, over recent years a body of evidence has accumulated indicating that the concurrent administration of chemotherapy and radiotherapy should be considered the new standard of care for the management of locally advanced cervical cancer. While an advance has been made, questions still remain regarding the optimal chemotherapy regimen to use in combination with radiation therapy. Attempts to answer this question will be the focus of future trials.

REFERENCES

Alvarez RD, Potter ME, Soong SJ *et al.* (1991) Rationale for using pathologic tumor dimensions and nodal status to subclassify surgically treated stage IB cervical cancer patients. *Gynecologic Oncology* 43: 108–112.

Barillot I, Horiot JC, Pegneux J *et al.* (1997) Carcinoma of the intact uterine cervix treated with radiotherapy alone: a French co-operative study: update and multivariate analysis of prognostics factors. *International Journal of Radiation Oncology, Biology and Physics* 38: 969.

Bundy B (2002) Chemoradiation for locally advanced cervical cancer: Does it help? *Journal of Clinical Oncology* 20: 891–893.

Byfield JE, Calabro-Jones P, Klisar I *et al.* (1982) Pharmacologic requirements for obtaining sensitization of human tumour cells *in vitro* to combined 5-fluorouracil and X-rays. *International Journal of Radiation Oncology, Biology and Physics* 59: 2422–2427.

Carde P, Laval F (1981) Effect of cis-dichlorodiammine platinum II and X-rays on mammalian cell survival. *International Journal of Radiation Oncology, Biology and Physics* 7: 922–933.

Cardenas J, Olguin A, Figueroa F *et al.* (1992) Neoadjuvant chemotherapy and radiotherapy versus radiotherapy alone in stage IIIB cervical carcinoma. Preliminary results. *Proceedings of the American Society of Clinical Oncology* 11: abstract 232.

Chauvergne J, Rohart J, Heron JF *et al.* (1990) Essai randomise de chimiotherapie initiale dans 151 carcinomes du col uterin localement eteridus (T2b-N1, T3b, M0). *Bulletin du Cancer (Paris)* 77: 1007–1024.

Chiara S, Bruzzone M, Merlini L *et al.* (1994) Randomised study comparing chemotherapy plus radiotherapy versus radiotherapy alone in FIGO stage IIB–III cervical carcinoma. *American Journal of Clinical Oncology* 17: 294–297.

Eifel PJ, Morris M, Wharton JT *et al.* (1994) The influence of tumor size and morphology on the outcome of patients with FIGO stage IB squamous cell carcinoma of the uterine cervix. *International Journal of Radiation Oncology, Biology and Physics* 29: 9–16.

Eifel PJ, Winter K, Morris M *et al.* (2002) Pelvic radiation with concurrent chemotherapy versus pelvic and para-aortic radiation for high-risk cervical cancer: an update of RTOG 90-01. *International Journal of Radiation Oncology, Biology and Physics* 54: 2 ASTRO 2002: 1.

Green J, Kirwan JM, Tierney JF *et al.* (2005) Concomitant chemotherapy and radiation therapy for cancer of the uterine cervix. *Cochrane Database of Systematic Reviews* 3 CD002225.pub2. DOI: 10.1002/14651858.CD002225.pub2.

Green JA, Kirwan JM, Tierney JF *et al.* (2001) Survival and recurrence after concomitant chemotherapy and radiotherapy for cancer of the uterine cervix: a systematic review and meta-analysis. *Lancet* 9284: 781–786.

Grigsby Petal W, Heydon K, Mutch DG *et al.* (2001) Longterm follow-up of RTOG 92-10: Cervical cancer with positive para-aortic lymph nodes. *International Journal of Radiation Oncology, Biology and Physics* 51: 982–987.

Grogan M, Thomas G, Melamed I *et al.* (1999) The importance of hemoglobin levels during radiotherapy for carcinoma of the cervix. *Cancer* 86: 1528–1536.

Kallman RF, Rapacchietto D, Zaghloul MS (1991) Schedule-dependent therapeutic gain from the combination of fractionated irradiation plus C-DDP + 5-FU or plus C-DDP + cyclophosphamide in C3H/Km mouse model systems. *International Journal of Radiation Oncology, Biology and Physics* 20: 227–232.

Keys HM, Bundy BN, Stehman FB *et al.* (1999) Cisplatin, radiation and adjuvant hysterectomy compared with radiation and adjuvant hysterectomy for bulky stage IB cervical carcinoma. *New England Journal of Medicine* 340: 1154–1161.

Kumar L, Kaushal R, Nandy M *et al.* (1994) Chemotherapy followed by radiotherapy versus radiotherapy alone in locally advanced cervical cancer: a randomized study. *Gynecologic Oncology* 54: 307–315.

Lanciano RM, Won M, Coia LR (1991) Pre-treatment and treatment factors associated with improved outcomes in squamous cell carcinoma of the uterine cervice: a final report of the 1973 and 1978 Patterns of Care Studies. *International Journal of Radiation Oncology, Biology and Physics* 20: 667–676.

Landoni F, Maneo A, Colombo A *et al.* (1997) Randomised study of radical surgery versus radiotherapy for stage IB–IIA cervical cancer. *Lancet* 350: 535–540.

Leborgne F, Leborgne JH, Doldan R *et al.* (1997) Induction chemotherapy and radiotherapy of advanced cancer of the cervix: a pilot study and phase III randomized trial. *International Journal of Radiation Oncology, Biology and Physics* 37: 343–350.

Leibel S, Bauer M, Wasserman T *et al.* (1987) Radiotherapy with or without misonidazole for patients with stage IIIB or stage IVA squamous cell carcinoma of the uterine cervix: preliminary report of a Radiation Therapy Oncology Group randomised trial. *International Journal of Radiation Oncology, Biology and Physics* 13: 541–9.

Logsdon MD, Eifel PJ (1999) FIGO stage IIIB squamous cell carcinoma of the uterine cervix: an analysis of prognostic factors emphasising the balance between external beam and intra-cavitary radiation therapy. *International Journal of Radiation Oncology, Biology and Physics* 43: 763.

Lorvidhaya V, Tonusin A, Sukthomya W *et al.* (1995) Induction chemotherapy and irradiation in advanced carcinoma of the cervix. *Gan Kagaku Ryoho* 22 (suppl. 3): 244–251.

Lowrey GC, Mendenhall WM, Million RR *et al.* (1992) Stage IB or IIA–B carcinoma of the intact uterine cervix treated with irradiation: a multivariate analysis. *International Journal of Radiation Oncology, Biology and Physics* 24: 205.

Monk BJ, Wang J, Im S *et al.* (2005) Rethinking the use of radiation and chemotherapy after radical hysterectomy: a clinical–pathologic analysis of a Gynecologic Oncology Group/Southwest Oncology Group/Radiation Therapy Oncology Group trial. *Gynecologic Oncology* 96: 721–728.

Morris M, Eifel PJ, Lu J *et al.* (1999) Pelvic radiation with concurrent chemotherapy versus pelvic and para-aortic radiation for high-risk cervical cancer. A randomized Radiation Therapy Oncology Group clinical trial. *New England Journal of Medicine* 340: 1137–43.

National Cancer Institute (1999) NCI Clinical Announcement. Bethesda, MD: United States Department of Health and Human Services, Public Health Service, National Institutes of Health, February 1999.

Nigro ND, Seydel HG, Considine B *et al.* (1983) Combined preoperative radiation and chemotherapy for squamous cell carcinoma of the anal canal. *Cancer* 51: 1826.

Pearcey J, Brundage M, Drouin P *et al.* (2002) Phase three trial comparing radical radiation therapy with or without cisplatin chemotherapy in patient with advanced squamous cell carcinoma of the cervix. *Journal of Clinical Oncology* 20: 966–972.

Peters W, Liu PY, Barrett RJ *et al.* (2000) Concurrent chemotherapy and pelvic radiation therapy compared with pelvic radiation therapy alone as adjuvant therapy after radical surgery in high-risk early-stage cancer of the cervix. *Journal of Clinical Oncology* 18: 1606–1613.

Phillips RA, Tolmach LJ (1966) Repair of potentially lethal damage in X-irradiated HeLa cells. *Radiation Research* 29: 413–432.

Piver MS, Howes AE, Suit HD *et al.* (1972) Effect of hydroxyurea on the radiation response of C3H mouse mammary tumours. *Cancer* 29: 407–412.

Rakovitch E, Fyles AW, Pintilio M *et al.* (1997) Role of mitomycin C in development of late bowel toxicity following chemo-radiotherapy for locally advanced cervical cancer. *International Journal of Radiation Oncology, Biology and Physics* 38: 979–987.

Rose PG, Bundy BN, Watkins EB *et al.* (1999) Concurrent cisplatin-based chemoradiation in locally advanced cervical cancer. *New England Journal of Medicine* 340: 1144–1153.

Rotman M, Pajak TF, Choi K *et al.* (1995) Prophylactic extended-field irradiation of para-aortic lymph nodes in stages IIB and bulky IB and IIA cervical carcinomas. Ten-year treatment results of RTOG 79-20. *Journal of the American Medical Association* 274: 387–393.

Sinclair W (1968) The combined effect of hydroxyurea and X-rays on Chinese hamster cells *in vitro. Cancer Research* 28: 198–201.

Souhami L, Gil R, Allan S *et al.* (1991) A randomized trial of chemotherapy followed by pelvic radiation therapy in Stage IIIB carcinoms of the cervix. *International Journal of Radiation Oncology, Biology and Physics* 9: 970–997.

Stehman FB, Bundy BN, Thomas G *et al.* (1993) Hydroxyurea versus misonidazole with radiation in cervical carcinoma: Long term follow-up of a Gynecologic Oncology Group trial. *Journal of Clinical Oncology* 11: 1523–1528.

Sundfor K, Trope CG, Hogberg T *et al.* (1996) Radiotherapy and neoadjuvant chemotherapy for cervical carcinoma. A randomized multicenter study of sequential cisplatin and 5-fluorouracil and radiotherapy in advanced cervical carcinoma stage IIIB and IVA. *Cancer* 77: 2371–2378.

Tattersall MHN, Larvidhaya V, Vootiprux V *et al.* (1995) Randomized trial of epirubicin and cisplatin chemotherapy followed by pelvic radiation in locally advanced cervical cancer. *Journal of Clinical Oncology* 13: 444–451.

Thomas G, Dembo A, Ackerman I *et al.* (1997) A Phase III study of concurrent 5-fluorouracil and/or partially hyperfractionated radiation in advanced cancer of the cervix. *Proceeding of 21st Annual Meeting of Society of Gynecologic Oncologists.*

Tierney JF, Stewart LA (2002) Neoadjuvant chemotherapy followed by radiotherapy for locally advanced cervix cancer: A meta-analysis using individual patient data from randomised controlled trials. *Proceedings of the 9th Biennial Meeting of the International Gynecologic Cancer Society*: abstract CV002.

Tierney JF, Stewart LA, Parmar MKB (1999) Can the published data tell us about the effectiveness of neoadjuvant chemotherapy for locally advanced cancer of the uterine cervix? *European Journal of Cancer* 35: 406–409.

Tobias EJ, Buxton G, Blackledge JJ *et al.* (1990) Neoadjuvant bleomycin, ifosfamide and cisplatin in cervical cancer. *Cancer, Chemotherapy and Pharmacology* 26 (suppl.): 59–62.

Whitney CW, Sause W, Bundy BN *et al.* (1999) A randomised comparison of fluorouracil plus cisplatin versus hydroxyurea as an adjunct to radiation therapy in Stages IIB–IVA carcinoma of the cervix with negative para-aortic lymph nodes. A Gynecologic Oncology Group and Southwest Oncology Group Study. *Journal of Clinical Oncology* 17: 1339–1348.

Withers HR, Taylor JM, Maciejewski B (1988) The hazard of accelerated tumor clonogen repopulation during radiotherapy. *Acta Oncologica* 27: 131–146.

Wong L, Choo Y, Choy D *et al.* (1989) Long-term follow-up of potentiation of radiotherapy by cis-platinum in advanced cervical cancer. *Gynecologic Oncology* 35: 159–163.

Wong LC, Ngan NYS, Cheung ANY *et al.* (1999) Chemoradiation and adjuvant chemotherapy in cervical cancer. *Journal of Clinical Oncology* 17: 2055–2060.

CHAPTER 44

Vaccines to prevent and treat human papillomavirus-associated anogenital disease

Ian H. Frazer and Sally Appleton

INTRODUCTION

Viral aetiology of anogenital cancer

Infection of the cervical and anogenital epithelium with human papillomavirus (HPV) is now recognised to be responsible for the majority of anogenital cancer and pre-cancer. Pioneering work by zur Hausen and colleagues in the 1980s, linking HPV infection with cervical cancer, led to extensive epidemiological studies, which have demonstrated that HPV is found in more than 99% of cervical cancers, and it is considered to be the primary carcinogenic factor (Wallboomers *et al.*, 1999; Bosch *et al.*, 2002). HPV infection of the anogenital epithelium is sexually transmitted, and at least 50% of sexually active women will have a genital HPV infection at some time during their lives (Xi *et al.*, 1997). HPV is considered to be the most frequently sexually transmitted virus, and is often present in the anogenital epithelium of women who have no cytological abnormalities in the cervix or visible disease elsewhere.

Cervical cancer is the second most common cancer among women worldwide, and the commonest cancer attributable to HPV infection, with over 500 000 new cases diagnosed annually worldwide, resulting in approximately 250 000 deaths. A higher prevalence is observed in developing countries, with the highest rates reported in Mexico and Central America (Hernandez-Avila *et al.*, 1997). Of the approximately 100 identified genotypes of HPV, seven account for more than 80% of invasive cervical cancer (Wallboomers *et al.*, 1999). HPV type 16 is found in 50%, and types 18, 31, 33 and 45 are identified as other major causative agents. Consequently, these types are referred to as high-risk types. While vulval cancer is much less common than cervical cancer, and presumably therefore a less common consequence of exposure to the widely prevalent high-risk HPV types, the majority of vulval intraepithelial neoplasia (VIN) and cancer of the vulva (Jones, 2001) is associated with high-risk HPV infection. HPV infection also causes benign epithelial warts in the vulval region as elsewhere in the anogenital tract. The causative agents of

greater than 95% of genital warts are two HPV types, 6 and 11, which are designated low-risk as they are not thought to promote malignancy.

Papillomavirus life cycle (see also Chapter 19)

HPVs replicate only in epithelial cells. They enter epithelial cell cytosol by attaching to one of a range of cell-surface receptors, including $\alpha_6\beta_4$ integrin, heparin-like glycosaminoglycan molecules and some Fc receptors (McMillan *et al.*, 1999; Da Silva *et al.*, 2001; Giroglou *et al.*, 2001). The cells initially infected are epithelial stem cells, or transit-amplifying cells. HPV establishes its genome extrachromosomally in the nucleus of these cells. As the infected cell divides, viral DNA is distributed between both daughter cells. There are three groups of viral genes, or viral transcription units (Peh *et al.*, 2002), involved in viral replication, and these sequentially produce virally encoded proteins in infected cells. The first transcription unit, comprising the E6 and E7 viral non-structural genes, promotes cellular proliferation and prevents cellular differentiation, ensuring a large pool of cells with viral episome. The second unit, comprising the E1, E2, and E4 non-structural genes, promotes viral episomal amplification while arresting replication of the infected cell in G2. The third unit, comprising the L1 and L2 capsid genes, is expressed most superficially and allows packaging of the viral genome. These proteins together provide the targets for vaccines designed to prevent or treat HPV infection.

In most HPV-associated anogenital cancers, HPV DNA has become integrated into host genetic material, rather than remaining as nuclear extrachromosomal elements. The viral integration site commonly occurs within the E1/E2 region, severing the E2-controlled regulation of E6 and E7 protein expression (zur Hausen, 1999). These proteins have the capacity to transform cells, and hence to promote the development of malignancy. E7 protein blocks retinoblastoma protein (pRb) tumour-suppressor function by binding to unphosphorylated pRb. This causes the release of a transcription factor, E2F,

609

which allows cell cycle progression at the G1/S border. E6 protein inactivates the tumour suppressor p53, the protein that would normally detain the cell in G1 to allow DNA repair, by binding it with a ubiquitin protein ligase and targeting it for degradation. E7 adds to E6 activity by binding proteins that p53 would act upon to arrest the cell in G1. In this way, E6 and E7 are able to immortalise cells, and become the targets for vaccines designed to treat established anogenital malignancy.

PROPHYLACTIC VACCINES FOR HPV-ASSOCIATED DISEASE

Basics of HPV prophylactic vaccine development

Vaccines to prevent viral infections induce the host immune system to produce neutralising antibody directed at structural determinants on the target virus. Generally, prophylactic vaccines comprise either inactivated or live attenuated virus. Inactivated virus or virus structural proteins are combined with aluminium hydroxide gel, which stabilises the antigen, provides a depot and promotes local inflammation, enhancing immune reactivity. Live attenuated vaccines would not be acceptable for oncogenic viruses such as HPV, because of the longer-term risk of reversion of an attenuated strain to a potentially oncogenic phenotype.

Papillomaviruses cannot be produced in large quantities *in vitro* for vaccine production, because their life cycle is tightly tied to the differentiation of the epithelial cells which are permissive for their replication, and hence standard tissue culture techniques are unable to permit replication of virus. Development of papillomavirus prophylactic vaccines therefore had to await the recognition that the major capsid proteins of papillomavirus, L1 and L2, could be expressed in eukaryotic cells, where they self-assembled into virus-like particles (VLPs) (Zhou *et al.*, 1991). L1 VLPs, produced in bulk in yeast or in insect cells using baculovirus expression vectors, have become the basis of vaccines currently under development to prevent HPV infection and cervical cancer (Fig. 44.1) (Stanley, 2002; Schiller *et al.*, 2001).

Natural immune responses to HPV following infection

Production of HPV VLPs of defined genotype, using recombinant viral capsid proteins, allowed measurement of papillomavirus-specific humoral immune responses. Infection with HPV generally results in the development of antibody

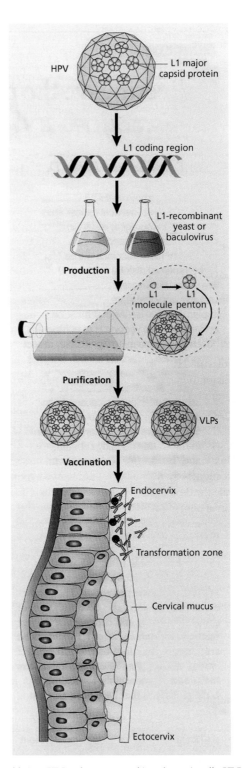

self-assemble into VLPs when expressed in eukaryotic cells. VLPs aim to protect against the development of cervical cancer; protection would be mediated by the induction of high titres of neutralising antibodies against the HPV genotypes in the vaccine that prevent the virus infecting the transformation zone of the cervix. This is where most pre-cancers and eventually cancers originate. From Schiller and Davies, 2004.

Fig. 44.1 (*right*) Schematic representation of the production of, and vaccination with, human papillomavirus (HPV) virus-like particles (VLPs). The HPV major capsid protein L1 can fold correctly and

to conformational epitopes of the viral capsid (Carter *et al.*, 1996). However, this immune response, which is virus type specific, is weak and inconstant when compared with the response observed following infection with the majority of viruses. Thus, though seroepidemiological studies confirm a strong association of capsid-specific antibody with cervical premalignancy and cancer (Dillner, 1999), serology cannot be used to confirm or exclude whether an individual has current or past infection with a particular PV. Whether the natural immune response to the HPV capsid following infection protects against future infection with the same PV types is unclear. Although recurrent episodes of PV-associated wart disease are held to represent reactivation of latent infection or alternatively new infection with a different PV genotype, new infection with a molecular variant of a previously encountered genotype is described (Mayrand *et al.*, 2000), suggesting that natural infection may not always invoke host protective immunity against future infection.

Development of VLP vaccines

Early studies of HPV VLPs as possible vaccines to prevent HPV infection demonstrated that VLPs were immunogenic, invoking antibody-recognising virus-specific determinants on the viral capsid (Christensen *et al.*, 1994). Several animal models of PV infection, including canine oral papillomavirus (Bell *et al.*, 1994), cottontail rabbit papillomavirus (Breitburd *et al.*, 1995) and bovine papillomavirus (Kirnbauer *et al.*, 1996) infection, were then used to study VLPs as possible vaccines. While the direct relevance of each of these PV infections to infection of human anogenital epithelium can be questioned, resistance to disease following viral challenge could be induced in each model by prior immunisation with appropriate L1 VLPs. Further, studies in these models have demonstrated that protection is mediated by antibody, is PV type specific, is long lasting and correlates with the induced titre of neutralising antibody directed to conformational epitopes on the viral capsid (Suzich *et al.*, 1995).

Human trials of VLP vaccines

The encouraging animal studies of VLP-based PV vaccines were followed by trials in humans. Phase I studies with HPV 11 and HPV 16 VLPs were designed to show safety and establish appropriate vaccine doses and regimens (Brown *et al.*, 2001; Evans *et al.*, 2001; Harro *et al.*, 2001; Emeny *et al.*, 2002; Williams *et al.*, 2002). These studies confirmed the inherent immunogenicity of papillomavirus VLPs, and high titres of neutralising antibody were observed in almost 100% of subjects immunised following a three-immunisation regime delivered over 6 months with as little as 10 µg of virus protein. Phase II randomised placebo-controlled efficacy studies of HPV 16 VLPs in young women without prior evidence

of HPV infection (Koutsky *et al.*, 2002) have shown that this VLP-based vaccine is 100% effective at preventing new persisting HPV 16 infection. In one study (Koutsky *et al.*, 2002) of 768 vaccinees, none developed persistent HPV 16 infection, whereas, among 765 placebo recipients, 41 new HPV 16 infections, including nine cases of HPV 16-associated cervical intraepithelial neoplasia (CIN), were observed. Similar numbers of incident infections with HPV types other than HPV 16 were observed in both groups, confirming type specificity of protection. A further phase II study of an HPV 16 and HPV 18 combined VLP vaccine (Cenvarix, GlaxoSmithKline) (Billich, 2003) has demonstrated equally encouraging results. In another study, Harper *et al.* (2004) reported on a randomised controlled trial using bivalent HPV 16 and HPV 18 VLPs, L1 capsid components derived from insect cells (baculovirus). A total of 560 women between 15 and 25 were vaccinated and compared with 553 placebo-treated cases. After 27 months it was shown that the efficacy in preventing HPV 16 and HPV 18 infection was 100%. There was a highly significant difference between this group and the placebo-treated group.

A larger phase II study of multivalent vaccines has been recently reported by Villa *et al.* (2005) and was designed to demonstrate that vaccines can protect against HPV types commonly associated with cervical cancer and genital warts, and can also prevent CIN. While these studies are focused on cervical disease, it is probable that a vaccine able to prevent significant HPV infection in the cervix will be efficacious against HPV infection elsewhere in the anogenital tract.

In the study reported by Villa *et al.* (2005), which was a randomised 'double-blind' placebo-controlled phase II study designed to assess the efficacy of a prophylactic quadrivalent vaccine which targeted the HPV types associated with 70% of cervical cancers (types 16 and 18) and with 90% of genital warts (types 6 and 11), 277 young women with a mean age of 20.2 years were randomly assigned to quadrivalent HPV VLP vaccine and 275 (mean age 20 years) to one of two placebo preparations at day 1, month 2 and month 6. The HPV types were represented in the vaccine as follows: type 6, 20 µg; type 11, 14 µg; type 16, 40 µg; and type 18, 20 µg. This composition is the vaccine now being trialled as Gardasil (Merck). Over a 36-month period, each young woman underwent a regular cervicovaginal sampling for HPV DNA, testing for serum antibodies to HPV and a gynaecological examination which included the taking of a Pap smear. The combined incidence of infection with HPV 6, 11, 16 or 18, or cervical or external genital disease, i.e. persistent HPV infection, HPV detection at the last recorded visit, the presence of CIN or cancer or external genital lesions that were caused by the HPV types in the vaccine comprised the primary endpoint. Combined incidence of persistent infection or disease with the relevant HPV types 6, 11, 16 or 18 fell by 90% (95% CI 72–97, $P < 0.001$) in those who were given the vaccine compared with those given the placebo. This study shows how targeting these four HPV types could substantially reduce the acquisition of infection and clinical disease caused by common HPV types.

A recent report (Lowndes and Gill, 2005) of the interim findings of a phase III study (FUTURE II), in which 12 166 women aged 16–26 years from 13 countries were randomised to receive a three-dose regime of either the vaccine (Gardasil, Merck) or placebo at day 1, month 2 and month 6 extended previous findings to look at prevention of clincial disease caused by high-risk HPV types. The 2-year analysis of protection against precancer and cancer provided by the quadrivalent recombinant vaccine against HPV types 6, 11, 16 and 18 showed that no cases of cervical precancer were observed in women randomised to the vaccine ($n = 5301$) compared with 21 cases in the placebo group ($n = 5258$), after an average follow-up of 17 months from completing the vaccination regime. The quadrivalent recombinant vaccine against these four HPV types prevented 100% of cases of high-grade CIN (CIN2–3) developing. The differences were highly significant ($P < 0.0001$). As discussed previously, types 16 and 18 are associated with approximately 70% of cervical neoplasia.

While these reported studies have focused predominantly on cervical disease, it is probable that a vaccine able to prevent significant HPV infection in the cervix will be efficacious against HPV infection elsewhere in the anogenital tract, as suggested by the findings in a interim analysis of a further phase III study of Gardisil (FUTURE 1; Mao *et al.*, 2006). This study also demonstrated high levels of neutralising antibody 3.5 years after completion of immunisation per protocol, suggesting that protection against HPV infection following immunisation might be expected to be long lived.

Other prophylactic vaccine systems

First-generation prophylactic vaccines against PV infection will probably be based on VLP technology, but these vaccines may be improved upon, particularly for the areas of the world where cervical cancer is common. Second-generation vaccines would ideally extend coverage beyond the two commonest types of PV infection associated with malignancy, and might optimally be delivered by a route other than intramuscular injection, or need fewer than three administrations for protection. Further, since it can be estimated that over 5 million women globally are destined to develop cervical cancer from already acquired PV infection, a second-generation vaccine might combine prophylaxis against future PV infection with a therapeutic component for current PV infection. Therapeutic vaccines will be discussed further in a later section of this review.

A number of approaches have been considered for second-generation vaccines. VLPs of other genotypes can be produced, though it is unknown how many could be incorporated in a single vaccine and still allow development of immunity against all types. Oral and other mucosal delivery routes for VLPs have been attempted in animals and humans, as yet without major

success. Polynucleotide L1 vaccines (Donnelly *et al.*, 1996) are cheap to produce and are held not to need a cold chain for effective delivery. Codon-modified L1 polynucleotide vaccines (Leder *et al.*, 2001; Liu *et al.*, 2001) produce capsid-specific neutralising antibody in animals, and can combine a prophylactic and therapeutic component by the admixture of genes expressing ubiquitinated and non-ubiquitinated proteins. However, in general, polynucleotide vaccines have yet to demonstrate efficacy in humans or other primates (Gurunathan *et al.*, 2000; Shedlock and Weiner, 2000). Vaccines based on the L2 capsid protein of PV have the potential to cover more PV genotypes since there appears to be some cross-reactivity between genotypes, both in animals and in early phase human studies (Kawana *et al.*, 2001), but the L2 protein is not particularly immunogenic either following natural infection or when delivered as a peptide vaccine in animals or humans. Thus it appears likely that current VLP technology will be the major thrust of PV prophylactic vaccine deployment over the next decade.

Prophylactic vaccine deployment strategies

A decrease in the prevalence of cervical cancer could be achieved through primary prevention of HPV infection of the cervix, and this approach is of particular relevance in developing countries, where screening programmes for cervical pre-cancer cannot be delivered or followed through. Social strategies that have been promoted for prevention of other sexually transmitted infections have included sexual abstinence, mutually monogamous sexual relationships between non-infected partners, and correct use of condoms, but these are not always easily implemented. Further, there is little evidence that these would be effective in controlling the spread of HPV infection, as the majority of primary infections are asymptomatic, and occur within 5 years of onset of sexual activity, while condoms are only partially effective at preventing transmission of HPV infection (Wen *et al.*, 1999). A vaccination campaign aimed at the prevention of cervical cancer would be likely to target teenage girls prior to or shortly after commencement of sexual activity. At this age, informed parental as well as patient consent would be likely to be required. To promote acceptance of the vaccine, public education of the relative benefits against risks will be required, and cultural and social factors would be significant in securing consent. Inclusion of the HPV genotypes associated with genital warts in a prophylactic vaccine may provide an added benefit to vaccinated subjects, and may also make vaccine deployment more acceptable to male recipients, though it is argued that the control of cervical cancer is as effectively achieved by targeting the HPV vaccine exclusively to females as to both males and females, where vaccine or resources for deployment are limited.

The question of which HPV type should be immunised against also raises interesting questions but reference to

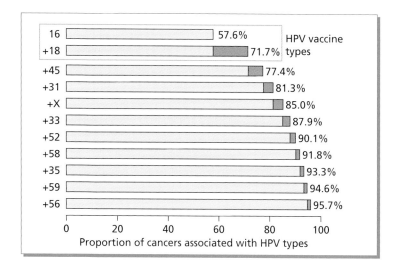

Fig. 44.2 HPV types in cervical intraepithelial neoplasia (CIN)2/3 and cervical cancer. Adapted from Muñoz *et al.*, 2003.

Figure 44.2 will show that vaccinating against types 16 and 18 could prevent just over 70% of cervical cancers (Muñoz *et al.*, 2003, 2004) (Fig. 44.2).

HPV THERAPEUTIC VACCINES

Why do we need one?

For individuals persistently infected with a virus, a prophylactic vaccine designed to produce neutralising antibody against the virus capsid is unlikely to be successful in eliminating infection, since the virus resides and reproduces within cells, and the viral proteins are in consequence not accessible to antibody (Frazer, 2004).

How might it work?

Host immune responses naturally eliminate the majority of viral infections. These encompass activation of innate (non-antigen-specific) immune effector mechanisms, including natural killer (NK) and NKT cells and their associated antiviral cytokines, including interferons, by cells responding through Toll-like receptors to pathogen pattern recognition molecules and to local cell death and necro-inflammatory products. Additionally, virus-specific T cells of helper (CD4) or cytotoxic (CD8) phenotypes are induced in the course of viral infection, following presentation of viral proteins as peptides to the immune system by suitably activated professional antigen-presenting cells (APCs). These adaptive immune responses help to control infection, generally by killing virus-infected cells.

A therapeutic vaccine, designed to eliminate a chronic viral infection, must achieve a type or magnitude of immune response which the host immune system has failed to achieve naturally in response to the same infection. It is therefore important, when planning an HPV therapeutic vaccine, to

understand why natural infection has failed to produce a host-protective immune response. It is also important to consider which viral proteins should be targeted by the vaccine.

Cellular immune responses to natural infection

Immune responses to PV proteins are hard to detect following PV infection, with the exception of the antibodies directed against the capsid proteins described above. This may be partly a methodological problem, as cellular responses to viral non-structural proteins are in general hard to detect in viral infection in humans, even when they are manifestly sufficient to eliminate infection. Antibody can be used as a surrogate marker for the cellular responses to viral protein that might be important in eliminating infection. The only consistent feature of the humoral immune response to viral proteins following anogenital HPV infection is development of antibody to the E7 protein of HPV 16 in patients with invasive cervical cancer (Jochmus-Kudielka *et al.*, 1989). However, there are tantalising suggestions of cellular immune responses to both E6 and E7 in patients with HPV-associated premalignancy (Höpfl *et al.*, 2000; Kadish *et al.*, 2002; Welters *et al.*, 2003) and evidence that E6-specific immunity may determine disease outcome (Welters *et al.*, 2006).

Reasons for a poor immune response to HPV infection

A lack of cellular immunity to viral non-structural proteins in patients with HPV infection may explain the persistence of PV infection, and it therefore becomes relevant to ask why so little immune response is induced naturally by infection (Frazer, 1996). As PV proteins are expressed only in small amounts, and in superficial epithelial cells, they are probably not presented much to T cells by APCs. Additionally, PV infection is non-lytic, and the local inflammatory response to cells killed by virus infection is one of the major stimuli necessary to evoke effective presentation to T cells by professional APCs. Finally, the epithelium secretes many cytokines designed to protect epithelial cells against immune damage, since epithelial integrity is a key component of host homeostasis. Thus PV infection distinguishes itself from many other chronic virus infections, including human immunodeficiency virus, hepatitis B and C viruses and herpes simplex virus, which are associated with easily measurable immune responses which are insufficient or of an inappropriate quality to eradicate infection.

Developing and testing vaccines for HPV therapy

A wide range of therapeutic modalities have been tested in an attempt to invoke PV-specific immunity capable of eliminating HPV-infected cells. A number of animal models have been used and in addition several clinical trials have been undertaken in humans. The animal models comprise:

• transplantable tumours [C2 (Tindle *et al.*, 1995), C3 (Feltkamp *et al.*, 1993), TC-1 (Lin *et al.*, 1996)] expressing one or more PV proteins, tested in syngeneic recipients, that can be immunised prior to tumour transfer, or immunised after tumour is established;
• mice transgenic for HPV proteins, generally targeted to skin; a variant of this is to transfer a skin graft from such an animal to a naive host (Dunn *et al.*, 1997).

Additionally, animals which develop disease following exposure to their natural papillomavirus infection can be studied, including:

• beagle dogs, which develop transient oral warts following infection with canine oral papillomavirus (Bell *et al.*, 1994);
• cottontail rabbits, which develop skin warts following challenge with cottontail rabbit papillomavirus (Christensen and Kreider, 1991); these warts can become chronic and can transform to carcinomas;
• cows, which develop transient skin warts and occasionally facial cancers following infection with bovine PV (Jarrett *et al.*, 1990);
• rabbits, which develop transient tongue warts following infection with rabbit oral papillomavirus (Embers *et al.*, 2002).

Data from animal models

Most immunisation regimes incorporating an adjuvant and PV antigens, when given prophylactically, prevent tumour growth in mice challenged with a transplantable tumour expressing a PV protein. This model is therefore unlikely to be discriminatory for vaccines which might be of use in humans, and will not be considered further here.

A rather more restricted set of immunogens are able to cause regression of established antigen-expressing transplantable tumours; these are effective when delivered as polynucleotide vaccines (Table 44.1), as recombinant viruses (Table 44.2) or as protein with adjuvants (Table 44.3). In this model, early rejection of established transplantable tumours relies on innate immunity, and can be assisted by CD8 T-cell-mediated adaptive immune responses, while tumours that are better-established (> 7 days) require antigen-specific CD8 T cells for elimination (Stewart *et al.*, 2003). Most polynucleotide immunisation regimes have required more than expression of the E7 protein for tumour control (Table 44.1), possibly because E7 is poorly expressed from polynucleotide constructs, and enhanced expression through modified codon usage improves CTL responses and eliminates the need for adjunct immunotherapy (Liu *et al.*, 2002). E7 as immunotherapy is however effective if delivered with a wide range of adjuvanting and enhancing systems (Tables 44.2 and 44.3).

Grafted E7 transgenic skin is more refractory than transplantable tumours to therapeutic treatment. While newly established grafts, like newly established transplantable tumours, are rejected following enhancement of innate immune responses, established grafts promote tolerance and do not respond to specific immunotherapy (Frazer *et al.*, 2001). Tolerance of HPV protein appears to be local in this model, as graft recipients will, following immunisation, reject an E7-bearing transplantable tumour. Rejection of grafted E7 transgenic skin can be achieved by activation of sufficient E7-specific CTL (Matsumoto *et al.*, 2004) and the challenge for successful immunotherapy in patients may be to work out how to induce sufficient CTL through immunisation to achieve elimination of infected cells.

Treatment studies of animal PV infections have demonstrated that the PV E1, E2, E6 and E7 gene products are all potential targets for immunotherapy of established infection, with some preference for E2 and E6 as monotherapy over the other proteins, and some preference for therapy with multiple proteins over monotherapy (Tables 44.1–44.3). A comparison of the location of expression of the early proteins of PV in the animal and human infections suggests that these proteins will be better presented in basal epithelium in the animal models. This may account for the near-complete natural spontaneous regression rate for animal PV infections, and suggests that therapeutic success in animal models of infection with particular PV proteins will not necessarily predict similar outcomes in humans.

Ultimately, vaccine development is driven empirically, mandating phase I and II clinical trials in infected human subjects of possible effective immunotherapeutics. In this regard, it is worth observing that there are no immunotherapeutic products in routine clinical practice, though immunotherapeutics for melanoma and a limited range of cancers have given encouraging results in early-phase trials. Further, studies to date have not revealed reliable surrogate markers of immune response predicting outcome of immunotherapy.

Table 44.1 Polynucleotide-based potential human papillomavirus therapeutic vaccine modalities employed in animal models.

Antigen	Model animal/tumour	Outcome	Reference
CRPV–E1, E2, E6, E7	Rabbit/CRPV	Partial protection against progression of established infection to cancer	Han *et al.*, 2000
CRPV–E7	Rabbit/CRPV	Partial protection against progression of established infection to cancer	Han *et al.*, 2002
COPV–E2, E6, E7	Beagle/COPV	Enhanced regression of tumours with E2 immunotherapy	Moore *et al.*, 2003
E7 + LAMP-1	Mouse/TC-1	E7/LAMP-1 fusions gave better regression of established metastatic tumour than E7 alone	Ji *et al.*, 1998; Chen *et al.*, 1999; Ji *et al.*, 1999
E7–MDV UL49 fusion	Mouse/TC-1	CTL induction and therapeutic effect	Hung *et al.*, 2002
E7 + calreticulin	Mouse/TC-1	CTL and tumour regression, calreticulin also effective as therapy when delivered as polynucleotide	Cheng *et al.*, 2001
E7 polytope + ubiquitin	Mouse/C3	CTL and tumour regression	Velders *et al.*, 2001a
E7 ± fusion with LAMP	Mouse/TC-1	CTL, partial therapeutic effect with E7 and with E7–LAMP	Smahel *et al.*, 2001
E7–membrane insertion protein from *Pseudomonas aeruginosa*	Mouse/TC-1	CTL, tumour regression	Hung *et al.*, 2001a
E7–VP-22	Mouse/TC-1	CTL, tumour regression, VP-22 also effective alone	Hung *et al.*, 2001b
E7–flt3Ligand	Mouse/TC-1	CTL, tumour regression	Hung *et al.*, 2001c
E6, E7	HLA A*0201 transgenic mouse/E7 and Ras-transformed A*0201 mouse tumour	CTL induction and reduction of tumour growth	Eiben *et al.*, 2002

COPV, canine oral papillomavirus; CRPV, cottontail rabbit papillomavirus; CTL, cytotoxic T lymphocyte.

Table 44.2 Virus-based potential HPV therapeutic vaccines tested in animal models.

Virus	Encoded protein	Test model	Outcome	Reference
Vaccinia	Listerolysin–E7	Mouse/TC-1	CTL and tumour regression in some animals; Vac–LLO–E7 better than Vac–LAMP-1–E7	Lamikanra *et al.*, 2001
Sindbis	E7 + VP-22	Mouse/TC-1	CTL and tumour regression	Cheng *et al.*, 2002
Alphavirus	E6–E7 fusion protein	Mouse	CTL induction and tumour regression	Daemen *et al.*, 2002
Alphavirus	E7–HSP-70	Mouse/TC-1	CTL, tumour regression	Hsu *et al.*, 2001
Venezuelan encephalitis	E7	Mouse/C3	CTL and tumour regression	Velders *et al.*, 2001b
Venezuelan encephalitis	E6, E7 polytope	HLA A*0201 transgenic mouse/E7 and ras-transformed A*0201 mouse tumour	CTL induction and reduction of tumour growth	Eiben *et al.*, 2002
Adeno-associated	E7–CTL epitope–HSP-70	Mouse/TC-1	CTL and tumour regression	Liu *et al.*, 2000
Adenovirus	E2	Rabbit/CRPV	Reduction in papilloma size and number post immunisation compared with control immunisation	Ferrara *et al.*, 2003; Brandsma *et al.*, 2004

CTL, cytotoxic T lymphocyte; CRPV, cottontail rabbit papillomavirus; HSP, heat shock protein.

Table 44.3 Other potential HPV therapeutic vaccines tested in animal models.

Delivery system	Antigenic proteins	Test model	Outcome	Reference
Salmonella typhimurium	HPV–L1 VLPs	Mouse/C3	Tumour regression after mucosal immunisation	Revaz *et al.*, 2001
Listeria	E7–listerolysin fusion	Mouse/TC-1	CTL, 75% tumour regression with LLO, no regression without	Gunn *et al.*, 2001
PV VLP capsomers	L1	Mouse/C3	CTL and regression	Ohlschlager *et al.*, 2003
Peptide + anti-CD137	E7–CTL peptide/Freunds	Mouse/C3, TC-1	CTL and tumour eradication; successful therapy required CD137 expression on the tumour	Wilcox *et al.*, 2002
Peptide + CpG	E7 peptides/CPG	Mouse/C3	Eradication of tumours	Zwaveling *et al.*, 2002
QS21 or MLP	E7	Mouse/TC1	CTL and tumour regression	Gerard *et al.*, 2001a
SBAS1 adjuvant	E7	Mouse/TC-1	CTL, Th1 response and tumour regression, in E7-tolerant transgenic mice tumour regression without CTL	Gerard *et al.*, 2001b
Dendritic cells	E7 peptides or tumour lysate	Mouse/MK16 transduced with E6/7	CTL, tumour regression	Indrova *et al.*, 2001
HSP fusion	E7	Mouse/TC-1	Regression, Th1 response, CTL,	Chu *et al.*, 2000
PROVAX adjuvant	E7	Mouse/E7 transduced melanoma	Slowing of growth, due to CD8 T cells	Hariharan *et al.*, 1998
Suicide gene modified cancer cells	E7	Hamster/E7 transformed cells	Regression of tumour due to bystander effect/immunity?	Vonka *et al.*, 1998
Transfer of T cells	E7	Mouse/C3	Early tumours controlled by NKT cells and other non-antigen-specific mechanisms; well established tumours respond to E7-specific T cells	Stewart *et al.*, 2003

CTL, cytotoxic T lymphocyte; HPV, human papillomavirus; NKT cells, natural killer T cells; VLP, virus-like particle.

Data from human studies

A number of potentially immunotherapeutic vaccines for persistent HPV infection have been trialled in humans (Table 44.4). Most have proven immunogenic, by one or more of a range of measures, in the majority of trial subjects. Immune responses have been more frequently observed in patients with premalignancy than in those with invasive cancer. Some trials have reported evidence of regression of, or stabilisation of, HPV-associated disease, though the majority of these early-phase trials have been conducted without placebo controls. No study has claimed that a particular measured immune response was predictive of vaccine efficacy, and trials of immunotherapy will therefore rely on clinical endpoints alone for the moment.

In most of the reported studies, only patients infected with the specific HPV type of the vaccine were treated, or the HPV type in the lesion was not recorded. In one study, however, an effect of immunotherapy with HPV 16 E7 on regression of HPV 6/11 warts was observed, suggesting that vaccine efficacy might include a component of activation of the innate immune system, as has been demonstrated relevant in animal models, and this observation suggests that adjuvant and delivery system control groups should be incorporated in early-phase trials.

While concerns have been raised about the safety of vaccines based on transforming viral proteins, these concerns are generally allayed for the clinical studies described by using mutated viral proteins, lacking oncogenic potential, and/or by using fusions that lack the functional configuration of the native proteins, as T-cell adaptive immune responses depend only on the linear sequence of the immunogen, and not on its tertiary structure.

Immunotherapy for other HPV-associated genital tract neoplasia

E6 and E7 proteins of high-risk PVs maintain the transformation of anogenital epithelial cells in intraepithelial neoplasia and cancer. A significant frequency of mutations is observed in the antigen-presenting machinery of the cells of HPV-associated invasive cancer, rendering these cells potentially resistant to immunotherapy (Davidson *et al.*, 2003). Thus, while there may be a place for adjuvant immunotherapy in the management of

Table 44.4 Clinical trials of HPV-specific immunotherapy.

Delivery system	Antigen	Disease group	Immunogenicity	Clinical outcome	Reference
Fusion protein (TA-CIN, Xenova)	HPV16–L2E6/E7 fusion (no adjuvant)	Healthy volunteers	Antibody, T cell proliferation, IFNγ ELISPOT all detected	Double-blind placebo-controlled; no HPV infections	De Jong et al., 2002
HSP fusion protein (HSP E7, Stressgen)	HPV16–E7	Genital warts	Not reported	Open-label uncontrolled; regression of warts: 3/14 CR; 10/14 PR; warts not HPV16	Goldstone et al., 2002
Encapsulated polynucleotide (ZYC101, Zycos)	HPV16–E7 peptide	Anal dysplasia; cervical dysplasia	Majority of subjects ELISPOT positive; induction of E2-specific immunity	Open-label uncontrolled; HPV type 16 by selection; regression of AIN: 3/12 PR; regression of CIN: 5/15 CR	Klencke et al., 2002; Sheets et al., 2003
Protein/saponin adjuvant (Cervax16, CSL)	E6/E7 fusion protein	CIN	Antibody/DTH/CTL	Randomised placebo-controlled; HPV type-specific reduction in HPV infection; 7/14 CR; 7/14 PR/no clinical regression	Frazer et al., 2004
Vaccinia virus (TA-HPV–Xenova)	E6/E7 fusion protein	Cervical cancer	CTL (1/8); antibody (3/8)	Open-label uncontrolled; outcome not documented	Borysiewicz et al., 1996
Vaccinia virus (TA-HPV, Xenova)	E6/E7 fusion protein	VIN	E6-specific cytokine responses (6/10)	Open-label uncontrolled; > 50% resolution in 5/12 subjects	Baldwin et al., 2003
Vaccinia virus (TA-HPV, Xenova)	E6/E7 fusion protein	VIN	Antibody or CMI in 13/18 subjects	Open-label uncontrolled; > 50% resolution in 8/18 subjects	Davidson et al., 2003
Peptide/oil+water adjuvant	E7 peptide	Cervical cancer	Not stated	Open-label uncontrolled; HPV16 by selection outcome 2/17 SD	Van Driel et al., 1999
Protein/algammulin adjuvant	E7–GST fusion protein	Cervical cancer	Antibody, DTH	Open-label uncontrolled; no alteration in natural history of disease	Frazer et al., 1999
Peptide + IFA	E7–A0201 peptide	VIN/CIN	CTL 10/16, no DTH	Open-label uncontrolled; HPV16 by selection 3/18 CR; 6/18 PR	Muderspach et al., 2000
VLPs	L1	Genital warts	Antibody and DTH	Open-label uncontrolled; regression of warts: CR 25/33	Zhang et al., 2000
Dendritic cells	Recombinant E7 protein	Cervical cancer	CMI (proliferation ELISPOT) in 4/11	Open-label uncontrolled; no objective responses	Ferrara et al., 2003
MVA	E2	CIN1–3 — mostly CIN1	Possible CTL response not clearly characterised	Open-label uncontrolled; regression of 34/36 lesions	Corona Gutierrez et al., 2004

AIN, anal intraepithelial neoplasia; CIN, cervical intraepithelial neoplasia; CR, complete regression; DTH, delayed-type hypersensitivity; GST, glutathione-S-transferase; MVA, modified vaccinia Ankara; PR, part regression; SD, stable disease; VIN, vulval intraepithelial neoplasia.

early-stage anogenital cancer, HPV immunotherapy is ideally targeted at premalignant disease, in which problems with antigen presentation have not been described. While the studies cited in this review confirm that therapeutic vaccines are immunogenic in humans, therapeutic vaccine technology is at a much earlier stage of development than HPV prophylactic vaccines. Efficacy trials of therapeutic vaccines as sole treatment for CIN3 are difficult to envisage, as this disease mandates conventional treatment. Vulval intraepithelial neoplasia is an attractive target disease for testing HPV-specific immunotherapy because it is frequently associated with HPV infection, there are few effective alternative therapies, spontaneous regression is not common, disease status is relatively easily assessed, and there is a defined risk of progression to neoplasia. Thus, trials in patients with VIN (Baldwin *et al.*, 2003; Davidson *et al.*, 2003) may provide the key to development and assessment of effective immunotherapy for the full spectrum of HP- associated anogenital malignancy.

Conclusions

Virus-like particle-based vaccines are designed to prevent infection with the 'high-risk' PVs thought to initiate cervical and lower genital tract intraepithelial neoplasias and cancer, by induction of neutralising antibody to the viral capsid proteins. These vaccines should be available within the next few years, as trials to date have shown efficacy at preventing cervical HPV infection. While these positive results are encouraging, there remains a possibility that dry squamous epithelium will be less effectively protected by neutralising antibody than the mucosal surfaces of the cervix. Post-marketing surveillance will demonstrate whether VLP-based vaccines are effective at preventing vulval HPV infections and consequent neoplastic changes. It is held unlikely that VLP-based prophylactic vaccines will be therapeutic for existing vulval HPV infection.

Therapeutic vaccines for existing HPV infection, based on viral non-structural proteins, are under development and there are encouraging animal and human data demonstrating immunogenicity, and hinting at efficacy in some HPV-associated disease. These vaccines are at an earlier stage of development than the prophylactic vaccines, and it is not currently possible to predict when such vaccines might be available for clinical use. If they prove efficacious for other HPV-infected sites, it is likely that they will also work for lower genital tract lesions, and as such VIN may be a preferred disease for which to demonstrate proof of principle efficacy for HPV therapeutic vaccines.

REFERENCES

Baldwin PJ, Van der Burg SH, Boswell CM *et al.* (2003) Vaccinia-expressed human papillomavirus 16 and 18 E6 and E7 as a therapeutic vaccination for vulval and vaginal intraepithelial neoplasia. *Clinical Cancer Research* 9: 5205–5213.

Bell JA, Sundberg JP, Ghim S *et al.* (1994) A formalin-inactivated vaccine protects against mucosal papillomavirus infection: A canine model. *Pathobiology* 62: 194–198.

Billich A (2003) HPV vaccine MedImmune/GlaxoSmithKline. *Current Opinion in Investigational Drugs* 4: 210–213.

Borysiewicz LK, Fiander A, Nimako M *et al.* (1996) A recombinant vaccinia virus encoding human papillomavirus types 16 and 18, E6 and E7 proteins as immunotherapy for cervical cancer. *Lancet* 347: 1523–1527.

Bosch FX, Lorincz A, Muñoz N *et al.* (2002) The causal relation between human papillomavirus and cervical cancer. *Journal of Clinical Pathology* 55: 244–265.

Brandsma JL, Shlyankevich M, Zhang LX *et al.* (2004) Vaccination of rabbits with an adenovirus vector expressing the papillomavirus E2 protein leads to clearance of papillomas and infection. *Journal of Virology* 78: 116–123.

Breitburd F, Kirnbauer R, Hubbert NL *et al.* (1995) Immunization with viruslike particles from cottontail rabbit papillomavirus (CRPV) can protect against experimental CRPV infection. *Journal of Virology* 69: 3959–3963.

Brown DR, Bryan JT, Schroeder JM *et al.* (2001) Neutralization of human papillomavirus type 11 (HPV-11) by serum from women vaccinated with yeast-derived HPV-11 L1 virus-like particles: Correlation with competitive radioimmunoassay titer. *Journal of Infectious Diseases* 184: 1183–1186.

Carter JJ, Koutsky LA, Wipf GC *et al.* (1996) The natural history of human papillomavirus type 16 capsid antibodies among a cohort of university women. *Journal of Infectious Diseases* 174: 927–936.

Chen CH, Ji H, Suh KW *et al.* (1999) Gene gun-mediated DNA vaccination induces antitumor immunity against human papillomavirus type 16 E7-expressing murine tumor metastases in the liver and lungs. *Gene Therapy* 6: 1972–1981.

Cheng WF, Hung CF, Chai CY *et al.* (2001) Tumor-specific immunity and antiangiogenesis generated by a DNA vaccine encoding calreticulin linked to a tumor antigen. *Journal of Clinical Investigation* 108: 669–678.

Cheng WF, Hung CF, Hsu KF *et al.* (2002) Cancer immunotherapy using Sindbis virus replicon particles encoding a VP22-antigen fusion. *Human Gene Therapy* 13: 553–568.

Christensen ND, Kreider JW (1991) Neutralization of CRPV infectivity by monoclonal antibodies that identify conformational epitopes on intact virions. *Virus Research* 21: 169–179.

Christensen ND, Höpfl R, DiAngelo SL *et al.* (1994) Assembled baculovirus-expressed human papillomavirus type 11 L1 capsid protein virus-like particles are recognized by neutralising monoclonal antibodies and induce high titres of neutralising antibodies. *Journal of General Virology* 75: 2271–2276.

Chu NR, Wu HB, Wu TC *et al.* (2000) Immunotherapy of a human papillomavirus (HPV) type 16 E7-expressing tumour by administration of fusion protein comprising *Mycobacterium bovis* bacille Calmette-Guerin (BCG) hsp65 and HPV16 E7. *Clinical and Experimental Immunology* 121: 216–225.

Corona Gutierrez CM, Tinoco A, Navarro T *et al.* (2004) Therapeutic vaccination with MVA E2 can eliminate precancerous lesions (CIN 1, CIN 2, and CIN 3) associated with infection by oncogenic human papillomavirus. *Human Gene Therapy* 15: 421–431.

Cromme FV, Airey J, Heemels M-T *et al.* (1994) Loss of transporter protein, encoded by the TAP-1 gene, is highly correlated with loss of HLA expression in cervical carcinomas. *Journal of Experimental Medicine* 179: 335–340.

Da Silva DM, Velders MP, Nieland JD *et al.* (2001) Physical interaction of human papillomavirus virus-like particles with immune cells. *International Immunology* 13: 633–641.

Daemen T, Regts J, Holtrop M, Wilschut J (2002) Immunization strategy against cervical cancer involving an alphavirus vector expressing high levels of a stable fusion protein of human papillomavirus 16 E6 and E7. *Gene Therapy* 9: 85–94.

Davidson EJ, Boswell CM, Sehr P *et al.* (2003) Immunological and clinical responses in women with vulval intraepithelial neoplasia vaccinated with a vaccinia virus encoding human papillomavirus 16/18 oncoproteins. *Cancer Research* 63: 6032–6041.

De Jong A, O'Neill T, Khan A *et al.* (2002) Enhancement of human papillomavirus (HPV) type 16 E6 and E7-specific T-cell immunity in healthy volunteers through vaccination with TA-CIN, an HPV16 L2E7E6 fusion protein vaccine. *Vaccine* 20: 3456–3464.

Dillner J (1999) The serological response to papillomaviruses. *Seminars in Cancer Biology* 9: 423–430.

Donnelly JJ, Martinez D, Jansen KU *et al.* (1996) Protection against papillomavirus with a polynucleotide vaccine. *Journal of Infectious Diseases* 173: 314–320.

Dunn LA, Evander M, Tindle RW *et al.* (1997) Presentation of the HPV16E7 protein by skin grafts is insufficient to allow graft rejection in an E7-primed animal. *Virology* 235: 94–103.

Eiben GL, Velders MP, Schreiber H *et al.* (2002) Establishment of an HLA-A*0201 human papillomavirus type 16 tumor model to determine the efficacy of vaccination strategies in HLA-A*0201 transgenic mice. *Cancer Research* 62: 5792–5799.

Embers ME, Budgeon LR, Pickel M, Christensen ND (2002) Protective immunity to rabbit oral and cutaneous papillomaviruses by immunization with short peptides of L2, the minor capsid protein. *Journal of Virology* 76: 9798–9805.

Emeny RT, Wheeler CM, Jansen KU *et al.* (2002) Priming of human papillomavirus type 11-specific humoral and cellular immune responses in college-aged women with a virus-like particle vaccine. *Journal of Virology* 76: 7832–7842.

Evans TG, Bonnez W, Rose RC *et al.* (2001) A phase 1 study of a recombinant viruslike particle vaccine against human papillomavirus type 11 in healthy adult volunteers. *Journal of Infectious Diseases* 183: 1485–1493.

Feltkamp MC, Smits HL, Vierboom MP *et al.* (1993) Vaccination with cytotoxic T lymphocyte epitope-containing peptide protects against a tumor induced by human papillomavirus type 16-transformed cells. *European Journal of Immunology* 23: 2242–2249.

Ferrara A, Nonn M, Sehr P *et al.* (2003) Dendritic cell-based tumor vaccine for cervical cancer. II. Results of a clinical pilot study in 15 individual patients. *Journal of Cancer Research and Clinical Oncology* 129: 521–530.

Frazer IH (1996) Immunology of papillomavirus infection. *Current Opinion in Immunology* 8: 484–491.

Frazer IH, Tindle RW, Fernando GJ *et al.* (1999) Safety and immunogenicity of HPV16 E7/Algammulin immunotherapy for cervical cancer. In: Tindle RW (ed.) *Vaccines for Human Papillomavirus Infection and Anogenital Disease.* Austin, TX: Landes Bioscience, pp. 91–104.

Frazer IH, De Kluyver R, Leggatt GR *et al.* (2001) Tolerance or immunity to a tumor antigen expressed in somatic cells can be determined by systemic proinflammatory signals at the time of first antigen exposure. *Journal of Immunology* 167: 6180–6187.

Frazer IH (2004) Prevention of cervical cancer through papillomavirus vaccination (Review). *Nature Immunology* 4: 46–54.

Frazer IH, Quinn M, Nicklin JL *et al.* (2004) Phase 1 study of HPV16-specific immunotherapy with E6E7 fusion protein and ISCOMATRIX trade mark adjuvant in women with cervical intraepithelial neoplasia. *Vaccine* 23: 172–181.

Gerard CM, Baudson N, Kraemer K *et al.* (2001a) Therapeutic potential of protein and adjuvant vaccinations on tumour growth. *Vaccine* 19: 2583–2589.

Gerard CM, Baudson N, Kraemer K *et al.* (2001b) Recombinant human papillomavirus type 16 E7 protein as a model antigen to study the vaccine potential in control and E7 transgenic mice. *Clinical Cancer Research* 7 (3 suppl.): 838s–847s.

Giroglou T, Florin L, Schäfer F *et al.* (2001) Human papillomavirus infection requires cell surface heparan sulfate. *Journal of Virology* 75: 1565–1570.

Goldstone SE, Palefsky JM, Winnett MT, Neefe JR (2002) Activity of HspE7, a novel immunotherapy, in patients with anogenital warts. *Diseases of the Colon and Rectum* 45: 502–507.

Gunn GR, Zubair A, Peters C *et al.* (2001) Two *Listeria monocytogenes* vaccine vectors that express different molecular forms of human papilloma virus-16 (HPV-16) E7 induce qualitatively different T cell immunity that correlates with their ability to induce regression of established tumors immortalized by HPV-16. *Journal of Immunology* 167: 6471–6479.

Gurunathan S, Wu CY, Freidag BL, Seder RA (2000) DNA vaccines: a key for inducing long-term cellular immunity. *Current Opinion in Immunology* 12: 442–447.

Han R, Cladel NM, Reed CA *et al.* (2000) DNA vaccination prevents and/or delays carcinoma development of papillomavirus-induced skin papillomas on rabbits. *Journal of Virology* 74: 9712–9716.

Han R, Peng X, Reed CA *et al.* (2002) Gene gun-mediated intracutaneous vaccination with papillomavirus E7 gene delays cancer development of papillomavirus-induced skin papillomas on rabbits. *Cancer Detection and Prevention* 26: 458–467.

Hariharan K, Braslawsky G, Barnett RS *et al.* (1998) Tumor regression in mice following vaccination with human papillomavirus E7 recombinant protein in PROVAX. *International Journal of Oncology* 12: 1229–1235.

Harper DM, Franco EL, Wheeler C *et al.* (2004) Efficacy of a bivalent L1 virus-like particle vaccine in prevention of infection with human papillomavirus types 16 and 18 in young women: a randomised controlled trial. *Lancet* 364: 1757–1765.

Harro CD, Pang YY, Roden RB *et al.* (2001) Safety and immunogenicity trial in adult volunteers of a human papillomavirus 16 L1 virus-like particle vaccine. *Journal of the National Cancer Institute* 93: 284–292.

zur Hausen H (1999) Papillomaviruses in human cancers. *Proceedings of the Association of American Physicians* 111: 581–587.

Hernandez-Avila M, Lazcano-Ponce EC, Berumen-Campos J *et al.* (1997) Human papilloma virus 16–18 infection and cervical cancer in Mexico: a case-control study. *Archives of Medical Research* 28: 265–271.

Höpfl R, Heim K, Christensen N *et al.* (2000) Spontaneous regression of CIN and delayed-type hypersensitivity to HPV-16 oncoprotein E7. *Lancet* 356: 1985–1986.

Hsu KF, Hung CF, Cheng WF *et al.* (2001) Enhancement of suicidal DNA vaccine potency by linking Mycobacterium tuberculosis heat shock protein 70 to an antigen. *Gene Therapy* 8: 376–383.

Hung CF, Cheng WF, Hsu KF *et al.* (2001a) Cancer immunotherapy using a DNA vaccine encoding the translocation domain of a bacterial toxin linked to a tumor antigen. *Cancer Research* 61: 3698–3703.

Hung CF, Cheng WF, Chai CY *et al.* (2001b) Improving vaccine potency through intercellular spreading and enhanced MHC class I presentation of antigen. *Journal of Immunology* 166: 5733–5740.

Hung CF, Hsu KF, Cheng WF *et al.* (2001c) Enhancement of DNA vaccine potency by linkage of antigen gene to a gene encoding the extracellular domain of Fms-like tyrosine kinase 3-ligand. *Cancer Research* 61: 1080–1088.

Hung CF, He LM, Juang J *et al.* (2002) Improving DNA vaccine potency by linking Marck's disease virus type 1 VP22 to an antigen. *Journal of Virology* 76: 2676–2682.

Indrova M, Bubenik J, Simova J *et al.* (2001) Therapy of HPV 16-associated carcinoma with dendritic cell-based vaccines: *in vitro* priming of the effector cell responses by DC pulsed with tumour lysates and synthetic RAHYNIVTF peptide. *International Journal of Molecular Medicine* 7: 97–100.

Jarrett WFH, O'Neil BW, Gaukroger JM *et al.* (1990) Studies on vaccination against papillomaviruses: The immunity after infection and vaccination with bovine papillomaviruses of different types. *Veterinary Record* 126: 473–475.

Ji HX, Chang EY, Lin KY *et al.* (1998) Antigen-specific immunotherapy for murine lung metastatic tumors expressing human papillomavirus type 16 E7 oncoprotein. *International Journal of Cancer* 78: 41–45.

Ji HX, Wang TL, Chen CH *et al.* (1999) Targeting human papillomavirus type 16 E7 to the endosomal/lysosomal compartment enhances the antitumor immunity of DNA vaccines against murine human papillomavirus type 16 E7-expressing tumors. *Human Gene Therapy* 10: 2727–2740.

Jochmus-Kudielka I, Schneider A, Braun R *et al.* (1989) Antibodies against the human papillomavirus type 16 early proteins in human sera: Correlation of anti-E7 reactivity with cervical cancer. *Journal of the National Cancer Iinstitute* 81: 1698–1704.

Jones RW (2001) Vulval intraepithelial neoplasia: current perspectives. *European Journal of Gynaecology and Oncology* 22: 393–402.

Kadish AS, Timmins P, Wang YX *et al.* (2002) Regression of cervical intraepithelial neoplasia and loss of human papillomavirus (HPV) infection is associated with cell-mediated immune responses to an HPV type 16 E7 peptide. *Cancer Epidemiology Biomarkers and Prevention* 11: 483–488.

Kawana K, Kawana Y, Yoshikawa H *et al.* (2001) Nasal immunization of mice with peptide having a cross-neutralization epitope on minor capsid protein L2 of human papillomavirus type 16 elicit systemic and mucosal antibodies. *Vaccine* 19: 1496–1502.

Kirnbauer R, Chandrachud LM, O'Neil BW *et al.* (1996) Virus-like particles of bovine papillomavirus type 4 in prophylactic and therapeutic immunization. *Virology* 219: 37–44.

Klencke B, Matijevic M, Urban RG *et al.* (2002) Encapsulated plasmid DNA treatment for human papillomavirus 16-associated anal dysplasia: a Phase I study of ZYC101. *Clinical Cancer Research* 8: 1028–1037.

Koutsky LA, Ault KA, Wheeler CM *et al.* (2002) A controlled trial of a human papillomavirus type 16 vaccine. *New England Journal of Medicine* 347: 1645–1651.

Lamikanra A, Pan ZK, Isaacs SN *et al.* (2001) Regression of established human papillomavirus type 16 (HPV-16) immortalized tumors *in vivo* by vaccinia viruses expressing different forms of HPV-16 E7 correlates with enhanced CD8+ T-cell responses that home to the tumor site. *Journal of Virology* 75: 9654–9664.

Leder C, Kleinschmidt JA, Wiethe C, Müller M (2001) Enhancement of capsid gene expression: Preparing the human papillomavirus type 16 major structural gene L1 for DNA vaccination purposes. *Journal of Virology* 75: 9201–9209.

Lin KY, Guarnieri FG, Staveley-O'Carroll KF *et al.* (1996) Treatment of established tumors with a novel vaccine that enhances major histocompatibility class II presentation of tumor antigen. *Cancer Research* 56: 21–26.

Liu DW, Tsao YP, Kung JT *et al.* (2000) Recombinant adeno-associated virus expressing human papillomavirus type 16 E7 peptide DNA fused with heat shock protein DNA as a potential vaccine for cervical cancer. *Journal of Virology* 74: 2888–2894.

Liu WJ, Zhao KN, Gao FG *et al.* (2001) Polynucleotide viral vaccines: codon optimisation and ubiquitin conjugation enhances prophylactic and therapeutic efficacy. *Vaccine* 20: 862–869.

Liu WJ, Gao FG, Zhao KN *et al.* (2002) Codon modified human papillomavirus type 16 E7 DNA vaccine enhances cytotoxic T-lymphocyte induction and anti-tumour activity. *Virology* 301: 43–52.

Lowndes CM, Gill ON (2005) Cervical cancer, human papillomavirus and vaccination. *British Medical Journal* 331: 915–916.

Mao C, Koutsky LA, Ault KA *et al.* (2006) Efficacy of human papillomavirus-16 vaccine to prevent cervical intraepithelial neoplasia: a randomized controlled trial. *Obstetrics and Gynecology* 107:18–27.

Matsumoto K, Leggatt GR, Zhong J *et al.* (2004) Impaired antigen presentation and effectiveness of combined active/passive immunotherapy for epithelial tumors. *Journal of the National Cancer Institute* 96: 1611–1619.

Mayrand MH, Coutlée F, Hankins C *et al.* (2000) Detection of human papillomavirus type 16 DNA in consecutive genital samples does not always represent persistent infection as determined by molecular variant analysis. *Journal of Clinical Microbiology* 38: 3388–3393.

McMillan NAJ, Payne E, Frazer IH, Evander M (1999) Expression of the α6 integrin confers papillomavirus binding upon receptor-negative B-cells. *Virology* 261: 271–279.

Moore RA, Walcott S, White KL *et al.* (2003) Therapeutic immunisation with COPV early genes by epithelial DNA delivery. *Virology* 314: 630–635.

Muderspach L, Wilczynski S, Roman L *et al.* (2000) A phase I trial of a human papillomavirus (HPV) peptide vaccine for women with high-grade cervical and vulvar intraepithelial neoplasia who are HPV 16 positive. *Clinical Cancer Research* 6: 3406–3416.

Muñoz N, Bosch FX, De San Jose S *et al.* (2003) Epidemiologic classification of human papillomavirus types associated with cervical cancer. *New England Journal of Medicine* 348: 518–527.

Muñoz N, Bosch FX, Castellsigue X *et al.* (2004) Against which human papillomavirus type shall we vaccinate and screen? *International Journal of Cancer* 111: 278–285.

Ohlschlager P, Osen W, Dell K *et al.* (2003) Human papillomavirus type 16 L1 capsomeres induce L1-specific cytotoxic T lymphocytes and tumor regression in C57BL/6 mice. *Journal of Virology* 77: 4635–4645.

Peh WL, Middleton K, Christensen N *et al.* (2002) Life cycle heterogeneity in animal models of human papillomavirus-associated disease. *Journal of Virology* 76: 10401–10416.

Revaz V, Benyacoub J, Kast WM *et al.* (2001) Mucosal vaccination with a recombinant *Salmonella typhimurium* expressing human papillomavirus type 16 (HPV16) L1 virus-like particles (VLPs) or HPV16VLPs purified from insect cells inhibits the growth of HPV16-expressing tumor cells in mice. *Virology* 279: 354–360.

Schiller JT, Davies P (2004) Delivering on the promise: HPV vaccines and cervical cancer. *Nature Reviews Microbiology* 2: 343–347.

Schiller JT, Lowy DR (2001) Papillomavirus-like particle based vaccines: cervical cancer and beyond. *Expert Opinion on Biological Therapy* 1: 571–581.

Shedlock DJ, Weiner DB (2000) DNA vaccination: antigen presentation and the induction of immunity. *Journal of Leukocyte Biology* 68: 793–806.

Sheets EE, Urban RG, Crum CP *et al.* (2003) Immunotherapy of human cervical high-grade cervical intraepithelial neoplasia with microparticle-delivered human papillomavirus 16 E7 plasmid DNA. *American Journal of Obstetrics and Gynecology* 188: 916–926.

Smahel M, Síma P, Ludvíková V, Vonka V (2001) Modified HPV16 E7 genes as DNA vaccine against E7-containing oncogenic cells. *Virology* 281: 231–238.

Stanley MA (2002) Human papillomavirus vaccines. *Current Opinion on Molecular Therapy* 4: 15–22.

Stewart TJ, Smyth MJ, Fernando GJ *et al.* (2003) Inhibition of early tumor growth requires J alpha 18-positive (natural killer T) cells. *Cancer Research* 63: 3058–3060.

Suzich JA, Ghim SJ, Palmer-Hill FJ *et al.* (1995) Systemic immunization with papillomavirus L1 protein completely prevents the development of viral mucosal papillomas. *Proceedings of the National Academy of Sciences of the USA* 92: 11553–11557.

Tindle RW, Croft S, Herd K *et al.* (1995) A vaccine conjugate of 'ISCAR' immunocarrier and peptide epitopes of the E7 cervical cancer-associated protein of human papillomavirus type 16 elicits specific Th1- and Th2-type responses in immunized mice in the absence of oil-based adjuvants. *Clinical and Experimental Immunology* 101: 265–271.

Van Driel WJ, Ressing ME, Kenter GG *et al.* (1999) Vaccination with HPV16 peptides of patients with advanced cervical carcinoma: Clinical evaluation of a phase I–II trial. *European Journal of Cancer [A]* 35: 946–952.

Velders MP, McElhiney S, Cassetti MC *et al.* (2001a) Eradication of established tumors by vaccination with Venezuelan equine encephalitis virus replicon particles delivering human papillomavirus 16 E7 RNA. *Cancer Research* 61: 7861–7867.

Velders MP, Weijzen S, Eiben GL *et al.* (2001b) Defined flanking spacers and enhanced proteolysis is essential for eradication of established tumors by an epitope string DNA vaccine. *Journal of Immunology* 166: 5366–5373.

Villa LL, Costa RL, Petta CA *et al.* (2005) Prophylactic quadrivalent human papillomavirus (types 6, 11, 16, and 18) L1 virus-like particle vaccine in young women: a randomised double-blind placebo-controlled multicentre phase II efficacy trial. *Lancet Oncology* May 6: 271–278.

Vonka V, Sobotkova E, Hamsikova E *et al.* (1998) Induction of anti-tumour immunity by suicide-gene-modified HPV-16-transformed hamster cells. *International Journal of Cancer* 77: 470–475.

Walboomers JM, Jacobs MV, Manos MM *et al.* (1999) Human papillomavirus is a necessary cause of invasive cervical cancer worldwide. *Journal of Pathology* 189: 12–19.

Welters MJP, De Jong A, Van den Eeden SJF *et al.* (2003) Frequent display of human papillomavirus type 16 E6-specific memory T-helper cells in the healthy population as witness of previous viral encounter. *Cancer Research* 63: 636–641.

Welters MJ, van der Logt P, van den Eeden SJ *et al.* (2006) Detection of human papillomavirus type 18 E6 and E7-specific CD4+ T-helper 1 immunity in relation to health versus disease. *International Journal of Cancer* 118: 950–956.

Wen LM, Estcourt CS, Simpson JM, Mindel A (1999) Risk factors for the acquisition of genital warts: are condoms protective? *Sexually Transmitted Infections* 75: 312–316.

Wilcox RA, Flies DB, Zhu G *et al.* (2002) Provision of antigen and CD137 signaling breaks immunological ignorance, promoting regression of poorly immunogenic tumors. *Journal of Clinical Investigation* 109: 651–659.

Williams OM, Hart KW, Wang ECY, Gelder CM (2002) Analysis of CD4+ T-cell responses to human papillomavirus (HPV) type 11 L1 in healthy adults reveals a high degree of responsiveness and cross-reactivity with other HPV types. *Journal of Virology* 76: 7418–7429.

Xi LF, Koutsky LA (1997) Epidemiology of genital human papillomavirus infections. *Bulletin de l'Institut Pasteur* 95: 161–178.

Zhang LF, Zhou J, Chen S *et al.* (2000) HPV6b virus like particles are potent immunogens without adjuvant in man. *Vaccine* 18: 1051–1058.

Zhou J, Sun XY, Stenzel DJ, Frazer IH (1991) Expression of vaccinia recombinant HPV 16 L1 and L2 ORF proteins in epithelial cells is sufficient for assembly of HPV virion-like particles. *Virology* 185: 251–257.

Zwaveling S, Mota SCF, Nouta J *et al.* (2002) Established human papillomavirus type 16-expressing tumors are effectively eradicated following vaccination with long peptides. *Journal of Immunology* 169: 350–358.

CHAPTER 45

Psychosocial aspects associated with cervical disease and neoplasia

Cornelius O. Granai

INTRODUCTION

Physicians are asked by patients and society to suggest medical treatments by which meaningful physical recovery from illness/disease is most likely. Few can doubt the remarkable contributions of science to health, or the physician's caring behind the evolution in medical knowledge. Still, and as the poets suggest, many aspects of well-being lie outside of clinical logic or medical prose.

Medical insights about DNA, protein, cells, organs, anatomy, physiology, pathology, symptoms, treatment and prognosis all contribute to meeting health care needs. But are not broader perspectives also pertinent to more fully serving patients' needs? The broader psychological impact on a woman undergoing hysterectomy or even Pap smear screening can be enormous and the clinician must appreciate and attempt to understand these effects (Summers, 1998; Groff *et al.*, 2000). From that vantage, consider the personal poetry of Cheryl Townsend writing about the (surgical) loss of her uterus/cervix (Townsend, 1999).

The uniquely female organs — breasts, uterus, ovaries, vagina, vulva and cervix — are deeply central to female identity — just as the penis and the testicles are to men (Bergmark *et al.*, 1999). A loss of these organs, even when rationally understood as logical or essential in the case of certain life-threatening diseases, is not without its unavoidable psychosocial consequences/anxieties (Burney, 1812; Casey, 1996). Some women report, and probably many more worry about, losing a sense of self after hysterectomy, and this is true regardless of childbearing intent (Williams and Clark, 2000). The reproductive organs are, after all, an integral part of identity. Their loss, especially with the associated loss of fertility, can have a powerful adverse effect on a person's reality (Lewis *et al.*, 2000). This, in turn, can bring sadness and grief, affecting sexual expression and intimacy and threatening primary relationships (Zegwaard *et al.*, 2000). What makes someone 'whole' is likely to always outdistance final understanding, but recognising the potential psychological problems caused by loss or destruction of the cervix and uterus can help the clinician to manage the often unknowable complexities of such surgery or radiation produce (Dell and Papagiannidou, 1999).

A NARROWER FOCUS: THE CERVIX

Systematically dividing the body in terms of anatomy and physiology has proven far easier than understanding the non-linear psychosocial effect of those divisions. While all 'body parts' can be assumed to have meaning to the individual, it is equally intuitive that all parts do not engender identical psychosocial impacts. One division by which discrepancy in the 'personal meaning' can be found is between those 'parts' which are visible and those which are not. The invisibleness of 'internal organs', often compounded by their vagueness of biological function, conveys them to a relative impersonalness (Richter *et al.*, 2000). This obscurity explains why, for example, the adrenal glands and omentum have far less psychosocial meaning to individuals than do more familiar structures like the nose, uterus and breasts with their well-known physiological roles (Richter *et al.*, 2000).

As well known as 'the cervix' is compared with most other internal organs, abstractness still remains. Even 'anatomical understanding' is blurry as the cervix is a subregion of the uterus. Many otherwise well-educated women (and men) imagine the cervix as distinct and separate from the uterus, though somehow related (Summers, 1998). Despite anatomical confusion, 'the cervix' is widely regarded as being important, both physiologically and personally. There are obvious reasons for those perceptions. While not directly visible, the cervix is readily palpable, giving it a tangible presence not possessed by true intra-abdominal organs. More importantly, the cervix is intimately associated with sexuality, the profoundness of achieving and maintaining pregnancy, and giving birth. Thus, in contemplating the cervix's psychosocial impact on women, the multidimensional and overlapping implications of cervico-uterine anatomy, reproduction, reproductive cycling, procreation, contraception, birthing, sexuality, sexual expression, sexual identity, and how these relate to being 'whole' as a female, all have relevance (Williams and Clark, 2000).

Because the cervix and uterus are inextricably linked anatomically, physiologically and in general perception, and because there is relatively little medical literature uniquely concerning the psychosocial impact of 'the cervix' per se, much of what can be said on the subject must be inferred from the broader information available on 'hysterectomy' (including the cervix). Even disregarding the less enlightened eras in western culture, when the very word 'hysterectomy' was associated with the popular, though absurd, misconception that 'psychosis' and 'the uterus' were linked, there remains a contemporary impression that removal of a woman's uterus and cervix often leads to depression, sexual dysfunction and a whole host of mental and physical disabilities (Alexander *et al.*, 1996). These views are probably rooted in belief structures formed long before a hysterectomy is contemplated (Everson *et al.*, 1995; Twinn *et al.*, 2002).

CULTURAL VIEWS

Substantial sociological literature exists documenting how different cultures view sexuality, being female and womanhood (Williams and Clark, 2000; Kidanto *et al.*, 2002; Twinn *et al.*, 2002). As might be surmised, major variations have been found. Still, all cultures hold female primacy in bearing children sacred. The remarkableness of females in procreation and the selfless nurturing seemingly embedded in that potential are universally valued by the men; but here too substantial differences exist between cultures. These complexities of perceptions, among many others, cannot help but cause psychosocial impact on concepts surrounding reproductive organs and self (Galavotti and Richter, 2000; Lewis *et al.*, 2000; Rannestad *et al.*, 2000).

Cultural conventions of reproductive biology and their representations to society have a formative effect on personal self-image. Prime examples of this phenomenon are seen in the way girls learn about menarche (Mingo *et al.*, 2000). Cultural rituals abound marking and celebrating this milestone in a girl's life (Frisbie, 1993). These experiences can strongly affect how girls, and later women, relate to their reproductive systems and sexual relationships. What girls are told, infer and assimilate about such matters carries over into their adult reactions and interpretations about their being. But the self-image women hold is not unilaterally induced by the females in a society; it is also influenced by the attitudes of the males (Groff *et al.*, 2000; Williams and Clark, 2000; Schover, 2003). For instance, anthropologists have long observed that women in certain African cultures are no longer defined (by men) as being 'female' if they have undergone hysterectomy. Indeed, some cultures hold that men are appropriately within their rights to permanently leave a hysterectomised spouse, even if the surgery was performed for life-saving reasons and child-bearing was no longer desired or possible (Bernhard *et al.*, 1992). Such examples begin to reveal the wide-ranging influences bearing on the potentially profound, but often unspoken, psychosocial responses women have to injuries, treatments and loss of their uterus and cervix (Lewis *et al.*, 2000; McKee *et al.*, 2002; Tishelman *et al.*, 2002).

Even within a single country — ostensibly possessing similar values — studies have found substantial differences in psychoso-

cial impressions, with implications for the cervix. Within the USA, for example, major differences in attitude exist between geographical regions, and to some extent between races, as pertains to hysterectomy. These differences may add to the matrix of reasons underlying the variability in the hysterectomy rates seen nationally, which can be fivefold (Haas *et al.*, 1993). At great risk of oversimplifying, comparing American women, empirical data suggest that less educated women are less concerned about negative notions of hysterectomy (Kjerulff *et al.*, 1993; Brett *et al.*; 1997; Groff *et al.*, 2000; Lewis *et al.*, 2000). Another example of the psychosocial discrepancies occurring within a single country can be found in the relatively greater belief held by African American males that hysterectomy results in negative changes in the male–female relationship (Richter *et al.*, 2000; Williams and Clark, 2000). This sense may contribute to why, in statistical proportions higher than for whites or Asians, black males seek a new female relationship after a spouse's hysterectomy. Awareness of such male tendencies would logically affect how the women in those relationships feel and act (or do not act), possibly to the detriment of their own health (Agency for Health Care Policy and Research, 1996; Groff *et al.*, 2000; Williams and Clark, 2000; Tishelman *et al.*, 2002).

Some explanations for the perplexing feelings held by men about a woman's loss of uterus/cervix have been documented to include a lack of accurate understanding of female anatomy and physiology, the sense that the woman is no longer whole without her uterus/cervix, a belief that sex won't be as good after surgery and that the man will not be able to 'plant his seed' (Lalos and Lalos, 1996; Williams and Clark, 2000). Add to these beliefs the fear that they may 'catch the disease which led to their wife's hysterectomy' — including STDs or, worse, cancer — and an overarching environment of negativeness, with corresponding psychosocial effects on women and men, becomes apparent (Sevin, 1999; Groff *et al.*, 2000; Shiffman and Castle, 2003).

As vast as these concerns (male and female) are, and as deep as cultural influence can be, most misguided concepts can be favourably altered by education (Frisbie, 1993; Kunz and Oxman, 1998; McKee *et al.*, 2002). Underlying myths can be systematically addressed and correct information given (Williams and Clark, 2000). Doing so has a mitigating effect, diminishing an otherwise negative psychosocial impact on women and their partners. Providing this education is an important role for health care providers, and is best started in childhood and continued throughout life (and surely before, during and after major health events, like those requiring hysterectomy) (Rudy and Bush, 1992; Callaghan and Li, 2002).

HYSTERECTOMY FOR NON-MALIGNANT REASONS

Hysterectomy is the most common non-obstetrical major surgery in the USA, with about 633 000 cases being performed annually (Lepine *et al.*, 1997). As mentioned, hysterectomy rates vary by geographical region, the south having the highest, the north-east the lowest (Bernstein *et al.*, 1993; Broder *et al.*, 2000). Overall, 37% of American women and 20% of women in the UK have had hysterectomy by age 66 (Coulter *et al.*, 1988). The peak incidence is at 40–49 years old. The vast majority of hysterectomies are done with quality of life as the indication, pain and bleeding being chief among the indicators (Bachmann, 1990; Maresh *et al.*, 2002). In sharp contrast to the widespread hearsay, 88% of women report improvement in their symptoms, hence in quality of life, consequent on hysterectomy (Carlson *et al.*, 1994; Everson *et al.*, 1995; Kjerulff *et al.*, 2000). And numerous studies have found that the performance of supracervical hysterectomy, leaving the cervix *in situ*, does not result in better post-surgical sexual function (Kikku *et al.*, 1981; Kikku, 1983, 1985; Zhang *et al.*, 2002), fewer urinary tract problems or any other advantages (Virtanen *et al.*, 1993; Schaffer and Word, 2002; Thakar *et al.*, 2002; Learman *et al.*, 2003) compared with total hysterectomy with removal of the cervix. Further, controlled trials have now shown that hysterectomy is able to bring symptomatic relief when more conservative interventions have failed, yielding significant improvements in overall mental health, sleep problems, sexual function and general health perceptions (Kupperman *et al.*, 2004). Despite the overwhelming scientific evidence to the contrary, there continues to be a small number of vocal advocates who persist in circulating anecdotal stories of weight gain, depression, facial hair growth and sexual dysfunction following hysterectomy (Groff *et al.*, 2000).

Despite the more critical studies documenting real improvement in the majority of women, the problem of post-hysterectomy sexual dysfunction is still real for some (Dinnerstein *et al.*, 1977; Poad and Arnold, 1994). The aetiology of postoperative sexual dysfunction is not always surgically induced and, whatever the cause, there are helpful remedies for most of these women. Sexual dysfunction following hysterectomy varies with age, menopausal status, oophorectomy, partner's attitude and level of pre-hysterectomy sexual functionality (Schover, 1999; Krychman and Carter, 2003). Studies have shown that, if non-anatomical sexual dysfunction existed pre-surgery, these women/couples will probably continue to have the same type of sexual dysfunction after hysterectomy (Eisemann and Lalos, 1999; Thakar *et al.*, 2002). In other words, anecdotal reports of sexual dysfunction and other problems after hysterectomy, often a subject for popular media, rarely control for the level of pre-existent dysfunction (Everson *et al.*, 1995; Williams and Clark, 2000). Unfortunately, the distribution of those flawed unilateral stories only helps to reinforce an environment of negative psychosocial impressions (Kunz and Oxman, 1998; Benson and Harz, 2000; Hoffman, 2003).

It is encouraging to know that full recovery after hysterectomy is possible, but this is not to suggest surgery as the first option in the management of symptoms. Indeed, non-surgical interventions are less expensive and frequently successful in obviating the need for hysterectomy (Hurskainen *et al.*, 2004). But when lesser therapies are unsuccessful and hysterectomy is required, the positive outcome reported in recent, well-controlled, prospective trials tell a story of optimistic potential, including the return of high rates of sexual satisfaction (Hurskainen *et al.*, 2004; Kupperman *et al.*, 2004; Pitkin and Scott, 2004). While the news here is good, the loss of uterus/cervix remains a major physical event with both real and mythical implications, which need to be addressed by health care providers if maximal recovery is to occur. The risk of sexual dysfunction after hysterectomy is not small (initially 40–60% in some series), but prospective contemporary evidence suggests that sexual dysfunction, or for that matter bladder and bowel function, is not negatively altered by hysterectomy when properly managed. Preoperative identification of problems in these areas and a frank yet optimistic discussion of realistic post-hysterectomy expectations can eliminate or at least reduce the destructive psychosocial impact of these symptoms and all of their ripple effects (Krychman and Carter, 2003; Weijmer Shultz and Van de Wiel, 2003).

HYSTERECTOMY FOR CANCER

Major as the psychosocial impacts of hysterectomy and recovery are in their own right, both are many times compounded when the indication for surgery is cancer (Lagana *et al.*, 2001). Fewer than 10% of hysterectomies in the USA are done for cancer, the majority being in older women with endometrial cancer (Guyatt and Rennie, 2002). Still, many women are treated with surgery, radiation and chemotherapy for cervical cancer in the USA, and multitudes more worldwide — especially in countries where cervical cancer screening programmes are less prevalent or non-existent (ACOG Practice Bulletin, 2002). Because cervical cancer has a younger age of onset, the likelihood of unfulfilled fertility desires is greater, further compounding the psychosocial effects (Nair, 2000; Covens *et al.*, 2001; Carter *et al.*, 2003).

Virtually all women with gynaecological cancers report some level of sexual dysfunction after treatment (Schover *et al.*, 1989; Anderson, 1990; Anderson *et al.*, 1997; Bergmark *et al.*, 1999). Anderson's studies found a 90% incidence of sexual dysfunction among gynaecology cancer patients (Anderson, 1990). This contrasts with the much lower rates following hysterectomy for non-malignant indications or even non-gynaecological malignancies (e.g. 25% sexual dysfunction rates after therapy for Hodgkin's disease) (Mumma *et al.*, 1992; Bloom *et al.*, 1993; van Tulder *et al.*, 1994). The magnified psychosocial effects caused by the diagnosis of cancer are readily understood as malignancy raises questions of life and death (Hagerty *et al.*, 2003). Add to these deep psychological concerns the physical changes, which are often quite substantial by virtue of the extensive nature of cancer treatment, and it is no wonder that sexual dysfunction becomes a nearly inevitable part of recovery (Auchincloss and McCartney, 1998; Butler-Manuel *et al.*, 1999; Zegwaard *et al.*, 2000; Lagana *et al.*, 2001). In a study of cervical cancer patients with early stage disease, a significant proportion had post-treatment sexual dysfunction attributed to severe dyspareunia caused by tissues altered by radical surgery or radical radiation (Cyranowski and Anderson, 1998; Bergmark *et al.*, 2002; Covens, 2003). In comparing these two primary oncological treatment modalities, common sense and various reports suggests less sexual dysfunction following radical surgery, especially if ovarian function is preserved (which is not possible if pelvic radiation is used) (Anderson *et al.*, 1989; Bruner *et al.*, 1993; Berclaz *et al.*, 2002; Grumann *et al.*, 2001).

RECOVERY/PSYCHOSOCIAL PERSPECTIVE

Central to the recovery of cancer patients following radical hysterectomy or radical radiation treatment of the cervix — in a way not fundamentally dissimilar to the recovery of all women undergoing removal of the uterus/cervix — is the physician's proactive awareness of the patient's and family's need for education and support (Plante *et al.*, 1997; Schover, 1999). Seventy-eight per cent of cancer patients report that they wish to speak directly with their physician about sexuality and sexual function as part of their overall recovery (Landcaster, 1993; Lagana *et al.*, 2001). However, most also say they are too shy or fearful to do so (Agency for Health Care Policy and Research, 1996). Instead, they wait for the subject to be raised by the physician, which usually does not occur (Singer and Schwartz, 2002). To the extent that the psychosocial aspects of recovery are discussed, female physicians are more likely to broach the subject (Groff *et al.*, 2000).

Hoping to begin to rectify this obvious omission in health care, it has been suggested that problems like 'sexual dysfunction' be accorded the status of major post-treatment morbidity, just like fever, infection and wound breakdown (Carter *et al.*, 2003). As such, the morbidity of sexual dysfunction, in some ways a marker for broader psychosocial concerns, should be routinely screened for by physicians and treated when encountered (Bloom *et al.*, 1993; Greimel and Freidl, 2000; Lagana *et al.*, 2001). After diagnosis, the ideal means of managing serious/complex sexual dysfunction is with the expertise of a multidisciplinary team including psychosexual interventions such as counselling and support (Nair, 2000; American Cancer Society, 2001; Lagana *et al.*, 2001; Capelli *et al.*, 2002; Petersen and Quinlivan, 2002). But the key to intervention, no matter how complex, is recognition of the problem in the first place. Often this has only to do with 'opening the door' to a conversation with the patient, which she will appreciatively enter and elaborate her problems and concerns. Successful overall rehabilitation can follow (Li *et al.*, 1999; Gergmark *et al.*, 2000; Zegwaard *et al.*, 2000). The responsibility of initiating this conversation appropriately falls to the primary surgeons/oncologists most involved with the woman's ongoing (cancer) treatment and long-term follow-up (Nair, 2000). Female nurses who are part of the treatment team may be easier for the patient to talk with and they should also introduce the question of sexual function during and after treatment with the patient. Physicians and all members of their teams need to be constantly alert for clues to their patient's psychosocial, as well as physical, morbidities, and to the long-term sequelae which can result if these morbidities are not addressed (Robison, 1998; Ganz *et al.*, 2000). The ones cited are but a few of those pertaining in life, here paradoxically revealed by the 'narrow focus' of the uterine cervix. And, although the poets remind us some things are destined for mystery, their consideration, and what naturally flows from it, is part of the best health care we wish for all patients. These mysteries may be even farther removed from this male author, incapable of knowing by first-hand experience. So, then, a gentle disclaimer:

> Writing on subjects, regardless their way
> best done by those who know what they say
> from learning from life and feeling what is
> rather than lectures, gold stars on a quiz,
> rather than quoting that published in bold
> data flat certain the facts are as told.
> Better to know from having lived where
> earnest the insights that common sense bares,
> yet here sits said 'author' to write what is real
> on matters of being that he cannot feel.
> But in the inversion might something be gleaned
> through kindness of others some parallels seen?

REFERENCES

ACOG Practice Bulletin (2002) Diagnosis and treatment of cervical carcinomas, number 35. *Obstetrics and Gynecology* 99: 855–867.

Agency for Health Care Policy and Research (1996) AHCPR funds studies on hysterectomy and alternative treatments for uterine conditions. *Research Activities* 198: 15.

Alexander DA, Naj A, Pinion SB *et al.* (1996) Randomized trial comparing hysterectomy with endometrial ablation for dysfunctional uterine bleeding: Psychiatric and psychosocial aspects. *British Medical Journal* 312: 280.

American Cancer Society (2001) *Sexuality and Cancer: For the Woman who has Cancer and her Partner.* American Cancer Society booklet, 98 pp.

Anderson BL (1990) How cancer affects sexual functioning. *Oncology* 4: 81–94.

Anderson BL, Anderson B, deProsse C (1989) Controlled prospective longitudinal study of women with cancer: sexual functioning outcomes. *Journal of Consultative and Clinical Psychology* 57: 692–697.

Anderson BL, Woods XA, Copeland LJ (1997) Sexual self schema and sexual morbidity among gynecological cancer survivors. *Journal of Consultative and Clinical Psychology* 65: 221–229.

Auchincloss S, McCartney DF (1998) Gynecologic cancer in Holland. *Psychoncology*. New York: Oxford University Press, pp. 359–370.

Bachmann GA (1990) Hysterectomy: a critical review. *Journal of Reproductive Medicine* 35: 839–62.

Benson K, Hartz AJ (2000) A comparison of observational studies and randomized, controlled trials. *New England Journal of Medicine* 342: 1878–1886.

Berclaz G, Gerber E, Beer K *et al.* (2002) Long-term follow-up of concurrent radiotherapy and chemotherapy for locally advanced cervical cancer: 12-year survival after radiochemotherapy. *International Journal of Oncology* 20: 1313–1318.

Bergmark K, Avall-Lundqvist E, Dickman PW *et al.* (1999) Vaginal changes and sexuality in women with a history of cervical cancer. *New England Journal of Medicine* 340: 1383–9.

Bergmark K, Avall-Lundqvist E, Dickman PW *et al.* (2002) Patient-rating of distressful symptoms after treatment for early cervical cancer. *Acta Obstetrica et Gynecologica Scandinavica* 81: 443–450.

Bernhard LA, Harris CR, Caroline HA (1992) Men's views about hysterectomies and women who have them. *Image* 24: 177.

Bernstein SJ, McGlynn EA, Siu AL *et al.* (1993) The appropriateness of hysterectomy: a comparison of care in seven health plans. *Journal of the American Medical Association* 269: 2398–2402.

Bloom JR, Fobair P, Gritz E *et al.* (1993) Psychosocial outcomes of cancer: a comparative analysis of Hodgkin's disease and testicular cancer. *Journal of Clinical Oncology* 11: 979–988.

Brett KM, Marsh JVR, Madans JH (1997) Epidemiology of hysterectomy in the United States: Demographic and reproductive factors in a nationally representative sample. *Journal of Women's Health* 6: 309.

Broder MS, Kanouse DE, Mittman BS, Bernstein SJ (2000) The appropriateness for recommendations for hysterectomy. *Obstetrics and Gynecology* 95: 199–205.

Bruner DW, Lanciano R, Keegan M *et al.* (1993) Vaginal stenosis and sexual dysfunction following intracavity radiation for the treatment of cervical and endometrial carcinoma. *International Journal of Radiation, Oncology, Biology and Physics* 27: 825–830.

Burney F (1812) A mastectomy. *The Journal and Letters.* Oxford: Oxford University Press, pp. 2798–2805.

Butler-Manuel SA, Summerville K, Ford AM *et al.* (1999) Self assessment of morbidity following radical hysterectomy for cervical cancer. *British Journal of Obstetrics and Gynaecology* 19: 180–183.

Callaghan P, Li HC (2002) The effect of pre-operative psychological interventions on post-operative outcomes in Chinese women having an elective hysterectomy. *British Journal of Health Psychology* 7: 247–252.

Capelli G, De Vincenzo RI, Addamo A *et al.* (2002) Which dimensions of health-related quality of life are altered in patients attending the different gynecologic oncology health care settings? *Cancer* 95: 2500–2507.

Carlson KJ, Miller BA, Fowler FJ Jr (1994) The Maine Women's Health Study. Outcomes of hysterectomy. *Obstetrics and Gynecology* 83: 556–565.

Carter J, Auchincloss S, Sonoda Y, Krychman M (2003) Cervical cancer: issues of sexuality and fertility. *Oncology* 17: 1229–1242.

Casey C (1996) Psychosexual morbidity following gynecological malignancy. *Irish Medical Journal* 89: 200–202.

Coulter A, McPherson K, Vessey M (1988) Do British women undergo too many or too few hysterectomies? *Social Science and Medicine* 27: 987–994.

Covens A (2003) The Carter/Auchincloss/Sonada *et al.* article reviewed. *Oncology* 17: 1239–1242.

Covens A, Rosen B, Murphy J *et al.* (2001) Changes in the demographics and perioperative care of stage IA(2)–IB(1) cervical cancer over the past 16 years. *Gynecologic Oncology* 81: 133–137.

Cyranowski JM, Anderson BL (1998) Schemas, sexuality, and romantic attachment. *Journal of Personal and Social Psychology* 74: 1364–1379.

Dell P, Papagiannidou S (1999) Hysterical talk? A discourse analysis of Greek women's accounts of their experience following hysterectomy with oophorectomy. *Journal of Reproductive and Infant Psychology* 17: 391–404.

Dinnerstein L, Wood C, Burrows GD (1977) Sexual response following hysterectomy and oophorectomy. *Obstetrics and Gynecology* 49: 92–6.

Eisemann M, Lalos A (1999) Psychosocial determinants of well-being in gynecologic cancer patients. *Cancer Nursing* 22: 303–6.

Everson SA, Matthews KA, Guzick DS *et al.* (1995) Effects of surgical menopause on psychological characteristics and lipid levels: the healthy women study. *Health Psychology* 14: 435–443.

Frisbie CJ (1993) *Kinaalda: A Study of the Navajo Girl's Puberty Ceremony.* Salt Lake City: University of Utah Press.

Galavotti C, Richter DL (2000) Talking about hysterectomy: the experiences of women from four cultural groups. *Journal of Women's Health and Gender Based Medicine* 9: S63–S67.

Ganz PA, Greendale GA, Peterson L *et al.* (2000) Managing menopausal symptoms in breast cancer survivors: results of a randomized controlled trial. *Journal of the National Cancer Institute* 92: 1054–1064.

Gergmark K, Avall-Lundqvist E, Steineck G (2000) A Swedish study of women treated for cervix cancer. Gynecologic cancer often affects sexuality. *Lakartidningen* 97: 5347–5355.

Greimel ER, Freidl W (2000) Functioning in daily living and psychological well-being of female cancer patients. *Journal of Psychosomatic and Obstetric Gynaecology* 21: 25–30.

Groff JY, Mullen PD, Byrd T *et al.* (2000) Decision making, beliefs, and attitudes toward hysterectomy: a focus group study with medically underserved women in Texas. *Journal of Women's Health and Gender Based Medicine* 9: S39–S50.

Grumann M, Robertson R, Hacker NF, Sommer G (2001) Sexual functioning in patients following radical hysterectomy for stage IB cancer of the cervix. *International Journal of Gynecolical Cancer* 11: 372–380.

Guyatt G, Rennie D (2002) *User's Guide to the Medical Literature: A Manual for Evidence-based Clinical Practice.* Chicago, IL: American Medical Association.

Haas S, Acker D, Donahue C, Katz ME (1993) Variation in hysterectomy rates across small geographic areas of Massachusetts. *American Journal of Obstetrics and Gynecology* 169: 150–154.

Hagerty RG, Butow PN, Ellis PA *et al.* (2003) Cancer patient preferences for communication of prognosis in the metastatic setting. *Journal of Clinical Oncology* 22: 1721–1730.

Hoffmann H (2003) Is my sex life normal? *The Female Patient*, pp. 16–17.

Hurskainen R, Teperi J, Rissanen P *et al.* (2004) Clinical outcomes and costs with the levonorgestrel-releasing intrauterine system or hysterectomy for treatment of menorrhagia: randomized trial 5-year follow-up. *Journal of the American Medical Association* 291: 1456–1463.

Kidanto HL, Kilewo CD, Moshiro C (2002) Cancer of the cervix: knowledge and attitudes of female patients admitted at Muhimbili National Hospital, Dar es Salaam. *East African Medical Journal* 79: 467–475.

Kikku P (1983) Supravaginal uterine amputation vs. hysterectomy: effects on coital frequency and dyspareunia. *Acta Obstetrica et Gynecologica Scandinavica* 62: 141–145.

Kikku P (1985) Supravaginal uterine amputation versus hysterectomy with reference to subjective bladder symptoms and incontinence. *Acta Obstetrica et Gynecologica Scandinavica* 64: 375–9.

Kikku P, Hirvonen T, Gronroos M (1981) Supra-vaginal uterine amputation vs. abdominal hysterectomy: the effects on urinary symptoms with special reference to pollakisuria, nocturia, and dysuria. *Maturitas* 3: 197–204.

Kjerulff KH, Langenberry PW, Guzinski GM (1993) The socioeconomic correlates of hysterectomies in the United States. *American Journal of Public Health* 83: 106.

Kjerulff KH, Langenberg PW, Rhodes JC *et al.* (2000) Effectiveness of hysterectomy. *Obstetrics and Gynecology* 95: 319–326.

Krychman ML, Carter J (2003) The sexual health service at the Barbara White Women's Health Center at Memorial Sloan-Kettering Cancer Center. In: *Update in Gynecologic Oncology: Quality of Life in the Gynecologic Cancer Patient*. New York: Memorial Sloan-Kettering Cancer Center, pp. 1–2.

Kunz R, Oxman AD (1998) The unpredictability paradox: review of empirical comparisons of randomized and non-randomized clinical trials. *British Medical Journal* 317: 1185–1190.

Kuppermann M, Varner RE, Summitt RL Jr *et al.* (2004) Effect of hysterectomy vs. medical treatment on health related quality of life and sexual functioning: the medicine or surgery (Ms) randomized trial. *Journal of the American Medical Association* 291: 1447.

Lagana L, McGarvey EL, Classen C *et al.* (2001) Psychosexual dysfunction among gynecological cancer survivors. *Journal of Clinical Psychology in Medical Settings* 8: 73–83.

Lalos A, Lalos O (1996) The partner's view about hysterectomy. *Journal of Psychosomatic and Obstetric Gynaecology* 12: 119.

Landcaster J (1993) Women's experiences of gynecological cancer treated with radiation. *Curaltonis* 16: 37–42.

Learman LA, Summitt RL Jr, Varner RE *et al.* (2003) A randomized comparison of total or supracervical hysterectomy: surgical complications and clinical outcomes. Total or Supracervical Hysterectomy (TOSH) Research Group. *Obstetrics and Gynecology* 102: 453–62.

Lepine LA, Hills SD, Marchbanks PA *et al.* (1997) Hysterectomy surveillance — United States, 1980–1993. *Morbidity and Mortality Weekly Report CDC Surveillance Summaries* 46: 1–15.

Lewis CE, Groff JY, Herman CJ *et al.* (2000) Overview of women's decision making regarding elective hysterectomy, oophorectomy, and hormone replacement therapy. *Journal of Women's Health and Gender Based Medicine* 9: S5–S14.

Li C, Samsioe G, Iosif C (1999) Quality of life in long-term survivors of cervical cancer. *Maturitas* 32: 95–102.

Maresh MJA, Metcalfe MA, McPherson K *et al.* (2002) The VALUE national hysterectomy study: description of the patients and their surgery. *British Journal of Obstetrics and Gynaecology* 109: 302–312.

McKee MD, Caban A, Burton W, Mulvihill M (2002) Women's knowledge and experience of atypical Pap results in a high risk community. *Women's Health* 36: 19–31.

Mingo C, Herman CJ, Jasperse M (2000) Women's Stories: Ethnic variations in women's attitudes and experiences of menopause, hysterectomy, and hormone replacement therapy. *Journal of Women's Health and Gender Based Medicine* 9: 27–39.

Mumma GH, Mashberg D, Lesko LM (1992) Long-term psychosexual adjustment of acute leukemia survivors: impact of marrow transplantation versus conventional chemotherapy. *General Hospital Psychiatry* 14: 43–55.

Nair MG (2000) Quality of life in cancer of the cervix patients. *International Clinical Psychopharmacology* 15 (suppl. 3): S47–S49.

Petersen RW, Quinlivan JA (2002) Preventing anxiety and depression in gynecological cancer: a randomized controlled trial. *British Journal of Obstetrics and Gynaecology* 109: 386–394.

Pitkin RM, Scott JR (2004) Evaluating gynecological surgical procedures: trials and tribulations. *Journal of the American Medical Association* 291: 1503–1504.

Plante M, Roy M (1997) Radical trachelectomy. *Operative Techniques in Gynecological Surgery* 2: 187–199.

Poad D, Arnold EP (1994) Sexual function after pelvic surgery in women. *Australian and New Zealand Journal of Obstetrics and Gynaecology* 34: 471–474.

Rannestad T, Eikeland O, Helland H, Qvarnstrom U (2000) Quality of life, pain, and psychological well-being in women suffering from gynecologic disorders. *Journal of Women's Health and Gender Based Medicine* 9: 897–903.

Richter DL, McKeown RE, Corwin SJ *et al.* (2000) The role of male partners in women's decision making regarding hysterectomy. *Journal of Women's Health and Gender Based Medicine* 9: S51–S61.

Robison JW (1998) Sexuality and cancer: breaking the silence. *Australian Family Physician* 27: 45–47.

Rudy DR, Bush IM (1992) Hysterectomy and sexual dysfunction: You can help. *Patient Care* 26: 67.

Schaffer JI, Word A (2002) Hysterectomy — Still a useful operation. *New England Journal of Medicine* 347: 1360–1362.

Schover LR (2003) The Carter/Auchincloss/Sonoda *et al.* article reviewed. The University of Texas, MD Anderson Cancer Center. *Oncology* 17: 1234.

Sevin BU (1999) Social implications of sexually transmitted cancer. *Journal of Women's Health and Gender Based Medicine* 8: 759–766.

Shiffman M, Castle PE (2003) Human papillomavirus. Epidemiology and public health. *Archives of Pathology and Laboratory Medicine* 127: 930–934.

Schover LR (1999) Counseling cancer patients about changes in sexual function. *Oncology* 13: 1585–1596.

Schover LR, Fife M, Gershenson DM (1989) Sexual dysfunction and treatment for early stage cervical cancer. *Cancer* 63: 204–212.

Singer S, Schwartz R (2002) Psychosocial aftercare of patients with endometrial or cervical cancer. *Zentralblatt für Gynäkologie* 124: 64–70.

Summers A (1998) Mental health consequences of cervical screening. *Psychology, Health & Medicine* 3: 113–127.

Thakar R, Ayers S, Clarkson P *et al.* (2002) Outcomes after total versus subtotal abdominal hysterectomy. *New England Journal of Medicine* 347: 1318–1325.

Tishelman C, Lundgren EL, Skald A *et al.* (2002) Quality of care from a patient perspective in population-based cervical cancer screening. *Acta Oncologica* 41: 253–261.

Townsend C (1999) *Here*. Stow, OH: Implosion Press. Also at www.agentofchaos.com/a20-poems.html (July 2002).

Twinn S, Shiu AT, Holroyd E (2002) Women's knowledge about cervical cancer and cervical screening practice: a pilot study of Hong Kong Chinese women. *Cancer Nursing* 25: 377–384.

van Tulder MW, Aaronson NK, Bruning PF (1994) The quality of life of long term survivors of Hodgkin's disease. *Annals of Oncology* 5: 153–158.

Virtanen HS, Makinen JI, Tenho T *et al.* (1993) Effects of abdominal hysterectomy on urinary and sexual symptoms. *British Journal of Urology* 72: 868–872.

Weijmer Schultz WC, Van de Wiel HB (2003) Sexuality, intimacy, and gynecological cancer. *Journal of Sex and Marital Therapy* 1: 121–128.

Williams RD, Clark AJ (2000) A qualitative study of women's hysterectomy experience. *Journal of Women's Health and Gender Based Medicine* 9: S15–S25.

Zegwaard MI, Gamel CJ, Durgis DJ *et al.* (2000) The experience of sexuality and information received in women with cervical cancer and their partners. *Verpleegkunde* 15: 18–27.

Zhang X, Gao Y, Yao Y *et al.* (2002) Effects of different operation modes and intervention on sexual life in the women who received hysterectomy. *Chinese Mental Health Journal* 16: 749–750, 757.

CHAPTER 46

Colposcopy training and accreditation

Charles W.E. Redman

INTRODUCTION

Colposcopy can be regarded as a test whose performance depends on the observer as well as on the clinical context in which it is used. Colposcopic findings are subjective and the related management decisions require problem-solving skills and experience. Both diagnosis and subsequent management require not only adequate training but also a sufficient workload to maintain those skills.

Generally there is increasing concern that patients receive high-quality and cost-effective care. The need to protect against inadequate practice is particularly relevant to colposcopy because of its subjective nature and because the large numbers of women who are examined are usually well. Performed correctly colposcopy minimises damage but performed badly the scope for needless damage is great. Whereas the indications for colposcopy may vary throughout the world, its primary objective is the same, namely to detect cervical disease, particularly preinvasive changes.

This chapter considers the argument for standards in colposcopy training and accreditation and partially details the experiences of the British Society for Colposcopy and Cervical Pathology (BSCCP) and the European Federation for Colposcopy (EFC) in tackling these issues. This is probably the first organised and formulated colposcopy training programme in existence. Although not specifically covered in this chapter, the exercise to establish quality standards in mammography screening in Europe might also usefully be looked at for guidance in establishing an approach (de Wolf and Perry, 1996).

In order to realise this goal it will be necessary to reach a common consensus on what is desired and how to go about it. A useful starting point would be to review the experience of others in similar ventures.

THE BRITISH (UK) EXPERIENCE

In the UK, colposcopy is performed as part of the National Health Service (NHS) Cervical Screening Programme (NHSCSP, 1996). Women aged between 20 and 65 are invited to have a cervical smear every 3–5 years, as a primary screen to select patients for further colposcopic assessment. Using a computerised call and recall system up to 93% of the targeted population, approximately 4 million women, are screened each year, of whom about 100 000 are referred for colposcopy. There are approximately 2000 practising colposcopists in the UK, 1800 (90%) of whom are members of the British Society for Colposcopy and Cervical Pathology and approximately 1600 (80%) registered with the BSCCP as certified colposcopists. Most colposcopists are doctors (95%), mostly gynaecologists, but there is an increasing number of nurse colposcopists.

Until recently, whereas cytological practice was subject to internal and external quality assurance with well-defined training requirements, colposcopy was practised on an *ad hoc* basis with minimal formal quality assurance.

In 1996 a working party involving the various parties involved in the NHSCSP recommended that there should be an agreed training programme. Responding to this recommendation the BSCCP launched an accreditation process and, in conjunction with Royal College of Obstetricians and Gynaecologists, introduced a structured training programme which all future colposcopists will need to complete successfully in order to practise as BSCCP-certified colposcopists.

BSCCP certification for colposcopy

The NHSCSP colposcopy quality standards require that all colposcopists are adequately trained and see sufficient patients to maintain their skills. The BSCCP has set the goal that all patients undergoing colposcopy are seen either by BSCCP-certified colposcopists or by trainees under supervision. At present certification occurs on a triennial basis and requires the colposcopist to demonstrate:

- a sufficient workload, which is defined as a minimum of 50 new patients per annum;
- commitment to audit;
- engagement in continued medical education, i.e. attendance at at least one BSCCP-recognised meeting every 3 years.

The BSCCP/RCOG (Royal College of Obstetricians and Gynaecologists) training programme

This programme is open to any qualified doctor or nurse who has attended a BSCCP-recognised basic colposcopy course. The trainee needs to identify a trainer, who must be a BSCCP-certified colposcopist, and then register with the BSCCP.

The training programme has an agreed curriculum and is structured and trainee centred. The trainee must see a total of 150 patients under supervision (the first 50 of these must be directly supervised and after that a formative assessment is carried out). In addition to completing a logbook the trainee is required to present 10 short case commentaries, on which their management is discussed. Successful completion of these requirements allows the trainee to be awarded the BSCCP/RCOG Colposcopy (D) diploma, i.e. in diagnostic colposcopy. There is an optional treatment module which allows the BSCCP/RCOG Colposcopy (DT) diploma, i.e. diagnosis and treatment.

Strengths of the programme

The training programme and accreditation process have been pragmatically created in an attempt to promote a degree of quality assurance without undue complexity or introducing unrealistic goals. This has been a notable achievement. There are a number of factors that have facilitated this initiative. The majority of UK colposcopy is practised within the NHS, which has during this period been increasingly concerned with audit, clinical governance and quality. The NHS is responsible for virtually all medical and nursing training in the UK.

Colposcopy forms part of the NHSCSP, which has helped to introduce a uniform strategy based on agreed quality standards. Through previously agreed national guidelines, the role of and indications for colposcopy have been well defined and there has been consultation with other professional bodies.

Weaknesses of the programme

While the training programme was formulated by those actively practising and teaching colposcopy, there was no formal educationalist input, although many accepted educational principles have been incorporated. It is a training programme that has minimal quality control and no objective assessment of the product, i.e. the trained colposcopist.

The quality of a training programme is dependent on the trainers. At present the only requirement to become a trainer is to be a BSCCP-certified colposcopist. Many trainers are unlikely to have received educational training and their abilities to train must vary. Apart from auditing some of the case commentaries (which in part may reflect the quality of training) there is no training quality assurance. Measures to address this shortcoming are being discussed, including seeking feedback from trainees and considering the possibility of some form of 'exit' assessment as occurs in other professional areas, such as obstetric ultrasound.

Lessons to be gained from the UK experience

In a relatively short space of time a comprehensive accreditation and training programme has been instituted. In many ways the scene was set for this to happen as throughout the NHS a quality assurance culture has emerged, responding to a political and public demand for cost-effectiveness and accountability. There appeared to be a high degree of consensus that these changes were right and necessary; consequently little opposition has been encountered.

Another factor that promoted the implementation of these initiatives was the uniformity of health care provision. Throughout the UK, colposcopy is a component part of the NHSCSP, and is usually undertaken as a secondary screening test on cases selected by cervical cytology, according to national guidelines. The screening strategy and its prosecution involves relatively few agencies, which have considerable influence on practice; once decisions are made they can be implemented relatively easily, illustrating the value of a recognised organisational structure.

The various changes introduced were kept simple with a view to increasing stringency and sophistication with time rather than bringing in wholesale a complicated package that would fail through impracticality.

The experience of the British (UK) system described above is at present being introduced to Europe via the auspices of the European Federation of Colposcopy. It is instructive to examine the steps by which this introduction has taken place, and study of these steps may provide a model for its employment in other countries.

DEVELOPMENT OF A EUROPEAN COLPOSCOPY TRAINING PROGRAMME

The growing opportunity for doctors within the European Union to train in one country and then to practise in another strongly indicates that common standards in training and clinical practice are needed. However, despite the self-evident value of sharing common standards for training and accreditation throughout Europe, the task of achieving this goal is immense. Not every country has the unifying factors that exist in the UK (the NHS, for example), and this hampers communication and obtaining a consensus. In addition, throughout Europe, apart from the obvious language difficulties, there are various systems of nomenclature and terminology which complicate discussion.

The need for organisation

Despite the need for a coordinating and organising body, it is also important to accept that there will be variation in practice from country to country for a variety of reasons. In addition, it is clear that the actual planning and provision of training is most effectively delivered using national bodies, such as individual colposcopy societies, which are in the best position to respond to the individual and varying national health care needs. However, not every country has a colposcopy society and the influence and significance of these societies varies immensely. There is clearly a need for a body that can promote standards in colposcopy at a European level by encouraging common standards in training and clinical practice.

The EFC is uniquely suited to this role. At its inception it was agreed that, while the standardisation of both training and clinical practice were important, the introduction of a common training programme had a fundamental significance.

Basic components of a training programme

A clinical training programme is not simply an educational course. It should have clearly defined aims and objectives which state what the programme will achieve and how the training is to be delivered. Assessment and quality assurance also need to be considered.

An initial survey of colposcopy training programmes in Europe, conducted in 2001, identified that there were only four existing national training programmes, despite the fact that colposcopy is performed throughout Europe. In other words, colposcopy societies have predominantly concentrated on scientific issues rather than supporting training. One of the key tasks for the EFC is to focus the attention of its member societies on training.

It is of interest to review the similarities and differences of the four programmes (Table 46.1).

From an educational point of view, three programmes were set up without formally identifying the aims and objectives (although the BSCCP/RCOG training programme did so in a later educational review). This emphasises how clinical training has, in general, lacked formal educational input. Formal assessment occurs in three of the four programmes but not in the UK, although there is some limited clinical and portfolio-type assessment. Differences in clinical practice are

apparent when comparing the workload criteria for trainers; for example, colposcopists in colposcopy training centres in Yugoslavia spend a greater proportion of their time undertaking colposcopy than clinicians in the UK. In addition, in the UK colposcopy training is predominantly part-time whereas in Yugoslavia it is full-time, which accounts for the difference in training duration.

There is clearly a need for greater unification in training. At the outset, it could not be assumed that all would agree on what colposcopy actually comprises and what should be included in a training curriculum. Therefore this needed to be addressed as an initial task. This could have been approached in a number of ways but a competence-based approach was used; in other words the emphasis would be on what is actually done rather than on theoretical or knowledge-based considerations.

Competence-based assessment and education

Competence-based education and training is an appealing concept. Its aim is to delineate, in explicit terms, the competences that an individual requires either at the end of an educational course or indeed those required to be able to continue to practice. The specialised nature of colposcopy naturally lends itself to competence-based studies, which can identify areas in which practitioners are lacking in complete competence and thus determine the priorities for a programme of structured continuing education.

How can competences be decided?

There are a number of options, which include:
- subject-centred or 'content knowledge' approach;
- task analysis;
- the Delphi technique.

The subject-centred or 'content knowledge' approach is the traditional approach by which almost all doctors have been and are being trained in the UK and Europe generally. The training methodology is theory dominated and demands factual knowledge at the expense of practical experience and clinical competence (i.e. abstract-rich and concrete-poor). The drawbacks of this approach are widely acknowledged.

Task analysis involves detailing all the functions that constitute the practice of colposcopy. One could then prepare a training programme founded on these activities. The obvious disadvantage of this approach is that it refers only to functional tasks and not how best to perform them. Such an exercise can only have doubtful worth.

The Delphi technique relies on the judgement of an expert panel or 'wise men'. This is one of the most commonly and successfully used mechanisms for identifying professional behaviour/competences. In brief an expert panel is identified. The number of these 'wise men' can vary but past practice has indicated that a minimum figure of 20 or so experts is appropriate.

Table 46.1 Comparison of current colposcopy training programmes.

Country	Aims[1]	Duration (months)[2]	Assessment[3]	Cases[4]	Trainer[5]
Belgium	x	6	√	150	x
Croatia	x	6	√	x	x
UK	√	18	x	150	50
Yugoslavia	√	3	√	x	900

1 Formally stated training aims and objectives.
2 Average duration of training programme.
3 Formal end of training assessment.
4 Stipulated minimum number of cases a trainee must see.
5 Stipulated number of cases a trainer must see in order to train.

These experts are interviewed individually and asked to complete the following tasks: (1) to define the general areas of knowledge, skills and attitudes needed for successful colposcopic practice; (2) to identify specific competences required within these general areas. These replies are collated confidentially into a single compilation incorporating all the items. This single list is then sent to all the participants with the request that they add to (or delete from) the appropriate section any competences they regard as necessary.

These returns are then collated and, if necessary, the process is repeated until a consensus is obtained. Eventually a final list is drawn up, based on the additions and deletions. This is then returned to the experts who are asked to indicate beside each one, using a five-point scale, how essential it is, in their opinion, that a colposcopist should possess that particular competence. These ratings are analysed and the results obtained indicate the principal competences necessary. This is then used as the basis for a training curriculum and a continuing education scheme.

European Federation for Colposcopy Delphi exercise

An important preliminary step was to agree the goal of the training programme. Currently colposcopy is practised in a number of different contexts throughout Europe. At the initial meeting of the EFC Training Sub-committee, held in Paris in October 2000, it was agreed that the goal of the training programme should initially focus on diagnosis and was defined as: 'To enable trainees to obtain the core knowledge and develop the necessary skills and the personal and professional attributes to enable them to be lifelong learners and compassionate colposcopists.'

The crucial decision was that the curriculum would be competence-based, comprising those core competences regarded as essential for the practice of colposcopy, and that the curriculum would be formed through consultation with experts throughout Europe using the Delphi technique.

The steering group drew up a list of possible core competences required for colposcopy and circulated it to all experts

Table 46.2 Minimum standards of training for colposcopy.

A Preliminary/preparatory	27 Recognise high-grade precancerous cervical abnormality
1 Understand the development of cervical pre-cancer and cancer	28 Recognise features suggestive of invasion
2 Take a relevant history	29 Recognise and assess vaginal intraepithelial neoplasia
3 Correctly position patient	30 Recognise and assess vulval intraepithelial neoplasia
4 Insert a speculum and visualise the cervix	31 Be able to determine extent of abnormal epithelium
5 Perform a smear, including with a cytobrush	32 Recognise acute inflammatory cervical changes
6 Perform bacteriological swabs	33 Recognise HPV infection
7 Perform samples for HPV sampling	34 Recognise condylomata acuminata
8 Practice complies with health and safety recommendations	35 Recognise condylomata plana
9 Understand National Cervical Screening guidelines	36 Recognise the changes associated with treatment
B Colposcopic examination	E Practical procedures
10 Use and adjust the colposcope	37 Recognise benign cervical polyps
11 Determine whether or not the TZ is visible	38 Administer local analgesia
12 Determine whether or not colposcopy is satisfactory	39 Determine where to take directed biopsies
13 Examine the TZ with saline and green filter	40 Perform a directed cervical biopsy
14 Examine the TZ using acetic acid	41 Perform a directed vaginal biopsy
15 Quantify and describe acetic acid changes	42 Perform a directed vulval biopsy
16 Use an endocervical speculum	43 Control bleeding from biopsy sites
17 Recognise abnormal vascular patterns	
18 Examine the cervix and the vaginal vault using iodine solution	F Administration
19 Examine the vagina using acetic acid	44 Document cervical findings satisfactorily
	45 Formulate and action appropriate management plans according to guidelines
C Normal colposcopic features	
20 Recognise original squamous epithelium	G Communication
21 Recognise columnar epithelium	46 Adequately answer patients' questions about abnormal smears and their management
22 Recognise metaplastic epithelium	47 Counsel patients prior to colposcopy
23 Recognise a congenital TZ	48 Obtain informed consent correctly
24 Recognise the effects of pregnancy	49 Counsel patients after colposcopy
25 Recognise the normal features of a postmenopausal cervix	50 Break bad news
	51 Communicate well with other health professionals
D Abnormal colposcopic features	
26 Recognise low-grade precancerous cervical abnormality	

HPV, human papillomavirus; TZ, transformation zone.

who had expressed an interest in taking part. The exercise was conducted as previously described, over four iterative rounds, and a list of core competences was identified, which serves as the objectives of the training programme (Table 46.2) (Redman *et al.*, 2004).

Colposcopy is a relatively narrow clinical field and it is perhaps surprising that there was significant modification to the original list of competences forwarded, which had been based on the established BSCCP/RCOG programme. A quarter of the original list of 42 was dropped and 20 of the final agreed 51 core competences were added by the panel. During the process the change in ratings suggested that there was increasing agreement between the experts. Nonetheless the adjustments to ratings had little impact on what would be included in the core curriculum; consensus as to what competences were deemed as core or not changed in only 10 instances. It could be argued that experts, by definition, are unlikely to alter their position significantly, though the number and nature of the changes reflected a spirit of cooperation. Participants varied considerably in the number of changes made but the most active ones were as inclined to move towards the consensus of the previous round as those who made fewer changes; there was therefore no evidence of 'tactical voting'.

Developing the training programme

Using the Delphi technique to identify the training objectives of the programme was an important initial step and has generated a spirit of group cooperation and achievement. The next step has been to agree the key features of the training programme and, to date, this process is nearing completion.

At the outset it was agreed that a programme is an extended period of experiential clinical training that requires at least one trainer. It was considered important that EFC training programmes should share common standards in the following areas:
- trainee caseload;
- trainer caseload;
- assessment.

National training programmes might vary from country to country but the intention is that they would receive reciprocal recognition by sharing common aims, objectives and programme standards.

The views of the 45 members of the expert panel who had participated in the Delphi exercise were sought and this report summarises the findings of this survey. By 1 October 2002, responses had been received from 17 experts, from 13 countries.

Trainee caseload

The survey indicated that the minimum number of cases a trainee will have to see in the course of their training should be

specified. On the basis of the survey it was recommended that trainees should see a minimum of 100 cases (see Table 46.3) but, equally importantly, the nature of the case mix should be specified (see Table 46.4). All agreed that the case mix should include new and old patients and it was recommended that, overall, a trainee should see a minimum of 100 cases, 50 of which must be new. In addition it was felt that 30% of the caseload should be related to high-grade abnormal smears, demonstrating at least moderate dyskaryosis (see Table 46.5).

Trainer caseload

The number of patients a trainer sees is also an important consideration as it necessarily influences training opportunities and the duration of training. This is an important issue

Table 46.3 Suggested size of trainee caseload.

Caseload size	No.	Representative countries
30	1	Croatia
100	4	Belgium, Hungary, Spain, UK
150	9	Austria, Czech Republic, Ireland, Netherlands, Portugal, UK, Yugoslavia
200	1	Spain
250	1	Denmark
300	1	Germany

Table 46.4 Trainee caseload case mix — % new patients.

% New patients	No.	Representative countries
25	2	Portugal, Spain
30	5	Austria, Belgium, Czech Republic, Netherlands, UK
50	5	Denmark, Ireland, Netherlands, UK
70	1	Hungary
75	1	Yugoslavia
> 50	1	Germany
Not stated	1	Croatia
No	1	Spain

Table 46.5 Trainee caseload case mix — % abnormal smears.

% Abnormal smears	No.	Representative countries
10	1	Spain
25	1	UK
30	7	Denmark, Hungary, Netherlands, Portugal, UK, Yugoslavia
50	2	Germany, Ireland
Not stated	3	Austria, Belgium, Croatia
No	1	Czech Republic, Netherlands, Spain

Table 46.6 Suggested size of trainer caseload.

Caseload size	No.	Representative countries
50	6	Austria, Netherlands, Portugal, Spain, UK
100	4	Belgium, Ireland, Netherlands, UK
150	1	Denmark
200	2	Czech Republic, Hungary
300	1	Germany
450	1	Yugoslavia
800	1	Spain
Not stated	1	Croatia

Table 46.7 Trainer caseload case mix — % abnormal smears and/or colposcopic abnormality.

% Abnormal smears	No.	Representative countries
20	1	Germany
25	1	Spain
30	1	Yugoslavia
80	2	Ireland, Portugal
90	1	UK
100	8	Austria, Czech Republic, Belgium, Hungary, Netherlands, UK
No	2	Denmark, Spain
Not stated	1	Croatia

Table 46.8 Trainer caseload case mix — % of new cases with high-grade abnormality (either cytological or colposcopic).

% New cases	No.	Representative countries
10	3	Austria, Germany, Spain
25	1	Portugal
30	6	Belgium, Ireland, Netherlands, UK
40	1	Czech Republic
50	1	Yugoslavia
No	2	Denmark, Spain
Not stated	3	Croatia, Hungary, UK

Table 46.9 Educational areas and related methods of assessment.

Mode of assessment	Educational area principally assessed
MCQ	Knowledge
Performance-based tests e.g. OSCE	Knowledge, clinical skills, attitude
Self-assessment	Clinical skills, attitude
Portfolios	Knowledge, attitude.

MCQ, multiple choice questions; OSCE, objective structured clinical examination.

because clinical resources and time are finite. In the USA, it is recommended that the training programme be completed with 12 months of the initial basic colposcopy course. In the UK trainees, in general, take up to 18 months to complete their training. About 20% do not complete training within this time for one reason or another, usually either lack of training opportunities or competing clinical commitments. It is recommended that training should last no longer than 24 months.

All participants in the survey confirmed that a trainer should see a stipulated minimum of cases (see Table 46.6).

The survey also considered whether it mattered what sort of cases the trainer saw, as common sense would suggest that there has to be sufficient clinical material in order to train adequately, in terms of both quantity and quality. Perhaps surprisingly, not everyone in the survey felt that caseload should be defined, probably for a variety of reasons, including practicality. However, after discussion it was felt that there had to be some caseload criteria for recognised trainers. On the basis of the survey responses, it was recommended that:

• every trainer should perform at least 100 colposcopies per annum;

• at least 50 of these cases should be new presentations with either abnormal cytology or abnormal colposcopic findings, 30% of which should be high grade (see Tables 46.7 and 46.8).

These recommendations will have important implications, as only a proportion of colposcopists will see sufficient numbers to meet these criteria and therefore be able to train.

Assessment

In general terms, any training programme should have some form of assessment to ensure that its aims and objectives are being achieved. Assessment not only assesses the product (the trainee) but can also enhance the training itself as it reinforces what is deemed important. Some colposcopists have argued that assessment is not needed, arguing that colposcopy is a narrow and simple area of clinical practice: if this were the case then the BSCCP would never have been formed nor would the pressure to provide a training programme have arisen. In clinical medicine the importance of assessment is undeniable, as it provides a safeguard that the trainee is fit to practise. Extensive assessments are performed in allied clinical areas such as in general obstetric and gynaecological training programmes and also as part of higher clinical skills such as training in the obstetric ultrasound training programme. As one of the aims of introducing a colposcopy training programme was to safeguard patients, some form of assessment would be desirable.

Assessment needs to be reliable, valid and feasible. There is a variety of different assessment methods which optimally assess different educational areas (Table 46.9). Of the four existing training programmes some form of assessment occurs in three,

Table 46.10 Possible methods of assessment in colposcopy training.

Competence area	Possible mode of assessment
Clinical skills	Clinical performance/trainer Portfolio (commentaries) Self-assessment
Image recognition	Image recognition — OSCE Portfolio (performance table)
Communication	Patient feedback Clinical performance/trainer
Administration	Clinical performance/trainer

though this primarily assesses knowledge (using MCQs) rather than clinical performance or image recognition. In the USA, the American Society for Colposcopy and Cervical Pathology assesses clinical performance using a checklist approach and formally assesses image recognition using computer-based colpophotographs.

At present the question of assessment within the specific EFC training programme is being addressed and it is not possible to state formally what form it will take. It is possible, though, to discuss some of the underlying principles. The EFC colposcopy training programme has a competence-based curriculum, which contains a defined list of core competences that serve as the training objectives. It follows that assessment needs to check if these training objectives are being delivered (Table 46.10).

The core competences fall into four main areas:
• clinical skills, i.e. ability to use a colposcope, position patient, determine management etc.;
• image recognition, i.e. ability to recognise and characterise normal and abnormal colposcopic findings;
• communication;
• administration.

It can be very difficult to assess clinical skills reliably other than by direct observation. The intimate nature of colposcopy precludes a simple OSCE approach, and practically the trainer is the only really feasible observer. This means that objectivity is a problem. Probably some form of checklist should be used

on a stipulated number of patients in order to introduce some objectivity. The use of a logbook and portfolio, which includes a number of clinical commentaries may enable assessment of understanding and clinical problem solving.

Image recognition is an essential area and is, in principle, easy to test, subject to the quality of image reproduction. The main considerations are logistical, such as whether this assessment should be undertaken in an exam setting (set place and time) or as part of self-assessment. Clinical results can be used to assess diagnostic ability but are subject to a number of confounding factors, including clinical guidelines.

Communication skills can be tested in a variety of ways. OSCE are increasingly used but are time consuming, expensive and not necessarily valid. Another approach is to systematically obtain patient feedback using exit questionnaires. Although this method is subject to a number of shortcomings, the findings are relevant in that the client group is involved and the method has the virtue of being simple and cheap to perform. However, some form of validation studies will be needed.

CONCLUDING COMMENTS

The recognised need for professional accountability and quality assurance is especially relevant to colposcopy. The advantages of having commonly agreed training standards within Europe are obvious, although achieving this will be a challenge. Success will depend on a wide variety of different factors but by far the most important of these will be the efforts of individual colposcopy societies and their ability to work together.

REFERENCES

de Wolf CJM, Perry NM (1996) *European Guidelines for Quality Assurance in Mammography Screening*, 2nd edn. Luxembourg: European Commission.

NHSCSP (National Health Service Cervical Screening Programme) (1996). *Quality Assurance Guidelines for the Cervical Screening Programme*. Sheffield: NHSCSP Publications.

Redman CWE, Dollery E, Jordan JA (2004) Development of the European Colposcopy Core Curriculum: use of the Delphi technique. *Journal of Obstetrics and Gynecology* 24: 780–784.

CHAPTER 47

The future — towards the elimination of cervical cancer

Henry C. Kitchener

INTRODUCTION

Before trying to look into the future there are always lessons to be gained from studying the past. What the past tells us is that cervical screening based on exfoliative cytology has undoubtedly saved many thousands of lives, but it is a complex activity and can only be afforded by countries with substantial investment in health care. So the most important consideration for the future is to develop affordable and sustainable means of preventing cervical cancer in developing countries. This will have a far greater impact on reducing death rates around the world than any changes made to existing programmes. The second fact that stands out is that, despite its complexity, cervical cytology has been both effective and cost-effective by the standards of societies with developed health care systems. Before changes are made to large programmes, future developments will need to improve significantly on cytology in terms of both effectiveness and cost efficiency. Therefore the evidence base for doing so needs to be extremely strong. Despite its relative shortcomings, the 'Pap test' or 'cervical smear' has become a standard part of gynaecological care and much faith is invested in it. For both developed and underdeveloped health care systems the way forward in the future may be different in the short to medium term. In the long term, however, the vision of human papillomavirus (HPV) vaccination preventing all forms of cervical neoplasia may eventually find a global role.

DEVELOPED HEALTH CARE SYSTEMS

The future goals of countries with established cervical screening programmes would be to continue to increase levels of protection afforded by cervical screening by identifying increasingly sensitive strategies and increasing population coverage. In addition it would be desirable to identify technologies which would enable cervical screening to become more automated and more robust, thus reducing our dependence on current levels of cytoscreeners.

Human papillomavirus testing

There is no doubt that, given our current understanding of HPV testing, this could play a dominant role in cervical screening. Before this can be considered for use in national screening programmes it needs to be subjected to very rigorous evaluation in direct comparison with cervical cytology. We need to understand how we could use it in conjunction with other forms of testing, such as reflex cytology or other markers. What would be the cost–utility of its use? How acceptable as a marker of risk would it be to women? There is no doubt that over the next 5 years we will develop more mature insights than we have at the moment and the role of HPV testing for primary cervical screening will have become clearer than it is now. Until that time, however, an uncontrolled introduction of HPV testing is unlikely to be helpful. In the meantime, HPV testing could well become implemented as a means of triaging low-grade cytological abnormality and also in treatment follow-up protocols. In these settings the negative predictive value of HPV testing is very powerful and is likely to be able to accelerate its return to routine screening. Equally, testing HPV-positive provides a logical basis for further investigation. Protocols which balance the competing demands of sensitivity and specificity and achieve satisfactory levels of positive predictive value will need to be developed.

Cell cycle markers

As our understanding of the molecular biology of the cervical cell increases, an increasing number of molecular markers that are associated with cervical intraepithelial neoplasia (CIN) will be discovered. It is unlikely that a marker will be discovered which uniquely identifies progression to invasive disease, but certain markers or combinations of markers may achieve an optimum model for sensitivity and specificity. Furthermore, a cell cycle marker which does not have the potential stigma of an HPV test may be preferred by many women. A number of markers have already been investigated but none has yet been subjected to sufficiently rigorous scrutiny to merit implementation in routine practice. This situation may well change over the next 5 years. Indeed HPV markers and non-HPV markers could be tested in combinations from a single liquid sample.

Electro-optical technology

A number of technologies have emerged which have the potential to discriminate between normal and abnormal cervical epithelium. These are attractive in concept as they may provide an instant indication of whether further investigation is necessary or the woman has screened negative. The basis for discriminating between normal and abnormal may, however, be insufficiently exact to achieve the necessary performance characteristics required for cervical screening. Again, if these technologies are to have an impact they will need to be shown, in convincing randomised clinical trials, to have greater effectiveness and cost-effectiveness than the existing forms of screening.

Prophylactic HPV vaccines

This is the great hope for the future and has been so for 20 years since papillomavirus was shown to be closely associated with cervical cancer. The advent of vaccines based on virus-like particles has been very exciting, and over the next 5 years the results of two global trials will attempt to demonstrate the effectiveness of these vaccines as a means of preventing cervical neoplasia. There are a number of challenges, which include the means of preventing infection by all the relevant oncotypes, acceptability to society and affordability, particularly as the diminishing burden of cervical cancer competes with many other new forms of treatment and technology in modern medicine. Nevertheless prophylactic HPV vaccines hold enormous promise as a public health measure, particularly if they could negate the need for screening.

UNDERDEVELOPED HEALTH CARE SYSTEMS

It is appropriate to complete this brief glimpse into the future with what is undoubtedly the most important issue: to reduce the enormous burden of disease and death from cervical cancer in developing countries. A number of very important developments are taking place which provide great hope. The first and probably most important is that the level of wealth in a number of very large and formerly poor countries is increasing at a rapid rate. Both India and China, which together account for one-third of the world's population, have seen enormous gains in economic development and as this continues in the future it will allow increased resources

for health care. This means that, whatever means of cervical screening are considered most beneficial, they will be more affordable than they are currently, which makes their implementation increasingly likely. Unfortunately, many countries, particularly in Africa, are likely to remain impoverished and dependent on aid for health care developments.

Despite the difficulties there have been impressive attempts made to investigate cervical screening in developing settings, particularly in South Africa, Thailand, India and South America. It is widely acknowledged that cervical screening by means of cytology is unlikely to be the way forward in many countries because of the complex infrastructure it requires. Visual inspection following the application of acetic acid, on the other hand, offers a low-tech means of identifying women at increased risk, although its poor specificity will require many women without significant cervical pathology to undergo some form of treatment. HPV testing could achieve higher levels of both sensitivity and specificity than a visual inspection using acetic acid but it will require more technical backup and it would be more expensive. Different countries are likely to adopt different protocols according to their resources and geography. Implementation projects in Thailand have been demonstrating the necessary infrastructure to introduce cervical screening and, although currently based on visual inspection, these infrastructures may be adapted to evolving strategies in the future. A very impressive trial has just been completed in India, which compared HPV testing, visual inspection and cervical cytology. Although there were differences in performance between the three arms, all three achieved high levels of CIN detection and showed that if the cost–utility that is required can be achieved programmes could be implemented.

Prophylactic HPV vaccines

There is no doubt that the hoped-for future for these countries is programmes of preventative vaccines, which would enable young adolescents to be protected from the effects of oncogenic papillomavirus infection. There is already evidence from hepatitis B vaccination programmes that the incidence of hepatocellular cancer is falling in high-incidence countries and there is no reason to believe that this should not apply to cervical cancer. In order to achieve what may be achieved there needs to be a political will that recognises cervical cancer as a disease that can be eliminated, and that identifies the resources required to do this as a priority. There will always be competing demands from other global disease, such as AIDS (aquired immune deficiency syndrome) and malaria, but in the future women should not have to worry about developing cancer of the cervix or die from its effects.

Index